D1165889

FUNDAMENTALS OF NURSING
Concepts and Procedures

Barbara Kozier, BSN, RN, MN

Glenora Lea Erb, BSN, RN

ADDISON-WESLEY PUBLISHING COMPANY

Medical/Nursing Division, Menlo Park, California

Reading, Massachusets • London • Amsterdam • Don Mills, Ontario • Sydney

Sponsoring Editor: James Keating
Production Editor: Pat Franklin
Cover Design: Michael A. Rogondino
Book Design: Linda S. Stinchfield
Artist: Jack Tandy
Photographers: George B. Fry, III, and Joe Greco

Library of Congress Cataloging in Publication Data

Kozier, Barbara Blackwood.
　　Fundamentals of nursing.

　　Bibliography: p.
　　Includes index.
　　1. Nursing. I. Erb, Glenora Lea, 1937–
joint author. II. Title.
RT41.K72　　　610.73　　　78-7776
ISBN 0-201-03904-4

ABCDEFGHIJ-MU-782109

The authors and publishers have exerted every effort to ensure that drug selection and dosage set forth in this text
are in accord with current recommendations and practice at the time of publication. However, in view of ongoing
research, changes in government regulations and the constant flow of information relating to drug therapy and
drug reactions, the reader is urged to check the package insert for each drug for any change in indications of dosage
and for added warnings and precautions. This is particularly important where the recommended agent is a new
and/or infrequently employed drug.

Addison-Wesley Publishing Company
Medical/Nursing Division
2725 Sand Hill Road
Menlo Park, California 94025

To the late Dr. Bertie Blackwood, M.B., B.S., M.R.C.S., L.R.C.P. (Lond.)
A loving father and physician who valued learning

This book for nursing students is intended to be used either as a text for fundamentals of nursing or as a core text throughout a nursing program. The emphasis is on clinical nursing practice.

Unlike many fundamentals texts, this book is both comprehensive in the scope of topics covered and complete in its detailed coverage of each topic. This kind of coverage offers students *two additional benefits:* it provides them with a single, self-contained text valuable for future reference, and it makes it unnecessary for them to purchase many additional supplements at this stage of their education.

Scientific concepts and principles from all areas of science are included to provide the student with a more complete understanding of the whys behind nursing actions. Principles underlying nursing are stressed and developmental variables relevant to nursing intervention are integrated. To help direct students in their study, each chapter begins with an outline and a list of learning objectives and ends with a summary, annotated selected readings, suggested learner activities, and list of references. (An instructor's guide is available for the teacher.)

Because nurses are seen to practice their professions in homes, in community agencies, and in hospitals, a broad spectrum of preventive and therapeutic aspects of nursing is presented. Considerable emphasis is placed on nursing care for sick people; however, the nurse's function in response to the needs of the family as well as his or her role as a health team member are also included.

Manual skills, which make up much of nursing practice, are described in table form. The principles underlying each step of the various procedures are also given. The text is supportive of these procedures

in that it provides an explanation of the nursing process, which nurses use in assessing, providing, and evaluating nursing care.

Unit I orients the student to nursing and provides sociologic and contemporary information that can be applied clinically.

Unit II introduces the student to concepts of "illness" and to the nursing process. Nursing tools for implementation of the process are also included. Two chapters (10 and 11) are devoted entirely to growth and development, covering all stages of life. These growth and development concepts are then integrated into subsequent chapters that apply nursing to all ages. Normals for each are provided comparatively, such as the normal pulse rates for each age group. Other integrating concepts include homeostasis, stress/adaptation, humanism, and ethnicity.

Unit III covers the physical needs and common problems of patients and their families.

Unit IV focuses on cognitive and emotional problems frequently encountered by patients and their families. Because of the increasing emphasis on communication and patient teaching, this unit is devoted entirely to communication concepts and techniques and emphasizes the nurse's role as a health educator.

Unit V gives comprehensive coverage of physiologic needs.

Unit VI gives considerable attention to intrapersonal and interpersonal needs with complete chapters on sexuality, spiritual preference, self-acceptance, stimulation, and accepting loss and death.

Unit VII covers special nursing measures for medications, preoperative and postoperative care

PREFACE

and tests and treatments.

The book is written and organized in a to-the-point approach that students will truly appreciate and is further enhanced by the design of the book. Hundreds of illustrations (including step-by-step procedures, which present motor skills in one column and the explanation for the action in another), are provided in addition to numerous tables and charts. To assist the student in understanding the concepts and procedures presented throughout the text, a glossary and extensive appendices (covering abbreviations, prefixes, suffixes, symbols, etc.) are provided at the end of the text.

For further insight into the nursing process and for a more thorough introduction to this text, please turn to Chapter 1.

Acknowledgments

We would like to express our appreciation to the many faculty and students with whom we have worked and from whom we have learned. In particular we wish to thank H. Mary Evans and Verna Kay Hankinson for their assistance with obstetrical nursing and fluid and electrolyte balance, respectively. Also, we thank Val Nicholson for her stimulating ideas and encouragement during the early stages of the book.

Our warmest thanks go to Doreen Watts who typed long hours over two years, correcting spelling and deciphering terms. We offered her a continual challenge, but she never lost her sense of humor. We also thank Helen Moore for the typing assistance that she provided. Harry Vaines' efforts with some of the photography is also appreciated.

Various people at the agencies and hospitals who assisted with photographs are also to be thanked: Lara Thordarson, City of Vancouver Health Department, who with Deirdre Giles and the nurses and patients of the South Vancouver Health Unit gave generously of their time; and Judy Staples, of the Midpeninsula Health Service, who worked many long hours with George B. Fry, III, and Joe Greco, photographers, in securing the photographs used throughout the text. Many of the photographs were taken at Stanford Hospital and at Children's Hospital at Stanford. The fine results would not have been possible without the gracious assistance of the patients and staff at both of these hospitals. Special thanks are deserved by Joyce Campbell and Jocelyn Howden, Lion's Gate Hospital, and to Diana Ritchie and Rosemary Webber of Mount Saint Joseph Hospital. We also appreciate the assistance of the staff from various hospitals who provided sample clinical records for inclusion in the book.

To all of the other people involved in the production of this book we are grateful: James Keating, Sponsoring Editor; Pat Franklin, Production Editor; and Jack Tandy, illustrator. We consider them a great team to work with.

We thank our respective families and friends for their patience while "the book" became a priority. In particular we are grateful to two puppies, Maurice and Muffet, who provided balance and relief during the days of writing.

Barbara Kozier
Glenora Lea Erb

CONTENTS IN BRIEF

UNIT I NURSING AND HEALTH NEEDS

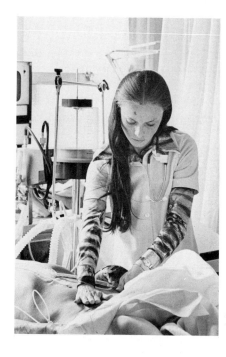

CONTENTS
IN DETAIL

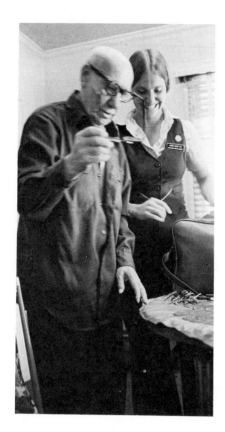

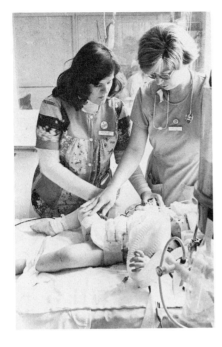

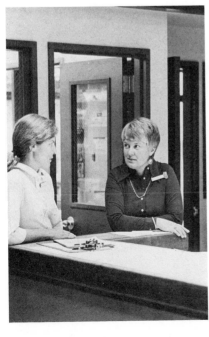

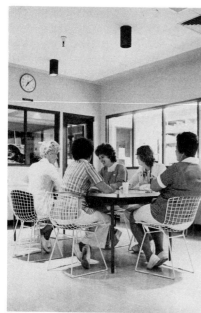

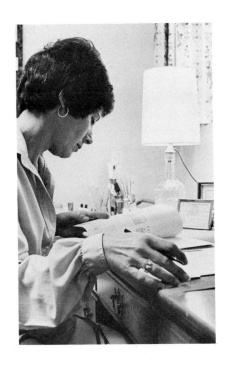

UNIT II   INTEGRATING CONCEPTS

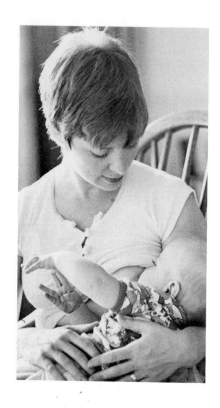

Chapter 8   STRESS AND ADAPTATION   114

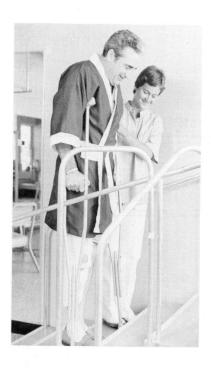

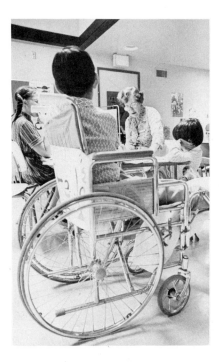

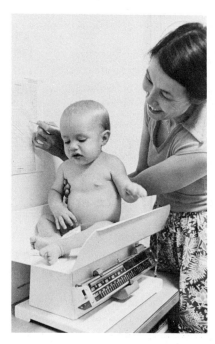

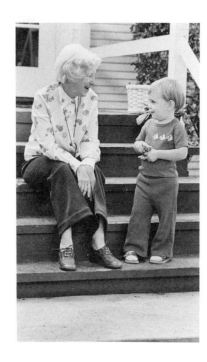

UNIT III   INTEGRATING SKILLS   216

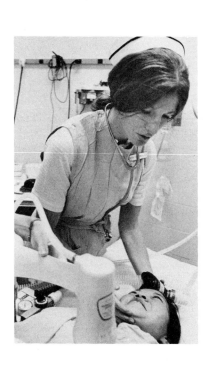

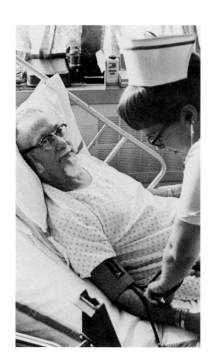

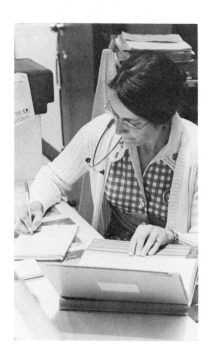

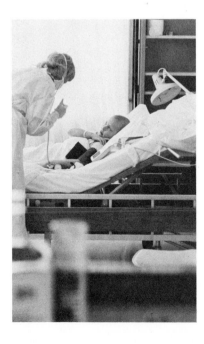

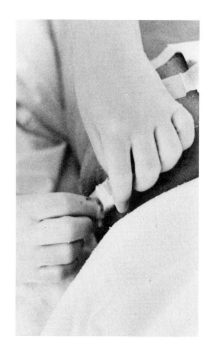

UNIT IV   THERAPEUTIC COMMUNICATION   396

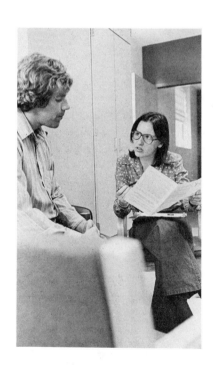

Chapter 18   COMMUNICATING EFFECTIVELY   398

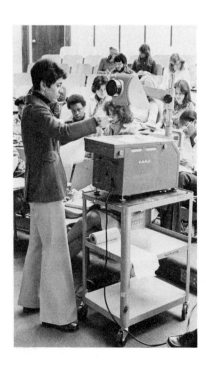

UNIT V PHYSIOLOGIC NEEDS

Chapter 20 PERSONAL HYGIENE

Contents in Detail

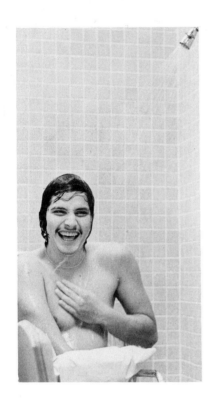

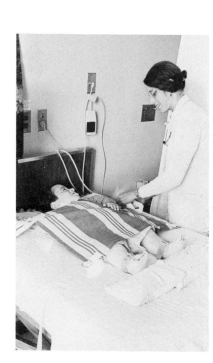

Chapter 21   PROTECTION   **478**

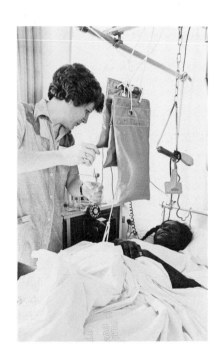

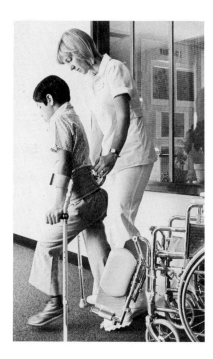

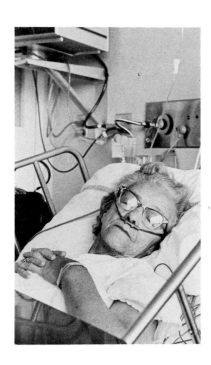

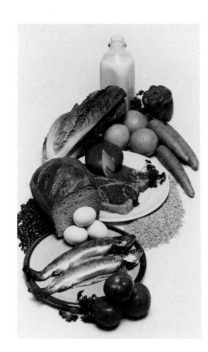

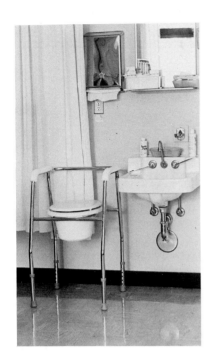

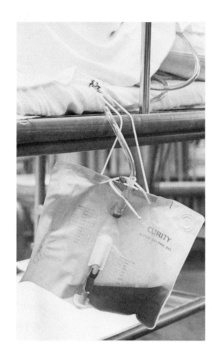

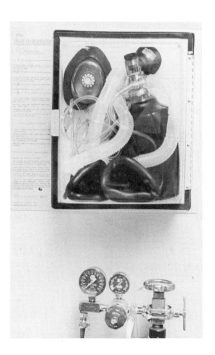

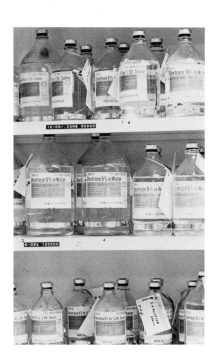

Chapter 30   FLUID AND ELECTROLYTE PROBLEMS   714

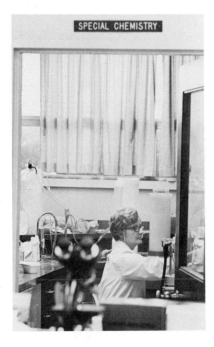

UNIT VI   PSYCHOSOCIAL NEEDS

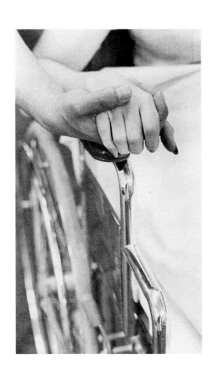

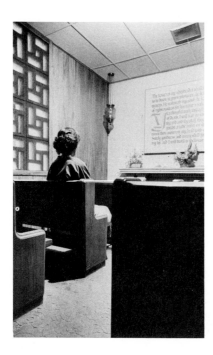

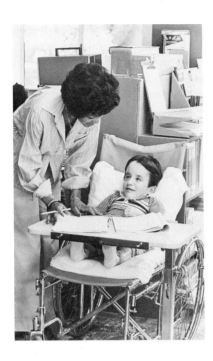

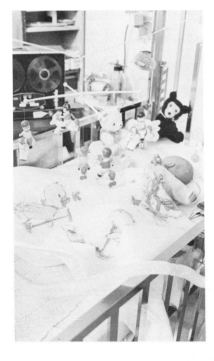

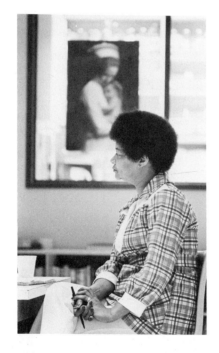

UNIT VII   SPECIAL NURSING MEASURES   822

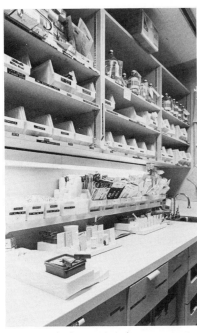

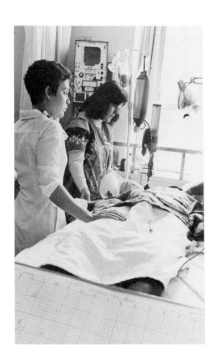

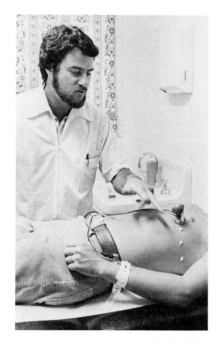

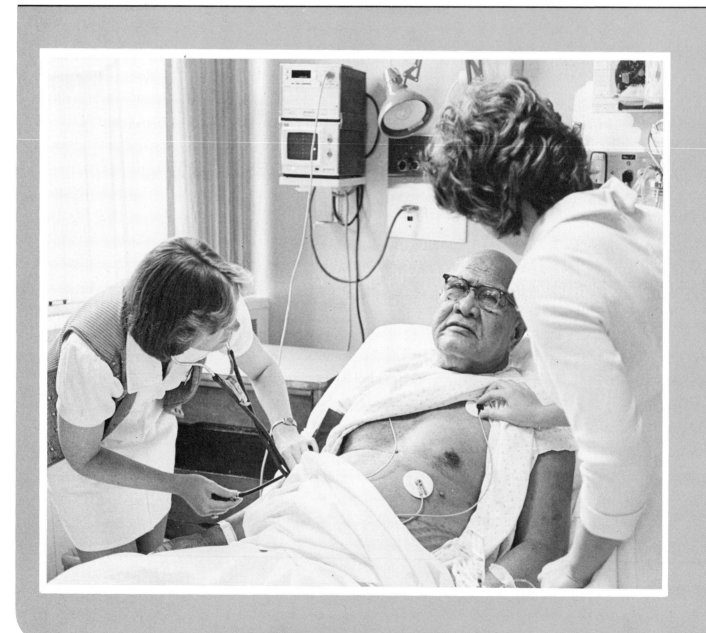

NURSING AND HEALTH NEEDS

CHAPTER 1

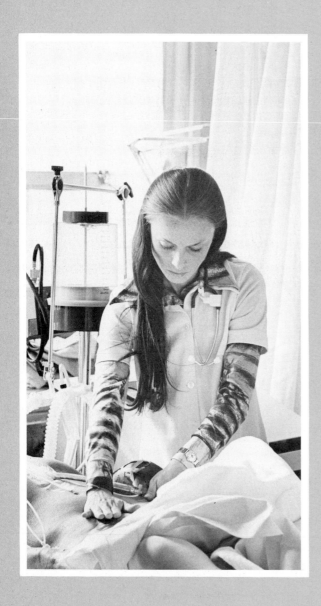

NURSING AND THE NURSE

OBJECTIVES

- Provide some definition of nursing and discuss the interrelated elements of nursing.
- Explain the components of nursing care.
- Describe the various settings for nursing practice.
- Describe some factors that influence nursing practice.
- Discuss the various trends in nursing practice and their significance.
- Describe the three roles of the nurse.
- Describe five methods of helping provided by nurses and give examples.
- Describe the various types of educational programs for nurses.
- Discuss the various professional nursing organizations and their functions.

WHAT IS NURSING?

Nursing is practiced with a vital concern for the science of health and the art of care. The profession involves a humanistic blend of scientific knowledge, nursing philosophy, and clinical practice—with an important measure of communications and social sciences added as well. As a result, today's nursing student must master an astounding number of professional concepts and skills. The purpose of this book is to help students meet that challenge by providing a comprehensive framework for holistic and humanistic nursing practice.

Our study will begin with an examination of the past and present of nursing, as well as future possibilities, by viewing roles and functions of the nurse, components of nursing care, and trends in nursing practice as these elements are influenced by various sociologic factors. In later chapters, these theories will serve as the structure on which to apply principles of clinical practice. By integrating concepts with skills, today's nurse becomes a realistic practitioner of both the art and science of this profession.

The Evolving Profession

Constantly evolving, the nursing profession owes much to the influence of Florence Nightingale (1820–1910), a woman with a vision. Emerging in an age when nursing was regarded with vehement contempt, Nightingale crusaded to change the world's view of the nurse. No longer is nursing held in the disreputable light of the 19th century. Nightingale's belief in education, her development of theories of nursing practice and hygiene techniques, and her campaign for an emphasis on prevention in health care are important facets of the nursing spectrum today.

However, earlier in this century, some of Nightingale's ideals were temporarily misplaced. Medicine, in its zeal to control disease, frequently emphasized cure rather than prevention. Nurses were trained rather than educated, frequently working long hours performing hospital chores rather than spending time and energy on patients. Nurses all too often were able to follow orders only rather than take an active part in patient care. Nightingale's intentions for the nursing profession were temporarily lost but fortunately not forgotten. Her vision was shared—and is shared—by nursing pioneers in the years that followed, and this vision is the motivating force behind the campaign for similar aims. This

in combination with our changing society, advances in medicine, and our goals for human rights serves to continue the evolving process of the nursing profession.

An Emerging Definition

Just as nursing today is different from the nursing practiced 50 years ago, it takes a vivid imagination to think about the nursing profession in the next 50 years to come. Ours is an ever-changing world. To understand present-day nursing and at the same time prepare for nursing in tomorrow's world, it is important not only to have an understanding of past events but also to have an understanding of contemporary nursing practice and the sociologic factors affecting it.

Let us begin by looking at definitions of nursing that have been set forth by various professional groups.

Nursing was defined by the International Council of Nurses (ICN) in 1972 as follows:

> The unique function of the nurse is to assist the individual, sick or well, in the performance of those activities contributing to health or its recovery (or to peaceful death) that he would perform unaided if he had the necessary strength, will or knowledge.

A further development was made in defining nursing by the American Nurses' Association (ANA) in 1973 in *Standards of Nursing Practice.* This official definition states: "Nursing practice is a direct service, goal oriented, and adaptable to the needs of the individual, the family and community during health and illness."

In both definitions certain ideas and goals are emphasized. Drawing from these important ideas, we have created a composite definition of nursing and expanded on the elements involved:

1. Nursing is nurturing, caring for and about people.
2. Nursing is a service to patients, their families, and communities. Examples of community nursing practice are found in well-baby clinics, mental health day-care centers, and parenthood classes.
3. Nursing can be either preventive or therapeutic. For example, a well child may need protection

against poliomyelitis, thereby requiring nursing services for immunization. A child ill with pneumonia may need nursing services while he is in bed at home (see Figure 1-1).

4. Nursing is a direct service, that is, one of direct contact between nurse and patient or nurse and family.

5. Nursing is adapted to the individual needs of the patient. Because each patient has characteristics and attributes that are unique, nursing must consider these in meeting patients' health needs.

Interrelated Elements

Nursing involves an interrelationship of many different people in many different settings concerned with many different ideas, techniques, and functions. Nursing involves a combination of elements, but emphasis frequently is placed on only one aspect of being a nurse. For example, a nurse may have excellent communication and patient care skills, but may be sadly deficient in procedures such as monitoring a patient's vital signs.

Today there is an emphasis on the whole person. This does not include just the whole patient; it also includes the whole nurse. We are not merely physical beings but are social, moral, psychologic, and spiritual beings as well. The whole nurse applies a network of skills to the practice of nursing a whole patient. The whole nurse in concerned also with the family and the community and is aware of the effects of these groups on the patients's well-being in addition to family and community well-being.

The whole nurse has a knowledge of the theory and philosophy of nursing, the science of the human body and health, and procedures of nursing care.

The whole nurse practices nursing on four different levels:

1. *Promotion of health:* assisting people who are either healthy, disabled or ill to increase their level of wellness (see "The Health Continuum," Chapter 2). An example would be the dietary advice required by an obese person.

2. *Prevention of disease or injury:* assisting people who are either healthy or ill to prevent disease, for example, providing immunizations against smallpox.

3. *Restoration of health:* assisting a patient to return to health after illness, for example, teaching a patient to protect an incision and to change the surgical dressing.

4. *Consolation of the dying:* assisting terminally ill patients of all ages to a peaceful death (see Figure 1-2).

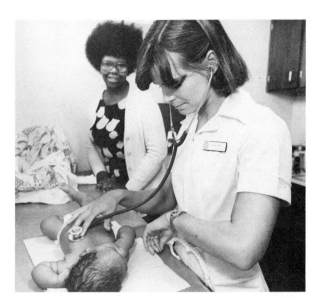

Figure 1-1. A nurse in a community clinic assesses an infant's health and offers a mother assistance with regard to care.

Even the nurse practicing in a highly specialized setting such as an intensive care unit or an elementary school employs these four levels of care. Each level is equally important in the total health picture of patient, family, and community.

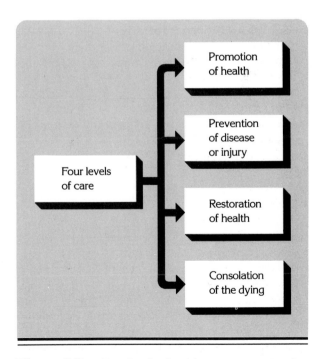

Figure 1-2. Four levels of nursing care are promotion of health, prevention of disease or injury, restoration of health, and consolation of the dying.

Components of Nursing Care

The nurse is that member of the health team who spends the most time with the patient and who has the most direct involvement. Besides other functions, the nurse is the watchful eye of the health team. The nurse, working with the physician and other staff or sometimes independently, assesses the patient physically and psychologically. Nursing plans are then based on this assessment, and care is implemented according to the plan. The nurse next assesses the patient's response to the implemented care and makes adjustments accordingly.

As Florence Nightingale wrote in *Notes on Nursing,* published in 1859:

> The most important practical lesson that can be given to nurses is to teach them what to observe—how to observe—what symptoms indicate improvement—what the reverse—which are of importance—which are none—which are the evidence of neglect—and of what kind of neglect.

The importance of observation has not diminished throughout the years. Indeed nursing care is based heavily on principles related to observation: *assessment, planning, implementation,* and *reassessment.*

With these principles in mind, let us look at the components of nursing care: (a) activities of care itself, (b) coordination of total patient care, (c) plans for continuity of care, (d) evaluation of patient care, and (e) direction of nursing care provided by others.

Activities of Nursing Care

Nursing care activities may include any or all of the following:

- Assisting the patient with basic needs
- Administering medications and treatments
- Observing the patient's response and adaptation to illness
- Observing the patient's response and adaptation to treatment
- Teaching self-care and counseling on health matters
- Supervising or guiding the patient in rehabilitative activities related to daily living
- Planning with the patient in such a manner as to develop a sense of trust, self-worth, and, ultimately, self-realization.

Nursing care activities can be described as either dependent or independent functions. *Dependent functions* are those activities carried out at the request of or with the guidance of the physician, for example, giving an antibiotic by injection to a patient every four hours. *Independent functions* are those activities carried out in the nurse's judgment and without the physician's direct order, for example, teaching a patient and her family how to give insulin. Although independent nursing activities are not the direct result of a physician's order, all nursing activities are interdependent with the activities of other members of the health team.

Coordination of Care

Coordination of total patient care involves helping all persons involved in a particular patient's care to work together as one unit toward a common goal. (See also "The Health Team," Chapter 2.) The nurse works with patient and family as well as other members of the health team. Because the nurse is with the patient more than other members of the health professions, and because of the nurse's relationship with a patient, this coordinating function is most effectively carried out by nurses. For example, by coordinating the time of laboratory and radiology tests, which may both require the patient to fast, the patient can be spared a delayed breakfast for one morning instead of two. In another situation, physician's orders may allow a patient to sit in a chair only three times a day for a brief period. The nurse then may plan this activity in conjunction with meal hours. This permits the patient the enjoyment of sitting up for meals and can also conserve the patient's energies.

Plans for Continuity of Care

The patient does not cease to require care just because his physical presence is no longer directly in the nurse's view. The nurse plans for continuity of care to further assist the patient to good health. Appropriate planning permits the patient to change physical setting, for example, from a hospital to home and family or from one hospital unit to another, with a minimum of disturbance to the patient personally and no disruption in care. Continuity is especially important when a patient requires care over a prolonged period of time. In this instance many different health personnel may be involved from time to time, thus making continuity planning a necessity. A systematic method of communication must be practiced; otherwise gaps may occur in patient care. For example, a patient may have an order to have activity increased as tolerated. Unless a plan is communicated, one nurse may interpret this to mean sitting in a chair for ten minutes twice a day, but another may expect the patient to walk to and from the bathroom. In a psychiatric nursing setting, it is particularly essential that a consistent approach be provided by all health workers involved in the patient's care. For example, if a patient has difficulty making decisions, each nurse, occupational therapist, recreational therapist, and other health workers involved in this patient's care should encourage and help the patient to make decisions.

Evaluation of Care

Evaluating patient care is a continuous nursing function. How is the patient adjusting and reacting? What does the patient see as needs? How does the patient see these needs changing? The answers to these questions assist the nurse to evaluate the effectiveness of the care with the patient. Patient care, then, needs to be flexible and responsive to the needs of the patient and family. A simple example of this would be rearranging a patient's exercise schedule to make time for visitors later in the day.

Direction of Care Provided by Others

The registered nurse is generally the member of the nursing team who delegates functions to the other nursing personnel or to the family. This delegation is done considering the particular needs of the patient and the skills of the nursing personnel or the family. After delegating these activities, nurses need to be available in case their assistance is required later. The nurse also makes a continuous evaluation of the effectiveness of the care given in terms of the patient's needs and the family's needs.

SETTINGS FOR NURSING PRACTICE

Nursing practice involves a variety of persons in a variety of situations. While people have many things in common, they also have many differences encompassing all aspects of life from age and physical shape to environment and political ideas. The patient (in some settings referred to as the *client*) may be a member of a *nuclear family*, that is, parent(s) and child(ren); or the patient's family may be the group of people with whom the patient lives regardless of their relationship. The similarities and differences of people—that is, both nurses and patients—will be discussed in detail in later chapters dealing with ethnicity, spirituality, and growth and age as well as later in this chapter (see "Current Influences" in this chapter).

These many different people are cared for by the nurse in many different settings, some of which allow the nurse to function more independently than others. There is a growing trend for nurses to take a more active part in treating patients in many settings.

These settings for nursing practice can be grouped broadly into (a) hospitals, (b) community agencies, and (c) physician's office. In addition, other settings of practice are becoming available to the nurse.

Depending on the setting, there are differences in the degree of autonomy of the nurse, the nursing tasks required, and the relationships to the physician and other health workers. Today's nurse has a variety of career choices and can pursue his or her personal and professional goals.

Hospitals

Hospitals are health institutions that vary in size and in the services they provide. General hospitals treat a variety of patients with different health problems and different socioeconomic backgrounds. They vary in size from the small hospital in a rural setting to the large metropolitan hospital of perhaps 2000 beds. A specialized hospital, on the other hand, may be of any size, but it restricts its services to special areas such as obstetrics, pediatrics, or psychiatry. Nurses who are employed in hospitals generally have limited autonomy in their functions, although nurses in psychiatric settings may have more autonomy than nurses in many areas of a hospital. Recently, however, nurses who work in specialty areas, such as intensive care units, have been functioning with increasing autonomy and with highly advanced skills.

Hospitals are *bureaucratic* organizations with regulations and policies that largely govern the activities of the employees. This is most obvious in large hospitals. The smaller institutions tend to be less formal and have more flexible and fewer policies. Nurses in hospitals are expected to fit into the system of the institution and to share its values as an organization. This expectation can be in conflict with the judgment of the nurse when assisting patients. For example, a patient who is accustomed to bathing in the evening may wish to continue this practice in the hospital as a relaxing measure to assist in sleep. The hospital, on the other hand, may not have sufficient nursing staff working in the evening to provide the patient with the assistance required for a bath.

In hospital settings, nurses interact with a number of physicians and a variety of other health personnel. They perform a variety of nursing tasks, often at the direction of the physician. These tasks, such as giving medications, are usually dependent, cure-related activities, and as such they frequently take precedence over independent activites, that is, those that are prescribed and initiated by nurses. An example of the latter might be counseling regarding dietary habits. However, as patterns of nursing education change, as hospital policies change, and indeed as state and provincial legislative regulations change, the independent functions of the nurse are changing as well. Today's nurse is growing in terms of responsibility.

Community Agencies

Nurses are also employed by community agencies for a wide range of nursing activities. A community can be a particular geographic area or a group of people brought together because of common interests. For example, a community might be a town, or it might refer to the teachers, students, and families associated with a specific school.

Community agencies include community clinics, public health agencies, industrial clinics, schools, home nursing services, and others. In these settings, nurses tend to function more independently than in hospitals. Their contact with the physician is episodic. In rural areas, contact with the physician may occur only when, in the nurse's judgment, a physician's advice or intervention is required.

Depending upon the purpose of the community agency, nurses' activites may include a mixture of care, cure, and coordinating activities. Generally, nurses use more independent judgment in these settings, and the activities tend to be less related to the physician's cure regimen than in the hospital.

Physicians' Offices and Clinics

In physicians' offices and clinics, nurses have a minimum amount of independent function. The physician is generally there when the patients are present, and many of the nurse's activities are largely in response to the physician's request. The nurse's function is related mainly to the physician's therapy in many of these settings (see Table 1-1).

Other Career Possibilities

More and more career possibilities are available for today's nurse. Besides nursing education, there are career opportunities in various clinical specialties. Also, as physicians and other health professionals develop group practices, the nurse joins the health team along with others (for example, social workers and technologists) as a vital part of this group devoted to a broad range of services and holistic health. In more and more states, nurses are developing their own practices; some private nurse practitioners work in association with a physician or health group, while others in poverty urban areas or isolated rural areas practice alone, referring patients who need additional care to physicians. In addition, the clinical lab-

Table 1-1   Areas of Registered Nurse Employment*

	United States†	Canada‡
Hospitals, nursing homes, and related institutions	529,677 (68.04%)	107,769 (83%)
Public health, occupational health, community health care, and related agencies	58,241 (7.48%)	9,346 (7.26%)
Nursing education	23,240 (2.98%)	3,678 (2.85%)
Physicians' offices, military services, family practice units, and other related services	65,722 (8.44%)	7,342 (5.70%)
Total	778,470 (100%)	128,675 (100%)

†United States: 1972 figures

‡Canada: 1974 figures

*Taken from American Nurses' Association. 1976. *Facts about Nursing 74–75*. Kansas City, Missouri, pp. 1–36, and Statistics Canada. 1975. *Nursing in Canada*. Ottawa, p 33.

oratory setting is opening up to nurses with many persons in the nursing profession entering research fields.

Career Patterns

A nursing career is flexible and open to personal and educational growth and expansion. Two differing but related career patterns, which include a broad range of nursing practice possibilities, are available to the nurse. One career pattern (episodic) emphasizes nursing practice that is essentially curative and restorative, generally acute or chronic in nature, and most frequently provided in the setting of the hospital and inpatient facility. The second career pattern (distributive) emphasizes the nursing practice that is designed essentially for health maintenance and disease prevention, generally continuous in nature, seldom acute, and most frequently operative in the community or in newly developing institutional settings (National Commission 1974:23).

These recommendations take into consideration the increasing complexity of nursing practice in a wide variety of settings and recognize that it is difficult for a nurse to function effectively in every setting.

FACTORS INFLUENCING NURSING PRACTICE

To understand nursing as it is practiced today and as it will be practiced tomorrow, one must not only have a historical perspective of nursing's evolution but must also understand some of the social forces presently influencing this profession. These forces usually affect the entire health care system, and nursing, as a major component of that system, cannot avoid the effects.

Historical Development

Nursing as an activity that provides help to the ill, to children, and to babies has existed since the earliest times. During the centuries prior to the early Christian period (1–500 AD), caring for the sick was chiefly done by women in their homes. Later, monastic orders provided nursing functions as part of their activities. The first nursing order, the Augustinian Sisters, was established in the Middle Ages. This was probably the first organized group to provide purely nursing services to people.

Prior to the Protestant Reformation in the sixteenth century, hospital facilities were organized chiefly by the Roman Catholic Church. With the Reformation, beginning in 1517, came a decline in the interest and support of people in the church and religion. This change resulted in a period in nursing history known as the "dark period." Hospitals were unsanitary places, dark and foreboding. Nursing was provided by women who were frequently described as drunk, heartless, and immoral. They were expected to carry out the housework of the hospital, wash the laundry, and do all the cleaning for very little reward. Nurses were not required to have any training, and it was not unusual for a nurse to work anywhere from 12 to 40 consecutive hours. This period of decline lasted until the middle of the nineteenth century.

The era of reform in nursing is marked by the work of the British nurse, Florence Nightingale, during the Crimean War (1854–1856). Nightingale's efforts made nursing once again a respectable vocation. However, Nightingale's reform activities did not stop at respectability; besides crusading for cleanliness and comfort in hospitals, Nightingale also worked toward educating the populace regarding health measures in an effort to stave off the diseases that were widespread because of poor conditions in the cities. Nightingale believed in prevention and in nursing the whole person, calling upon her fellow nurses to make sure patients always had fresh air, good water, proper medication, quiet, mobility, and knowledge of caring for themselves in the future. Many of Nightingale's ideas are now standards of patient care. Education of nurses was a major goal of this reformer. Among her many other accomplishments was the establishment of the Nightingale School of Nurses at St. Thomas' Hospital, London, in 1860. This school is credited with providing the first planned educational program for nurses. She also assisted in the establishment of the first organized home nursing services.

In North America, the establishment of nursing and health services was slow prior to the American Revolution (1775–1783). One notable organization was The Nurse Society of Philadelphia, which gave women minimal instruction in obstetrics in order for them to provide maternity nursing services in home settings.

The late 1800s showed rapid reform of nursing services in the United States and Canada. Schools of nursing with planned educational programs were started. From these schools a number of nurses graduated who became the early leaders in the profession.

Elizabeth Hampton Robb had been a young school teacher in Canada. She decided to change her profession and entered the Bellevue Hospital Training School in New York. After graduation she became superintendent of the Illinois Training School at 26 years of age and three years later went to Baltimore to organize a new school in connection with Johns Hopkins Hospital. Among her many accomplishments was a nursing textbook, which was recognized as a standard text for nursing schools in America.

Mary Adelaide Nutting, also from Canada, was in the first class at Johns Hopkins. After graduation she established a course of training for students prior to ward experience at Johns Hopkins. Later she reduced the nursing students' hours from 12 to eight and lengthened the nurses' training to three years.

Mary Agnes Snively graduated from Bellevue. She returned to Canada to be in charge of the nurses' training at Toronto General Hospital. She is credited with being largely responsible for the direction of Canadian nursing education and was the first president of the Canadian Nurses' Association.

Two American graduates from the New York Hospital, Lillian D. Wald and her friend, Mary Brewster, were the first to offer trained nursing services to the poor in the New York slums. What began as their home among the poor on the upper floor of a tenement is now famous as a center of public health nursing (the Henry Street Settlement). Soon after, school nursing was established as an adjunct to visiting nursing. Again Wald was involved along with Lina L. Rogers.

American's first trained nurse, Linda Richards, graduated in 1873 in Boston. She is credited with nursing reform in 12 major hospitals, some of which were specialized mental hospitals. She initiated training schools for students in mental health nursing, which included a period of training in general hospitals. She also founded the first training school for nurses in Japan.

These pioneers in nursing developed many standards of nursing practice, health care, and assistance for the poor, elderly, and mentally ill. Others followed them, and the nursing profession evolved with the modern technologic world.

From those early days up to and including the present, nursing has undergone change in every area. Rapid strides have been made in nursing education programs and in a wide variety of hospital and community nursing services. While these changes have occurred, nursing has always continued to provide a stable helping service to people.

Current Influences

North America is anything but a desert island. While it may be possible to retreat into some of the remote areas of the United States and Canada in an attempt to escape from civilization, sooner or later some vestige of modern culture is bound to appear—an airplane straying overhead, a power line, a tire track. The point is that it is difficult to escape the influences of society, science, and technology. Nursing, as a profession deeply involved with people, certainly cannot escape influence at all. There are many factors influencing the individual nurse, nursing practice, and, of course, patients. To function effectively in this world of media bombardment, rapid systems of communications, and advances in research, the nurse must develop in relation to outside influences. The current major factors of influence can be grouped into eight broad areas: (a) consumer demands and participation, (b) changing family structure, (c) economics, (d) science and technology, (e) legislation, (f) demography, (g) the nursing profession, and (h) the women's liberation movement.

Consumer Demands

Consumers of nursing services (the public) have become an increasingly effective force in changing nursing practice. On the whole, people have become better educated and have more knowledge about health and illness than in the past. This is to no small measure because of television and the news media. Consumers also have become more aware of the needs of others for care. The ethical and moral issues associated with poverty and neglect have caused people to be more vocal in regard to the needs of minority groups and the poor.

The public's concept of health and nursing has also changed. People now believe that health is a right of all people, not just a privilege of the rich. People are also bombarded with the message by the media that individuals must assume responsibility for their own health by obtaining a physical examination once a year; checking for the seven danger signals of cancer; and maintaining mental well-being by balancing work and recreation. Interest in health and nursing services is therefore greater than it has ever been. Furthermore, many people now want more than freedom from disease; they want energy, vitality, and a feeling of wellness.

Increasingly, the consumer has become an active participant in making decisions about health and nursing care. Planning committees concerned with providing nursing services to a community have active consumer membership. An example is the White Cross Center, a branch of the American and Canadian Mental Health Associations.

Family Structure

The need for and provision of nursing services is being influenced by new family structures. An increasing number of people are living in family structures other than those of the extended family and the nuclear family, and the breadwinner is no longer necessarily the husband. An extended family consists of parents, children, grandparents, and sometimes aunts and uncles; a nuclear family consists only of parents and their children.

There are now many single-parent families of single men or women raising children and many two-parent families in which both parents work. It is also common for young parents to live at great distances from their parents. These familes need support services such as day-care centers. Such families as well as nuclear families do not have grandparents or other relatives who would be easily available to help in times of illness or who would give advice about childrearing and child health. The advice these parents get about their children may come from physicians and nurses as well as other sources.

Similarly, grandparents, who now may live alone and far away from other members of the family, require homemaker and visiting nurse services when they are ill to take the place of the care that used to be provided by younger members of the family.

Economics

Another factor that has increased the demand and need for nursing services is the greater financial support provided through health insurance programs in the United States and Canada. Medicare, Medicaid, and other govenment programs as well as other public and private financing agencies have increased the need for broad nursing services. Thus health services that often were not used when people could not afford the expense of new eyeglasses, hospitalization, or an annual medical examination, for example, are now being increasingly utilized. Federal governments have recognized this need and have markedly increased their budgets in the past ten years for health care services. Along with this increase in expenditure is an increase in the number of people who provide health services. In nursing alone, the number of practicing nurses in the United States grew from 722,000 in 1970 to 857,000 in 1974, an increase of approximately 19% (ANA 1976:1). In Canada, there was also an increase in the number of practicing nurses during a similar period (Statistics Canada 1975:55).

Science and Technology

Discoveries in science and the related technologies, such as control of many of the infectious deseases, have affected nursing. The invention of the vaccine for poliomyelitis has made the nursing skills required to assist the acutely ill patient with poliomyelitis in the 1950s largely a matter of history. Advances in science also have an indirect effect upon nursing. For example, as the physician acquires new knowledge and skills in cardiac surgery, the nurse must also acquire additional knowledge and skills to complement those of the physician.

In some settings, technologic advances have required that nurses become highly specialized. It has frequently become necessary for nurses to utilize sophisticated equipment for patient monitoring or treatment. As technologies change, nurses' education changes as well, with some nurses requiring advanced training to effectively perform as a member of the health team.

The appearance on the market of new pharmaceuticals affects nursing practice. The invention of lithium carbonate used to control the manic state of manic-depressive illness is another example. It has changed the role of the nurse from one of psychologically assisting the patient with his mania to one of counseling about effective use of the medication.

New facts are being discovered in every field associated directly or indirectly with nursing. The social sciences are enabling a better understanding of human behavior and are building a knowledge of interrelatedness between the mind and the body. Advances in technology are exemplified by the many machines now used to help patients maintain life. There seems to be no end to the discoveries and the knowledge explosion of the twentieth century.

With this knowledge explosion, unfortunately, has also come the charge by many that medicine—and some health professionals—have become dehumanized. As science and technology develop methods of treating disease, it is the responsibility of all health professionals to temper technology, to remember that patients are human beings requiring warmth, care, and acknowledgement of self-worth. The nurse in daily dealings with patients is in an ideal situation to humanize technology as much as is possible.

Scientific developments have led to other changes in the nursing profession by indirectly affecting human health. For example, some industries have proven to be hazardous to employees because of the dangerous equipment involved or because of harmful chemical residues. Trauma (injury) and disease are frequently the direct result of advanced technology; the classic example of this is the statistic that automobile accidents are among the top five causes of death in North America. In addition, our advanced society frequently produces much stress and diminished mental health. These problems created by technologic change present new challenges to the health team.

Legislation

Legislation in regard to nursing practice and in relation to health matters affects the public and nursing. In Chapter 6, legislation governing nursing is discussed. However, changes in legislation affecting health also affect nursing. For example, recent legislation broadens the laws governing abortions in some states and in Canada. This change in the law has lowered the birth rate significantly and has increased the need for nursing care associated with abortions.

Demography

Demography is the statistical study of the population. It includes the distribution of the population (a) by age and (b) by place of residence as well as (c) *mortality* (death) and (d) *morbidity* (incidence of disease) statistics. From demographic data, needs of the population for nursing services evolve. For example:

1. The total populations in both the United States and Canada have increased since 1900. Furthermore, the proportions of elderly people have also increased in both populations, creating an increased need for nursing services for this group. For further information on population, see "Health Problems: Patterns and Trends," Chapter 2.

2. Another study of the population indicates a shift of the primary residence of people from rural (country) settings to urban (city) settings. In 1970, in the United States, 73.5% of the population lived in metropolitan areas in contrast to 64.0% in 1950 (US Department of Commerce 1974b:110–112). Thus most nursing services were provided in urban settings.

3. Mortality rates in the United States reflected a steady decrease from 1900 to 1971, thereby adding 22 years to the average life span at the time of birth (US Department of Health, Education, and Welfare [US DHEW] 1974:7). Much of this decrease can be attributed to the control of infectious diseases such as smallpox and diphtheria. For additional mortality statistics, see Figure 1-3 and Chapter 2.

4. Morbidity studies indicate (a) higher incidence of long-term illness; (b) increase in venereal disease, alcoholism, and drug addiction; (c) increase in lung cancer and heart disease; (d) increase in automobile accidents; (e) increase in homicide; especially among nonwhite men; and (f) high infant mortality (Somers 1971:18–20).

The Nursing Profession

Members of the nursing profession are also actively influencing nursing services. Increasingly they have assumed more responsibility and accountability for nursing activites. They also have established areas of function for nurses outside of hospitals, such as community clinics and home nursing. More recently the American Nurses' Association has published a list of nursing standards in an attempt to determine the quality of nursing care provided to the public (see "Trends in Nursing Practice" in this chapter). Beyond these activities, some members of the nursing profession are involved in health politics. Many are working with legislative committees to develop licensing standards for new branches of the nursing profession, such as nurse practitioners or nurse midwives. Others are developing programs in continuing education or specialized areas of nursing.

Women's Liberation Movement

The women's liberation movement has brought public attention to women's rights and all human rights. Persons are seeking equality in all areas, particularly

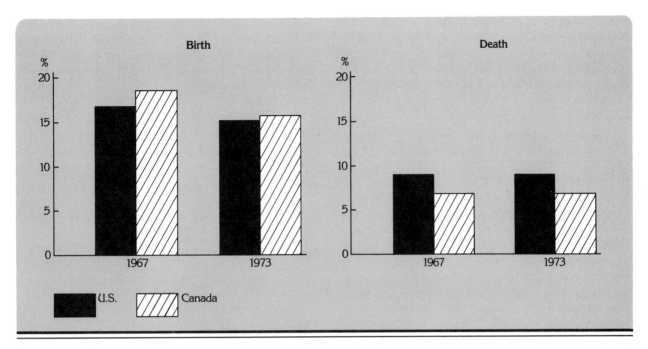

Figure 1-3.   Birth and death rates in the United States and Canada, 1967 and 1973. (From the U.S. Department of Commerce, Bureau of Census, 1974. *Population of the United States trends and prospects: 1950–1990* and Statistics Canada, 1973. *Population.* Ottawa.)

educational, political, economic, and social areas. Because the majority of nurses are women, there has been an effect upon the perspectives of nurses in regard to economic and educational needs. As a result, nurses are increasingly asserting themselves as professional people who have a right to equality with men. Nurses are demanding more responsibility in patient care and are becoming equal members of the health team.

TRENDS IN NURSING PRACTICE

Some trends in nursing practice are subtle and are emerging slowly, while others are obvious and seem to have surfaced quickly. Not all the trends complement each other; some are divergent if not in conflict. Over a period of time, some aspects of nursing practice will emerge as prevailing trends; others may be modified by social forces. As nursing is responsive to societal conditions, some of the following trends in nursing practice will gain in emphasis.

Broadened Focus of Care

The focus of care has broadened from care of the ill to care of people in sickness and in health, and from the patient to the patient and his family. In the past, the nurse's role was chiefly concerned with caring for people who were ill. Nursing care was disease and illness oriented. However, more emphasis is now being placed upon promoting health and preventing disease. It has been predicted that one day all diseases, including heart disease and cancer, will be conquered. At that time the nurse will be chiefly concerned with assisting people to attain their *optimum level of health.* Nursing care is also broadening to include a family focus. The assistance for a family might be directly related to the needs of the patient, or it might be concerned with totally different health problems. For example, the family may need assistance in providing economical but nutritious meals to growing teenagers.

Modern nursing care also includes a holistic

focus. Today's nurse deals with patients as emotional and social beings as well as physical beings. Care is provided not just for a particular disease or wound but for the health of the whole body. The broadened focus of care requires an integration of skills and concepts.

Increasing Scientific Basis

In the past, nursing care was largely *intuitive* or *empirical*. *Empirical* refers to relying upon experience or observation rather than upon science. The nurse sensed the measures that would assist the patient frequently through trial and error, and many nurses, through experience, became highly skilled in providing care in this manner. With research and the resultant knowledge, most nursing care now has a scientific base in the biologic, physical, and social sciences. Some nursing practice today is still intuitive, but as more knowledge is gained, nursing care will have an increasing scientific basis.

Increasingly Complex Technologic Skills

At one time nursing care was chiefly "ministering to the patient, wiping the fevered brow." Nursing care, particularly in hospitals, increasingly necessitates using highly complex machines such as cardiac monitors, respirators, and computers. The focus of nursing care remains the patient, but technologic advances affect the methods used to provide this care.

Increased Independence

Nursing practice increasingly includes areas that use the independent judgment of nurses. At one time nursing practice was entirely dependent, that is, it was a result of a physician's order. Although these activities are still a part of nursing practice, more and more the nurse is functioning in areas that require independent judgment such as teaching dietary practices to pregnant women or providing these women with primary prenatal care.

New Roles

The emergence of new roles for the nurse is a fifth trend. The *nurse clinician* functions in many hospitals today. This nurse had advanced skills in a particular area of nursing practice, for example, psychiatric nursing. The clinician serves as a consultant to the nursing staff and assists them with particular problems they may have in identifying or meeting a patient's needs.

Another new role for the nurse is the expanded role in *primary care*. Primary care refers to the first contact a patient has with the health care system. In the past the first person a patient usually met was the physician. In primary care the nurse takes medical histories and carries out physical examinations traditionally thought of as solely those of the physician.

Primary care nursing has also been adopted in some hospitals. In this situation the patient is assigned to one nurse upon admission. This nurse is totally responsible for the care of three or four patients 24 hours of the day during their hospital stay. This nurse is responsible for establishing the nursing care plan for the patient. The plan is then carried out by other nursing personnel when the nurse is off duty. By using the primary nursing care concept in a hospital, the patient has one nurse in particular who is responsible for communication and care during the entire hospital stay. For the nurse, this method of organzation fosters independent nursing action and greater responsibility and accountability for patient care.

Another innovation is the *independent nursing practitioner*. This nurse usually has an office in the community and functions independently. That is, patients come to the office for nursing care. Some nurses, as independent practitioners, work closely with a group of physicians.

Community Nursing Services

Another trend is the movement of nursing practice to the community. At one time nurses worked only in institutions looking after the sick; however, nursing services now are being provided in the community, often in homes and in clinics. These nursing activities assist not only those who are ill, but they also assist those who are healthy to maintain wellness. This is one of the major areas of growth in the nursing services.

Development of Nursing Standards

One of the most recent developments in nursing is the establishment of standards for nursing practice.

Table 1-2   Standards of Nursing Practice*

Standard	Rationale	Standard	Rationale
1. The collection of data about the health status of the client/patient is systematic and continuous. The data are accessible, communicated, and recorded.	Comprehensive care requires complete and ongoing collection of data about the client/patient to determine the nursing care and needs of the client/patient. All health status data about the client/patient must be available for all members of the health care team.	5. Nursing actions provide for client/patient participation in health promotion, maintenance, and restoration.	The client/patient and family are continually involved in nursing care.
2. Nursing diagnoses are derived from health status data.	The health status of the client/patient is the basis for determining the nursing care needs. The data are analyzed and compared to norms when possible.	6. The nursing actions assist the client/patient to maximize his health capabilities.	Nursing actions are designed to promote, maintain, and restore health.
3. The plan of nursing care includes goals derived from the nursing diagnoses.	The determination of the results to be achieved is an essential part of planning care.	7. The client/patient's progress or lack of progress toward goal achievement is determined by the client/patient and the nurse.	The quality of nursing care depends upon comprehensive and intelligent determination of nursing's impact upon the health status of the client/patient. The client/patient is an essential part of this determination.
4. The plan of nursing care includes priorities and the prescribed nursing approaches or measures to achieve the goals derived from the nursing diagnoses.	Nursing actions are planned to promote, maintain, and restore the client/patient's well-being.	8. The client/patient's progress or lack of progress toward goal achievement directs reassessment, reordering of priorities, new goal setting, and revision of the plan of nursing care.	The nursing process remains the same, but the input of new information may dictate new or revised approaches.

*From American Nurses' Association. 1973. *Standards of nursing practice.* Kansas City, Missouri. Reprinted with permission.

These standards provide patients and nurses with exact criteria against which care can be measured in terms of effectiveness and excellence. Basic to the development of these standards are the following needs:

1. The need of patients and their families to have the assurance that they are receiving a safe and good standard of care.

2. The need of patients and health administrators to know that the standard of care is efficiently provided at an acceptable level. Both the consumer and the health administrator have become increasingly concerned about the cost of all health care.

3. The need of nursing personnel to have precise standards against which they can measure the care they provide, thus protecting themselves and the patients.

Nursing standards (see Table 1-2) clearly reflect the specific functions and activities that nurses provide, as opposed to those functions of other health workers. The standards are written after the nursing activites are identified and classified within an organizational framework.

THE NURSE AS A PROVIDER OF HEALTH CARE

The Roles of the Nurse

Nursing is a system of interrelated people, skills, and concepts, and the roles of the nurse are interwoven throughout this system. The nurse has three main roles in relation to the care of patients and their families, and the emphasis of each role varies with the situation. These interrelated roles are basic to the whole nurse who adapts skills and modes of care as needs arise. The three main roles are (a) therapeutic (instrumental), (b) caring (expressive), and (c) socializing.

The Therapeutic Role

The therapeutic role has the function of curing. This role is illustrated most vividly by the nurse who works in acute patient settings in hospitals, for example, in a coronary care unit. Here the patients are acutely ill, and most of the nurse's activities—dispensing medications, evaluating vital signs, and other such activities—are oriented toward assisting the patients along the road of recovery.

The Caring Role

The caring role is difficult to define specifically. It is the role of human relations. The chief goal of the nurse in this role is to provide support, an intangible that should not be confused with dependence. The nurse supports the patient by attitudes and actions that show concern for patient welfare and accepts the patient as a person, not merely a chart. The nurse recognizes that many people have different backgrounds and different ideas, many of which may be counter to the nurse's views. Nevertheless, the nurse provides care and maintains a harmonious environment to assist the patient's recovery. Through these activities the patient's motivational equilibrium is maintained, thus facilitating the therapeutic function. It is important that these functions also support the therapeutic goals of the patient. For example, if one of the objectives for the patient is to regain independence in activities, then the caring functions must not foster dependence under the guise of support. Also, the nurse is careful not to make decisions for the patient but encourages patient and family participation in planning care. The nurse needs to carry out these caring functions with the welfare of the patient in mind.

This role of the nurse is magnified in the care of people who have long-term illnesses. These patients and their families have time to develop a relationship with nurses and often require supportive, caring functions more than therapeutic functions.

The Socializing Role

The socializing role of the nurse is the one often forgotten. For patients who are separated from their families and their normal activites, socializing offers distractions and respite from the focus on illness. Patients do not always want a therapeutic conversation; sometimes they just want news of another world and conversation they can enjoy. This is particularly true of patients with long-term illnesses.

How Nurses Help

For the nurse, providing assistance is a matter of course. Helping is a fundamental of the nursing profession. Some methods of assisting are more effective than others, and some patients are more willing to receive assistance than others. The situations vary; people have different wants and needs, and the nurse must be flexible enough to adapt. Assistance must be given in a manner that does not destroy the patient's sense of self-worth.

Nursing practice involves helping the patient, family, or both either directly or indirectly. *Direct activities* are those carried out in the presence of the patient or family. Some activities are carried out on the patient's behalf but not in the patient's presence; these are *indirect activities* and include such things as a meeting between nurse and physician to discuss a change in medication for a patient. As that member of the health team who is closest to the patient, the nurse assumes the role of patient advocate, acquainting the physician with the patient's physical and emotional responses to treatment.

The choice of the method of assistance to be used by a nurse depends upon the particular situation. In providing nursing care the nurse needs to be sensitive to the patient on many levels and must be aware of change, selecting a method of help according to the requirements of the situation. Five methods of assisting are

1. Acting for or doing for another.

2. Guiding another.

3. Supporting another.

4. Providing an environment that promotes personal development in one's ability to meet the present or future demands for action.

5. Teaching another (Orem 1971:72).

Acting for or Doing for Another

In this method the nurse's own abilities (physical and mental) are used so that the patient's needs are met. When a patient is unconscious, the care plan is carried out using the nurse's judgment and without the patient's participation. For a nurse to act for a patient who is conscious, however, the patient must legally agree. In most situations, patients can assist in planning their care even if they cannot physically participate in it.

Doing for the patient occurs in a number of situations when it is not possible for the patient to care for himself. Examples are (a) certain physical illnesses, (b) incompetency, and (c) being very young or old.

Guiding Another

In this method of helping, the nurse guides the patient, either verbally or by action. The patient must be willing to accept the guidance or the instruction, and the nurse must be able to provide it. An example would be suggesting to a patient who was up in her chair for the first time after surgery that she return to bed for a rest before becoming too tired. In this situation the nurse is guiding the patient using knowledge of the patient's health and strength.

Supporting Another

A person may be supported either physically or emotionally by a nurse. Often both types of support are given at the same time. For example, when a patient who has had a fractured hip gets out of bed for the first time, he may need physical support because of weakness and encouragement and emotional support to allay his fear of falling. Support may often be the first step in helping a patient toward independent functioning.

Providing a Developmental Environment

In this type of assistance, nurses provide an environment that helps a patient set appropriate goals and meet those goals. For example, a patient who has had an operation and is recovering well may be introduced to a patient who is anticipating the same type of surgery. A child may be taken to a play room and encouraged to exercise his arms by providing toys that will help him accomplish this purpose. A severely depressed person may require surroundings that are sunny, cheerful, and decorated attractively as well as an atmosphere that is safe, simple, and unconfusing.

Teaching Another

Teaching is another way in which nurses can assist patients to develop skills and obtain knowledge. For learning to take place, the patient needs to be ready to learn and to want to learn.

Often, for effective learning, appropriate activities need to be arranged. For example, for a pregnant woman to learn prenatal exercises, she usually needs an opportunity to carry out the exercises while the nurse is present to assist her.

EDUCATION FOR NURSES

The nurse's function today is sufficiently complex that a nursing student requires knowledge in the biologic, physical, and social sciences. It is no longer possible for a nurse to acquire a safe level of skill through empirical means alone. Specific knowledge and skills are required that can only be gained through an organized nursing curriculum.

The traditional orientation of nursing education has been toward learning skills that are required in hospitals. However, considerable evidence exists that there is an increased need for community and home services; there are also some negative aspects of hospitalization, such as separation from a family which in many situations should be avoided. As a result, nursing curricula are now focused more broadly upon health and illness needs, and hospital-community needs, as well as the appropriate knowledge from the biologic, social, and physical sciences.

State laws in the United States and provincial laws in Canada recognize two types of nurses: the licensed practical (vocational) nurse (LPN or LVN) and the registered nurse (RN).

Licensed Practical Nurse Programs

Approved practical nursing programs are provided by community colleges, vocational schools, hospitals, and a variety of health agencies. These courses are usually a year in length and provide both classroom and clinical experiences. At the end of the program the graduate takes examinations to obtain a license as a practical nurse. In some states and provinces, applicants for licensure are assessed on the basis of their nursing experience rather than upon their formal education in an approved school. Licensed practical nurses are employed in hospitals and in community services such as home nursing. Their skills are basically those required for bedside nursing under the guidance of a registered nurse, who has the knowledge and skills to make more accurate nursing judgments.

Registered Nurse Programs

The registered nurse programs are of three general kinds:

1. Diploma programs generally sponsored by hospitals are usually three years in length.
2. Associate degree programs provided by junior and community colleges and some technical institutes are usually two calendar years or three academic years in length.

3. Baccalaureate degree programs provided by universities and senior colleges are usually four years in length.

After graduation from an approved program, the nurse takes examinations to become a licensed RN.

In some areas of the country a ladder type of education exists. This means that the students can move from the practical nurse program to the associate degree and then to the baccalaureate without repeating courses and by obtaining full credits for previous education. Some other variables in nursing programs are the varying emphasis on biologic or social sciences, manual skills or communication skills, and professional education or liberal education. In each approved RN program, however, the students receive appropriate instruction in five areas of nursing: medical, surgical, pediatric, obstetric, and psychiatric nursing.

Certain changes are taking place in the types of programs available. In North America there has been in recent years a continual decrease in the number of diploma programs and an increase in the number of associate degree and baccalaureate programs. In Canada most diploma programs have been transferred into community colleges. Three provinces, Quebec, Ontario, and Saskatchewan have accomplished the change; British Columbia, Alberta, and Manitoba have only partially transferred their nursing programs. The four Atlantic provinces continue to operate diploma programs in hospitals. The educational

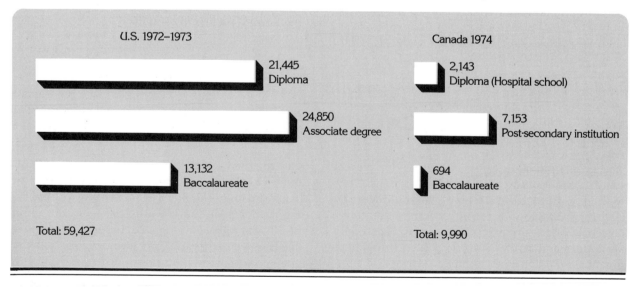

Figure 1-4.   The numbers of nursing graduates from three types of education programs in the United States and Canada. (From the American Nurses Association. 1976. *Facts About Nursing 74-75,* Kansas City, Missouri, p. 66, and Statistics Canada, 1975. *Nursing in Canada,* Ottawa, p. 72.)

institutions offer diplomas rather than associate degrees. See Figure 1-4 regarding graduates from different types of nursing programs in the U.S. and Canada.

Continuing Education Programs

Continuing education programs are also conducted by a variety of educational institutions and health agencies. These programs are usually designed to meet one or more of the following purposes:

1. To keep nurses abreast of newly developed techniques and knowledge.
2. To assist nurses to attain expertise in a specialized area such as intensive care nursing.
3. To provide nurses with information essential to

nursing practice, for example, the legal aspects of nursing.

Education for Expanded Nursing Roles

Expanded roles of nurses such as the nurse clinician and nurse practitioner have been briefly discussed earlier in this chapter. Courses are available at universities to prepare nurses for the independent nurse practitioner role.

Courses to prepare the nurse clinician are offered in many universities at a masters' level. In these courses nurses obtain special skills and knowledge in a selected nursing area. There are also courses available that can assist the nurse to handle the clinical specialist role (Oda, 1977:374).

NURSING AND HEALTH ORGANIZATIONS

Nursing and health organizations bring together *health practitioners* with the intention of improving the health and nursing services of people within their jurisdictions. Nursing organizations are organized at the international, national, and local levels.

International Council of Nurses (ICN)

Illness and disease do not stop at the boundaries of countries. Although different areas of the world and even perhaps different countries have their own health problems, it is often in their mutual interest to cooperate in health and nursing matters. Because of the ease with which people can now travel around the world, problems in India can quickly become problems in North America. More frequently, people traveling abroad return home only to be stricken by an illness rarely seen in this country. As the world grows closer through technologic advances and people travel more, we must become increasingly concerned and involved with health matters of people all over the world. In 1973 the International Council of Nurses stated in the Code for Nurses:

> The need for nursing is universal. Inherent in nursing is respect for life, dignity and rights of man. It is unrestricted by considerations of nationality, race, creed, color, age, sex, politics or social status.

The ICN was established in 1899. Nurses from both the United States and Canada are listed among the founding members. The Council is a federation of national nurses' associations such as the American Nurses' Association and the Canadian Nurses' Association. In 1974 there were 79 national associations from different countries affiliated with the ICN.

The purpose of the ICN is to provide a medium through which national nursing associations can work together and share common interests. By membership in the national association a nurse is automatically a member of the ICN. The functions of the ICN are:

1. To promote the organization of national nurses' associations and advise them in their continued development.
2. To assist national nurses' associations to play their part in developing and improving (a) health service for the public, (b) the practice of nursing, and (c) the social and economic welfare of nurses.
3. To provide means of communication between nurses throughout the world for mutual understanding and cooperation.
4. To establish and maintain liaison and cooperation with other international organizations and to serve as representatives and spokesmen of nurses at the international level.

5. To receive and manage funds and trust which contribute to the advancement of nursing or for the benefit of nurses.

6. To do all such things as may be incidental or conclusive to the attainment of the objective of the ICN (ICN 1973 *b*).

The World Health Organization (WHO)

WHO is one of the special agencies of the United Nations. It is an intergovernmental agency formed in 1948 whose primary aim is to bring all people in the world to the highest possible level of health. As of 1974, 143 countries were members of WHO. Its major activities are to provide assistance to countries in terms of such activities as improving health standards, education, and training, and fighting disease and water pollution.

Nursing makes an essential contribution to the activities of WHO. American and Canadian nurses are frequently requested to go to countries that require assistance in nursing education and in public health. About 300 nurses are at present working for WHO in countries other than their own.

National Nursing Organizations

American Nurses' Association (ANA)

The ANA is the national professional association in the United States as the Canadian Nurses' Association (CNA) is in Canada. The ANA is composed of the nurses' associations from the fifty states, Guam, Virgin Islands, Puerto Rico, and the District of Columbia. These state associations are divided like the provincial associations into regional and local chapters.

The objectives of the ANA are to foster high standards of nursing practice and to promote the education and welfare of nurses so that all people can have better nursing care.

National League For Nursing (NLN)

The League is an organization of both individuals and agencies. The object of the NLN is to foster the development and improvement of all nursing services and nursing education. People who also have an interest in nursing services, for example, hospital administrators, can be members of the League.

The League has a broad range of activities, some of which are to provide educational services such as workshops, recruitment assistance for nursing programs, and a testing service for both registered and practical nurses for licensure.

Nursing Student Organizations

In the United States the National Student Nurses' Association (NSNA) is the official preprofessional organization for students of nursing. It functions under the aegis of the ANA and NLN; however, it is autonomous in that it is financed and run by nursing students.

The purpose of NSNA is "to aid in the development of the individual student and to urge all students of nursing, as future health professionals, to be aware of and contribute to, improving the health care of all people" (NSNA 1972:3).

The NSNA speaks for students of nursing when this is indicated, and it has other activities such as the recruitment of minority groups into nursing and participation in programs related to student suicide and the use of drugs on campus. Members of NSNA also attend the ANA and ICN meetings to meet with nursing students from other states and countries.

In Canada, nursing students have a similar organization (CSNA), and the students attend provincial, national, and international meetings. The provincial Student Nurses' Associations also have programs related to the needs of nursing students and the concerns within the health field in general.

Other Organizations

In addition to these organizations, there are alumni associations for most nursing schools to which the graduates of the particular school can belong. These associations generally have programs of particular concern to the graduates and often have fund-raising activities to support nursing students.

There are other organizations such as the Red Cross, the National Black Nurses' Association, and specialized groups such as the Association of Operating Room Nurses and the American Association of Nurse Anesthetists. For the nurse who qualifies for membership, these organizations also offer services and programs.

THE NEW WORLD OF NURSING

We live in a world of cultural borrowing. Our ideas, philosophies, and technologies are blends of concepts from all over the globe. This borrowing of culture and knowledge has demanded that the professions evolve with the developing world and recognize that everything is part of one vast whole earth—which is but one part of an even greater universe.

Humanity is a part of nature, and the practice of nursing is a part of humanity. As Florence Nightingale asked many times, "Can there be any greater work than this?" Indeed, were she alive today, she might add, "Can there be any greater time to do this work?" Nursing has come a long way. No longer disreputable and no longer a position of servitude, nursing is now an important career choice for many men and women who are vitally interested in preserving health. With a genuine emphasis on such goals as wellness, prevention, and humanism, today's nurse is immersed in the needs and rights of all persons.

It is the purpose of this book to present concepts important for nurses, including basic physiology, fundamental nursing skills, and a means to integrate these three types of knowledge. The book will discuss problems of legality, rights of patients, and rights of nurses as well as such aspects as ethnicity, sexuality, and basic human needs. The differences in persons at various ages and various stages of development will be discussed in both physiologic and psychologic terms. Nursing skills will be presented in the text and will also be summarized in *Procedures* tables. Not any one skill or any one idea makes a whole nurse. This book will take these concepts apart and piece them back together again, integrating one with another in an attempt to provide a framework for a holistic, humanistic professional—today's nurse.

As science and civilization continue to develop, the role of the nurse will change. An even greater emphasis will be placed on disease prevention and health maintenance. Some branches of nursing will achieve greater autonomy and will provide more direct services in patient care. At all times and through whatever complex change, however, the most important aspect of nursing will be very simple: people.

SUMMARY

The nurse in today's world faces the challenge of blending technology with humanity. As a constantly evolving profession, nursing has combined some of the reform concepts of Florence Nightingale with scientific advances of the past few decades. Therefore, a definition of nursing requires input from many sources on many different levels. Contemporary definitions describe the nurturing (caring) function of the nurse as well as the helping functions, which require knowledge and skills on the part of the nurse. The goal of nursing is to assist individuals who are healthy or ill to achieve their optimal levels of functioning. Nursing is a service that involves direct contact, considers the individual differences of people, and serves individuals, families, and communities. Many interrelated elements comprise the practice of nursing. The whole nurse integrates concepts with skills to nurse patients as complete human beings. The whole nurse practices on four different levels: promotion of health, prevention of disease or injury, restoration of health, and consolation of the dying.

Nursing practice has five components. The nurse provides nursing care such as assisting the patient with basic needs, administering medications, and teaching self-care. Some of these activities are *dependent functions*; others are *independent functions*. The nurse also coordinates the care given by other health professionals, plans for continuity of care, evaluates care, and directs others in giving nursing care.

Three broad settings for nursing practice are hospitals, community agencies, and physician's offices (clinics). The degree of autonomy of the nurse, the nursing activities performed, and the relationships the nurse has with other health workers varies within these settings. The nurse may function more independently and may require more judgment skills in some settings than in others. New practice settings are becoming available to the nursing professional, including private practice and nursing research.

Vast changes have taken place in nursing in the past 50 years. Many factors have influenced these changes. The consumer of nursing services is increasingly active in exerting more pressure for health care rather than disease cure. Changes from large extended families to small nuclear families or single-parent families have increased the need for homemaker and day-care services. Decreases in morbidity and mortality, changes in government legislation, and advances in technology all affect needs for nursing services.

Future trends in nursing practice are predictable to some degree by current social and economic forces. Nurses need to have increasing knowledge that is scientifically based and involves preventive health care. New roles and changes in old roles are emerging to meet the demands for service and to maintain a high standard of care. Some of these are the expanded role in primary care, the new role of the nurse clinician, and the new role of the independent nurse practitioner.

Three main roles of the nurse are categorized as therapeutic, caring, and socializing. In the former two roles particularly, the nurse needs to select specific ways of helping patients and families. If the patient is dependent, the nurse must act for or do for the patient. For others who are less dependent but lacking in judgment, knowledge, or energy, the nurse needs to guide or support the patient. Provision of a developmental environment is also essential to the safety, growth, and security needs of patients. Finally, teaching is necessary to help patients acquire necessary knowledge to achieve or maintain health. It is the nurse's responsibility to be sensitive and attuned to which method of helping is warranted in a given situation.

Nurses need knowledge in the biologic, physical, and social sciences. Well-planned curricula in nursing education must include these as well as consider the future health and illness needs of consumers. At present, two types of nurses are recognized in the state and provincial laws of the United States and Canada: the LPN and the RN. Nurses need to participate actively in continuing education programs and in their professional nursing associations to keep abreast of changes and to ensure provision of the best standards of nursing services to people.

In the years to come, nursing will continue to evolve. The modern nurse will continue to integrate concepts with skills, concentrating on humanistic care for the whole person.

SUGGESTED ACTIVITIES

1. In a clinical setting, observe the activities of a licensed practical nurse, an orderly, and a registered nurse. List the functions you observed. In a group discussion, compare these observations with those of other group members and prepare a composite list for each person.

2. In an appropriate clinical setting, observe a head nurse, a community nurse, and a clinical nurse specialist. List the functions you observe, and discuss these functions as they relate to the five components of nursing practice discussed in this chapter.

SUGGESTED READINGS

Cooper, Signe S. 1968. Continuing education: an imperative for nurses. *Nursing Forum* 7(3):289–297.

This author supports the demands of the times, which emphasize ongoing educational commitment by responsible people. Because of rapid scientific advancement, a person who is best equipped for the future is one who strives to keep current as changes occur.

Hannah, Kathryn J. September, 1976. The computer and nursing practice. *Nursing Outlook* 24:555–558.

The author presents information on the use of computers in health care with particular reference to the implications for nurses.

Kreuter, Frances Reiter. May, 1957. What is good nursing care? *Nursing Outlook* 5:302–304. Reprinted in Myers, Mary E. 1971. *Nursing fundamentals.* Dubuque, Iowa: William C. Brown Co., Publishers, pp 25–31.

This 1957 article discusses nursing care as a component of nursing practice. Included is a definition of nursing and Kreuter's concept of nursing care.

Phillips, Michael. December, 1975. Nursing MANpower. *The Canadian Nurse* 71:23–25.

The scarcity of male nurses as role models for psychiatric patients was solved to some degree by the Clarke Institute of Psychiatry.

Smith, Dorothy W. 1970. Change: how shall we respond to it? *Nursing Forum* 9(4):391–399.

In this article the author discusses pressures from society, from other professional groups, and from within the nursing profession itself.

SELECTED REFERENCES

American Nurses' Association. 1973. *Standards of nursing practice.* Kansas City, Missouri.

———. 1976. *Facts about nursing, 74–75.* Kansas City, Missouri.

Bachand, Sr. M. May, 1974. Wanted: a definition of nursing practice. The *Canadian Nurse* 70:26–29.

Barritt, E. R. 1973. Florence Nightingale's values and modern nursing education. *Nursing Forum* 12(1):6–47.

Bayer, Mary, and Brandner, Patty. January, 1977. Nurse/patient peer practice. *American Journal of Nursing* 77:86–90.

Bullough, Bonnie. September, 1976. Influences on role expansion. *American Journal of Nursing* 76:1476–1481.

Eisenman, Elaine Pivnick. October, 1976. Primary care in a mental health facility. *Nursing Outlook* 24:640–645.

Fasano, Marie A. April, 1976. From LVN to RN in one year. *Nursing Outlook* 24:251–253.

Henderson, Virginia. October, 1969. Excellence in nursing. *American Journal of Nursing* 69:2133–2137.

———. 1972. *ICN basic principles of nursing care*. Geneva: International Council of Nurses.

International Council of Nurses. 1973a. *Code for nurses*. Geneva, Switzerland.

———. 1973b. *Constitution and regulations*. Geneva, Switzerland.

Lenburg, Carrie B. July, 1976. The external degree in nursing: the promise fulfilled. *Nursing Outlook* 24:422–429.

Manthey, Marie. January, 1973. Primary nursing is alive and well in the hospital. *American Journal of Nursing* 73:83–87.

Michelmore, Ellen. August, 1977. Distinguishing between AD and BS education. *Nursing Outlook* 25:506–510.

Millis, John S. July, 1977. Primary care: definition of, and access to . . . . *Nursing Outlook* 25:443–445.

Mussallem, Helen K. March, 1969. The changing role of the nurse. *American Journal of Nursing* 69:514–517.

National Commission For the Study of Nursing and Nursing Education. Summary report and recommendations. In Lysaught, Jerome P. 1974. *Action in nursing: progress in professional purpose*. New York: McGraw-Hill Book Co.

National Student Nurses' Association, 1972. *Bylaws*. New York.

Nightingale, Florence. 1859. *Notes on nursing*. London: Harrison.

Nightingale, Florence. 1860. In Bishop, F. L. A., and Goldie, Sue. 1962. *A bio-bibliography of Florence Nightingale*. London: Dawsons of Pall Mall.

Oda, Dorothy. june 1977. Specialized role development: a three-phase process. *Nursing Outlook* 25:374–377.

Orem, Dorothea E. 1971. *Nursing: concepts of practice*. New York: McGraw-Hill Book Co.

Radtke, Maxine, and Wilson, Alan. March, 1973. Team conferences that work. *American Journal of Nursing* 73:506–508.

Sims, Elsie. February, 1977. Preparation for independent practice. *Nursing Outlook* 25:114–118.

Skipper, James K. 1965. The role of the hospital nurse: is it instrumental or expressive. In Skipper, James K., and Leonard, Robert C., eds. *Social interaction and patient care*. Philadelphia: J. B. Lippincott Co.

Smoyak, Shirley A. Nov., 1976. Specialization in nursing: from then to now. *Nursing Outlook* 24:676–681.

Somers, Anne R. 1971 *Health care in transition: directions for the future*. Chicago: Hospital Research and Educational Trust.

Statistics Canada. 1973. *Population*. Ottawa.

———. 1975. *Nursing in Canada: Canadian nursing statistics*. Ottawa.

US Department of Commerce, Bureau of the Census. Nov., 1974a. *Social and economic statistics administration. Current population reports*. Washington, DC.

———. 1974b. *Population of the United States: trends and prospects*. Series 23, No. 49. Washington, DC.

US Department of Health, Education, and Welfare, Public Health Service. 1974. *Facts of life and death*. Rockville, Maryland.

Williams, Carolyn A. April, 1977. Community health nursing—what is it? *Nursing Outlook* 25:250–254.

CHAPTER 2

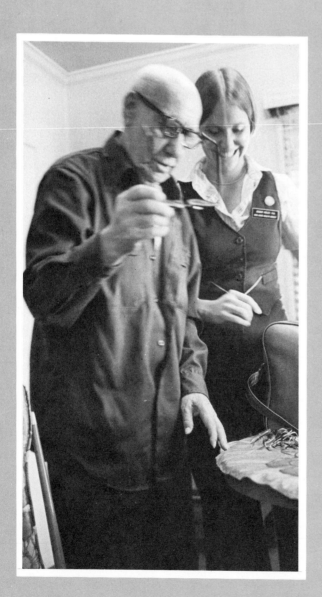

HEALTH AND HEALTH PROBLEMS

PROBLEMS IN THE PRESENT HEALTH-ILLNESS CARE DELIVERY SYSTEM

Fragmentation of Care

Increased Cost of Health-Illness Services

Outdated Knowledge and Skills of Health Practitioners

Needs of Ethnic and Poverty Groups

Special Needs of the Elderly

Uneven Distribution of Health Services Nationally

THE USE OF HEALTH AND ILLNESS SERVICES

FINANCING HEALTH AND ILLNESS SERVICES

OBJECTIVES

- Explain the definition of health and the concept of the health continuum.

- Discuss the general trends in health problems.

- Describe what services are involved in health and illness care.

- Describe the various health care agencies.

- Explain the difference between an official agency and a voluntary agency.

- Discuss some problems in the present health care delivery system.

- Describe how consumers use health services.

- List the six general ways in which health care is financed.

Health or wellness is a much sought after state; it is a highly desirable state for most people and yet, to many it remains elusive. Health can be described as being of sound body, mind, and soul; yet this description does not really explain specifically what health is, much less how people can attain it. Nurses need to know more explicitly the characteristics or behavior identified with a healthy body and a healthy mind before unhealthy conditions can be recognized. An understanding of health must include an understanding of the differences among individuals as well as the process of continually changing health as described in the health continuum.

The health team provides a wide variety of assistance to people who are healthy and who are ill or injured. The former activities are receiving increasing stress in the present day health care system. Most members of the health team function under the supervision of an agency. These agencies are of a wide variety and have different emphases and different functions.

People use health services in various ways. To a large degree the way agencies are used and the amount they are used are the measures of their effectiveness. Sometimes health services do not meet the needs of the people in the community. The nurse may see situations of unmet needs and wonder why such situations exist. Knowledge of the enormous financial support required to provide health services in addition to the enormous financial burden borne by the people of the country for health yields some measure of understanding. Failure to meet patients' needs, however, is difficult to condone, no matter what the reason.

The patterns and trends of health problems reveal how far health services have come and how far they have yet to go in preventing disease. An understanding of this will assist nurses to prepare for their future roles in the health care system and to better understand contemporary change.

A complete health care system has four parts: health promotion, disease prevention, diagnosis and therapy, and rehabilitation. Nurses function in all these areas and need to be aware of the health problems of people, whether they are obvious or hidden.

DEFINITIONS OF HEALTH

Health is a highly individualized perception. It has many meanings for some people and can mean different things to different people. Some people think of health in terms of being able to carry out their normal daily tasks: a woman goes to her employment and accomplishes her usual amount of work; a youngster goes to school and plays baseball at noon. Other people consider themselves healthy only when they have vitality in their daily living and a feeling of wellness. However, definitions of wellness can vary also. One person may consider herself well only when she functions with a high energy level. Another person may never have that amount of energy, yet he may consider himself well.

Meanings and descriptions of health can also vary in relation to geography and to culture. Health in a highly industrialized nation such as the United States is quite different from health as it is described in some of the more deprived nations. In the latter situations, the presence of skin lesions may be considered normal and part of the health picture, whereas the absence of lesions may be considered uncommon.

In summary, there is no absolute definition for health. There is no certain knowledge as to how to attain an ultimate level of health, nor can health itself be measured.

The World Health Organization in 1947 proposed a broad definition of health: "*Health* is a state of complete physical, mental and social wellbeing, and not merely the absence of disease or infirmity" (WHO 1947:1). At that time this definition was considered by some to be impractical; however, more and more it is being viewed as a possible goal for all people.

Health has also been defined as "the state of optimum capacity of an individual for the effective performance of his roles and tasks" (Parsons 1972:107). An emphasis in this definition is the "capacity" of the individual rather than a commitment to roles and tasks. A person by this definition may not wish to go to work, but this does not mean that the individual is not healthy. Another example is that people who have diabetes, epilepsy, or paraplegia can be considered healthy if they can perform roles and tasks effectively within their capacity.

In a study it was found that people have three distinct criteria by which they consider themselves to be ill. These are:

1. The presence or absence of symptoms, such as a fever or pain.

2. Their perceptions of how they feel; for example, good, bad, sick.

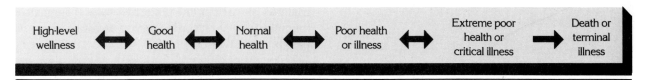

Figure 2-1.   The health continuum from peak-level wellness to death.

3. The ability of the person to carry out daily activities, such as a job or schoolwork (Bauman 1965:206).

The Health Continuum

Wellness and illness can be thought to be on the opposite ends of a health continuum. From the peak level of wellness on the right side of the continuum, a person's condition can move through high-level wellness, good health, normal health, poor health, and extremely poor health, eventually to death. Persons move back and forth within this continuum day by day. There is no distinct boundary across which people move from health to illness or from illness back to health. How persons perceive themselves and how others see them vis-a-vis health and illness will also affect their placement on the continuum. There is considerable range in which people can be considered healthy or ill (see Figure 2-1).

One's state of health is never constant; it is always changing. For example, a man may wake up in the morning with a headache; by noon he feels better, and by evening he feels quite well.

HEALTH PROBLEMS: PATTERNS AND TRENDS

Demographic statistics on the age of the population, mortality, and morbidity reflect trends and needs in the health and illness care system.

Population

Statistics that reflect an increase in the total population over the years indicate the need for an increased number of health and illness services. In both the United States and Canada there have been tremendous population growths, particularly since 1945 (see Figure 2-2). A breakdown of the population reflects an increase in the number of elderly in both populations. In 1975, it was estimated that the total number of people in the United States over the age of 65 years was 21.4 million (US DHEW 1975:181). By the year 2000 it is estimated that there will be an increase to 30 million (US DHEW 1975:195). In Canada a similar increase in the number of older people is anticipated: from 1.7 million in 1974 (Statistics Canada 1974:74) to 3.2 million by the year 2000 (Canada Department of National Health and Welfare 1974:60).

The increased life expectancy rate, reflecting the fact that the average man and woman live longer than they did in years past, is largely due to the success with which many acute diseases are treated today. The reasons for the longer life span of women are multiple. Authorities believe that females have a biologic advantage that requires more research to explain. Other factors contributing to increased relative longevity for women are the lower maternal death rate in women and the higher rate of cardiovascular renal diseases in men. Two other factors affecting the male-to-female population balance are higher accident rates among males and the successful detection and treatment programs for breast and uterine cancer in women. The latter compare to the less successful records for lung cancer in men. From these it can be seen that the increasing number of elderly in the population is reflected in the prevailing kinds of disease. Although the chronic (persisting over a long time) diseases can affect people in all age groups, the elderly show the highest incidence of these conditions in the population. Together with their dependency needs, the elderly require financial, housing, and health care assistance in ever-increasing numbers. Within this elderly group, the ratio in the United States is 100 women to 76 men in the over-65 age group (Somers 1974:16). In Canada in 1974 the life expectancy at birth for males was 69.5 years and for females 77.1 years (Canada Department of National Health and Welfare 1976:58).

In both the United States and Canada the other age group that requires the most health services is the very young, and it also makes up a sizable proportion

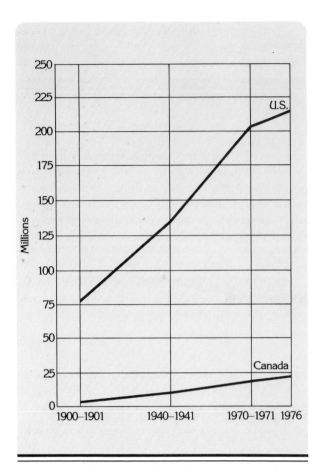

Figure 2-2.   The increases in population in the United States (1900) and Canada (1901) to 1976. (From the U.S. Department of Commerce, April, 1977. *Estimates of the Population of the United States to March 1, 1977.* Series P.25, No. 700, p. 1. U.S. Bureau of the Census *Current Population Reports.* Series P.25, No. 643. *Estimates of the Population of the United States by Age, Sex and Race. July 1, 1974 to 1976.* U.S. Government Printing Office, Washington, D.C. 1977, p.1. *Census of Canada Population:* Geographic Distributions Catalogue 92-801, Bulletin 1.2.)

of the population. In the United States in 1975 there were almost 41 million children under the age of 15. In Canada in the same year there were about 6 million under the age of 15 (United Nations 1976).

Mortality

Mortality means death, and mortality statistics are stated as a ratio of the population. The mortality rates of infants are falling but are still high for an indus-

trialized country. In the United States it is estimated that within the first six days of life, 16 babies of every 1000 born will die.

The major causes of death in these early days are attributed to immaturity, lack of oxygen, and other generally defined conditions. During the first year of life the four most important causes of death are congenital malformations, accidents, influenza, and pneumonia. Deaths from ages one to four years are chiefly due to accidents. During the ages of four to fourteen years, deaths are rare. However, the rate in the fifteen to nineteen age period increases again, with accidents as the major cause of death. The death rate from then on increases with age, and until age thirty-five years, accidents continue to be the major cause of death. After that time, cardiovascular-renal disease and malignant neoplasms become the major cause of death until the end of the life span. The major causes of death in the general population are shown in Table 2-1.

In Canada, ischemic heart disease and cerebrovascular accidents together accounted for 41.3% of the total mortality in 1971 (see Table 2-2).

Table 2-1   Three Leading Causes of Death in the United States by Age Group (1970)*

Age	Cause	Number
1–4 years	Accidents	4,300
	Congenital anomalies	1,331
	Influenza and pneumonia	1,043
5–14 years	Accidents	8,203
	Malignant neoplasms	2,429
	Congenital anomalies	901
15–24 years	Accidents	24,336
	Homicide	4,157
	Suicide	3,128
25–44 years	Accidents	23,970
	Diseases of the heart	18,238
	Malignant neoplasms	17,841
45–64 years	Diseases of the heart	176,618
	Malignant neoplasms	121,000
	Cerebrovascular disease	31,193
65 years and over	Diseases of the heart	538,417
	Malignant neoplasms	185,280
	Cerebrovascular disease	170,051

*From US, Department of Health, Education, and Welfare, Public Health Service, Health Resources Administration, National Center for Health Statistics. 1974. *Facts of life and death.* Publication no. (HRA) 74–1222 (Washington, D.C.).

Table 2-2   Major Causes of Death in Canada, All Ages (1971)*

Cause	Percentage of all deaths	Predominant ages
Ischemic heart disease	31.1%	40 years and over
Cerebrovascular disease	10.2%	65 years and over
Respiratory diseases and lung cancer	10.0%	Under 1 year and 55 years and over
Motor vehicle and all other accidents	7.6%	All ages
Cancer of the gastrointestinal tract	5.1%	50 years and over
Cancer of the breast, uterus, and ovary	3.1%	40 years and over
Diseases specific to the newborn	2.1%	Under 1 week
Suicide	1.6%	15 years to 65 years
Congenital anomalies	1.3%	Under 1 year

*From Canada, Department of National Health and Welfare. 1974. *A new perspective on the health of Canadians: a working document.* Ottawa, p. 22.

Morbidity

Morbidity statistics describe the incidence of disease in the population and are more difficult to obtain than mortality statistics. Illness is usually not reported except for certain contagious diseases, and it is often treated in the home. One source of morbidity data is the number of days patients spend in hospitals. These figures have limitations in that they generally reflect severe cases and not diseases such as colds and influenza that do not require hospitalization.

Using patient hospital-days for morbidity statistics in Canada reflects the following: heart disease accounted for 9.0% of all causes for hospitalization, followed by accidents and respiratory diseases (see Table 2-3). It is recognized, however, that the major morbidity in Canada, which does not necessarily involve hospitalization, includes alcoholism, venereal disease, dental disease, and psychologic illnesses (Canada Department of National Health and Welfare 1974:24–25).

Mental health problems are an ever increasing morbidity statistic. Patients with mental health problems occupy half of the hospital beds in the United States. Although there has been a major effort to establish community services for the mentally ill in recent years, the problem does not appear to have diminished.

Trends and Problems

In assessing health statistics, it is possible to summarize some significant trends and problems in the health of people in the United States and Canada. These are:

1. A high infant mortality rate with special reference to nonwhite babies.

2. Increasing death rate from the chronic diseases, for example, heart disease.

3. Recent increase in venereal disease in some areas of both countries.

4. Steady increase in alcoholism and drug addiction.

5. Increase in the death rate from lung cancer.

6. Increase in mortality from automobile accidents.

7. Decline in the incidence of acute contagious disease.

8. Rapid rise in the incidence of homicide and suicide.

Table 2-3   Patient-Days by the Ten Leading Causes of Illness in Canada, All Ages (1973)*

Cause	Number of days	Percent
1. Heart disease	3,725,130	9.0
2. Accidents	3,277,061	7.9
3. Respiratory diseases	3,069,400	7.4
4. Cerebrovascular disease	2,610,115	6.3
5. Mental disorders	2,573,827	6.2
6. All deliveries	2,160,397	5.2
7. Diseases of the nervous system	2,019,026	4.9
8. Diseases of the musculoskeletal system	1,827,948	4.4
9. Other diseases of breast and female genitalia	1,087,825	2.6
10. Cholelithiasis	1,041,273	2.5

*From Canada, Department of National Health and Welfare. 1976. *Health field indicators, Canada and provinces.*

THE HEALTH CARE DELIVERY SYSTEM

The health care delivery system in North America provides two general types of services: illness care services (restorative) and health care services (preventive). Illness care services help people who are ill or injured. Health care services provide for the promotion of better health for people and for the prevention of disease and accidents. Although most facilities within the system, for example, hospitals, clinics, and physicians' offices, provide both types of services, illness care services heavily predominate. In fact, most services are oriented around illness care; preventive care is very much a secondary activity. One exception to this generalization might be the community nurse in some areas of the country whose major service is immunization, mother and child counseling, and general health promotion.

The health care facilities have been influenced in the past largely by the needs of the people providing the service. For example, hospitals have developed in relation to medical and technologic advances and generally reflect the needs of physicians. People have also expected that health care facilities would be available to help them primarily when they were ill or injured. As a result, preventive health care facilities have been slower to develop. This can be attributed to three major factors:

1. The physician is largely illness oriented in his or her practice.

2. The consumer is less well aware of preventive and health promotion requirements.

3. The nurse's role as the chief provider of health care has been slow to evolve, and frequently the illness care activities take precedence over preventive health care activities.

Comprehensive Health and Illness Care

Comprehensive health and illness care services should encompass four areas: health maintenance; prevention of disease and injury; diagnosis and treatment of disease and injury; and rehabilitation. None of these services is necessarily independent of the other; frequently they operate at the same time and overlap in their effects. For example, a patient receiving a diagnostic test, such as a chest radiograph for tuberculosis, might also be acquiring knowledge that will help her prevent disease; or a patient who is receiving iron pills in order to restore his hemoglobin level may at the same time learn to prevent the problem by a nutritious diet. In looking at the concept of total health and illness care, both physical (somatic)

and mental health and illness are included. *Physical* (or *somatic*) health and illness refer to the human body, whereas *mental* health and illness refer to the mind as distinct from the body. *Psychosomatic,* also referred to as somatopsychophysiologic, refers to the mind and the body and the interrelationship of the two in a person, which, for example, can occur when mental or emotional problems result in bodily symptoms such as a headache.

The World Health Organization stated that a comprehensive health service should encompass care in the following five categories: health maintenance, increased risk stage, early detection stage, clinical stage, and rehabilitation.

Health Maintenance

Health maintenance will probably become one of the fastest growing areas of the health-illness care system in the future. As people become increasingly aware of good health and as the diseases are conquered, more and more emphasis will be placed upon this area. At the present time, health promotion is the major function of the community nurse and community health workers generally. At this time, programs in health promotion are directed toward five major areas: (a) maternal and child health, (b) mental health, (c) environmental health (physical fitness), (d) nutrition, and (e) dental health.

Prevention of Disease and Injury

Prevention of disease has long been emphasized with reference to the infectious diseases. The longer life expectancy and lowered mortality figures of the nineteenth and early twentieth centuries can be almost completely attributed to effective preventive programs in relation to diphtheria, smallpox, typhus, typhoid fever, and tuberculosis. More recently there have been effective preventive programs for poliomyelitis.

Prevention of disease goes beyond infectious diseases. Research is underway in regard to the prevention of long-term diseases such as malignant neoplasms and cardiovascular diseases. On national, state (provincial), and local levels, prevention programs in recent years have been aimed at assisting with obesity problems and publicizing, through the news media, the dangers of smoking, alcoholism, and drugs.

Today, prevention programs appear to be of four major kinds:

1. Crisis programs to prevent mental health problems on an individual and family basis.

2. Early detection programs for chronic disease, for example, cardiovascular diseases.

3. Safety programs aimed at both industrial and automobile accidents.

4. Environmental programs to prevent pollution and destruction of the environment (water, air, forests, natural life).

Preventive health programs are generally oriented to the family and a community. The individual approach of immunization programs is still practiced and is essential to maintain control of the infectious diseases; however, the broader approach is being utilized increasingly in order to assist more people to prevent disease and injury.

The World Health Organization describes an increased-risk stage as the time when preventive measures can be taken to protect an individual who for some reason is particularly susceptible to disease. An example might be the administration of tetanus antitoxin to a person who has a contaminated wound.

Diagnosis and Treatment of Disease and Injury

The diagnosis and treatment of disease and injury has long occupied the forefront position in the health care service. Essentially, this area is the prerogative of the physician, and patients usually seek help at their own initiative.

In addition, there are diagnosis and treatment programs on a broad basis. Community-wide programs are now conducted to detect tuberculosis, venereal disease, cancer, hypertension, glaucoma, sickle cell anemia, and diabetes. Advertising in these areas tells people what symptoms to look for as well as the importance of consulting a physician. Mobile units visit local communities and offer several services, usually free of charge. Early detection is emphasized together with appropriate treatment.

The early detection stage is the time when early symptoms of disease begin to appear. At this stage, detection and appropriate treatment can often prevent more serious problems; for example, the importance of early diagnosis and treatment of a breast growth cannot be overemphasized.

The clinical stage is the treatment stage for illness and injury. At this time, the typical symptoms are exhibited by the patient and the physician's therapy is prescribed.

Rehabilitation

Rehabilitation applies to all aspects of health, both physical and mental. It presupposes that a person can return to an optimal level of functioning. Not only does it include the reeducation of muscles so that a person with a walking disability can become mobile again, it also includes the acquisition of an emotional status congruent with fulfilling social roles for the emotionally ill patient. Rehabilitation starts at the point of the first encounter of the patient with a health team member. It continues until that person is functioning as self-sufficiently as possible. Often rehabilitation is thought of narrowly as relating to a physical disorder and to a physiotherapy department, but rehabilitation as it exists today frequently involves a patient, a family, and perhaps a total community. It no longer applies only to physical disorders but to social and emotional factors as well. Rehabilitation focuses on the principle that the adult functions independently and is able to meet personal needs as well as the needs of dependents. In rehabilitation this goal provides the direction for the activities; the capacity of the individual establishes the level of the functioning.

HEALTH CARE AGENCIES

A wide variety of facilities and agencies provide illness and health care in the average community. Some of these are:

1. Physicians' offices and clinics
2. Hospitals
3. Day-care centers
4. Home nursing services
5. Rehabilitation services
6. Nursing homes (in some places called extended-care hospitals or facilities)

Physicians' Offices and Clinics

The physician's office is one of the major sources of illness care in North America. The majority of physicians either have their own offices or work with several other physicians in a group practice. People go to a physician because they consider themselves ill, or because a relative thinks the patient is ill, or because the patient feels the need of medical advice.

The physician with an office practice is chiefly illness oriented. The average time the physician spends directly with a patient in an office visit is very short— 6.1 minutes in one study (Somers 1971:9). In this time the physician is mainly concerned with the diagnosis and therapy pertaining to the patient's immediate illness or injury.

Hospitals

Hospitals are the main institutions through which restorative care to the ill and injured has been provided. They vary in size from the 12-bed rural hospital to the 1500-bed metropolitan hospital with a 50-bed day surgery center. Hospitals can be classified according to their ownership or control and according to the services they provide. According to ownership and control, hospitals are classified as governmental (public) and nongovernmental (private). Governmental (public) hospitals are either federal, state, city, or county hospitals in the United States and federal or provincial hospitals in Canada. In both countries governments have traditionally provided hospital facilities for veterans, the merchant marine service, and individuals with long-term illness. The government in the United States provides approximately 70% of the hospital beds in the country. General hospitals admit patients requiring a variety of facilities, including medical, surgical, obstetric, pediatric, and psychiatric services. Other hospitals offer only specialty services such as psychiatric or pediatric.

Although hospitals are chiefly thought of as institutions that provide care, they also have other functions such as providing resources for health-related research and teaching. In these two aspects, the hospital personnel may actually conduct research and educational programs, or they may provide resources for other personnel such as teachers from a university to carry out research and teaching responsibilities.

Nongovernmental or private hospitals are generally owned or controlled by churches, industry, private groups of physicians or citizens, or fraternal orders.

Hospitals can be further described as acute or chronic. An acute hospital provides assistance to patients who are acutely ill or whose length of illness and need for hospitalization is relatively short, for example, one day to perhaps one month as a maximum length for stay. Long-term hospitals provide health services for people on a longer time basis, sometimes for years or the remainder of the patient's life.

The traditional organization within a hospital has been departmental. Departments such as medical, nursing, dietary, laboratory, maintenance, pharmacy, or purchasing carry out their functions, which may be directly or indirectly related to patient care. One of the limitations of this organizational pattern is the isolation of each department and the subsequent discrepancies in personnel utilization and efficiency.

A more recent organizational structure for hospitals is the arrangement of the departments into systems and programs, each of which has a common characteristic. The systems provide a commonality among diverse functions; for example, the business system would include the functions of the business office, the accounting office, and the payroll office. Some or all of these might have been separate departments in the more traditional organizational pattern. The programs are the means of coordinating the resources of the various systems into care, teaching, and research functions. For example, in an ambulatory care program for patients, assistance is received from the four systems of business, quality control, patient care, and professional services in this manner:

1. Business system collects fees.
2. Quality control system establishes medical records.
3. Patient care system supplies nursing personnel and social services.
4. Professional service system provides physicians' services.

With the expansion of knowledge and skills in the health field together with the increasing costs in health care, flexible organizational patterns will be seen as a means of providing a diversity of services efficiently and effectively.

Day-care Centers

Day-care centers are either attached to hospitals or operate independently to provide health service during daytime hours. Often these agencies provide a specific service as, for example, the community mental health center for patients who have emotional problems but who do not require hospitalization, and the day surgery centers. The latter admit children or adults who require minor surgery to the center (often in a hospital) in the morning. After the surgery, the patient returns to the center where members of the family often assist with nursing care. The patient returns home the same day. These centers have two advantages: they permit the patient to continue to live at home while at the same time obtaining needed health care and they free costly hospital beds for the more seriously ill patients.

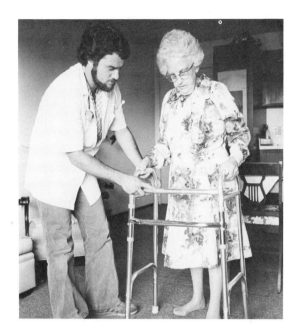

Figure 2-3. Home nursing services provide assistance to an individual who is learning to walk.

Home Nursing Services

Home nursing services operate out of hospitals and community agencies. In both instances a variety of nursing services can be provided to patients and to families. Some of these services are: well-baby visits to new parents to assist with the initial care of the baby; bedside nursing for the chronically ill; the administration of medications, for example, insulin to diabetics; and mental health assistance for patients and families who have emotional problems. As a counterpart of these home nursing services there are now laboratory visiting services in some metropolitan areas. Through this service, patients who are confined to their homes can have specimens such as blood taken and submitted to a laboratory for analysis (see Figure 2-3).

Rehabilitation Centers

Rehabilitation involves assisting a person who is disabled to achieve optimum levels of physical, social, and vocational functions. Rehabilitation frequently includes working with the family and the community as well as the patient. Rehabilitation centers often exist as departments within hospitals and provide services to patients admitted to the hospital and to patients who come to the center on an appointment basis. Some rehabilitation centers also exist as separate health agencies with inpatient, outpatient, and home visiting services. These centers often combine the services of physical therapists, occupational

therapists, social workers, and nursing personnel. Specialists such as speech and recreational therapists and vocational counselors may also be on the staff of such a center.

Nursing Homes (Personal Care Homes)

Nursing homes are usually owned by individuals or groups of individuals, for example, physicians or ethnic groups, or by governments. A wide variety of institutions can be called nursing homes, and they offer a considerable variety of services. Generally speaking, they provide care on a long-term basis in contrast to the community hospital. Because long-term illness occurs with the highest frequency among the elderly, many nursing homes have programs that are oriented to the needs of this age group.

The type of care provided to the patients varies considerably. Some homes admit and retain only residents who can dress themselves and are ambulatory. Other homes provide bed care for patients who are more incapacitated. Nursing homes can, in effect, become home to people, and consequently the people who live there are frequently referred to as residents rather than patients.

Official and Voluntary Agencies

Agencies in the community that provide illness and health care services are financed and operated either by the government (official agencies) or chiefly through contributions from the people in the community (voluntary agencies).

Official Agencies

Official agencies are established at the local, state (provincial), and federal levels. Local health departments (county, bicounty, or tricounty) have the responsibility traditionally for (a) developing programs that are responsive to the health needs of the people, (b) providing the necessary staff and facilities to carry out these programs, and (c) continually evaluating the effectiveness of the programs and monitoring changing needs. State health organizations (approximately 60 different organizations) are responsible for assisting the local health departments. In some remote areas of a state, these departments also provide direct services to people.

The Public Health Service (PHS) of the US Department of Health, Education, and Welfare is an official agency at the federal level. Its functions include:

1. Research and training in the health field.
2. Assistance to communities in planning and developing health facilities.
3. Assistance through financing and provision of trained personnel to states and local communities.

The federal governments in both the United States and Canada maintain responsibility for health matters of seamen and those related to interstate and interprovincial transportation. Otherwise, health matters through legislation are generally the responsibility of states in the United States and of the provinces in Canada.

Voluntary (Nonofficial) Agencies

Voluntary health service agencies are supported by the people in a community. They are non-profit-making organizations that rely on donations and, in some cases, government grants for support. They are usually formed by volunteers in response to a specific recognized need such as day care for the mentally retarded. Often they supplement official agencies' functions. Some voluntary agencies are oriented to the care of special groups in the community, others to special programs such as pollution control.

Once a voluntary agency has pointed out a need in a community, an official agency may well take over some of the voluntary agencies' functions. One example of this is the Cancer Society, which funded treatment for cancer. The treatment functions were taken over by official government agencies such as hospitals, and the Cancer Society retained its nontreatment functions such as fund raising. Other examples are the National Heart Associations and Visiting Nurse Services (Associations).

THE HEALTH TEAM

The health team consists of a group of people from different disciplines who coordinate their particular skills in order to assist a patient and/or family. The personnel who comprise a particular team will depend upon the needs of the patient. In the present system of health care in North America the personnel commonly include physicians, nurses, dietitians, physiotherapists, social workers, occupational therapists, paramedical technologists, pharmacists, and inhalation therapists.

The Physician

In a hospital setting, the physician is responsible for the medical diagnosis and for determining the therapy required by a person who is ill or injured. In a community setting the physician may also be involved in diagnosis and therapy, or in a more consultative role. An example of the latter is the physician who specializes in public health and who serves as a consultant to the school nurse in regard to children who have health problems.

A *physician* is a person who is legally authorized to practice medicine in a particular jurisdiction. The physician will have successfully completed a course of medical studies.

The Nurse

A number of nursing personnel may be involved in the health team and may have their own nursing team (see "The Nursing Team"). Sometimes nurses may find it necessary to provide some of the services normally ascribed to other members of the team. This often happens in settings other than large metropolitan hospitals where all the health services required by a patient are not available. An example of this might be assisting a patient who has had a cerebral vascular accident (stroke) with remedial exercises to regain function of his left arm. In an urban hospital these exercises would generally be taught by a physiotherapist; however, in a rural setting a physiotherapist's services are often not available, so the nurse frequently provides this assistance.

The Dietitian or Nutritionist

When dietary and nutritional services are required, the dietitian or nutritionist may also be a member of a health team. Dietitians in hospitals design special diets, for example, for a child who has diabetes mellitus, and they supervise the preparation of the meals according to the diet. The nutritionist in a community setting recommends healthy diets for people and is frequently involved in broad advisory services in regard to the purchase and preparation of foods.

Because of the institutional setting for the activity, the dietitian in the hospital is mostly involved with therapeutic diets. The nutritionist in the community may more often function at the level of promoting health and preventing disease, for example, advising families about regular balanced diets for growing children and during pregnancy.

The Physiotherapist

The physiotherapist (physical therapist) provides assistance to a patient who has problems related to his musculoskeletal system. The physiotherapist's functions can be described as:

1. Assessing mobility and strength.
2. Providing therapeutic measures, for example, exercises and heat applications to improve mobility and strength.
3. Teaching patients new skills, for example, how to walk with an artificial leg.
4. Teaching patients measures to prevent illness, for example, teaching deep breathing to a patient before surgery as a preventive measure against postoperative pneumonia.

Most physiotherapists provide their services within hospitals; however, independent pratitioners are establishing offices in communities and providing a service to patients either at an office or in the patient's home.

The Social Worker

The patient and his/her family are assisted by the *social worker* with such problems as finances, rest home accommodation, counseling on marital problems, and adoption of children. It is not unusual for health problems to produce problems in living. For example, an elderly woman who lives alone and has a stroke resulting in impaired walking may find it impossible to continue to live in her third-floor apartment.

The Occupational Therapist

The occupational therapist assists patients with some impairment of function to gain skills as they relate to activities of daily living (ADL) and/or helps people with a skill that is therapeutic and at the same time provides some satisfaction. An example of teaching an activity of daily living might be teaching a man who has severe arthritis in his arms and hands how to adjust his kitchen utensils so that he can continue to cook. The same man could be taught a therapeutic skill such as weaving, which could be a recreational activity for him but also assists him to exercise his arms and hands. Occupational therapists coordinate their activities closely with those of other members of the health team.

The Paramedical Technologist

Laboratory technologists, radiologic technologists, and nuclear medicine technologists are just three kinds of paramedical technologists in an ever expanding medical technology field. *Paramedical* refers to some connection with medicine. Laboratory technologists examine and study specimens such as urine, feces, blood, and discharges from wounds in order to provide the physician with exact information that can facilitate the medical diagnosis and the effectiveness of a therapeutic regimen. The radiologic technologist assists with a wide variety of x-ray procedures, from the simple chest radiograph familiar to most people to the more complex fluoroscopy and radiography of the patient's stomach using a contrast medium. The nuclear medicine technologist is a more recent member of the technology group. Through the use of radioactive materials, the nuclear medicine technologist can provide diagnostic information about the functioning of a patient's liver and can also provide therapeutic doses of radioactive materials as part of a therapeutic regimen. These technologists have highly developed skills and specialized knowledge, which is important to patient care.

The Pharmacist

The *pharmacist* prepares and dispenses pharmaceuticals in hospital and community settings. The role of the pharmacist in monitoring and evaluating the actions and effects of medications on patients is becoming increasingly prominent. Pharmacists are also actively involved in preparing individual dosages for patients in some hospitals that employ the Unit Dose System, and in some settings they prepare and add medications for intravenous therapy.

The Inhalation Therapist

The *inhalation therapist* or respiratory technologist is skilled in therapeutic measures used in the care of patients with respiratory problems. These therapists are knowledgeable about oxygen therapy devices, intermittent positive pressure breathing respirators, artificial mechanical ventilators, and accessory devices used for inhalation therapy. Frequently they are involved in diagnostic procedures such as pulmonary function tests. Programs in inhalation therapy are offered in post-secondary educational institutions and are usually of two or three years duration.

THE NURSING TEAM

The *nursing team* is composed of personnel who provide nursing services to a patient and/or family. The membership of the team will vary depending upon the needs of the particular patient. Generally speaking, the leadership of the nursing team is provided by a registered nurse. The team leader is responsible for the delegation of duties to other members of the team and for the care given to the patients. A team can include registered nurses from baccalaureate, diploma, and associate degree programs as well as nurse clinicians (often in a consultative role), community nurses, vocational nurses (practical nurses), and non-nurse personnel. This latter group may include orderlies, aides, nursery workers, and nursing assistants.

The members of the nursing team have a wide variety of educational backgrounds and nursing skills. The function of a particular member in a patient's care is dependent upon the patient's and/or family's needs and the knowledge and skill of the individual team member. The patient is the focus of the team whose members collaborate on a patient care plan. Whenever possible, it is desirable for the patient and family to also be active participants in both planning and implementation of care. In some situations, when the patient's family members are absent, other persons such as friends may assume the role of family members. The degree of a patient's participation will be determined by physical and mental capacity needed at that particular time.

PROBLEMS IN THE PRESENT HEALTH-ILLNESS CARE DELIVERY SYSTEM

Currently there are several problems in the health-illness care system as it exists in North America. Many of the problems are a result, or partially a result, of the enormous change that has taken place in health-illness care during the past 30 years. The major advances in the medical field, in fact in an entire technologic world, have brought a better quality of care to many people. However, along with this improved care, there are problems such as the fragmentation of care, the cost of the health-illness service, and the outdated knowledge and skills of some practitioners in the health field.

Other problems have always existed with health-illness delivery systems and are still present today. Some of these are the needs of poverty groups for care, the needs of minority groups for particular assistance, the needs of the illiterate, semiliterate, and poorly educated for information and knowledge, and the needs of an increasingly large group of the elderly. Another problem is the uneven national distribution of health-illness services, that is, the limited resources available in rural areas and in the inner-city areas as contrasted with the services available in urban-suburban areas. The consumer is becoming increasingly aware of these problems and is exerting increasing pressure to correct them, but corrections are gradual and have to occur within the economic and political framework of the country.

Fragmentation of Care

Along with the highly developed skills and the new knowledge that has resulted largely in the past 30 years of research, an ever increasing number of health workers are being used to provide these services. They may be highly specialized technicians or technologists who have relatively narrow but exacting skills, such as respiratory technologists, biomedical electronic technologists, and nuclear medicine technologists, to name just a few. Increased specialization has also taken place among physicians. The ratio of physicians practicing primary care dropped from 94 per 100,000 population in 1931 to 73 per 100,000 population in 1967 (US Bureau of the Census 1976). All this specialization means fragmentation of care and sometimes less than desirable total care. To patients, it may mean they will be assisted by from perhaps five to 30 people during their hospital experience. This seemingly endless stream of personnel is often confusing and frightening. The patient often feels like a cog in the wheel and asks, "Who really cares about me?" and "Who is really responsible?" With the increasing number of health workers there are also problems with the smooth flow of information and plans to help the patient. Again, the patient wonders, "Will someone forget to order my medication?" "Will someone help me get my meals when I return home from the hospital?" The concept of total care is more difficult to implement when so many people are involved.

Increased Cost of Health-Illness Services

The problem of financing the health-illness services is an ever increasing one. There are six major reasons for these increased costs:

1. Existing equipment and facilities are continually becoming obsolete as research uncovers new and better methods in health-illness care.
2. Additional space and sophisticated equipment are required in order to provide the newest of diagnostic and treatment methods.
3. Inflation increases all costs.
4. The total population has grown.
5. People increasingly recognize that health is a right of *all* people, hence larger numbers of people are seeking assistance in health matters.
6. The number of people who provide health-illness services has increased.

Despite the programs that assist individuals to pay for their services (see "Financing Health and Illness Services") it is estimated that between 30 and 40 million people in the United States have no health insurance coverage, and another 60 million have inadequate coverage. The rising costs of health-illness care have a very personal meaning to many of the nation's population.

Outdated Knowledge and Skills of Health Practitioners

With the many discoveries in the health field, graduates rapidly become out of date in their skills unless they make a concentrated effort to update themselves through continuing education programs of various sorts. Many professional groups are well aware of this problem, and steps are being taken to ensure that practitioners are current and show evidence of updating their skills in order to maintain their licenses. In some states, continuing education units (CEUs) are mandatory as a requisite for licensure (for example, Florida).

Needs of Ethnic and Poverty Groups

There is a cultural lag in reference to the provision of health-illness services to ethnic groups within the community. The more sophisticated and impersonal the health services become, the further they are removed from groups who are inwardly oriented and who have a strong family tradition. These groups tend to rely upon the private physician. They prefer the personalized care of someone who understands them and their family. In fact, many such people look upon the modern health care system with distrust.

It has also been mentioned that there is a group of people in the United States who have no health insurance coverage. For the very wealthy, health insurance is no problem, but most people without insurance require assistance in order to maintain their health. Along with poverty, there is frequently fear and ignorance: fear of what might happen if help were requested and ignorance about how and when to obtain health care.

Quasi-practitioners are sometimes sought by these groups in lieu of scientifically oriented health practitioners. Quasi-practitioners are nonmedical healers who use a wide variety of methods that are not validated by scientific means. Among them are the faith healers, the magical healers, and the practitioners of folk medicine. Examples of the latter are the Spanish-American *medicastro* (quack) and *curandero* (Healer, medicine man) of the southwestern United States. There is little question that these groups meet some needs of people; however, the danger is that while people are being treated in this manner, diseases that could possibly be cured by science become incurable. The emotional appeal of these quasi-practitioners is not restricted to the lower socioeconomic groups. Their appeal is broad, but they are less accepted by people who have some scientific education.

Special Needs of the Elderly

Because people over 65 are becoming an increasingly large group in the population, their health needs deserve special concern. The long-term illnesses are most prevalent in this group, and with these illnesses frequently come special needs for housing, treatment services, and financial support. The elderly particularly need to feel they are still part of a community even though they are approaching the end of the life span. Feelings of being useful, wanted, and productive citizens are essential to their health. Special programs are being designed in communities in order that many of the talents and skills of this group are still used and not lost to society. These programs, for example, partial employment, are designed with the capacity of the elderly person in mind.

Uneven Distribution of Health Services Nationally

Serious problems exist in the distribution in health services in both the United States and Canada. Two facets of this problem in the provision of care by physicians are: (a) the uneven distribution of physicians as evidenced by the relatively high ratio of physicians to population in Washington, D.C., of 318 per 100,000 as compared to 69 to 100,000 in Mississippi (some rural areas in fact have no physicians) and (b) the increase in the number of specialists as compared to the number of primary-practice physicians. The same problems exist for other health care workers such as nurses and physiotherapists (Somers 1971:7).

THE USE OF HEALTH AND ILLNESS SERVICES

In the United States and Canada more and more people are seeking personal help for health problems. In 1963, in the United States alone, approximately 65% of the population saw a physician at least once. Of this group over 8% were admitted to a hospital, and half of them had some surgical procedure (Anderson and Andersen 1972:387).

The hospital is the fastest growing part of health services. The admission rate increased from 59 per 1000 population in 1935 to 130 per 1000 population in 1971. With this rising increase in use, there has also been a rising increase in cost. It is estimated that the average bed in an acute general hospital cost $75 per day in 1971. With the advent of hospital insurance, more people are now admitted to hospitals than before. The length of stay of the average patient in 1975 was 7.8 days (US DHEW 1977). This shortening of the hospital stay period can be explained by the change in the medical concept of care to early ambulation of patients as well as the increase in the number of patients admitted to hospitals with minor conditions. An additional factor in the shortening of the hospital stay is the use of utilization review committees that adhere to criteria for average length of stay for patients with various conditions.

Physicians' services are also being called upon increasingly. Young people tend to go to the physician because of acute diseases, for example, upper respiratory infections, and the elderly because of long-term and chronic conditions. The elderly use physicians' services at the highest rate.

Dental service utilization remains relatively low in the United States although it has increased with the past generation. In 1930, 21% of the population saw a dentist at least once a year; this increased to approximately 40% by 1970. Studies show that more females use dental services than males and that the highest age of utilization is the 6- to 17-year-old group (Anderson and Andersen 1972:395).

Preventive health services in the community can be thought of in three levels:

1. Primary services, which prevent disease, for example, immunization to stop diphtheria.

2. Secondary services, which check the development of a disease, for example, middle ear infection.

3. Tertiary services, which manage a disease that is neither curable nor preventable, for example, diabetes mellitus.

An annual physical examination by the physician can be considered a preventive health service to people. In 1964 a survey indicated that approximately half of the population had undergone a physical examination within the year. The reasons that caused people to obtain examinations were almost evenly divided: the person was experiencing illness symptoms; the examination was required, for example, for a job; or the annual physical was a preventive measure (Anderson and Andersen 1972:396–397).

FINANCING HEALTH AND ILLNESS SERVICES

Health has been described as the fastest growing industry in the United States. The federal governments in both the United States and Canada have increased their budget allocations for health services in recent years. In 1970, the expenditures in the United States were about 73 billion dollars, and it is estimated that by 1980 the costs may well run as high as 200 billion dollars.

There are five general types of financing of health illness care:

1. voluntary insurance (private insurance)
2. social insurance (public insurance)
3. industry
4. personal payment
5. charitable resources

Voluntary Insurance

Health-illness care costs are covered by private insurance plans. It is estimated that approximately 85% of the people in the United States under the age of 65 years have some health insurance. The costs of these insurance plans, for example, Blue Shield and Blue Cross, are borne by the individual, or in some situations they are shared by the employer.

A type of voluntary health insurance is the prepaid group plan. In these plans, participants pay for the services of physicians who participate in the plan and the facilities arranged for in the plan. An example of this method of financing is the Kaiser Permanente Medical Care Program in California and other states. Prepaid group plans provide for services required by the participants 24 hours per day. The basis is that, by advanced payment, the individual takes out insurance against any health requirements in the future. These plans place heavy emphasis upon the promotion of health and prevention of disease and injury of the participants. Prepaid plans are sometimes referred to as Health Maintenance Organizations (HMOs).

Social Insurance

This includes insurance programs such as Medicare, which provides for the costs of hospitalization; related care is financed through the Old Age Survivors and Disability Insurance. It covers most people who are over 65 years of age. Medicaid, on the other hand, provides for the payment of physicians' services and certain health services. Participation in it is voluntary, and it is primarily designed for the elderly, although as of 1976 people under 65 years who are disabled can also participate. The monthly fee is divided between the person participating and the government. In Canada the government has financed hospital care since 1957 and physicians' services since 1968.

Industry

In many settings, industry provides for hospital care and/or medical care and related services for employees and families. The rationale behind this is that healthy workers are more productive workers. In America, industry sometimes provides financial support to the hospital itself, especially in some isolated mining and lumbering centers. By the provision of hospitals, workers and their families are more likely to be attracted to these centers and to stay there.

Personal Payment

Another method of payment of health care is through personal payment. Until the last ten years, this was the major method of payment of hospitalization costs in the United States, and it is still used by some people. At present, personal payment is the major method for paying for dental care, medicines, and ambulatory care.

Charitable Resources

Charitable resources for medical payments are supported by donations from individuals or groups of individuals or through bequests. Charitable donations are still made by some philanthropic organizations to assist the poor and to support some innovations. On the whole, however, charitable donations as a means of paying for health care are declining in importance.

SUMMARY

There is no absolute definition of health. Some people think that as long as they can work they are healthy; others think that health is the absence of disease. Increasingly, however, greater emphasis is being placed on health as being the optimum level of wellness that can be acquired for any particular individual. This definition suggests that even without a disease process a person may not be healthy or that people with some diseases such as diabetes can be healthy. In addition, health is a dynamic, not a static state. The degree of wellness of a person changes constantly along a continuum on which high-level wellness is at one extreme and illness and death are at the opposite extreme.

Common health problems in North America and the required health services are reflected in demographic statistics such as age of the population, mortality, and morbidity. Increases in total population demand increased health care services. Successes in treating acute diseases and lower maternal death rates are two factors that have increased longevity. As a result, the incidence of chronic diseases in the elderly such as heart disease has increased. Of note are the age extremes of the population, that is, the very young and the elderly. These groups require the most health services.

Mortality statistics indicate differences in causes of death among various age groups. The predominant cause of death is heart disease in individuals over 40 years, whereas accidents are the major cause in all other age groups. In the adolescent and young adult age group the incidence of homicide and suicide is high. Morbidity statistics reveal a high incidence of alcoholism, drug addiction, venereal disease, dental disease, and psychologic illnesses. The one obvious decline is in the incidence of acute contagious diseases.

Two general types of health care services are provided in North America. These are the restorative care services for people who are ill and the preventive care services for healthy people to maintain health and avoid disease and injury. The former service predominates. A comprehensive health care delivery system should encompass four interdependent areas: health maintenance, prevention of disease and injury, diagnosis and treatment of disease and injury, and rehabilitation. Both physical and mental health and illness must be included. Health maintenance programs will probably receive greater emphasis in the future.

A wide variety of health care agencies exists in most communities. These include physicians' offices or clinics, hospitals, day-care centers, home nursing services, rehabilitation services, and nursing homes. These agencies can be classified as official agencies or voluntary agencies. The former are financed and operated by government, the latter by contribution from interested individuals in the community.

The health team consists of a wide variety of health personnel, each offering a specialized service to patients. The membership of the health team for each patient differs in accordance with the particular needs of the patient and his/her family. Some may require the service of a social worker; others may need a dietitian. Almost all patients require services from physicians and nurses. The nursing team itself is comprised of various personnel with varied educational backgrounds and skills. The leadership of the nursing team is generally entrusted to a registered nurse.

Six major problems exist in the current health-illness care system in North America. First, the care provided is fragmented. Because of increased specialization, the patients can no longer see a family doctor for all of their ailments. Many patients may have a half dozen specialists and get bewildered and worried about which health practitioner really cares about them as total persons. Second, the cost of health care is very high, necessitating programs to assist individuals to pay for health services. The cost to the public as a whole nonetheless remains exorbitant. Third, the rapid changes in medical science and technology quickly outdate the skills of health practitioners. Fourth, the services to poverty and minority groups are inadequate. Fifth, the special needs of the elderly are expanding. Last, health services are distributed unevenly. The number of primary practice physicians is decreasing, and rural areas have low ratios of health workers per capita compared to urban settings. Despite these problems, more and more people are seeking help for health problems and are using the available health services.

Health services can be regarded as the fastest growing industry in the United States. Five general types of financing for these services include voluntary health insurance plans, social insurance programs, payments by individuals, payments by industry, and charitable donations.

SUGGESTED ACTIVITIES

1. Visit and compare the activities of two different kinds of health care agencies.

2. Select a family (your own or another) and list the health care services that have been utilized by each of its members in the year. Consider whether other services could have been used.

3. Interview a few friends of different age groups and elicit their perceptions of when they consider themselves healthy and when they consider themselves ill.

SUGGESTED READINGS

Bullough, Bonnie. September, 1976. Influences on role expansion. *American Journal of Nursing* 76:1476–1481.

This article discusses some of the factors that affect the expansion of the nurse's role, including the women's liberation movement and medicine.

Brickner, Philip W., et al. May, 1976. Outreach to welfare hotels, the homebound, the frail. *American Journal of Nursing* 76:762–764.

For those people who cannot or will not use the current health care system, special programs have been established to provide professional services to "medically unreached groups."

Kinoy, Susan K. September, 1969. Home health services for the elderly. *Nursing Outlook* 17:59–62.

A social worker explores ways of securing a continuum of home health services for the elderly in an urban setting in accordance with their needs.

McCarthy, Elaine. October, 1976. Comprehensive home care for earlier hospital discharge. *Nursing Outlook* 24:625–630.

This coordinated home care program provides less expensive care for the patients and to the insuring agencies. It outlines the staff responsibilities, the criteria for admitting a patient to the agency, and the results of the program.

Pender, Nola J. June, 1975. A conceptual model for preventive health behavior. *Nursing Outlook* 23:385–390.

This article analyzes the factors that promote or inhibit an individual's motivation to protect his own health. People do not always take advantage of preventive health services, even when they are readily available.

Roemer, Milton I. June, 1971. Health care financing and delivery around the world. *American Journal of Nursing* 71:1158–1163.

The methods of financing health care in various countries of the world are discussed. Included in the article is a description of the five methods of financing health care and some conclusions regarding these payment methods.

SELECTED REFERENCES

Anderson, Odin W. 1972. Health services systems in the United States and other countries: critical comparisons. In Jaco, E. Gartly, ed. *Patients, physicians and illness,* 2nd ed. New York: The Free Press.

Anderson, Odin W., and Andersen, Ronald M. 1972. Patterns of use of health services. In Freeman, Howard E., et al., eds. *Handbook of medical sociology,* 2nd ed. Englewood Cliffs, New Jersey: Prentice-Hall, Inc.

Antonovsky, Aaron. 1972. Social class, life expectancy and overall mortality. In Jaco, E. Gartly, ed. *Patients, physicians and illness,* 2nd ed. New York: The Free Press.

Atwater, J. B. May, 1974. Adapting the V. D. clinic to today's problem. *American Journal of Public Health* 64:433–437.

Bauman, Barbara. 1965. Diversities in conceptions of health and physical fitness. In Skipper, James K., Jr., and Leonard, Robert C., eds. *Social interaction and patient care.* Philadelphia: J. B. Lippincott Co.

Brown, M. A. February, 1973. Adolescents and VD. *Nursing Outlook* 21:99–103.

Canada Department of National Health and Welfare. 1974. *A new perspective on the health of Canadians: a working document.* Ottawa.

———. 1976. *Health field indicators, Canada and provinces.* Ottawa.

Consumer speaks out about hospital care. Sep., 1976. *American Journal of Nursing* 76:1443–1444.

Demographic Year Book 1975. 1976. New York: United Nations.

Finnegan, L. P., et al. April, 1974. Care of the addicted infant. *American Journal of Nursing* 74:685–693.

Jamann, J. S. May, 1971. Health is a function of ecology. *American Journal of Nursing* 71:970–973.

Krepick, D. S., et al. March, 1973. Heroin addiction: a treatable disease. *Nursing Clinics of North America* 8:41–52.

Leininger, Madeleine. 1975. Health care delivery systems for tomorrow: possibilities and guidelines. In Leininger, Madeleine, ed. *Barriers and facilitators to quality health care* Philadelphia: F. A. Davis Co.

Lewis, L. W. July, 1975. The hidden alcoholic: a nursing dilemma. *Nursing 75* 5:20–27.

Orque, Modesta S. May, 1976. Health care and minority clients. *Nursing Outlook* 24:313–316.

Parsons, Talcott. 1972. Definitions of health and illness in the light of American values and social structure. In Jaco, E. Gartly, ed. *Patients, physicians and illness,* 2nd ed. New York: The Free Press.

Sims, Mary, et al. March, 1973. Drug overdoses in a Canadian city. *American Journal of Public Health* 63:215–226.

Somers, Anne R. 1971. *Health care in transition: directions for the future.* Chicago: Hospital Research and Educational Trust.

Statistics Canada. 1974. *Population projection for Canada and the provinces.* Ottawa.

US Bureau of the Census. 1976. *Statistical Abstract,* 97th ed. Washington, DC.

US, Department of Health, Education, and Welfare, Public Health Service, Health Resources Administration, National Center for Health Statistics. 1974. *Facts of life and death.* Publication HRA 74–1222. Washington, D.C.

———. 1975. *Health United States.* Publication HRA 76–1232. Washington, D.C.

US, Department of Health, Education, and Welfare. 1975. *Toward a comprehensive health policy for the 1970s: A white paper.* Washington, DC.

———. 1977. *Utilization of short-stay hospitals: Annual summary for the United States, 1975.* Series 13, No. 31. Rockville, Maryland.

World Health Organization. 1947. *Constitution of the World Health Organization. Chronicle of the World Health Organization 1.* Geneva, Switzerland.

CHAPTER 3

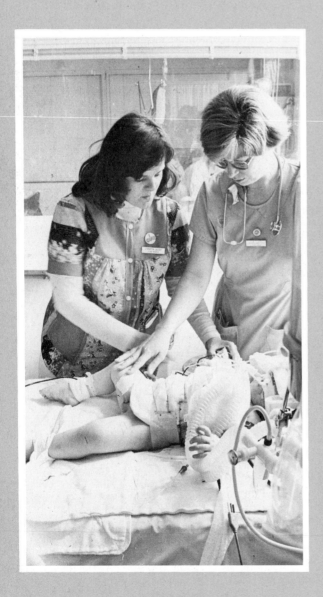

THE PATIENT AND ILLNESS

ETIOLOGY OF DISEASE

Genetic Factors

Microorganisms and Parasites

Chemical and Physical Factors

Psychologic Factors

Cultural and Social Factors

Ecologic Factors

OBJECTIVES

- Describe and compare illness and disease.
- Discuss the five stages of illness and the significance of each stage.
- Describe some typical behaviors of the sick role.
- Explain how illness can affect family roles and functions.
- Discuss the various factors that cause disease.

Illness is a universal phenomenon. Everyone at one time or another has experienced some illness, even if it was just a common cold. Illness has many connotations to people; thus different factors can affect both a nurse's and a patient's perspective on illness. Just as a patient's beliefs are influenced by cultural and social backgrounds, so are a nurse's. To really assist and understand a patient, it is important for a nurse to have self-awareness of personal perspectives and beliefs, particularly those which may differ from the patient's.

The sick person assumes a role. A *role* is defined as "a pattern of behavior corresponding to a system of rights and duties and is associated with a particular position in a social group" (Wilson 1949:208). A person in the sick role in North America has certain rights and certain responsibilities, which are accepted by society. The sick person will experience certain emotions related to being ill, which may affect behavior. Therefore, caring for an ill person requires an understanding of how this particular person and family can and do react to illness.

In discussing the etiology (cause) of disease it is now accepted that a number of factors are involved. Not only must the necessary cause, such as bacteria, be present, but so must other sufficient factors, such as fatigue or malnutrition. These latter factors vary from one person to another.

The nurse's role in illness has been described in various ways by nurses and social scientists. It also varies from setting to setting and from patient to patient, reflecting the needs of the patient and family.

ILLNESS DEFINED

Illness has been defined in a number of ways; it has been described as sickness or as a deviation from a healthy state. More recently, sociologists have defined illness in such a way as to differentiate it from disease. Illness in this context is considered to be a highly personal state in which the person feels ill; for example, the person feels pain or nausea and as a result tends to modify behavior in some way. Illness can be defined as "a state of disturbance in the normal functioning of the total human individual, including both the state of the organism as a biological system, and of his person and social adjustments" (Parsons 1972:107). This definition includes illness of organic or somatic origin (biologic disturbances) and illness of psychologic origin (personal and/or social changes).

Disease, on the other hand, is solely a biologic entity; it is something that alters the function of the body in some way, such as an obstruction in a blood vessel or a tumor in the liver. With reference to these definitions it is apparent that a person may feel ill and yet there is no disease present; on the other hand, a disease might be present but the person may or may not feel ill. Generally speaking, illness can be considered to be any condition that causes a person to seek advice from a physician. Illness behavior, then, is the behavior in this context.

Illness Behavior Is Learned

The illness behavior of a person is a culturally and socially learned response. Cultures differ widely in their responses to illness. Different subcultures within a society such as the United States demonstrate these differences. For example, Jewish and Italian patients often respond to pain in emotionally expressive ways that tend to exaggerate the pain experienced, while Anglo-Americans tend to be stoic and less expressive. The Irish, on the other hand, tend to deny the existence of the pain (Mechanic 1972:120).

These cultural differences are learned from early childhood. For example, if a child cries whenever he is hurt and as a result receives help and comfort, he learns that crying will bring him the help and comfort he wishes. At the other extreme, a child who is repeatedly ignored when she cries, learns this does not bring her comfort but perhaps other types of behavior will. This child may learn that by being stoical she gets comfort and support from the family, who sees this behavior as admirable.

Social conditioning also affects illness behavior. For example, older children are usually more stoical than younger children; boys are socialized to react less to hurt or pain than girls. These stereotypical socialization patterns are changing, however. And although generalizations can be made in regard to culturally learned behavior, there are wide variations within a culture that mitigate against predictive behavior assessment.

Even within the same culture there can be a wide variety of responses between people to the same illness condition. One person might dismiss a condition and not let it alter his life, while another may show considerable change socially and emotionally to the same condition. Often the way persons react is related to other stresses and problems or coping difficulties that they have at that time rather than to the illness itself. Everyone can understand that illness is stressful and that the total number of stresses one has influences illness behavior. From this the nurse should be aware that even a minor complaint about illness may be a patient's way of seeking help for another problem.

Illness behavior can obtain some advantages. For example, for a man who lives alone in a cold room during the winter, illness and subsequent admission to a hospital may have many obvious advantages in terms of food, warmth, being cared for, and escape from worry and maintaining life in his own environment. This is an extreme example of the secondary advantages of illness. More commonly the nurse will encounter simpler mechanisms, as for example, the woman who develops a severe headache just before she is expected to go to the dentist, thus avoiding a visit she has dreaded for some time. Sometimes a reaction such as this is symptomatic of an underlying problem, which manifests itself in this manner.

STAGES OF ILLNESS

Five stages of illness have been described:

1. the symptom experience stage
2. assumption of the sick role
3. medical care contact stage
4. the dependent/patient role stage
5. the recovery or rehabilitation stage (Suchman 1972:145)

The Symptom Experience Stage

This stage of illness is the transition stage. During this period patients come to believe something is wrong. Either a person close to them mentions that they look unwell, or patients experience some symptoms, which can appear insidiously. Initially persons often go through a phase of denial and continue to function as if they felt well. During this period, they may not want to bother their family or doctor with something that seems to be trivial. This situation delays treatment, which is an unwise practice.

There are three aspects of this symptom experience stage: the physical experience of symptoms such as pain or fever; the cognitive aspect, that is, the interpretation of the symptoms in terms that have some meaning to the person; and the emotional response of fear or anxiety relative to the experience.

During this period unwell persons usually consult with a significant person or persons close to them about their symptoms or feelings. People will validate, for example, with their spouses or partners that the symptoms are real and obtain support to seek a physician's advice. Sometimes at this stage sick persons will try home remedies such as laxatives or cough medicines obtained from the neighborhood drugstore.

Assumption of the Sick Role

This stage can be referred to as the state of acceptance of the illness. At this time individuals decide that their symptoms or concerns are sufficiently severe to suggest that they are sick. Persons will seek confirmation of the illness from family and friends and will then assume the sick role (see "The Sick Role"). Some people seek professional help quickly, but others continue self-treatment, often following the suggestions of family and friends.

In this stage sick persons are usually afraid, but now accept that they are ill even though they may not be able to accept the possible reasons. In conferring with people close to them, sick persons are not only seeking advice, they are also seeking support that perhaps they should give up some of their activities, and, for example, stay home from work.

At the end of this stage sick persons will experience either one of two outcomes. They may find that the symptoms have changed and that they are feeling better. Still they will seek confirmation of this from the family, and if family members support the patients' perceptions they will no longer be considered or consider themselves sick. As a result persons must then resume normal obligations such as returning to work or attending a school concert. On the other hand, if the symptoms persist or increase and if this is validated by family or significant others, then sick persons know they should seek a physician's advice.

Medical Care Contact Stage

Sick persons seek the advice of a physician either on their own initiative or that of the family. When people go for medical advice, they are really asking for three types of information.

1. Validation of real illness.

2. An explanation of the symptoms in understandable terms.

3. Reassurance that they will be all right or prediction of what the outcome will be.

If the physician does not validate illness, persons have two recourses: to return to normal activities or to seek another physician's advice. If the symptoms disappear, persons will perceive that they really are not ill. If symptoms continue, persons will return to the physician or go to a second physician for medical care. It is at this stage that some people who are repeatedly told that they are not ill seek out quasi-practitioners. This is often done as a last resort in an attempt to obtain some alleviation for the perceived symptoms. Some people will go from physician to physician until they find someone who will provide a diagnosis that more closely fits their own perceptions.

The Dependent Patient Role Stage

At this stage when the physician has validated that the person is ill, the individual then becomes a patient, dependent upon the physician for help. During this stage sick persons may or may not be reluctant to accept a physician's recommendations. They may go through a period of vacillation about what is best for them and alternately accept and reject the physician's suggestions. People vary greatly in the degree of ease with which they can give up their independence, particularly in relation to life and death. Entering into this conflict for the patient are often role obligations such as those required as a wage earner, as a father, as a mother, or for the student as a baseball team member or singer. It is also at this time that the meaning of the illness to the patient may differ from that of the physician unless complete and open communication exists. During this stage a nurse can often provide the patient with additional information, which may allay some fears, and/or provide data that augments the physician's diagnosis. Misconceptions can result from limited information that patients place in their own frame of reference. For example, a patient may be told by the physician that he has a small encapsulated growth in his right groin and surgical removal is advised. The patient's mother died years before after being told she had a growth in her breast. The patient may therefore assume that he is also going to die as a result of this growth.

Most patients generally accept their roles as being dependent upon the physician, although peo-ple will retain varying degrees of control over their own lives. For example, some patients will request precise information about their diseases, their treatment, and the related problems and reserve the decision about accepting the treatment until they have all this information. Other patients prefer that the physician proceed with whatever treatment is considered appropriate and do not request additional information.

During this period, sick persons gradually become more passive and accepting. They require an environment that is predictable and one where the people are genuinely concerned about them. In addition to being concerned about themselves, some sick persons' behavior will regress to an earlier stage in their development. As a result, patients will have fewer *coping mechanisms* (physical and emotional adaptive or defensive abilities) and will tend to react similarly in different situations. This is important because frequently patients' reactions are related to previous experiences and to misconceptions about what will happen.

Children are accustomed to being dependent for some of their needs, although this does depend upon age and home situation. For example, 1-year-old children are accustomed to being bathed and to having help eating, so when they are ill, this assistance is not a major adjustment. An adult, however, is usually unaccustomed to this assistance, and if it is required during the illness, it can be an area of independence that is difficult to relinquish. People have varying dependency needs. For some, illness may meet dependency needs that have never been met and thus provide satisfaction to the patient. Other people have minimal dependency needs and thus do everything possible to return to independent functioning. A few may even try to maintain independence to the detriment of their recovery.

The Recovery or Rehabilitation Stage

During this stage the patient learns to give up the sick role and return to former roles and functions. For patients who have acute illnesses, the time as a patient is generally short, and recovery is usually rapid. Thus they find it relatively easy to return to their former lifestyles. For people who have long-term illnesses and who have to make adjustments in lifestyles, this recovery stage is more difficult. This is particularly true for people who have to learn new skills such as walking or talking.

During this stage, readiness for social functioning lags behind physical functioning. Patients may find themselves physically able to go out to dinner but may perceive that functioning socially provides stress with which they are not ready to cope.

It is during this stage that nurses can assist patients to function with increasing independence. By planning with patients as to those functions they can accomplish by themselves and those with which they feel a need for assistance, the nurse can foster a sense of independence and the attainment of skills for living. Important also is that the nurse convey an attitude of hope and support. Each person, even an infant, needs this in order to return to health.

THE SICK ROLE

The sick role is assumed by people when they accept illness and when their illness has been validated by a physician. It describes the typical patient's behavioral orientation, but it is not intended to describe every patient's orientation. The sick role has been described as having four aspects:

1. Patients are not held responsible for their condition.
2. Patients are excused from certain social roles and tasks.
3. Patients are obliged to try and get well as quickly as possible.
4. Patients or the family are obliged to seek competent help (Parsons 1964:436–437).

The patient in North American society is not held responsible for incurring the illness. Illness is considered to be undesirable and yet beyond a person's control. In some subcultures illness can be viewed as punishment from God, and therefore in that sense the persons are responsible because of their sins. This is the case in the Spanish-American culture, in which God is believed to be primarily in charge of health and illness. Some of this folk belief is held over in American society. Often one hears a patient say, "What have I done to deserve this?" This remark reflects punishment. Today, however, people increasingly are being held responsible for their illness, as for example, the cardiac patient who smokes or the overweight person who acquires diabetes.

The sick person is also excused from some normal duties. This is true regardless of whether the person has a cold or requires surgery. Social pressures or expectations exerted upon sick people depend upon the prognosis and the severity of the illness. People who are severely ill and whose prognosis is poor or uncertain are permitted to be dependent and are treated as dependents. Other people, however, who are not seriously ill and whose prognosis is good are more likely to be encouraged to fulfill personal and social responsibilities. In this context the person with a cold may still be expected to give a scheduled speech or to write an examination. For people who are chronically ill there may be permanent exemption from some duties or activities; for example, the father confined to bed is not expected to attend his daughter's field hockey games. In this type of situation, arrangements will usually be made within the family for another member to fulfill this role while the father is unable to do so.

A third aspect of the sick role is the obligation of the person to get well as quickly as possible. The sick role is a dependent role in at least some aspects. For the person who fears dependency, assuming a sick role and seeking help may be threatening. This person might well ignore advice despite the most serious consequences. On the other hand, some people find the dependency situation of being sick gratifying. Most people are familiar with the sense of relief that comes when they are able to withdraw even for a day from the pressures of the job. Carried to the extreme, some patients find the dependency so satisfying that they perpetuate the sick role and do not try to get well, or even after they are physically well they continue to complain of symptoms. Some people in the dependent stage also find it satisfying to control others through excessive demands. Regardless of these exceptions, most people do try to get well as quickly as possible.

The fourth aspect of the sick role is seeking competent help. This presupposes that this competent help is available to the patient. It should also be recognized that what the patient considers to be competent help may not agree with the opinion of the general population. For example, a man with a whiplash injury as a result of an automobile accident becomes dissatisfied with his physician's treatment because of his slow recovery and goes to a healer who uses hypnotism. A second example is that of a young lady who has mannerisms that others find unpleasant. She talks a great deal and orders others around. Because of these two characteristics, among others, she is unable to keep a job for more than two months. Someone suggests that she discuss this matter with her physician with a view to therapy. She decides instead to join a cult of young people, considering the members of the cult to be competent help.

Behavior Changes of Sick Persons

Fearfulness

A person usually becomes fearful as a result of assuming the sick role. Generally, the person is afraid of reduced functioning and/or of changed social relationships or of death. The person worries about the outcome of the illness, particularly when the diagnosis is uncertain. The individual also worries about the meaning of reduced functioning: "Will this mean a lower family income?" These changes often mean that patients must change their concept of themselves, such as from a capable wage earner to a part-time employee. Persons also worry about possible changes in social relationships. For example, if the wife becomes the major wage earner, how will this affect the husband–wife relationship?

Regression

Persons who are threatened by illness will feel anxious. In order to cope with anxiety they may *regress* in their reactions to those more appropriate of an earlier stage of maturation. For example, the 8-year-old may bedwet or suck his thumb; the adult may seek attention by constant demands. As a part of this regression, the patient will show a number of kinds of behavior: egocentricity, an exaggerated concern over small matters, narrowed interests, emotional overreaction, and some changes in the perception of people in the environment.

Egocentricity

Egocentricity is a concern about oneself. When patients become egocentric, they are preoccupied with themselves and the illness. They usually do not want to hear about someone else's operation; they want to talk about their own operation or their own pain. Egocentricity is often more apparent when patients are in a hospital. In this setting, isolated from their families and their activities, patients have more time to think about themselves. In addition, when they encounter people with whom to talk, in particular

physicians and nurses, often the conversation is restricted to their pain or illness.

Concern over Small Matters

An exaggerated concern over small matters occurs also as patients become preoccupied with themselves. Patients may concern themselves with matters that normally are of little concern to them. Concern about a wrinkle in a bedspread or an intolerance of delays are examples of this type of behavior. Most people, when they are ill, however, are sufficiently aware of the situation around them and are considerate of others most of the time. Nurses need to encourage expression of the exaggerated concerns of patients and understand that most of these are related to the sick role.

Narrowed Interests

Narrowed interests occur chiefly when patients are hospitalized or ill for a long period of time. This narrowing of interests may be due in part to the reduced perceptions of ill persons that accompany stress and to a lack of energy on the part of patients, who may be weakened and who need all their energy to get well. Contributing to this problem is also the fact that patients have been relieved of many of their responsibilities because of the illness. For these reasons, ill people are not necessarily interested in everything that usually interests them when they are well.

On the other hand, patients in hospitals may be seen taking an interest in something they normally would not be interested in. This observation can be made, for example, at World Series time when someone who normally does not watch baseball becomes an avid follower of the series. This change in behavior usually has two reasons: the sharing of the experience with other patients and the distraction that it offers for a short time without the need to be highly emotionally involved.

Emotional Overreactions

Emotional overreactions are common in people who are ill; they cry more easily, become angry quickly, and mostly have an increased need for affection and attention from others. For the patient who has family and friends, this need for attention is generally met largely by the family and friends; but for the patient who does not have visitors, this support is provided chiefly by nurses. This is the caring aspect of nursing, the genuine concern for the person frequently referred to as TLC (tender loving care). To the child, this caring offers the reassurance that is usually provided by parents. To the adult this need for affectionate, caring actions is also present but is not as pronounced.

Perceptual Changes

Changes in perception of others are often experienced when people are ill. Shifts occur in their perceptions of the people around them. The physi-cian often becomes all powerful in the patient's eyes. The nurse may be seen as in a mothering role, that is, comforting, supporting, and providing security. These perceptions may be unconscious or conscious to the patient. Sometimes these perceptions are the cause of frustration to the patient, however, as when the nurse directs attention to other patients. This may be obvious on the children's units of a hospital when a child who does not receive the nurse's attention all the time expresses frustration with an angry outburst.

THE EFFECTS OF ILLNESS UPON FAMILY MEMBERS

When any member of a family is ill, there is some effect upon the entire family. The kind of effect and its extent are chiefly dependent upon three criteria: which member of the family is ill, the seriousness and the length of the illness, and the cultural and social customs operating in that particular family.

The changes that can occur within a family can include:

1. Role changes.
2. Task reassignments.
3. Increased stress due to anxiety about the outcome of the illness for the patient and conflict in regard to the number of responsibilities.
4. Financial problems.
5. Loneliness as a result of separation and pending loss.
6. Change in social customs.

Each member of the family is affected differently depending upon whether it is a grandmother, the father of a nuclear family, or a teenager who is ill. Each of these people has a different role in the family, and each performs different tasks related to the support of the family. Each person also has a different social value to society. For example, elderly persons have made a contribution to society in terms of employment or raising a family. At this time in life it is unlikely that they are assuming many responsibilities other than for themselves and perhaps for a marital partner.

The amount of change that family members experience is often related to their dependency needs in relation to the sick person. For example, when a child is ill, there are few changes other than the respon-sibilities directly related to the child. But when the mother is ill, many changes are often necessary in the lives of the family members in order to assume her functions.

The Sick Elderly Person

When an elderly person is ill, the role change most frequently required is for a son or daughter to assume the parental functions to the parent. Because of the dependency needs of the sick elderly person, sons or daughters may find it necessary to provide housing facilities, meals, and assistance with daily needs over a prolonged period of time. Thus in order to protect and care for the elderly sick person, the parent-child roles are frequently reversed. This role reversal may only be temporary during the time of the illness, or it may become permanent. Since elderly people usually have few responsibilities, task reassignment is usually restricted to direct care for the sick person. The stress related to concern about the outcome of the illness is present for all the family, in particular, for a spouse. Younger persons in the family often deal with serious illness in an elderly person by stating that "he has led a good life" or that "she has had so much pain the past years," so they are able to prepare themselves for that person's death. This same reasoning is rarely applied to a child or younger adult who is ill.

When an elderly person is ill, the sons and daughters, who are adults, may be faced with conflicts in relation to their responsibilities. A daughter of the elderly person who lives some distance away needs to maintain her job and look after her own family, but at the same time her parents need her in another city. How often should she visit? How should she fulfill her responsibilities? These questions pose problems for a family separated by miles.

The financial problems of the sick elderly can be a major problem for a family as well as a community. Because illness in this age group tends to be chronic, the costs of illness tend to be prolonged and considerable.

Loneliness as a result of separation from or pending loss of an elderly person is usually felt most by a marital partner. When a marriage has lasted for 50 or 60 years, elderly people find it difficult to envisage what it will be like without a husband or wife. Older people generally recognize that they are at the end of their life spans, but separation and loneliness are prominent concerns. Grandchildren also experience anxiety regarding the outcome of a grandparent's illness, particularly if they have had long and pleasant ties and experiences. Primary ties are generally in the nuclear family (parents and children), however, and often the elderly person lives in another setting or in another city. When an elderly person is ill or hospitalized, the normal employment is maintained by family members. The family lifestyle generally has minimal disruption. Most changes occur in the social practices of family members, chiefly as a result of visiting the sick person.

The Sick Parent

When the sick person is a parent, the amount of change experienced by a family is to some degree related to the kinds of responsibilities the individual has and the number and age of dependents under the person's care. For example, when a father is ill for a long period of time, his roles are usually taken over by other members of the family, frequently his wife. Tasks related to the house or to attending a child's basketball games, for example, are either reassigned or not performed at all. The anxiety of family members in relation to the outcome of a parent being ill is usually high, and this is especially true if the parent is the wage earner. The implications of prolonged illness or death can affect the family in almost all areas of living because of the needs of the dependents.

The prolonged illness of the mother can also have serious consequences and be particularly disruptive if an outsider is employed to perform many of the tasks formerly carried out by the mother. Children, particularly young ones, in this situation suffer a loss in affection and feel insecure when their mother is away or is too ill to function as usual. Often a lack of understanding about why their mother is in the hospital coupled with a feeling of loneliness and not being wanted present problems. Sometimes the mother's functions are taken over by grandparents or by aunts and uncles as well as by the husband. When serious illness of unknown outcome is experienced by a young mother, worrisome problems are faced by a husband and family as to how they will manage over a long period of time. Most arrangements have financial implications and also involve role changes for the husband and children. In this situation the husband may have to function as both father and mother and give up many of his normal social activities. The children may also need to assume more housekeeping functions.

The Sick Child

Because a child is dependent upon parents for so many daily needs, an ill child and the family encounter fewer role adjustments as compared to the changes necessary for the sick adult. Task reassignments are also generally minimal. Sometimes a younger sibling takes over a paper route for a sick brother or sister, and home chores will be shared by all the members of the family.

Anxiety will be experienced by all members of the family if the outcome of the illness is in doubt. If the child is to be permanently handicapped in some manner, this can have implications for the parents in terms of schooling, future employment, and future needs. The financial responsibility for this is often a serious one for young parents to assume. In this particular situation, other children may feel neglected if an unusual amount of attention is given to the ill child. Husband and wife may also expend most of their energies visiting the hospital and have little time for each other. This situation if extended over a long period of time can place additional stress upon a marriage.

When a child is admitted to the hospital, parents and siblings may experience some sense of loss; however, children usually continue with their daily activities, and there is minimal disruption to the home setting.

ETIOLOGY OF DISEASE

Etiology is the study of the factors that cause disease. Today it is generally accepted that a disease process is the result of more than one etiologic (causative) factor and that it is the interaction of these factors that results in the disease process. Early theories describing disease had a number of orientations. Three of these are as follows:

1. Disease is the result of the presence of a microorganism. Although pathogenic organisms are now known to be the causative organisms behind some infectious diseases, this theory does not explain the long-term diseases that are particularly prominent among the elderly.

2. The mind and body are entirely separate of one another. People who held to this belief saw the mind and the body as entirely separate entities, to be considered and treated separately. This is an obsolete belief, since it is now known that the mind and body do interact and that one does affect the other. For example, stress over many years can produce a stomach ulcer.

3. The cause of a disease always comes from outside a body. Modern and primitive man have considered disease to be external to the body. Disease has been referred to as bad or evil by primitive man—an evil spirit that entered the body from the outside. In modern society, disease is often also viewed as external to a person, but it can also arise from the inside, for example, a tumor.

Modern theories of the causation of disease largely rest upon the concept of stress and a person's adaptation. A person is seen as a total entity who is constantly interacting with the environment in order to maintain a state of biologic, psychologic, and sociologic equilibrium. When people's coping mechanisms are such that they are unable to regain equilibrium, illness or disease occurs. The factors that cause the stress are referred to as *stressors*, which are found in both the external and internal environment (within the person) (see Chapter 8).

Of the factors that interact to produce disease, one factor, the *necessary cause*, must be present to produce the disease. However, just because it is present, the disease process may not occur unless other factors referred to as *sufficient factors* are also present. An example is the occurrence of herpes simplex, the common cold sore. These sores are due to the presence of a virus in the individual, which is usually acquired in early life and stays present in the body. For the sores to occur, other factors must also be present, such as overexposure to sunlight, a cold, or emotional stress. These latter factors can be considered to be the sufficient factors, and the virus in this case is the necessary cause.

The necessary factors that are injurious to man can be placed in six groups: (a) genetic factors, (b) microorganisms and parasites, (c) chemical and physical factors, (d) psychologic factors, (e) cultural and social factors, and (f) ecologic factors. Some authorities include *neoplasms* as an additional cause; however, the specific cause of neoplasms is unknown.

Genetic Factors

The *chromosome* is the nuclear structure responsible for transmitting genetic information. It influences the growth and development of the individual, including vulnerability to stress and ability to cope with disease. An abnormal gene product results in impaired cellular metabolism, producing an inborn error in metabolism. These errors result in structural and physiologic abnormalities. Some of these genetic abnormalities are apparent at birth, for example, tetralogy of Fallot (a cardiac defect) and spina bifida (a defect of the bony spinal canal); others appear later in life, such as sickle cell anemia, which is seen in 1–2% of the black population and can manifest itself either in childhood or during adult life.

The degree to which genetic inheritance affects life can be highly variable depending to a large degree upon environmental factors. For example, the person who inherits a short, plump stature may be inclined to be obese. This condition can predispose a person to heart disease and to psychologic stress relative to the appearance. However, if persons control their weight through exercise and a suitable diet, they may well prevent the heart disease and the anxiety that could accompany obesity.

Microorganisms and Parasites

Microorganisms are minute living organisms. Included in the group are bacteria, rickettsiae, viruses, moles, yeasts, and protozoa. *Parasites* are plants or animals that live upon or within another living organism to the disadvantage of the latter.

Microorganisms and parasites are highly variable in their ability to produce disease. Some microorganisms, such as the smallpox virus, are acutely infectious, producing disease in any person who is unprotected (has not been vaccinated successfully), twelve days after the person has contacted it. *Mycobacterium tuberculosis*, on the other hand, is more likely to produce disease in a person who is poorly nourished rather than a healthy, well-nourished person.

In order that microorganisms and parasites produce disease in a person, one or more of the following conditions are likely to exist:

1. The person is susceptible to the organism; that is, has not been protected by immunization.

2. The appropriate route of entry to the person's body is available. For example, the tetanus bacillus enters through a break in the skin.

3. The person has a lowered resistance due to fatigue, poor nourishment, or emotional stress.

4. The person has a predisposing condition such as diabetes mellitus that makes the individual prone to infections.

Chemical and Physical Factors

Included in this group of factors that cause disease are external mechanical forces that can cause bodily injury and substances such as poisons, radiation, heat, and drugs, which can damage tissues of the body. A practical example is overexposure from the sun's rays, which can cause painful burns.

Within the body some chemical substances can be produced in abnormally large or small amounts, thus causing injury to the body systems and tissue. Examples are the excessive secretion of the gastric juices, which contributes to occurrence of ulcers in the stomach, and the decreased production of insulin, which results in the disease process known as diabetes mellitus.

Psychologic Factors

Psychologic stressors originate either in the external or internal environment of the person. Initially they affect the mind and are perceived as stressful; then physiologic changes may follow. There are three major psychologic factors that produce disease. These factors are listed in the following column:

1. Loss or the fear of loss of something or someone who is valued. The death of a spouse or partner, loss of employment, or even the loss of facial beauty due to an automobile accident are three examples. The effect of these losses is highly individualistic. Whereas one person may value physical beauty highly, another may not experience a similar degree of loss in the same situation.

2. The experience of injury and pain or the threat of it. These experiences are somewhat related to the sense of loss. For example, if a person is injured in an automobile accident and as a result has facial scars, this may mean the loss of a long-anticipated modeling job.

3. Frustration of drives. A *drive* can be defined as a force that activates human behavior, such as hunger. When a drive is frustrated, that is, when it is blocked so that satisfaction is not achieved, a person experiences stress. If an appropriate outlet for expression of the drive is not found, the person is frustrated and could possibly become ill. An example would be a man who is highly desirous of making a great deal of money (drive). He works hard and does make money (behavior), but then he loses all of it (dissatisfaction). As a result he becomes acutely depressed (illness).

The degree to which frustration of drives can lead to illness is to a large degree dependent upon the individual's total life situation. The person who has a happy, satisfying personal life is less likely to become ill as a result of thwarted drives than is the otherwise unhappy, dissatisfied person.

Cultural and Social Factors

Cultural and social factors can also contribute to illness. The *culture* of a person includes the customs, traditions, the patterns of interaction between classes of people, and the techniques of providing approval and disapproval to the members of the culture. Cultural factors contributing to illness may be seen where people live in two cultures that are in conflict. An example would be a closely knit Italian family who move to the United States and maintain their old-country culture within the larger American culture. A conflict might arise when the daughter of the family wishes to marry outside the Italian community when the custom of that particular culture is that she marry a man of her father's choice within the community. This conflict can bring stress to the entire family and even illness to particular members.

Cultural taboos can also be the source of illness or prevent a person from receiving appropriate treatment. In a situation where discussing sexual matters is taboo, a person who has a venereal disease may not ask for information or seek treatment.

Social factors can also cause or contribute to illness and disease. Conditions of poverty, overcrowding, and loneliness in the cities all contribute to disease and illness. The stress of upward mobility in a middle-class family can incur its toll in terms of illness. For example, a successful businesswoman who continually receives promotions moves her family from one city to another with each promotion. As a result, current social contacts need to be terminated, new friendships formed, and an unfamiliar environment adjusted to. These increased social stresses can incur illness.

Ecologic Factors

Ecology is the study of the environment and life history of organisms. Human ecology is the study of the interaction between people and the environment. We read every day about maintaining the balance between humans and nature. This balance can be upset by pollution of water by the deposit of industrial wastes into the rivers or by pollution of the air, which in extreme instances has caused deaths. As a result of technologic advances, the environment can be disturbed in such a manner that disease to humans results. (See Chapter 20, "Environmental Sanitation.")

SUMMARY

The term *illness* no longer refers to the sole biologic entity called disease, but rather to a highly personalized state in which an individual feels unwell. When feeling unwell, the person behaves in various ways in accordance with culturally and socially learned responses. Crying, stoicism, attention seeking, or denial are some responses that may have been learned.

Five stages of illness generally occur. The first, a transition stage, occurs when the person experiences some symptoms. These may be denied and often need validation from others. During the second stage, the sick role is accepted and assumed. Medical care is sought if spontaneous recovery does not occur. The third stage involves confirmation of illness by the physician. In the fourth stage, once illness is verified, the sick person then becomes dependent upon the physician's help. Recommendations of the physician may or may not be accepted. The final stage is recovery or rehabilitation, which may require adjustments in lifestyles. The nurse's role throughout these stages varies in accordance with the needs of the patient.

The sick role has four aspects in North American society. Although sickness is considered undesirable, the patient is generally not held responsible for incurring the illness. The second aspect is that the sick person is excused from his normal duties. However, the patient is obliged to get well as soon as possible, and he is expected to seek competent help.

Associated with the sick role are certain behavioral changes. Generally, persons are anxious and fearful of reduced functioning, changed social relationships, and death. Often regression occurs and may be seen in a number of behavioral ways. Preoccupation and concern about oneself (egocentricity), exaggerated reactions to trivia, narrowing of interests, and changes in the patient's perceptions need to be accepted with understanding by the nurse.

When one member of a family is ill, all other members are affected. The stress incurred and the worry associated with it are dependent in large part on the seriousness of the illness. The roles and functions of the ill person may be reassigned. Financial problems, separation from the family, and changes in social relationships need to be handled. The more dependent the family members are upon the ill person, the greater the adjustments needed. Nurses need to be aware of the effects of illness on family members as well as on the patient. These changes often create additional stress to the patient.

Modern theory of the etiology of disease rests largely upon the concept of stress and adaptation. Authorities believe that both necessary causes and sufficient factors must be present to produce disease. Six necessary factors are classified: genetic factors, microorganisms and parasites, chemical and physical factors, psychologic factors, cultural and social factors, and ecologic factors. Sufficient factors can induce fatigue or malnutrition.

SUGGESTED ACTIVITIES

1. Talk with a patient and determine:
   a. Why and when he or she sought medical advice.
   b. How the doctor explained the illness.
   c. How long the patient expects to be ill.
   d. What role adjustments have been necessitated by the patient and family.
2. Select a patient and list all the factors that caused and contributed to the illness.
3. In a group discuss some behavioral changes that you have personally experienced when ill.

SUGGESTED READINGS

Craven, Ruth F., and Sharp, Benita H. 1972. The effects of illness on family functions. *Nursing Forum* 11(2):187–193.

This article describes the effects of illness upon the contemporary American family and how nurses can assist in supporting the functions of the family.

Galton, Lawrence. April, 1977. Questions patients ask about health and how you can answer them. *Nursing 77* 7:(4):54–59.

This author has compiled some typical patient questions and provides answers that have been supported by studies.

Luckmann, Joan, and Sorensen, Karen Creason. February, 1975. What patients' actions tell you about their feelings, fears and needs. *Nursing '75* 5(2):54–61.

Some common responses of patients to illness are discussed. These responses can reveal their fears and needs and thus require understanding on the part of the nurse. Specific ways for the nurse to handle these responses are included.

Martin, Harry W., and Prange, Arthur J. March, 1962. The stages of illness—psychosocial approach. *Nursing Outlook* 10:168–171.

This article discusses three stages of psychosocial illness: the stage of transition, the stage of acceptance, and the stage of convalescence. The nurse has a clearly defined role in each stage and needs to learn more about the psychologic aspects of illness to fulfill the nursing role satisfactorily.

VanKaam, Adrian L. December, 1959. The nurse in the patient's world. *American Journal of Nursing* 59:1708–1710.

This article discusses how a seriously ill person's world narrows and becomes a lonely place. Communication with a nurse who understands the person can relieve this loneliness in the patient's world of illness.

SELECTED REFERENCES

Coe, Rodney M. 1970. *Sociology of medicine.* New York: McGraw-Hill Book Co.

Crawford, Charles O., ed. 1971. *Health and the family: a medical-sociological analysis.* New York: The MacMillan Co.

Duff, Raymond S., and Hollingshead, August B. 1968. *Sickness and society.* New York: Harper and Row.

Graham, Saxon, and Reeder, Leo G. 1972. Social factors in the chronic illnesses. In Freeman, Howard D., et al., eds. 1972. *Handbook of medical sociology,* 2nd ed. Englewood Cliffs, New Jersey: Prentice-Hall, Inc.

Kassebaum, Gene G., and Baumann, Barbara O. 1972. Dimensions of the sick role in chronic illness. In Jaco, E. Gartly, ed. 1972. *Handbook of medical sociology,* 2nd ed. Englewood Cliffs, New Jersey: Prentice-Hall, Inc.

King, Stanley H. 1972. Social-psychological factors in illness. In Freeman, Howard E., et al., eds. 1972. *Handbook of medical sociology,* 2nd ed. Englewood Cliffs, New Jersey: Prentice-Hall, Inc.

Mechanic, David. 1972. Response factors in illness: the study of illness behavior. In Jaco, E. Gartly, ed. 1972. *Patients, physicians and illness,* 2nd ed. New York: The Free Press.

Parsons, Talcott. 1972. Definitions of health and illness in the light of American values and social structure. In Jaco, E. Gartly, ed. 1972. *Patients, physicians and illness,* 2nd ed. New York: The Free Press.

Parsons, Talcott. 1951. *The social system.* New York: The Free Press.

Suchman, Edward A. 1972. Stages of illness and medical care. In Jaco, E. Gartly, ed. 1972. *Patients, physicians and illness,* 2nd ed. New York: The Free Press.

Vincent, Pauline. July, 1975. The sick role in patient care. *American Journal of Nursing* 75:1172–1173.

Wilson, Logan, and Kolb, William L. 1949. *Sociological analysis: an introductory text and case book.* New York: Harcourt, Brace, and Company.

CHAPTER 4

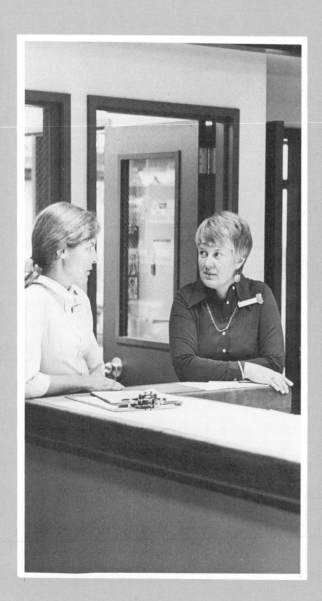

ETHICAL ASPECTS OF NURSING

RESPONSIBILITY

ETHICAL PROBLEMS OF NURSES

Conflicts between Professional Role and Personal Values

Problems between the Nurse and Peers

Problems between the Nurse and Patient and/or Family

Conflicts between the Nurse and an Agency

Problems of Conflicting Responsibilities

OBJECTIVES

- List the purposes of nursing ethics.

- Discuss specific aspects of the established nursing codes of ethics cited in this chapter.

- Differentiate between ethics and personal values.

- State how personal values can conflict with professional responsibilities.

- Explain the concept of accountability.

- Explain ways in which one can convey an attitude of responsibility.

- Discuss some ethical problems that nurses face and some of the appropriate actions that can be taken.

Nurses are becoming more responsible and accountable for their own professional actions. This has occurred concurrent with the expansion of the nurse's role. Both legal and ethical considerations apply in accountability. This chapter discusses nursing ethics and cites the International Council of Nurses and the American Nurses' Association codes of nursing ethics, which offer students and graduates guidelines for professional behavior.

The fact that one's personal values may or may not be compatible with nursing ethics is considered; however, just as other values are learned, those required for nursing can be learned. The aspects of accountability are outlined, that is, to whom is one accountable, for what is one accountable, and how is accountability measured.

A section on ethical problems that nurses may face is included in a situation-and-question format. Answers to these questions are intentionally not provided in order to encourage discussion and consideration by learners.

ETHICS DEFINED

Ethics are the rules or principles that govern right conduct. They deal with what is good and bad and with moral duty and obligation. Ethics are not unlike the law in that each deals with rules of conduct, which has underlying principles relating to right and wrong and codes of morality. Ethics are designed to protect the rights of human beings.

Ethics are part of the culture of a society. They have existed in every society since the Greek era. The word *ethics* has its origin in the Greek word *ethos*, meaning custom or guiding beliefs. Greek ethical speculation has its foundations in the moral tradition and attitudes of the Greek people. Modern ethics, on the other hand, have developed with the influence of the Christian church.

In health delivery systems, ethics are characteristic of professions. In nursing, ethics provide professional standards for nursing activities, which protect the nurse and the patient.

CODES OF ETHICS

A code of ethics is essential to a profession. It provides a means whereby professional standards of practice are established and by which they are maintained and improved. Codes of ethics are formal guidelines for professional action. They are shared by the persons within the specific professions and should be generally compatible with a person's personal values.

A code of ethics gives the members of the profession a frame of reference for judgments in complex nursing situations. No two situations are identical, and nurses are frequently in situations in which judgment is required as to which course of action should be taken. A code of ethics serves as a guide in many of these situations.

When people enter the nursing profession, other members of the profession assume that they accept the established nursing codes of ethics. New nurses inherit the trust and the responsibility to carry out ethical practices and to exhibit ethical conduct.

The International Council of Nurses, American Nurses' Association, Canadian Nurses' Association, and state and provincial associations have established codes of nursing ethics. If a nurse violates the code, the association may expel the nurse from membership. Increasingly, professional nursing associations are taking an active part in both improving and enforcing standards.

Purposes

Purposes of nursing ethics can be outlined as follows:

1. Providing a basis for regulating the relationship between the nurse, the patient, co-workers, society, and the profession.

2. Providing a standard basis for excluding the unscrupulous nursing practitioner and for defending a practitioner who is unjustly accused.

3. Serving as a basis for professional curricula and for orienting the new graduate to professional nursing practice.
4. Assisting the public in understanding professional nursing conduct.

In 1973, the International Council of Nurses (ICN) adopted the code of ethics that follows. The code is meant as a guide for nurses, and it is intended that it be understood, internalized, and used by nurses in all aspects of nursing practice. The code should be considered together with the relevant data of each situation; thus it provides assistance in setting priorities and in taking action. For the nurse practitioner, the code specifically provides assistance in making judgments and in the development of attitudes appropriate to nursing.

ICN CODE FOR NURSES*
Ethical Concepts Applied to Nursing

The fundamental responsibility of the nurse is fourfold: to promote health, to prevent illness, to restore health, and to alleviate suffering.

The need for nursing is universal. Inherent in nursing is respect for life, dignity, and rights of man. It is unrestricted by considerations of nationality, race, creed, color, age, sex, politics or social status.

Nurses render health services to the individual, the family and the community and coordinate their services with those of related groups.

Nurses and People

The nurse's primary responsibility is to those people who require nursing care.

The nurse, in providing care, promotes an environment in which the values, customs and spiritual beliefs of the individual are respected.

The nurse holds in confidence, personal information and uses judgment in sharing this information.

Nurses and Practice

The nurse carries personal responsibility for nursing practice and for maintaining competence by continual learning. The nurse maintains the highest standards of nursing care possible within the reality of a specific situation.

The nurse uses judgment in relation to individual competence when accepting and delegating responsibilities.

The nurse when acting in a professional capacity should at all times maintain standards of personal conduct which reflect credit upon the profession.

Nurses and Society

The nurse shares with other citizens the responsibility for initiating and supporting action to meet the health and social needs of the public.

Nurses and Co-workers

The nurse sustains a cooperative relationship with co-workers in nursing and other fields. The nurse takes appropriate action to safeguard the individual when his care is endangered by a co-worker or any other person.

Nurses and the Profession

The nurse plays the major role in determining and implementing desirable standards of nursing practice and nursing education.

The nurse is active in developing a core of professional knowledge.

The nurse, acting through the professional organization, participates in establishing and maintaining equitable social and economic working conditions in nursing.

*International Council of Nurses. 1973, *ICN Code for Nurses: ethical concepts applied to nursing*. Geneva: Imprimeries Populaires. Reprinted with permission of the ICN.

The American Nurses' Association adopted a Code of Ethics in 1950, and it was revised in 1968 and 1976. This code is designed to provide guidance for nurses by stating principles of ethical concern. The following section presents the code and a commentary on each of its parts.

ANA CODE OF ETHICS*

1. The nurse provides services with respect for human dignity and the uniqueness of the client unrestricted by considerations of social or economic status, personal attributes, or the nature of health problems.

Illness is a universal phenomenon; therefore the need for nursing is also universal. Because nursing is required by the broad spectrum of people who make up society, the nurse should be free of value judgments about "good people and bad people"; it is necessary to accept each person, as well as the person's attitudes, customs, and beliefs. In this way nurses can best provide support to people of varied backgrounds.

2. The nurse safeguards the client's right to privacy by judiciously protecting information of a confidential nature.

It is clearly the nurse's responsibility to keep confidential any information received from the patient, only conveying details about illness or the physical, social, or personal situation of the patient to other persons who are also professionally concerned directly with the patient's care.

In some instances, the nurse may be required to provide testimony in a court. In these instances, the court will advise the nurse as to what is admissible and to what the nurse must testify.

Because people can be seriously harmed and embarrassed by a breach in confidence of the nurse, all nurses must use good professional judgment in what they say, being sure that it is stated to the correct person and that what is conveyed could be of value in promoting the health of the patient. The basis of this ethical principle is also found in the law (see Chapter 6, "Invasion of Privacy").

3. The nurse acts to safeguard the client and the public when health care and safety are affected by the incompetent, unethical, or illegal practice of any person.

Nurses themselves are responsible for maintaining their own competence, updating their knowledge and skills as it is appropriate. Not to do so would imply that a nurse could not provide as high a standard of practice as the profession considers necessary.

4. The nurse assumes responsibility and accountability for individual nursing judgments and actions.

The nurse has a responsibility to report to the appropriate authority or to the professional association any conduct of other nurses or physicians that endangers patients. The priority of the nurse is the patient, patient safety, and patient care.

5. The nurse maintains competence in nursing.

Maintaining competence in nursing practice is essential; nurses must keep abreast of new developments to ensure the best standards of patient care. An essential quality of the nurse is a zest for continued study, since knowledge and skills for nursing need to be continually updated. The nurse who pursues knowledge independently is undoubtedly more effective in practice than one who does not.

6. The nurse exercises informed judgment and uses individual competence and qualifications as criteria in seeking consultation, accepting responsibilities, and delegating nursing activities to others.

Nurses need to recognize their own areas of competence and incompetence; they have a right to refuse to carry out responsibilities that they consider unethical. Policies of agencies and the law assist the nurse as to what practices are considered to be within the nurse's area of responsibility. In addition, if a nurse is not familiar with some nursing activity, it is the nurse's right to explain this and to refuse to carry it out.

7. The nurse participates in activities that contribute to the ongoing development of the profession's body of knowledge.

Increasingly, nurses are becoming involved in research activities as individual practitioners and as employees of hospitals and community health agencies. Nurses themselves are conducting research into nursing practice as well as are a variety of health personnel such as physicians and biochemists.

The nurse who plans to participate should first make sure that the patient understands and agrees to be part of the research; second, the nurse should make sure that the research proposal has the approval of the agency research committee or the appropriate approving authority of the agency. For further information see "Ethics of Nursing Research."

8. The nurse participates in the profession's efforts to implement and improve standards of nursing.

Peer review and established nursing standards assist in improving nursing. The nurse has a responsibility to participate in these activities as well as to participate in educational programs.

Standards for practice must always change as the health care system changes. The professional nurse has a responsibility to assist in making these changes and implementing them.

9. The nurse participates in the profession's efforts to establish and maintain conditions of employment conducive to high quality nursing care.

Each nurse, acting through the professional organization, needs to be concerned with the economic and general welfare of the members of the profession. These are important factors in both recruiting nursing students and in retaining nurses in the work force. Through the nursing association, nurses assist in the establishment of employment practices and in bargaining for economic and general benefits.

10. The nurse participates in the profession's effort to protect the public from misinformation and misrepresentation and to maintain the integrity of nursing.

Nurses are generally held in respect by members of the public, who have confidence in their knowledge and their advice. Often when a nurse speaks, it is assumed that the opinion given is the opinion of all nurses. For example, to advertise or recommend a product might be harmful or misleading to the public. The nurse appears to have knowledge that the particular product is better than others on the market; this may not be true because that knowledge is usually beyond the nurse's qualifications and authority.

11. The nurse collaborates with members of the health professions and other citizens in promoting community and national efforts to meet the health needs of the public.

A professional nurse, with specialized knowledge and skills, has a responsibility to contribute in such a manner as to assist people to meet the health needs of the community. Citizens are increasingly concerned and becoming involved in planning health care. A nurse can offer such a group information that would be pertinent and helpful. Nurses also have a responsibility to act on committees with other health members and other professionals such as teachers and social workers in meeting the health problems of the people in the community.

*American Nurses' Association. 1976. *Code for nurses.* Kansas City, Missouri: American Nurses' Association. Reprinted with permission.

ETHICS OF NURSING RESEARCH

As a profession committed to the improvement of health services to society, nursing is obligated to develop new knowledge as well as to utilize available knowledge and skills. Such a commitment to the development of nursing theory and to the improvement of nursing practice presupposes a commitment to research. There is, then, an obligation for nurses to undertake studies that produce broad theoretical constructs as well as studies that are directed toward more immediately tangible outcomes.

The ethics of nursing research must be consistent with the ethics of nursing practice. Nurses must not knowingly permit their services to be used for purposes inconsistent with the ethical standards of their profession.

Since nursing research necessarily involves human subjects directly or indirectly, its activities must be guided by certain ethical considerations. The following statements prepared by the Canadian Nurses' Association are intended to identify some basic ethical principles that serve as guides for the nurse researcher.

CNA ETHICS OF NURSING RESEARCH*

THE SUBJECT

Respect for the value of human life, for the worth and dignity of human beings, and their rights to knowledge, privacy, and self-determination must underlie research practices in nursing as in other health disciplines. The legitimacy of involving human subjects in nursing research must be assessed within the context of these values. The right of the subject to informed consent, confidentiality, positive risk value, and competence of the investigator must be assured.

Free and Informed Consent

When individuals are involved as subjects of research, the researcher must obtain free and informed consent. Informed consent implies that every effort be made to have the subject understand the purpose and nature of the research and the use or uses to which the findings will be put, in such a way that he can appreciate the implications of participation or non-participation. He must also be informed that if any significant change in purpose, nature, or use of findings is contemplated, he will also be informed and have the right to consent or refuse to participate further.

Free consent means that the relationship between the researcher and the subject, and persons or institutions involved in his care will not place him under any obligation to agree or take part in the project against his own personal inclinations. It also means that his refusal to take part, or his withdrawal after having once consented, should not lead to any repercussions or recriminations. Free consent implies informing the subject that he has the right to withdraw at any point during the research.

If the nature of the research is such that fully informing subjects before the study would invalidate results, then this fact must be stated to the subject, together with whatever explanations can be given. There must be provision for appropriate explanation to the subject on completion of the study.

If the subject for any reason is unable to appreciate the implications of participation, informed consent must be obtained from the legal guardian or an impartial committee acting on behalf of the subject. If the research should impinge on the privacy or other rights of any third party, such as the spouse of the subject, this person's consent must also be obtained.

Confidentiality

Subjects must be assured that confidentiality will be respected. Where anonymity is promised, it must be provided. Hidden coding to enable the researcher to identify individuals must not be resorted to. Every effort must be made to ensure that individuals and institutions cannot be identified.

Injury, Risk, and Priorities

Research subjects must be assured protection against physical, mental or emotional injury. Should the research involve risk of injury, such risks must be weighed against the good to be achieved. Should the risk outweigh the positive value of the research, the project must not be pursued.

Where there is conflict between the rights of the subject and the needs of the researcher for freedom of inquiry, the conflict must be resolved with priority given to the concerns and rights of the subject.

THE RESEARCHER

In order to maintain high ethical standards, the nurse researcher must possess knowledge and skills compatible with the demands of the investigation to be undertaken. The researcher has responsibility to acknowledge personal limitations and to correct misrepresentations made by others. The researcher is obligated to develop the design and procedures appropriate to the study.

The researcher is accountable in varying ways to those participating in the investigation. The purpose of the research must be honestly represented, and any uses to which the findings may be put, made known to persons or institutions involved. In order to justify the investigation, the researcher must ensure that the purposes and anticipated outcomes are compatible with the financial investment and the people and resources used.

In order to ensure the integrity of the investigation, the researcher must present the project for review to a group of professional peers. With certain studies, ongoing reviews by a peer group may be mandatory.

THE SETTING

The milieu in which an investigation is to be conducted must be assessed in terms of the potential for a nurse researcher to conduct a study that is consistent with these guidelines. While the board and/or administrators of an institution or agency may require approval by its research committee of a nursing study as well as of any other proposal, any such approval body should include nursing representation. There should be ongoing provisions for coping with setting-related ethical problems during the course of the investigation.

Nurse researchers ought to be the principal investigators in the study of nursing problems and must be collaborators with other researchers in the study of interprofessional problems of health care. This interprofessional involvement indicates that a common code of ethics for health research should be developed to facilitate research in nursing and its related professions.

*Canadian Nurses' Association, 1972. Ethics of nursing research. *The Canadian Nurse* 68(9):23–25. Reprint with permission.

PERSONAL VALUES

A *value* can be defined as something of worth, a belief held dearly by a person. A value is a personal belief about the worth, truth, or desirability of a particular idea, object or behavior (Czmowski 1974:194). This definition is important in that it indicates that a value is personal, whereas codes of ethics belong to a profession or to society as a whole.

Most authorities agree that values are formed from personal experiences. Values form a basis for a person's behavior; a person's real values are shown by consistent patterns of behavior. Once one is aware of one's values, the values become an internal control for behavior.

Values have both intellectual and emotional components. The person is intellectually convinced about a value, holds it dearly, and is prepared to defend it.

People start to learn their values at home, and values continue to develop throughout life. When a student chooses to become a professional nurse, that student brings to nursing certain values which have already developed. Many of these values are probably compatible with nursing ethics, but some may not be compatible. However, values can be learned, and in order to practice as a professional nurse, a nurse's values should be compatible with the profession's code of ethics. Values such as respecting the dignity of people without bias, safeguarding a person's right to privacy, and accepting responsibility for one's own actions are manifested in behaviors such as conscientiously performing delegated activities and reporting errors such as a drug omission. Valuing the right of privacy is frequently seen in such behaviors as curtaining off areas for patient activities of bathing, treatments, or draping procedures or providing a conference area for patient consultation with a priest or grieving family members. Other values are honesty, gentleness, punctuality, respect, and feeling for others.

A personal philosophy serves to integrate a person's spiritual, professional, social, and esthetic values, all of which produce a composite for a pattern of living.

Because of a nurse's experiences, some ethical values that are considered basic to nursing practice may not be a part of the nurse's value system. An example of this might be safeguarding a person's right to privacy. This value can be learned through understanding the needs of the patients and by being sensitive to their feelings. A nursing student may not have had the opportunity to learn this, and yet it is an ethical value basic to nursing, which the nursing student can learn.

Conflict of Personal Values and Professional Duty

With the changing scope of nursing practice and medical technology, there is an increasing chance that more and more nursing responsibilities will come into conflict with personal values of an individual nurse. This is true today when issues of life and death are the subject. On the one hand, employers have needs and expectations for service from nurses; on the other hand, nurses have the right to be permitted to be guided by their own personal values. An example of an area of conflict in the contemporary nursing scene is assisting with therapeutic abortions. Nurses have the right to refuse to participate in those areas of nursing practice which are against their personal values and nurses' positions should not be jeopardized as a result. It is essential, however, that the patient's welfare not suffer as a consequence.

Other common considerations are those related to euthanasia, prolonging the life of nonresponsive patients by machines, and withholding blood transfusions because of an individual's religious convictions. The future, no doubt, promises many more lifesaving situations that may conflict with personal values.

ACCOUNTABILITY

Accountability is being answerable. In nursing, this means that nurses should be answerable for all their professional activities. They must be able to explain their professional actions and accept responsibility for them. Three questions naturally arise.

First, to whom is the nurse accountable? As a nurse, there is accountability to the patient; as an employee, there is accountability to the employer; as a professional person, there is accountability to the professional association; and, as the nurse involved in the care that is provided, there is accountability to the patient's physician. Often, if nurses can determine to whom they are responsible, they can then decide which directive to follow. In one situation the nurse may be first accountable to the physician; in another, it may be to the patient or the employer. An example might be the nurse who provides medications to a patient that are ordered by the physician,

lists these medications for the billing office of the hospital, and supports the patient and assists with worries regarding the illness. In the first instance, the nurse's primary accountability is to the physician; in listing the medications, the primary accountability is to the hospital; and in the third instance, helping the patient, the nurse's chief accountability is to the patient.

Second, for what are nurses accountable? Nurses are accountable for all their professional nursing activities. Some of these are readily measured or observed; others remain elusive.

Third, how is the nurse accountable? By what criteria is accountability measured? The nurse's actions are evaluated against standards that are objective, realistic, and desirable. One standard might be the charting done by the nurse; another standard could be the plan of nursing intervention.

RESPONSIBILITY

To be *responsible* means to be reliable and trustworthy. This attribute indicates that the professional nurse carries out required nursing activities conscientiously and that the nurse's actions are honestly reported.

When the patient becomes aware that the nurse is a responsible person with the knowledge and skills appropriate to the setting, then a sense of trust develops in the patient, thereby relieving the anxiety that occurs when patients are unsure about the nurse's integrity and competence.

There are several ways in which you as a nurse can communicate this quality of being a responsible person:

1. Convey a sincere interest in the patient.
2. Always follow through with activities. If you are delayed in doing something the patient expects, provide an explanation about the delay.
3. Address the patient in a manner that conveys respect.
4. Talk with the patient about subjects the patient desires, rather than your own interests.
5. Do not discuss other patients in a derogatory manner or convey confidential information about them.
6. Accept any criticism from the patient, and try to see the patient's point of view.

ETHICAL PROBLEMS OF NURSES

An analysis of the results of a study of the ethical problems of nurses categorized the results into three types of problems (Allen 1974:22–23):

1. A question of to whom the nurse is responsible.

2. A question of what course of action to take while knowing what should be done.

3. A question of what can be done about an unsatisfactory level of nursing care.

Ethical problems faced by nurses can also be placed in five broad areas:

1. Conflicts between professional role and personal values.

2. Problems between the nurse and peers and/or other health professionals.

3. Problems between the nurse and the patient and/or the family.

4. Problems between the nurse and the agency.

5. Problems of conflicting responsibilities.

Conflicts between Professional Role and Personal Values

In these problems, the nurse knows what should be done, but for various reasons either acts differently or withdraws from the situation. In all cases the nurse could have an ethical problem.

In one example, a nurse's personal value system does not support abortion. This nurse has begun to develop a good personal relationship with a 13-year-old girl who has been admitted to the hospital for a legal abortion. The girl is in conflict within herself about having the abortion; because of her conflicting feelings and her fear of the procedure, she wants to have the nurse's personal support. The nurse, in her professional role, needs to support the girl in going ahead with the abortion; however, as a person, the nurse's value against the abortion makes it difficult for her to give the girl her complete support. Question: Should the nurse play a strictly professional role and give the girl support only for the abortion, or should she reveal that her personal value is against abortion?

A second example might be that of a nurse who is asked to teach birth control and whose personal value system does not agree. Question: Does the nurse do the teaching, or does the nurse refuse?

A third example is that of a white nurse who is afraid to correct a black nurse for an error because he is afraid that the black nurse will report him to the Human Rights Commission. Question: Does the white nurse correct the black nurse and risk labor problems and possible firing?

In each of these situations the nurse knows the correct action to take for the patient; however, either the nurse's own values or fear of the problems of a legal inquiry provide ethical conflicts.

Problems between the Nurse and Peers

When a nurse is faced with a problem in relation to peers or other health professionals, the nurse may or may not know the course of action to take.

The first example would be a nurse who sees another nurse steal medications from the nursing unit drug cupboard. The nurse who was discovered cries and explains that she must have the sleeping pills in order to sleep during the day while her three children are home from school. She only uses them when she is on night shift. She is the sole supporter of her children and needs the job. Question: Does nurse number one report nurse number two for stealing, or does she ignore the matter?

A second situation involves a nurse newly employed at a hospital who requests Christmas time off because he says his father is dying and he wants to spend his last Christmas with him. Under the special circumstances, the nurse is granted the time. Another nurse on the unit finds out that the first nurse's father is not dying and that he plans to spend Christmas vacation skiing with a friend. Question: Does nurse number two report nurse number one's plans to the nursing supervisor, or does he forget the information?

In a third situation, a surgeon, the chief of staff of surgery, comes on a hospital nursing unit one evening to see a patient before surgery, and a nurse smells alcohol on the surgeon's breath. Question: Does the nurse report this or ignore it?

A fourth situation involves a nurse who is employed on a community mental health team. Another nurse discovers that nurse number one spends most of the time at home looking after an ill mother and fabricates reports about visiting patients in their homes. Question: Does nurse number two present this information to the members of the community team, or does nurse number two discuss this with nurse number one?

Problems between the Nurse and Patient and/or Family

In these situations, the nurse has ethical problems that involve a patient, family, or both. In one instance, a patient requests an abortion. Her husband agrees, but he tells the nurse that he will always be tormented with the thought that he agreed to destroy a human being he helped to create. The wife tells the nurse that her husband really was not the father of the unborn baby. Question: Should the nurse tell the father, or the physician, or the nursing supervisor?

In a second example, a young patient who believes he is dying tells the nurse that he wants to die with a clear conscience and confesses to the fact that at age 15, three years previously, he had held his brother's head under water until he drowned. He further states that his parents believe that his brother drowned accidentally. Question: Should the nurse tell the physician, the nursing supervisor, or the parents?

A third example involving patients and their families is that of a nurse who is caring for a woman injured in an automobile accident. The husband, also in the accident, was admitted to another hospital unit and dies. The nurse is constantly questioned by the patient about the husband. The physician directs the nurse not to tell the patient but to make up answers; the physician gives no reason. Question: Should the nurse fabricate answers for the patient, report the matter to the supervisor, and/or tell the patient the truth?

Conflicts between the Nurse and an Agency

In these problems, the nurse's professional and personal ethical values come into conflict with agency policy.

In one situation, the nurse is asked by a dying patient not to call a clergyman, but the hospital policy is that the clergy are called for all dying patients.

Question: Should the nurse call a clergyman or discuss this with the patient and family?

In a second example, a hospital has a policy that all sedative medications are counted at the end of each shift. The nurse has already been reprimanded for staying overtime to do this. Question: Should he not count the tablets but just subtract what he has given for the count, or should he do the count and neglect a patient who requires a change of dressing?

A third situation is that of a nurse who is employed in a home visiting nursing service. While she is visiting a woman who has multiple sclerosis, the husband comes home and asks the nurse to have sexual relations with him and says he will pay the nurse well. Question: Should the nurse accept or refuse? Should she tell the wife, the physician, and/or the nursing supervisor, or say nothing?

In the fourth situation, a teenager who is emotionally upset requires information about how to obtain an abortion. The agency's policy is not to discuss abortions. Question: Should the nurse give the information to the patient or follow the agency's policy?

Problems of Conflicting Responsibilities

Nurses are repeatedly faced with divided responsibility. On the one hand, the nurse is frequently an employee responsible to a hospital or health agency. On the other hand, the nurse is a professional person responsible to the professional ethics of an association and the standards of nursing practice of the profession. Last, the nurse is responsible to and for patients and is taught to respond to their needs in a therapeutic manner.

As an example, a nurse is asked by a physician not to keep a record of all the supplies used for a particular patient because the patient will have difficulty paying the bill; on the other hand, the physician wants the patient to have good care. Question: Should the nurse report the matter to the hospital or follow the physician's request?

In a second situation, a nurse on the evening shift is asked by a nursing supervisor to administer an intramuscular antibiotic to the supervisor, using the nursing unit stock. Question: What should the nurse do? To whom is the nurse responsible?

SUMMARY

Ethics are the rules and principles that guide right conduct. Ethical codes are characteristic of professions, including the nursing profession. With the rapid advance in medical technology, nurses are increasingly being faced with ethical issues such as abortion, euthanasia, organ transplants, and issues in daily functioning.

Nursing ethics have four broad purposes:

1. They regulate the relationships between the nurse, the patient, co-workers, society, and the profession. This is done for the protection of individuals and to assist people to function within the relationships.

2. They provide standards that serve to exclude the unsafe or dishonest practitioner and to protect the practitioner who has been unjustly accused of a wrongdoing. As such, ethics help protect the public from unsafe nursing practices and protect the competent and ethical nursing practitioner.

3. They serve to orient the new graduate and the nursing student to nursing practice. Through familiarity with nursing ethics, the nursing student is assisted in the assumption of the nursing role.

4. Ethics assist the public to understand professional nursing conduct and thereby help patients and their families in their expectations of the nurse. Ethical codes thus provide some guidelines for behavior, which become predictable to people.

Various codes of nursing have been drawn up in order to assist nurses in the performance of their nursing activities. Two codes, those of the International Council of Nurses and the American Nurses' Association, are discussed.

Special and increasing concern is being given to the ethics involved with nursing research. Many nurses become involved in research, and this research generally involves patients. In order to assist nurses in the responsibilities to patients and at the same time assist with research, the Canadian Nurses' Association prepared a paper, "Ethics of Nursing Research." Points of emphasis include free and informed consent on the part of the patient and family; confidentiality of the data, even to the extent of securing the patient's anonymity if this is desired; the protection of the patient from any kind of injury; and the priority of the welfare of the patient over the needs of the researcher wherever these are in conflict. The re-

searcher's responsibilities and accountability are also described together with the setting for the research.

Personal values are learned, and as such, people start learning these early in life in the home. A nursing student can learn values for nursing practice even if they have not been a part of the student's value system previously. There may be instances in which a nurse's personal values may be in conflict with professional duty as in instances of abortion or euthanasia.

Accountability and responsibility are important aspects of ethical practice. Accountability is being answerable; responsibility means to be reliable and trustworthy. It is important to patients and their families that the nurse convey the sense of being a responsible person. There are six ways in which the nurse can help to convey this.

Nurses face a number of ethical problems in their daily nursing activities. These have been placed in five broad categories. Examples of the types of problems have been given in order to encourage thought and discussion about them.

For some of the problems presented it is difficult to establish right or wrong for others. The right action is evident, but the problems surrounding such an action make it more difficult.

SUGGESTED ACTIVITIES

1. Review the section in this chapter entitled "Ethical Problems of Nurses," pages 65 and 66. Discuss with a group of nursing students what you would do in these ethical situations.

2. Discuss with others your impressions of the responses to the survey on ethical issues reported in the *Nursing '74* articles listed in the "Suggested Readings" section.

3. List some of your own personal values and consider whether they are compatible with the nursing ethics cited in this chapter.

SUGGESTED READINGS

Nursing ethics the admirable professional standards of nurses: a survey report. September, 1974. *Nursing '74* 4(9):35–44.

This article reports on a survey of responses by nurses to ethical and interpersonal problems. It includes what some nurses feel about distasteful patients, challenging doctors' orders, drug addiction, and sexual involvements.

Nursing ethics the admirable professional standards of nurses: a survey report. Part 2: Honesty, confidentiality, termination of life, and other decisions in nursing. October, 1974. *Nursing '74* 4(10):56–66.

This article is a continuation of the above survey and includes the subjects of charting, pilferage, confidentiality, abortion, and terminal illness.

Rodriguez, Dorothy Batton. 1971. Moral issues in hemodialysis and renal transplantation. *Nursing Forum* 10(2):201–220.

This author concludes that nurses are obligated to study the controversial ethical and moral problems of organ transplantation. Many of the questions, she says, must be worked out cooperatively by medicine, law, religion, and society.

SELECTED REFERENCES

Allen, Moyra. February, 1974. Ethics of nursing practice. *The Canadian Nurse* 70:22–23.

American Nurses' Association. 1972. *Accountability of the nurse.* Speeches presented during the 48th convention, American Nurses' Association, Kansas City, Missouri.

American Nurses' Association. 1976. *Code for nurses with interpretive statements.* Kansas City, Missouri.

Beauchamp, Joyce M. 1975. Euthanasia and the nurse practitioner. *Nursing Forum* 14(1):56–73.

Brown, Norman, et al. July 1971. How do nurses feel about euthanasia and abortion? *American Journal of Nursing* 71:1413–1416.

Canadian Nurses' Association. September, 1972. Ethics of nursing research. *The Canadian Nurse* 68(9):23–25.

Cawley, Michele Anne. May, 1977. Euthanasia: should it be a choice? *American Journal of Nursing* 77:859–861.

Churchill, Larry. May, 1977. Ethical issues of a profession in transition. *American Journal of Nursing* 77:873–876.

Creighton, Helen. 1975. *Law every nurse should know,* 3rd ed. Philadelphia: W. B. Saunders Co.

Czmowski, Marie. 1974. Value teaching in nursing education. *Nursing Forum* 13(2):192–206.

Fagin, Claire. April, 1971. Accountability. *Nursing Outlook* 19:249–251.

Gortner, Susan R. December, 1974. Scientific accountability in nursing. *Nursing Outlook* 22:764–768.

International Council of Nurses. 1973. *ICN Code for Nurses, ethical concepts applied to nursing.* Geneva: Imprimeries Populaires.

Jacobson, Sharol F. 1973. Ethical issues in experimentation with human subjects. *Nursing Forum* 12(1):58–71.

Johnson, Priscilla. May, 1977. The gray areas—who decides? *American Journal of Nursing* 77:856–858.

Lestz, Paula. May, 1977. A committee to decide the quality of life. *American Journal of Nursing* 77:862–864.

Levine, Myra E. May, 1977. Nursing ethics and the ethical nurse. *American Journal of Nursing* 77:845–849.

Lewis, Edith P. May, 1972. Accountability: how, for what, and to whom? (Editorial). *Nursing Outlook* 20:315.

National League for Nursing. 1976. *Accountability: accepting the challenge.* Pub. No. 16. New York.

Rapp, J. Douglas. 1976. Implications of moral and ethical issues for nurses. *Nursing Forum* 15(2):168–179.

Romanell, Patrick. May, 1977. Ethics, moral conflicts and choice. *American Journal of Nursing* 77:850–855.

Yeaworth, Rosalee C. May, 1977. The agonizing decisions in mental retardation. *American Journal of Nursing* 77:864–867.

CHAPTER 5

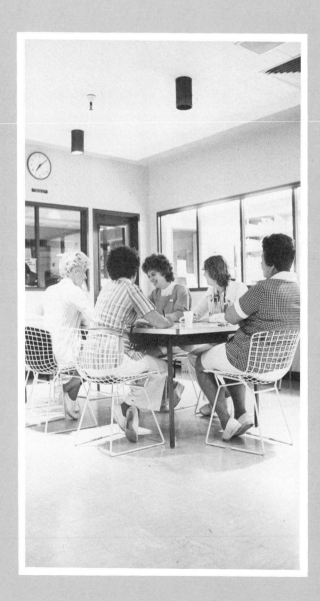

RIGHTS OF PATIENTS, NURSES, AND STUDENTS

OBJECTIVES

- Explain some reasons for the development of statements of rights.

- Describe the Patient's Bill of Rights established by the American Hospital Association and the Canadian National Consumers' Association.

- Refer others to special lists of rights such as rights for the handicapped, the mentally retarded, the dying, the elderly, and the pregnant patient.

- Refer others to guidelines available from professional associations for nurses who participate in research projects.

- Explain your own rights as a student and as a nurse.

Patients' rights are the product of both the legislation of the country and the ethical standards of society. They are recent developments. In the past the patient and family were often denied fundamental rights, such as those of privacy, courtesy, and information at a time of illness. They often felt as if they were the least important of all the people involved in the situation.

The American Hospital Association (AHA) approved a Patient's Bill of Rights in 1973; the United Nations adopted the Declaration of the Rights of Disabled Persons in December, 1975. Bills are being passed that provide for the rights of patients in some states and provinces. Since the publication of the AHA Bill, a number of other rights statements have been made public, notably for the handicapped, the dying, the retarded, and the elderly.

These statements regarding the rights of patients appear to have been influenced by several factors. The first is the increased awareness on the part of the consumer about the right to health care and increasing participation in planning that care. The second is the increasing number of malpractice suits that are receiving publicity and thus coming into the public's awareness. As a result of these, the consumer is increasingly concerned about rights, often in a protective sense.

The third factor that has influenced concern about patients' rights is the legislation that has been created in other previously protected relationships, such as the employee-employer relationship and the human rights and equal rights legislation to protect people from discrimination.

Last, patients' rights bills are partly a product of concern of the consumer about the increasing amount of research that is being conducted in the health field and increasing use of patients by a number of disciplines for educational purposes. Although patients and their families are generally willing to participate in research and educational programs, the question is frequently asked, "Do I have to?" In addition, some patients wonder, if they do not agree to participate, whether their care will suffer as a consequence. (See Chapter 4 for Canadian Nurses' Association "Ethics of Nursing Research.")

Increasing attention is also being given to nurses' rights and students' rights. Some of these rights are included in this chapter.

PATIENTS' RIGHTS

Consumers of health services are increasingly vocalizing their concerns about the type of service they want and need. Most desire more accessible services, more coordinated services, more information about their illness and care, more participation in their care, and more personalized service. In response to the public demands, bills of rights have been developed and widely distributed. Two of these are (a) A Patient's Bill of Rights, developed by the American Hospital Association in 1973, and (b) Consumer Rights in Health Care, published in Canada by the National Consumers' Association (follows Patient's Bill of Rights).

A PATIENT'S BILL OF RIGHTS*

1. The patient has the right to considerate and respectful care.

According to this right, a patient is entitled to an acceptable standard of care and to consideration during the provision of that care. Included is the right of the patient to an explanation about what is happening, the why and the when, and the opportunity to participate in the planning whenever this is feasible. It has been advocated by the Department of Health, Education, and Welfare in the United States that health institutions establish the mechanisms whereby patients' grievances can be heard and investigated.

A trend that follows in this general area is that of the patient advocate, a role assumed by nurses in some settings. The patient advocate represents the patient and works on the patient's behalf. Frequently nurses function as patient advocates in situations in which they arrange, for example, for the services of another community agency. However, in some settings a specific health professional is designated the patient's advocate by title and function. This person serves as an educational consultant for patients and for staff. Explanations can often assist a patient to accept some particular treatment to which, for example, she has previously objected. When a patient com-

plains that the hospital has lost his clothing, or that a nurse intentionally hurt him, then the patient advocate represents the patient in investigating the claims and coming to some solution. Sometimes a patient advocate can assist the administration of an agency to change policies that patients find objectionable and that the agency can amend.

2.   The patient has the right to obtain from his physician complete current information concerning his diagnosis, treatment, and prognosis, in terms the patient can be reasonably expected to understand. When it is not medically advisable to give such information to the patient, the information should be made available to an appropriate person in his behalf. He has the right to know by name the physician responsible for coordinating his care.

By this statement the patient has a right to understand the diagnosis, treatment, and prognosis. This means that the patient needs to have an understanding of some medical terminology such as prognosis in order that what the patient learns has meaning. Just as patients have a right to accurate information about their health, they also have a right not to be informed if it is considered that the information would have negative effects upon them, such as an acute depressive reaction or an acute anxiety reaction. The physician is responsible for making this decision and informing the appropriate member of the family if it is indicated.

3.   The patient has the right to receive from his physician information necessary to give informed consent prior to the start of any procedure and/or treatment. Except in emergencies, such information for informed consent should include but not necessarily be limited to the specific procedure and/or treatment, the medically significant risks involved, and the probable duration of incapacitation. Where medically significant alternatives for care or treatment exist, or when the patient requests information concerning medical alternatives, the patient has the right to such information. The patient also has the right to know the name of the person responsible for the procedures and/or treatment.

Consent is a free, rational act that presupposes knowledge about the thing to which consent is given by a person who is legally capable of consent. Informed consent includes:

1.   Explanation of the condition.

2.   Explanation of the procedures to be used and the consequences.

3.   Description of alternative treatments or procedures.

4.   Description of the benefits to be expected (not assured).

5.   Answers to the patient's inquiries.

6.   Understanding that the patient has not been coerced to agree and may withdraw if he changes his mind (Kelly 1976:28).

Patients have the right to an informed consent, that is, the right to consent to any treatment or procedures, after being fully informed. Patients also have a right to know, to question, and to understand therapies such as medications they are receiving. They have a right to a specific answer to questions. This is a relatively recent change based upon changes in both the common and the statutory laws. Consumers at one time felt that they were at the mercy of health professionals and that they had no right to ask questions or to ask for explanations about what they did not understand. These responsibilities belong to the physician; however, frequently they will be delegated to the nurse in both the hospital and the community settings.

Patients also have the right to know the name of the physician who is coordinating care. A number of physicians often look after one patient in some medical centers, and the patient sees several physicians in the course of a hospital day, often none of whom are the patient's own general practitioner. The reasons for this are probably twofold: the education programs for physicians that are conducted in many large centers and the trend toward specialization in medical practice. As a result, the patient can be confused by the number of faces and really not know who is primarily responsible for care and its coordination.

4.   The patient has the right to refuse treatment to the extent permitted by law and to be informed of the medical consequences of his action.

Patients can change their minds and refuse a treatment and/or procedure. They may do this in writing, verbally, or both. If the patient tells the nurse that he or she refuses a treatment, the nurse has two responsibilities, (a) not to go ahead with the treatment and (b) to inform the hospital or agency authorities and the patient's physician. It then becomes the physician's responsibility to explain to the patient the medical consequences of this decision.

5.   The patient has the right to every consideration of his privacy concerning his own medical care program. Case discussion, consultation, examination, and treatment are confidential and should be conducted discreetly. Those not directly involved in his care must have the permission of the patient to be present.

Patients have the right to be examined or seen by only those essential to their care or therapy. Others must obtain permission from the patient. Although it is the physician's responsibility to obtain this consent, it is also often delegated to nurses. For example, for an examination by an intern or medical student or for a consultation by a consulting physician, the nurse needs to ensure that the patient has given consent before the examination or consultation. If the patient has not done so freely, the nurse must report this to the hospital authorities and to the physician.

The right to privacy has many facets. See also p. 89. Individuals differ in their needs for privacy and in the violations or exposures that threaten these needs. Some request the restriction of visitors. Some need to be alone and withdraw while expressing feelings such as when crying. Most, however, like their bodies covered from exposure and prefer private enclosures for bathing or toileting. Participation in research or educational endeavors may or may not be of concern to patients. Nonetheless, such participation requires verbal or written consent. Even after death the right for privacy persists. The right to not be observed, exposed, or touched by the unauthorized or to not receive an autopsy are examples. Rights of privacy after death move to the surviving relatives.

6.   The patient has the right to expect that all communications and records pertaining to his care should be treated as confidential.

Confidentiality regarding information about patients and their families is discussed on p. 90, "Privileged Communication." This right presents several challenges to the nurse's discretion and judgment. Receiving confidential information is a straightforward matter, but how to handle this information is less so. A certain amount of this information must be communicated to other health workers to provide continuity in the patient's care. The patient needs to know how the information will be handled and what information needs to be shared with others. The degree of the patient's illness and the type of information influence the nurse's decisions. In some situations the patient may object.

It is legally recognized that the patient's record is the property of the health agency, but nine states allow patients access to the information in the record.

7.   The patient has the right to expect that within its capacity a hospital must take reasonable response to the request of a patient for services. The hospital must provide evaluation, service, and/or referral as indicated by the urgency of the case. When medically permissible, a patient may be transferred to another facility only after he has received complete information and explanation concerning the needs for and alternatives to such a transfer. The institution to which the patient is transferred must first have accepted the patient for transfer.

8.   The patient has the right to obtain information as to any relationship of his hospital to other health care and educational institutions insofar as his care is concerned. The patient has the right to obtain information as to the existence of any professional relationships among individuals, by name, who are treating him.

Rights 7 and 8 refer chiefly to the responses of hospitals and to referrals to other health agencies. In the latter instance, the patient is provided with the right to information about the relationships of the hospital with educational institutions such as universities and other health-care agencies, such as privately owned hospitals. In addition, the patient has the right to know whether the owner of a private hospital is related to the physician in the institute to which the physician is being transferred.

9.   The patient has the right to be advised if the hospital proposes to engage in or perform human experimentation affecting his care or treatment. The patient has the right to refuse to participate in such research projects.

Nurses are often involved in research conducted with the participation of patients. In 1966, the US Department of Health, Education, and Welfare articulated a series of regulations in regard to experimentation. These regulations include:

1. Voluntary, specific consent to participate in the research, with a clear explanation of the experiment, including possible dangers.

2. Complete freedom to refuse on the part of the patient.

3. The qualifications of the researcher and the researcher's responsibilities.

4. The relationship between the value of the research and its political values.

Furthermore, the American Nurses' Association and the Canadian Nurses' Association have published guidelines for nurses who participate in research projects. These are designed to protect both the patient and the nurse.

10. The patient has the right to expect reasonable continuity of care. He has the right to know in advance what appointment times and physicians are available and where. The patient has the right to expect that the hospital will provide a mechanism whereby he is informed by his physician or a delegate of the physician of the patient's continuing health.

Consumers of health care are also demanding a reasonable standard in the continuity of care. They are asking that while in hospital, they be adequately informed in order to maintain a program of health care after discharge. Teaching the patient and family appropriate health care often becomes the nurse's responsibility.

11. The patient has the right to examine and receive an explanation of his bill regardless of source of payment.

Many agencies provide detailed documentation of costs of services and supplies. Nurses may or may not be involved in recording some of these, such as the number and kinds of dressings or the type and quantity of medication. In some situations it may be the nurse's responsibility to offer the explanation of the bill or certain aspects of it.

12. The patient has the right to know what hospital rules and regulations apply to his conduct as a patient.

Rules, regulations, and policies of the hospital that are of concern to the patient need to be explained. Some agencies distribute information pamphlets to patients that include regulations about smoking and visiting and information about the availability of televisions, telephones, cafeteria services, and chaplain services. The nurse is frequently the person who receives questions about these matters. It is the nurse who also is responsible for informing patients about special regulations such as no smoking in rooms where oxygen is being administered.

*American Hospital Association. 1973. A patient's bill of rights. *Nursing Outlook*. 21:82 and 24:29. Reprinted with the permission of the American Hospital Association.

CONSUMER RIGHTS IN HEALTH CARE*

I. Right to be informed:

— about preventive health care including education on nutrition, birth control, drug use, appropriate exercise.

— about the health care system, including the extent of government insurance coverage for services, supplementary insurance plans, and referral system to auxiliary health and social facilities and services in the community.

— about the individual's own diagnosis and specific treatment program, including prescribed surgery and medication, options, effects and side effects.

— about the specific costs of procedures, services and professional fees undertaken on behalf of the individual consumer.

II. Right to be respected as the individual with the major responsibility for his own health care:

— Right that confidentiality of his health records be maintained.

— Right to refuse experimentation, undue painful prolongation of his life or participation in teaching programs.

— Right of adult to refuse treatment, right to die with dignity.

III. Right to participate in decision making affecting his health:

— Through consumer representation at each level of government in planning and evaluating the system of health services.

— The types and qualities of service and the conditions under which health services are delivered.

— With the health professionals and personnel involved in his direct health care.

IV. Right to equal access to health care (health education, prevention, treatment and rehabilitation) regardless of the individual's economic status, sex, age, creed, ethnic origin and location:

— Right to access to adequately qualified health personnel.

— Right to a second medical opinion.

— Right to prompt response in emergencies.

Canadian Consumer, April, 1974, published by the Consumers' Association of Canada (CAC).

RIGHTS OF SPECIAL GROUPS

Special groups in the country have recently had lists of rights made public. Some of these groups are the handicapped, the dying, the retarded, and the elderly. These lists of rights are a result of the increased awareness of the consumer regarding his rights in general and his specific rights as a member of a group.

In the Declaration on the Rights of Disabled Persons adopted by the General Assembly of the United Nations in December, 1975, thirteen points are made. This declaration includes in the definition of *disabled*, "... deficiency, either congenital or not, in his or her physical or mental capabilities."

The rights stated in this declaration do not have the force of law; however, many do have a basis in the laws of some countries. For example, statement 2 refers to the application of these rights to all people without discrimination on the basis of race, color, sex,

language, or religion. This statement is similar to human rights legislation found in many countries today.

Also in 1975, the Dying Person's Bill of Rights was created at a workshop on The Terminally Ill Patient and The Helping Person. This workshop took place in Lansing, Michigan, and was sponsored by the Southwestern Michigan Inservice Education Council. Amelia J. Barbus, associate professor of nursing at Wayne State University, Detroit, conducted the workshop.

The Declaration on the Rights of the Mentally Retarded was adopted by the United Nations in 1971.

Following are the declarations of rights for the handicapped, mentally retarded, dying, and pregnant patient.

DECLARATION ON THE RIGHTS OF DISABLED PERSONS*

1. The term "disabled person" means any person unable to ensure by himself or herself wholly or partly the necessities of a normal individual and/or social life, as a result of a deficiency, either congenital or not, in his or her physical or mental capabilities.

2. Disabled persons shall enjoy all the rights set forth in this Declaration. These rights shall be granted to all disabled persons without any exception whatsoever and without distinction or discrimination on the basis of race, colour, sex, language, religion, political or other opinions, national or social origin, state of wealth, birth or any other situation applying either to the disabled person himself or herself or to his or her family.

3. Disabled persons have the inherent right to respect for their human dignity. Disabled persons, whatever the origin, nature and seriousness of their handicaps and disabilities, have the same fundamental rights as their fellow-citizens of the

same age, which implies first and foremost the right to enjoy a decent life, as normal and full as possible.

4. Disabled persons have the same civil and political rights as other human beings; article 7 of the Declaration of the Rights of Mentally Retarded Persons applies to any possible limitation or suppression of those rights for mentally disabled persons.

5. Disabled persons are entitled to the measures designed to enable them to become as self-reliant as possible.

6. Disabled persons have the right to medical, psychological and functional treatment, including prosthetic and orthetic appliances, to medical and social rehabilitation, education, vocational education, training and rehabilitation, aid, counselling, placement services and other services which will enable them to develop their capabilities and skills to the maximum and will hasten the process of their social integration or re-integration.

7. Disabled persons have the right to economic and social security and to a decent level of living. They have the right, according to their capabilities, to secure and retain employment or to engage in a useful, productive and remunerative occupation and to join trade unions.

8. Disabled persons are entitled to have their special needs taken into consideration at all stages of economic and social planning.

9. Disabled persons have the right to live with their families or with foster parents and to participate in all social, creative or recreational activities. No disabled person shall be subjected, as far as his or her residence is concerned, to differential treatment other than that required by his or her condition or by the improvement which he or she may derive therefrom. If the stay of a disabled person in a specialized establishment is indispensable, the environment and living conditions therein shall be as close as possible to those of the normal life of a person of his or her age.

10. Disabled persons shall be protected against all exploitation, all regulations and all treatment of a discriminatory, abusive and degrading nature.

11. Disabled persons shall be able to avail themselves of qualified legal aid when such aid proves indispensable for the protection of their persons or property. If judicial proceedings are instituted against them, the legal procedures applied shall take their physical and mental condition fully into account.

12. Organizations of disabled persons may be usefully consulted in all matters regarding the rights of disabled persons.

13. Disabled persons, their families and communities shall be fully informed, by all appropriate means, of the rights contained in this Declaration.

*Adopted by the General Assembly of the United Nations, December, 1975.

THE DYING PERSON'S BILL OF RIGHTS*

I have the right to be treated as a living human being until I die.

I have the right to maintain a sense of hopefulness however changing its focus may be.

I have the right to be cared for by those who can maintain a sense of hopefulness, however changing this might be.

I have the right to express my feelings and emotions about my approaching death in my own way.

I have the right to participate in decisions concerning my care.

I have the right to expect continuing medical and nursing attention even though "cure" goals must be changed to "comfort" goals.

I have the right not to die alone.

I have the right to be free from pain.

I have the right to have my questions answered honestly.

I have the right not to be deceived.

I have the right to have help from and for my family in accepting my death.

I have the right to die in peace and dignity.

I have the right to retain my individuality and not be judged for my decisions which may be contrary to beliefs of others.

I have the right to discuss and enlarge my religious and/or spiritual experiences, whatever these may mean to others.

I have the right to expect that the sanctity of the human body will be respected after death.

I have the right to be cared for by caring, sensitive, knowledgeable people who will attempt to understand my needs and will be able to gain some satisfaction in helping me face my death.

*The dying person's bill of rights. 1975. *American Journal of Nursing* 75:99.

DECLARATION ON THE RIGHTS OF MENTALLY RETARDED PERSONS*

1. The mentally retarded person has, to the maximum degree of feasibility, the same rights as other human beings.

2. The mentally retarded person has a right to proper medical care and physical therapy and to such education, training, rehabilitation and guidance as will enable him to develop his ability and maximum potential.

3. The mentally retarded person has a right to economic security and to a decent standard of living. He has a right to perform productive work or to engage in any meaningful occupation to the fullest possible extent of his capabilities.

4. Whenever possible, the mentally retarded person should live with his own family or with foster parents and participate in different forms of community life. The family with which he lives should receive assistance. If care in an institution becomes necessary, it should be provided in surroundings and other circumstances as close as possible to those of normal life.

5. The mentally retarded person has a right to a qualified guardian when this is required to protect his personal well-being and interests.

6. The mentally retarded person has a right to protection from exploitation, abuse and degrading treatment. If prosecuted for any offence, he shall have a right to due process of law with full recognition being given to his degree of mental responsibility.

7. Whenever mentally retarded persons are unable, because of the severity of their handicap, to exercise all their rights in a meaningful way or it should become necessary to restrict or deny some or all of these rights, the procedure used for that restriction or denial of rights must contain proper legal safeguards against every form of abuse. This procedure must be based on an evaluation of the social capability of the mentally retarded person by qualified experts and must be subject to periodic review and to the right of appeal to higher authorities.

*Adopted by the United Nations, December, 1971.

THE PREGNANT PATIENT'S BILL OF RIGHTS*

1. The Pregnant Patient has the right, prior to the administration of any drug or procedure, to be informed by the health professional caring for her of any potential direct or indirect effects, risks or hazards to herself or her unborn or newborn infant which may result from the use of a drug or procedure prescribed for or administered to her during pregnancy, labor, birth or lactation.

2. The Pregnant Patient has the right, prior to the proposed therapy, to be informed, not only of the benefits, risks and hazards of the proposed therapy but also of known alternative therapy, such as available childbirth education classes which could help to prepare the Pregnant Patient physically and mentally to cope with the discomfort or stress of pregnancy and the experience of

childbirth, thereby reducing or eliminating her need for drugs and obstetric intervention. She should be offered such information early in her pregnancy in order that she may make a reasoned decision.

3. The Pregnant Patient has the right, prior to the administration of any drug, to be informed by the health professional who is prescribing or administering the drug to her that any drug which she receives during pregnancy, labor and birth, no matter how or when the drug is taken or administered may adversely affect her unborn baby, directly or indirectly, and that there is no drug or chemical which has been proven safe for the unborn child.

4. The Pregnant Patient has the right if cesarean section is anticipated, to be informed prior to the administration of any drug, and preferably prior to her hospitalization, that minimizing her and in turn, her baby's intake of nonessential preoperative medicine will benefit her baby.

5. The Pregnant Patient has the right, prior to the administration of a drug or procedure, to be informed of the areas of uncertainty if there is no properly controlled follow-up research which has established the safety of the drug or procedure with regard to its direct and/or indirect effects on the physiological, mental and neurological development of the child exposed, via the mother, to the drug or procedure during pregnancy, labor, birth or lactation (this would apply to virtually all drugs and the vast majority of obstetric procedures).

6. The Pregnant Patient has the right, prior to the administration of any drug, to be informed of the brand name and generic name of the drug in order that she may advise the health professional of any past adverse reaction to the drug.

7. The Pregnant Patient has the right to determine for herself, without pressure from her attendant, whether she will accept the risks inherent in the proposed therapy or refuse a drug or procedure.

8. The Pregnant Patient has the right to know the name and qualifications of the individual administering a medication or procedure to her during labor or birth.

9. The Pregnant Patient has the right to be informed, prior to the administration of any procedure, whether that procedure is being admin-

istered to her for her or her baby's benefit (medically indicated) or as an elective procedure (for convenience, teaching purposes or research).

10. The Pregnant Patient has the right to be accompanied during the stress of labor and birth by someone she cares for, and to whom she looks for emotional comfort and encouragement.

11. The Pregnant Patient has the right after appropriate medical consultation to choose a position for labor and for birth which is least stressful to her baby and to herself.

12. The Obstetric Patient has the right to have her baby cared for at her bedside if her baby is normal, and to feed her baby according to her baby's needs rather than according to the hospital regimen.

13. The Obstetric Patient has the right to be informed in writing of the name of the person who actually delivered her baby and the professional qualifications of that person. This information should also be on the birth certificate.

14. The Obstetric Patient has the right to be informed if there is any known or indicated aspect of her or her baby's care or condition which may cause her or her baby later difficulty or problems.

15. The Obstetric Patient has the right to have her and her baby's hospital medical records complete, accurate and legible and to have their records, including Nurses' Notes, retained by the hospital until the child reaches at least the age of majority, or alternatively, to have the records offered to her before they are destroyed.

16. The Obstetric Patient, both during and after her hospital stay, has the right to have access to her complete hospital medical records, including Nurses' Notes, and to receive a copy upon payment of a reasonable fee and without incurring the expense of retaining an attorney.

It is the obstetric patient and her baby, not the health professional, who must sustain any trauma or injury resulting from the use of a drug or obstetric procedure. The observation of the rights listed above will not only permit the obstetric patient to participate in the decisions involving her and her baby's health care, but will help to protect the health professional and the hospital against litigation arising from resentment or misunderstanding on the part of the mother.

*From Doris B. Haire, author, and the International Childbirth Education Association, Publisher.

SUMMARY OF NURSING RESPONSIBILITIES

From the foregoing it is possible to summarize the responsibilities of nurses in regard to recognizing and protecting the rights of patients:

1. Respect the dignity of each patient and family.

2. Respect the patient's right to refuse any treatment, procedure, or medication and to report refusals to the physician and appropriate persons of the agency.

3. Respect the right of each patient and family to confidentiality of information.

4. Answer, when delegated by the physician, the patient's questions and provide the information normally provided by the physician.

5. Listen carefully to patients and report their concerns to the appropriate person.

NURSES' RIGHTS

More recently the idea of nurses' rights has arisen and is receiving considerable attention. Initially this attention was focused upon the right of the nurse to refuse to carry out a specific service such as assisting with an abortion or giving a medication that the nurse considered dangerous for the patient. Now nurses' rights are being described in positive terms. Fagin lists seven rights of nurses (1975:82–85).

1. The right to find dignity in self-expression and self-enhancement through the use of our special abilities and educational background.

2. The right to recognition for our contribution through the provision of an environment for its

practice, and proper, professional economic rewards.

3. The right to a work environment which will minimize physical and emotional stress and health risks.

4. The right to control what is professional practice within the limits of the law.

5. The right to set standards of excellence in nursing.

6. The right to participate in policy making affecting nursing.

7. The right to social and political action on behalf of nursing and health care.

STUDENTS' RIGHTS

In 1974 in the United States, the Family Educational Rights and Privacy Act (Buckley Amendment) was passed by Congress. In it two major propositions are evident: that the records of students should be open to the student concerned and that the records are private.

The specific records open to the student are the educational records, not the health records or the private files of teachers. Permission to see the student's file is limited to those who have a real reason related to the educational process, a nursing instructor who is teaching the student, or the registrar.

In addition, letters of recommendation can be kept from the student only if there is a waiver signed by the student, giving up the right to see the letter. Students do not have the right to see confidential materials obtained from parents, such as financial statements.

Students have the right to give or withhold permission for references based on information in their files. When the teacher, for example, must go to the central file to provide reference information about graduates, the student has the right to give consent before this can be done. References given without the use of the file do not require permission.

According to the Buckley Amendment, students have the right to challenge factual information, and a conciliation or hearing can subsequently take place.

Students also have other general rights directly involved in their nursing education. They have the right to expect that the curriculum described in the school brochure or calendar is followed. They have a right to competent instruction in the hospital. Because students are accountable to patients for care, they must receive sufficient assistance and instruction in order that the patient care they give is safe.

SUMMARY

Patients' rights are increasingly being recognized and publicized. Several factors have influenced the development of these rights, notably consumer demands and involvement in the planning and provision of health care services. Consumers are expressing needs for personalized services, for active participation in health care planning, for greater accessibility and coordination of services, and for knowledge about their current individual health status and outcomes of health care. They expect higher standards of care, the right to refuse recommended therapies, the right to volunteer for or refuse participation in human experimentation projects, and accountability for costs incurred for services.

In addition to generalized rights for all patients, the rights of special groups of consumers are being considered. These groups include the handicapped, the pregnant patient, the mentally retarded, and the dying. Emphasized in lists of rights for these groups is consideration for their special needs and protection against exploitation and discrimination.

SUGGESTED ACTIVITIES

1. Select a patient in the clinical area and determine whether, in your opinion, the patient's rights, as stated by the American Hospital Association or the Canadian National Consumers' Association, have been considered.

2. Talk with someone in the community and find out what this person considers to be rights as a patient.

3. Find out whether statements of students' rights have been published within your locality or by your provincial or state student nurses' association.

SUGGESTED READINGS

Fagin, Claire M. January 1975. Nurses' rights. *American Journal of Nursing* 75:82–85.

Dr. Fagin discusses rights generally, moving from human rights and women's rights to nurses' rights.

Kelly, Lucie Young. January 1976. The patient's right to know. *Nursing Outlook* 24:26–32.

This article describes changes leading to the recognition of patients' rights. Also included is information in regard to informal consent, sharing records with the patient, and research.

Porter, Anne, et al. January 1977. Patient needs on admission. *American Journal of Nursing* 77:112–113.

A random study of adult medical-surgical patients indicated that information on hospital regulations and the hospital environment was what they wanted most.

Smith, Dorothy W. March 1969. Patienthood and its threat to privacy. *American Journal of Nursing* 69:509–513.

The line between maintaining a patient's privacy and providing continuity of care is explored. Although it is a privilege for the nurse to receive a patient's confidences, it presents many challenges to the nurse's judgment and discretion.

SELECTED REFERENCES

American Hospital Association. 1973. A Patient's Bill of Rights. *Nursing Outlook* January 1976, 24:29 and February 1973, 21:82

American Nurses' Association. 1968. *The nurse in research: ANA guidelines on ethical values.* New York.

American Nurses' Association. 1975. *Human rights guidelines for nurses in clinical and other research.* ANA publication code no. D-46 5M 7/75. Kansas City, Missouri.

Bandman, Elsie, and Bandman, Bertram. May, 1977. There is nothing automatic about rights. *American Journal of Nursing* 77:867–872.

Consumer rights in health care. April, 1974. *Canadian Consumer* 4:1.

A consumer speaks out about hospital care. September, 1976. *American Journal of Nursing* 76:1443–1444.

Dying Person's Bill of Rights. 1975. *American Journal of Nursing* 75:99.

Nations, Wanda C. June, 1973. Nurse-lawyer is patient-advocate. *American Journal of Nursing* 73:1039–1041.

Pollok, Clementine S., et al. April, 1976. Students' rights. *American Journal of Nursing* 76:600–603.

Pollok, Clementine S., et al. April, 1977. Faculties have rights, too. *American Journal of Nursing* 77:636–638.

Thorner, Nancy. January 1976. Nurses violate their patients' rights. *Journal of Psychiatric Nursing and Mental Health Services* 14(1):7–12.

United Nations. December 20, 1971. *Declaration on the Rights of Mentally Retarded Persons.* New York: United Nations Publications.

United Nations. December 9, 1975. *Declaration on the Rights of Disabled Persons.* New York: United Nations Publications.

CHAPTER 6

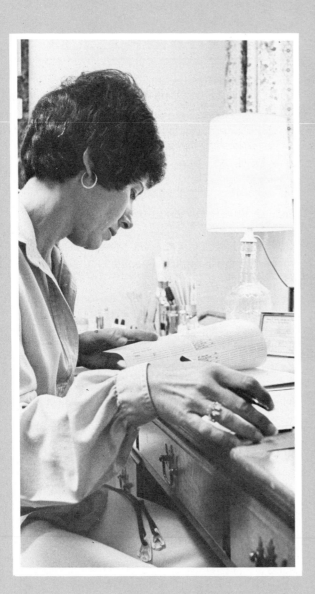

LEGAL ASPECTS OF NURSING

INVASION OF PRIVACY

LIBEL AND SLANDER

PRIVILEGED COMMUNICATION

ASSAULT AND BATTERY

GOOD SAMARITAN ACTS

PROFESSIONAL LIABILITY INSURANCE

Instructor and Student Protection

THE NURSE'S RESPONSIBILITIES RELATING TO THE LAW

OBJECTIVES

- Explain the functions of the law and the steps in the judicial process.
- Explain the concept of licensure as it applies to nursing.
- Discuss what a contract is and how nurses are involved in contracts.
- Explain the nurse's function in regard to wills.
- Compare negligence and malpractice and cite examples of nursing negligence and malpractice.
- Describe libel, slander, privileged communication, and assault and battery.
- Explain what is involved in the Good Samaritan Act.
- Describe the function of professional liability insurance.
- Explain the nurse's responsibilities in relation to the law.

Law is becoming increasingly complex in today's society. As such, its interpretation is generally a matter for experts, that is, for lawyers who specialize within the field of law. A nurse cannot be expected to have a complete understanding of the law. It is important, however, to understand the legal rights of nurses as well as those of patients and their families in order to understand the judicial process and to know when it is wise to consult a lawyer. By understanding these basic concepts, nurses can protect themselves from lawsuits and criminal prosecution.

THE LAW

Nearly every society has rules and regulations, which are developed and promulgated by the society itself. These rules and regulations are the laws of the country, and they provide one aspect of social control for people. Laws can be thought of as having four basic functions in a society:

1. To define relationships among the members of a society and to state which activities are permissible and which are not permissible.
2. To describe what force may be applied to maintain law and by whom it is to be applied.
3. To provide for the solution of trouble.
4. To redefine relationships between persons and groups when conditions of life change.

The legal systems in both the United States and Canada have their origins in the English common law system. The *common law* has its source in the courts. Once a judge has made a decision, the decision becomes a part of the common law of the court's jurisdiction, for example, state or locality. The courts follow a precedent system: a lower court, for example, a local court, must follow the decisions of a higher court, for example, a state or federal court.

Civil law (private law) is that law which derives from codes enacted by the legislature. It also deals with relations among people and is also called private law. *Criminal law* deals with actions against the safety and welfare of the public, such as homicide and robbery. Criminal law is a part of *public law*. The latter deals with the relationship between an individual or individuals and the state.

There are two main sources for the law. The first source is the enactments of a legislative body, such as the Congress of the United States or the Parliament in Canada, which passes federal laws. The laws passed by legislatures, whether federal, state, or provincial are called *statutory laws*. The second source of law is the court system. The laws that come from this source are called *decisional laws.*

There are two kinds of legal action: civil action and criminal action. *Civil action* deals with the relationships between individuals in society, for example, when a person takes a suit against a second person whom he believes cheated him. A *criminal action* deals with disputes between an individual and the society as a whole, as for example, when a person shoots another and society brings her to trial. Actions that might be of concern to nurses are those relating to wills and the estates of deceased persons. These cases are civil actions and are known specifically as probate proceedings.

The judicial process primarily functions to settle disputes peacefully and in accordance with the law. A lawsuit has strict procedural rules. There are generally five steps:

1. A document called a complaint is filed by a person referred to as the *plaintiff*, who claims that his or her legal rights have been infringed upon by one or more persons, referred to as *defendants*.
2. A written response, referred to as an *answer*, is made by the defendants.
3. There are pretrial activities, referred to as *discovery*, by both parties in an effort to gain all the facts of the situation.
4. In the *trial* of the case, all the relevant facts are presented to a jury or a judge for a decision or verdict.
5. If the decision is not acceptable to one of the parties, an *appeal* can be made for another trial.

During a trial, a plaintiff must offer some evidence of wrongdoing. This is called the *burden of proof*. An additional aspect of this burden of proof is that the plaintiff must have a greater amount of convincing evidence than the defendant if the plaintiff is to win.

NURSING LICENSURE

Licenses are legal documents that permit persons to offer their skills and knowledge to the public in a particular jurisdiction or area covered by the license. In order for an organization to obtain the right to licensure, it generally must meet three criteria:

1. There is a need to protect the public's safety or welfare.
2. The occupation must be clearly delineated as a separate distinct area of work.
3. The association must be suitable in its ability to assume the obligations of the licensing process (Sarner 1968:14).

There are two types of licensure: mandatory and permissive. *Mandatory licensure,* in the case of nursing, requires that anyone who practices nursing must be licensed. The only exceptions are: (a) in the case of an emergency, (b) practice by nursing students as part of their education, and (c) nurses employed by the federal government. In *permissive licensure,* the titles *RN* and *LPN* are protected, but the practice of nursing is not prohibited by others who are not licensed.

Nursing Practice Acts

The first nursing practice acts were adopted in the United States in 1903 in New York, New Jersey, North Carolina, and Virginia. Each state in the United States and each province of Canada currently has nursing practice acts, which protect the nurse's professional capacity and legally control nursing practice through licensing. Nursing practice acts define professional nursing, and because of the number of acts there are many definitions. In 1961, the American Nurses' Association recommended the following definition of nursing in respect to professional nursing practice acts:

> The practice of professional nursing means the performance for compensation of any act in the observation, care and counsel of the ill, injured or infirm, or in the maintenance of health or prevention of illness of others, or in the supervision and teaching of other personnel, or in the administration of medications and treatments as prescribed by a licensed physician or dentist; requiring substantial specialized judgment and skill and based on knowledge and application of the principles of biological, physical and social science. The foregoing shall not be deemed to include acts of diagnosis or prescription of therapeutic or corrective measures.

This definition of nursing has three important points:

1. It defines nursing as performance for compensation.
2. It states what nursing is.
3. It states what nursing is not.

In recent years there has been some discussion regarding whether the nursing graduates from 2-year programs in the general education system and diploma graduates are professional nurses. In May, 1973, the Board of Directors of the ANA voted "to recognize all registered nurses as professionals" (ANA 1973:1135). This statement then clarifies that in nurse practice acts, the term *professional nurse* refers to all registered nurses unless otherwise specified.

The states and provinces also license practical nurses in much the same way as professional nurses. The major difference between the two kinds of nurses is that through education and training the registered professional nurse has more refined skills and knowledge and can make better judgments in relation to assessment and the interpretation of data and thence in the determination and provision of the required nursing care.

Revoking a License

The nursing association in each state and province has a committee such as a board of examiners, which has the power to revoke licenses for just cause. Licenses can be revoked because of incompetency in nursing practice, conviction of a crime such as selling drugs, alcoholism or drug addiction, obtaining licensure through deception, falsifying school records, or hiding a criminal history; in some areas, the law specifies aiding in a criminal abortion. In each situation all the facts are generally reviewed by a committee at a hearing. In most places the nurse is entitled to be represented by legal counsel at the hearing. If the nurse's license is revoked as a result of the hearing, an appeal can be made to the court, or in some states, another agency is designated to review the decision before any court action is initiated.

CONTRACTS

A *contract* is an agreement between two or more competent persons, upon sufficient consideration, to do or not to do some lawful act. A contract may be written or oral; however, a written contract cannot be changed legally by an oral agreement. If two people wish to change some aspect of a written contract, this needs to be written into the contract, because one party cannot hold the other to an oral agreement that differs from the written one.

A contract is the basis of the relationship between a nurse and an employer, for example, a nurse and a hospital or a nurse and a physician. It is also the basis of the relationship that a nurse has with a patient. This latter is true whether the nurse is employed directly by the patient and family or by an agency.

A contract is considered to be *expressed* when the two parties discuss and verbally agree for a nurse to work at a hospital for a stated length of time and under certain conditions. An *implied* contract is one in which there has been no discussion between the parties, but the law considers that one exists. An example of this is a situation in which an unconscious patient receives an intravenous infusion from a nurse; the law will state that an agreement is implied between the nurse and the patient that the patient must pay for the infusion and for the nurse's services.

A nurse who is employed by a hospital works as an agent of the hospital, and the contract with the patients is an implied one. However, a nurse who is employed directly by a patient, for example, a private-duty nurse, may have a written contract with that patient in which the nurse agrees to provide professional services for a certain fee. If the patient is dying, the nurse can be protected by a written contract that allows the collection of the fee from the estate.

A nurse might be prevented from carrying out the terms of the contract because of either illness or death. However, personal inconvenience and personal problems, for example, the nurse's car breaking down, are not legitimate reasons for not fulfilling a contract. A nurse cannot be held to a contract if the terms of the contract were misrepresented. An example of this might be of a private-duty nurse who agrees to look after a patient who has just had an operation; the patient, however, is also an alcoholic and is experiencing delirium tremens. Because this latter information was withheld from the nurse at the time the contract was made, the nurse would not be held legally to the contract.

WILLS

A *will* is a declaration by a person as to how the person's property is to be disposed of after his or her death. In order that a will be valid, the following conditions are necessary:

1. The person making the will must be of sound mind, that is, able to understand and retain mentally the general nature and extent of his or her property, the relationship of the beneficiaries as well as those relations to whom none of the estate will be left, and the disposition the person is making of the property. A person therefore can be seriously ill and unable to carry out business functions and yet be able to make a will.

2. The person must not be unduly influenced by anyone for a will to be valid.

Sometimes a patient might be persuaded by a person close to the patient at that particular time to make that person a beneficiary. Patients sometimes are persuaded to leave their estates to a person looking after them rather than to their relatives. Frequently, the relatives will contest the will in this situation and take the matter to court claiming undue influence.

Nurses may be requested from time to time to witness a will. In most states and provinces a will must be signed in the presence of two witnesses. In some situations a mark can suffice if the person making the will cannot write a signature.

In most settings it is a requirement that both witnesses be present at the same time when the person is signing the will. A person who is a witness to a will should not be a beneficiary because in most jurisdictions it affects the right to take part of the estate. If a nurse is a witness to a will, it would be wise to note on the patient's chart the fact that a will was made as well as the nurse's perception of the physical and mental condition of the patient. This record will serve to provide the nurse with accurate information if at a later date the nurse is called as a witness. The record could also be helpful if the will is contested. If a nurse does not wish to act as a witness, for example, if in the nurse's opinion undue influence has been brought on the patient, then it is the nurse's right to refuse to act in this capacity.

CRIMES AND TORTS

Crimes

A *crime* is an act committed in violation of societal law and punishable by a fine and/or imprisonment. A crime does not have to be intended in order to be a crime. For example, a nurse may accidentally give a patient an additional dose of narcotic to relieve a patient's discomfort, but the dose may be lethal.

In most states and provinces, crimes are classified as either felonies or misdemeanors. *Felonies* are crimes of a serious nature, such as murder, and are punishable by terms in prison. *Misdemeanors* are of a less serious nature and are more usually punishable by fines or short-term prison sentences or both. First-degree murder and second-degree murder are felonies. The former involves the intent to murder, while the latter is without previous intent. In some areas second-degree murder is referred to as manslaughter.

If a nurse carries out an illegal practice and the patient dies, the nurse can be guilty of manslaughter. An example is the nurse who performs a therapeutic abortion and as a result the patient dies. Other crimes that are considered to be misdemeanors or felonies are robbery, blackmail, and rape.

Torts

A *tort* is a wrong committed by a person against another person or against the other's property and is usually punishable by a fine. It is independent of a contract. Torts, if serious, can be tried as both a civil and criminal action. A nurse who loses a patient's teeth or who gives a patient a hot-water bottle which burns him commits a tort. Both negligence and malpractice are torts that result either from carrying out an unreasonable act or failing to carry out a reasonable act.

Fraud

Fraud can be described as the false presentation of some fact or facts with the intention that it will be acted upon by the other person. For example, if a person presents false records of education to a nursing school in order to gain admission, this is fraud. Another example of fraud would be a nurse who upon application to a hospital for employment is asked to list the previous five employers. The nurse, however, omits two of the employers from the list for personal reasons and does not inform the employer to whom the nurse has applied.

Negligence and Malpractice

Negligence is "the omission to do something that a reasonable person, guided by those ordinary considerations which ordinarily regulate human affairs would do, or doing something which a reasonable and prudent person would not do" (Creighton 1975:119). *Malpractice* is one part of the law of negligence as applied to the professional person. It is, in effect, any professional misconduct, unreasonable lack of skill, or lack of fidelity in professional duties (Sarner 1968:11).

It is not always understood that nurses are responsible for their own actions even though they may be employees of a health agency. In the descriptions of both negligence and malpractice, good intentions are not mentioned. It is not pertinent whether the person intended to be negligent. If a nurse gives an incorrect medication, even though it is done in good faith, the fact that the nurse failed to read the label correctly indicates malpractice. Another significant aspect of negligence and malpractice is that both omissions and commissions are included. That is, a person can be guilty of malpractice by forgetting to give a medication as well as by giving the wrong medication.

Whether an action is negligence or malpractice depends upon whether it is a lay or professional action. If a nurse performs a professional function, it is a matter of malpractice, whereas if the action is that usually provided by lay people, then it is negligence. Nurses are held responsible for their own actions.

Types of Negligent Actions

Sponge Counts

Sponges may be left inside a patient during an operation. In this kind of situation the nurse either failed to count the sponges before the surgeon closed the incision, or the nurse counted the sponges incorrectly. In either case a sponge is left inside the patient, and the nurse whose responsibility it was to count the sponges can be held liable for negligent actions.

Burns

Another relatively frequent negligent action attributed to nurses is a patient burn of one kind or another. Burns may be caused by hot-water bottles, heating pads, and solutions that are too hot for application. In these situations it does not require a professional education to know that hot objects can burn people. A nurse may also be negligent by leaving a patient without taking precautions to warn or protect the patient, for example, from a steam vaporizer.

Falls

Another type of accident that occurs commonly is a fall by a patient, sometimes with resultant injury. Side rails are used on cribs and beds for babies and small children and when necessary for adults as a preventive measure. If a nurse leaves the rails down or leaves a baby unattended on a bath table, then that nurse is guilty of negligence if the patient falls. Most hospitals and nursing homes have policies regarding the use of safety measures such as side rails and restraints. A nurse needs to be familiar with these policies and to use the precautions indicated to prevent this type of accident.

Failure to Observe and Take the Appropriate Action

In some instances nurses are guilty of negligence when a patient's complaints are ignored. If the nurse does not report a patient's complaint of acute abdominal pain, the nurse is negligent, and the ensuing appendix rupture and death may be ruled to be the result of the nurse's negligence. As another example, a nurse fails to take the blood pressure and pulse and check the dressing of a postoperative patient who has just had a kidney removed. The nurse is negligent, and if the patient hemorrhages and dies, the death may be held to be the result of the nurse's negligence.

Wrong Medicines, Wrong Dosage, Wrong Concentration, Wrong Route of Administration

Another common group of errors occur in the administration of medications. With the large number of medications on the market today and the variety of methods of administration, these errors may well be on the increase. Nurses are negligent in not reading the label on the medication, misreading or incorrectly calculating the dosage, not identifying the correct patient, or administering a medication prepared for oral administration intravenously. Some medication errors are very serious, and some can cost the patient's life. If, for example, a nurse gives dicumarol to a patient recently returned from surgery, the patient could hemorrhage as a result. Nurses need to always check medications very carefully. If a patient states he had not had a green pill before, the nurse would be very wise to check the order and the medication again before giving it to the patient.

Mistaken Identity

Identifying patients correctly is a problem, particularly in busy hospital scenes. It is not unknown for a nurse to prepare the wrong patient for an operation, and as a result the wrong patient has a gallbladder removed. These negligent actions can frequently be costly to a patient and place the nurse in a position of negligence.

Failure to Communicate

There have been additional instances of negligence on a nurse's part when a complaint from a patient or the family is not communicated to a physician or investigated by the nurse. Nurses should always take the statements of a patient and a family seriously and follow up with further investigation and reporting as appropriate. To ignore or forget a patient's complaint of pain can be a negligent action on the part of a nurse.

Loss of or Damage to Patient's Property

Items of property such as jewelry, money, and dentures are a constant concern to hospital personnel. Today hospitals are taking less responsibility in this area and are generally requesting patients upon admission to sign a form relieving the hospital and the employees of any responsibility for property. There are, however, situations in which the patient cannot sign and the nursing staff must follow prescribed policies regarding the care of the patient's property. On hospital units, dentures are often a major problem; they are lost in bedding or left on a meal tray. Nurses are expected to take reasonable precautions in regard to a patient's property. The nurse can be held liable for the loss or damage of patient's property if reasonable care is not taken.

Types of Malpractice Actions

Malpractice is a part of negligence as it applies to a professional person. Whereas the examples of acts of negligence are based upon activities any normal, reasonable person could carry out, malpractice relates to knowledge and skills acquired by the professional

person in his education. The line between malpractice and negligence is not distinct, and authorities differ in their interpretation of some situations. Some authorities consider malpractice and professional negligence to be synonymous. In one interpretation, malpractice includes activities that are *beyond* the level of the particular professional person, as for example, in the case of a nurse who independently diagnoses and treats a patient using procedures that are the prerogative of the physician. Another situation of malpractice could occur if a nurse administered silver nitrate drops of 25% strength into a newborn baby's eyes when it is a common, reasonable expectation for a nurse to know that 1% strength silver nitrate solution is used.

INVASION OF PRIVACY

The right to privacy of persons is the right that individuals have to withhold themselves and their lives from public scrutiny. The action of invasion of privacy is a direct wrong of a personal nature. It injures the feelings of the person and does not take into account the effect of specific information upon the standing of the person in the community.

The right to privacy can also be described as the right to be left alone. In this context there is the delicate balance between the need of a number of people to contribute to the diagnosis and treatment of a pa-

tient and the patient's rights to privacy. In most situations necessary discussion about a patient's medical condition is considered appropriate, but unnecessary discussions or gossip are considered an invasion of privacy.

A patient has a right to privacy and a right to refuse to participate in clinical demonstrations for medical and nursing personnel. In teaching hospitals it is important that the patient's consent be obtained prior to any demonstration or teaching conference in order to respect the right of privacy.

LIBEL AND SLANDER

Both libel and slander come under the heading of defamation, which is also a wrongful action. *Defamation* is communication that is injurious to the reputation of a person. *Libel* is defamation by means of print, writing, or pictures. *Slander* is defamation by the spoken word, stating unprivileged or false words by which a reputation is damaged. A nurse has a qualified privilege to make statements that could be considered defamatory about a patient, both orally and in writing, but only as a part of nursing practice and only to a physician or another health-team member who is looking after the patient. Even if a nurse is

providing the truth, this is not a defense against libel or slander. A nurse, for example, may recall that a particular patient had been admitted to a hospital for venereal disease a year earlier. This information can be appropriately conveyed to the patient's physician, but it would be grounds for slander if the nurse gave this information to nurses from another ward.

For nurses to be protected against claims of slander and libel, comments about patients need to be kept to a minimum and made only to people entitled to have them.

PRIVILEGED COMMUNICATION

Privileged communication refers to that information given to a professional person such as a physician. Historically under common law a physician who, for example, learned that a patient had a history of mental illness, could be made to reveal this in a court. As a result, patients withheld some information from their physicians, which was not always in their best interests. Most states and provinces solved this problem by enacting legislation that overrode the common law and provided that under certain circumstances, the physician cannot be compelled to reveal confidential information. Some of these acts were later amended to include the clergy and spouses. As of 1968, three states, New York, Arkansas, and New Mexico, had extended these statutes to include nurses.

Legislation regarding privileged communication is highly complicated. A nurse would be unwise to encourage a patient or advise a patient in regard to the subject. The privileged communication law is for the benefit of the patient; a nurse who is given confidential information should convey this to the physician and answer questions fully and honestly if required to testify in a court of law. If the law of privileged communications is to be applied, the attorney for the patient will object to the question and resolve the problem.

The matter of privileged communication is referred to in the ANA *Code for Nurses*. It advises the nurse to seek legal counsel in regard to privileged communication in order to be familiar with the rights and privileges of the patient and the nurse (ANA 1976).

ASSAULT AND BATTERY

The terms *assault* and *battery* are often heard together, but each has its own meaning. *Assault* can be described as the attempt to touch another person or the threat to do so, both of which are unjustified. *Battery* is physical harm to a person. It includes not only willful and negligent touching of a person, but also touching the person's clothes.

Every person has the legal right to refuse physical contact with another. While receiving health care, a patient has the right to refuse physical contact, as for example, an injection or an operation; otherwise, the personnel can be the recipients of a suit for assault and battery.

Technical assault differs from criminal assault in that the latter is usually carried out with the intent to injure. If a person is touched and has not given his consent, a lawsuit based upon technical assault can result. Consent to treat a patient is therefore required.

Three groups of persons cannot provide consent. In most areas in order for minors to obtain treatment, consent must be given by a parent or guardian. The same is also true of an adult who has the mental capacity of a child.

The second group consists of persons who are unconscious or injured in such a way that they are unable to give consent. In these situations the consent is usually obtained from the closest adult relative. If it is a true emergency and consent cannot be obtained from the patient or a relative, then the law generally agrees that consent is assumed.

The third group consists of mentally ill persons. States and provinces generally provide in mental health acts or similar acts definitions of mental illness and the rights of these people under the law as well as the rights of the staff caring for the patient.

GOOD SAMARITAN ACTS

Good Samaritan Acts are designed to protect medical practitioners, such as physicians and in some states also nurses, who provide assistance at the scene of an emergency. The medical practitioners in this legislation are protected against claims of malpractice

unless it can be shown that there was willful wrongdoing on their part. Although not all acts mention nurses, there is general agreement that when acts refer to practitioners of the healing arts, this includes nurses.

Even if a nurse is not familiar with the legislation in a certain state or province, it is generally believed that a person who renders help in an emergency, at the same level of helping as that provided by any reasonably prudent person under similar circumstances, cannot be held liable. The same reasoning is also true of nurses, who may be the best-prepared people at the scene of the accident. If the level of care a nurse provides is the same caliber as that provided by any other nurse, then the nurse will not be held liable.

PROFESSIONAL LIABILITY INSURANCE

Because of the increase in the number of malpractice lawsuits against professional people in the health field, nurses are advised in many areas to carry their own liability insurance in order to protect themselves. *Liability* is the legal responsibility of a person to account for wrongful acts by making financial restitution. In most instances, hospitals have liability insurance, but few hospitals cover their employees. Even if a hospital does protect its employees, there could be instances when the nurse is under the direct supervision of the physician and could be considered temporarily in his/her employ. Although a physician or a hospital could be sued because of the negligent conduct of a nurse, the nurse can also be sued and held liable for negligent or malpractice actions.

Liability insurance generally covers all costs of defending a nurse, including the costs of retaining an attorney. The insurance also covers all costs incurred by the nurse up to the face value of the policy, including a settlement made out of court. In return, the insurance company has the right to make the decisions in regard to the claim and the settlement.

Instructor and Student Protection

Instructors of nursing and nursing students are also vulnerable to lawsuits. In hospital nursing education programs, instructors and students are often specifically covered for liability by the hospital. This does not mean that an instructor, however, cannot in turn be sued by a hospital in cases of negligence and malpractice. If a nursing student makes an error, the student is responsible for this action; however, the instructor is also responsible for assigning the student activities that are within the student's capabilities. Courts in the United States have recently found that nursing students must be competent practitioners in their activities. This finding will protect the patient who is in a health education environment.

Students and teachers of nursing employed by community colleges and universities are less likely to be covered by the insurance carried by hospitals and health agencies. It is advisable that these people check with their employers as to the coverage that applies to them. Increasingly, instructors are carrying their own malpractice insurance in both the United States and Canada. In the United States this can be obtained through the American Nurses' Association or private insurance companies; in Canada it can usually be obtained through provincial nurses' associations. Nursing students in the United States can also obtain insurance through their national students' association.

THE NURSE'S RESPONSIBILITIES RELATING TO THE LAW

A nurse has a number of responsibilities relating to the law. The first is that as an individual, the nurse can be held liable for nursing acts. Even if a nurse is directed by a physician, the responsibility for the nursing activity is the nurse's. Second, an employer, physician, or hospital can be held responsible for the negligence of the employee. The nurse, however, cannot be held responsible for the negligence of an employer. Third, if a nurse is requested to carry out an activity that the nurse believes will be injurious to the patient, the nurse's responsibility is to refuse to carry out the order. Fourth, a nurse will be acting illegally by diagnosing illness or treating a patient for an illness such as a tumor. These functions are within the scope of a physician's practice. Fifth, a nurse has a legal responsibility not to commit any criminal act such as assisting with criminal abortions or taking tranquilizers for personal use from a patient's supply. Sixth, a nurse should not reveal confidential information other than to an appropriate person. Seventh, a nurse also has a responsibility to explain nursing activities to a patient but not to comment on medical practice in such a way as to disturb the patient or cause problems for the physician. The latter is not within the scope of the nurse's professional responsibility.

SUMMARY

There are different types of law in society; among them are common law and civil law. Common law is the accumulation of law as a result of court decisions; it is made by judges. Civil law refers to a statutory law that affects the relations between people. It derives from the legislature. Criminal law deals with the actions of individuals against the welfare of society, and as such it is a part of the public law.

The judicial process has five distinct steps: filing of a complaint, reception of an answer, pretrial activities, trial, and a decision, which may or may not be acceptable. If the decision is not acceptable, an appeal can subsequently be made. The trial is the formal examination of an issue in a court.

There are two types of licensure: mandatory and permissive. With the former, a license is required in order that a nurse can practice the nursing profession. With permissive licensure, the law does not require a license in order to legally practice. Nursing practice acts of each state and province legally control the practice of nursing within their jurisdictions.

A nurse enters into a contract with an employer when the nurse obtains employment. It is important that the nurse fulfill the terms of the contract. Exceptions to this are made when the nurse is ill or dies or if the contract has been misrepresented. A contract is also binding upon an employer.

A nurse may be asked to witness the signing of a will. A will is a declaration made by a person as to how the person's property is to be disposed of after death. Nurses would be wise to know of any particular conditions that would govern their action as witnesses.

A crime is an act committed in violation of societal law. A tort is a wrong committed against another person or the person's property. Fraud is the misrepresentation of facts. Negligent acts and malpractice need also to be understood by nurses. Negligence applies to everyone, whereas malpractice applies to a professional person. In trials of malpractice, a nurse may be called as an expert witness. As such, the nurse is expected to testify as to what is reasonable or unreasonable under the particular circumstances.

A privileged communication is information given to a professional person such as that information given to a physician by a patient. Nurses are advised to seek legal counsel in their own jurisdiction in regard to this aspect of the law as it applies in the nurse-patient relationship. Good Samaritan Acts also protect nurses. These acts are designed to protect people who act in an emergency such as at the scene of a highway accident.

Liability is the legal responsibility of a person to account for wrongful acts by making financial restitution. Because nurses can be held responsible for their own actions, many have liability insurance to protect themselves from negligent acts and from malpractice costs.

In summary, the nurse has seven responsibilities relating to the law. The nurse is responsible for his or her own actions which must be within the law and within the behavioral norms of the role.

SUGGESTED ACTIVITIES

1. Obtain information from your local nursing association as to the type of malpractice insurance available to you.

2. Select an anonymous patient's record and list all the data on the chart that would be considered privileged information. Discuss your findings with a group of other nursing students.

3. Discuss with a group of nursing students how the following situation might be appropriately handled:

A physician's wife is a patient on the gynecology unit of a hospital. As a nursing student on the unit, you have been instructed by her doctor to make sure that information in the patient's record is not available to anyone except the patient's physician and nursing staff. The patient's husband is a well-known physician in the hospital and asks a nursing student for his wife's record.

SUGGESTED READINGS

Facing a grand jury. March, 1976. *American Journal of Nursing* 76:398–400.

The unnamed nurse/author describes a personal experience as a witness in an abortion issue. Included in the article are eight final recommendations for nurses to follow in order to protect themselves.

Perry, Shannon E. March, 1977. If you're called as an expert witness. *American Journal of Nursing* 77:458–460.

The author explains the procedure involved when one is called as an expert witness. The purpose of being called as an expert witness together with some of the rules involved in the process are explained.

Shannon, Mary Lucille. August, 1975. Nurses in American history: our first four licensure laws. *American Journal of Nursing* 75:1327–1329.

This article cites the first four licensure laws passed in 1903. They are regarded as only a beginning and are of interest particularly when viewed in the time when women did not vote. They provided an opening for the improved laws of today.

Williams, Brooke N. January, 1976. Malpractice: how good is your insurance protection? *Nursing 76* 6:3, 6–7.

This author provides some legal definitions and discusses insurance protection, sources from which to acquire a policy, differences between coverage based on occurrence or claims made, supplement "umbrella" policies, and other tips for assuring adequate protection.

SELECTED REFERENCES

American Nurses' Association. 1976. *The Code for Nurses.* Kansas City, Mo.

American Nurses' Association. July, 1973. ANA issues statement on diploma graduates. *American Journal of Nurses* 73:1135.

American Nurses' Association. 1961. *Legal definition of nursing.* Kansas City, Mo.

American Nurses' Association. 1975. *Human rights guidelines for nurses in clinical and other research.* Publication no. D-46 5M 7/75. Kansas City, Mo.

Bolton, Michael. 1976. *Civil rights in Canada.* Vancouver, Canada: International Self-Counsel Press, Ltd.

Creighton, Helen. 1975. *Law every nurse should know,* 3rd ed. Philadelphia: W. B. Saunders Co.

Kelly, Lucie Young. January, 1976. The patient's right to know. *Nursing Outlook* 24:26–32.

Good, Shirley, and Kerr, Janet C. 1973. *Contemporary issues in Canadian law for nurses.* Toronto: Holt, Rinehart and Winston of Canada, Ltd.

Murchison, Irena A., and Nichols, Thomas S. 1970. *Legal foundations of nursing practice.* New York: The MacMillan Co.

Sarner, Harvey. 1968. *The nurse and the law.* Philadelphia: W. B. Saunders Co.

UNIT II

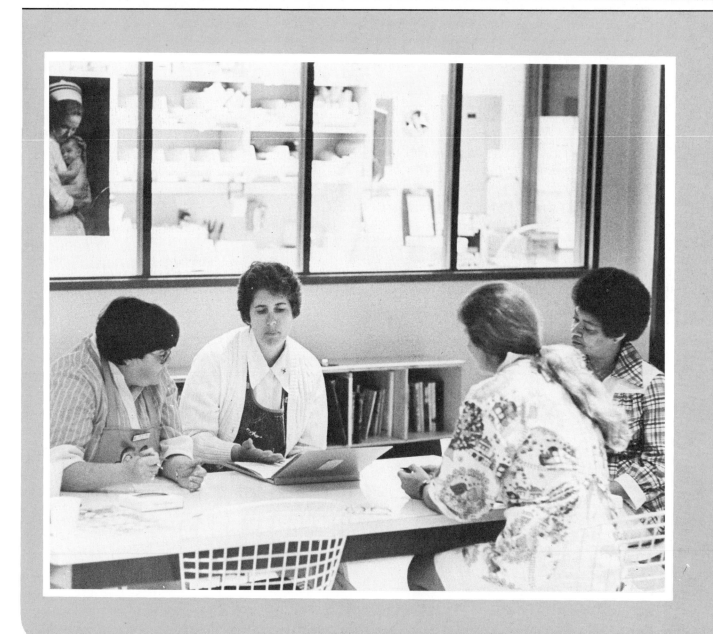

INTEGRATING CONCEPTS

CHAPTER 7

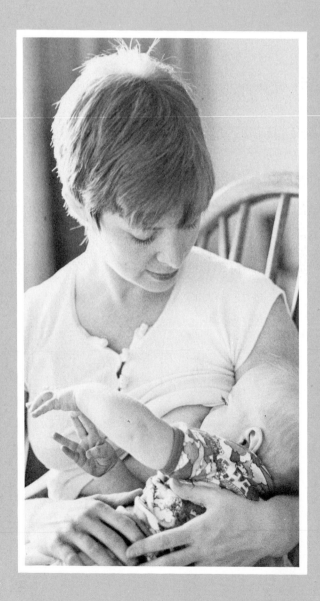

HOMEOSTASIS AND HUMAN NEEDS

CHARACTERISTICS OF PEOPLE WHOSE NEEDS ARE MET

Physical Well-being

Mental Well-being

OBJECTIVES

- Explain the concept of homeostasis and the four main characteristics of homeostatic mechanisms.

- Describe how three major glands and two major systems of the body maintain the body's biologic homeostasis.

- Discuss some prerequisites for the development of psychologic homeostasis.

- Define the term *basic human need* and discuss some general characteristics of all human needs.

- Compare Maslow's categories of needs with Kalish's categories of needs.

- Describe specific needs within the framework of human needs outlined in this chapter.

- Describe characteristics of people whose needs have been met.

This chapter is about homeostasis and basic human needs. Since it is a basic health concept, homeostasis will be referred to often throughout this book. An understanding of the physiologic and psychologic homeostatic mechanisms will assist nursing students to understand people, especially patients, as integrated human beings.

Basic human needs provide an organized ap-proach to understanding the behavior of people. Maslow's categories and hierarchy of human needs as adapted by Kalish provide a framework for discussion. Needs that fall within each of the categories are discussed with particular reference to information of value to nurses. Characteristics that describe a person whose physical and psychologic needs are met are also included.

HOMEOSTASIS

Homeostasis is the state of balance or constancy of a person. In daily life there are changes that require physiologic and psychologic adjustments in order to maintain a state of homeostasis. When a person is in homeostasis or equilibrium, the person is said to be in a state of health. When factors either external or internal to the body produce a disequilibrium, the person is considered not to be healthy. The human body is extremely sensitive to any changes and automatically brings into play powerful regulating mechanisms in order to maintain a state of balance. This state of balance operates within a narrow range. Each mechanism of the body that maintains homeostasis has the following parts:

1. A *receptor* or sensor, which can receive a message (input, stimulus) or sense a change in the internal and external environment.

2. A *circuit*, which transmits the message to an effector organ.

3. An *effector organ*, which acts (produces output) to alter the internal environment and return it to the normal homeostatic range.

Homeostatic mechanisms have four main characteristics. First, they are self-regulating. That is, they come into play automatically in the healthy person. However, if a person is ill, or if an organ such as an adrenal gland is damaged, the homeostatic mechanisms may not be able to respond to the input as they would normally. Second, homeostatic mechanisms are compensatory: they tend to counteract conditions that are abnormal for the person. An example is a sudden drop in the temperature. The compensatory mechanisms come into play as follows: the peripheral blood vessels constrict, thereby diverting most of the blood internally. There is also increased muscular activity and shivering to create heat. Through these mechanisms the body temperature remains stable despite the cold. A third characteristic of homeostatic

mechanisms is their tendency to be regulated by negative feedback systems. This negative feedback system is a common control mechanism for hormone levels. *Negative feedback* is a mechanism in which deviations from normal are sensed and negated. The deviations from normal may be either in excess of normal or less than normal. By the negative feedback mechanism the biologic system is directed or adjusted back to normal. To exemplify, an increase in the production of parathyroid hormone is stimulated by a drop in serum calcium, but when parathyroid hormone is increased and raises the level of serum calcium, its production is then inhibited. Not all, but many hormones are controlled by this negative feedback effect. A fourth characteristic is that in order to correct one physiologic imbalance, several negative feedback systems may be required. For example, with hypoxia (shortage of oxygen), characteristic of people who live in very high altitudes, red blood cells will increase and heart rates will be faster in order to transport the blood and available oxygen around the body.

Physiologic Homeostasis

Although all systems and organs of the body, with the exception of the genitals, are involved in homeostatic maintenance, there are three major glands and two systems that largely maintain the body's biologic homeostasis. They are the pituitary gland, the adrenal glands, the parathyroid gland, the respiratory system, and the renal-cardiovascular system (see Figure 7-1).

The Pituitary Gland

The pituitary gland, although only the size of the tip of the little finger, releases several hormones in re-

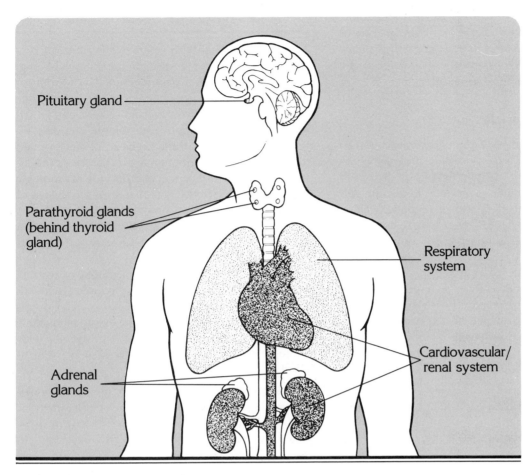

Figure 7-1. The three major glands and the three major systems of the body that maintain homeostasis.

sponse to the body's needs. Some of these are secreted by the anterior part of the pituitary gland under the stimulus of the *hypothalamus.* Others are stored in the posterior part of the pituitary gland *(neurohypophysis).* These latter hormones are secreted by the nervous system and stored until needed in the neurohypophysis.

Two major hormones secreted from the anterior pituitary are *adrenocorticotropic hormone* (ACTH) and *thyrotropic hormone* (or thyroid-stimulating hormone, TSH). ACTH stimulates the adrenal cortex to produce steroids. TSH stimulates the secretion of thyroxin from the thyroid gland. The major function of thyroxin is to control the body's rate of metabolism.

From the posterior pituitary gland the homeostatic hormone stored and released is *antidiuretic hormone* (ADH). ADH controls water reabsorption in the kidney tubules and thus prevents the body fluids from becoming overly concentrated. An increase in the amount of water in the blood stream causes the blood pressure to rise; thus ADH is sometimes re-

ferred to as a vasopressure drug when it is given therapeutically.

The Adrenal Glands

The adrenal glands produce two very different types of hormones. The inner part of the adrenal glands, the medulla, which is part of the sympathetic nervous system, produces adrenalin and norepinephrine. These are discussed in Chapter 8. The outer part of the adrenal glands, the cortex, secretes two kinds of homeostatic hormones. Under the stimulus of pituitary ACTH, *aldosterone,* a mineralocorticoid, is secreted, which induces sodium retention by the kidneys and potassium excretion. Aldosterone is therefore an important hormone in regulating the body's electrolyte levels (see Chapter 29). Other hormones, *hydrocortisone* and *cortisone,* are also secreted by the adrenal glands. These hormones, referred to as glucocorticoids, affect the metabolism of fat, protein, and glucose and subsequently the production of energy for the body. Hydrocortisone is by far the most abundant glucocorticoid. Another major function of the glucocorticoids is to increase a person's resistance to physical stress. See Chapter 9 on the endocrine adaptive response.

The Parathyroid Glands

These glands secrete *parathyroid hormone* (PTH) which maintains the levels of calcium and phosphate ions in the blood and body fluids. Although knowledge about this hormone as it relates to calcium and phosphorus metabolism is still incomplete, PTH is considered invaluable for the body's homeostasis. Both calcium and phosphorus are necessary for healthy bones and teeth. Calcium is also necessary for blood coagulation when the body is injured and for proper transmission of nerve impulses. A dramatic example of low calcium levels in the body is tetany, a condition in which all the body's muscles are hyperirritable and in spasm. When spasm of the laryngeal muscles occurs, respiratory obstruction and death can ensue.

The Respiratory System

The respiratory system regulates the intake of oxygen and the exhalation of carbon dioxide. Oxygen is essential for metabolism and hence the production of energy. Elimination of carbon dioxide is also essential to maintain the body's acid-base balance, which is a very precise control system. (See Chapter 30.)

The Renal-Cardiovascular System

The kidneys are responsible for the excretion and reabsorption of many by-products of metabolism. Their role in maintaining the homeostasis of body fluids, body electrolyte levels, and the body's acid-base balance is vital. The cardiovascular system as a transport system is essential in providing and removing essential elements for all body cells.

Psychologic Homeostasis

This type of homeostasis refers to emotional or psychologic balance or a state of mental well-being. Psychologic homeostasis is maintained by a variety of mechanisms. Each person has certain psychologic needs, such as love, security, and self-esteem, which must be met to maintain psychologic homeostasis. When one or more of these needs is not met or when it is threatened, certain mental mechanisms are activated to protect the person and provide psychologic homeostasis. The motivation that results in the use of these mechanisms is unconscious to the person, not consciously determined. For further information about mental mechanisms see Chapter 8, "Psychologic Adaptation."

Psychologic homeostasis is acquired or learned through the experience of living and interacting with others. In addition, the influence of societal norms and culture on behavior cannot be overlooked. Some prerequisites therefore are needed to develop psychologic homeostasis. These factors can be summarized as:

1. A stable physical environment in which the person feels safe and secure. For example, the basic needs for food, shelter, and clothing must be provided consistently from birth onward.

2. A stable psychologic environment that also commences when the person is an infant so that feelings of trust and love are developed. Growing children and adolescents also need kind but firm and consistent discipline as well as encouragement and support to be their own unique selves.

3. A social environment that includes adults who are healthy role models. From these individuals, the customs and values of society are learned.

4. A life experience that provides satisfactions. Throughout life many frustrations are encountered, which are better dealt with if enough satisfying experiences have occurred to counterbalance the frustrating ones.

HUMAN NEEDS

Despite the fact that each individual has characteristics unique to that person, certain basic needs are common to all people. For this textbook, *basic human needs* are defined as those necessary things which are required by human beings in order to maintain physiologic and psychologic homeostasis.

The following characteristics are applicable to the basic needs of people:

1. All people have the same basic needs; however, each person's needs are modified by the culture in which the individual lives. A person's perception of a need will vary as a result of learning and the standards of the culture. An example is the importance or unimportance of achievement in a particular culture or subculture.

2. People meet their own needs relative to their own priorities. For example, during a flood, a mother might give up her share of water and die in order that her child may have sufficient water to live.

3. Although basic needs generally must be met, some needs can be deferred. An example is the need for independence, which an ill person can defer until well.

4. Failure to meet needs results in one or more homeostatic imbalances, and this can eventually result in illness.

5. A need can be aroused as a result of either external or internal stimuli. An example is the need for food. A person may experience hunger as a result of thinking about food (internal stimulation) or as a result of seeing a beautiful cake (external stimulation).

6. When a need is perceived, a person has a wide variety of responses from which to choose in order to meet the need. The choice a person makes is largely a result of learned experiences and the values of the culture within which the person lives. For example, the professional woman who comes home from work feeling tired may meet the need for relaxation by having a cocktail. This response reflects her experience and culture.

7. Needs are interrelated. Some needs cannot be met unless related needs are also met. The need for hydration can be seriously altered if the need for elimination of urine is not also met. Likewise, the need for security can be markedly altered if one's need for oxygen is threatened as a result of a respiratory obstruction.

Abraham Maslow's model of human needs includes both physiologic and psychologic needs. In addition, it provides a hierarchical framework for needs that are critical to survival and for needs that are less critical. The following are Maslow's five categories of needs (1970:37):

1. physiologic needs
2. safety and security needs
3. love and belonging needs
4. need for self-esteem
5. need for self-actualization

Maslow's highest level, that of *self-actualization*, is the apex of the fully-developed personality; accordingly, few people are fully self-actualized (1968:204).

Kalish (1977:32) has adapted Maslow's hierarchy and suggests an additional category of needs between the physiologic needs and safety and security needs. This category includes sex, activity, exploration, manipulation, and novelty (see Figure 7-2). Kalish emphasizes that children need to explore and manipulate their environments in order to achieve optimal growth and development. He notes that adults, too, will often seek novel adventures or stimulating experiences before considering their safety or security needs. Maslow, on the other hand, includes the pursuit of knowledge and aesthetic needs in the category of self-actualization.

In this chapter the basic human needs are subdivided into six categories similar to those of the Kalish model. They are adapted, however, to correspond with the textbook material as follows: (a) physiologic needs, (b) stimulation needs, (c) protection needs, (d) love and belonging needs, (e) esteem needs, and (f) spiritual needs. Because spiritual beliefs are helpful in times of stress, this latter category is considered to be important for nurses. Within each of these categories specific needs are discussed with emphasis on the nurse's role in understanding and meeting the needs of people who are healthy or ill. Finally, the characteristics of the fully self-actualized person are considered.

Physiologic Needs

The physiologic needs encompass the basic survival requirements of humans in order to maintain biologic homeostasis, and in fact life itself. Generally, when these needs are not met, other needs, such as activity and affection, are not aroused. For most adults, being unable to meet their own needs for food and water can be distressing and can sometimes produce feelings of helplessness. For anyone, the inability to acquire sufficient oxygen, to feel suffocated, is a frightening experience.

Nurses are frequently called upon to assist patients of all ages to meet their physiologic needs. In terms of nursing priorities, survival needs of patients generally take precedence over other needs, such as

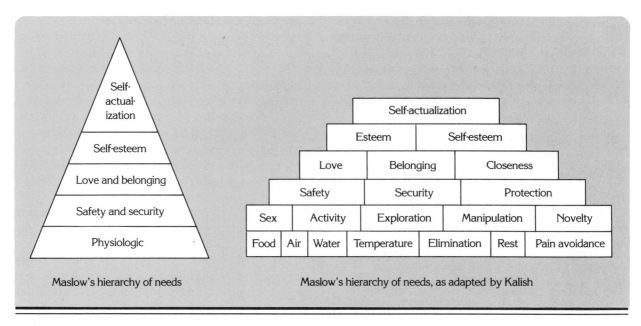

Maslow's hierarchy of needs

Maslow's hierarchy of needs, as adapted by Kalish

Figure 7-2.   Maslow's hierarchy of needs and Maslow's needs as adapted by Kalish. (Adapted from Maslow, Abraham H. 1943. "A Theory of Human Motivation," *Psychological Review* 50:370–396. Copyright © 1943 by the American Psychological Association, Inc. Reprinted by permission. From Kalish, Richard A. 1966. *The Psychology of Human Behavior,* Monterey, California: Brooks/Cole Publishing Company. Reprinted by permission of the publisher. Copyright © 1973 by Wadsworth Publishing Company, Inc.)

those included in the psychologic needs category. Nurses, however, need to be sensitive to the patients' feelings when assisting them with their physiologic needs. For the adult patient in particular, the inability to meet one's own needs in this area usually represents a disturbing and sometimes embarrassing degree of dependency upon others. The needs included in this category are oxygen, water, food, elimination, rest and sleep, pain relief, exercise, and temperature regulation.

The Need for Oxygen

Man cannot survive without oxygen in normal circumstances for more than four to five minutes without the occurrence of irreversible brain damage. Nursing measures to ensure the free passage of oxygen into the body and subsequently to all tissues of the body are emergency measures. If a patient is unable to inhale because of an obstructed trachea or if a patient is hemorrhaging from any part of the body, essential oxygenation of the body tissues cannot be maintained.

Oxygen is vital to all the cells of the body for their metabolic activities, which provide energy. An adequate supply of oxygen to the body tissues relies upon an intact respiratory system, nervous system, and cardiovascular system. A cardiac arrest is another example of an emergency situation related to oxygenation: the heart fails to pump the blood and hence deliver oxygen to body cells. There are also countless situations that are not considered emergencies but that also interfere with the oxygen supply; for example, in anemia the capacity of the blood to deliver oxygen is reduced because of the reduced supply of the red blood cells to carry oxygen.

The Need for Water

Water is second only to oxygen as a requirement for life. In health, water is obtained for the body from the fluids people take and from the food that they ingest. Therefore, impairment in the availability of either or both of these sources can seriously affect a person.

Water is a universal solvent, that is, it is the basic solvent for all the chemical reactions that take place in the human body. In infants a higher proportion of the body is water than is that of the adult. Therefore, the effects of dehydration in infants can be dramatic and serious.

Under normal conditions of activity and climate, adults have been known to survive as long as 18 days without water. However, this is an abnormally long time, and as a general rule three to five days is considered to be the maximum time adults can function without water.

The Need for Food

Although people can live without food for a number of weeks, the need of the human body for food should not be underestimated. When external food sources are not available to a person, the body will use its own internal resources. Carbohydrate reserves (for example, glycogen in the liver) are used first, followed by the fat reserves, which are stored as fat deposits in characteristic locations of the body, and last, protein reserves are called upon. It is thought that the liver is the first place protein is stored; however, the amount of protein stored in the liver and elsewhere is limited and quickly becomes depleted.

The length of time that a person can survive without food depends to a large degree upon the person's own physical status. It is doubtful that a person would survive ten weeks without food. Specific nutrients are also essential needs. Lack of vitamin D is evident in a child who has the skeletal deformities of rickets.

The type of food a person is accustomed to depends largely upon cultural norms, subgroup norms within a society, and individual idiosyncrasies. For example, people of the Chinese culture are usually accustomed to rice; some people in North America enjoy snails, while others would become nauseous at the thought of eating them. Individual idiosyncrasies abound; some like onions, others not; some people like white bread, others eat only brown bread. The importance of good nutrition cannot be overstated. Normal growth and development depend upon it, and both physical and mental health suffer from inadequate nutrition.

The Need for Elimination

In order that a person's body may function efficiently, it is necessary that food residues and gases be eliminated from the gastrointestinal tract and that the waste products of metabolism be detoxified and/or eliminated from the body. The organs involved in elimination are the kidneys, the large intestine, the lungs, and the skin. Complete malfunction of the kidneys (kidney shutdown) is a life-and-death matter.

Nurses will also see patients who have difficulty eliminating carbon dioxide through the lungs. The accumulation of carbon dioxide in the body increases the acid content of the blood. Because body cells survive in an alkaline medium, death ensues when carbon dioxide is not eliminated adequately.

People usually have their own individual pattern for bowel evacuation. The patient who is able to maintain this pattern, for example, evacuating the bowels once a day after breakfast, is less likely to become constipated. Nurses can assist patients by helping them become aware of their normal habits and facilitate the continuance of these habits whenever possible. Occasional irregularities brought about by a change in daily routines need not be a cause for alarm. Changes in diet or increased stress normally alter bowel evacuation.

One less obvious function of the bowels (large intestine) is to reabsorb water. This is an essential function necessary to preserve the body's fluid and electrolyte balance. The occurrence of diarrhea in illness is an example of the excessive elimination of both fluids and electrolytes.

The skin of a person eliminates water as perspiration with small amounts of salt (NaCl). This ability of the skin is an important mechanism in maintaining the body's temperature within a normal range.

The Need for Rest and Sleep

Much is still to be learned about the mechanisms and the functions of sleep. What is known is that without sufficient sleep, mental concentration and memory recall are reduced; a person becomes irritable and less able to cope with psychologic stress. With prolonged sleep deprivation, *hallucinations* while awake can occur. To *hallucinate* is to perceive through the senses something unreal, for example, seeing elephants dancing on the wall.

Insomnia (the inability to sleep) is a relatively common problem in today's society. Frequently a nurse will be called upon to assist a patient with supportive measures to help the patient sleep. People have individual needs for sleep and hours of sleep. Often people will have ritualistic habits such as a glass of warm milk or a tub bath before retiring. Being able to continue these habits whenever possible will assist patients greatly to sleep.

The Need for Avoidance of Pain

The avoidance of pain is considered to be another basic need of humans. However, since pain is the most common symptom of illness, few patients are able to avoid the experience. As a result, many nursing activities are centered around providing relief measures for pain. Pain can temporarily disrupt several basic needs, such as nutrition, exercise, or security. However, the goal of nursing activities is usually to provide for comfort, rest, or sleep.

The Need for Exercise

The benefits and functions of exercise are well recognized today and well publicized. Although people can survive without exercise, exercise even for the immobilized improves health and prevents problems.

The right amount and kind of physical activity will exercise the heart by increasing its rate. As a result, deeper respirations take place, the lung expansion is increased, and increased cardiopulmonary circulation occurs. Exercise also improves muscle tone and frequently increases the range and ease of movement of the joints.

For exercise to be effective, it should be regular and sustained. Generally, exercising at least three times per week is advised. People today are increasingly aware of the need for exercise as a means to improved health and to the prevention of health problems. Activities such as jogging and bicycling are taking on greater importance to people of many ages.

The Need for Temperature Regulation

A relatively constant body temperature is required for body cells to function effectively. If a body temperature becomes extreme, death will occur. Since heat is always being produced in the body by metabolic processes, mechanisms are required for an equal amount of heat to be lost. The skin is one organ responsible for maintaining the body temperature at an optimum level by the processes of evaporation and perspiration. Heat is transferred from the deeper tissues to the blood stream and thence to the skin. Some heat is also lost in expired air, feces, and urine.

Nurses frequently need to assist patients when the body's homeostatic mechanisms for temperature control are not able to copy effectively with temperature changes. Specific nursing interventions will be discussed later in the book.

Stimulation Needs

Stimulation needs arise from stimuli that rouse the mind or spirit or incite a person to activity or towards an incentive. As a category for basic needs of people, *stimulation* is used here in a broad sense, referring to stimulation of the emotions, the cognitive processes, and the senses. A number of activities can provide

stimulation. Any change can be stimulating to a person provided that the degree of change is appropriate for that person. One person might find that moving to another city is a stimulating experience that affords new opportunities to learn new life experiences; however, another person making the same move may well be overwhelmed and, rather than finding the move stimulating, may experience acute feelings of insecurity. Changes of a lesser degree, such as a new book, a new hat, or a different restaurant, can also be stimulating.

Stimulation can also come from a hobby or an activity in which a person is interested. This type of stimulation can serve to balance the routine of daily life and the problems a person faces. Sensory stimulants such as a movie, the smell of newly-baked bread, a beautiful sunset, or the sound of certain music can also add interest to life.

Not all stimulation that a person receives is pleasant. An adult might be bombarded by acoustic stimuli that he finds unpleasant when a teenager turns the music to a high volume. Unpleasant sensory stimuli are familiar to all of us. However, even this stimulation can provide interest, and it can help to meet some people's basic needs.

In this section two basic stimulation needs are considered: the need for activity and the need for exploration, novelty, and change. Sexual needs are discussed with the need for love.

The Need for Activity

Activity in this context is used to mean physical and mental activity. Every person has a need for some activity. Often the kind and the amount is determined by the person's physical and mental status. Physical activity such as playing a game of tennis or walking along a beach in the cool of the evening can be stimulating activities for a person both mentally and physically. A person often feels that vitality is restored and the mind is rested, and thoughts of the experience often return to give pleasure. Activities such as hobbies, knitting, and picture puzzles can also serve to stimulate a person's mental activity and interests.

Nurses will often be challenged to assist patients to meet their needs for both physical and mental activity. The means by which these needs can be met are often affected by illness. The patient who is restricted to a hospital bed from which there is no view can often lack the stimuli that most people in daily life take for granted. To such people the television is often a therapeutic diversion and interest. The elderly person who is in the hospital and whose thoughts and words frequently come slowly, for a busy nurse, is very much in need of assistance for stimulation.

One of the functions of a nurse is to socialize with patients; this can assist in meeting needs for stimulation. Discussions about a patient's interest in cooking or in sports often are helpful. It is important, however, that the socializing is oriented to helping a patient meet the patient's needs, not the nurse's needs.

The Need for Exploration, Novelty, and Change

The need for exploration is particularly evident in the development of a child. Through exploration of the environment, a five-year-old child learns to climb trees and to pick apples; the child learns what a flower is and where the rain comes from. This need to explore which all children have is basic to much of their learning and their interests.

Novelty or newness can also offer stimulation to people. The expression on the face of a child who goes to his first circus or a baseball fan who attends her first World Series are just two examples of meeting this need for novelty. Imagine how boring it is for a long-term patient who never has a new experience during a whole year. The patient sees the same people, talks about the same subjects, and frequently begins to lose interest in the surroundings and perhaps in life itself.

Change is not unlike novelty; it can refer to newness or to another way of doing something. For some patients who are in the hospital for several months, a change in the position of a bed in order to obtain another view from a window can be stimulating.

Protection Needs

The Need for Safety

Safety needs are needs to protect oneself from physical harm. The threats to the safety of the person can be categorized as mechanical, chemical, thermal, and bacteriologic. Generally, adults meet their own safety needs in daily life, and seldom, except under unusual circumstances such as war, are they considered survival needs. In illness, however, persons are frequently less able to protect themselves; their resistance to infection can be lowered, or they may be immobilized.

Patients are not always aware of the threats of injury in a hospital or health agency. Nurses there-fore need to be aware of situations in which patients could be injured. Explanations to patients and taking appropriate safety measures generally will protect a person adequately. These measures not only include those that prevent accidents but also those that maintain cleanliness and maintain body alignment.

1.   Measures for Cleanliness. The emphasis people place on cleanliness in North America often surpasses that which is necessary for safety. However, good hygienic practices facilitate the maintenance of skin integrity and the health of mucous membranes. Intact skin and mucous membranes provide a tough barrier to chemical and bacterial invasion. Much time is spent by nurses in assisting people with the hygienic practices of bathing and care of hair, teeth, and nails. Infection control measures are also frequently employed when the skin is broken as with a surgical incision or a burn.

Cleanliness can also be discussed in an environmental context. Sanitation measures for sewage disposal and measures taken to prevent air pollution, infestation of insects, and vermin all protect people from environmental hazards.

2.   Measures to Maintain Body Alignment. Good body alignment requires minimal muscular effort. It does not place strain on muscles, ligaments, or joints and favors proper functioning of all the body systems. Helping patients to maintain body alignment is of particular importance in clinical situations. Incorrect alignment can produce contractures of the ankle, knee, or hip joints, which can lead to disturbances in both posture and gait.

Often people who are ill are unable to maintain suitable body alignment. Because of weakness, pain, or disorientation, nurses frequently need to assist patients to healthy positions and provide supports in order that they can maintain these positions.

The Need for Security

The need for security can be regarded in two ways, in a physiologic context and in an interpersonal relationship context. The former relates to anything that poses a threat to a person's body or to life itself. The threat may be either real or imagined. For example, illness, excruciating pain, a physical attack, or acute anxiety can all bring about reactions of a protective nature.

In the second context, people need to have feelings of interpersonal security. Interpersonal security is dependent upon many factors. Some of these are consistency from others, awareness of the expectations or limitations of others, familiarity with people and the environment, the ability to control matters concerning self, the ability to communicate, and the need to know or understand. With consistency, people are able to predict to some degree what to expect. When expectations and limitations are clear, behavior patterns that are acceptable in a relationship are understood. The structure or rules offer security to a person. It becomes obvious that familiarity with people or places facilitates security when one experiences the opposite feelings that accompany meeting new people or living in strange places. Aligned with familiarity is the ability to communicate in a similar language with others.

The unknown often produces feelings of anxiety and insecurity. For example, think of the patient who is having surgery for a tumor that could be cancerous. Until the diagnosis is known, the person's security is threatened. In institutionalized health care settings, people also temporarily lose their rights to control matters concerning themselves. For example, the time and type of bath that a patient has is often prescribed by the policies of a hospital instead of the person's own preference.

Love and Belonging Needs

The Need for Love and Affection

The need for love is so basic that it has been described as the bony structure of man's whole emotional life (Caprio 1965:16). So much has been written on the subject of love by philosophers, poets, novelists, and behavioral scientists that the meaning of love is not always clear. To define love is difficult. There are many kinds of love, such as mother love, romantic love, love between friends and family members, and love of God. Perhaps it is enough to understand that love is accomplished with the heart and not the mind, that love is a feeling—an acting response rather than an intellectual process. Love is also a strong positive feeling that is not possessive. Some characteristics of love are outlined as follows:

1. Love is not only a subjective feeling that a person has (an emotion) but also a series of acts by which one person conveys to another the feeling that someone is deeply involved and profoundly interested in the person and the person's welfare.

2. Love is unconditional; it makes no bargains but conveys that one person is concerned for another person, that someone is there to give support and to contribute to the other's development as best

as possible because the one values the other for what he is and as he is.

3. Love is supportive; it conveys to the other that you will always be present when the person most needs you, that you will neither condemn nor condone but that you will be there to offer your sympathy and understanding. Whatever the other needs as a human being, she shall have. It is tolerant but not dependent (Montague 1974:15).

The need for love is met in many ways. Sexual union can be one of the most personal expressions of love between couples. For infants, the physical closeness and warmth offered by a mother during feeding times can be an expression of love. In fact, the fulfillment of the need for love in small children is essential for healthy emotional development. A person's basic security comes from being loved when one is very small. Experiments have shown that young animals and children who lack love can exhibit unusual behavior patterns (Hurlock 1968:157).

In some situations, nurses can become the surrogate parents for young children who are in the hospital by supplying them with the affection and the physical closeness they need. With adults and elderly people the role of the nurse is less concrete. However, in all instances an interest in the welfare of people and a caring and supportive attitude need to be communicated. These can be conveyed in many ways: by touching, by staying with a patient when the patient is frightened, and by listening and communicating in a friendly manner.

The Need for Sex and Intimacy

Although the sexual act is essential to survival of the human species, the character of the need for sex embraces much more than a reproductive function. Already mentioned is the fact that the sexual act can be an expression of the need to give and receive love. The whole field of sexuality and sexual relationships is now being recognized and talked about. Literature abounds on the subject.

In the health field, sexuality, as it relates to a person's body image and self concept has many implications. In many illnesses, patients are unable to satisfy their sexual needs in the usual way. The needs may therefore be either sublimated or expressed in flirtations or other kinds of behavior that require understanding on the part of the nurse. For both men and women, changes in body image brought about by surgical intervention or disease processes can threaten sexual relationships. For example, it is not uncommon for the woman who has had a radical mastectomy to feel anxiety about how well her love partner will accept the change. For men whose sexual organs have been removed or even repaired, the psychologic trauma can be severe. The male self-image throughout the ages has always emphasized potency and virility. Even when sexual organs are not involved as in the case of long-term illness, the sexual needs of patients should be considered. In many situations the nurse can be instrumental in assessing and identifying patients' sexual problems. For patients having surgery, answering questions and explaining the effects of the surgical procedure can be helpful. For long-term patients, nurses can plan to provide privacy for patients to be with loved ones. In many situations the nurse may refer the patient to other health professionals who are experienced interviewers and counselors in sexual matters.

The Need to Belong

The need to belong can be vividly portrayed by teenagers and their peer groups or by adults who join lodges and clubs of various kinds. This desire to affiliate with others for friendship or companionship and to share common activities, language, and dress, offers a sense of identity and prestige to some people. Being a member of a group can give the individual the prestige or recognition that is given to the group as a whole. This may be more recognition than the person could ever attain alone.

The need to belong is being recognized as important in some health care settings. Rather than differentiating staff members from patients by dress in some mental health centers, the staff uniform has been abandoned. In addition, evidence of belonging is emphasized by referring to the patients as members, thus affording them an equal status to the staff in the mental health group. Whatever the setting, the nurse can encourage a sense of belonging to patients and their families by involving them in planning their care.

Esteem Needs

The Need for Self-esteem

Self-esteem is often referred to as self-respect, self-approval, or self-worth. Whatever the label that is used, all people need to think well of themselves. Some psychologists believe that persons need to respect themselves before they can respect others. To possess self-esteem, persons must respect what they

have done and what they can do. That is, people need to think they are all right, needed, and useful.

A person's self-esteem is dependent upon other basic needs being met. If needs such as love or security are not met satisfactorily, then the basic need of self-esteem is also threatened.

People's self-esteem is often influenced considerably by their feelings of dependence or independence. Few, if any, humans are entirely independent or completely self-sufficient, but some have stronger needs for independence than others. Dependency and independency needs vary within the same person at different stages or times in life. For example, at birth there is little choice other than to depend upon others. As growth occurs, one learns to become more independent and to balance dependency needs upon the environment and others with one's own self-directive or self-sufficient abilities.

Illness almost always alters dependency and independency needs. Even temporary limitations on the activities a person normally carries out can decrease self-respect. It often becomes the nurse's responsibility to make decisions with the patient about balancing needs for dependence and independence in order to hasten recovery. It is important to allow the person as much control of self and environment as possible to maintain self-esteem.

Changes in the body image brought about by surgery or a disease process also seriously affect a person's self-worth. For example, a patient who is paralyzed or who has had an amputation of her legs is required to change her self-concept. No longer will she appear as she did before or be able to do all the things she was accustomed to doing.

Most people have feelings of inferiority and lack self-confidence from time to time. People may react in ways that are attempts to bolster their self-esteem but that can alienate others. Criticism at this time tends to exaggerate the person's behavior. A nonreactive but accepting behavior on the part of the nurse is most helpful. Acceptance differs from approval. A person's behavior can be accepted by another person, but that does not mean that the person's behavior is approved. Although the concept of acceptance may be easy for a nurse to understand, it is not always easy to apply. For example, it is not unusual to encounter behavior from a patient that the nurse considers offensive, as when a patient uses sarcastic or obscene language. In these situations many nurses find it difficult to accept the patient and his or her behavior and not react to it. Frequently, this kind of behavior is an attempt on the part of a person to gain attention in order to meet some personal needs. The person may not be aware of the reason behind the behavior. In these instances, a nonreactive response from the nurse and an accepting attitude toward the person are required. The nurse can reply in a natural way with words such as "Your words offend me and they are not necessary; how can I help you?" From experience, nurses will find that the person's behavior frequently changes to more socially acceptable patterns.

The Need for Recognition

All people require social approval and recognition for what they achieve. In Western cultures much emphasis has been placed on a person's occupational role and on the acquisition of material possessions. For an individual this feeling of achievement may be oriented chiefly to a series of promotions or to the acquisition of more expensive houses and swimming pools. This achievement value is partly influenced by the norms of the society in which the person lives and partly by personal experiences. For example, a son who has a father who was very successful playing football may as an adult strive to make a million dollars in order to show his father he also can be successful even though he did not play football well. A feeling of achievement can also be gained in the performance of other roles, such as being a mother or working mother or being a responsible father and a family man.

In health settings nurses have many opportunities to provide recognition for patients' achievements. Even brief statements such as "It's nice to see you again" or inquiring about family members can be satisfying to some patients by recognizing them as worthwhile persons. Other patients, because of a basic lack of a sense of accomplishment, may behave in ways puzzling to a nurse in order to acquire some attention and recognition. For example, a person may refuse to carry out activities he is capable of doing such as shaving or feeding himself. Often by anticipating a person's needs and offering praise for small achievements, these behavioral symptoms usually disappear.

Spiritual Needs

The spiritual needs of humans are largely met by the system of beliefs of individuals and by religious organizations in society. From these, people find answers to such questions as "Who am I?," "Why am I here?," and "Who controls my destiny?" Spiritual needs are not entities unto themselves. Close relationships exist between them and the physical and psychologic needs of people. All these needs must be considered in understanding the person as a whole. Two major spiritual needs to be considered by nurses are the need of a person to believe and the need to hope.

The Need to Believe

Beliefs vary among different cultures and even among individuals in the same culture. However, the universal need exists for people to believe in someone or something, whether it is a supreme being (a supernatural entity) or something above and beyond oneself. Beliefs entrust faith, confidence, and reliance in the divine or godlike person or concept. Every system of beliefs evolves a set of rituals for people to follow and concepts that guide a person's behavior in order to achieve its highest goal and give life some meaning.

In health and in illness, people require acceptance by others of their own particular religious values and beliefs. It is a common practice nowadays for hospitals to include a chaplain as a member of the health team. Nurses are in a position to identify spiritual needs and should include these needs of patients in care planning. It is not uncommon for the elderly in particular to have a greater need for religion as they come to terms with what life means to them toward the end of their life span.

The Need to Hope

To hope is to long for or desire something with the expectation that it will come to fulfillment. It is closely aligned to faith and trust. Hope is future oriented, suggesting that the future will be better than the present or the past. In the health care setting, hope is a common need. People hope that their surgery will be successful, or that their recovery will be speedy, or that loved ones will not suffer unnecessary discomfort. Even when the criteria of medical science suggest a poor prognosis for a patient, the person still hopes for something better. The will to live and to recover is often associated with the need to hope. People who lack hope can delay their recovery or even die prematurely. Nurses may find themselves in a paradoxical situation at times in helping patients fulfill this need. It is an easy matter when the nurse and patient hold the same degree of hope in a situation, but when the patient is hopeful and the nurse holds the opposite viewpoint (or vice versa), the nurse must still recognize and understand the patient's need.

CHARACTERISTICS OF PEOPLE WHOSE NEEDS ARE MET

Many descriptions can be written of the characteristics of people whose basic human needs are met. If the needs are met, the person may broadly be described as having a state of physical and mental well-being or health.

Physical Well-being

A state of physical well-being encompasses fulfillment of all the previously discussed physiologic and protective needs. Lists of characteristics describing these are developed in subsequent chapters of the book. For example, how does one determine that a person is well nourished or well hydrated or physically fit? Examples of criteria that are included subsequently follow:

1. The well-hydrated person is said to have moist mucous membranes, straw-colored urine, and stable weight from day to day (see Chapter 29).
2. The well-aligned person in a standing position can be described as having toes pointed forward, head erect, and normal vertebral curves present (see Chapter 22).

Mental Well-being

There are many approaches and definitions of mental health or mental well-being. Mentally healthy people can be considered to be people who are able to meet their own essential psychologic needs and cope successfully with changes related to these needs. The feeling of mental well-being is a need of all people, although some people may be unaware of this. People who lament its lack desperately seek ways to acquire the feeling.

Mental health is frequently thought of by people as happiness, peace of mind, or satisfaction with life. Mental health is involved in every person's daily life. More specifically, it refers to how people relate and get along with other people, such as family members, neighbors, associates, and the people in the community. It also involves the manner by which a person melds ambitions, desires, abilities, ideas, and feelings in order to function effectively and meet the problems of life.

The lists of criteria for mental health or the feeling of mental well-being are numerous. Some people consider that self-actualization is the essence of mental health. The following is a summary of the major characteristics of a fully self-actualized person.*

1. Realistically oriented, a good judge of people and quickly judges them.
2. Accepts self and others and the world for what they are, not hypocritical.
3. High degree of spontaneity, natural in behavior, may appear unconventional.
4. Problem-centered, not self-centered, not very introspective.
5. Inclined to be detached, not entirely dependent upon others, can amuse self, great need for privacy at times.
6. Autonomous within self and independent, serene.
7. Fresh appreciation of people and the world, not dulled.
8. Capable of profound inner experiences, seems detached from the world sometimes.
9. Truly interested in the welfare of man.
10. Has a few special friends, highly selective in friends, easily moved by children.
11. Can relate to and learn from rich and poor, race or position not important.
12. Focuses on ends, strongly ethical and highly moral, though may differ with popular idea of right and wrong.
13. Inner motivated sense of humor, does not laugh at cruelty, sees jokes in everyday things spontaneously.
14. Tremendous capacity to be creative, fresh way of doing things.
15. Open to new experiences and resistant to conformity.

Approaches by other professionals are summarized on the following page.

*Specified material from pp. 28–29 in *Adult Psychology,* 2nd Edition by Ledford J. Bischof. Copyright ©1976 by Ledford J. Bischof. By permission of Harper & Row, Publishers, Inc.

109

Carl R. Rogers

Rogers writes about the "fully functioning person." The good life to which he refers is a process rather than a state of being. By this he means that it is constantly changing but moving in a direction selected freely by the person. Rogers' characteristics of the good life process can be summarized as:

1. Openness to new experiences.
2. Tendency to live fully in each moment. The experiences then of that moment help form future activities.
3. Trust in one's own judgments and reactions (Rogers 1961:183–196).

Marie Jahoda

Marie Jahoda suggests the following as criteria of a mentally healthy person:

1. The attitudes of persons toward themselves are positive. That is, persons are self-reliant, self-confident, and self-accepting.
2. Persons can become aware of the meanings of their actions through introspection. By this the person's behavior is accessible to the consciousness.
3. A person's self-concept is similar to that which others have of the person.
4. Persons can accept themselves.
5. Persons have a sense of identity, that is, they know who they are and at the same time have a few doubts about it.
6. Persons change and grow throughout life.

7. Persons act in a unified manner, that is, their behavior is consistent throughout their life (Jahoda 1958:82–95).

William Glasser

William Glasser (1965:5–41) states there are two needs that are fulfilled by the mentally healthy person: the need to love and be loved and the need to feel that one is worthwhile to self and to others. A person fulfills these needs by doing that which is realistic, responsible, and right. Realistic behavior is that which the person chooses by reasoning and by considering the remote as well as the immediate consequences to self and others.

Glasser defines responsibility as the ability of the person to fulfill personal needs and at the same time not deprive others of being able to fulfill their needs. In this sense a responsible person is motivated to strive and to endure privation if necessary to attain self-worth. In contrast, an irresponsible person will suffer or will cause others to suffer at some point in time. Glasser further proposes that happiness occurs most often in people who are willing to take responsibility for their own behavior.

In the same context, what is right is behavior that is compatible with a satisfactory standard of behavior. People need to consistently evaluate their behavior and act to improve it when it is below an acceptable standard. In the event a person does not do this, the person will be unable to meet his or her own needs to feel worthwhile. There are degrees of mental health, and no one person has all the characteristics of mental health all the time.

SUMMARY

When a person is in a state of homeostasis, the person is regarded as being healthy. This means that the person's basic human needs are satisfied, including both the physiologic and the psychologic needs, and that the internal environment of the body remains relatively constant. Physiologic homeostasis operates within a narrow range by sensitive regulating mechanisms. These homeostatic mechanisms contain a receptor, a circuit, and an effector organ.

There are four main characteristics of all homeostatic mechanisms. They are self-regulating, are compensatory, and are generally operated by a negative feedback system. In addition, several negative feedback systems may be required to correct one physiologic imbalance.

Three major glands (pituitary, adrenals, and parathyroids) and two body systems (respiratory and renal-cardiovascular) are largely responsible for maintaining man's physiologic homeostasis. The *adenohypophysis* secretes ACTH and TSH, which in turn regulate the adrenal cortex to produce steroids and the thyroid gland to produce thyroxin. The body's rate of metabolism is maintained by thyroxin. The *neurohypophysis*, on the other hand, is involved in maintaining the volume and concentration of body fluids through its release of ADH. The *adrenal cortex* secretes two major homeostatic hormones, the mineralocorticoids and the glucocorticoids. Aldosterone, the primary mineralocorticoid, causes sodium retention, thereby maintaining the body's total quantity of sodium and other electrolytes. Hydrocortisone, the primary glucocorticoid, is involved in regulating the body's fat protein and glucose metabolism. The *parathyroid glands* and PTH are essential in maintaining the body's calcium and phosphorous levels. The importance of the respiratory system and renal-cardiovascular systems in maintaining homeostasis are more obvious. The regulation of oxygen for metabolism, the transportation of all nutrients to the cells, and adequate elimination of metabolic by-products by the lungs and the kidneys are vital in maintaining homeostasis.

Psychologic homeostasis is equally important in maintaining a person's mental health. The psychologic homeostatic mechanisms referred to as mental mechanisms are learned through life experiences and interactions with others. Prerequisites for the development of psychologic homeostasis include a safe and secure physical environment, a trusting and loving psychologic environment, a social environment that provides healthy adult role models, and sufficiently satisfying life experiences.

Satisfaction of specific basic human needs is essential for people to maintain homeostasis and their optimal levels of well-being. The hierarchy of human needs developed by Abraham Maslow is widely recognized and with Kalish's adaptation can be useful for nurses. Six categories of needs are outlined in this chapter. The first category, physiologic needs, includes oxygen, water, food, elimination, rest and sleep, avoidance of pain, exercise, and temperature regulation. All of these needs with the exception of exercise are basic to survival. Second, the stimulation needs of activity, exploration, novelty, and change are necessary to achieve optimal growth and development and curiosity. Third, the protection needs of safety and security emerge. These have physiologic and psychologic components. Love and belonging needs, which include sex and intimacy needs, are the fourth category. Satisfaction of these needs provides the basis for fulfillment of higher needs such as esteem needs, the fifth category, and finally the development of a self-actualized personality. The spiritual needs of believing and hope were included as a separate category, since they tend to become prominent in times of stress or illness.

Although categorization of needs is suggested, people often meet their own needs relative to their own priorities. Other characteristics of needs are also recognized. One of these is that all needs are interre-

lated. Another is that individuals choose a variety of ways to meet their needs, modifying them in accordance with their culture or unique idiosyncrasies. Failure to meet needs, however, results in homeostatic imbalances and eventually illness. A major function of the nurse is to assist people who are healthy or ill to meet their basic needs. In times of illness the satisfaction of some needs is deferred temporarily, and a priority of needs has to be determined with the patient when possible in view of the illness situation.

Few people achieve self-actualization. However, optimal mental well-being can be attained. Characteristics of the self-actualized person and of mentally healthy persons are included as a guide for consideration. Generally when one is mentally healthy, one feels comfortable about oneself, feels right about other people, and is able to meet the demands that life presents.

SUGGESTED ACTIVITIES

1. Select one or two basic human needs from each category discussed in this chapter and determine how well one of your patients is succeeding in fulfilling these needs or getting assistance to do so. Include whether the patient is required to alter his or her ways of meeting these needs.

2. Compare the various descriptions of mental well-being and determine in a group discussion with other students which criteria you find helpful in assessing mental health.

3. Consider patients who might require particular help meeting stimulation and security needs, and ways in which the nurse can assist them.

SUGGESTED READINGS

Byrne, Marjorie L., and Thompson, Lida F. 1972. *Key concepts for the study and practice of nursing.* St. Louis: The C. V. Mosby Co., pp 9–13.

Humans as a set of human needs are discussed within the broader context of people and behavior. A classification of needs is suggested.

Langley, L. L. 1965. *Homeostasis.* New York: Reinhold Book Corp.

This book provides an in-depth discussion of the concept of homeostasis. A historical perspective, general principles, and the specific homeostatic processes of body temperature, body weight, blood pressure, respiration, body fluid, hormones, and movement are included.

SELECTED REFERENCES

Bischof, Ledford J. 1976. *Adult psychology,* 2nd ed. New York: Harper and Row.

Caprio, Frank S. 1965. *The power of sex.* New York: The Citadel Press.

Chodil, Judith, and Williams, Barbara. 1973. The concept of sensory deprivation. In Auld, Margaret E., and Birum, Linda Hulthen. *The challenge of nursing: a book of readings.* St. Louis: The C. V. Mosby Co.

Glasser, William. 1965. *Reality therapy.* New York: Harper and Row.

Guyton, Aurthur C. 1976. *Textbook of medical physiology,* 5th ed. Philadelphia: W. B. Saunders Co.

Hurlock, Elizabeth B. 1968. *Developmental psychology,* 3rd ed. New York: McGraw-Hill Book Co.

Jacob, Stanley W., Francone, Clarice Ashworth, and Lossow, Walter J. 1978. *Structure and function in man,* 4th ed. Philadelphia: W. B. Saunders Co.

Jahoda, Marie. 1958. *Current concepts of positive mental health.* New York: Basic Books, Inc.

Kalish, Richard A. 1977. *The psychology of human behavior,* 4th ed. Belmont, California: Wadsworth Publishing Company, Inc.

Maslow, Abraham H. 1968. *Toward a psychology of being,* 2nd ed. New York: Van Nostrand Reinhold Co.

Maslow, Abraham, H. 1970. *Motivation and personality,* 2nd ed. New York: Harper and Row.

Montague, Ashley. 1975. A scientist looks at love. In Montague, Ashley, ed. *The practice of love.* Englewood Cliffs, N.J.: Prentice-Hall, Inc.

Morgan, Arthur James, and Moreno, Judith Wilson. 1973. *The practice of mental health nursing.* Philadelphia: J. B. Lippincott Co.

Rogers, Carl R. 1961. *On becoming a person: a therapist's view of psychotherapy.* Boston: Houghton Mifflin Co.

Selye, Hans, 1956. *The stress of life.* New York: McGraw-Hill Book Co.

Selye, Hans. 1974. *Stress without distress.* Philadelphia: J. B. Lippincott Co.

CHAPTER 8

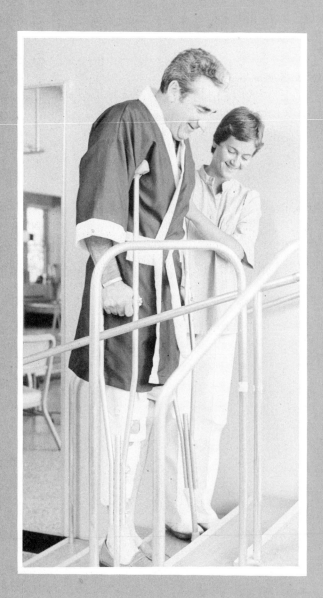

STRESS AND ADAPTATION

PHYSIOLOGIC ADAPTATION

The Endocrine Adaptive Response

The Neurologic Adaptive Response

The Inflammatory Adaptive Response

The Immunologic Adaptive Response

PSYCHOLOGIC ADAPTATION

Mental Defense Mechanisms (Adaptive Coping Processes)

ASSISTING PEOPLE TO ADAPT TO STRESS

CRISIS

Types of Crises

Crisis Intervention

OBJECTIVES

- Discuss the concept of stress and how the body responds to stress according to Selye's adaptation syndromes.

- Describe four variables influencing the degree to which stressors can affect individuals, and provide examples for each.

- Identify and explain the physiologic and psychologic signs and symptoms of stress.

- Describe four physiologic adaptive mechanisms of the body: neurologic, endocrine, inflammatory, and immune.

- Describe five types of inflammatory exudates and give common examples of where they occur in the body.

- Differentiate between the healing processes of regeneration and of replacement with fibrous tissue formation.

- List and explain the factors that promote tissue healing.

- Differentiate between natural and acquired types of immunity.

- Describe the four divisions of acquired immunity, including antigen-antibody sources and the duration of immunity.

- Identify the purposes of mental mechanisms and describe them.

- Describe ways that can assist a person to adapt to stress.

- Discuss the concept of crisis.

In recent years stress has become a household word. Parents refer to the stress of raising children, working people to the stress of their jobs. In fact, the 1970s have been described as the decade of stress. Familiarity with the word *stress* is largely due to the publications of Hans Selye. His books, such as *The Stress of Life*, are widely read by the public.

The concept of stress is important because it provides a way of understanding the person as a unified being who responds in totality (mind and body) to a variety of changes that may take place in daily life. Stress is a universal phenomenon. All people experience stress.

Recall that homeostasis refers to conditions of the body that constantly vary and yet maintain constant stability. As the person encounters any stress, various systems of the body are brought into play in order to adjust and maintain homeostasis.

Adaptation means adjustment. In the sense that it is used in this chapter, it refers to adjustment to stress. People adapt on a number of levels, physiologically, mentally, and emotionally. Each of these concepts, stress and adaptation, is further discussed in this chapter.

STRESS

Definition

Stress was defined by Selye as "the state manifested by a specific syndrome which consists of non-specifically induced changes within the biologic system" (1956:54). Selye had made a number of observations about disease, which resulted in the above definition. First he noted that, although there were characteristic or different signs and symptoms of numerous diseases, they all had many signs and symptoms in common (there was a specific syndrome). Also, there was no common cause (they were nonspecifically induced). Stressors that usually result in illness were described on pages 51 to 53. A *stressor* is any factor that produces stress; that is, it is a factor that disturbs the body's equilibrium.

Because stress is a state of the body, it can only be observed by the changes in the body that it produces. This response of the body is specific; that is, there are common and definite signs and symptoms, such as pain, fever, and loss of appetite. Selye further concluded that these common symptoms, or stress, are a part of every disease process.

Body Response to Stress

The response of the body to stress Selye referred to as the stress syndrome or *general adaptation syndrome* (GAS). This is a general response of the body, created by the release of certain adaptive hormones within the person's body (see "Physiologic Adaptation, The Endocrine Adaptive Response"). The GAS, Selye found, occurred whenever an organism underwent prolonged stress. Body organs affected by stress are the gastrointestinal tract, the adrenals, and the thymus. In addition to a general adaptation syndrome, that is, generalized manifestations of stress, it was also proposed that the body can react by a local response. One organ or a part of the body can react alone. This is referred to as the *local adaptation syndrome*, or LAS. One example of the LAS is inflammation (see "Physiologic Adaptation, The Inflammatory Adaptive Response").

A state of stress is necessary for life; without it a person would not exist. Stress is necessary for both life and growth; that is, it is necessary for the human body constantly to adapt to its environment in order to survive. The state of stress, however, is intensified when a person is required to change activity or to increase the pace of activity in order to adapt. This process of adapting is frequently referred to as *coping*.

Stages of GAS and LAS

Selye proposed that both the GAS and LAS had three stages (1956:31): (a) the alarm reaction, (b) the stage of resistance, and (c) the stage of exhaustion.

The Alarm Reaction

This is the initial reaction of the body, the body's defenses against the stressor, which might be heat, bacteria, or a verbal or physical attack from someone. The defenses of the whole body are mobilized and prepared to act in order to protect the body. This stage Selye divided into two parts: the shock phase and the countershock phase.

During *the shock phase*, the stressor may be perceived consciously or unconsciously by the person. In any case the autonomic nervous system reacts, and large amounts of adrenalin and cortisone are released into the body's system. The person is then ready for fight-or-flight. This primary response is short lived, lasting from one minute to 24 hours.

The second part of the alarm reaction is called *the countershock phase.* During this time the body changes produced during the shock phase are reversed. It is therefore during the shock phase of the alarm reaction that a patient is best mobilized to react.

The Stage of Resistance

During this second stage in the GAS and LAS syndromes the body's adaptation takes place. It is during this stage that the body attempts to cope with the stressor. Attempts are made to limit the stressor to the smallest area of the body that can deal with it. See pages 123 to 126.

The Stage of Exhaustion

During this stage the adaptation that the body made during the second stage cannot be maintained. This means that the ways used to cope with the stressor become exhausted. As a consequence, the stress effects may spread to the entire body. At the end of this stage the body may either rest and then return to normal, or death may be the ultimate consequence. The choice of the end of this stage will depend largely upon the adaptive energy resources of the individual, the severity of the stressor, and whatever external adaptive resources, such as blood, are provided (see Figure 8–1).

The reaction to stress described by Hans Selye referred particularly to the physiologic process of the body in reaction to acute stressors. However, in long-term stress, the psychologic as well as physiologic reactions of a person to stress are of concern. Adaptive reactions of humans may be ineffective, that is, maladaptive. The total person and the person's life situation could have a negative influence upon the choice

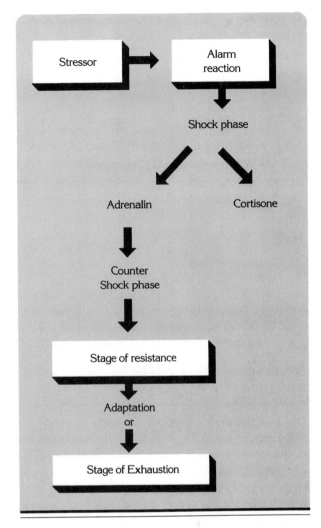

Figure 8-1.   The three stages of adaptation to stress: the alarm reaction, the stage of resistance, and the stage of exhaustion.

of the adaptive channel to take. For example, a businessman might take a highly competitive position in a company because of the money and status it brings, although he is personally unsuited to a competitive situation.

STRESSORS

Stressors are found in the internal environment (within the body) and in the external environment (outside the body). An example of a stressor within the body would be a tumor of the stomach; an example of a stressor outside the body would be an angry remark from a friend.

Stressors can also be both physiologic and psychologic. Examples of physiologic stressors would be a knife wound, an overdose of heroin, or the influenza virus. Psychologic stressors include an alcoholic spouse, fear of an operation, or grief over the death of a loved one.

The degree to which stressors affect individuals is dependent on:

1. Nature of the stressor.
2. Number of stressors to be coped with at one time.
3. Duration of exposure to the stressor.
4. Past experiences with a comparable stressor (Byrne 1972:48).

Nature of the Stressor

The nature of the stressor has two components: (a) what the stressor means to the person, and (b) the magnitude of the stressor.

To one person, an inoculation with smallpox vaccine produces a high state of stress, but for another, the injection is not a stressor. The second component, the magnitude of the stressor, also affects the person's response. The pain from a cut on a finger may elicit little stress, whereas the pain of an inflamed appendix may produce a much greater state of stress.

Number of Stressors to be Coped with at One Time

The number of stressors one is coping with at one time can greatly affect one's response. This often explains why a stressor that the nurse considers to be small can elicit a disproportionate response. For example, a patient in the hospital who is coping with separation from her family, the unknown in regard to the outcome of her illness, and financial problems, can react angrily when the nurse brings her the wrong fruit juice. Normally, this woman would not care which juice she was served; however, she is using up her energies on the aforementioned problems and has little left to cope with this incident. This is also a good example of how a state of high stress can become a stressor itself. A patient reacts angrily and feels more stress because of this reaction. Another example would be a student who is highly anxious

(stressed) about an examination. This student then gets a cold, an illness he rarely has and would not likely have acquired if he had not been in such a state of stress.

Duration of Exposure to the Stressor

Duration of exposure to the stressor can also affect a person's reaction. A person's resistance to a stressor is low during the stage of alarm, higher during the resistance stage, when the coping mechanisms are brought into action, and then drops below normal during the stage of exhaustion. Therefore, if one's stage of resistance is extended beyond one's coping powers by the duration of the stressor, one becomes exhausted and can eventually die. An example of this would be a patient who is admitted to hospital with a fractured femur. The patient survives the surgery and is healing well when he develops an acute pain in his gallbladder, necessitating another operation. By this time this particular patient's energy reserves have been used up, and, although the operation was successful, the patient develops an infection, which delays his return home.

Past Experience with a Comparable Stressor

Past experiences of a person with a comparable stressor can be particularly significant for patients entering a hospital. For some people, their only contact with hospitals has been related to dying friends and relatives. To such patients the act of entering the hospital is particularly stressful, as they worry about whether they will die. The patients' worries in this case are completely unrelated to the reason for admission.

See Table 8–1 for ratings or units applied to changes in life situations. The degree of stress a person experiences can be determined to some extent by the readjustment required for certain situations or life events.

SIGNS OF INCREASED STRESS

A person who is experiencing an increased state of stress brought on by any stressor exhibits certain signs and symptons. These stressors can be of a physiologic or a psychologic nature. Regardless of which kind of stressor is affecting the body, it responds in similar ways.

Physiologic Signs and Symptoms

1. Pupils dilate for serious threats to the body to increase visual perception.
2. Sweat production (diaphoresis) is increased to control elevated body heat due to increased metabolism.

Table 8-1   Stress Units for Life Events*

Family constellation	Mean value	Individual changes	Mean value
Death of spouse	100	Jail term	63
Divorce	73	Personal injury or illness	53
Separation	65	Death of a close friend	37
Death of close family member	63	Outstanding personal achievement	28
Marriage	50	Revision of personal habits	24
Marital reconciliation	45	Minor violation of the law	11
Change in family member's health	44	**Employment and/or school**	**Mean value**
Pregnancy	40		
Gain new member to family	39	Fired at work	47
Sexual difficulties	39	Retirement	45
Arguments with spouse	35	Business readjustment	39
Children leaving home	29	Change in job	36
Trouble with in-laws	29	Change in work responsibility (promotion	29
Change in living conditions	25	or demotion)	
Move or change in residence	20	Spouse begins or stops work	26
Change in schools, recreation, and church	20	Begin or end school	26
activities		Trouble with boss	23
Change in social activities	19	**Financial**	**Mean value**
Change in sleeping habits	16		
Change in number of family get-togethers	15	Change in financial status	38
Change in eating habits	15	Mortgage or loan over $10,000	31
Vacation	13	Foreclosure	30
Holidays	12	Mortgage or loan under $10,000	17

Suggested Score Interpretation

150–199	Mild stress. Thirty-seven percent of the population will become ill.
200–299	Medium stress. Fifty-one percent of the population will become ill in two weeks.
300 and over	High stress. Seventy-nine percent of the population will become physically ill soon.

*Burgess, Ann Wolbert, and Lazare, Aaron. 1976. *Community mental health: target populations*. Englewood Cliffs, New Jersey: Prentice-Hall, Inc., p. 59. © 1976. Reprinted by permission of Prentice-Hall, Inc.

3. The heart rate increases, which leads to an increased pulse rate to transport nutrients and by-products of metabolism more efficiently.

4. Skin is pallid due to constriction of peripheral blood vessels, an effect of norepinephrine.

5. Blood pressure is elevated due to the constriction of blood flow to the brain and muscles.

6. The rate and depth of respirations are increased. Adrenalin dilates the bronchioles, assisting hyperventilation.

7. Urinary output is either frequent or decreased. The former is thought to be an automatic nervous response, whereas the latter may be due to the antidiuretic hormone.

8. The mouth may be dry.

9. Peristalsis of the intestines is decreased, resulting in possible constipation and flatus.

10. Mental alertness is improved for serious threats.

11. Muscle tension is increased to prepare for rapid motor activity or defense.

Behavioral (Psychologic) Signs and Symptoms

The key to the response of a person behaviorally (psychologically) is the perception of the individual. If a person perceives (a) that an event is harmful or potentially harmful and (b) that the person's skills to cope with the event are inadequate, then stress is experienced.

The psychologic responses to stress that are manifested clinically are:

1. Reduced intellectual processes.
2. Increased self-sensitivity.
3. Decreased ability to cope with or master tasks.
4. Decreased sense of personal effectiveness.

Each of these can be observed by the nurse. It should be remembered, however, that each person has different ways of responding and may manifest only one or more of the above in a pronounced way.

Reduced Intellectual Processes

Several alterations in mental processes of the stressed individual have been noted. They can be summarized as (a) decreased ability to use or remember incoming information, (b) reduced ability to think clearly, and (c) difficulty in making decisions. These responses are familiar to all of us. Most people can readily recall their responses to the stress of driving in a busy six-lane freeway. The stress of getting into the appropriate lane for an exit absorbs one's thoughts. Any other information offered at that time such as a companion's joke or a comment about the surrounding scenery will not be appreciated or used. The same holds true for a student in a sociology class studying for a microbiology exam scheduled for the next period. If the teacher asks the student to answer a question at this time, the response is likely to be "Would you please repeat the question?" or "I don't know the answer" or an acknowledgment that the student wasn't listening. Because of this reduced ability to use incoming information, some health agencies provide simple, direct statements for patients in written form. Common examples are the provisions of written information about diagnostic tests, expectations in preparation for surgery, or services provided by the hospital or health agency.

Decision making and the ability to think clearly are also difficult for stressed individuals. Nurses will frequently encounter this with patients. Some may have difficulty deciding what to eat for dinner or how to deal with an alcoholic partner. Others may question whether to keep a newborn out of wedlock, or delay needed surgery or an annual medical examination.

Increased Self-sensitivity

Stress causes an increase in one's sensitivity to self, both physically and psychologically. The simple act of blushing is a common example. One manifestation the nurse may note can be a person's preoccupation with body functions such as headache or constipation. The latter is often of particular concern to elderly patients. When one's sense of self is heightened, one's perception of the environment is reduced and may even be distorted. This can be seen in situations when a patient may express feelings of being talked about when a group of doctors or nurses is seen conferring in the nursing station, or when a patient feels neglected about being the last one in a room to receive care by the nurse.

Minor events that would normally be accepted by a person become magnified and out of proportion to the stressed person. Events such as an open window, a medication ten minutes late, or apple juice for breakfast when orange juice was ordered can produce stress responses of tears, anger, and annoyance. It must be remembered that, because behavior is extremely complex, the above are only examples. Responses are highly individualized and must be considered as such. Only by analyzing each situation precisely can the specific reasons for responses be understood.

Decreased Ability to Cope with Responsibilities or Master Tasks

Stress also alters one's ability to mobilize one's own resources necessary to cope with responsibilities or to master new tasks. Some of the first responsibilities that are frequently set aside by stressed individuals are social obligations. For example, the student who is moving from home to an apartment and who has several assignments to complete, an examination forthcoming, plus boyfriend or girlfriend problems may well not be able to contend with cooking, cleaning, shopping, and visiting friends in the usual manner. On the other hand, if social obligations have priority, then the assignment suffers or the examination is poorly written.

The perceived decrease in the ability to master tasks is related to some degree to the reduced mental processes already discussed. People having difficulty learning new tasks confront the nurse frequently. For example, the diabetic patient may be too stressed to cope with the task of injecting her own insulin or the colostomy patient with caring for his own colostomy. It is important to realize that increasing expectations beyond that which a person feels capable of doing will only increase the problem and may well result in failure to achieve the task.

Decreased Sense of Personal Effectiveness

Closely aligned to the difficulties in achieving tasks may be feelings of worthlessness, incompetence, helplessness, bewilderment, or loss. All of these feelings suggest that one regards oneself as ineffective. As a result, often one's relationship with others deteriorates and family ties become strained. Examples are (a) the young, active mother with anemia who feels tired and irritable and unable to take care of her three preschool children, or (b) the young executive who is barely coping with her work role but who feels a total failure in her mother and wife roles.

PHYSIOLOGIC ADAPTATION

Adaptation, for human beings, refers to the whole range of protective adjustments in response to stressors. There are two interrelated levels of adaptation, physiologic and psychologic. Physiologic adaptation refers to changes of the body. Physiologic stressors either change or threaten to change the physiologic balance of the body.

There are a large number of physiologic responses of the human body to stressors. The major adaptation mechanisms are discussed here; others are integrated throughout the chapters of the book. The most common mechanisms are:

1. the endocrine adaptive response
2. the neurologic adaptive response
3. the inflammatory adaptive response
4. the immunologic adaptive response

The Endocrine Adaptive Response

The endocrine system consists of a series of glands located in different parts of the body. Endocrine glands secrete chemical substances called *hormones.* Some hormones can be classified as *local hormones,* that is, they stimulate cells near the endocrine gland itself. Examples are histamine and the gastrointestinal hormones. The other group of hormones are considered *general hormones.* They are secreted directly into the blood stream and circulated through the body, consequently affecting cells and organs throughout the body. Although each hormone has specific functions, in general, hormones have the following functions:

1. Regulation of the secretion of other hormones.
2. Regulation of cellular metabolism.
3. Regulation of fluid and electrolytes in the body.
4. Regulation of tissue growth.
5. Regulation of the sexual function and sexual attributes in both males and females.

The stress syndrome of the GAS, according to Selye, relies largely upon two coordinating systems, the endocrine and the nervous. Both systems have balancing forces, those which are prodefensive and those which are antidefensive. In the former, the body responses attack the stressor; in the latter, the body responses retreat from the stressor. Specific regulators are the brain, nerves, pituitary, thyroid, adrenals, liver, kidney, blood vessels, connective tissue cells, and white blood cells (Selye 1956:113). The endocrine response involves primarily the pituitary and the adrenal glands. When the alarm signal announcing a stressor reaches the pituitary gland from the hypothalamus, three hormones are released from the adenohypophysis (anterior pituitary gland): adrenocorticotropin (ACTH), thyrotropin (TTH), and somatotropin (STH).

ACTH stimulates the adrenal cortex to produce substances that Selye refers to as *anti-inflammatory corticoids* (A-C). The commonly known A-C is cortisone, which has been used effectively for patients with rheumatoid arthritis and other inflammatory conditions. Cortisone is also referred to as a glucocorticoid, since it elevates the blood sugar (glucose) level.

Several changes are brought about in the body by the A-Cs, particularly in the stages of alarm and exhaustion. During the stage of resistance, corticoid activity falls. The LAS replaces the body's generalized reaction. Some changes produced by the A-Cs are as follows:

1. White blood cells (eosinophils and lymphoid cells) are destroyed. Thus allergic and immune responses are inhibited.
2. Minute arteries of the kidneys are constricted, which increases the secretion of renal pressor substances. This results in generalized constriction of blood vessels throughout the body and an elevated blood pressure.
3. Inflammation in connective tissue is inhibited.
4. The adrenal cortex enlarges and increases in activity.
5. The thymus gland atrophies (shrinks) as well as other lymphatic structures such as the spleen and lymph nodes.

6. Gastrointestinal ulcers develop, particularly in the stomach and duodenum.

During stress, TTH is also significant. It stimulates the thyroid gland to secrete thyroxin. Thus the metabolism of all body organs is accelerated to meet the increased demands of stress. The function of the third anterior pituitary hormone, STH, is less understood. It is believed that STH either stimulates *proinflammatory corticoid* (P-C) production by the adrenal cortex or that it assists the P-Cs to stimulate inflammation at the local site. The proinflammatory corticoids are the mineralocorticoids, which conserve sodium in the body and excrete potassium. Aldosterone is an example.

Selye believes that the proportion between A-Cs and P-Cs is normally maintained in balance. During periods of stress, however, the A-Cs tend to predominate under the influence of ACTH (Selye 1956:107). The important issue is that the body's resistance and hormonal adaptation to stressors is a three-part mechanism consisting of a balance of three factors:

1. The direct effect of the stressor on the body.
2. The physiologic responses that stimulate defense by the tissues, that is, the proinflammatory corticoids.
3. The physiologic responses that inhibit defense by the tissues, that is, the anti-inflammatory corticoids.

The effects of these adaptive hormones can be modified by other factors such as adrenalin, diet, or heredity. When corticoid production becomes excessive or insufficient, various diseases of adaptation develop. Examples of disease due to excessive proinflammatory hormones are arthritis, allergy, and asthma.

The posterior pituitary gland (neurohypophysis) is also activated during stress. Antidiuretic hormone (ADH) stimulates the kidneys to retain fluid for the body. This mechanism is important when the body fluids, particularly in the intravascular compartment, are depleted in situations such as dehydration or hemorrhage. Oxytoxic hormone (oxytocin) is also released by the neurohypophysis. This substance causes the uterus to contract and is specifically required for the stress of birth (see Figure 8–2).

The Neurologic Adaptive Response

The second system involved in the body's adaptation to stress is the autonomic nervous system. This system has two divisions, (a) the parasympathetic nervous system and (b) the sympathetic nervous system.

In most instances the two divisions innervate the same organs. The parasympathetic system can stimulate one organ at a time, whereas the sympathetic system usually stimulates (innervates) all organs at once. Daily activities of a person usually require parasympathetic stimulation of single organs for adjustment. When extra activity is required, in instances such as a quick departure, the sympathetic nervous system comes into action, causing widespread stimulation of body organs.

Both aspects of the autonomic nervous system operate involuntarily and control many of the internal functions of the body, such as the heart and respiratory rates. The autonomic nervous system is stimulated by the cerebral cortex. There are a number of discrete centers, particularly in the prefrontal lobes and temporal regions of the cortex, that excite the autonomic nervous system through the hypothalamus. Some stimulation of the cortical centers can result from external sensory input to the cerebrum. Seeing a car accident or placing one's hand on a hot stove are examples. Other stimulation can originate in the cerebrum itself from such intellectual activity as thinking about a forthcoming date. In either case the stimulation is transmitted to centers in the hypothalamus, the pons, or the mesencephalon. From one of these centers stimuli then travel through nerves to the adrenal medulla, the central portion of the adrenal gland. Recall that stressors at the same time are stimulating the endocrine system by way of the pituitary gland and the adrenal cortex.

The adrenal medulla is stimulated to secrete the *adrenalins* (nerve hormones), epinephrine and norepinephrine. These hormones are secreted into the circulating blood stream and are distributed to all parts of the body. They have almost the same action as direct sympathetic stimulation. The effects of the adrenalins are often referred to as the fight-or-flight response.

The physiologic responses of the adrenalins are frequently observed by the nurse in clinical situations. Pain, a common stressor in patients, can often be assessed by the autonomic nervous system responses. Patients will have beads of perspiration on their foreheads and appear pale. Increased muscle tension may be noted by patients pacing the floor, clenching their fists, or by facial grimacing. Increased vital signs, particularly hyperventilation, may also be noted.

The antagonist of the adrenalins is *acetylcholine.* This hormone is secreted only at nerve endings rather than through the general circulation. An example of the opposing effects of the adrenalins and acetylcholine is seen in localized inflamed areas.

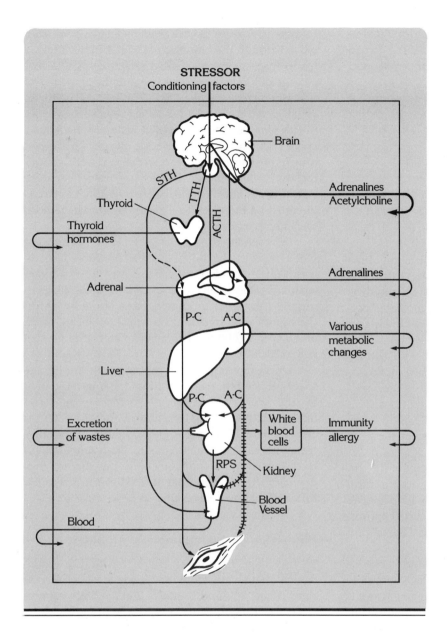

STRESSOR
Conditioning factors

Brain

STH

TTH

ACTH

Thyroid

Thyroid hormones

Adrenalines
Acetylcholine

Adrenal

Adrenalines

P-C   A-C

Various metabolic changes

Liver

P-C   A-C

Excretion of wastes

White blood cells

Immunity allergy

RPS

Kidney

Blood Vessel

Blood

Figure 8-2. The endocrine adaptive response. (From *The Stress of Life*, revised edition, by Hans Selye. Copyright © 1976 by Hans Selye. Used with permission of McGraw-Hill Book Company.)

Acetylcholine assists the inflammatory process by dilating the blood vessels, whereas the adrenalins inhibit inflammation by producing vasoconstriction.

The Inflammatory Adaptive Response

Inflammation is the response of the tissues of the body to injury. It is an adaptive mechanism invoked to destroy or dilute the injurious agent, to prevent further spread of the injury, and to promote repair of damaged tissue. It is characterized by the five signs of pain, swelling, redness, heat, and impaired function of the involved part. Commonly, conditions with the suffix *-itis* refer to an inflammatory process. For example, appendicitis refers to inflammation of the appendix; gastritis refers to inflammation of the stomach. Inflammation is a local reaction and may be equated to Selye's local adaptation syndrome (LAS).

Injurious stressors (inflammants) to body tissues can be categorized as physical agents, chemical agents, and microorganisms. Physical stressors include mechanical agents causing trauma to tissues, excessive heat or cold (a burn or frostbite), and radiation. Chemical stressors include external irritants such as strong acids, alkalis, poisons, irritating gases, and internal irritants or substances manufactured within the body, such as the products of altered metabolism, for example, excessive hydrochloric acid in the stomach. Microorganisms include the broad groups of bacteria, viruses, fungi, protozoa, and rickettsia.

The inflammatory response involves a series of dynamic events or defenses of the tissues, which can be subdivided into:

1. cellular and vascular changes

2. formation of inflammatory exudate

3. repair of tissues

Cellular and Vascular Changes

In this first stage, there is initially constriction of the blood vessels at the site of injury, lasting only a few moments. This momentary response is followed by (a) dilatation of small blood vessels, (b) increased permeability of the blood vessel walls, (c) slowing of blood flow, and (d) mobilization of leukocytes.

Dilatation of small localized blood vessels occurs as a result of histamine, which is released by the injured cells. Thus much blood flows to the injured area, bringing with it large numbers of leukocytes. This marked increase in blood supply is referred to as *hyperemia* and is responsible for the characteristic signs of redness and heat.

Vascular permeability is simultaneously increased at the injured site. This is thought to occur in response to necrosin, which is released by damaged cells, and other chemical mediators called kinins, such as bradykinin. The result of this altered permeability is an outpouring of plasma and blood substances such as leukocytes, erythrocytes, and platelets into the interstitial spaces. This stage is responsible for the characteristic sign of swelling (edema) and is in part responsible for the associated pain of inflammation, since pressure is created on nerve endings. Too much fluid pouring into such areas as the pleural or pericardial cavities can seriously affect organ function. In other situations, such as fluid in a joint, mobility is impaired.

Slowing of blood flow occurs in the dilated vessels. This altered rate of flow facilitates the mobilization of leukocytes and their movement into the tissue spaces along with other substances.

Mobilization of leukocytes includes the two processes of (a) margination and (b) emigration. Normally blood cells (erythrocytes, leukocytes, and platelets) flow along the center of a blood vessel, while a cell-less stream of plasma flows around the cells against the wall of the blood vessel. When the blood flow slows, leukocytes aggregate or line up along this inner surface of the blood vessels. This

process is known as *margination*. Leukocytes then move through the blood vessel wall into the affected tissue spaces, a process called *emigration*. The actual passage of blood corpuscles through the blood vessel wall is referred to as *diapedesis*. The reason leukocytes are attracted to injured tissue has been described by the term *positive chemotaxis.* The action of chemotaxis is not fully understood, but basically, cells are drawn toward the source of chemicals released in the tissues (positive chemotaxis), or they are propelled away from the chemical (negative chemotaxis). Leukotaxine released by injured cells is thought to have positive chemotaxic properties.

In response to the exit of leukocytes from the blood vessels, the bone marrow produces and releases large numbers of leukocytes into the blood stream *(leukocytosis).* The exact mechanism stimulating this increase is unknown, but it is another cardinal sign of inflammation. A normal leukocyte count of 7,000 to 10,000 per cubic millimeter of blood can rise to 20,000 or more.

Once having gained entrance to the tissue spaces, the leukocytes then attack the injurious agent by the process of *phagocytosis.* Macrophages (reticuloendothelial cells) present in the tissue spaces also assist the leukocytes in phagocytosis. Antibodies from plasma also come to the site. Their function will be discussed in more detail later in this chapter. Suffice it to say for now that antibodies can make the inflammant more susceptible to phagocytosis.

Formation of the Inflammatory Exudate

In this stage of inflammation, the fluid and substances that escape from the blood vessels, as well as dead tissue cells and products that they release, produce the inflammatory *exudate.* A plasma protein called fibrinogen (activated by necrosin) and thromboplastin, a product released from injured tissue cells, and platelets together form an interlacing network of fibrin or a clot. This fibrin mesh or clot walls off the area in an attempt to localize the inflammation. It also provides the framework for the reparative stage.

Types of Exudate

The nature and amount of exudate vary in accordance with the tissue involved and the intensity and duration of the inflammation. The major types of exudate are categorized as serous, catarrhal, purulent, fibrinous, and hemorrhagic.

A *serous exudate* is comprised chiefly of serum derived from the blood and serous membranes of the body, such as the peritoneum, pleura, pericardium, and meninges. It is watery in appearance and has few cells and little or no fibrin. An example is the fluid in a blister from a burn.

Catarrhal is a term used to describe the inflammatory discharge of mucous membranes such as the nasopharynx or intestines. A well-known example is the common cold. The exudate is similar in appearance to serous exudate except for the presence of mucus.

The *purulent exudate* is a thicker fluid than the serous exudate due to the presence of pus. It consists of leukocytes, liquefied dead tissue debris, and dead and living bacteria. The process of pus formation is referred to as *suppuration,* and bacteria producing pus are called pyogenic bacteria. Examples are the exudates of a boil and an abscess. Purulent exudates can differ in color, some acquiring tinges of green or yellow. The colors depend to some degree upon the specific causative organism. Formation of pus takes time, so this exudate is not seen in the acute stage of infections. Other inflammatory agents, such as turpentine in subcutaneous tissues, can also support pus formation. Nurses need to be specific about color and consistency when recording the presence of purulent exudates.

A *fibrinous exudate,* as the name denotes, contains large amounts of fibrin. Fibrin is produced when large amounts of the plasma protein fibrinogen combine with the thromboplastin of injured cells and blood platelets. This type of exudate occurs in severe acute inflammations, indicating sufficient permeability and damage to capillaries to allow the escape of the large protein molecule. Excessive amounts of fibrin may form sticky membranous coatings on tissue surfaces, causing them to adhere. This is the beginning of the formation of adhesions, which most frequently develop on serous surfaces of the pleura and peritoneal membranes of the intestines.

Another term for *hemorrhagic exudate* is *sanguineous exudate.* It consists of large amounts of red blood cells, thus indicating damage to capillaries that is severe enough to allow the escape of red blood cells from plasma. This type of exudate is frequently seen with surgical incisions, bruises, or open wounds. Nurses often need to distinguish whether the sanguineous exudate is dark or bright. For example, a bright sanguineous exudate from a surgical incision indicates fresh bleeding and trauma, whereas dark sanguineous exudate can denote smaller and older trauma.

In many instances the nurse will observe *mixed* types of exudates. For example, a mucopurulent exudate can occur from the upper respiratory tract, and this indicates the presence of excessive mucus and

pus. A serosanguineous exudate is also commonly seen with surgical incisions and denotes serous and sanguineous exudate.

Repair of Tissues: The Healing Process

The reparative phase begins when the injurious agent has been overcome and the debris cleared away by lymphatic drainage. Injured tissues can be repaired by (a) regeneration or (b) replacement with fibrous tissue (scar) formation.

Regeneration is the replacement of destroyed tissue cells by cells that are identical or similar in structure and function. It involves not only replacement of damaged cells one by one, but also organization of these cells so that the architectural pattern of the tissue and function is restored.

The *stroma* is the tissue which forms the framework (connective tissue) or ground substance of an organ. The *parenchyma* is the essential functional elements of an organ. Functional cells must have proper relationships between stroma and parenchyma, and between the blood vessels, lymph vessels, nerves, and ducts. All must take place concurrently. If one component lags behind the other, a normal product will not be formed. The villain, fibrous (scar) tissue, frequently wins, since it has the capacity to proliferate under the unusual conditions of ischemia and altered pH.

The ability to reproduce cells varies considerably from one type of tissue to another. For example, epithelial tissues of the skin and of the digestive and respiratory tracts have a good regenerative capacity, provided that their underlying support structures are intact. The same holds true for osseous, lymphoid, and bone marrow tissues. Tissues that have little regenerative capacity include nervous, muscular, and elastic tissues. These are highly specialized tissues that cannot be replaced by identically organized cells, but rather are replaced by scar tissue. Unfortunate examples are the damage to the brain in a stroke victim or the damage to the heart muscle in a cardiac patient. These tissues cannot be replaced.

When regeneration is not possible, repair occurs by *fibrous tissue substitution.* The inflammatory exudate with its interlacing network of fibrin provides the framework for this tissue to develop. Damaged tissues are replaced with the connective tissue elements of collagen, blood capillaries, lymphatics, and other tissue ground substances. In the early stages of this process the tissue is called *granulation tissue.* It is a fragile, gelatinous-like tissue, appearing pink or red because of the many newly formed capillaries. Later in the process when the tissue shrinks (the capillaries are constricted, even obliterated) and collagen fibers contract, a more firm, fibrous tissue remains. This tissue is called a *cicatrix* or scar.

Although scar tissue has the positive attribute of repairing the injured area, it also can present some problems. It can reduce the functional capacity of the involved tissue or organ. For example, scar tissue in cardiac muscle renders that area weaker. Mechanical obstructions can also arise, such as may occur in the healing of a duodenal ulcer. Sometimes the pyloric sphincter becomes stenosed in the stage of contraction of scar tissue.

Factors that Favor Tissue Healing

1.   Minimum of injury. The less the injury, both in terms of extent and time, the more rapid is the healing process. If few cells and blood vessels are damaged, for example, less time is required to replace the destroyed tissue.

2.   Adequate blood supply. Because the blood provides the needed products for healing, any factor restricting blood flow to the injured area hinders the healing process. Damaged or occluded arteries and restrictive bandages can inhibit blood flow. The presence of gross edema can also hinder the transport of substances in the tissue spaces.

3.   Good nutritional status. Protein and vitamin C are the nutrients principally involved in healing of wounds. Protein is essential for the formation of new tissue. Vitamin C is thought to be necessary for the maturation of collagen fibers in the later stages of healing.

4.   Youth. Healing is more rapid in young people than in the elderly.

5.   Absence of other stressors. The presence of infection, foreign bodies, diabetes, or other stressors can delay healing. Radiation is said to slow the healing process after five to six days.

6.   Adequate immune mechanisms. For injuries that are induced by bacteria, the presence of appropriate immune mechanisms, facilitating phagocytosis and clearing of debris in the exudative phase, will hasten the healing process.

7.   Balance of adrenocortical hormones. According to Selye, proinflammatory and anti-inflammatory hormones exist. The latter hormones are the glucocorticoids. An excess of these hormones inhibits the inflammatory process, thereby slowing the healing process. Cortisone is thought to decrease the formation of collagen fibers.

The Immunologic Adaptive Response

The immune response is a more specific response of the body than the inflammatory response. It is a response to foreign protein materials in the body, such as bacteria or tissues of another person, or, in some situations, even the body's own proteins. Foreign proteins in the body are called *antigens* and are considered as invaders. If the proteins originate in one's own body, the antigen is referred to as an *autoantigen.* Protective substances in the body that are produced to counteract antigens are called *antibodies.* Antibodies are highly specific molecules of gamma globulins produced in response to contact with antigens. Antibodies are said to be highly specific because an antibody that is formed against a particular antigen will generally react only with that antigen.

Antibodies (Immunoglobulins)

Antibodies are also referred to as *immune bodies* or *immunoglobulins.* Immunoglobulins are part of the body's serum proteins, specifically the gamma globulins. Laboratory methods (electrophoresis) have isolated five different immunoglobulins in serum. These are designated by the leters G, A, M, D, and E, and are usually written as IgG, IgA, IgM, IgD, and IgE. Each of the five has different structures and functions. Table 8–2 indicates some of these functions. IgG is the most abundant immunoglobulin, constituting about 75% of the immunoglobulins in serum. IgA and IgM constitute about 25%, and IgD and IgE comprise less than 1%.

Table 8-2   Antibodies and Their Functions

Antibody	Function
IgG	Provides antiviral, antitoxic, and some antibacterial antibodies; it is the only one to cross the placental barrier
IgA	Protects mucous membranes of gastrointestinal and respiratory tracts; found in tears, saliva, colostrum, and intestinal and bronchial secretions
IgM	Provides A, B, and O blood groups' isoantibodies and antibodies to gram-negative microorganisms
IgD	Unknown
IgE	Provides allergic and anaphylactic antibodies

Sources of Antibodies

The major cells producing antibodies are called plasma cells. They are located in lymphoid tissue. In addition, reticulum cells and lymphocytes located in the bone marrow, spleen, and liver produce small amounts of antibodies. In recent years the function of the thymus gland in the development of the immune mechanism has been discovered. The thymus gland is the original site that produces most of the antibody-forming cells.

Immunity

Immunity is the specific resistance of the body to infection (pathogens or their toxins). There are two major types of immunity, natural and acquired.

Natural immunity is that resistance which is endowed by heredity. It is inborn and ready made. This type of immunity may be considered at the individual, species, and racial levels. Some species are more resistant than others to specific pathogens. Humans, for instance, are resistant to distemper virus, a morbid ending for cats and dogs. Racial differences also exist. For example, black people have more resistance to malaria than do white people. Even at the individual level, observations indicate that some persons are more resistant to certain infections than other persons.

Acquired immunity is that which occurs only after the person has been exposed to a disease agent. It can be an active or passive process of the body (see Figure 8–3), each of which may be naturally or artificially induced. Thus there are four divisions of acquired immunity (see Table 8–3).

Active Immunity

Active immunity is that which results when one (the host) produces one's own antibodies in response to microorganisms or their toxins in the body. It takes time to develop and usually provides permanent or lifelong immunity.

In *naturally acquired immunity*, antibodies are actively produced within the body in response to an active infection such as scarlet fever or chickenpox. The infectious process may be so mild (subclinical) that it goes unrecognized by the person, yet a specific active immunity results.

Artifically acquired immunity occurs when antigens are intentionally, by artificial means, administered to the host. The body actively produces antibodies in response to this stimulus. Antigens are administered in the form of vaccines or toxoids.

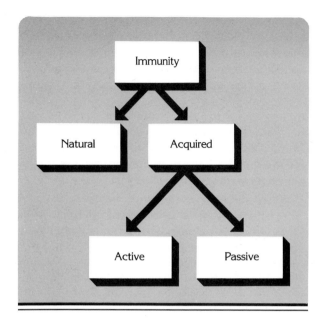

Figure 8-3.   The types of immunity.

Table 8-3   Types of Acquired Immunity

Type	Antigen or Antibody Source	Duration
Active	Antibodies are produced by the body in response to infection.	Long
a. Natural	Antibodies are formed in the presence of active infection in the body.	Lifelong
b. Artificial	Antigens (vaccines or toxoids) are administered to the person to stimulate antibody production.	Many years; must be reinforced by booster inoculation
Passive	Antibodies are produced by another source, animal or human.	Short
a. Natural	Antibodies are transferred naturally from immune mother to baby through placenta or colostrum.	6 months to 1 year
b. Artificial	Immune serum (antibody) from an animal or another human is injected.	2 to 3 weeks

Vaccines are composed of living organisms, a live vaccine, or dead organisms, referred to as killed vaccines. The use of live vaccines imitates nature's way of producing immunity. When the vaccine is administered, a very mild or subclinical infection is produced, which stimulates active antibody production. Some of these live vaccines are *attenuated* (weakened), that is, they are altered by exposure to unnatural growth conditions in order to render them less virulent. Examples of attenuated vaccines are the Sabin polio and BCG (tuberculosis) vaccines.

Dead suspensions, or killed vaccines, are produced by subjecting virulent bacteria or viruses to an excess of heat, ultraviolet light, or certain chemicals such as phenol, formaldehyde, or alcohol. The most common types of bacteria used are typhoid and whooping cough. Killed vaccines also include viruses. Two of the best-known ones are the Salk vaccine for poliomyelitis and the influenza vaccines.

In contrast to the two preceding methods, *toxoids* are also administered, which do not employ the use of microorganisms, living or dead. In some diseases the primary damage to the body is produced not by the bacteria themselves, but by the exotoxins that are produced. Examples are diphtheria and tetanus. Because these toxins are highly toxic, they are usually altered or inactivated by heat or chemicals prior to inducing immunity. The resulting product is called a toxoid, which is simply a neutralized toxin.

Active immunity that is artificially acquired is not as lasting as active immunity that is naturally acquired. After a period of time antibody levels in the serum drop. This is why booster inoculations are required. For additional information on recommended routine immunization schedules, see Tables 21–5 and 21–6.

Passive Immunity

Passive immunity is that which occurs when a person receives antibodies that have been produced in the bodies of other animals or persons. Occasionally people contract diseases, such as tetanus, diphtheria, or snake bite, that are serious and require immediate lifesaving responses in the form of ready-made antibodies. There is no time for the person to develop antibodies. This person must receive preprepared antibodies before too much damage occurs. In other situations, a person may not be ill but has been exposed to an infectious disease.

Naturally acquired passive immunity involves the diffusion of antibodies from the mother's blood across the placenta into the circulation of the unborn child. The immunoglobulins type G are small enough to pass through placental walls. Postnatally antibodies are passed to the infant in colostrum (the first milk secreted after birth). The infant's body does not participate in antibody production. It passively receives antibodies synthesized in the mother's tissues. This type of immunity is effective, but not lasting (up to one year).

Artificially acquired passive immunity is achieved when antibodies produced in other humans or animals are administered in an unnatural way. Again, since the body does not participate in the antibody production, this type of immunity is short lived (two to three weeks). Antibodies that are administered artificially are referred to as *immune sera* or *antisera*.

Common antisera are those against diphtheria, tetanus, gas gangrene, rabies, and botulism. Human gamma globulin is occasionally administered for the treatment of measles, hepatitis, and poliomyelitis.

Although the antisera used in passive immunity have the advantage of providing an immediate immune response, they have the potential disadvantage of producing *hypersensitive reactions* or allergies. Because the antisera frequently used are of animal origin and are proteins, they can act as foreign material like an antigen to a recipient. Very severe reactions can occur to foreign sera with subsequent injections. This is referred to as *anaphylactic shock*.

PSYCHOLOGIC ADAPTATION

Mental adaptive processes and behavior patterns called *mental defense mechanisms* or *coping mechanisms* are used daily by everyone as a means of adapting to life's situations. These processes and mechanisms serve to protect a person's self-esteem and sense of security. Just as the body through its biochemical and physical processes serves to maintain a physiologic equilibrium or homeostasis, the personality through automatic and unconscious processes endeavors to maintain a psychologic stability.

A healthy personality requires the development of those behavioral processes which are necessary for adapting to life. Examples of these are the communicative and problem-solving behaviors, that is, language and thought processes, which are necessary for human adaptation. These adaptive processes are acquired through learning just as are the mental mechanisms by which the personality attempts to defend itself, enhance itself, mediate conflicting drives, and allay tensions. Knowledge of these processes and mechanisms and their associated behavior patterns will help the nurse better understand the fears and anxieties of people and how he or she can best help them.

Mental Defense Mechanisms (Adaptive Coping Processes)

Mental mechanisms are acquired during the development of the personality as an attempt to defend itself, establish compromises between conflicting impulses, and allay inner tensions. A conflict can be thought of as the struggle between two parts of the personality. An example would be a girl who does not want to go to school one day in order to go to a movie and yet knows that she should go to school.

Conflict produces anxiety. *Anxiety* is a state of tension, indicating impending disaster, or a feeling of helplessness and fear in regard to future events. *Fear*, on the other hand, is an emotional response to an actual present danger. Once the danger is eliminated, the fear disappears. During development of the personality, mental mechanisms evolve to protect the person from anxiety.

Adaptive defense mechanisms are generally employed by a person unconsciously. Even though the mechanisms may seem maladaptive to the nurse, they have probably been employed in order to control anxiety and thereby maintain psychologic homeostasis. As a result, the nurse should be careful not to interfere with the mechanisms because if the patient is without them at that time, the patient's anxiety may well be immensely increased. Since emotions such as anxiety and anger are discussed in later chapters, this chapter is restricted to a description of the mental mechanisms.

Repression

Repression is one of the commonest mental mechanisms used to deal with conflicts. By repression, desires, impulses, thoughts, and strivings that conflict with the image we have of ourselves or are disturbing to us, are put out of the consciousness. They cannot be recalled or recognized, and thus we are protected from anxiety. Experiences that involve guilt, shame, or lowering of self-esteem are most apt to be repressed.

As an example, a young man was engaged to be married. His fiancee terminated the engagement; the man found this to be embarrassing and repressed the fact that his fiancee had broken the engagement and instead believed he had terminated the relationship himself. Another example is that of a patient who could not control her urine postoperatively. The patient urinated in her bed and felt ashamed and embarrassed. As a result, she completely repressed the incident so that she did not remember it upon leaving the hospital.

Identification

Identification is an important mental mechanism in the growth of an individual. A young boy will take over the attitudes and behavior patterns of both parents, especially his father, whereas a young girl will frequently adapt chiefly those of her mother. Both will also adapt the behavior and attitudes of other people who are significant to them. In identification a person admires the qualities of significant people and aspires to be like them. In the developmental context, successive identifications finally evolve into adult individuation, that is, a firm personal identity.

Identification can also be used as wish fulfilling for a person. An example would be a person who confesses falsely to a crime. This confession is generally based upon the desire of the person to commit the crime. This mechanism is also used by people with poorly organized personalities who attach themselves to other persons in whom they see desirable qualities.

In another sense, identification is projected onto another person. Again, unconsciously a person places certain traits on another person. For example, certain traits of a person might remind a nurse of a disliked relative. The other person is then quite unconsciously disliked, just as the relative is.

Empathy is a healthy form of identification. In this case, the identification is limited and temporary, but it enables one person to feel for and understand the feelings of another.

An example of identification is a teenage patient who changes her hair style so that it is like the style of a nurse whom she admires. In another example, a young boy swears just as his father swears.

Reaction Formation

Reaction formation is the behavior of a person that is the exact opposite of what the person would tend to show. For example, a person shows great concern for a person about whom she is actually hostile, or an aggressive person demands his rights continually who is really defending himself against feelings of insecurity.

Compensation

Compensation is really a substitute phenomenon. Physiologically the body frequently compensates for pathologic conditions; for example, a person with a heart valve stricture will often have a hypertrophied heart muscle. In this case, the heart tries to overcome the blockage and pump blood through the valve by increasing the size of the muscle.

In behavior, a person acts in such a manner as to compensate for some characteristic. An example is the person of short stature who shows aggressive, dominating traits. The manner this person has adopted is to suggest strength and authority, which the person's size does not convey. Extremes in this behavior are called overcompensation.

Compensating behavior can also be highly commendable socially. For example, a boy who cannot participate in athletics compensates by studying hard and attaining high grades. Another example is that of a blind person and the highly acute hearing she develops to compensate for the loss of sight.

Rationalization

Rationalization is one of the commonest mechanisms; it is designed to maintain the self-respect of a person and prevent feelings of guilt. This mechanism provides rational, intellectual reasons for behavior that really has been prompted by unrecognized motives. Allied to rationalization is the sour-grapes mechanism. In this defense persons disparage some goal, which in reality they would like to attain. For example, the student who really wanted to be class president states that she wouldn't take the job if it were offered because it is a lot of work and no fun. Another example of rationalization is the patient who comes to the hospital for an operation and states that he is really pleased to come in order to obtain a good rest.

Substitution

Substitution is a mechanism used to reduce one's tension when one is frustrated. (To be frustrated is to be blocked from attaining a goal.) In substitution, one chooses alternate goals, which are attainable and which have comparable gratification. When one is unable to attain a goal, such as being a physician, one has three choices: (a) to continue to strive for and overcome obstacles to the goal, (b) to avoid the goal or flee from it, or (c) to choose a substitute goal.

Substitution in the case of the student who wishes to be a physician might be to choose dentistry, which is an attainable goal for the student.

Displacement

Displacement is an anxiety-reducing device. In this mechanism, an emotional feeling is transferred from the actual object to a substitute. Feelings such as love and hate are apt to be displaced. For example, hostility toward a parent by a child is redirected to a teacher because it is too threatening and socially unacceptable to hate a parent. Thus the child verbalizes hostility toward this teacher, who does not produce as much anxiety.

Restitution

Restitution is a mechanism by which one relieves one's mind of guilt by restitutive (restorative) acts. For example, a boy breaks his sister's toy, then feels guilty and offers to give the sister his prize frog to make up for the broken toy.

Projection

Projection is a mechanism by which one attributes to others characteristics that one does not want to admit are one's own. That is, persons criticize others for traits that in effect the persons themselves possess. This is frequently seen in daily life, as for example, a man who criticizes his neighbor for being a terrible gossip when in fact it is the man himself who gossips but is not aware of it.

Symbolization

Symbolization is the use of objects to represent ideas or emotions that may be too painful to express. To the conscious mind of the person, the symbol is not a symbol but is real in itself. Examples might be a woman whose cat is an unconscious symbol of her child who died at birth, or a teenager who wears clothes his mother dislikes, the clothes symbolizing rebellion against his mother.

Regression

By *regression* an individual adopts behavior that was comforting earlier in life. One example is a six-year-old child who starts bedwetting after his mother returns home with a new baby. In this example, the child unconsciously returns to an earlier behavior pattern in order to obtain his mother's attention. Another example would be a patient in the hospital who becomes more dependent upon the nurse for her needs than is physically necessary. Again, the patient is returning to an earlier level of dependency, which at one time in her life was comforting.

Denial

Denial is a mechanism by which consciously intolerable thoughts, wishes, facts, and deeds are disowned by an unconscious denial of their existence. An example is a patient who is told he has cancer; he finds this to be an intolerable fact and denies it unconsciously as if he had never been told.

Sublimation

Sublimation is a mechanism by which energy inherent in unacceptable impulses is redirected into socially useful goals. The person finds outlets for the energy from the anxiety that results from these unacceptable needs and impulses. In sublimation the energy is frequently transformed to channels such as a vocation, art, music, or other endeavors that provide a richer life for the person and often the social group. Examples might be the physician who devotes all her energies to her practice, when at home she has a husband who is an alcoholic, or a man who devotes most of his time to charitable endeavors, rather than recognize his loneliness in his home.

Suppression

Suppression can be considered as the opposite of repression in that one willfully and consciously puts a thought or feeling out of one's mind. An example is

the man who forgets and misses an appointment to the dentist. He feels threatened by the event, and by refusing to think about it, he relieves his anxiety.

Introjection

Introjection is the opposite of projection, but it is also an unconscious mechanism. The character traits of another person are taken into oneself. These traits that are made part of oneself may be desirable or undesirable. Children develop a healthy conscience in this manner by taking in the advice and warnings of parents. On the other hand, feelings of hatred about a person that are turned inward can create depression and suicide.

Conversion

Conversion is the mechanism of transforming (converting) a mental conflict into a physical symptom. Shameful feelings or painful emotions are first repressed and then converted into physical symptoms such as numbness or pain. The resulting physical discomfort is often accepted by the person without much distress. Thus, in reality, one is punishing oneself.

Fantasy

Fantasy is likened to make-believe and daydreams. Wishes and desires are imagined as fulfilled. Imagination makes life more acceptable and is helpful when used to determine constructive action and thought. Past experiences can be relived, everyday problems solved, and plans for the future made. However, the person who uses fantasy to excess and who retreats from reality is using this mechanism in an unhealthy way.

ASSISTING PEOPLE TO ADAPT TO STRESS

Stress accompanies every disease and illness. It is therefore important that nurses be able not only to recognize stress but that they be able to assist people to adapt to stress.

It has already been mentioned that stress is highly individualistic; a situation that to one person is a major stressor may not affect another. The following are methods by which stress can be reduced. Some will be effective for one person, others for another. A nurse who is sensitive to a patient's needs

and reactions can choose those methods which will be most effective to a person.

1. The nurse is sensitive to specific situations and experiences that increase stress for patients.

Two examples of this might be an adult who appears highly stressed each time he receives an intramuscular injection and a child who appears frightened and highly stressed when her parents arrive at the hospital to visit her.

Often a careful remark about the stress will elicit information that the nurse or physician can use to assist the patient. In the first example, the patient's stress may be reduced by information about the injection and the technique by which it is given. Perhaps this patient was under a misconception about the content of the intramuscular syringe, the function of the drug, or the technique of administration. Specific knowledge in this case may allay his apprehension. In the second situation, that of the child, the nurse may learn, after establishing a relationship of trust with the child, that her parents mistreat her at home and that her parents neglect her because of their own needs. In this case, the nurse can convey this information to the physician, who may request the assistance of an agency in the community to investigate the conditions of the home.

2. The nurse orients the patient to the hospital or agency.

In this situation the nurse can help both the patient and family or circle of friends in their adjustments. In a hospital, the patient is assisted in the role change from that, for example, of an independent wage earner to that of a relatively dependent patient in a hospital. The family of the patient are assisted in their adjustment by knowledge of the visiting hours and of what they can do to best assist the patient.

3. The patient and family can be supported at a time of illness.

By the nurse conveying caring and understanding of their positions, the nurse can assist patients to reduce their stress. To feel that there is someone else who helps and cares is supportive to people who are stressed. Often families require time to ventilate their worries and their anxieties in order to feel assured and less stressed.

4. The patient is provided with time to ventilate his or her feelings and thoughts.

As part of the plan of care, nurses need to allow for time for patients to describe their feelings and worries if they wish. Some people find it relatively easy to describe their feelings, while others may prove hesitant to do so. The nurse needs to be sensitive to the patient's needs and neither to probe with questions nor to be too busy to listen.

5. The patient in a hospital is provided with some way of maintaining identity.

One's name and clothes are important parts of one's uniqueness as an individual. Nurses can assist patients by calling them by their correct names and by assisting them to wear their own clothes in a hospital setting when this is possible. In the community, a nurse can help patients maintain their identity also by recognizing a new shirt or recently styled hair. All of these assist people to feel they are individuals and to maintain their identities.

6. The patient is encouraged to participate in the plan of care.

One's stress is frequently reduced by the feeling that one has some input into one's own care and what is going to happen. The loss of the right to determine their own destiny can be particularly stressful to some people, particularly adults who function independently or who assume responsibility for others in their daily lives.

Both adults and children can be included in formulating plans for their medical therapy and their nursing care. Not only does this activity reduce stress, it also results in patients complying with their care and feeling they are persons of worth, which is important for their self-concept.

7. Information is repeated when the patient has difficulty remembering.

People who have a high level of stress frequently have difficulty remembering information and using the information when necessary. Nurses can assist patients by repeating information when it is requested and assisting people to apply it when they so desire. This problem is particularly true of elderly people who are stressed as a result of the change of setting as well as their illness.

8. Relating to a hospital admission, stress can be reduced by deferring as many questions as possible until later on in the stay, rather than at admission.

A hospital admission is in itself a stressor, which further heightens a person's stress. Questions at this time can be difficult for a person to answer; recall is more difficult because of stress. Therefore, any questions that can be deferred until later will help patients reduce their stress.

9. Physical activity can dissipate stress.

If a person is able, physical activity such as folding linen can reduce stress. For patients who are restricted to bed, such activities as leather work or knitting can be helpful.

10. Expectations should be within the patient's capabilities.

Whatever the activity, the nurse should make sure that it is possible for the patient to accomplish. If an activity, whether it be an exercise or recreation, is beyond the patient's ability, the patient will not be able to achieve the goal and is likely to be more stressed. Frustration and depression may result. Being able to meet goals helps a patient feel personally effective, thus helping self-image.

11. Nurses can assist patients and their families by bringing them into contact with people in community agencies who can help them make valid plans.

People such as social workers are familiar with planning and arrangements that may need to be made by a patient. Their advice and assistance will enable the patient to make plans that are most likely to be valid and that can be carried out. Often people are stressed needlessly because they do not know what help is available to them in the community. Plans that have a reasonable chance of being successful are highly desirable for a stressed person. Disappointment is likely to elevate the stress state and disappoint a patient and family.

12. Reinforcement of positive environmental factors and recognition of negative ones help to reduce stress.

A nurse can also help a patient's return to homeostasis by reinforcing those factors in the environment which are helpful and by recognizing but not reinforcing factors that are prohibitive. A person's thoughts can dwell upon problems and difficulties, which increases stress, rather than focus positively upon what can be accomplished, which usually decreases stress.

13. Providing information when the patient has insufficient information can reduce stress.

Fear of the unknown and incorrect information can frequently cause stress. A patient may be told a fact, but the terms can be misunderstood. Additional information or clarification of information can allay misunderstanding.

14. The nurse can reduce stress by assisting a patient to make a correct appraisal of a situation.

Sometimes through a lack of knowledge or through a misinterpretation of a sequence of events, incorrect conclusions are made by people. As an example, the results of a breast biopsy are not back from the hospital laboratory in two days. The patient may assume that something is seriously wrong because it has taken two days, even though that length of time may be dictated by the specific test. Information from the nurse as to the length of time that biopsy specimens normally take for diagnosis will often relieve a patient's stress and facilitate homeostatic balance.

15. Providing an environment in which a person can function independently to some degree without assistance helps to reduce stress.

Most adults in North America are accustomed to functioning independently and interdependently, often caring for dependents at the same time. For an adult to assume the dependent patient role even for a short time is difficult and stress producing. If patients can have some degree of independent functioning, such as by using eating utensils that have been adapted in order that they can feed themselves, patients' stress will be lowered. Patients will have an improved self-concept and will feel that they are not totally helpless. This feeling of helping oneself is important for mental health and for morale. Persons who feel they are a bother are often distressed patients.

16. Arranging for other patients with similar experiences to visit may help to reduce stress.

Patients who have a medical condition such as a colostomy may be highly stressed and feel that they will never be able to live a normal life again. To meet another person who has a colostomy and who has successfully adjusted to this condition can lower the stress of patients greatly. Not only are the patients reassured, they may also gain information that will assist them in rehabilitation.

17. Nurses and paramedical personnel need to communicate competency, understanding, and empathy rather than stress and anxiety.

The patient and family or circle of friends look upon the nurse as a source of knowledge and skill. If this person conveys stress or anxiety, a patient and family will be stressed about the nurse's competency and ability to function where the patient's health and life are involved. Nurses need to know themselves well and be able to function in an undefensive manner that conveys competence and empathy in order to reduce the patient's stress level.

CRISIS

A *crisis* is a sudden event in one's life that disturbs a person's homeostasis. If the event is such that the normal coping mechanisms of a person cannot resolve the problem and the disequilibrium continues from a few hours to a few days, the disruption is called a crisis. Persons who have a crisis in their lives experience three main signs and symptoms:

1. Heightened feeling of stress.
2. Inability to function in the usual organized manner.
3. Signs that indicate unpleasant emotional feelings.

When people have crises in their lives, there can be three outcomes. First, previously developed coping mechanisms may be sufficient to return the person to the same level of emotional homeostasis as before. Second, the person's coping mechanisms may be insufficient, which results in less emotional stability than previously. Third, the person's coping mechanisms may be such that as a result of the crisis the person gains emotional strength and stability.

A crisis has been described as having four phases:

1. The person experiences feelings of stress and uneasiness. The person therefore tries emergency problem-solving methods to solve the crisis. These are found to be ineffective.
2. The person then experiences increased tension and disorganization due to the continual impact of the crisis and ineffective coping.
3. By the third phase, the person is experiencing even more tension and is mobilizing both internal and external resources.
4. In the fourth phase, the person experiences major disorganization and thus true emotional homeostatic imbalance.

Before the fourth phase or the crisis phase, the problem may be resolved in one of the following ways:

1. The person uses emergency, problem-solving methods.
2. The person changes from unattainable goals to attainable goals.
3. The problem itself is removed or is dissipated.
4. The problem is defined in another manner.

Types of Crises

Crises are generally of two types: internal (developmental) and external (coincidental).

Internal (Developmental) Crises

Developmental crises occur at critical points in the development of the person. Erik Erikson formulated four stages in the development of a person. These are infancy, childhood, adolescence, and adulthood. He further identified eight developmental crises, which must be resolved. These are, in order, basic trust versus mistrust, autonomy versus shame and doubt, initiative versus guilt, industry versus inferiority, identity versus role confusion, intimacy versus isolation, generativity versus stagnation, and ego integrity versus despair. These developmental crises are anticipated in the life of a person, and therefore the person has the opportunity to prepare for them before they occur. A person who does not cope successfully with one or more of these developmental crises is described as having a fixation, which can lead to a personality defect. (See Chapter 10.)

External (Coincidental) Crises

External crises occur at any time in a person's life. They include stress such as may be due to loss of a job, loss of an income, or an accidental death of a loved one. Nurses may see crises of people as a result of the occurrence of illness, the admission of a child to a hospital, or the death of a member of a family, for example.

Crisis Intervention

A basis of crisis intervention is the problem-solving method or the nursing process. This involves four steps: assessing the problem, planning the intervention, intervening, and evaluating the results. When a person's crisis is in the first phase, environmental manipulation can be an effective method of intervening. At this stage the problem for patients may be removed, for example, by changing the environment or by providing persons with detailed information about the medications they are receiving. At the second stage, general support is effective. The nurse listens, expresses warmth and empathy, and is nonjudgmental.

At the third level, the intervention involves dealing with those areas in which there is enough knowledge so that the nurse knows what steps are needed to help the patient resolve the precrisis situation. An example might be helping a patient who has been told he must have heart surgery with information about what to expect.

At the fourth level, the nurse applies intervention to the person by learning the person's particular needs and problem. The patient often needs to be assisted to understand the *why* of the situation and given a choice of options as to how to solve the problem.

Crisis intervention is oriented to help persons solve a problem that they have not been able to solve themselves. Through it persons can learn skills, such as establishing options, which can assist them throughout life.

SUMMARY

All stressors to the body evoke common adaptive responses regardless of whether they arise from within or without the body, whether they are pleasant or unpleasant, or whether they are real or imagined. For this reason, Selye defines stress as a state manifested by a specific syndrome that is nonspecifically induced. The body's response to stress is referred to as the general adaptation syndrome (GAS) and the local adaptation syndrome (LAS). Both the GAS and the LAS have three stages: (a) the alarm reaction, (b) the stage of resistance, and (c) the stage of exhaustion. These adaptive reactions described by Selye are physiologic ones. However, individuals also respond with psychologic adaptive reactions. All adaptive reactions may be considered as effective or ineffective.

The degree of response to stressors depends upon four factors. First, the nature of the stressor influences the response by its magnitude and its specific meaning to a person. Second, the number of stressors to be coped with at the same time is significant; the more stressors, the greater the response. Third, duration of exposure to the stressor affects the reaction. The longer a person endures the stressor, the more exhausted become the person's powers of resistance. Fourth, the past experiences of a person with comparable stressors alters response to them.

Common signs and symptoms of stress can be observed. Some physiologic responses are diaphoresis, increased heart and respiratory rate, skin pallor, and urinary frequency. The psychologic responses noted are usually reduced intellectual processes, increased self-sensitivity, decreased ability to cope with or master tasks, and a decreased sense of personal effectiveness.

Four major physiologic adaptive mechanisms are the endocrine, the neurologic, the inflammatory, and the immunologic. The endocrine response involves the adaptive hormones from the pituitary gland and the adrenal cortex. ACTH stimulates the production of antidefensive hormones by the adrenal cortex (anti-inflammatory corticoids). Cortisone is the commonly known one. The A-Cs effect changes in organs throughout the body. Some documented by Selye are inhibition of inflammation, development of gastrointestinal ulcers, and inhibition of immune responses. In contrast, prodefensive hormones (proinflammatory corticoids) are also released. The commonly known P-C is aldosterone, which, by mechanisms not fully understood, facilitates the inflammatory process at the local site. The body's adaptation and resistance during stress relies upon a balance between the A-Cs and the P-Cs. Other hormones that are activated during stress are TTH by the adenohypophysis and ADH by the neurohypophysis.

The neurologic adaptive response involves the autonomic nervous system. It operates simultaneously with the endocrine response. In this case, hormones (adrenalins) are secreted by the adrenal medulla. The physiologic responses of the adrenalins are commonly referred to as the fight-or-flight responses, which prepare the body for defense or attack.

The inflammatory adaptive response is a major example of the LAS. Its purpose is to destroy and to localize three injurious agents and to repair resulting damage to the tissues. Three stages of this process are (a) cellular and vascular change, (b) formation of inflammatory exudate, and (c) repair of tissues. The first stage is characterized by hyperemia and the observable signs of swelling, redness, heat, pain, and impaired mobility. Blood vessels dilate and become more permeable, plasma moves into the tissues, blood flow slows, and the leukocytes marginate, emigrate, and attack the stressor by phagocytosis. The second stage produces the exudate, consisting of fluid and other substances from the blood vessels, dead tissue cells, and their by-products. The inflammation is localized by the formation of a fibrin mesh or clot. Exudates vary in accordance with the tissue involved and the intensity and duration of the inflammation. Major types of exudate are serous, catarrhal, purulent, fibrinous, and hermorrhagic. The third and final stage of inflammation is repair of the tissues by either regeneration or fibrous tissue substitution. The latter process involves the formation of granulation tissue and cicatrix (scar tissue).

Several factors influence the character and speed of tissue healing. Included are the degree of injury, the adequacy of the blood supply, the nutrients available, the age of the person, the presence of other stressors, the adequacy of immune mechanisms, and the balance of A-Cs and P-Cs.

The immunologic response is a highly specific adaptive response, involving the formation of antibodies (immunoglobulins) to counteract foreign proteins in the body called antigens. Five immunoglobulins designated by the letters G, A, M, D, and E have been isolated, each having different functions. Immunity of humans is either natural or acquired. The former is a species resistance, while the latter involves exposure to disease agents. Acquired immunity is referred to as active when the host produces his or her own antibodies either naturally or artificially in response to vaccines or toxoids. It is referred to as passive immunity when antibodies that are produced by other animals or persons are administered. Passive immunity can be naturally acquired by a fetus or newborn from antibodies synthesized by the mother. Artificial means to produce passive immunity are immune sera or antisera. Active immunity has the advantage of a longer duration, but passive immunity has the advantage of immediate or rapid immunity.

Psychologic adaptive responses are referred to as mental defense mechanisms or coping mechanisms. They protect the person by relieving inner tensions or conflicts and anxiety. The behavioral responses are primarily employed by unconscious means. They may be regarded as effective or as ineffective in terms of adapting to life situations. In other words, each mechanism can be considered in terms of healthy use or unhealthy use.

Nurses must not only be able to recognize stress but must also be able to assist people to adapt to stress. Several methods can be selected in accordance with the needs of the person at any given time. The nurse first needs to be sensitive to specific situations that increase the person's stress. Some general measures to reduce stress include orienting patients to the hospital or the agency, providing time for patients to ventilate their feelings and thoughts, preserving the patient's identity, encouraging participation in the plan of care, repeating information, encouraging physical activity, and arranging for other patients with similar experiences to visit.

The term *crisis* is increasingly being used to describe sudden events that disrupt a person's equilibrium to the point where assistance is required to help the coping mechanisms. Two types of crises are classified: internal (developmental) and external (coincidental). The nurse can be instrumental in helping patients to identify and to plan ways to deal with a crisis.

SUGGESTED ACTIVITIES

1. Try to assess your own level of stress within the past few months according to Table 8–1 in this chapter, and determine your individual stress score.

2. Select a friend or patient who you think is undergoing physical and psychologic stress, and compare the signs and symptoms he or she is experiencing or manifesting with those described in this chapter.

3. In a clinical or home situation, select a person and apply some of the methods suggested to help a person adapt to stress. Then evaluate their effectiveness.

4. In a clinical setting, select a patient with an inflammation. Assess the patient's signs and symptoms and determine what factors are facilitating or hindering the healing process.

5. With a group of students, describe and share examples of situations in which patients, family members, friends, and yourself have used specific mental mechanisms.

SUGGESTED READINGS

Martin, Harry W., and Prange, Arthur J., Jr. March, 1962. Human adaptation—a conceptual approach to understanding patients. *The Canadian Nurse* 58 (3): 234–243.

The ways in which stress affects individuals and the adaptive techniques are discussed. Special consideration is given to the stress that accompanies people who are ill.

Peterson, Margaret H. September, 1972. Understanding defense mechanisms programmed instruction. *American Journal of Nursing* 72(9): 1651–1674.

This programmed instruction provides the nursing student with a means by which to learn human defense mechanisms. Situations are described in which mechanisms are employed, and the student is asked to identify the mechanism.

Shields, Leona. September–October, 1975. Crisis intervention: implications for the nurse. *Journal of Psychiatric Nursing and Mental Health Services,* 13(5): 37–42.

The author describes the four phases of crisis with examples of the four levels of intervention.

SELECTED BIBLIOGRAPHY

Burgess, Ann Wolbert, and Lazare, Aaron. 1976. *Community mental health—target populations.* Englewood Cliffs, N.J.: Prentice-Hall, Inc.

Byrne, Marjorie L., and Thompson, Lida F. 1972. *Key concepts for the study and practice of nursing.* St. Louis: The C. V. Mosby Co.

Engel, George L. 1962. *Psychological development in health and disease.* Philadelphia: W. B. Saunders Co.

Kempf, Florence., and Useen, Ruth Hill. 1964. *Psychology dynamics of behavior in nursing.* Philadelphia: W. B. Saunders Co.

Kolb, Lawrence C. 1977. *Modern clinical psychiatry,* 9th ed. Philadelphia: W. B. Saunders Co.

Levine, Seymour. 1971. Stress and behavior. In *Readings from Scientific American: physiological psychology.* San Francisco: W. H. Freeman and Co.

Morgan, Arthur, and Moreno, Judith Wilson. 1973. *The practice of mental health nursing: a community approach.* Philadelphia: J. B. Lippincott Co.

Sedgwick, Rae. September–October, 1975. Psychological responses to stress. *Journal of Psychiatric Nursing and Mental Health Services.* 13(5): 20–23.

Selye, Hans. 1974. *Stress without distress.* Scarborough, Ont., Canada: The New American Library of Canada, Ltd.

Selye, Hans. 1956. *The stress of life.* New York: McGraw-Hill Book Co.

CHAPTER 9

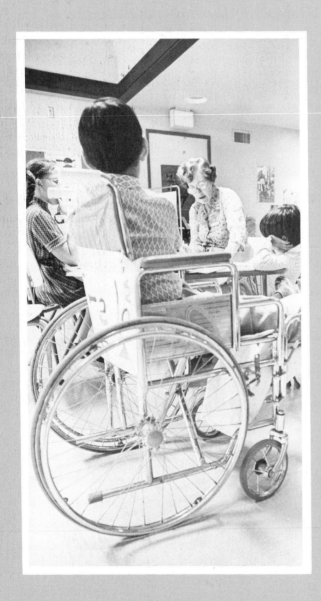

HUMANISM AND ETHNICITY

OBJECTIVES

- Explain the importance of humanism and ethnicity in the provision of nursing care.

- Discuss the difference in incidence of some diseases among different ethnic groups.

- Identify some problems unique to ethnic minorities in the provision and use of physical and mental health-care services.

- Discuss some general commonalities among minority ethnic groups in relation to health care.

- Describe some specific differences in beliefs, habits, and customs of selected ethnic groups that have implications in the provision of nursing care.

Humanism and ethnicity are of particular importance in the United States and Canada, where there are a large number of cultural groups. Nurses need to understand that human values and beliefs are often culturally determined, and thus a patient may not see things the way the nurse does. In this chapter, five of the many North American ethnic groups are considered with specific reference to their health care needs and perspectives:

> Native Americans (American Indians)
>
> Blacks
>
> Chinese

Jewish people

Chicanos (Mexican-Americans)

Issues in regard to humanistic values and health have not been fully explored or resolved. For example, recent legislation in regard to abortions in the United States and in Canada is still being challenged by some cultural and religious groups who contend that the rights of an unborn child are being violated through abortion. With advances in technology as well as other social changes, nurses will be challenged to preserve human values of the diverse ethnic groups while providing needed nursing care.

HUMANISM

Humanism refers to man's human attributes, to those characteristics which are considered human. Some of these attributes can be considered to be universal, that is, they occur in all cultures. Examples are feelings of empathy, compassion, and sympathy toward other people and a respect for life.

Many characteristics of humanism, however, rather than being universal are related to a person's culture, and they vary from one culture and from one subgroup to another. They involve beliefs and values that are learned during a lifetime.

American and Canadian societies are multicultural in that they have many diverse cultural groups within them. American society in its humanism is person-centered, and it includes a human rights concept. This means that individual people are autonomous and have certain rights and freedoms; in fact, each person has the right to be treated as an individual. This can be contrasted with some other societies in which the tribe or the family is the primary orientation of values and rights, not the person. Other characteristics of American humanism—though not necessarily unique to American humanism—are: helping the poor and helping those who are suffering. In addition it is expected that people will respect the ways and values of others, even if these differ from their own.

Ethnoscience

Ethnoscience refers to "the systematic study of the way of life of a designated cultural group with the purpose of obtaining an accurate account of the people's behavior and how they perceive and interpret their

universe" (Leininger 1970: 168). Anthropologists have for years studied cultural groups' own perceptions of and knowledge about their world. However, ethnoscientists use a more rigorous method of systematic data collection to provide an accurate collection and analysis of data. Ethnoscientists attempt to provide an inside view of a culture from the way the people of the culture talk about it. They study and classify data about a cultural or subcultural group so that their report is meaningful to both the people within the culture and the people outside of the culture who try to understand it. Emphasis is placed upon the person's point of view, the person's vision, and the person's world.

Nurses can apply much of the knowledge gained by ethnoscientists, specifically about the health-illness systems of behavior of people from cultural backgrounds different from their own. In the past decade or more the patient's personal view of illness has received recognition and emphasis. Nurses have, as a result, implemented methods to discover how well patients understand their illness, how patients perceive they can be helped by health personnel, and how illness has affected them and their family. In recent years the person's cultural views affecting health practices and beliefs have been receiving greater recognition. The fact that beliefs and practices about health vary among different cultures and the implications this has for nursing have also been receiving greater recognition. In order to provide effective nursing services to patients, data about both the patient's personal and cultural views regarding health and illness are needed. Nursing care plans need to give consideration to the patient's world and his experiences; nurses need to attempt to see and hear the world as their patients hear it and see it. Specific cultural data can provide scientific generalizations about wellness and illness behavior among different cultures. Patients needs and behavior can then be dealt with according to their particular health norms.

MULTICULTURAL CONSIDERATIONS FOR HEALTH CARE

The provision of quality health care to all North Americans is a desired goal. Because of the multicultural nature of the American society it is essential that consideration is given to the unique health needs of ethnic minority groups. Following are some general considerations that can help in developing an awareness and sensitivity to some of these specific needs.

Physical Health

Studies have shown that some ethnic groups are prone to certain diseases more than to others. These diseases may be inherited or acquired, that is, environmentally induced. The incidence of specific diseases will be discussed subsequently with selected ethnic groups.

Acquired diseases that are common to most ethnic minority groups are malnutrition, tuberculosis, parasitosis, neoplasms, and diseases of the digestive tract. Other diseases have a higher incidence in specific ethnic groups. Some of these are the following:

1. *Sickle cell anemia* occurs in about one out of every 400 black Americans.

2. *Gout* has a higher incidence in Puerto Ricans and Filipinos. This is a disease in which uric acid levels increase in the blood stream, resulting in the deposition of uric acid crystals in the joints or other tissues. Swelling, inflammation, and pain occur.

3. The tendency toward *hypertension* is higher in Filipino males, Jewish people, and blacks.

4. *Lactase deficiency* occurs more often in black Americans and Orientals.

5. *Acatalasia* occurs mostly in Orientals such as the Japanese, Koreans, and Chinese. This is a rare inherited deficiency of catalase in body tissues, particularly in the erythrocytes, bone marrow, liver, and skin. It results in an increased susceptibility to tissue damage by normal microbial flora and is most often first detected in the mouth.

6. *Coccidioidomycosis* (valley fever), a fungal infection acquired by the respiratory route, is more common in blacks and Filipinos.

7. *Sarcoidosis* occurs ten times more frequently among blacks than among whites. The term *sarcoid* means fleshy. Sarcoidosis is a granulomatous disorder of unknown cause. It is characterized by epithelioid cell granulomas that affect any part of the body. Most frequently the lymph nodes, spleen, lungs, skin, eyes, and small bones of the hands and feet are involved.

Mental Health

In current psychiatric therapy, emphasis is placed upon one's responsibility to oneself to be comfortable, to grow, and to be competent and successful (Osborne 1976:20). Individualism is stressed. However, for most people of minority-groups, the basic concern and usual interactions are with the family and friendship groups. They do not place individualism above family and friends. They often want other people whom they can depend upon for support and stress the social component of the human race. Therapies are therefore needed that include significant other people in the environment, especially the family. The term *family* is not restricted to the American nuclear family of a couple and their children, but often also includes the extended family, such as aunts, uncles, and grandparents. These people provide the primary support system for minority-group clients. Of the many systems of therapy, those which are often or always done in groups, such as encounter therapy and transactional analysis, may be more effective modes of therapy for those people.

In mental health therapy for minority cultures, the racial identity and unique cultural experiences of the clients cannot be ignored. Sometimes the predisposing and precipitating causes of the illness may be rooted in the problems of the race or culture. On the other hand, the problems may be related to the person's human qualities such as socialization and to interpersonal relationships with others, even within the person's own cultural group. Some problems may be related to a composite of the two, for example, racial or cultural and individual or humanistic. Therefore nurses require special understanding of the unique differences of cultural groups.

Some patients belonging to certain ethnic groups may not possess the qualities required for some psychiatric therapies, and this needs consideration. For example, many therapies rely upon particular personality and intellectual characteristics such as good verbal skills, adequate ego strength for introspection, and the ability to delay gratification (Leininger 1970:168). Not all ethnic groups may value or possess these qualities. It is said as a result that minority-group clients are more frequently the recipients of physiologic or custodial therapies than the majority white American group. Even the definitions and conceptions of mental health and mental illness can vary. For example, majority-group people who are professionals may think in terms of self-actualization, whereas minority-group people may think in terms of survival.

The use of mental health services and the availability of these to minority groups is variable. Some ethnic groups consider it bad form to discuss their personal problems with strangers, including therapists and nurses. Others may view therapeutic resources as irrelevant to their specific needs and even inaccessible. For example, many psychiatrists operate on a fee-for-service basis. These fees are out of reach to many members of minority groups. Even if a resource is accessible and is utilized, the minority group's ideas about the usefulness of the resource can be questionable, particularly if the therapist or nurse is representative of the majority group society.

When members of racial minorities do come to mental health therapists, certain feelings and behaviors are of value to bear in mind in conducting therapy. These feelings and behaviors are not unique to minority groups and may not be experienced by all minority-group clients, but they are appropriate for consideration. These common feeling and behavior patterns are:

1. feelings of inferiority and inadequacy
2. incompetent behaviors
3. anger and hostility
4. withholding and withdrawal
5. selective inattention
6. overcompensation (Osborne, 1976:22–24)

Feelings of inferiority and inadequacy can be operant as a result of prejudice and racism in a society. The effects of racism are often inappropriate distribution of resources such as housing, education, jobs, and health services, which limit the achievement of aspirations of the minority group. Feelings of inferiority then arise in members of the disadvantaged group in specific situations such as when they are competing for a job with members of the majority group.

Incompetence is the behavioral outcome of feelings of inferiority and inadequacy. The person may be unable to perform certain activities or may manifest behaviors that do not achieve the desired goal. Judgments of incompetency are made again in situations in which a minority person is competing against majority-group people, in situations that are ruled by the majority group. For example, a minority-group person may be judged by a criterion such as an IQ test which has racial and cultural biases.

Anger is generated from reflections about judgments of incompetence and feelings of inferiority, but because the minority-group person fears retribution by the majority, this anger is frequently suppressed rather than expressed. Suppressed anger results in hostility, which has a corrosive effect upon the person, diffusing into and marring many of the person's relationships. A great deal of energy is expended to keep this anger suppressed. Occasionally it is expressed but not toward the threatening oppressors; rather the anger may be expressed toward inanimate objects in the environment or toward people who cannot retaliate. Hostility may be expressed as paranoid ideas which reinforce the idea that members of the majority group have feelings of hostility toward the minority-group person. Feelings of hatred, on the other hand, are usually focused more on specific persons or objects.

Withholding and withdrawal are behaviors that eventually occur when feelings of anger accumulate. Withholding refers to not sharing feelings and experiences with others. Withdrawal behavior denies the existence of a situation or that help available is relevant to the person.

Selective inattention, also referred to as cognitive screening, is another form of behavior that oppressed people may manifest. In this behavior one learns to remove from one's awareness situations and events that are frustrating or insulting. The advantage of this is that one can then pursue one's goals without expending energy on or reacting to situations that provoke feelings of inferiority or inadequacy. On the other hand, overuse of this mechanism can lead to muted emotional responses.

Overcompensation is a form of behavior that can occur with some minority persons. It is an attempt to perform in a way superior to that of the majority of the population. In other words, the person concludes that in order to succeed in this society he or she must perform better than is expected of the white person. This can lead to family problems if, for instance, the job requires much time and effort. It may even create more conflict with the white majority colleagues who do not have the motivation to perform as well.

Social Considerations

Each cultural group establishes norms, values, and beliefs that assist the functioning of that particular group. In North America there is a tendency to make the assumption that anything that differs from one's own culture is inferior. Yet there is richness and value in each culture. Although the ways and reasons underlying certain practices may not always be clear, nurses need to appreciate and to accept these differences, to view these differences as positive elements, and to modify nursing intervention accordingly. The ways and practices of each culture are deeply rooted and have worked effectively through time for each particular group. Nurses need to capitalize on every experience with people from different cultures in order to learn their unique characteristics.

Although each culture has its own unique differences (see subsequent sections), some general similarities can be considered. These are

1. language barrier
2. food habits
3. perception of illness
4. illness practices
5. time orientation
6. concept of family
7. male/female norms

Language Barriers

Some patients may not speak English fluently enough to express their needs or wishes or to understand all that is said to them. This can be particularly frustrating and anxiety producing when a person is ill and can neither express problems nor understand instructions. Also, it is most difficult for people to convey their feelings about situations in a second language, a crucial problem in cases of emotional and psychiatric illness.

Food Habits

Food habits and foods ingested vary considerably from one culture to another. Hospitalized patients often have very little choice about types of food served. Family members could be encouraged to bring in special meals within the limitations of the patient's diet. Instructions about meal planning for special diets at home may have to be given to younger family members who are more fluent in the English language, or they may have to be given by a health worker who is of the same culture and who can act as an interpreter.

Perception of Illness

How illness is viewed is also determined to a large degree by one's culture. Some cultures view illness as punishment from God for sinful acts. Others may regard illness as the work of malevolent persons who want to see them suffer. Still others are convinced that illness is caused by evil spirits, and as a result they can receive help only from spiritualists or witch doctors.

Illness Practices

Ways of curing illness are often closely allied to the way the cause of illness is perceived. For those who believe their illness is God's punishment, pain killers and even some nursing care may be refused, since these patients believe they must atone for their sins. Other practices may include bargaining or atonement rituals with God or specific saints, such as repeating rosary prayers a specified number of times. Penitence may be done by fasting for a number of days or walking on one's knees to a certain cathedral. Efforts on the part of health personnel to convince some patients that their mental illness may be due to a biochemical imbalance or that physical illness may be due to an infectious process can be futile in these instances. Some patients may prefer a spiritualist to a physician, for example.

Time Orientation

In contrast to the majority North American culture which places great value on the future, many minority groups place more value on the present, the here and now. It is important that nurses recognize this concept and plan nursing interventions with a here-and-now orientation. Instruction about long-term goals or health needs cannot be overlooked, however. It presents a challenge to health professionals to educate people to look into the future as a realistic concept.

Concept of Family

The concept of family can differ from that of white middle-class culture. The minority group family may include the *nuclear family* plus uncles, aunts, grandparents, cousins, and godparents—the *extended family*. When health care is offered to persons with this concept, it is important to consider the total family needs. It has been known that some family members' needs may take priority to the detriment of the patient. For example, a mother may not think that purchasing elastic stockings for her own ankle edema is as important as purchasing food for a distant relative who is unemployed. The public health nurse in this instance may have to see that the distant relative's needs are taken care of before the mother's needs can be dealt with.

Associated with this concept that family members are most important and must be helped at all costs is the belief that personal and family information must stay within the family. Some cultural groups are very reluctant to disclose family information to outsiders, including physicians and nurses. This can present difficulties for psychiatrists and mental health workers in particular.

Male/Female Norms

In some cultures men must be strong and brave. They cannot cry or complain of discomfort and must always maintain control of emotions such as fear. For women, modesty is valued. Some cultures dictate that females cannot have their bodies inspected or touched by a strange man, which includes physicians. If a female holding such a belief must be examined by a male physican, a female nurse should be present. This modesty is often manifested even in the presence of other women. Care must be taken to cover female patients as much as possible during examination procedures.

AMERICAN INDIANS (NATIVE AMERICANS)

The total American Indian population in the United States in 1970 was 792,730 (U.S. Bureau of the Census 1976) and in Canada in 1974 it was 276,436 (data obtained from the office of the Minister of Supply and Services of Canada, 1977). In both countries the responsibility for the health services for Indians rests with the federal government.

Because over 300 different tribes of Indians exist in the United States, each with its own language, folkways, religion, mores, and patterns of interpersonal relationships, caution needs to be taken about the Indian culture. Further complicating this matter is the dilution of each purely Indian ethnic group that has occurred with generations of contact with non-Indians. In terms of health care this variability needs to be considered. For example, the native American who lives in isolation on a reservation may hold to traditional beliefs of cure provided by the medicine man, while the urban native American who lives away from the reservation may respond more to the values of modern medicine provided by the white man. It is not uncommon for Indians to accept both kinds of health practices concurrently.

What consititutes a native American's cultural identity can no longer be determined by physical appearance. Some persons who are only one-eighth Indian by blood may view themselves as more traditionally Indian than persons who have less dilution of ancestry. For this reason Indians are sometimes classified as "functional" or "nonfunctional" (Spruce 1972:6). One is a functional Indian if one has an intimate understanding of one's people gained through socialization from childhood. One's behavior is dictated by the accepted patterns of one's Indian neighbors. One thinks of oneself as being Indian and is considered by the group to be an Indian. In contrast, one is a nonfunctional Indian if one appears to be full-blooded but knows little or nothing about the traditions of culture of the Indian people. Nonfunctional Indians believe in accordance with the majority white culture and consider themselves non-Indian. Despite these variables, some similarities of all Indian cultures can be considered and are discussed in the following sections.

Illness Beliefs and Practices

Native Americans tend to value a harmonious relationship with the world around them. Each rock, tree, animal, flower, and person is equally respected and all are seen to coexist in harmony. Thus illness is viewed in terms of an imbalance between the person who is ill and the natural or supernatural forces around the person rather than in terms of an altered physiologic state. Causes of illness relate to this concept. Native Americans believe that if one interferes with this harmony by abusing another person or thing, one may become ill. Bad thoughts or wishes of jealousy or anger by another person may also cause illness. In addition, supernatural or spiritual forces may be involved.

Various curative and preventive rituals may be conducted to restore the balance. Some of these may be carried out by medicine men, others by family members. Sacred foods such as cornmeal may be sprinkled on one's shoulder before one enters a home to prevent flu or cold germs from entering the home. This sacred food may also be sprinkled around an ill person's bed for a period of time. It is important for nurses to provide privacy for such ceremonies and to inquire about the length of time this food should be left in place, how to dispose of it, and, if it must be disturbed, exactly how and where the nurse may do so. Other items such as herbs or other mixtures are frequently placed near the patient on the bedside stand or on the bed, or some may be worn by the patient. Permission needs to be acquired should these need to be removed.

Healing ceremonies, sometimes referred to as *sings* or *prayers,* may be requested. These vary in length from one-half hour to nine days. Space and privacy need to be provided for such ceremonies. Usually in the hospital the sing is less than an hour. A medicine man may also be requested to perform specific curative rituals that vary in accordance with the signs and symptoms of the patient.

Death or Loss

American Indians are less concerned with the future than are whites. The quality of life in the here and now is more important than longevity. There is no belief in a life hereafter. Native Americans accept that they will die as part of the life cycle and do not worry about how or when or why. They know they will join another world of long-ago ancestors when the Spirit intends. Funerals generally take place in the home and are associated with a large feast and gifts for relatives of the deceased. Proper burial rituals according to tribal tradition are important to American Indians. Associated with burial is the belief of wholeness. Thus when limbs are amputated, Indians may want to

reclaim them and retain them for appropriate burial when the person dies.

Eye Contact

Native Americans sometimes are labeled as being nonmotivated, disinterested, or shifty-eyed because they may not look directly into the eyes of another person. This practice is based on their respect for the other person's privacy and the other person's soul. It is believed that direct eye contact is disrespectful and may even take the other's soul away.

Kinship

The family, relatives, and friends are important to Indians. During illness the patient is comforted when many relatives and friends visit. This conveys caring. Being present is generally more important than talking, and it is not uncommon for large numbers of people to congregate. More often one person likes to remain near the patient for long periods. The native American kinship system can be confusing to nurses of other cultures. A child, for example, may have several mothers or several sets of brothers or sisters who are not direct-line relatives but according to the tribe are considered as such. These people are all important to the patient who is ill. The aged, particularly, are looked upon for counsel and wisdom. Friendship ties are strong and can become as meaningful as those of the family or extended family.

Time

Native Americans tend to be casual about time as compared to people of other cultures. Their lives are less rigidly controlled by the clock. An Indian will sleep when tired, eat when hungry, and disregard a health appointment during the fishing season. This has many implications when health care instruction is given, such as prescribing medications to be given every 6 hours or every 4 hours.

Health Problems

The special health problems of American Indians include the following:

1. The suicide rate is twice as high as that of other races.
2. The homicide rate is 3.3 times greater.

3. Mortality in relation to alcohol is 6.5 times greater.

4. Emotional problems of children are increasing.

5. Otitis media is replacing tuberculosis as a major health problem.

6. Nutritional deficiencies are common.

7. Infant illness and death during the first year are higher than in the white population (US PHS 1972:13–17).

Recent data also suggest that the clinical picture for some diseases such as diabetes, hypertension, and alcoholism is different for American Indians. For example, the diabetic Indian patient who has a blood sugar of 500 mg/ml may remain asymptomatic. The normal blood sugar is 80–100 mg/ml (West and Kalbsleisch 1970:656–663). Indian youths also acquire hypertension, gastric ulceration, and liver cirrhosis at earlier ages than do whites.

BLACKS

With the arrival of the first African slaves in Jamestown, Virginia, in 1619, over three centuries ago, a history of deprivation on this continent began for blacks. Both children and adults served as personal servants or helpmates to white children and adults. Because black slaves were assigned to work in the fields and the homes of the slave master, black children missed the usual childhood activities. Often the black children were assigned as personal servants to white children for 24 hours a day and would sleep on the floor beside the beds of these white children.

Even after slavery was abolished, blacks have endured the effects of white racism—economic and social deprivation. Nevertheless, many blacks are now members of the middle-class; many are professionals. In some parts of America, however, some blacks still live in shacks that may not have running water, toilets, or heat. In some city ghettos, families live in crowded, dilapidated tenements that may be infested by rats or cockroaches. Basic necessities such as food and clothing are sometimes scarce.

It is not uncommon for both black parents to work to cope with their economic problems. As a result black children are often left to take responsibilities for younger children, to run errands, help with housework, and perhaps do the shopping. Many children by the age of 8 or 9 years have odd jobs to support the family income. It is little wonder that their priority system in living is often described in terms of survival. Health care may, in many instances, not be a priority, if food is scarce.

Malnutrition can be a major health problem among blacks. It has been noted, for example, that black women as compared to white women have a higher incidence of anemia and other complications during pregnancy due to unbalanced diets and inadequate medical care. Infant mortality rates as a result are high.

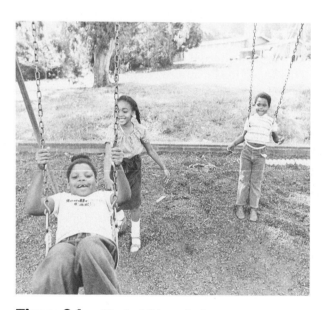

Figure 9-1.   Black children playing.

In the 1970 census, blacks were cited as comprising 11.1% of the total United States population. In the ten largest cities their percentage of the population ranges from 17.9% in Los Angeles to 71.1% in Washington, D.C. (Dudley and Smith 1970:23–25). In Canada in 1971, blacks made up of 0.2% of the population (Fawcett 1977).

According to some surveys almost 50% of black high school students do not believe that whites can be trusted (Comer and Poussaint 1975:288). They are disillusioned with the image of democracy and the lack of progress in solving racial problems. In contrast, smaller percentages of the older black population hold this belief. This attitude has implications for health care delivery, since many of the providers of health care belong to the white race, particularly physicians and registered and public health nurses.

Habits and Beliefs

Food habits are influenced by heritage in part and by economic factors. Hogs, chickens, corn, and beans were native products in the early history of the South. The land did not lend itself to pastures for grazing cattle. Parts of the hog that were not considered desirable to the white masters were given to the black slaves to eat. These included the head, feet, brain, chitterlings (intestine), maw (stomach), and fatback (layers of fat). Today many blacks still prefer these meats as well as chicken because they are economical and because of their cultural heritage.

Some blacks believe that certain combinations of foods or drugs can cause severe illness or even death. A few examples are:

1. Eating fish and milk or ice cream at the same meal.

2. Drinking milk when one (particularly a child) has a high fever.

3. A penicillin injection after drinking whiskey (Martin 1976:54).

Voodoo and *witchcraft* practices still exist to a minor extent. Thus the cause of illness may be thought of as the result of a *hex*. Spiritualists or *sorcerers* may sometimes be consulted, or some patients may vacillate for treatment between Western physicians and witch doctors or spiritualists who can remove spells.

Health Problems

The life expectancy of the black population is lower than that of the white population. In 1970 the average life expectancy for the black male was 61.3 years as contrasted with 68.3 years for the white male; for the black female it was 69.4 years as contrasted with 75.7 years for the white female (Dudley and Smith 1970:57). Other 1970 statistics reveal:

1. The death rate of black mothers at childbirth is 8½ per 10,000 live births as compared to 2 per 10,000 for white mothers.

2. The infant mortality rate for blacks is double that of the white population (see Chapter 2).

3. The death rate from childhood diseases is six times greater in black childrem (McVeigh 1970:45–49).

Some specific diseases are more common among blacks due to environmental and hereditary factors.

1. Tuberculosis is three times greater in blacks than in whites.

2. Hypertension is high in incidence.

3. Sickle cell anemia occurs in 1 per 500 blacks, but 1 in every 12 carries the trait.

4. Uterine cancer is twice as common in black females as compared to whites.

5. Malnutrition has been previously mentioned.

CHINESE

The Chinese in the United States and Canada are largely concentrated on the west coast of both countries. The Chinese population can be thought of as divided into three groups: (1) the people who were born in rural villages in China and immigrated to North America 40 to 50 years ago; (2) the new immigrants who have come within the past 20 years, from several Asian countries and Hong Kong; (3) Chinese born in North America who are descendants of 19th century immigrants. Chinese in the first group are still largely oriented to Chinese folk medicine, while those in the third group are oriented to Western medical practices but still may be influenced by their elders in regard to health care.

Prior to the revolution in China, the Chinese family was *patriarchal* and *patrilineal*. Respect for one's ancestors and for one's parents was important, and obedience to the family was practiced. The Chinese family was frequently an extended one with several generations living in one household. Family clans were strong social organizations and were formed of people of the same bloodline with the same surnames. People who came to North American 40 to 50 years ago set up the same traditional family based on associations to which they were accustomed in China.

Following the revolution, traditional family practices and superstitions became less evident. Family ties continue to be strong; however, the nuclear family now is seen more commonly in Chinese society.

Health

Chinese folk medicine originated with *Taoist* philosophy. It proposes that health is regulated by two forces, the *yin* and the *yang*. The yin is a negative, female force; some of its characteristics are darkness, cold and emptiness. The yang represents positive force. It also represents the male, light, warmth, and fullness. When these two energy forces are in balance, health exists. When one has too much yin, one is nervous and is predisposed to digestive disorders. Too much yang, on the other hand, causes dehydration, fever, and irritability.

Chinese folk medicine is practiced with the use of herbs and with *acupuncture*. A folk medicine diagnosis is made chiefly by observation, questioning, listening to the body, and taking the pulse. The prescription is a combination of herbs, which are obtained from a Chinese pharmacy. Acupuncture is used chiefly to treat muscular and skeletal disorders. Needles are inserted into the body at specific points along certain internal channels, which are called meridians. The internal organs are believed to be connected to the skin points and to the meridians; the acupuncture assists to balance the energy that flows within them.

The concept of yin and yang is also involved in a balanced meal. Yin is cold and includes fruits, vegetables, and cold drinks. Yang includes hot food, for example, soups, scrambled eggs, and ginger. A Chinese patient who is ill with a hot disease, for example, an eye infection, will want treatment with cold foods rather than hot foods in order to get well.

Chinese people of the older generations may also believe that their blood is not replaceable. Therefore, they are often very reluctant to give their blood even for just a blood test. Like many other people, the elderly Chinese often believe that a hospital is a place to go to die rather than to get well.

There are also specific health problems that are found among the Chinese population: eye problems, tuberculosis, dental caries, malnutrition, and mental illness. Some of these health problems are directly related to the poor environmental conditions of North American Chinatowns rather than to an inherited predisposition.

Some patients will follow both Western and Chinese medical advice at the same time. This can produce problems if the therapies are not correlated. For example, a patient may be receiving the same drug from a herbal pharmacy that is prescribed by the Western physician, thus taking a double dose. Chinese patients should be encouraged to tell a doctor whether they are taking or receiving other therapy.

Folk medicine practices are often carried out during pregnancy. For example, soy sauce may be restricted in its use so that the baby's skin will not be very dark, or a mother may refuse to take iron because it will harden the bones and make the delivery of the baby difficult.

Following are some differences between Western practice and Chinese folk medicine:

1. One dose of an herbal medicine is thought to cure a person or make the person feel better. Thus, the vast number of medicines prescribed by some Western physicians is puzzling to them.

2. Herbs are generally boiled in water for a prescribed time before being ingested rather than prepared as capsules or pills.

3. Chinese patients may change physicians during an illness in order to find the best cure.

4. When Chinese patients change physicians they may not tell the former doctor because they do not want the doctor to lose face.

JEWISH PEOPLE

A Jew, by Israeli law, is any person born of a Jewish mother or anyone who is converted to Judaism through the appropriate strict and elaborate ritual. This definition applies only to people living in Israel; however, there are people in the United States and Canada whose lifestyle and reactions to illness are similar to those of Jews in Israel.

There are approximately 6 million people in the United States and 275,000 people in Canada who consider themselves Jews (Statistics Canada 1971). There are three main groups: the Orthodox, the Conservative, and the Reform Jewish groups. All these groups accept the first five books of the Old Testament as to the origin of the world as written by Moses. However, the groups do differ in their acceptance of the other books of the Old Testament and in their acceptance of later writings of Jewish writers and rabbis. These later writings are referred to as the *Talmud*.

The Talmud covers a wide range of subjects and provides instructions on social behavior. In effect, the Talmud has a major role in regulating the lifestyle of the Jewish people. The lifestyles of Conservative and Reform Jews differ from those of Orthodox Jews.

The Orthodox Jews accept the writings in the Talmud and rabbinical laws as well as the laws in the first five chapters of the Old Testament. They follow the 613 commandments. Of these commandments, 213 are concerned with medical matters.

Laws

There are a number of laws relating to health matters, which may well be of concern to nurses.

The Sabbath

The Sabbath is an important day in the life of Jewish people. The commandment is: "Six days shall you labor and do all your work: but the seventh day is a Sabbath unto the Lord your God, in it you shall not do any manner of work . . . for the Lord blessed the Sabbath day and sanctified it" (Exodus 20:9–11). Orthodox Jews who observe this commandment will want to carry out certain practices and restrict certain activities.

1. A Jewish woman will wish to light two candles on Friday at sunset. If candles are prohibited because of fire regulations, electric lights are acceptable.
2. Jewish people will not travel or handle money on the Sabbath. Therefore admission to the hospital and discharge should be arranged for another day. The exception would be when a Jewish person's life is in danger; then Jews are expected to do whatever is necessary to save their life.

Dietary Laws

There are dietary laws, which prohibit eating of certain foods and which describe the preparation of certain foods. *Kosher* means proper or in accordance with religious law and is used to describe food that has been appropriately prepared.

The meat from animals that have cloven hoofs and that chew their cud is acceptable for eating. This includes cattle, sheep, goats, and deer. Hogs are not acceptable. Chicken, turkey, geese, and ducks are also permitted for food. Part of the law requires that the animals be slaughtered according to a specific ritual and that meat be salted and soaked in order to remove any remaining blood.

An Orthodox Jew will also eat fish that has both scales and fins. Therefore, a Jew will eat salmon or cod, for example, but not shrimp, oysters, or crabs.

A further dietary restriction involves the serving of dairy foods and meat. The eating of dairy foods must be separated by three to six hours from the eating of meat for the Orthodox Jewish patient.

Abortion

The Talmud states that an abortion, no matter what the age of the fetus, is mandatory if the life of the mother is threatened. However, abortion for other reasons such as economics or personal preference is prohibited. Jewish law permits the use of contraceptive pills but at the same time encourages large families.

Death

In Jewish law euthanasia is prohibited, but withdrawal of medical equipment is permitted if it is certain that withdrawal will shorten the period of dying and not take a life. This law supports the practice if the patient is expected to die within three days.

Death is defined for the Orthodox Jew as the absence of spontaneous respiration. This differs from some medical and legal definitions. After death, the law relates to two aspects of the death: the support of the living relatives and mourners and respect for the body.

Autopsies are generally prohibited for the Jewish dead; however, it is permissible for an autopsy to take place when it is possible that the findings of an autopsy can help another patient.

Circumcision

On the eighth day after birth all Jewish males are circumcised. This is done by either a qualified rabbi or a surgeon. Upon the performance of the circumcision the child has entered into a covenant with God, and he receives his name. If the baby is premature or has health problems, the circumcision can be postponed.

Diseases

There are a number of disease conditions that are known to occur more frequently in Jewish people. Thus a nurse who is working in a Jewish community needs to be aware of these and to observe for early symptoms. The diseases generally believed to affect Jews more than other people are diabetes mellitus, Buerger's disease, Tay-Sachs disease (a lipid disorder), obesity, ulcerative colitis.

CHICANOS

Chicanos (Mexican-Americans) belong to one of perhaps 20 groups of people who come from countries where Spanish is the dominant language. Many Mexican-Americans entered the United States during the early 1900s and brought with them the values, beliefs, and practices of rural Mexico; other Mexican-Americans are more recent immigrants. Folk concepts of health and illness that they had when they came to the United States continue to affect the thinking of some second- and third-generation Chicanos today. Among these beliefs are those concerning disease, some of which are:

1. *Mal de ojo* (evil eye). This disease is caused by another person's admiring a part of a person's body, for example, the eyes. The victim can lose the admired part or fall ill. In some places *mal de ojo* is thought to be prevented by touching the admired person, or it can be cured with eggs in a specific ritual. The symptoms of *mal de ojo* include headaches, fever, fatigue, and prostration.

2. *Empacho.* This disease, primarily seen in children, produces swelling of the abdomen as a result of intestinal blockage. It can be caused by overeating certain foods such as soft bread or bananas.

3. *Susto.* This is a disease of emotional origin. It is fright caused by natural phenomena such as lightning or loud noises. The symptoms have been described as insomnia, restlessness, and nervousness. It is a common folk disease that is difficult to cure, but it can be treated with herbal tea.

4. *Espanto.* This disease has symptoms similar to *susto.* It is fright caused by seeing supernatural spirits or events, and in the American slang, can be likened to being "spooked."

5. *Coraje.* This is rage, a response to a particular situation. The victim may continually scream, cry, or yell and display excessive hyperactivity.

Many Chicanos, when they are ill, may believe a folk medicine diagnosis rather than a Western diagnosis even though they may also seek help from a Western physician.

Health Superstitions

Chicanos believe to some degree a number of health-related superstitions. Three of these are the following:

1. There are specific foods that help good health and other foods that can produce poor health. An example of the former is tea made from fresh orange leaves; examples of the latter are rice and coffee, which should not be taken during an evening meal.

2. For a person to maintain good health the person must be in tune with God. Thus a person who is chronically ill is believed to have offended God and is therefore being punished.

3. Health to many Chicanos means being free of pain and being robust, even obese, rather than thin.

Chicanos are generally proud people, and those who are socially and economically deprived may well have low self-esteem and be reluctant to accept care for which they cannot pay. Therefore, Chicano patients in the hospital may not ask for help when they have pain; a young Mexican-American male may react with hostility rather than passivity because of his perception of self.

Chicanos also look upon the hospital as a place to die. Thus they may avoid hospitals when they can and may only enter with great fear and with the feeling that death is imminent.

Illness is generally regarded as not a personal affair but as a family affair. Therefore, when a person is ill, many relatives will generally gather around and visit. Restricting visitors can cause mistrust and needs to be dealt with in the context of illness as a matter for the entire family.

For nurses to be able to provide the Chicano patient and family with the care they require, it is important also to understand that as a cultural group they are very modest. Usually they consider bathing, defecating, and urinating to be very personal matters, and they may be shy about asking a nurse to leave at such times.

Diet

In folk tradition, food was thought of as either hot or cold, and certain illnesses were also considered to be either hot or cold. Herbs are also used for hot and cold problems.

Traditionally Chicanos eat food such as beans and tortillas. For hospitalized patients who are on a specific diet, this can present problems in menu planning. The reasons for a special diet should be thoroughly explained to the patient and the family.

SUMMARY

Although humanism is universal, its specific characteristics are learned and vary from one culture to another. Since North American society is composed of many cultural groups, it is important that nurses recognize the specific beliefs and values of different ethnic groups that relate to health and illness.

Several physical health problems are common to most ethnic minority groups. These include malnutrition, tuberculosis, neoplasms, and some digestive diseases. Other diseases that are not unique to any ethnic group occur with greater frequency among specific groups. Examples are the higher incidence of sickle cell anemia in blacks, gout in Puerto Ricans, and hypertension in Jews.

Variables also need to be considered in the provision of mental health care to individuals of ethnic minorities. Therapies provided often need to include not only the immediate family but also extended family members. Because behavior has individual and cultural components, both facets must be considered when assessing predisposing and precipitating causes of illness. Some feeling and behavior patterns are common to racial minority groups but are not necessarily unique to them. These include feelings of inferiority, which result in inadequate behavior compared to the dominant culture, and feelings of anger, which are generally withheld and suppressed. Many oppressed people will resort to selective inattention and overcompensation.

Social factors must also be considered in providing health care. General considerations for ethnic groups include possible language barriers, different food habits, and unique views of illness and methods of cure. Time orientations and male/female norms also vary. All of these factors directly influence the effectiveness of nursing care provided. Awareness of the specific differences in health-related beliefs and practices of various ethnic groups is also essential to nurses. Five large ethnic groups of North America are the Native Americans (American Indians), the blacks, the Chinese, the Jewish, and the Chicanos (Mexican-Americans). Each group is unique in relation to family orientation, concept of time, life and death, beliefs about cause of illness, curative rituals for illness, dietary habits, and specific health problems. The importance of understanding and accepting differences from one's own beliefs is emphasized.

SUGGESTED ACTIVITIES

1. With a group of nursing students of various ethnic and socioeconomic backgrounds, discuss and list some of the health practices or folk beliefs that you learned from your family or friends.

2. Select a patient in a clinical area that is of a different ethnic background from your own.

    a. Attempt to learn more about his or her unique customs and beliefs.

    b. Determine how the nursing care could be adjusted or accommodated to his or her differences.

3. Discuss with a group of people your attitudes about spiritualism and witchcraft practices as a means of treatment for health problems.

SUGGESTED READINGS

Campbell, Teresa, and Chang, Betty. April, 1973. Health care of the Chinese in America. *Nursing Outlook* 21(4):245–249.

This article includes some insights into Chinese beliefs and customs such as yin and yang, food habits, relationship of food to disease, practices during pregnancy, and attitudes about medications and hospitalization.

Berkowitz, Philip, and Berkowitz, Nancy S. November, 1967. The Jewish patient in the hospital. *American Journal of Nursing* 67:2335–2337.

This article explains some of the practices of Judaism in relation to the Sabbath, holy days, dietary laws, and synagogue practices.

Kniep-Hardy, Mary, and Burkhardt, Margaret A. January, 1977. Nursing the Navajo. *American Journal of Nursing* 77:95–96.

Suggestions are offered for adapting and individualizing nursing care for a Navajo patient. Several beliefs and customs are included.

Primeaux, Martha. January, 1977. Caring for the American Indian patient. *American Journal of Nursing* 77:91–94.

This article describes some common cultural beliefs that pertain to health care for Native Americans. Included are health rituals, child-rearing practices, and many other specific values and beliefs.

SELECTED REFERENCES

Beeson, Paul B., and McDermott, Walsh, eds. 1975. *Textbook of medicine*, 14th ed. Philadelphia: W. B. Saunders Co.

Brink, Pamela J., ed. 1976 *Transcultural nursing a book of readings*. Englewood Cliffs, New Jersey: Prentice-Hall, Inc.

Bush, Mary T., Ullom, Jean A., and Osborne, Oliver H. March–April, 1975. The meaning of mental health: a report of two ethnoscientific studies. *Nursing Research* 24(2):130–138.

Clark, Margaret. 1970. *A community study: health in the Mexican-American culture*, 2nd ed. Berkeley, Calif.: University of California Press.

Comer, James P., and Poussaint, Alvin F. 1975. *Black child care: how to bring up a healthy black child in America, a guide to emotional and psychological development*. New York: Simon and Schuster.

Dudley, Lavinia P., and Smith, John J., eds. 1970. *The American annual*. New York: Americana Corp.

Fawcett, Margot J., ed. 1977. *The Corpus almanac of Canada*. Toronto: Corpus Publishers Services.

Gonzalez, Hector Hugo. 1976. Health care needs of the Mexican American. In *Ethnicity and health care*. New York: National League for Nursing.

Leininger, Madeleine M. 1970. *Nursing and anthropology: two worlds to blend*. New York: John Wiley and Sons, Inc.

Leininger, Madeleine. 1974. Humanism, health and cultural values. In Leininger, Madeleine, ed. *Health care dimensions*. Philadelphia: F. A. Davis Co.

Martin, Betty J. W. 1976. Ethnicity and health care: Afro-Americans. In *Ethnicity and health care*. New York: National League for Nursing.

McVeigh, Frank J. May, 1970. The life conditions of Afro-Americans. *Afro-American Studies* 1:45–49.

Murillo-Rhode, Ildaura. 1976. Unique needs of ethnic minority clients in a multiracial society: a socio-cultural perspective. In *Affirmative action: toward quality nursing care for a multiracial society*. Kansas City, Missouri: American Nurses' Association.

Osborne, Oliver H. May–June, 1969. Anthropology and nursing: some common traditions and interests. *Nursing Research* 18(3):251–255.

Osborne, Oliver H. 1976. Unique needs of ethnic minority clients in a multiracial society: a psycho-social perspective. In *Affirmative action: toward quality nursing care for a multiracial society*. Kansas City, Missouri: American Nurses' Association.

Parreno, Sister Heide. 1976. Unique needs of ethnic minority clients in a multiracial society: a biological perspective. In *Affirmative action: toward quality nursing care for a multiracial society*. Kansas City, Missouri: American Nurses' Association.

Rotkovitch, Rachel. 1976. Ethnicity and health care—the Jewish heritage. In *Ethnicity and health care*. New York: National League for Nursing.

Spruce, Beryl B. 1972. The cultural patterns and values of the American Indian and their relation to health and illness. In *Becoming aware of cultural differences in nursing* (speeches presented during the 48th convention). Kansas City, Missouri: American Nurses' Association.

US Bureau of the Census. 1976. *Statistical Abstract of the United States*, 97th ed. Washington, D.C.

Wang, Rosalind M. 1976. Chinese Americans and health care. In *Ethnicity and health care*. New York: National League for Nursing.

West, Kelly, and Kalbsleisch, John. 1970. Diabetes in Central America. *Diabetes* XIX(5):656–663.

Wood, Rosemary. 1976. The American Indian and health. In *Ethnicity and health care*. New York: National League for Nursing.

CHAPTER 10

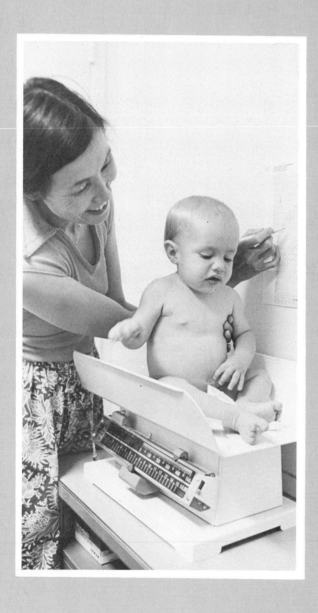

EARLY GROWTH AND DEVELOPMENT

THE PRESCHOOLER (FOUR AND FIVE YEARS)

Physical Development

Behavior

Needs

THE SCHOOL-AGE CHILD (SIX TO TWELVE YEARS)

Physical Development

Behavior

Needs

OBJECTIVES

Discuss some of the theories and classifications of human development.

- Discuss the fundamental principles of growth and development.

- Describe the growth cycles.

- Explain the pertinent physical growth changes and developmental processes that occur during the intrauterine stage and on to childhood.

- Describe the nurse's role in meeting the needs of people during these selected life stages.

- Discuss ways that the nurse can assist or help people to prevent various health problems that are more likely to occur during these stages.

A knowledge of growth and development is essential for nurses. The terms *growth* and *development* are often used interchangeably, but they are different. *Growth* refers to an increase in weight and height, an increase in physical size. *Development* is the increasing capacity and skill of a person to function. *Maturation* is a type of development referring specifically to the development of traits, which are passed on from one generation to another by the genes.

Each person demonstrates an individual *rate* of growth. The *pattern* of growth, on the other hand, is more predictable; for example, infants stand before they walk. Growth and development include physical, social, mental, emotional, sexual, and spiritual aspects, all of which are interrelated.

Growth and development in this chapter and the next will be discussed in the following stages:

Intrauterine
The Neonate (Birth to 28 Days)
The Infant (One Month to One Year)
The Toddler (One to Three Years)
The Preschooler (Four and Five Years)
The School-Age Child (Six to Twelve Years)
The Adolescent
Adulthood
  The Young Adult
  The Pregnant Woman
  The Middle Aged Adult
The Elderly Person

STAGES OF DEVELOPMENT

A great deal has been written regarding human development. The intention of this chapter and the next is to provide nursing students with a brief overview of some of the theories of development and with the essential knowledge associated with growth and development that is considered important for nursing students. The student is referred to the suggested readings and references at the end of both chapters for additional information.

Theories of Development

Piaget

Jean Piaget has developed theories that are chiefly concerned with cognitive or intellectual development. Piaget proposes that cognitive development is an orderly process in which the person builds four successive stages. Each of the four developmental stages is formed through three primary methods: assimilation, accommodation, and adaptation.

Assimilation is the process whereby humans are able to encounter and react to new situations by using the mechanism they already possess. In this way people are able to acquire new knowledge and skills as well as insights into the world around them.

Accommodation is a process of change whereby the person's cognitive processes have matured sufficiently so that they can adjust and therefore solve problems that were unsolvable before. This adjustment is possible chiefly because of new knowledge that has been assimilated.

Adaptation or coping behavior occurs when the person possesses the ability to handle the demands made by the environment.

Piaget's cognitive developmental process is divided into four major stages: the sensorimotor stage, the preoperational stage, the concrete operations stage, and the formal operations period. A person develops through each of these stages, and each stage has its own unique characteristics (see Table 10-1).

Freud

Sigmund Freud, whose writings and research were very popular in the 1930s, developed a number of concepts and stages of development that are still used today. The concepts of the unconscious mind, defense mechanisms, and the id, ego, and superego are Freud's. The *unconscious mind* refers to the mental life of a person of which the person is unaware. This concept of the unconscious was one of Freud's major contributions to the field of psychiatry. *Defense mechanisms*, or *adaptive mechanisms* as they are more commonly called today, are the result of the conflicts between inner impulses as well as the subsequent anxiety which develops. The *id* is the source of instinctive and unconscious urges, which Freud considered chiefly sexual in nature. The id is also the source of all pleasure and gratification. The *ego* is

Table 10-1.   Piaget's Developmental Stages (Cognitive)

Stage	Ages	Significant Behavior
Sensorimotor	0 to 2 years	Preverbal behavior; coordinates simple motor actions; perceives through different senses
Preoperational	3 to 7 years	Egocentrism; associates objects representative of concepts; elaborates concepts; asks questions
Concrete operations	7 to 11 or 12 years	Solves concrete problems; begins to understand relationships such as size; understands right and left; cognizant of viewpoints
Formal operations	11 to 15 or 16 years	Lives in the present and the nonpresent; concerned about the possible; capable of scientific reasoning; can use formal logic

formed by the person in order to make effective contact with these social and physical needs. Through the ego, the id impulses are satisfied. The third system in the personality, according to Freud, is the *superego.* This is the conscience of the personality, and it forms the control to inhibit the id. The action of the superego can result in a person's feelings of guilt, shame, and inhibition. See Chapter 8, "Stress and Adaptation," for additional information on adaptive processes and mental mechanisms (pages 121 to 131).

Freud's stages of development are:

1. oral—the first year
2. anal—the second and third years
3. phallic—the fourth and fifth years
4. latency—the school-age years (6 to 12 years)
5. pregenital and genital—adolescence and adult years (12 years and after)

He proposed that the underlying motivation to human development is an energy form or life instinct, which he called *libido.*

Each of these stages of development during the first five years is defined in terms of the ways of reaction of a part of the body. During the first or *oral stage,* the mouth is the principal area of activity. It is the main source of pleasure, primarily as a result of eating. It is also at this time that feelings of dependency arise, and they tend, according to Freud, to persist throughout life. The *anal stage* occurs during the second and third years, when the child is learning toilet training. Many character traits such as creativity, stinginess, and cruelty are said to have their sources during this stage. The *phallic stage* is the time when sexual and aggressive feelings associated with the genital organs come into focus. Masturbation offers pleasure at this time, and the Oedipus or Electra complex occurs. The *Oedipus complex* consists of the male child's attraction for his mother and hostile attitudes toward his father. The *Electra complex* consists of the female child's attraction for her father and hostility toward her mother. The *latency stage* consists of the quiet years during which impulses tend to be repressed. Following this comes adolescence and the reactivation of the pregenital impulses. The person usually displaces these impulses and subsequently passes into the final stage of maturity of an adult, the *genital stage.*

Erikson

Erik H. Erikson has described eight stages of development (see Table 10-2). These stages specifically relate to psychosocial development. Life is pictured as a sequence of levels of achievement. Successful achievement of these developmental levels can be supportive to the person's ego; failure to achieve can be damaging. The ego is the conscious core of the personality.

Erikson further stated that although one stage may be attained, the person may fall back and need to approach it again. His eight stages reflect both positive and negative aspects of the critical life periods. The resolution of the conflicts at each stage enables the person to function effectively in society.

Havighurst

Robert J. Havighurst established six periods or stages of development. The developmental tasks which he includes are both psychosocial and motor. There are also a number of tasks (nine or ten) delineated for each age period. Havighurst, unlike Erikson, proposes that once a task is mastered, the person retains it

Table 10-2.   Erikson's Eight Stages of Development

Age	Conflict	Some Positive Behavior
1. Early infancy (birth to 1 year)	Basic trust versus mistrust	Shows affection, gratification, recognition
2. Later infancy (1 to 3 years)	Autonomy versus shame and doubt	Dependent upon parents but views self as a person apart from parents
3. Early childhood (4 to 5 years)	Initiative versus guilt	Shows imagination, imitates adults, tests reality, anticipates roles
4. Middle childhood (6 to 11 years)	Industry versus inferiority	Has sense of duty, develops social and scholastic competencies, undertakes real tasks
5. Puberty and adolescence (12 to 20 years)	Identity versus role confusion	Is self-certain, experiences sexual polarization, is role experimenter, has ideologic commitment
6. Early adulthood (20 to 40 years)	Intimacy versus isolation	Shows capacity to commit oneself to others and capacity to love and work
7. Middle adulthood (41 to 64 years)	Generativity versus stagnation	Productive and creative for self and others
8. Late adulthood (65 years on)	Integrity versus despair	Appreciates continuing of past, present and future, accepts life cycle and style, accepts death

Table 10-3.   Havighurst's Six Periods of Developmental Tasks

Period	Tasks
1. Infancy and childhood	Learning to walk; learning to talk; learning to take solid foods; learning to control the elimination of body wastes; learning sex differences and sexual modesty; achieving physiologic stability; forming simple concepts of sound and physical reality; learning to relate oneself emotionally to parents, siblings, and other people; learning to distinguish right and wrong and developing a conscience
2. Middle childhood	Learning physical skills necessary for ordinary games; building wholesome attitudes toward oneself as a growing organism; learning to get along with age mates; learning an appropriate masculine or feminine social role; developing fundamental skills in reading, writing, and calculating; developing concepts necessary for everyday living; developing conscience, morality, and a scale of values; achieving personal independence; developing attitudes toward social groups and institutions
3. Adolescence	Accepting one's physique and accepting a masculine or feminine role; developing new relations with age mates of both sexes; achieving emotional independence of parents and other adults; achieving assurance of economic independence; selecting and preparing for an occupation; developing intellectual skills and concepts necessary for civic independence; preparing for marriage and family life; acquiring values and ethical systems in harmony with an adequate scientific world picture; desiring and achieving socially responsible behavior
4. Early adulthood	Selecting a mate; learning to live with a marriage partner; starting a family; rearing children; managing a home; getting started in an occupation; taking on civic responsibility; finding a congenial social group
5. Middle age	Achieving adult civic and social responsibility; establishing and maintaining an economic standard of living; assisting teenage children to become responsible and happy adults; developing adult leisure-time activities; relating oneself to one's spouse as a person; accepting and adjusting to physiologic changes of middle age; adjusting to aging parents
6. Later maturity	Adjusting to decreasing physical strength and health; adjusting to retirement and reduced income; adjusting to death of spouse; establishing an explicit affiliation with one's age group; meeting social and civic obligations; establishing satisfactory physical living arrangements

for a lifetime. He also states that the developmental tasks must be achieved in order for the person to be successful with later tasks (Havighurst 1967:2).

Havighurst's six periods of development are:

1. infancy and early childhood
2. middle childhood
3. adolescence
4. early adulthood
5. middle age
6. later maturity

See Table 10-3 showing the periods and the related developmental tasks.

Duvall

Duvall presents developmental tasks in eight categories through the family life cycle. The eight stages are: married couple, childbearing years, pre-school-age years, school-age years, teenage years, families as launching centers, middle-aged parents, and aging family members. The developmental tasks in these categories are largely family oriented.

Principles of Development

There are a number of principles of development, which are fundamental to understanding growth and development.

1. Growth is a continual process determined by maturation, which is predetermined for the individual. Each person normally passees through each successive stage of development. On occasion there may be individual exceptions, usually minimal, which are usually due to environmental influences.

2. All humans follow the same pattern of growth and development, but each person does so in his or her own way. These individual differences are due chiefly to three broad factors: the rate or way in which the maturational process takes place, inherited factors, and environmental influences, which include learning.

3. Human development is the result of both learning and maturation. Learning can either help or hinder the maturational process depending upon what is learned. Maturation is the growth of the functional aspects of the body. The maturation of a person is chiefly dependent upon the genes, which are inherited. Therefore the maturational rate is inherited, although it can be affected by a number of factors such as nutrition and parental attitudes.

4. Each stage in life has certain traits that are typical of that stage. For example, Piaget suggests that in the sensorimotor stage (birth to two years) children learn to coordinate simple motor tasks (see Table 10-1).

5. During infancy and early childhood basic attitudes, lifestyles, traits, and patterns of growth are formed. It is believed that during the early years basic personality patterns are formed, and the role the child plays in the family largely determines whether the child becomes a leader, a follower, or a nonresponder in life. The person's physical and psychologic traits have their bases in the early stages of living.

6. As children develop they are faced with the need to master certain skills and to learn certain behavior patterns; these are called *developmental tasks.* Some of the tasks they need to learn are pertinent to survival, such as learning to take solid food (see Table 10-3). Others are secondary to survival but pertinent to living in a society, such as learning to get along with peers. The expectations of the culture to which the individual person belongs change with each stage of development. For example, a two-year-old child is not expected to be able to write with a pencil, but a six-year-old child is expected to learn this skill.

7. The readiness of a child to learn is dependent upon the maturation process. The body must mature sufficiently before a person can perform certain skills. For example, fine motor coordination must already be developed before a child can learn to write. Eyesight must also be sufficiently developed before the child can read.

8. Development proceeds generally from the head downward, and from the trunk of the body to the extremities. Thus before a child walks, the child can first hold her head up and then sit up without assistance.

9. Reactions of a person are initially gross and undifferentiated and then become more specific. For example, a baby's initial response is one of crying; however, it gradually becomes more specific in that the child learns to laugh and to cry and then to speak words.

10. Development is unevenly paced. For example, a child's physical growth is accelerated during the first year and again in the preadolescent period.

11. Culture, ethnicity, and race can affect growth and development. For example, Oriental and black children tend to be smaller than white children of the same age. In addition, cognitive development differs greatly in various subcultures. For example, American Indian children are often not raised with sched-

ules, and thus the concept of time is often slower to develop in them than it is for white children. The latter are usually raised with the day marked by specific activities, which they learn to associate with time.

There is a tendency for children to be preoccupied with the skills they are learning at that particular time. For example, when children are learning to talk, they will talk a great deal, thus practicing word pronunciation.

GROWTH CYCLES

Growth is a predictable rhythmic progression; it does not occur regularly, but it does occur in cycles. There are four distinct growth periods, two in which there is rapid growth and two in which there is slow growth. The first occurs from birth and lasts until about two years; this is a period of rapid growth. The

second period, terminating at about puberty, is a period of slow growth. The third period is one of rapid growth again, beginning between 8 and 11 years and terminating at about 16 or 17 years. The fourth is a slow growth period from 17 years until maturity (about 21 years).

INTRAUTERINE DEVELOPMENT

Intrauterine development extends for approximately 9 calendar months (10 lunar months) or 38 to 40 weeks, depending upon the method of calculation. (A lunar month is 28 days.) If the time is calculated from the day of conception, this stage of life is considered to be 38 weeks or 9½ lunar months. If the time is calculated from the first day of the last menstrual period, its average length is 10 lunar months or 40 weeks. This time span is not precise, however. Many pregnancies terminate within one or two weeks before or after the estimated date. To determine an expected day of confinement (EDC) according to Nägele's rule, count back three calendar months from the first day of the last menstrual period and add seven days. For example, if the last menstrual period began on April 5, count back three months to January 5 and add seven days. The EDC is then January 12 of the next year.

For conception to take place, the ovum leaves its graafian follicle (ovulation). It is surrounded by a mucopolysaccharide fluid and is propelled along the fallopian tube by cilia of the tube. An ovum is capable of fertilization within 24 to 48 hours after ovulation. At the time of ovulation the viscosity of the cervical mucus is reduced. This facilitates the penetration of the spermatozoa.

The normal ejaculation of semen of a male contains several million spermatozoa. These spermatozoa move by flagella and reach the cervix of the uterus within 90 seconds. The spermatozoa cluster around the ovum, and hyaluronidase is released,

which dissolves the corona radiata, part of the mucopolysaccharide fluid. One sperm penetrates the cell membrane of the ovum, resulting in conception. (For additional information on conception, see Chapter 31.)

Important in intrauterine development is the formation of the placenta, which normally starts at about the third week. Amniotic fluid surrounds the fetus in utero. A pregnant woman usually has about 30 ml of fluid at 10 weeks and perhaps 1000 ml at 38 weeks, although this is variable.

The intrauterine stage of life can be divided into two phases, the embryonic and the fetal (Vaughan et al. 1975:17). The embryonic phase is the period during which the fertilized ovum develops into an organism that has most of the features of the human form. This period is considered to extend for either the first eight weeks, or the first 12 weeks or first trimester of pregnancy. Those authorities who consider the embryonic phase to be 12 weeks believe that some organs do develop after eight weeks.

This embryonic phase derives its name from the Greek word *embryo*, meaning "swell." The fetal phase extends from the first eight or 12 weeks until birth. The term *fetus* is Latin, meaning "young one." From about 20 weeks on, the fetus is considered viable, that is, able or likely to live if born. Before this time the fetus is considered previable or unlikely to live if born.

Traditionally pregnancy has been divided into three periods called *trimesters*, each of which is about three months in length. Each trimester marks certain landmarks for developmental changes in the mother and the fetus. The phases of intrauterine life, therefore, can also be considered in trimestral terms. The embryonic phase is the first trimester, and the fetal phase includes the second and third trimesters.

Embryonic Phase (Eight Weeks or First Trimester)

The rapidity of cell division and differentiation of the fertilized ovum (zygote) is remarkable. By 12 weeks the fetus weighs 15 to 20 gm and is about 7.5–9.0 cm (3–3.5 inches) long. It has a sex that can be distinguished, a heartbeat, and a definite human form. The head is very large, limbs are small with identifiable fingers and toes, facial features such as nose, mouth, and ears are distinct, and some ossification of the bones has started.

Within the first three weeks of life, tissues differentiate into three layers—the *ectoderm* (outer layer), *mesoderm* (inner layer), and *endoderm* (inner layer). The ectoderm and endoderm are formed in the second week; the mesoderm forms in between these two in the third week. From these layers are formed all of the body's complex organs and systems as a series of outpouchings, inpouchings, foldings, and tubular formations. Examples follow:

1. The ectoderm: Nervous system
   Sensory organs
   Epidermis, including hair
   Nails and teeth enamel
   Glands
2. The mesoderm: Dermis
   Skeleton
   Connective tissue
   Vascular system
   Genitourinary system
   Spleen
   Most muscles (skeletal and smooth)
3. The endoderm: Lining of respiratory and digestive tracts
   Bladder
   Liver
   Pancreas
   Thyroid and parathyroids
   Thymus gland
   Eustachian tubes

Concurrently during this phase of development three other events occur:

1. The embryo is implanted.
2. Placental function starts. The *placenta* is a flat disc-shaped organ, which is highly vascular. It normally implants in the upper segment of the muscular wall of the uterus. Its functions are to exchange nutrients and gases between the fetus and the mother.
3. The fetal membranes differentiate.

A summary of this embryonic phase follows:

Lunar month	Lunar week	Developmental occurrences
1	4	Cells divide actively from zygote. Endoderm and ectoderm form (second week). Mesoderm forms (third week). Heartbeat begins (fourth week). Digestive tract begins to form.
2	8	Brain develops and neurologic activity begins (eighth week). Isolated local muscle responses can be stimulated. Fetus weighs 1 gm (eighth week). Length is approximately 2.5 cm (1 inch). Embryo has unmistakable human form.
3	12	Some swimming motions occur. Fingers and toes are differentiated. Fetal circulatory system develops its final form (tenth week). Sex is determinable (twelfth week). Rudimentary kidneys form. Urine is excreted into bladder. Bile flow begins. Sockets develop in the jawbone for baby teeth. Fetus weighs 15–20 gm (twelfth week). Length is approximately 9 cm (3½ inches). Eyelids develop and fuse.

Fetal Phase

This phase of development is characterized by a period of rapid growth in the size of the fetus. Haase's rule offers a guide for estimating the approximate size of the fetus in centimeters each month of the intra-uterine life. For the first five months, the length of the fetus is determined by squaring the number of lunar months. For example, a three-month fetus is approximately 9 (3 × 3) cm long, and a five-month fetus is 25 (5 × 5) cm long. After the fifth month the size is estimated by multiplying the month by five. Thus a seven-month fetus is 35 (5 × 7) cm long, and a nine-month fetus is 45 (5 × 9) cm long.

At the end of the second trimester or six lunar months, the fetus resembles a small baby, 30 cm (12 inches) long and weighing about 0.67 kg (1.5 lb). Because very little fat is present beneath the skin, the skin appears wrinkled, red, and transparent. Underlying vessels are visible. A protective covering called *vernix caseosa* begins to develop over the skin. This is a white cheeselike substance that adheres to the skin and can become ⅛ inch thick by birth. *Lanugo*, a fine downy hair, also covers the body. It is during this period (five months) that the mother first perceives movement by the fetus and the first fetal heartbeat may be heard. The amount of activity varies among fetuses. There is some evidence that activity may be related to the mother's emotions by the transfer of epinephrine and other hormones through the placenta. Of the fetuses that are born before or at the end of six months, very few survive.

At the end of the third trimester (9½ lunar months) the fetus has developed to approximately 50 cm (20 inches) and 3.2–3.4 kg (7.0–7.5 lb). Newborn infants that are black, Indian, or Oriental often have lower birth weights than whites. The lanugo has disappeared, and the skin is a more normal color and appears less wrinkled. More subcutaneous fat makes the baby look more rotund; in fact, the latter two months in utero are largely devoted to accumulating weight. The fetus born in the last trimester prior to full term has varying chances for survival. Those born at seven months weigh about 1.1 kg (2.5 lb) and have approximately a 10% chance of survival; at eight months the fetus weighs about 1.8 kg (4 lb) and has a 75% chance.

Following is a summary of the fetal phase of development during the second and third trimesters:

Lunar month	Lunar week	Developmental occurrences
4	16	Nail growth on fingers and toes begins. Swallowing movements can be noted. Flowing movements can be produced by stimulation.
5	20	Respiratory movements may be seen, but alveolar structures are not well developed. Grasp reflex is evident. Lanugo covers the entire body. Heartbeat is strong (fetal heart sound may be heard). Meconium (intestinal contents) is present. Movement is now perceived by mother.
6	24	Skin develops vernix caseosa. Weak phonation may accompany respiratory movements. Fetus is able to protrude and purse both lips.
7	28	Fetus can actively suck. Grasp reflex is well developed. Earliest signs of Moro reflex can be elicited.
8	32	Skin is red and wrinkled. Vernix caseosa and lanugo are still present.
9	36	Subcutaneous fat deposition increases. Body becomes more rotund. Lanugo disappears.
10	40	Development is same as for ninth lunar month.

THE NEONATE (BIRTH TO 28 DAYS)

During the first 28 days of life the chief task of neonates is to adapt to their new environment. The first step in this process is the establishment of maintenance of breathing, an accomplishment that must occur within 30 seconds of birth if asphyxia is to be avoided. At birth neonates are completely dependent upon others for their life; they have no voluntary control over their movements, and their only emotion is a state of excitement. Their life is chiefly dominated by reflexes.

Physical Development

Appearance

Newborn babies appear in reality different from the usual pictorial newborns (see Figure 10-1). They usually have puffy eyelids and a flattish, broad nose. The lower jaw appears small and the neck very short. The shoulders slope, and the abdomen appears large and rounded with a protruding umbilical stump. The legs are bowed and appear short and out of proportion to the head, which makes up 21% of the total body surface. The arms appear long in proportion to the rest of the body. Lanugo may be apparent, particularly on the shoulders, back, and extremities. The vernix caseosa is obvious in the skin folds but will rub off naturally after a few days.

The skin of newborns is thin and appears delicate and often pink or reddish. They may have milia, which are small white spots on the nose and forehead. These are collections of sebaceous secretions, and they usually disappear about three weeks after birth.

Black, Oriental, and dark-skinned babies usually have bluish brown areas on their lower back called Mongolian spots. These will fade without treatment. Physiologic jaundice of the newborn generally occurs between three and four days after birth because of excess red blood cells in the baby's blood, which are left over from fetal life. This jaundice normally disappears by two weeks. Jaundice that occurs within 24 hours of birth, however, must be monitored carefully because it may be caused by an incompatibility between the baby's blood and the mother's blood.

Newborn babies can be assessed by the Apgar scoring system. It provides a numerical indicator as to

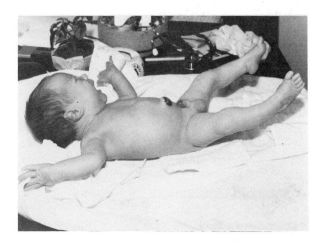

Figure 10-1.   A newborn baby showing the short bowed legs, protruding abdomen, and the drying umbilical cord. (Courtesy City of Vancouver Health Department.)

physical status, that is, to the baby's capacities to adapt to extrauterine life. Each of five signs has a maximum score of 2, so that the total score achievable is 10. A score under 7 suggests that the baby is having difficulty, and a score under 4 indicates that the baby's condition is critical. Apgar scoring is usually carried out 60 seconds after birth and is repeated in 5 minutes. Those with very low scores require special resuscitative measures and care. See Table 10-4.

Weight

The birth weight of approximately two thirds of babies born at full term is from 2.7–3.8 kg (6.0–8.5 lb). They generally double their birth weights by four to

Table 10-4.   Apgar Scoring System to Assess the Newborn

	Score		
Sign	0	1	2
1. Heart rate	Absent	Slow (below 100 per minute)	Above 100 per minute
2. Respirations	Absent	Slow, irregular	Regular rate, crying
3. Muscle tone	Flaccid	Some flexion of extremities	Active movements
4. Reflex irritability	None	Grimace	Cries
5. Color	Body pale or cyanotic	Body pink (for black babies, pink mucous membranes), extremities blue	Body completely pink in whites, pink mucous membranes in blacks

Table 10-5. Average Normal Vital Signs and Measurements of Newborns

Weight	3.4 kg or 3400 gm (7.5 lb)
Length	50 cm (20 inches)
Head circumference	34–36 cm (13.5–14.5 inches)
Heart rate	120–140 beats/min
Blood pressure	40–70 systolic
Temperature	36.5–37° C (97.7–98.6° F)
Respiratory rate	30–40/min

six weeks of age; by two years they approximately quadruple their birth weights. For example, a 2.7 kg (6 lb) baby at birth can be expected to weigh 5.4 kg (12 lb) by six months and about 10.8 kg (24 lb) at two years. There are a number of factors that can affect birth weights, such as the mother's nutrition and maternal age.

Initially after birth, a baby loses weight due to fluid loss and the excretion of meconium from the intestines. This weight loss is normally regained in about one week, and the loss is perfectly normal. From that time on a baby usually gains weight. For normal average measurements and average vital signs see Table 10-5.

Length

The average newborn in the United States is about 50 cm (20 inches) long. The usual range is from 47.5 to 52.5 cm (19 to 21 inches). Female babies are on the average smaller than male babies.

Head Growth

The head of the newborn is normally measured just above the eyes and around the occipital protuberance. A knowledge of the head measurements is important in assessing the normalcy of head growth. On an average a newborn's head will measure from 33.7 to 35.0 cm (13.5 to 14 inches) in circumference. Interestingly the chest circumference is generally about an inch less.

There are six fontanelles at birth, two of which are palpable. A *fontanelle* is an unossified area of the cranium. The anterior fontanelle lies midline between the two frontal bones and the two parietal bones. It is the largest, and it normally closes at about one year (10 to 18 months). The posterior fontanelle

lies between the parietal bones and the occipital bone, also in the midline. It closes between four and eight weeks after birth. For additional information see Chapter 14, pages 272 to 273.

Teeth

Newborn babies are normally born without visible teeth. At about five to six months the first teeth will appear, and at the end of two years babies are likely to have between 16 and 20 (all) of their deciduous teeth. It is during this period as well that the permanent teeth begin to calcify with the exception of the second and third molars.

Vital Signs

Newborns have unstable vital signs. Their temperature fluctuates from 36.1–37.8°C (97–100°F) because their heat regulating system is not fully developed. The pulse of the baby at birth ranges from 120–160 beats/min. Respirations are irregular, shallow, and quiet, ranging from 35–50/min. Blood pressure of the newborn normally ranges from 40–70 mm Hg (millimeters of mercury) systolic (see Table 10-5).

Meconium

Meconium is the first fecal material passed by the newborn. It normally appears up to 24 hours after birth and is black, tarry, odorless, and sticky. Transitional stools, which follow for about a week, are generally greenish yellow; they contain mucus and are loose.

Senses

The newborn infant is sensitive to touch. Through this the newborn perceives warmth, love, and security as well as the converse of these. The newborn is also sensitive to temperature extremes and pain; however, babies react diffusely and cannot isolate the discomfort. The pain of an open safety pin in the buttock, for example, will not be isolated to the buttock.

Visual abilities at birth are present; the newborn can follow large moving objects and can react to changes in the intensity of light. The baby blinks in response to bright light and to sound.

The pupils of the newborn respond slowly, and the eyes cannot focus on close objects. Hearing is indistinct at birth. This is because of the retention of fluid in the middle ear. The newborn does not differentiate sounds for some time but will have a startle reaction (Moro reflex) to a loud noise (see "Reflex

Ability"). The senses of smell and taste are not developed, although the newborn reacts to acid, bitter, salt, and sweet tastes by grimacing.

Reflex Ability

The reflexes of the newborn are unconscious, involuntary responses. They are neither learned nor consciously carried out. They are nervous system reflexes as a result of a number of stimuli. The degree of stimulation that is required to produce a reflex, for example the sucking reflex, varies considerably between individual newborns. Some newborns respond with vigor to the slightest stimulus, some babies respond slowly, and others are somewhere in between.

Nine main reflexes are normally present at birth. In addition, actions such as yawning, stretching, sneezing, burping, and hiccupping are all present at birth. Other reflexes are rooting, sucking, swallowing, Moro, palmar grasp, plantar, tonic neck, placing, and stepping.

The *rooting and sucking reflexes* are both involved in the feeding process. The former is elicited by touching the baby's cheek; this causes the baby's head to turn to the side that was touched. The sucking reflex occurs when the baby's lips are touched. The swallowing reflex can be observed in that the infant will swallow any liquid obtained from sucking.

The *Moro reflex* (startle reflex) is often assessed in order to estimate the maturity of the central nervous system. A loud noise, a sudden change in position, or an abrupt jarring of the crib elicits this reflex. The infant reacts by extending both arms and legs outward with the fingers spread, then suddenly retracting the limbs. Often the infant cries at the same time.

The *palmar grasp reflex* occurs when a small object is placed against the palm of the hand, which causes the fingers to curl around it. The plantar grasp reflex is similar in that an object placed just beneath the toes causes them to curl around it.

The *tonic neck reflex* (TNR) or fencing reflex is a postural reflex. When a baby turns his head to the right side, for example, while lying on his back, the left side of the body shows a flexing of the left arm and the left leg. This reflex is observed during the first week after birth.

The *placing reflex* occurs when a baby is held vertically with one leg away from the other. The other leg is then moved to touch the edge of a table. The baby automatically flexes her knee and tries to place her leg on the surface of the table.

The *stepping reflex* (walking or dancing reflex) can be elicited by holding the baby upright so that the feet touch a flat surface. The legs then move up and down as if the baby were walking. This reflex usually disappears at about two months.

A newborn baby also has a positive *Babinski reflex.* When the sole of the foot is stroked, the big toe raises and the other toes fan out.

Infant reflexes disappear during the first year of life. After this period the infant exhibits a negative Babinski, that is, the toes curl downward unless brain damage is evident.

Behavior

Motor Development

Motor development refers to the development of the baby's ability to move and to control the body. Movement begins before birth at about the third month when the fetus is able to move arms and legs spontaneously. After birth, activity increases gradually to include sucking, breathing, swallowing, and uncoordinated body movement. Newborn babies defecate and urinate with no controls.

Language and Speech Development

After birth babies cry when they are uncomfortable, usually because they are hungry. By one month they begin to make cooing sounds.

Sleep

Newborns can be expected to sleep from 18 to 22 hours a day. It is normal during sleep for them to suck and move their arms around. They usually awaken about every four hours, eat, and then go back to sleep.

Emotional Development

In newborn babies the capacity to react emotionally is already present. The first sign of emotion is usually that of excitement in response to a strong external stimulus, for example, a loud noise. This response becomes differentiated into a response of pleasure and one of displeasure. Pleasure can be elicited by rocking or patting, while displeasure can be elicited by an abrupt change of position.

At one month the emotional responses are generally restricted to tension and occasional panic. The latter is exhibited by crying, arching the back, and flexing and extending the extremities. The infant also experiences satisfaction chiefly from nourishment and when cuddled, held, and rocked. Newborn babies have no concept of body image. This starts later, often when they first see themselves in a mirror.

Learning Mental Mechanisms

Mental mechanisms are behavioral responses that are learned. They assist a person to adjust to the environment, and they assist in emotional development. Neonates have not learned any mental mechanisms. When babies are born, they are neither moral nor immoral. They are, in fact, nonmoral in that their behavior has been neither guided nor influenced by moral standards. A person can acquire morals only by identifying with a definite religion or philosophy. People learn morals from their parents, siblings, peers, and other significant persons.

Needs

Neonates have five special needs after their respirations are established. These are stabilization of body temperature, eye care, cord care, protection against infections, and nourishment.

Stabilization of Body Temperature

After birth a newborn's body temperature drops, usually due to the lower temperature of the delivery room as compared to that inside the uterus. Failure to provide warmth at this time can result in an increased metabolic rate, which, if prolonged, can result in an increased consumption of glucose, subsequent hypoglycemia, and consequent brain damage. The provision of external heat by using hot-water bottles or an incubator will assist newborns to establish a normal temperature. They continue to require protection from abrupt temperature changes because their temperature regulation is poorly developed. A room temperature of between 20.0–24.4°C (60–76°F), free of drafts, is considered to be appropriate.

Eye Care

After the baby is born, it is customary in most places to treat the eyes with a germicide that will destroy the gonorrhea organism that can be present in the baby's eyes if the mother is infected. The traditional germicide used is a 1% solution of silver nitrate, two drops in each eye. After a few minutes the eyes are irrigated with a warm normal saline (physiologic salt) solution to remove the excess silver nitrate and precipitate the remaining silver nitrate. Today penicillin is also used. It is administered as an ophthalmic ointment to the eye or intramuscularly.

Cord Care

During the first 24 hours of life the cord needs to be observed for bleeding. The cord usually heals in about one week by dry healing. It is customary to cleanse the cord daily with a 60% alcohol solution to facilitate the healing process and prevent infection.

Protection Against Infection

Although newborns have some protective antibodies from their mother, they have very little resistance to infection. For this reason it is customary for nurses to wash their hands before handling a baby, and in some areas masks are also worn. If a person has a respiratory infection or a skin infection, contact with a newborn baby is normally avoided.

Nourishment

Newborn babies may become hungry shortly after they are born, or they may not develop an appetite for one or two days. Behavior such as restlessness, crying, and moving the head can indicate hunger. For information on infant feeding see Chapter 25.

THE INFANT (ONE MONTH TO ONE YEAR)

The period of infancy is one of tremendous growth. This is the initial stage in the growth of a child. See Table 10-2 for common terms used to describe growth stages. One-year-old babies should weigh about three times their birth weight and may be able to walk with help.

Physical Development

Weight

Infants are twice their birth weight by six months and three times their birth weight by 12 months.

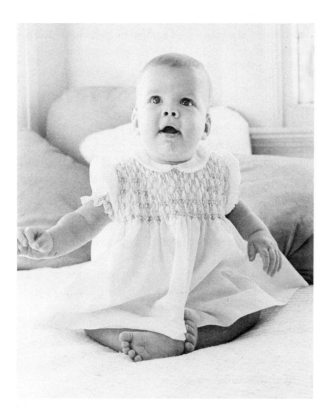

Figure 10-2. An infant sits without support at six months of age.

Height

By six months they gain another 13.75 cm (5.5 inches). By 12 months they add another 7.5 cm (3 inches). This increase is largely influenced by the baby's size at birth and by nutrition.

Head Growth

By 12 months head circumference has increased about 33% over the birth size.

The posterior fontanelle between the parietal bones and the occipital bone closes from four to eight weeks after birth. The anterior fontanelle (between the frontal and parietal bones) closes between 10 and 18 months.

Teeth

At about five to six months the infant's first teeth appear.

Vital Signs

Pulse averages 120–150/min at one month and 100–140/min at 12 months. Respirations are 30–60/min at one month and 20–40/min at 12 months. Temperature is between 36.1 and 37.8°C (97–100°F).

Senses

By three months vision develops so that both eyes are coordinated both horizontally and vertically. At four months the infant recognizes familiar objects and follows moving objects.

Behavior

Motor Development

By three months infants can raise the head from a prone position, and by six months they can sit without support. See Figure 10-2. They can turn the pages of a book and stand alone for a moment at 12 months. They also walk with help at 12 months and help with dressing.

Language Development

By one month an infant coos with pleasure and starts to babble a little by the second or third month. By six months they are chattering with nonsensical syllables, and this continues into the second year. By 12 months some children can say a few words they have heard, such as "Mummy" and "Daddy."

Sleep

By four months it is normal for infants to sleep eight hours or more at one period, and they require 16 to 18 hours each day. At six months the average amount of sleep required is about 12 hours at night and three to four hours during the day. At 12 months they sleep about 14 out of 24 hours, including one or two naps.

Social Development

By the second month infants enjoy playing with objects and with people. They vocalize in response to their mother's voice. By six months infants begin to recognize strangers, and by nine months they interact by playing peek-a-boo and similar games. By 12 months they recognize the meaning of "yes" and "no." Infants are still egocentric, concerned only with themselves.

Cognitive and Intellectual Development

Cognitive refers to such processes as remembering, thinking, perceiving, abstracting, and generalizing. It is the development of a logical method of looking at the world and utilizing perceptual and conceptual abilities. *Intelligence,* on the other hand, is the ability of the person to learn. *To learn* is to acquire knowledge, to retain knowledge, and to respond to new situations and to solve problems.

From four to eight months infants begin to have perceptual recognition. By six months they respond to new stimuli, and they remember certain objects and look for them for a short time. By 12 months infants have a concept of both space and time. They experiment to reach a goal such as a toy on a chair.

Emotional Development

At one month the emotional response of infants is generally restricted to tension and occasional panics. The latter are exhibited by crying, arching the back, and flexing and extending the extremities. Infants also experience satisfaction chiefly from nourishment and when they are cuddled, held, and rocked. At three months they need to suck in order to meet emotional needs and by six months other members of the family are important in meeting their emotional needs. At six months infants smile at their mother and family members, and they are able to wait a short time when they are hungry. By six months infants have a beginning sense of self and may often be seen pulling at their toes as they identify themselves.

Moral and Religious Development

At this early stage of development children associate right and wrong with pleasure and pain. What gives them pleasure is right, since they are too young to reason otherwise.

Needs

The needs of infants are primarily nutrition, sleep, play, immunizations, accident prevention, and mothering.

Nutrition

The early nourishment of infants is entirely liquid. Human milk is considered to be the ideal food for babies, and it is gradually supplemented with vitamins and more solid foods. The nurse is referred to Chapter 25 for further information on nutrition.

Sleep

Sleep is an important need of infants in that the bones, muscles, senses, nervous system, and internal organs develop during sleep. The sleep requirements of infants were discussed earlier in this chapter. The nurse is also referred to "Developmental Variables of Rest and Sleep," see Chapter 24.

Play

Infants occupy themselves, playing with their toes and hands and assuming many positions. Colorful hanging toys, particularly those which move, are important from birth to about three months. After that infants require toys they can grasp and put into the mouth but cannot swallow. Examples include a large wooden spoon, stuffed toys, and small plastic animals. By the time they are one year old, they want to pull things apart, such as building blocks, and move them around. They also enjoy playing in the sand or dirt where they can fill and dump small loads of sand. When infants begin to walk, they like push-and-pull toys such as wagons and pounding toys such as drums.

Immunizations

Immunizations are needed to protect infants from specific communicable diseases: diphtheria, pertussis, and tetanus. They are provided in a combined form (DPT)—diphtheria and tetanus toxoids and pertussis vaccine. Infants also require protection against poliomyelitis by the administration of oral polio vaccine. In the United States and Canada it is usual for infants to receive DPT and polio vaccine at approximately two, four, and six months. At one year of age, measles-rubella or a combined measles-mumps-rubella vaccine is recommended as well as a tuberculin test for contact with the tuberculosis bacillus. In some areas, smallpox vaccine is also given between the third and twelfth months. See Chapter 21 for further information.

Accident Prevention

Accidents are the leading cause of morbidity and mortality of children. Drowning, poisoning, suffocation, and falls are the major types of accidents experienced by infants. A baby may roll off a table when left alone. Thus infants need vigilant surveillance, since they are unable to protect themselves.

Mothering

Mothering is the sum total of care usually provided by a mother, but which can be provided by another person. It involves loving care, handling, stroking, and cuddling the child. From the third to the fifteenth month this mothering is essential, otherwise both physical and intellectual growth are impaired. Infants deprived of mothering in this stage of development will not learn to form significant relationships or to trust others. Erikson sees this stage as being characterized by the conflict of basic trust versus mistrust (Table 10-2). Sometimes infants who are institutionalized for a long period suffer maternal deprivation and fail to grow even though there is no organic reason. The effect of the deprivation will depend upon many factors, including the age of the child when deprived and the length of the deprivation. Maternal deprivation does not always cause a child to grow up as a delinquent or as an adult with many problems. People can learn and adapt to their environments in spite of this trauma.

THE TODDLER (ONE TO THREE YEARS)

Toddlers develop from having no voluntary control to being able to both walk and speak. They also learn to control their bladder and bowels, and they acquire all kinds of information about their environment.

Physical Development

Appearance

Two-year-old children lose the baby look (see Figure 10-3). Their growth rate slows from the previous rate. Toddlers are usually chubby. The face appears small in comparison to the skull; but as the toddler grows, the face appears to grow from under the skull and appears to be better proportioned. The brain has accomplished 70% of its growth by age two years.

Growth

During the second year the growing rate usually slows and toddlers may gain only another 11.25 cm (4.5 inches). At two years of age toddlers are likely to have between 16 and 20 (all) of their deciduous teeth. It is also during this period that the permanent teeth begin to calcify with the exception of the second and third molars.

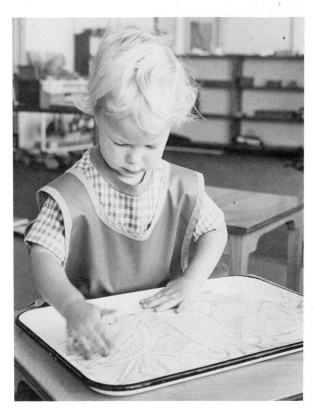

Figure 10-3.   This toddler enjoys finger painting.

Vital Signs

At two years the toddler's temperature is more stable at 37.8°C (100°F), which is considered normal. Respirations have slowed to 25–35 per minute, and the heartbeat averages 80–140 per minute. The blood pressure of the two-year-old averages 80–90 mm Hg systolic. By three years the temperature is 37.1°C (98.9°F), the pulse is 110 beats/min, and the respirations are about 25–35/min. The three-year-old's blood pressure will normally be 90 mm Hg systolic and 60 mm Hg diastolic.

Weight

Two-year-olds can be expected to weigh approximately four times their birth weight. At three years toddlers will weigh about 15 kg (33 lb).

Senses

At two years of age visual acuity is comparable to that of an adult. Hearing, taste, and smell are also well developed.

Posture

Toddlers have a pronounced lumbar lordosis and a protruding abdomen. With growth the abdominal muscles gradually develop, thus flattening the abdomen.

Behavior

Motor Development

At the age of 18 months babies can pick up small beads and place them in a receptacle. They can also hold a spoon and a cup and walk upstairs with assistance. They will probably crawl down the stairs.

At two years toddlers cannot only hold a spoon but can also put it into their mouth correctly. They are able to run; their gait is steady; and they walk with a lumbar lordosis and a less protuberant abdomen. Two-year-old toddlers can also balance on one foot and ride a tricycle.

By three years of age most children are toilet trained, although there still may be the occasional accident when playing or during the night.

Language and Speech

Most children learn to imitate words in the second year when sufficient cortical maturity has taken place. By two years they will usually be able to arrange several words into a sentence. Three-year-olds speak almost constantly. They practice speaking in bed and during play. They imitate adults and can express their feelings, thoughts, desires, and problems in words. Logic is elusive, so not all their words at any one time will relate to the same activity.

Sleep

Rest and sleep continue to be important to toddlers. They still require 12 hours of sleep at night during the second year as well as a nap of several hours during the day, making a total sleep requirement of about 15 or 16 hours per day. Three-year-olds also require a similar amount of sleep, anywhere from 9 to 13 hours each night, perhaps a reduction of one to two hours from their need at two years. Three- and four-year-olds may also have dreams and nightmares that awaken them.

Social Development

At two years children are very possessive of their toys. They are dependent upon their parents and strongly react to separation from them. By the time toddlers are three years old they are learning to play with their peers.

Cognitive Development

By two years children have developed considerably in terms of cognitive and intellectual skills. They have learned about the sequence of time. They have some symbolic thought, for example, a chair may represent a place of safety while a blanket symbolizes comfort. Concepts start to form in late toddlerhood. A concept develops when the child learns a number of words, all of which represent a class of objects or a thought. An example of a concrete concept would be *table*, representing a number of articles of furniture, which are all different kinds of tables. Between the ages of three and five years death becomes a concern. Death as a concept is thought of as someone leaving, such as when an uncle leaves the house.

Emotional Development

At 18 months toddlers imitate their parents and play games. They indicate displeasure over a wet diaper. By two years the rituals of routine are very important as displayed by crying when disturbed by change. Toddlers' emotions of love and hate are often extreme.

One way toddlers begin to develop their sense of autonomy is by asserting themselves with the frequent use of the word *no*. They are often frustrated by restraints to their behavior; as a result, between ages one and three years children may display temper tantrums. However, they slowly gain control over their emotions, usually with the guidance of their parents.

The period that centers around the development of a sense of autonomy (one to three years) is a time when children expand their social contacts. They are curious, and they ask many questions. Children at this age are often creative although the products of this activity may not be perfect.

Learning Mental Mechanisms

In infancy and toddlerhood a number of mental mechanisms are used to mediate anxieties. Three of these are symbolization, incorporation, and displacement.

Symbolization occurs when a mental image is created to stand for something. For example, being fed symbolizes security and pleasure. *Incorporation* occurs when people or objects are internalized by a person and become a part of understanding. For example, "mother" is internalized, and this then be-

170

comes the basis for the separation anxiety that infants normally experience at about age nine months. *Displacement* exists when emotions are transferred from the original person or object to another; for example, infants admitted to the hospital transfer the emotions they had for mother to the nurse.

Moral and Religious Development

During the second year of life children begin to know that some activities elicit affection and approval. They also recognize that certain rituals such as repeating some phrases from prayers also elicit approval. This provides children with feelings of security. By two years of age toddlers are learning what their parents' attitudes are in relation to religious and moral matters. By the time they are three years old children may repeat short prayers at bedtime.

Needs

The needs of toddlers are primarily sleep, accident prevention, and nutrition.

Sleep

Sleep for toddlers has been discussed earlier in this chapter. It is an important need of children two and three years old.

Accident Prevention

Accidents are a leading cause of morbidity and mortality of toddlers. Drowning, poisoning, suffocation, and falls are major types of accidents experienced by toddlers. For example, a toddler may get into bottles and put the contents in his mouth.

Nutrition

Toddlers' nourishment is basic to their health and growth. During their second year of life, the average toddler will gain 3–4 kg (6.6–8.8 lb) (Robinson et al. 1977:315). Because of their growth and activity, toddlers' food needs are proportionately greater than an adults' by body size. For additional information, see Chapter 25.

THE PRESCHOOLER (FOUR AND FIVE YEARS)

The preschool years include the ages 4 and 5 years. It is at this time that children begin to become social beings.

Physical Development

By the time children are four or five years old they appear taller and thinner than toddlers. This is because children tend to grow more in height than in weight. (See Figure 10-4.)

Weight

Preschool children's growth is generally slow. By five years they have added only another 3–5 kg (7–12 lb) to their three-year-old weight, bringing it to somewhere between 18.1 and 20.4 kg (40 and 45 lb).

Height

During the preschool years children grow about 5 to 6.25 cm (2.0–2.5 inches) each year. Thus by six years of age they have doubled their birth length to 100 cm (40 inches).

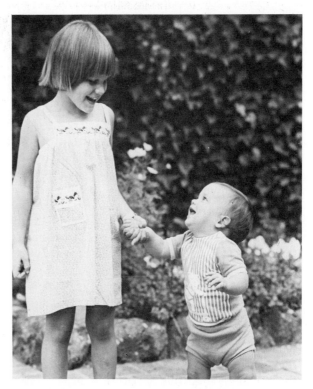

Figure 10-4. The preschool child appears taller and slimmer than the toddler.

Body Proportions

The preschooler's brain will have reached almost its adult size by five years. The extremities of the body will grow more quickly than the body trunk, thus giving the child a somewhat out-of-proportion appearance.

Vital Signs

The vital signs of preschoolers are normally a pulse rate of 90–110 beats/min, respiratory rate of about 20/min, and blood pressure 85 mm Hg systolic and 60 mm Hg diastolic. Body temperature will be between 37.2 and 37.0°C (100° and 98.9°F).

Vision

Preschool children are generally far sighted (hyperopic). As the eye grows in length, it becomes emmetropic (eye refracts normally). If the eyes become too long, the child then becomes myopic (near sighted).

Posture

The posture of preschoolers gradually changes. The posture becomes transformed as the pelvis is straightened and the abdominal muscles become stronger.

Behavior

Motor Development

By five years of age children are able to wash their hands and face and brush their teeth. They are self-conscious about exposing their body and go to the bathroom without telling others.

Typically preschool children run with increasing skill each year. By five years of age they run skillfully and jump three steps. Preschoolers can balance on their toes and can dress themselves without assistance.

Language and Speech

By four years of age children tend to believe that what they know is right. They tend to be dogmatic in their speech. Four-year-olds love nonsense words such as "jump-jump" and can string them out much to an adult's exasperation. At four children are aggressive in their speech, and they are capable of lengthy conversation, often mixing fact and fiction.

By five years of age, speaking skills are well developed. Children use words purposefully, and their questions are asked in order to acquire information. They do not merely practice speaking as three- and four-year-olds do but speak as a means of social interaction. Exaggeration of speech is common among five-year-olds.

Exercise and Rest

Preschoolers are still a bundle of energy. During nap time in the afternoon, they are more likely to rest than to sleep. When they sleep during the night, they are likely to sleep more peacefully than toddlers.

Social Development

Preschool children gradually emerge as social beings. At the age of three or four they learn to play with a small number of their peers. They gradually learn to play with more people as they grow older.

Cognitive and Intellectual Development

Concepts start to form in late toddlerhood or the early preschool years. Preschoolers become concerned about death as something inevitable, but they do not explain it. They also associate death with others rather than in relation to themselves.

Most children at the age of five years can count pennies; however, the opportunity to spend money usually does not occur until they attend school. Reading skills also start to develop at this age. Young children like the classic books for children, such as *The Three Bears*, and they like books about animals and other children.

Relationships

Preschoolers participate more with their family than they did previously; however, they also start to play with their peers. In associations with neighbors, family guests, and baby sitters, too, they learn about relationships.

Within the family the close emotional relationship that the child had with both parents changes to the phase Freud referred to as the Electra or Oedipal Complex (Engel 1962:90–104). At this time the child focuses feelings of love chiefly toward the parent of the opposite sex, and the parent of the same sex may receive some hostile feelings. It is also at this time that sexual development becomes an interest. The child becomes interested in clothes and hair styles.

Emotional Development

In Erikson's stages of development the major problem of preschoolers is attaining a sense of initiative: they must learn what they can do. As a result, preschoolers imitate behavior, and their imagination and creativity take them to vigorous pursuits.

Preschoolers also become increasingly aware of themselves. They play with their bodies largely out of curiosity. They need to know where the body begins and ends as well as the correct names for the different parts. By five years of age they are able to draw a person including all the features. Preschoolers also learn about their feelings; they know the words "cry," "sad," "laugh" and the feelings related to them. They also begin to learn how to control their feelings and behavior.

Learning Mental Mechanisms

During the preschool years, four mental mechanisms are learned: identification, introjection, imagination, and repression. *Identification* occurs when one perceives oneself as being similar to another person and behaving like that person. For example, a boy internalizes the attitudes, behavior, and gender of his father. *Introjection* is similar to identification. It is the assimilation of attributes of others such as values and attitudes. When preschoolers observe their parents, they assimilate many of their values and attitudes.

Imagination is an important part of preschoolers' life. The preschooler has an active imagination and fantasizes in play; for example, a chair becomes a beautiful throne to a girl and she is the ruler. *Repression* is pushing from one's awareness experiences, thoughts, and impulses. Thoughts related to the Oedipal or Electra conflict are generally repressed by the preschooler.

Moral and Religious Development

Preschool children hear others discuss moral and religious topics, but they learn best from the example set by their parents rather than from what they hear. Children accept the religion of parents without thought because parents are the people to whom they look for guidance. Many parents send their preschool children to Sunday School. Children will be aware of religious holidays more for the parties than for their meanings.

Preschoolers usually have a well-developed conscience and behave well with very little prompting.

Needs

The needs of the preschooler are primarily accident prevention, nutrition, dental care, play, and guidance.

Accident Prevention

Accidents continue to be the major cause of mortality among preschool children. These children are active and often clumsy, therefore predisposing themselves to injury. Accidents can be prevented with two approaches: control of the environment and education of the child. Control of the environment is carried out in many ways such as by keeping matches out of the child's reach, putting toys away when they are not being used, and maintaining a swimming pool in an enclosed area that will keep small unsupervised children out of the area. The education of the preschooler involves many aspects of daily living. Three of these are learning how to cross streets, learning traffic signals, and learning bicycle safety practices.

Nutrition

Preschool children still need milk in addition to a balanced diet of fruit, vegetables, bread, cereals, and meat or fish daily. Children eat much like adults except that they need smaller quantities. Generally they eat one tablespoon of each food type for each year, for example, four tablespoons of a vegetable for a 4-year-old.

Preschoolers also require sufficient protein for the growth of new tissues. A child who weighs 13.6 kg (30 lb) requires 37 gm of protein as well as 30 mg of vitamin C. The latter is found in fruits, fruit juices, and some vegetables. One medium orange contains 55 mg of vitamin C.

Preschool children also require snacks, usually in the morning, afternoon, and evening. A snack might be a glass of milk and a sandwich. When they eat, they eat one food at a time, and often dislike coarse-textured foods and strong-tasting foods.

Dental Care

Regular dental examinations are essential at this age because caries develop quickly in young children. Examinations usually are initiated at about 2½ years. It has been estimated that decay can be found in the teeth of 80% of children. Deciduous teeth guide the entrance of permanent teeth, and therefore abnormally placed or lost deciduous teeth can affect the alignment of permanent teeth. Dental care also involves brushing teeth after each meal and before retiring. For additional information on dental care, see Chapter 20.

Play

Preschoolers spend most of the day playing. Play serves a number of purposes:

1. Children learn to cooperate with others.
2. Focus changes from family to peers.
3. Children develop strength and coordination.
4. Abundant energy is dispersed.

5. Children have an avenue to express initiative and imagination.

Play is also fun to preschoolers. They take it seriously but express joy and pleasure during play. Play at this age is loosely organized.

Guidance

Guidance is an essential need of preschoolers. They require both guidance and discipline that is consistent and fair. Through guidance, they gain a sense of security and the feeling that their parents care about them. It is important that parents follow through with the discipline that they have explained, for example, insisting that a preschooler spend an hour in her room alone.

THE SCHOOL-AGE CHILD (SIX TO TWELVE YEARS)

The school-age period starts at about 6 years of age and includes the preadolescent period, which usually begins between nine and ten years. The school-age period ends at about 12 years with the onset of puberty. Puberty is the age at which the reproductive organs become functional and when secondary sex characteristics develop. See Table 10-6 for growth stages. Skills learned during this stage are particularly important in relation to work later in life and willingness to try new tasks (see Figure 10-5).

Starting school is significant for a number of reasons; for one, children are able to compare themselves with their peers in regard to skills. They also receive impressions of the perceptions of their teachers, school nurse, and peers in relation to skills. These can be supportive to a child's self-image or can weaken feelings of being an important person. All in all the period from 6 to 12 years is one of rapid and dramatic change.

Physical Development

Appearance

School-age children at seven years gain more weight and thus appear less thin than previously. Children have a growth spurt prior to puberty, girls usually ahead of boys. By 12 years of age, girls are often still taller than boys of the same age. Individual differences due to genetic influences and environment are generally obvious at this time.

Weight

At six years of age, boys tend to weigh about 0.5–1.0 kg (1–2 lb) more than girls. Schoolchildren gain an average of 3.2 kg (7 lb) each year. Thus by 12 years of age they weigh between 35.4 and 38.6 kg (78 and 85 lb).

Table 10-6.   Growth Stages

Stage	Ages
Infancy	Birth to 1 year
Toddler	1 to 3 years
Preschool	3 to 5 years
Juvenile (schoolchild)	6 to 9 years
Preadolescence (prepubescence)	Girls 10 to 12 years; boys 12 to 14 years
Puberty	Girls 12 to 14 years; boys between 14 and 18 years
Adolescence	Girls 12 to 18 years; boys 14 to 20 years

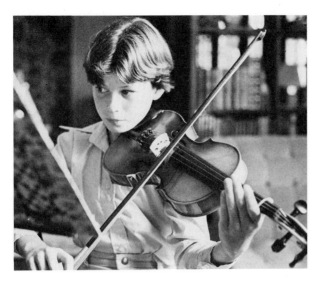

Figure 10-5. School-age years are a time for industry.

Height

At six years both boys and girls are about the same height, 115 cm (46 inches). They are about 140 cm (56 inches) by 12 years. Before puberty children of both sexes have a growth spurt, girls between 10 and 12 years and boys between 12 and 14 years. Thus girls may well be taller than boys at 12 years although the boys will have greater strength. The extremities of the body tend to grow more quickly than the body trunk, thus giving a somewhat out-of-proportion appearance to the person.

Teeth

Permanent teeth start to appear between six and seven years of age, and dental caries also can appear. Thus regular dental checkups are needed. By the age of 12 or 13 years children have most of their permanent teeth with the exception of their third molars, which erupt between 21 and 25 years of age. Sometimes the second permanent molars come later at about 14 years.

Vital Signs

By 12 years of age the body temperature, pulse, and respirations are similar to those of an adult. Body temperature averages 37°C (98.6°F). A boy's pulse will be between 65 and 105 beats/min and a girl's between 70 and 110 beats/min when resting. The respirations are between 18–30/min and blood pressure will measure from 95–108 mm Hg systolic and 56–68 mm Hg diastolic.

Vision

The eyesight of children six to eight years of age is accurate as to depth and distance perception. They can focus both eyes on an object at the same time because they have coordinated eye muscles. By later childhood it is not uncommon for a child to be myopic, that is, only able to see clearly objects that are close. This problem is generally corrected by glasses.

Posture

By six years the thoracic curvature starts to develop, and the lordosis disappears. Full adult posture is not assumed, however, until the complete development of the skeletal musculature during the adolescent period.

Reproductive and Endocrine Systems

Very little change takes place in the reproductive and endocrine systems until the prepuberty period. At this time, about ages eight to 12 years, endocrine functions slowly increase. This can result in increased perspiration and more active sebaceous glands. As a result acne may develop, particularly on the face, neck, and back.

Certain physical changes occur in the prepuberty period for both the boy and the girl. Some of the changes are as follows.

For the boy:

1. The testes increase in size.
2. The skin over the scrotum changes color; it becomes reddened and stippled.
3. There may be slight hypertrophy of the breasts, which disappears in a few months.
4. Pubic hair is sparse and downy and first appears around the genitals at about age 13 years. This hair darkens about one year later.
5. The penis enlarges in both width and length at about the same time.

For the girl:

1. The pelvis broadens.
2. The breast tissues develop. At first the nipple is slightly elevated at seven and one-half to eight years of age. The areola becomes somewhat protuberant between the ages of nine and 11 years.

3. Fat is deposited on the hips, thighs, and breasts.

4. The initial growth of pubic hair occurs at about 10½ years.

5. Vaginal secretions become milky and change from an alkaline to an acid pH (Murray et al. 1975:128; Scipien et al. 1975:172).

Behavior

Motor Development

During the middle years (six to ten), children perfect their muscular skills and coordination. By nine years, most children are adding to their skills by games of interest such as football or baseball. These skills are often associated with school, and many of them are learned there. By nine years, also, most children have sufficient fine motor control for activities such as building models or sewing.

Language and Speech

Sentence length increases for most children until the age of nine and one-half years, at which time it tends to remain at that length or decrease a little. Boys tend to lag behind girls in their speech development. They usually speak with shorter sentences, and their grammar is less correct.

Boasting generally takes place between 8 and 12 years, often with the intent of winning peer approval. Name calling also takes place between 8 and 12 years. It is done frequently to gain attention and to impress others with the child's superiority. Another type of speech is tattling, a form of criticism in which children use projection and blame their own shortcomings upon someone else. Tattling is considered by children to be one of the worst childhood crimes, and peer censure is generally severe.

Exercise and Rest

By the time children go to school, they probably do not need a nap in the afternoon. Sleep needs also are less. A six-year-old may require only 11 hours of sleep, while an 11-year-old may need only nine hours.

Exercise is important for school-age children who need it in order to build their muscles and develop fine motor coordination. It is at this age that parents can often introduce children to heathful and enjoyable physical activities. For example, the 10-year-old boy who plays golf with his parents not only

obtains good exercise but also is able to share an activity with persons who are important to his life.

Social Development

As they grow older, schoolchildren learn to play with more children at one time. Usually the six- or seven-year-old is a member of a peer group. This group replaces children's families in teaching attitudes and in influencing them. During late childhood, children join a gang, a small group of peers, which is formed by the children themselves. It is usually informal and transitory, and the leadership changes from time to time. It is during this period of socialization with others that children gradually become less self-centered and selfish and more cooperative and conscious of the group.

Cognitive and Intellectual Development

A concept that gains meaning for children when they start school is that of money. By the time they are seven or eight years old, children usually know the value of most coins.

The concept of time is also learned at this age. By six years of age, children enter school and the schedule in school helps them to learn time periods, but it is not until nine or ten years of age that children are able to understand the long periods of time in the past. Knowing the time of day and the day of the week are relatively easy for children because they have specific activities typical of the time to assist them. For example, a child goes to school Monday through Friday, plays on Saturday, goes to Sunday School on Sunday morning, and goes out with her father in the afternoon. Children can usually read a clock by the time they are six years old.

Later in childhood reading skills are pretty well developed, and what a child reads is largely influenced by the family. Later, at about 10 or 11 years, the child's tastes in reading change. Boys are more likely to enjoy adventure or science stories, and often girls prefer romance and real-life stories. Children from lower socioeconomic groups usually read more comic books than other books.

By nine years of age most children are self-motivated. They compete with themselves, and they like to plan in advance. By 12 years they are motivated by inner drive rather than by competition with peers. They like to talk and to discuss different subjects, and they like to debate.

During school-age years, the child learns to identify with the parent of the same sex and learns the behaviors associated with the role of that parent. At this time, the child probably will have some conflict with siblings, although this will be less so than it was for the preschooler, who often feels jealous when a new baby came into the family. Again the school-aged child may feel resentful at the appearance of a baby, and may also feel resentful about the freedom given older brothers and sisters. If parents compare siblings' accomplishments and talents, this can be further cause for resentment and rivalry.

Emotional Development

According to Erikson's stages of emotional development, from six to 11 years the conflict is industry versus inferiority.

In school, children have the restraints of the school system imposed on their behavior, which assists them in developing controls. At this time children compare their skills with those of their peers in relation to a number of areas, including motor development, social development, and language. This also assists in the development of self-concept. School-children can sometimes be cruel in their honesty, and teachers often need to intercede to assist children who have limitations.

Learning Mental Mechanisms

The schoolchild develops a number of mental mechanisms that serve to assist with adaptation. Four of these are regression, malingering, rationalization, and ritualistic behavior.

Regression is returning to a form of behavior that was suitable at an earlier age. For example, the child who is anxious about starting school may start bed-wetting at night or perhaps revert to baby talk. *Malingering* is a familiar mechanism to schoolchildren. It is pretending to be ill rather than face something unpleasant, such as the child who feels sick the morning before a test.

Rationalization is an attempt to justify behavior by logical reason and explanation. When a girl does not make the swimming team she may rationalize to her parents by saying she really did not try hard because she doesn't want to detract from her piano lessons.

Ritualistic behavior is exemplified by school-children in many settings. On the street a child may walk down the sidewalk without stepping on a crack. It is also seen in the type of rituals clubs and gangs have for their members. These rituals become very important to schoolchildren even though they usually do not persist for a long period of time, as for example the boy who must have a shower every morning yet forgets this ritual after a few weeks.

Moral and Religious Development

During the school years children may see God as a human being. They expect that when they pray, their requests will be answered. They may ask many questions about God and religion in these years and will generally believe that God is good and is always present to help. In the period just before puberty, children become aware that their prayers are not always answered and become disappointed. At this age some children drop religion from their lives, while others continue to accept it. This decision is largely influenced by the parents. If a child continues with religious training, the child is ready to use reasoning rather than blind believing in most situations.

Needs

Immunizations

During the years of childhood, boosters are indicated for those immunizations given in infancy. Generally they are given against tetanus, diphtheria, and poliomyelitis. Local health departments have their own recommended schedules, which are revised regularly in light of medical advances. See the schedules in Chapter 21.

It is recommended by some physicians that girls receive the rubella vaccine before puberty to prevent the acquisition of rubella and the subsequent formation of congenital defects in children they may have. Boys need to be protected against mumps, thus preventing subsequent sterility, which can occur as a result of acquiring mumps later in life.

Nutrition

Schoolchildren have greater nutritional requirements than do most adults. At six years of age they will require about 80 kilocalories per kilogram daily, but after 10 years this will decrease to perhaps 15–25 kilocalaries/kg/day, although the total daily calorie intake may increase from 1800 kilocalories at six years to 2800 kilocalories by 11 years for boys (Scipien 1975:199–200). As the child gets older the serving sizes increase. They may eventually be equal to an adult's serving or ever larger, depending upon the individual child's needs.

Play

School-age children have more friends than the preschooler. In early school years they are interested in playing roles with which they are familiar, such as those of a policeman or a teacher. By the age of nine or ten years, they become more interested in skill games such as football or baseball. Boys and girls separate for their play activities about this age. It is also about this age that the preadolescent gangs form and membership in the gang is strictly regulated. Often membership in a gang or club involves some sort of skill, such as tying knots, or endurance tests, such as bleeding a finger without acknowledging pain. It is also at this age that a child has a best friend. This is usually someone of the same sex, and it is with this person that the child shares feelings, thoughts, and activities.

Accident Prevention

See accident prevention for the preschooler in Chapter 21.

Guidance

Schoolchildren can discuss matters of discipline with their parents. They may need several alternative courses of action and probably more guidance than discipline. It is important that children not be embarrassed by being disciplined in front of others. Children also may be confused if a parent provides two messages at once. This happens when a parent tells a child something but then does another thing. For example, when a father tells his son that he should not lie, but then lies in front of the child, the child receives two messages.

SUMMARY

Through a knowledge of growth and development the nurse should be able to:

1. Assess the developmental needs of people.
2. Anticipate developmental stressors of people.
3. Determine the growth and developmental capacities of people.

There are a number of approaches to growth and development. A brief overview of some of these is given early in the chapter. With each stage there are developmental tasks or problems of people. Failure to master these tasks can result in impaired development and often impaired functioning in life; for example, the infant who fails to develop basic trust may have difficulty establishing close relationships later in life.

The first stage of growth and development is intrauterine development. It is initiated with conception and normally terminated with the birth of a baby 10 lunar months (9 calendar months) later. The intrauterine life can be divided into two phases, the embryonic and fetal. During these stages the tissue layers are laid down, and the development of a human being occurs.

The neonatal stage occurs from birth to 28 days. It is during this period that the baby adapts to the environment and establishes basic physiologic processes such as respiration and digestion. Assessment of the newborn is done with the Apgar scoring system. This system assesses heart rate, respirations, muscle tone, reflex irritability, and color, providing each with a numerical value of 0, 1, or 2.

The infant stage occurs from the age of one month to one year. It is during this time that Basic Trust needs to be developed. During this period the infant's birth weight will triple, and at one year of age the infant may be walking with help. The infant has many needs, such as nutrition, sleep, play, immunization, protection from accidents, and mothering.

Toddlerhood extends from one to three years of age. The toddler learns to control bladder and bowels. The basic need is to develop a sense of Autonomy. Toddlers are normally curious about their environment, but they need assistance so that this curiosity does not result in injury. Because of growth and activity at this age, nourishment is important. Another important need of the toddler is for sleep. It is during sleep that tissues form.

Preschoolers run and jump; they are a bundle of energy. Their developmental need, according to Erikson, is to show Initiative. The preschooler's posture changes from that of the toddler, and language and speech continue to develop. Preschoolers often believe that what they know is right. Preschoolers develop healthy routines and master other skills such as eating, climbing, and learning healthy emotional expressions.

The school-age stage starts at six years and terminates with puberty. The important task during this period is Industry. Permanent teeth start to appear between six and seven years, and most permanent teeth with the exception of the third molars are present by the age of 12. About the ages of eight and 12 years endocrine functions slowly increase and prepubertal physical changes occur. The child's particular needs during this period include immunizations, nutrition, play, and the prevention of accidents.

Social and emotional development are particularly significant during the school years. Children gradually learn to be less self-centered and more cooperative through social relationships with peers. Emotional development is demonstrated with increasing control. Through feedback from peers children are assisted in the development of their self concepts.

SUGGESTED ACTIVITIES

1. Visit a playground, school yard, or beach where there are children of various ages. Select several children to observe, and describe their activities in terms of their developmental stages.

2. Visit a newborn baby at home. Describe the baby following the outline presented in the textbook.

3. Visit a preschooler or a school-aged child who is a patient in a hospital. Assess the child's particular needs, including health needs and developmental needs.

4. Visit a classroom of a school where most of the children are about the same age. Observe the children for developmental differences.

SUGGESTED READINGS

Comer, James P., and Poussaint, Alvin F. 1975. *Black child care: how to bring up a healthy black child in America.* New York: Simon and Schuster, Inc.

The book describes the developmental needs with particular reference to black children. The sections include the infant, the preschool child, the black child in school, the elementary school-aged child, and adolescence.

Ilg, Frances L., and Ames, Louise Bates. 1955. *The Gesell Institute's child behavior from birth to ten.* New York: Harper and Row, Publishers.

This pocket book provides information about how a child grows; ages and stages and individuality are stressed. Part Two deals with specific subjects such as eating behavior, sleeping, and dreams and fears.

SELECTED REFERENCES

Bischof, L. J. 1976. *Adult psychology,* 2nd ed. New York: Harper and Row, Publishers.

Breckenridge, M. E. et al. 1969. *Growth and development of the young child,* 8th ed. Philadelphia: W. B. Saunders Co.

Duvall, E. M. 1977. *Marriage and family development,* 5th ed. Philadelphia: J. B. Lippincott Co.

Havighurst, Robert J. 1952. *Developmental tasks and education,* 2nd ed. New York: David McKay Co., Inc.

Hymovich, D. et al. 1973. *Family health care.* New York: McGraw-Hill Book Co.

Engel, George L. 1962. *Psychological development in health and disease.* Philadelphia: W. B. Saunders Co.

Erikson, Erik H. 1963. *Childhood and society,* 2nd ed. New York: W. W. Norton & Co., Inc.

Mitchell, John J. 1973. *Human life: the first ten years.* Toronto: Holt, Rinehart and Winston of Canada, Ltd.

Murray, R. et al. 1975. *Nursing assessment and health promotion through the life span.* Englewood Cliffs, New Jersey: Prentice-Hall Inc.

Piaget, Jean. 1963. *Origins of intelligence in children.* New York: W. W. Norton & Co., Inc.

Robinson, C. H. et al. 1977. *Normal and therapeutic nutrition,* 15th ed. New York: Macmillan Publishing Co., Inc.

Scipien, G. M. et al. 1975. *Comprehensive pediatric nursing.* New York: McGraw-Hill Book Co.

CHAPTER 11

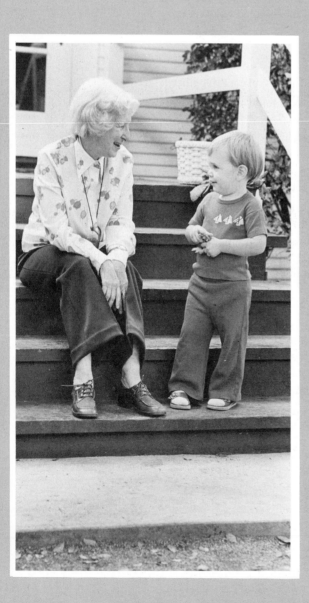

DEVELOPMENT FROM ADOLESCENCE TO OLD AGE

THE MIDDLE-AGED ADULT

Physiologic Changes

Needs

Common Problems

THE ELDERLY PERSON

Physical Changes

Psychosocial Development

Needs of Elderly People

OBJECTIVES

- Describe the pertinent physical growth changes and developmental processes that occur within adolescence, young adulthood, pregnancy, middle adulthood, and old age.

- Discuss the nurse's role in meeting the needs of people from adolescence through senescence.

- Discuss the various health problems that are prominent in adolescence, adulthood, pregnancy, and old age.

- Describe ways that the nurse can assist people to prevent some developmental health problems.

THE ADOLESCENT

Adolescence is a critical period in development. Its length varies from one culture to another. In America the period appears to be longer than in some cultures, extending to 18 years of age for girls and to 20 years for boys. Adolescence by definition is a period of time in which the person becomes physically and psychologically mature. At the end of adolescence the person is ready to enter adulthood and to assume the responsibilities of an adult.

Puberty is a period within the stage of adolescence in which many physiologic changes take place and the sex organs mature. In boys the maturing process takes about 2 years or more, while in girls it takes about 6 months. For girls it normally starts between 12 and 14 years and in boys between 14 and 18 years.

Physical Development

Appearance

The adolescent period is preceded by the prepuberal period, during which the second growth spurt has started. The first growth spurt was from birth to one year. This physical growth continues into the adolescent period. During this growth spurt, the bony structure grows faster than the muscles and internal organs. As a result, then, the young adolescent is clumsy and poorly coordinated. The feet and hands grow early, giving them an ungainly appearance. Often the adolescent feels tired because the heart and lungs have not sufficiently developed to service the body's needs for oxygen.

In boys, secondary sexual characteristics develop as well as other physical changes. Some of these in order of appearance are:

1. Sweating from the axillae.
2. Enlargement of the testes and the penis.
3. Appearance of facial hair at about 14 or 15 years.
4. Voice change at about 14 or 15, shortly after the appearance of the facial hair.

The maximum rate of growth for boys takes place at about 14 years, and the maximum height is reached at about 18 or 19 years. In their twenties men sometimes add another 1 or 2 cm to their height as the vertebral column gradually continues to grow.

Physical growth is greatly influenced during adolescence by a number of factors. Some of these are hereditary influences, nutrition, medical care, illness, physical and emotional environment, family size, and culture. Generally the people in the United States have grown taller in recent years. This is thought to be largely due to many of the above factors.

In girls a number of physical changes take place during adolescence:

1. The menarche occurs 9 months to one year after the peak growth rate has passed, between 12 and 13 years. It is usually another year to 18 months before the ovulatory cycle has sufficiently matured so that a girl can conceive.
2. The breasts continue to develop until about 13 years.
3. Pubic hair appears at about 11 years, and axillary hair appears later.

Girls reach their fastest growing rate at about 12 years and reach their maximum heights at about 15 to 16 years.

Both sexes will experience increased secretions from the *apocrine glands* in the skin during adolescence, resulting in acne. This was mentioned in Chapter 10 as starting in prepuberty.

Vital Signs

During adolescence the pulse rate drops in both boys and girls, although there is more of a drop in boys. The boy's pulse rate at 14 years of age can be expected to be between 60 to 100 beats/min, and by 18 years it will be about 50 to 90 beats/min. A girl's pulse rate will be between 65 and 105 beats/min at 14 years and 55 to 95 beats/min by 18 years.

The blood pressure increases through adolescence and then levels off at about 14 or 15 years of age. Girls appear to have a peak elevation of about 145/90 at about 11 years and boys 145/80 at 13 years (Vaughan et al. 1975:1003, 1098).

Behavior

The adolescent is faced with seven major psychologic tasks during this period:

1. Relating with the family.
2. Establishing a self-concept that remains stable.
3. Adjusting to his or her sexual role.
4. Establishing a value system that is appropriate for life.

5. Making a career or vocation choice.

6. Cognitive development.

7. Relating with a peer group.

Family Relationships

About the age of 15 years many adolescents gradually draw away from the family and gain independence. This need for independence and the need for family support sometime result in conflict within the adolescent and between the adolescent and the family. The young person may appear hostile or depressed at times during this painful process.

At this age adolescents prefer to be with their peers rather than their parents, and when they require advice they might well go to an adult other than their parents. Parents sometimes are bewildered at this stage of development and instead of reducing controls they increase them, which results in rebellion by the adolescent.

Adolescents also have to resolve their ambivalent feelings toward the parent of the opposite sex. In this endeavor they may have brief crushes on adults outside the family—a teacher or neighbor, for example. In these crushes, adolescents sometimes adopt some of the attributes of the other person. This can be helpful in the maturing process.

Some of the discord in the family at this time is due to the generation gap. The values of the adolescent may differ from those of the parents, and this may be difficult for the parents to understand and to accept.

Adolescents still need guidance from their parents although they appear neither to want it nor to need it. However, adolescents need to know that their parents care about them and that they want to help them. Restrictions and guidance need to be presented in such a manner that adolescents feel that they are loved. They need consistency in guidance and fewer restrictions than previously. They should have the independence they can handle and know that their parents will assist them when they feel the need for help.

Stable Self-concept

During this period, the body changes rapidly. This makes the adolescent's problem of developing a stable identity difficult. Adolescents are usually concerned about their bodies, their appearances, and their physical abilities. Hair styling, skin problems, and clothes become very important.

The adolescent needs to learn an accurate self-concept; one that accepts both personal strengths and weaknesses. Adolescents need to learn to build upon their strengths and not be preoccupied by defects, such as acne. They gain self-concepts largely from the impressions that others have of them. If others can accept defects, for example, a lost finger, this will help the adolescent accept this loss.

Sexual Role Adjustments

Sexual identification is begun at about 3 or 4 years of age and is established during adolescence. Adolescents are active sexually. Masturbation, heterosexual activity, and even homosexual activity are not uncommon. Boys have a higher sex drive than girls in late adolescence and therefore often become more experienced.

The number of pregnant unmarried adolescents has increased in recent years. In one counseling situation in Hawaii, 25% of the 400 women who had had abortions were adolescents (Gedan 1974:1856). Adolescents from the lower socioeconomic groups participate in more different kinds of sexual activities than do adolescents who enter college (Murray et al. 1975:177).

This is also a time when adolescents are forming their ideas about what kind of a mate they want. It is at this time that they put together the criteria they can use later in the selection process.

Establishing a Value System

During adolescence persons examine values, standards, and morals in terms of what they want to adopt. Adolescents may discard the values they have adopted from parents in favor of values they consider more suitable.

By the age of 16 years the adolescent is most likely to have made a decision about religion. At this age the church is the place where some teenagers meet others of the same age. Youth groups in this instance serve social and recreational as well as religious purposes.

Career Choice

In North America most adolescents are free to choose a vocation. In high school the initial steps are taken by selection of the program of studies that will lead to the career of one's choice.

The career choice is important not only in terms of type of employment but also in terms of lifestyle, status, and economic compensation. Many young people continue their education in college, and it may be at that time that they choose a specific career.

Cognitive Development

During this period the adolescent becomes more informed about the world and environment. The adolescent uses the new information to solve everyday problems and can generally communicate with adults on most subjects.

The mental ability of adolescents indicates that this is the time when they can best learn and use knowledge. They can be highly imaginative and learn to reason. Another skill is learning to learn, which adolescents develop and continue to use throughout life. Adolescents also develop their own areas for learning; they explore interests, and from some of these may evolve a career plan.

At one time, a boy may have taken an interest in special areas such as auto mechanics and spent hours polishing his car and taking it apart to repair it. A girl may have been more likely to develop an interest in hobbies such as sewing clothes. In recent years, however, male-female interests are melding.

Peer Group Relationships

During adolescence peer groups assume great importance. The peer group has a number of functions. It provides a sense of belonging, pride, social learning, and sexual roles. Most peer groups have well-defined modes of behavior that are acceptable for both boys and girls. In adolescence the peer groups change with age. They start as a group for one sex and evolve to heterosexual groups and finally to paired couples who share activities.

Dating helps prepare adolescents for marriage by teaching them how to act with members of the opposite sex. In the United States dating starts early, often by 11 years for girls and later, perhaps 15, for boys, although this varies with culture and social class and the subsequent pressures from society. Some adolescents initially date in groups of couples and eventually progress to dating more as single couples.

Needs

Nutrition

At this particular time nutritional needs increase. The boy has a greater need for nourishment now than at any other time in his life; the girl's nutritional needs are only greater when she is pregnant. Adolescents have tremendous appetites; a boy may need as many as 3070 kilocalories at 16 to 19 years, and girls need 2490 kilocalories between 13 and 15 years. Their requirements are lower after 16 years (Mitchell

1976:296). There is an increased need for protein, calcium, and vitamin D because of the growth rate during adolescence.

For an adequate diet the adolescent needs 1 qt of milk per day as well as meat, the vegetable-fruit group, and bread and cereals (see Chapter 25). The adolescent also requires greater quantities of food than the child.

Rest and Sleep

Most adolescents require 10 hours of sleep per day. This is needed to prevent undue fatigue and the possible subsequent acquisition of infections. Sometimes during the day a teenager also needs to rest. Often quiet activities such as reading are good respite from the physically active life.

Sexual Education

Teenagers want to know about sex. In one study 417 high school students participated to assess what they believed their needs were and what knowledge they already possessed. Most of the students had obtained their first information from friends or from reading while in grade school. The family and school were the other major sources of information (Inman 1975:217–219).

Some teenagers wanted sex information from both parents, and some wanted the church to also be involved. White students had more formal knowledge than nonwhite, and Protestants and boys had more informal knowledge than Catholic students and girls.

The subjects that the teenagers indicated to be the most important for inclusion in sex education were:

1. Venereal disease.
2. Biology of sexes and reproduction.
3. Pregnancy.
4. Birth control (requested by boys).
5. What boys think of girls and development of a sexual code of conduct (requested by girls).

Common Problems of the Adolescent

Obesity

Obesity is a common problem of the preadolescent period and it continues to be a problem in the adolescent period. It is estimated that between the ages of 10 and 19 years, 10%–16% of adolescents are obese.

Obese adolescents are frequently discriminated against in many ways. They are usually rejected by their peers, badgered by their parents, and laughed at on television and in the movies. Many feel ugly and unacceptable in social activities. Depression is not unusual among obese adolescents.

Treatment of obesity in this age group includes education on nutrition as well as assessment of psychosocial problems that may produce overeating.

Acne

Acne is a common problem of the preadolescent and adolescent periods due to increased activity of the sebaceous glands in the skin. Noninflammatory acne appears as open and closed whiteheads and blackheads. The inflammatory type appears as inflamed skin together with *pustules* and *papules*. A pustule is a visible collection of pus within the epidermis. A papule is a superficial circumscribed elevation of the skin. With this latter type there is a tendency for scarring to occur.

Thorough cleansing of the skin is important in the treatment of acne. A well-balanced diet and avoidance of fatigue, stress, and excessive perspiration are also desirable. Teenagers who find acne a problem are advised to consult a physician.

Accidents

The major cause of death during the adolescent period is accidents, in particular motor vehicle accidents. Obtaining a driver's license is an important event in the life of an adolescent in the United States and Canada, but the privilege is not always wisely handled. Motorcycles also contribute to the cause of injury and death in teenagers. Head injuries and fractures are frequent outcomes of accidents involving automobiles and motorcycles.

Adolescent Pregnancy

Unplanned pregnancies during adolescence are not uncommon. Education about contraceptive measures is recommended for adolescents. Pills, devices such as diaphragms, intrauterine devices (IUDs), the rhythm method and condoms are preventive measures (see Chapter 31, "Sexual Needs"). The incidence of abortion is notable among this group, and those who choose to carry through with their pregnancies have unique needs and problems. Rearing a child as an unwed single parent or placing a child for adoption are events of a crisis nature.

Venereal Disease

Venereal diseases are transmitted through sexual intercourse. Syphilis and gonorrhea are the most common, and the latter has been continually on the increase since 1957. More than half of the people who are reported to have gonorrhea are between 15 years and 24 years old. The increase appears to be due to two major factors, the changing sexual mores among young people and the increase in male homosexuality.

Because the term *venereal disease* conjures up feelings of guilt, shame, and fear in many people, medical help is frequently not sought as early as it should be. Table 11–1 describes the early symptoms of gonorrhea and syphilis.

Syphilis and gonorrhea are generally curable if the person receives the prescribed treatment, usually a regimen of penicillin injections.

Gastric Problems

It is not unusual for adolescents to complain of indigestion and gastric problems. These complaints may

Table 11-1.   Symptoms of Gonorrhea and Syphilis

	Male	**Female**
Gonorrhea*	Painful urination; urethritis with watery white discharge, which may become purulent	May be asymptomatic; or vaginal discharge, pain, urinary frequency
Syphilis†	Chancre, usually on glans penis, which is painless and heals in 4–6 weeks; secondary symptoms in 6 weeks to 6 months after chancre heals—skin eruptions, general lymphadenitis, low-grade fever	Chancre on cervix etc., heals in 4–6 weeks; secondary symptoms same as male

*Symptoms usually appear in 3–9 days after contact. Gonorrhea is usually treated with aqueous procaine penicillin.
†Symptoms usually appear in 10–60 days after contact. Syphilis is usually treated with benzathine penicillin or procaine penicillin G in oil.

well be due to the increase in gastric acidity that takes place during adolescence. Occasionally a gastric ulcer will develop as a result of the rise in acidity as well as the stress problems of the teenager.

Drug Abuse

Emotional swings and problems in adolescence are common. Drug abuse is one increasing problem of teenagers, some of whom have emotional problems. Many adolescents take drugs for the experience, in order to belong to a group, thus relieving loneliness, or to prove that they are courageous. Some of the drugs used are alcohol, glue and similar substances, barbiturates and amphetamines, hallucinogens, and marijuana. Marijuana is used widely by both adolescents and adults. Its use is a controversial issue at present, and there are advocates who believe it should not be grouped with the more dangerous drugs.

When teenagers habitually use drugs, this is a problem not only to the teens but also to the people with whom they associate. Help may be needed from the physician and in some cases from specialists such as psychiatrists who specialize in adolescent problems.

ADULTHOOD

The adult phase of development encompasses the years from the end of adolescence to retirement. Because the developmental tasks of adults in the early years differ from the later years, adulthood is often considered in two phases—the young adult phase and the middle-aged adult phase. In this book young adulthood will encompass the years from approximately 20 to 40 and middle age from 40 to 65. In addition, a section is included about the pregnant woman, although pregnancy is not unique to this period of development.

The state of remaining single is also recognized, since it is becoming the lifestyle of more and more North Americans. Many people choose to remain single to pursue an extensive education and then perhaps to have the freedom to pursue their chosen vocations.

The single status does, however, present some problems for a person. Social pressures for persons in their twenties and thirties are directed toward getting married. Often young single persons as well as older single adults need support for their single status and verification that they are contributing members of society.

Because single adults often live alone or with other adults who are employed, problems can present themselves when single persons are ill. Finding someone to drive them to a hospital or to help with shopping and meals during recuperation can be major challenges. A support system for a single adult may take more organization than that of a married person.

THE YOUNG ADULT

Physical Development

Persons in their early twenties are in their prime years physically. The skeletomuscular system is well developed and coordinated. This is the period when athletic endeavors reach their peak as is seen in many hockey, tennis, or football players. Indeed, after 40 years, most athletes are referred to as old.

All other systems of the body are also functioning at peak efficiency. The circulatory system is well developed so that pregnant women, for example, are able to develop additional blood supplies to the placenta. The reproductive system is fully developed. The woman's menstrual cycle is regular, and sexual organs are sufficiently mature to cope with childbearing. The man's sexual maturity, reached in adolescence, remains at a peak so that the sexual urge remains high throughout this phase. In summary, in this period of life physical change, with the exception of pregnancy, is minimal as compared to psychologic development. Changes that occur during pregnancy will be subsequently discussed.

Psychologic Development: Before Marriage

Young adults face a number of new experiences and changes in lifestyle. They must now make decisions for themselves rather than have them made for them, and many of the decisions made plant the seeds for the lifestyle to follow in years to come. The expectations of the young adult are often taken for granted, since they are well defined in most cultures. Choices must be made about getting an education and employment, about whether to marry or remain single, about starting a home, and about rearing children. Social responsibilities include forming new friendships and assuming some community activities.

Selecting Education and Employment

Getting a substantial general education is encouraged these days to ensure broader employment opportunities, to ensure a broad orientation to living one's life, and to ensure one's economic existence. Occupational choice and education are largely inseparable. The kind of education one has influences the occupational opportunities; conversely, the occupation chosen can determine the type of education to be acquired.

In the past, priority has been placed on encouraging young men more than young women to pursue advanced education, particularly college education. Traditionally for young women, education was deemed unnecessary for the roles of wife and mother. Today the role of the woman is changing, and many now choose to assume more active, civic roles in society prior to marriage, during marriage, and in later years.

Choosing a Mate

Deciding on a mate is no easy task. It is in many ways more complex and confusing than other tasks required of the young adult. In North America there is emphasis on the concept of falling in love as a basis for mate selection and marriage. However, the multifaceted shades of love make it difficult for some people to recognize and to know the meaning of love. Numerous definitions of love are available in literature, but the one important aspect of love is that it is lasting. Love survives times of frustration, strained relationships, and sadness, as well as times of happiness and achievement. It evolves out of interaction and requires adjustments and readjustments of the personalities of the two people involved. There is a desire to do all one can to make the other person's life meaningful. In contrast, infatuation is sexually stimulating and exciting but is too shallow to nurture total personal growth of either partner and tends to last only a short time.

Theories About Mating.   Multiple factors other than love influence mate selections, such as age, religion, race, social class, and common interests. Several theories exist that explain why people choose certain partners:

1. nearness or proximity
2. concept of the ideal mate
3. complementary needs
4. homogamy
5. compatibility (Kaluger et al. 1974:248)

Proximity is said to be a major influencing factor. People usually meet other people through the association of work, school, church, or recreational activities. Because of familiar associations, the gravitation of people toward each other is facilitated.

The *concept of the ideal mate* also guides choice of mates. The ideal or desired characteristics of what makes a good husband, wife, father, or mother are consciously or unconsciously met by the selected person. Some people are able to list these desired qualities.

In the theory of *complementary needs*, persons are attracted to others who have different characteristics. Each partner wishes to have the characteristics of the other and believes one member of the couple can help the other to be the kind of person he or she wants to be—or at least one partner can complement the other.

Homogamy is widely recognized as a theory of why certain mates are chosen. *Homogamy* refers to people who have similar social, racial, religious, and economic characteristics.

Couples who are *compatible* share a wide variety of commonly enjoyed activities together and have similar value systems. They communicate and respond deeply to each other. The partners understand and accept each other and are thus said to be supplementary rather than complementary.

Getting Engaged.   Many questions arise when the young adult contemplates becoming engaged. Some of these are "What does engagement really mean?," "Why get engaged?," "When should a couple become engaged and for how long?," and "What behavior is expected when one is engaged?" There are no universal answers to many of these questions. The answers rest largely with each individual couple and common practices within the social sphere.

The purposes of engagement for the partners have been outlined as:

1. Placing themselves as a couple in the eyes of themselves and the eyes of both families and friends.

2. Working through systems of communication that encourage exchange of confidences and increase the degree of empathy and the ability to predict each other's responses.

3. Planning for the marriage that lies ahead in relation to where and how their life together will be lived (Duvall 1971:385).

Engagement is a time when the couple can become introduced to and familiar with in-laws and share as a couple social activities with their respective families.

Getting Married

Most but not all people are married at least once in their lifetime. Although the traditional type of marriage is between a man and a woman, other forms of marriage are emerging, such as the communal or group marriage in which all members are married to each other and all of them become parents to all the children. Another type of marriage is the homosexual marriage, which may or may not produce a family through the adoption of children. The traditional family of husband and wife is the one largely accepted by society and law. The discussion in this book, therefore, will be restricted to this latter type of marriage while recognizing that change can and does occur.

The marriage contract is a legal one. Certain legal prerequisites are necessary prior to marriage, which are different in various states and provinces. There are minimum age requirements for men and women. Generally the age for women is lower than for men. Prior marriages must be dissolved, and no one can marry close blood relatives. The marriage relationship is allowed by the issuance of a marriage permit and formalized by a ceremony, but by law it can also exist without formal entry into a marriage contract. The latter is the common-law marriage.

Why People Marry.   There are several reasons why people get married, such as love, desire for children, escape from loneliness, economic security, sexual attraction, common interests, and social position. A few nonscientific theories about why people marry are provided in a less serious note with tongue in cheek (Kaluger 1974:244):

1. The Name-of-the-Game Theory. The game of life is to get married, so all one's plans and efforts are directed to that end. Man (and woman) needs more than bread alone to exist—a helpmate.

2. The Tom Cat Theory. Get married to stabilize sex relations.

3. The Avoidance Theory. Get married to avoid social and emotional unpleasantries.

4. The Contagious Disease Theory. This occurs in college dormitories. When one couple exchanges engagement presents, everyone wants to do the same.

Perhaps the important issue in getting married is not so much the reason why as the issue of what ingredients predict a successful marriage. Many studies have been done to establish predictors of good marriages, but many variables exist among individual marriages. One significant determinant for the success of new couples is the happiness of the parents in their marriage. Other factors include personal happiness in childhood with consistent discipline, being acquainted with each other for over a year, parental approval, common interests and cultural background, desire for children, and a sense of equality in relationships or at least clearly differentiated roles. The degree of sexual education and experiences premaritally are not significant factors.

Psychologic Development: After Marriage

When the honeymoon is over, if one is taken, newlyweds are faced with many adjustments in their demanding roles of husband and wife. The couple's developmental tasks are as follows:

1. Find a home of their own.

2. Decide on a system for getting and spending money.

3. Divide the routine household tasks.

4. Develop satisfactory sex relationships.

5. Learn to live together as a couple.

6. Work out relationships with relatives.

7. Find new friends.

8. Plan for children.

9. Develop a philosophy for living (Duvall 1971:169).

Learning to Live Together

New couples are generally reasonable and considerate of each other. Adjusting to each other may necessitate giving up some old habits and developing different ways or different times for doing things. For example, one partner may be an early riser and like to shower in the morning, but the other is accustomed to staying up late and likes a bath in the evening. Accommodating to food preferences, meal hours, sleeping with the window open or closed, taking time to relax or read the paper, sharing the television, entertaining others, and going out or staying in are other examples.

The marriage relationship cannot be easily described as an equal give-and-take situation. In most instances one partner gives more in certain aspects than in others. A major factor in determining the success of a marriage relationship is the quality of adjustments that are made by each for the other. Couples need to recognize marriage as a state of continual adjustments and as a partnership in which all things will *not* be agreed upon. Conflicts of interest and opinion inevitably arise. Learning to accept and understand each other as persons and learning to communicate and solve problems together is essential for success in marriage.

Communicating in mature and healthy ways is easier for some couples than others. Most couples tend to develop a private intimate communication system of words, gestures, and symbols. Words of endearment, gestures of affection, and symbols such as a favorite song become the couple's own language with a meaning known only to the two involved. However, it is more difficult for most to develop effective ways of handling negative feelings such as anger and disappointment. Being silent or sullen, withdrawing in anger, disintegrating into tears, or pretending that a problem does not exist are common patterns of behavior used when conflicts arise. However, little progress is made in solving problems by such patterns of behavior. The problem tends to be perpetuated unless a system of caring and communicating is developed together. Although it is difficult to be objective when feelings are intense, young couples can learn constructive ways of coping with cooling-down periods and effective ways to talk about their problems. Mutually-agreed-upon solutions can then be considered.

In developing a philosophy for living, the young couple need not take the same stand on every issue that arises. For example, the husband and wife may have opposing views on a recent political issue and need to act according to their own convictions in voting. Countless issues arise in which the couple weaves a philosophy of life, including racial issues, religious issues, childrearing practices, civic responsibilities, ways of dealing with the neighbors and the mailman, and the way the house is maintained.

Deciding about Household Tasks and Finances

Today the division of household responsibilities is clearly a decision of the couple themselves. Traditionally the roles of the man and woman were outlined for them. The husband was the sole breadwinner, and the wife was the housekeeper. The trend today involves the sharing of many tasks; the wife is often a wage earner along with the husband, particularly before children are born. The husband is now often involved in many of the household tasks such as cooking, grocery shopping, cleaning house, and washing the dishes. The division or sharing of tasks, however, involves mutual decision making and examination of past and present influences. Who looks after the garbage? Who washes the car? Who mows the lawn? Who does the laundry? Who pays the bills? Who feeds the dog? Flexibility in division of tasks is often necessary for working couples. Even though a general pattern of tasks is decided upon, temporary adjustments may often become necessary. For example, a husband and wife whose employment involves shift work may switch tasks periodically.

Financing the household also requires discussion and planning. The traditional role of the husband holding the purse strings and the woman knowing little about the amount of income is rare today. Often joint bank accounts are established, and decisions about what to spend for food, furniture, rent, or home mortgages, for example, are made cooperatively. Long-term and short-term budgets can present a challenge to the young couple who strive to stretch the dollar and realize some of their dreams.

Developing Satisfying Sexual Relations

Sexual drives and attitudes differ among individuals. The frequency of sexual intercourse is variable as is the nature of the love-making ritual. For example, sensitivity to touch, levels of arousal, length of orgasm, and visual and oral actions are all variable among individual people. Attitudes influence and preferences dictate the kinds of activities a couple performs. Some desire more tactile or oral stimulation prior to copulation; others prefer only direct copulation. The environment itself may be important to some, such as dim lighting, quiet surroundings, or soothing music. Specific aromas can arouse some people, hence the use of certain perfumes. The sexual act can be a most intimate, fulfilling form of communication between couples and is one that deserves effort in learning to give and receive love. Couples who care to learn about their partners' desires and preferences and to accept differences can usually achieve mutual fulfillment in sexual relations. It is important for couples to realize that lovemaking need not always include intercourse and orgasm.

Planning for Children

Planned parenthood and birth control measures are predominant customs nowadays. (For additional information on birth control see Chapter 31.) Most couples, however, have their first child within the first few years of marriage, and some are conceived before marriage. There are also some couples who are not interested in having children.

The advantages of planned parenthood become magnified when one considers the unplanned or unwanted baby. For a couple required to make adjustments as newlyweds, the unplanned baby can create a crisis. Educational goals, economic plans for a home, financial independence from parents, and time to enjoy each other at leisure can all be disrupted. Little time is allowed for the psychologic preparations required to assume the role of parent.

Promoting Relationships with Relatives and Friends

Frequently social ties established prior to marriage are interrupted for one or both partners after marriage. The wife may move to a new location with her husband or vice versa. Even if the couple does not move, the single-person activities and associations prior to marriage are not maintained with the same frequency. New social activities for the couple need to be found. These are often chosen on the basis of common interests with other couples, the social prestige the activities offer, such as a membership in a country club, the amount that can be afforded in entertainment, and the occupational contacts of the husband or wife. Having the boss and his or her spouse over for dinner or going to the company dance may take precedence over going to dinner and a dance alone, a common courting procedure prior to marriage. Simultaneously the couple undergoes a change in family orientation. They are each no longer a member of one family but are now a member of three—his, hers, and their own. Some couples retain close family ties, whereas others go their separate ways and see parents only occasionally. However, most couples assume some responsibility for keeping in touch with their families, and many receive help financially or with child care or other assistance. The role changes required for the son and the daughter to now become husband and wife can create some frustrations and conflicts in the early years of marriage. The wife is now the husband's first concern and not his parents, and similarly the husband comes before the daughter's parents. Most couples develop effective relationships with parents-in-law. What is family becomes larger in essence for both partners although the roles are different—increasingly independent.

THE PREGNANT WOMAN

The announcement of the first baby can be a joyful experience. The husband and wife feel the pride of knowing they can conceive and anticipate the expectancy period with pleasure. Pregnancy is not welcomed by all couples, however. The child may be unwanted or untimely or may induce many fears in one or both partners. Even for those who feel positively toward a pregnancy, psychologic adjustments are required in becoming a mother and a father. The demands of being a parent differ significantly from the demands of being a husband or wife. The young couple must now prepare for the expected baby, adjust present living arrangements, and learn how to care for a baby (see Figure 11–1).

Pregnancy is a shared responsibility of the couple. The expectant wife can do much to include the husband in this event. The husband can be encouraged to help select a physician, to participate in clothing purchases for his wife and the baby, and in general to share plans. The question of whether to breast feed is desirably decided upon together. Many educational programs are offered for prospective parents. Both husband and wife have the opportunity to share knowledge about medical services for pregnancy and childbirth, care of the pregnant woman and newborn, physical and mental changes associated with pregnancy, and what each prospective parent can do to have a child successfully. Husbands can

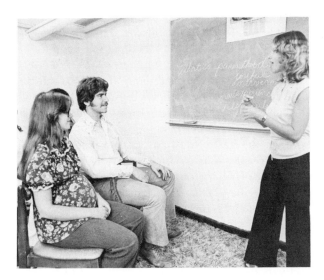

Figure 11-1. Early adulthood is a time to learn about parenting.

be helpful in supporting their wives through pregnancy. They can help them with good health practices and be tolerant of the physical and emotional changes that occur during pregnancy.

Physical Changes of Pregnancy

Cessation of Menses

Normally the high levels of estrogen and progesterone produced during the menstrual cycle drop rapidly, causing the lining of the uterus to slough off in menstrual flow. During pregnancy, however, these hormones are maintained at high levels after fertilization has occurred in order to retain the rich lining of the uterus. Thus menses do not occur. Menstrual periods can be missed for many reasons other than pregnancy, such as the stress of a final exam or severe physical illness. When two menstrual periods are missed, however, pregnancy is more probable.

Uterine Changes

During pregnancy, the uterus becomes enlarged, anteflexed, and soft. Softening of the cervix (Goodell's sign) occurs due to increased vascularity about the time the second menstrual period is missed. Normally the cervix is the consistency of the tip of a person's nose, but during pregnancy it feels soft like one's ear lobe or lips. The *isthmus* (the lower part of the body of the uterus between the cervix and the

fundus) softens more than the cervix (Hegar's sign) by about the sixth week and is another valuable sign of pregnancy. By bimanual examination (two fingers of one hand inserted into the vagina and the other hand palpating the abdomen) the lower uterine segment can be compressed relatively easily against the abdominal wall so that the examiner's internal and external fingers almost touch each other.

Braxton Hicks contractions of the uterus occur throughout pregnancy. These are painless intermittent contractions that may or may not be consciously recognized by the pregnant woman until 35 to 36 weeks. They occur at intervals of 5 to 10 minutes throughout pregnancy and often account for the experience of false labor. The purpose of the contractions is to enlarge the uterus. The contracting and relaxing muscles enlarge, and estrogen stimulates this enlargement.

Vaginal Changes

The mucous membrane of the vagina becomes bluish or violet in color because of an increased blood supply (Chadwick's sign). Normally it has a pink tint. This color change occurs at about four weeks but the discoloration remains after delivery; therefore it is helpful in diagnosing pregnancy only in a primigravida (a woman who is pregnant for the first time). In addition, the acidity of the vagina increases to protect against invading pathogens, and the vaginal secretions become thick and more profuse. In the cervical canal a thick, tenacious mucous plug forms, another protective device against pathogens throughout pregnancy. This mucous plug is expelled during labor and is referred to as *show.*

Breast Changes

Pregnant women experience sensations of tingling, fullness, stretching, throbbing, and even soreness in their breasts as they enlarge. Increased pigmentation of the nipple and of the area surrounding the nipple (areola) occurs and is particularly extensive in brunette women. The areola also becomes puffy and widens about an inch in diameter. Sebaceous glands in the areola enlarge during pregnancy and become protruded and prominent. These are referred to as *Montgomery's glands.* The breasts in preparation for breast feeding begin to secrete small amounts of colostrum, the watery precursor of milk. Blood vessels not noticed before pregnancy tend to become prominent as pregnancy advances, an indication that the blood supply is richer.

Skin Changes

Striae gravidarum, which in lay terms are referred to as *stretch marks,* frequently appear on the abdominal wall, the breasts, the buttocks, and the thighs. These appear as pink or reddish streaks and are caused by hormonal changes. The extent of striae formation varies considerably in women, and a very few women do not develop any. After labor the pink coloration of striae changes to the commonly known glistening white appearance of a scar. Striae are seen in conditions other than pregnancy that distend the abdominal wall.

Weight Gain

A total weight gain of 10.9 to 12.7 kg (24 to 28 lb) occurs steadily throughout each trimester of pregnancy, although wide individual variations exist. This additional weight is attributed to the causes shown in Table 11–2. As pregnancy progresses there is an increased tendency toward salt retention and concomitant water retention. Normally this fluid and salt are eliminated after delivery. For some women, sudden or rapid increase in this fluid retention in the last trimester is an indication of the onset of toxemia of pregnancy.

Other Changes

Many other changes occur in the pregnant woman to adapt to the needs of the fetus. The total blood volume increases by approximately one-third, and the production of red blood cells by the bone marrow is increased. The latter places extra demands on the

Table 11-2.   Weight Gain in Pregnancy

	Kilograms	Pounds
Uterine growth	1.1	2.5
Breast increase	1.4	3.0
Protein retention	1.8	4.0
Increased blood volume	1.5	3.5
Conception products	5.1	11.2
Interstitial water	2.0	4.5
Total	12.9	28.7

From Hellman, L.M., and Pritchard, J. 1975. *Williams obstetrics,* 15th ed. New York: Appleton-Century-Crofts.

body's iron reserves for hemoglobin formation. The increase in blood volume also has its effect on the cardiac output, since more blood per minute must be pumped.

Gastrointestinal functions are altered to some degree during pregnancy by progesterone, which slows the action of smooth muscle. Increased fluid absorption thus occurs, and constipation is enhanced. Pressure on the gastrointestinal tract also leads to the common symptoms of constipation, heartburn, and flatulence. Urinary output is increased and has a lower specific gravity than usual. Because of endocrine influences and pressure from the expanding uterus, the ureters soften and dilate. As a result the ureters do not propel urine as satisfactorily, and urinary stasis is common. The bladder itself functions effectively throughout pregnancy.

Metabolic changes also occur during pregnancy, particularly in carbohydrate metabolism. Usually the fasting blood sugar levels are lower and the pancreas secretes increased amounts of insulin. The renal threshold for sugar is often lowered during pregnancy and may result in elevated levels of sugar in the urine. This occurrence, however, should always be reported to the physician.

Several endocrine changes occur during pregnancy. The placenta, in addition to diffusing substances from mother to fetus, is the major endocrine gland during pregnancy. *Human chorionic gonadotropin* (HCG) is produced in the first trimester from chorionic villi, which are part of the basic formation of the placenta. This normally persists up to the twelfth week of pregnancy. HCG stimulates the ovaries to continue the production of estrogen and progesterone by the corpus luteum, both of which are needed to maintain the endometrium. Because HCG is excreted in the urine in the first trimester, its presence in the urine is used as a basis for the immunologic pregnancy test.

By the sixteenth week of pregnancy the placenta is formed, and it becomes the major source of estrogen and progesterone. When estrogen and progesterone are metabolized, they are excreted as estriol and pregnanediol. The presence of these substances in the urine indicates that the fetal and maternal well-being and placental diffusion are satisfactory. Both estrogen and progesterone are known to influence the growth of the uterus and the changes of the body and the breasts. The placenta also secretes *human placental lactogen* (chorionic somatomammotropin), which influences growth of fetal cells and prepares the breasts for lactation.

Oxytocin is released by the posterior pituitary

gland. This hormone is a strong uterine muscle stimulant that helps the uterus to contract before, during, and after delivery and thus reduces the possibilities of hemorrhage. Oxytocin also produces the letdown reflex in ejection of milk from the breasts. Stressors can inhibit the production of oxytocin, resulting in less milk production. Therefore minimizing stress is an important consideration for nursing mothers.

The adrenal cortex enlarges during pregnancy. A significant increase is noticed throughout pregnancy in the production of aldosterone, which regulates the retention of sodium by the kidneys. This sodium retention along with water can result in hidden or obvious edema.

Emotional Changes of Pregnancy

Ambivalence

Emotional changes of pregnancy parellel the physiologic changes. In the early months of pregnancy it is not unusual for the expectant mother to have some mixed feelings of pleasure and displeasure. Initially it takes time to accept the surprise of being pregnant. Even when a child is wanted and planned for, there is no best time to become prepared. For some, the timing may be awkward. School or a job may need to be interrupted or postponed for the wife. Nurses can often encourage expectant mothers to express their feelings of ambivalence and reassure them that the feelings are perfectly normal. These feelings of ambivalence are usually eventually resolved.

Mood Swings

Rapid emotional swings from sadness to happiness occur largely as a result of hormonal changes. Increased irritability and sensitivity need to be understood and accepted by both marriage partners. Very trivial remarks from the husband may cause the wife to burst into tears for no reason other than that she is pregnant.

Change in Body Image

In the second trimester the pregnant woman suddenly notices that her abdomen is bulging and that her clothes feel snug. Some women feel increasingly uncomfortable and unattractive with these changes. It is important for the husband and family to help the woman with these feelings. These can be compounded by her need for increased love and affection. Again the husband can be instrumental by demonstrating his love and by helping her as much as possible.

Passivity and Introversion

Passivity and introversion characteristically occur about the second trimester and reach a peak by approximately the seventh month. The wife fantasizes about her baby and begins to spend more time thinking about herself and less about others (introversion), and she is less active in making decisions and doing things (passiveness). She would rather others did things for her. She wants to receive instead of to give.

Changes in Sexual Desire

It is important for the husband and wife to be aware of changes in sexual desire. In the first trimester there may be little difference in sexual activity or there may be less activity, since one or both partners may fear abortion. This can be considered as a protective mechanism for the embryo. In the second trimester there may be an increased sexual desire. The wife may want more frequent copulation, and she may experience more orgasms as compared to her prepregnant state. Sexual interest may then decrease in the third trimester in both partners. Sexual activity is not contraindicated at this time, but fears of harming the baby may exist from erroneous knowledge sources. Because this vacillation occurs it is important for the couple to have some understanding of what is happening.

Needs of the Pregnant Woman

Pregnant women have needs relevant to their pregnancies: nutrition, rest, and exercise.

Nutrition

During the first two trimesters of pregnancy, a woman's caloric needs vary minimally from the prepregnancy stage. For moderately active women these caloric needs are about 2000 kilocalories per day. During the third trimester, however, the woman needs to have an additional 300 kilocalories per day, while lactating women require an additional 500 kilocalories per day. Adequate calories preserve protein for tissue growth.

The types of foods ingested to meet these increased caloric needs are of greater importance.

Throughout the antenatal period, protein requirements need to be doubled, and other specific nutrients such as iron, calcium, and vitamins A, B, and C need to be increased (see Chapter 25 for additional dieting information during pregnancy).

Rest

Rest is of particular importance during pregnancy and in particular during the last six weeks. This may be difficult for the woman who has young children, but planned rest periods are important. During the last six weeks, the unborn baby will probably feel heavy to the woman, since she will be carrying additional weight. This added weight and the other discomforts of pregnancy such as swollen ankles, varicosities, and backache increase the need for planned rest periods and exercise. During the last few weeks of pregnancy urinary frequency may interrupt sleep.

There are specific positions that can be assumed to assist relaxation and promote rest. One of these, the semiprone position, is discussed in Chapter 22. Other positions and exercises to promote rest and relaxation are discussed in Chapter 23.

Exercise

Exercise is important during pregnancy, and the usual daily activities generally suffice. Walking is en-

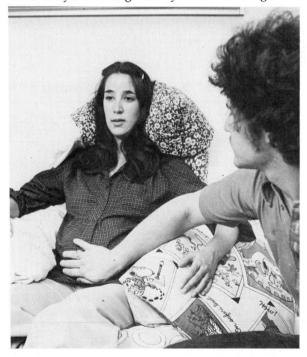

Figure 11-2 Expectant couple learns prenatal exercises.

couraged, however, because it stimulates the blood circulation. Normally, activity is not restricted except upon the physician's advice. (See Figure 11–2.)

Common Problems of Pregnancy

Most of the problems encountered in pregnancy are related to the physiologic changes that occur and are therefore often referred to as discomforts without pathology. Not all women experience all problems or have them to the same degree.

Nausea and Vomiting

About 50% of women experience nausea and vomiting, particularly in the first trimester of pregnancy. This problem is often referred to as *morning sickness*, since the symptoms frequently occur when the woman gets up in the morning. The symptoms are not restricted to this time of day, however. The cause of nausea and vomiting is unknown. Some think it is because of the high levels of progesterone, estrogen, and chorionic gonadotropin, particularly the former two hormones, since some women on birth control pills experience the same problem. A few others believe that they have a base in emotions such as ambivalence about pregnancy. Morning sickness has been known to occasionally occur in the husband along with the wife. Still others think it may be due to the lowered blood sugar or to an increase in saliva called *ptyalism*. Mouth secretions become more acidic during pregnancy, and the salivary glands are stimulated to produce large quantities of saliva. The nurse may recommend the following:

1. Eat smaller, more frequent high-protein meals to prevent the stomach from becoming empty.

2. Keep crackers or an apple at the bedside, and eat them before rising. This is an attempt to elevate the blood sugar level.

3. After arising, eat some foods high in carbohydrates.

4. Ginger ale or cola drinks may settle the stomach but have limited nutritional value.

5. Seek the advice of the physician. Some medications may be prescribed.

Breast Soreness

Breast soreness is due to the changes induced by progesterone and estrogen. Suggestions by the nurse can include:

1. Wear a good supportive brassiere with wide shoulder straps that supports the breasts upward and inward.

2. Anticipate buying a larger brassiere. Both bra and cup size usually enlarge two sizes.

3. Pad the inside of the bra with soft cotton or the like for nipple soreness.

Fatigue

Most women feel some fatigue particularly in the early months of pregnancy because of the metabolic changes. In later pregnancy, the extra weight and postural changes are largely responsible. Extra rest is required by planning an earlier bedtime hour and by resting throughout the day as needed. Learning to conserve energy when carrying out household tasks is also helpful. For example, it is less tiring to sit occasionally rather than stand for ironing.

Urinary Frequency

The need to urinate more frequently is common in the first trimester. This is understandable since the enlarging uterus is posterior to the bladder and creates pressure upon the bladder. There is little that can be done about this problem. Fortunately it resolves itself when the uterus rises into the abdominal cavity. Urinary frequency again occurs after *lightening* in the third trimester. Lightening is the descent of the uterus into the pelvic cavity. It usually occurs two to three weeks before the onset of labor.

Constipation

Constipation is a common problem of pregnant women commencing in the second trimester. Contributing factors are the pressure of the expanding uterus on the bowel and the increased reabsorption of water. Both contribute to alterations in bowel motility and stool consistency (drier stools).

Suggestions for relief are as follows:

1. Increase the fluid intake.

2. Obtain adequate exercise.

3. Ingest foods containing roughage.

4. It is advisable to avoid the use of mineral oil, since it interferes with the absorption of fat-soluble nutrients and to avoid enemas and laxatives because premature labor can be induced.

Flatulence is often associated with constipation. The avoidance of gas-forming foods such as fried foods, parsnips, corn, and sweet desserts and the ingestion of small amounts of food and the thorough chewing of food are helpful suggestions. Small amounts of yogurt are helpful.

Heartburn

Slight regurgitation of the acid contents from the stomach into the esophagus occurs during the second and third trimesters. The acid irritates the esophageal mucosa, resulting in a burning sensation. Remedies include the following:

1. Drink milk between meals.

2. Take small, frequent meals.

3. Avoid highly spiced or fried foods.

Food Craving

Craving for certain foods is referred to as *pica* and may be caused by physiologic, psychologic, or social factors. It is a well-known event often humorized in literature and movies. The stories about the husband getting up in the middle of the night to purchase strawberries or pickles are exaggerations of this situation. Some women in the southern United States are influenced by culture to ingest dirt or large amounts of starch. Nurses can provide counseling in regard to food cravings. Intervention may be necessary if a woman is not receiving a nutritionally balanced diet.

Backache

Bachache during pregnancy is due in large part to changes in body mechanics, change in posture, and overexertion. In the first trimester backache is associated with stretching of the uterosacral ligaments. Helpful preventive measures are as follows:

1. Pay continual attention to posture.

2. Wear supportive shoes with low heels.

3. Take rest periods after standing for long periods.

4. Do the pelvic rock exercise frequently (see Chapter 23).

Muscle Cramps

Spasmodic, painful muscle cramps in the legs sometimes occur as a result of fatigue, tension, chilling, or the excessive ingestion of milk. Relief can be obtained by straightening the leg (push down on the knee) and by stretching the toes upward. Frequent elevation of the legs and adequate warmth may prevent cramps to some extent. Excessive quantities of milk contribute to increased phosphorus absorption, which results in cramping. One solution is to reduce milk consumption, although additional calcium intake may then be necessitated by pills. Another solution is to take aluminum hydroxide with the milk to remove some of the phosphorus.

Edema

Some swelling of the lower extremities is common during the third trimester. It is aggravated by hot weather, by standing for long periods, and by the presence of varicose veins. Relief is usually obtained by elevating the limbs frequently.

Edema that is pronounced in the early morning and that involves the face or other parts of the body should be brought to the physician's attention. This latter situation could be the beginning of *preeclampsia,* a condition characterized by increasing hypertension, albumin in the urine, and generalized edema. It can occur during pregnancy or early in the puerperium.

The Puerperium

The *puerperium* is that period of time from delivery to about six weeks after delivery. A number of changes take place during this time that involve the reproductive tract, the breasts, and the woman's emotions.

Reproductive Tract Changes

During this period the uterus, which after delivery can be felt at the level of the umbilicus, becomes smaller and descends in the pelvic cavity. Usually by the tenth day postpartum, it will be below the level of the symphysis pubis. This decrease in the size of the uterus is called *involution.*

Also during this time, the lining of the uterus re-forms. The top layer sloughs off, and the endometrium regenerates. This is generally almost complete by six to ten days with the exception of the placental site, which takes about six weeks to heal. The old layer of the uterus that is sloughed off is discharged from the body as *lochia.*

Lochia has three stages:

1. *Lochia rubra* is the reddish to pinkish red discharge from the day of delivery to the third or fourth day postpartum.
2. *Lochia serosa* is a pink to brown discharge that occurs from about the fourth to the tenth day postpartum.

3. *Lochia alba* is a discharge of white or yellow appearance. It appears at about the tenth day and may last three to six weeks.

Breast Changes

The woman's breasts are normally soft the first two days after delivery. About the third day they become fuller and firmer. This is called *engorgement;* it is caused by the hormone prolactin, which is formed in the anterior pituitary gland. This hormone causes the production of milk, which together with increased lymph and blood circulation to the breasts causes the engorgement.

Emotional Changes

During the puerperium, the emotional changes can be divided into two stages: the taking-in phase and the taking-hold phase (Rubin 1961:753–755).

During the *taking-in phase,* which lasts two or three days after delivery, the woman appears passive and dependent. She will make few or no decisions, and most of her needs are expressed in terms of herself. Not only does she often show preoccupation for food, but she also needs at this time to repeat the details of the delivery frequently. In this way she integrates the experience of the delivery with the reality of her living.

The *taking-hold phase* is one in which the woman appears more decisive and autonomous. She appears interested in her baby and in people around her. It is at this time also that she will be concerned that her own body functions properly. For example, bowel control can be a problem. The mother requires reassurance at this time that she is performing well as a mother and that her bodily problems are normal if in fact they are. This period lasts about ten days.

The *postpartum depression* is another emotional reaction, which can occur about the third day or just after the woman comes home. She will state that she has a let-down feeling, and she will cry more readily for no reason that is apparent to her. There are a number of theories as to the cause of this depression but as yet there is no known proven cause. At this time, the woman needs understanding and attention from nurses as well as increased affection from her family. Usually this emotional reaction passes without serious consequences.

Learning mothering is a gradual process, and mothers need time to adjust to their new babies. Being at home alone with a new baby is a reality of recent generations. Previously mothers had parents and grandparents to share the care of newborns and household responsibilities. Postpartum groups are now established to assist new mothers in adjusting to the demands required by their role as wife and mother. These groups encourage a reality orientation for mothers who cannot feasibly do everything, such as, some household tasks which have to be postponed.

Needs of the Woman During the Puerperium

The major physical needs of the woman during the puerperium are nutrition and protection from infection, which involves breast care and perineal care.

Nutrition

If the woman is lactating (feeding her baby breast milk), her nutritional needs are changed. The diet is not dissimilar to that of the pregnant woman. The woman will require in addition to a well-balanced diet an additional 1000 kilocalories per day for the production of milk. She will also need additional protein (20 gm), bringing the total protein requirement to about 98 gm daily. Another additional requirement is for added fluids to 3000 cc daily. For additional information see Chapter 25, "Pregnancy and Lactation."

Protection from Infection

Breast Care. Breast care for the nursing mother involves two primary aspects: support of the breasts between feedings and nipple care.

A mother will require a supportive brassiere after delivery. Generally, it is worn 24 hours a day. If the woman does not have a brassiere, a breast binder can suffice.

For the woman who does not plan to breast feed, ice bags are generally applied to the breasts to reduce the heat. In some instances, fluids are also restricted and analgesics may be indicated.

For the breast-feeding mother, care of the nipples is of utmot importance. Nipples need to be kept clean and exposed to the air for ten minutes after feedings to maintain their dryness. A heat lamp may be applied a few times a day to ensure drying. Creams can be applied after nursing to help keep the nipple soft. At the first indication of cracking of the nipple, nipple shields are advised to prevent undue irritation from feeding.

Perineal Care. Care of the perineum includes observations of the lochia and the perineum itself. The lochia has already been described earlier in this chap-

ter. The amount of lochia discharged is generally about 200 gm. Initially, the flow may indicate the need of two perineal pads, which are changed every hour. The amount can be described as heavy, moderate, or light. A moderate flow is indicated when one perineal pad is relatively covered in about an hour.

The perineum needs to be observed for any contusions. The suture line, if there is one, needs to be observed for approximation of the skin edges, any bulging, edema, or undue redness. For information on perineal care, see Chapter 20.

Common Problems During the Puerperium

During the puerperium, a number of common problems may occur. Three of these are painful perineal sutures, constipation, and hemorrhoids.

Perineal Sutures

Painful perineal sutures can be a source of discomfort to a patient and may induce a reluctance to exercise because of anticipated pain. Heat lamps or peri-lights can often be used both to provide comfort and to hasten healing (for information on infrared lamps and heat lamps, see Chapter 17).

Sitz baths are also used to assist the healing process. They are used frequently by postpartum patients both in the hospital and upon their return home (see Chapter 17).

Constipation

It is not uncommon for women to have difficulty defecating after delivery of a baby. During the pregnancy, the intestines were crowded by the enlarged uterus, but after delivery the intestines are able to occupy their normal position within the body. In occupying this larger space, the muscle tone of the intestines is greatly reduced, hence constipation can result. Fecal softeners are frequently ordered by the physician together with an enema or a suppository about the third day.

Hemorrhoids

Hemorrhoids are frequently aggravated and can become painful during the puerperium because of pressure upon the rectum by the baby during delivery and the expulsive pushing efforts of the mother during delivery. A number of measures can be used to relieve this discomfort: warm compresses, sitz baths, anesthetic ointments, and witch hazel.

197

THE MIDDLE-AGED ADULT

The middle years in this context are considered to be from 40 to 65 years. This period has been called the years of stability and the years of consolidation. It is a time in most people's lives when children have grown and have moved or are in the process of moving away from home. Thus husbands and wives generally have more time for and with each other and time to pursue interests that may have been deferred for years.

Physiologic Changes

A number of changes take place during the middle years. At 40, most adults can function as effectively as they did in their twenties. However, during the 40 to 65 period, physical changes do take place. Some of these are as follows:

1. Gray hair appears.
2. Crease lines appear at the lateral aspects of the eyes (laugh lines).
3. Fatty tissue is redistributed in men and women; men tend to develop fat on their abdomens, and women also deposit fat around the middle of the body.
4. Energy is more slowly recovered and more quickly expended.
5. Hearing acuity decreases and sight dimishes, usually requiring reading glasses or bifocals.
5. Skeletal muscle bulk decreases at about 60 years; however, vigor and endurance start to deplete at about 40 years.
7. General slowing of metabolism results in weight gain.
8. Hormonal changes take place in both men and women (see following section).

Hormonal Changes

Both men and women experience decreasing hormonal production during the middle years. The *menopause* refers to the so-called change of life in women. It is the period when menstruation ceases. The *climacteric* (andropause) is used to refer to the change of life in men when sexual activity decreases. Sometimes *climacteric* is also used to refer to women as the time when reproduction is no longer possible.

The menopause usually occurs anywhere between 40 years and 55 years. The average is about 47 years. At this time, the ovaries decrease in activity

until ovulation ceases. There are a number of menstrual patterns that can reflect the menopause. Four of these are as follows:

1. Period flow will decrease in amount of blood, but periods remain regular.
2. Periods will come irregularly with some periods missed.
3. Menstrual flow will abruptly cease.
4. Menstrual flow will occur irregularly with irregular amount of blood flow.

During this time the ovaries decrease in size, and the uterus becomes smaller and firmer. With the depletion of the ovaries, progesterone is not produced, and the estrogen levels fall. Although the pituitary gland continues to produce the luteinizing hormone (LH) and the follicle-stimulating hormone (FSH), the ovaries do not respond. As a result of the terminated feedback influence, the pituitary gland increases the production of the gonadotropins, in particular FSH. This disturbed endocrine balance accounts for some of the symptoms of the menopause. Common symptoms are hot flushes, chilliness, a tendency of the breasts to become smaller and flabby, and a tendency to become obese. Insomnia and headaches also occur with relative frequency. Psychologically, the menopause can be an anxiety-provoking time, especially if childbearing is an integral part of the woman's self-concept.

In men there is not a change comparable to the menopause in women. Androgen levels decrease very slowly; however, men can father children even in late life. The psychologic problems that men experience are generally related to the fear of getting old and to problems related to retirement, boredom, and finances.

Needs

The age of middle years has four major needs: nutrition, rest and sleep, psychosocial adjustments, and acceptance of the changing self-image.

Nutrition

The major object in nutrition during the middle years is to maintain a balanced diet and at the same time decrease the caloric intake. Decreased metabolism together with decreased activity are reflected in a decreased need in caloric intake. Between age 45 and 75 years individuals require 200 kilocalories less than at age 25 years (Robinson et al. 1977:99).

Rest and Sleep

Rest and sleep are important in the middle years. During these years, adults have less vitality than previously and tire at a time when in their twenties they would continue to be physically active. Regular exercise must be balanced with rest and sleep. Exercise slows the aging process, assists in maintaining joint mobility, and promotes blood circulation to body tissues. The emphasis in exercise is that it needs to be taken regularly and that it needs to be appropriate to the person's physical condition.

Psychosocial Adjustments

At this time, adults are usually faced with a number of adjustments in relation to their relationships and their activities. Husbands and wives generally have more time for leisure activities. Relationships with families change. Children move away and marry and have children of their own. Parents are elderly and often have additional needs. Thus people in their forties and fifties often find themselves as grandparents, enjoying their grandchildren but with few responsibilities for them and at the same time assisting with the care of their own elderly parents. It is at this time that people often face the fact of the death of a parent and as a result come to terms with their own aging and inevitable death.

For adults who are career oriented, these years often represent the peak professional and occupational performance. Adults have many experiences behind them, which, together with intellectual skills, permit them to be effective in many areas such as financial and career endeavors.

During middle age, one is often faced with refresher courses and other courses that help one keep up with the many changes going on. It is at this time that previous training and education can become obsolete, requiring initiative in reeducation.

Self-image

At this time, the person looks older and will feel older. People usually accept the fact that they are aging; however, a few will try to defy the years by their dress and even their actions. It is at this time that some men and women will have extramarital affairs and even marry younger partners. For well-adjusted adults, these years are accepted for their values and their pleasures with no effort to appear younger than they really are.

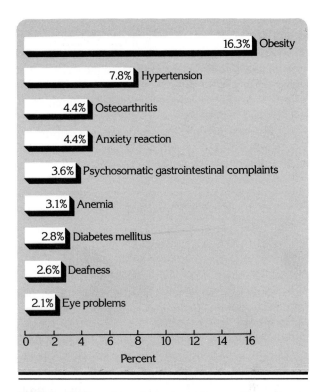

Figure 11-3. Disorders of middle age. (From Smith, David W. and Bierman, Edwin L.: *The Biologic Ages of Man,* © 1973 by the W. B. Saunders Company, Philadelphia, Pa.)

Common Problems

There are a number of common problems of the middle adult years that are chronic as well as frequently seen. Some of these are obesity, osteoarthritis, excessive use of alcohol, depressive disorders, and cardiovascular diseases (see Figure 11–3).

Obesity

Obesity is a common but preventable problem and one that is intimately associated with other problems such as atherosclerosis and digestive disorders. Reference has been made earlier in the chapter to the need for fewer calories as people age. Regular exercise is also advisable, not only as a means of weight control but also to improve cardiorespiratory functions.

Osteoarthritis

Complaints of arthritis increase in the middle years and continue to increase with age. Stiffness of joints, swelling, and pain are common complaints that a nurse hears. Obesity frequently accompanies this type of arthritis.

199

Excessive Use of Alcohol

The excessive use of alcohol presents a multifaceted problem to the individual and to society. The use of the drug is part of the lifestyle of many Americans and Canadians. Excessive use can result in unemployment, disrupted homes, accidents, and diseases. It is estimated that in the United States there are four million people who are dependent upon alcohol and can be considered alcoholics.

Depressive Disorders

At this period in life, men and women face a number of psychologic stresses. Women have the menopause and thus termination of the childbearing ability. Their children are grown and usually leave home, leaving some women with more time than they had previously. The woman who is married now focuses upon her husband and her own desires and ambitions. Sometimes these challenges result in depression or anxiety related to the question of her usefulness and to role changes.

Men also face stressors that can provide problems. Economic security, retirement, and the quality of the husband-wife relationship can produce problems. All of these areas require adjustments and may create anxiety as they are encountered.

Cardiovascular Diseases

These diseases are the leading cause of death during middle age in the United States (see Figure 11–4). Included in this group are coronary heart disease, atherosclerosis, and other vascular diseases. Preventive measures include regular exercise, keeping an appro-

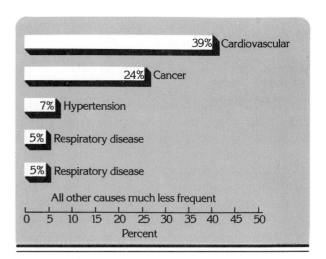

Figure 11-4. Common causes of death in middle age. (From Smith, David W. and Bierman, Edwin L., *The Biologic Ages of Man*, © 1973 by the W. B. Saunders Company, Philadelphia, Pa.)

priate weight, balanced diets, and abstinence from smoking.

Neoplasms

Growths account for considerable mortality and morbidity in both men and women (between a quarter and a third of the deaths). In women ages 45 to 64 years, breast neoplasms are the most frequent cause of death from malignancies. They are followed by cancer of the uterus (cervix) in incidence. In men, malignancy of the lung is the leading neoplasm causing death, followed by cancer of the prostate gland.

THE ELDERLY PERSON

In the twentieth century, about the 1930s, new and scientific investigations on aging were initiated. It was then that the term *gerontology* was adopted. Gerontology is the scientific study of the problems of the aging in all its aspects—biologic, psychologic, sociologic, and clinical. Since then literature and conferences on the subject of gerontology in all its aspects have abounded. As a result much has been learned about the process of human aging, including the physical and psychosocial changes, illness in later years, and dying.

Physical Changes

Different parts of the human body begin to decline at different ages and deteriorate at different rates. The basic mechanisms underlying the decline and deterioration are not known.

The Integument

Obvious changes occur in the *integument* (skin, hair, nails) with age, which often present concerns in rela-

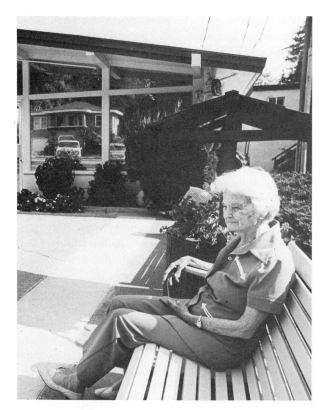

Figure 11-5. Elderly people often find changes in housing arrangements necessary.

tion to self-image more than acute physical problems. These changes include baldness or thinning and graying of the hair, wrinkles, loss of fullness, dryness, and increased itchiness of the skin. The skin also becomes paler and blotchy and loses its elasticity. Fingernails and toenails become thickened and brittle, and in women over 60 years, facial hair increases on the chin.

The reasons for these skin changes relate to progressive losses of underlying adipose and muscle tissue and loss of elastic fiber. Initially adipose tissue is redistributed from the extremities to the hips and abdomen in middle age. Generalized loss of adipose tissue progresses along with muscle atrophy, giving the wrinkled and wasted appearance of the elderly. Bony prominences become visible, a double chin develops, and lower eyelids appear puffy. In elderly women the breasts become smaller and may sag, if large and pendulous, giving rise to chafing where the skin surfaces touch. Loss of subcutaneous fat also decreases the elderly person's tolerance of cold.

Increased itchiness of the skin occurs due to dryness and to some deterioration of the nerve fibers and sensory endings. Decreased capillaries cause pallor and blotchiness along with reduced exposure to fresh

air and exercise. Evidence suggests that wrinkles on the face begin to form early in life from the lengthy use of facial expressions. They also are increased by prolonged exposure to the sun. Thus the characteristic wrinkles on the lateral sides of the eyes are sometimes referred to as *laugh lines.*

The causes of baldness and graying of the hair are unknown. Baldness is thought to be due to genetic factors, hormone changes, and racial tendencies. The way people respond to these changes varies among individuals and cultures. For example, one person may feel more distinguished with gray hair, while another may feel embarrassment. Most women regard female facial hair as repugnant because it does not reflect the feminine cultural image in North America.

Body Temperature

Body temperature is lower in the older person due to a decrease in the metabolic rate. It is not uncommon for an older person to have a temperature of 35°C (95°F), particularly in the early morning when the body's metabolism is low. This has implications for nursing when assessing the elderly for fever. For example, a temperature of 37.5°C (99.5°F) can represent a marked fever in some elderly people although it only represents a mild fever in young adults. It is important that the normal temperature of each individual person is known as a guideline in assessing changes.

One of the body's normal compensating reactions to a fall in heat production is the contraction of the surface blood vessels and shivering. Because the older person has a poorer shivering reflex and does not produce as much body heat from metabolic processes, prolonged exposure to cold is poorly tolerated. At the other extreme, higher body temperatures are usually compensated for by slowing down muscular activity to produce less heat and by dilating surface blood vessels and sweating to increase losses of body heat. Older people, however, have sluggish sweating and circulatory mechanisms and therefore cannot cope with heat as well as younger people. For example, they do not tolerate working in moderately high temperatures for prolonged periods.

The Skeleton

Slight loss in overall stature occurs with age due to atrophy of the discs between the spinal vertebrae. This can be exaggerated by muscular weakness resulting in a stooping posture and kyphosis or humpback of the upper thoracic spine. Osteoporosis, a decrease in bone density, along with increased brittleness of bone makes the elderly person prone to serious fractures, some of which are spontaneous. Since the incidence of osteoporosis is higher in elderly women, the effects of the menopause upon the skeleton are being investigated. Frequently female hormones are given to women to treat this problem. Other causes of osteoporosis are thought to be lack of activity and inadequate calcium intake or inability to use calcium.

In the joints some degenerative changes occur, which make movement stiffer and more restricted. This is aggravated by inactivity; for example, if persons sit too long, their joints become stiff and they have difficulty standing and walking. Although these skeletal changes do restrict the activity of the elderly, prevention of severe disability is possible.

The Muscles

With aging there is a gradual reduction in the speed and power of skeletal or voluntary muscle contractions. The capacity for sustained muscular effort is also decreased. Great individual differences are apparent throughout life in muscular efficiency. Exercise can improve muscles that have become weakened, and up to about the age of 50 years the skeletal muscles can increase in bulk and density. After that time there is a steady decrease in muscle fibers until the typical wasted appearance of the very old person occurs. Thus the elderly often complain about their lack of strength and how quickly they tire. Activities can still be carried out but at a slower pace. Prolonged muscular efforts may be sustained by older people provided that there are judicious uses of rest pauses and their capacity or peak performances are avoided.

The effects of age on the smooth or involuntary muscles such as the stomach, the colon, the respiratory tubes, and the bladder are small in contrast to the effects on the skeletal muscles, with the exception of the blood vessels. These muscles function relatively normally until late senescence.

The Senses

Vision.　Obvious changes around the eye are the shrunken appearance of the eyes due to loss of orbital fat, the slowed blink reflex, and the looseness of the eyelids, particularly the lower lid because of poorer muscle tone. Other changes result in loss of visual acuity, less power of accommodation to react in darkness and dim light, loss of peripheral field of vision, and difficulty in discriminating similar colors.

As the lens of the eye ages it becomes more opaque and less elastic. By the age of 80 all elderly people have some lens opacity (cataracts) reducing their visual acuity. Surgical removal is common at this age. Accompanying this are changes in the ciliary muscles (which control the shape of the lens) that reduce the power of the lens to accommodate to various distances. It is thought that the age changes in the nervous system play a part in reducing the diameter of the pupil, thereby restricting the amount of light entering the eye. This slows the reaction time for the elderly to any decreases in light or illumination, a problem compounded at night with driving. Because of arteriosclerotic changes in the blood supply, retinal function can be altered also. Reduced peripheral vision is thought to also be a result of arteriosclerosis.

Many of the aged require eyeglasses for close work. It is not uncommon for some to shop in department stores for glasses that have magnifying lenses because of their low cost. They need to be encouraged to have routine eye examinations by a physician and receive appropriate glasses. Many places now offer free eye examinations and glasses for elderly people.

Hearing.　Loss of hearing is usually gradual with aging, and it is more common in men, perhaps because of their exposure to noisy occupational situations. Loss is also greater for the left ear than the right. The elderly have more difficulty compensating for hearing loss than the young, who pay closer attention to the lip movements of the speaker. The hearing loss is greater for higher tones than lower tones, and thus speakers with distinct low voices are usually heard more easily. These changes occur as a result of changes in nerve tissues of the inner ear and thickening of the eardrum.

Other Senses.　Older persons have a poorer sense of taste and smell resulting in a reduced arousal by food. Taste buds in the tongue are reduced in number, and the olfactory bulb at the base of the brain atrophies. The olfactory bulb is responsible for smell perception.

The sense of balance is decreased with age, resulting in the greater incidence of falls and accidents in the elderly. Changes occur also in the sensations of pain and temperatures, as evidenced by the increased tolerance of the older person to these sensations.

The Voice

Vocal changes occur throughout life as a result of hardening and decreased elasticity of the laryngeal cartilages. These processes are completed by middle age. As age progresses the laryngeal muscles atrophy and vocal folds slacken. The voice becomes more highly pitched and grows less powerful and restricted in range. These changes are generally unnoticed unless greater demands on capacity such as for singing or public speaking are made. The noticeable changes such as slower speech and eventually slurring are the result of central nervous system changes rather than the local mechanisms.

Respiration

Respiratory efficiency is reduced with age. The lungs contain a smaller volume of air due to the musculoskeletal changes in the chest wall that reduce the size of the chest. There is a greater volume of residual air left in the lungs after expiration and a decreased capacity to cough efficiently because of weaker expiratory muscles. Mucous secretions tend to collect more readily in the respiratory tree due to the decreased activity of cilia. Thus susceptibility to respiratory infections is notable in the elderly.

Dyspnea occurs frequently with increased activity such as running for a bus or carrying heavy parcels up stairs. This dyspnea occurs in response to an oxygen debt in the muscles. Intense exercise without breathing is followed by short, heavy, rapid breathing, which is an attempt to replace this oxygen debt in the muscles. Although this is a normal response, it occurs more quickly in the aged, since delivery and diffusion of oxygen to tissues is often diminished by changes in both respiratory and vascular tissues.

Circulation

The working capacity of the heart is diminished. This is particularly evident when increased demands of the heart muscle are required such as during periods of exercise or emotional stress. The valves of the heart tend to become harder and less pliable, resulting in reduced filling and emptying abilities. In addition, the pumping action of the heart is reduced due to changes in the coronary (cardiac) arteries, which supply progressively smaller amounts of blood to the heart muscle. These changes are noticed in increasing shortness of breath on exertion and pooling of blood in the systemic veins.

Changes in the arteries occur concurrently. The elasticity of smaller arteries is reduced by the thickening of their walls and increased calcium deposits in the muscular layer. This often results in diminished blood supply to various body parts such as the extremities or the brain, resulting in pain on exertion in the calf muscles and dizziness, respectively.

Blood pressure measurements often indicate increases in both systolic and diastolic pressures in response in part to the inelasticity of the systemic arteries. Variations in the pulse rate of the aged also occur (70 to 80 beats/min is quite usual).

Digestion and Elimination

The digestive system is significantly less impaired by aging than other body systems. Previously mentioned were the diminished sense of taste and smell, which contribute in part to a lack of appetite. Gradual decreases in digestive enzymes occur; examples are ptyalin in salivary secretions, which converts starch, pepsin and trypsin, which facilitate protein digestion, and lipase, a fat-splitting enzyme. Yet digestive functioning and absorption of food is relatively unimpaired. The common complaints of heartburn, gas, and indigestion are largely due to other disease processes or dietary excesses of highly spiced or fried foods.

The majority of the elderly have poor teeth or have dentures and therefore may have difficulties with mastication. Foods that require extensive chewing such as meat and fresh vegetables or fruit may as a result be avoided, leading to nutritional deficiencies.

Constipation is a common complaint of older people. However, the aging process has little if any effect on the bowels, which retain their ability to function normally. Thus constipation is usually a result of poor fluid intake, inadequate roughage in the diet, and insufficient exercise.

The excretory functions of the kidney are diminished with age but usually not significantly below normal levels unless a disease process intervenes. Blood flow can be reduced by arteriosclerotic changes so that renal function is decreased. With age the number of functioning nephrons (the basic functional units of the kidney) is reduced to some degree, thus affecting the kidney's filtering abilities.

More noticeable changes are those related to the bladder. Complaints of urgency and frequency are common. In men these signs are often due to an enlarged prostate gland and in women to weakened muscles supporting the bladder or weakness of the urethral sphincter. The capacity of the bladder and its ability to empty completely are diminished with age. This explains the need for the elderly to arise during the night to void (nocturnal frequency) and the retention of residual urine, predisposing to bladder infections.

The Sexual Organs

In men degenerative changes in the gonads are very gradual. The ability of the testes to produce sperm remains into old age, although there is a gradual decrease in the number of sperm produced. The ability to copulate also remains until late in life, and therefore satisfying sexual activities need not be altered. However, a gradual reduction in the frequency of sexual intercourse occurs. In contrast, the degenerative changes in the ovaries of women are noticed by the abrupt cessation of menses in middle age during the menopause.

Changes in the gonads in elderly women result from the reduction of the ovarian hormones. Some changes go unnoticed such as the shrinkage in size of the uterus and ovaries. Other changes are obvious. The breasts atrophy without the effect of ovarian hormones, and lubricating secretions of the vagina are reduced. The latter is the cause of painful intercourse, which often necessitates the use of artificial lubricating jellies.

The Nervous System

The idea that a person's intellectual capacities decrease with age is a fallacy. The elderly are able to partake of desired intellectual pursuits. Many colleges and universities now provide special lecture series for elderly people in a variety of subjects. Although it is not common, grandparents have been known to graduate from universities at the same time as their grandchildren.

As age advances the person's reaction time is slowed because of the diminished conduction speed of nerve fibers. Reaction time can be delayed further by decreased muscle tone from diminished physical activity. The elderly compensate for this reaction difference by being exceptionally cautious as is obvious from their driving habits, which may exasperate some impatient young drivers. Because sensory nerve endings in the skin are also changed with age, old people are less easily aroused, and safety precautions are necessary when heat such as from a hot-water bottle is applied.

Psychosocial Development

The developmental tasks of elderly people can be summarized as:

1. Finding a satisfying home for later years.
2. Adjusting to retirement income.
3. Establishing comfortable household routines.
4. Nurturing each other as husband and wife.
5. Maintaining contact with children and grandchildren.
6. Keeping an interest in people outside the family.
7. Finding meaning in life.
8. Caring for elderly relatives.
9. Facing bereavement and widowhood (Duvall 1971:453).

Housing for Elderly People

An ancient Chinese saying states that the house with an old grandparent harbors a jewel. However, in North American society most aging people live in their own dwellings. Most think it unwise to live with married sons and daughters, since overcrowded and tense situations with children can arise. It is also difficult for some elderly people to relinquish the authority they have had with their own children and to allow them the opportunity to become independent when living with them.

Deciding where to live in the retirement years is a very individual matter, influenced by many factors, but to a large degree it is based upon five main ones:

1. Amount of income.
2. Closeness of family and friends.
3. Convenience to transportation services, medical services, shopping areas, and recreational pursuits.
4. Loss of a spouse.
5. Degree of health and independence.

Many aging couples prefer to retain their own homes so that children and grandchildren can return for holiday occasions. Others change from larger to smaller homes, even apartments after their children are financially independent. Sometimes large homes are a burden in cost and physical effort for aging couples. It is not uncommon for people to move to warmer climates. Many regions, such as Florida, Arizona, and southern California, are becoming retirement meccas. Moving to a new area may have the disadvantage of isolating oneself from family and friends. It is interesting to note, though, that some retired couples meet several of their old friends when they do move to a popular retirement region. New environments also require adjustments to new and unfamiliar settings, which is beneficial for some people but not to all. Coping with change is more difficult as age advances. For example, some persons prefer to retain their familiar butcher and hairdresser than to look for a new one.

Good housing for the elderly requires the following considerations:

1. One-floor houses are ideal for people who may have cardiac disease.

2. Stairways need solid handrails, and bathtubs should be equipped with hand bars.

3. Good lighting is essential, since the older person's eyes adjust less quickly to changes in light. Particular attention should be paid to hallways, stairways, closets, and the bedside.

4. A well-heated and draft-free home is needed to accommodate their intolerance to temperature changes. Thermostat and humidity controls are recommended.

5. Doors need to be wide enough for wheelchairs.

6. Throw rugs should be avoided or tacked down, and nonskid material should be put into bathtubs and shower stalls.

7. An outside sitting area that is sheltered partly from sun and wind is useful.

8. Access to shopping areas, church, and transportation services are essential to many.

9. Homes need to offer privacy and a certain degree of quiet, although some older people need increased auditory input, particularly those with visual loss. Noise to the visually impaired provides much of their sensory input.

10. Homes should be near others and near to medical services.

When the elderly become increasingly dependent upon others, the use of institutional lodgings becomes essential. These lodgings vary in many ways, according to the degree of independence of the person. All provide meal service but vary in the other services provided such as assistance with hygiene, dressing, physical therapy or exercise, recreational activities, transport services, and medical and nursing supervision. Many of these lodgings are costly and require that younger family members support the cost. Governments now are increasingly recognizing the need to provide additional low-cost lodging services for elderly people.

Retirement

The majority of elderly people are now unemployed after 65 years of age, a sharp contrast from the early 1900s when the majority continued to work. For most men and women retirement is mandatory according to the industry or professional policies. Some who are self-employed continue to work until ill health intervenes. Work offers these people a better income, a sense of self-worth, and the chance to continue long-established routines. For some the need to work exists for economic reasons.

With retirement many adjustments are required for both husband and wife. These adjustments include:

1. Adapting to a lower income.

2. Establishing new ways to keep active.

3. Adjusting to being home together all day.

4. Maintaining social relationships.

Lowered Income.   Some of the financial needs of elderly people diminish considerably. Less money is needed for clothing that before was required for entertainment and work, and many have planned ahead so that homes are free from debts. On the other hand, costs continue to rise, and for some it is difficult to make ends meet. For some people, essential nutritious foods and increasing medical needs create a financial burden. It is said that when older people speak about their greatest need, it is not happiness, not health, but money. This allows them to be independent and look after themselves.

Sources of income vary from state to state or province to province. Generally speaking the elderly person derives money from independent income if working, from social security plans, from investment incomes, from retirement pensions, and from private pensions. There are additional income supplements for those in need in many states and provinces. Other specific incomes are allocated for widows, for example. It is estimated that many pensioners are existing at near poverty levels of $2000 to $3000 yearly. As a result, young people are being encouraged to start savings schemes for retirement as early in life as possible.

Special benefits are increasingly being offered to elderly people in many areas. Some of these include bus passes and theater passes at reduced costs. Some areas even provide free health services.

Keeping Active.   Retirement can be a time when desired projects or recreational activities that have been put off for a long time can be pursued. Pensioners are no longer governed by an alarm clock and can be more leisurely about getting up in the morning. The enjoyment of staying up later is another luxury. Few elderly people, however, spend much time resting or sleeping. Being accustomed to activity most of their lives, most elderly find many opportunities open to them that are not mandatory but of interest. These can be of an occupational nature, a community project, a volunteer service, an intellectual or recreational pursuit, or a specific hobby such as stamp collecting or fishing. Travel opportunities are expanding.

The beginning of the lifestyle in later years is to a large degree formulated in youth. This was recognized long ago in the words of Robert Browning: "Grow old along with me!/The best is yet to be,/The last of life, for which the first was made." People who attempt to refocus and enrich their lives all of a sudden at retirement usually find themselves in difficulty. Those who learned early in life to live well-balanced and fulfilling lives are generally more successful in retirement. The woman who has spent most of her life being concerned about the tidiness of the house and the accomplishments of her children or the man who has spent all of his time being concerned about the paycheck and his job status can be left with a vacant emptiness when children leave and the job no longer exists. The later years can be ones of integrity that is continuity of a fulfilling life, or they can be years of despair.

Being Home All Day.   Most couples have some trepidations about the thought of both husband and wife being home all day. The husband may wonder what he is going to do and how to keep from tripping over his own feet. The wife may have similar concerns and may wonder how she is going to manage with her husband around all day particularly in her kitchen. For some wives who have all their lives been primarily homemakers, the household routines of washing, ironing, and cooking remain much the same. Thus statements are frequently made that a woman's job is never done and a woman never retires. The retired man, however, does not have this established routine. Disposing of the garbage and doing odd repair jobs do not fully occupy his time. Adjustments therefore are often required in looking after household activities during retirement. Tasks may be shifted or shared. Many men may assume some of the dishwashing and cooking responsibilities, and the women may share some of the gardening activities. With the constant concerns regarding failing health, this shifting of tasks and sharing of responsibilities can be advantageous if one spouse becomes ill. One can then function relatively independently.

Maintaining Social Relationships.   The social life of older people varies considerably. Married couples and members of higher socioeconomic groups tend to be socially more active than the widowed or those of lower socioeconomic status. Aging also influences social life. The span of social relationships narrows with age as an individual relies more heavily on the family for companionship. This narrowness is due largely to loss of work associates, poor health, and eventual death of friends, relatives, and spouse.

Many communities offer socializing activities to meet the social needs of elderly people. Clubs such as the Golden Age Club, lodges, and churches provide many opportunities for the elderly to maintain old friendships and to establish new ones.

Younger family members can do much to enhance the social stimulus of the elderly. The joy of being a grandparent can be of mutual benefit to the old and to the young. Without the pressures of parenthood many grandparents find their new role as grandparent more satisfying than the role of parent. It is often more acceptable to offer favors and to brag and express pride to others about grandchildren than it is with one's own children. Close and meaningful family relationships are rewarding and fulfilling experiences for aging people.

Facing Bereavement and Dying

Well-adjusted aging couples thrive on companionship. Many couples rely increasingly upon their spouses for this company and may have few outside friends. Great bonds of affection and closeness can develop during this period of aging together and nurturing each other through sickness and health.

When a mate dies, the remaining spouse inevitably experiences feelings of loss, emptiness, and loneliness. Many are capable and manage to live alone, however, reliance on younger family members increases as age advances and ill health occurs. Some widows and widowers remarry, particularly the latter perhaps because widowers are less inclined to maintain a household than widows.

Women more often need to face bereavement and solitude, since their life spans are usually longer. The brevity of life is constantly reinforced with the passing of other dear friends. It is a time when one's life is reviewed with happiness or regret. Feelings of serenity or guilt and inadequacy can arise. Often the degree of independence that was established prior to loss of a spouse facilitates this adjustment period. For example, a person who has some meaningful friendships, economic security, ongoing interests in the community, or private hobbies and a peaceful philosophy of life copes more easily with bereavement. Successful relationships with children and grandchildren are also of inestimable value. Facing death and dying is discussed in Chapter 35.

Needs of Elderly People

The needs of elderly people are influenced by the physical changes that occur with age and the developmental tasks that arise with living the last years of life. Following is a brief summary of these needs. Each need is discussed in more detail in respective chapters, for example, Chapter 24 on Rest and Sleep, Chapter 25 on Nutrition, and Chapter 35 on Dying.

Physical Needs

Protection.   Accident prevention is a major consideration for elderly people. Because vision is limited, reflexes are slowed; and because bones are brittle, climbing stairs, driving a car, or even walking require caution. The older person needs a well-lighted home. Many other safety measures should be implemented in the home, such as handrails on stairways, hand bars in bathtubs, nonskid throw rugs, and nonskid surfaces in bathtubs.

When driving a car particularly at night, caution must be exercised because accommodation to light is impaired and peripheral vision is diminished. Older persons need to learn to turn the head before changing lanes when driving, for example. Side vision should not be relied upon for example, when crossing a street. Driving in foggy or other visually hazardous conditions should be avoided.

Because the memory fails with advanced age, fires are not uncommon. The wife may forget that the iron or stove is left on, or the husband may not extinguish a cigarette appropriately.

Because of the reduced sensitivity to pain and heat, care must be taken to prevent burns when running baths or using artificial heating devices. The elderly are also intolerant to cold and need to wear clothing that is warm and may often require a blanket over their extremities. Insulation provided by woolen socks is safer for cold feet at night than hot-water bottles.

Nutrition.   A well-balanced diet is needed for aging people. However, smaller servings with fewer calories are required to balance the reduction in metabolic rate and exercise. A diet high in protein, moderate in carbohydrates, and low in fat is recommended. Malnutrition is not uncommon in elderly people because of poor teeth, the rising cost of food, particularly protein foods, and eating alone. Appetite can be further reduced by poor taste buds and a dulled sense of smell.

Elimination.   Constipation is not at all infrequent among the elderly. For some a cup of hot water or tea taken at a regular hour in the morning is helpful. For most, an assessment of fluid intake, exercise, and diet will help in deciding which solution to implement. Adequate roughage in the diet, adequate exercise, and six to eight glasses of fluid daily are essential preventive measures for constipation.

Nocturnal frequency is also a common problem. Many older people learn to deal with this by restricting their fluid intake in the latter part of the evening, particularly of those fluids which stimulate voiding, such as coffee or alcohol. Eventually most men require prostatic surgery to relieve increasing urinary frequency throughout the day, and some women require vaginal surgery for *cystoceles* or *rectoceles*. A cystocele is a protrusion of the urinary bladder through the vaginal wall. A rectocele is the protrusion of part of the rectum through the vaginal wall. Both of these conditions produce pressure and reduce bladder capacity, thereby creating the urgency and frequency to void.

Exercise and Rest.   A regular program of moderate exercise is recommended for the elderly. Walking, golfing, gardening, bowling, and bicycling are common activities. These can be achieved at a leisurely pace. It is important that exercise is not too strenuous and that rest periods are taken as needed. The rapid breathing and accelerated heart beat should disappear within a few minutes after exercise is terminated. Exercise should refresh rather than fatigue a person. For people who are more disabled and who cannot engage in active exercise, a program of isometric exercises can be implemented to maintain joint mobility and muscle tone (see Chapter 23). Exercise is also essential to maintain bone calcification.

More rest is required for older people, since they tire more easily. Often sleep habits change. Naps may be frequently taken throughout the day, and they often have difficulty sleeping at night. Measures to promote rest are discussed in Chapter 24. By encouraging plenty of fresh air and exercise, sleep at night is often facilitated.

Hygiene.   Daily bathing should be avoided for older persons, since their skin is dry and thin. Attention needs to be given to bony prominences if pressure is on them and to skin folds, which increase with loss of adipose tissue and can cause abrasion from friction of skin surfaces. Soothing creams and oils can be applied for dryness. Excessive hair on the face of elderly women needs removal. Nails that become brittle, particularly the toenails, may require the services of a podiatrist. A podiatrist is an individual who specializes in the care of the feet.

Sex.   Sexual drives remain active into the seventh, eighth, and ninth decades of life provided good health is retained and there is an available and interested partner. Drives are more active in men than women. However, the frequency of sexual activity declines with age. Sometimes a chronic cardiac or respiratory illness interferes with sexual energy, and counseling may be required from a physician or nurse about sexual restrictions.

Health Promotion.   Health care for elderly people includes medical supervision and dental supervision. Cardiovascular and respiratory diseases are common. Routine eye tests are needed to check for the presence of glaucoma, cataracts, and arteriosclerotic changes of the retina. Audiometric (hearing) studies are usually also included. For those who have eyeglasses and hearing aids, correct functioning of these needs to be checked at regular intervals. Regular dental supervision can help the older person to keep his or her teeth in good shape or to be fit with dentures.

Health services available to the elderly vary from place to place. Some elderly people's organizations routinely offer free eye examinations. Some nursing homes do not have dental services. Some communities offer comprehensive services through neighborhood geriatric clinics, visiting nurse services, and social services. The nurse who is aware of the available community resources can be instrumental in informing and referring people for appropriate care.

Psychologic Needs

Independence.   Most elderly people thrive on independence. It is important to them to be able to look after themselves even if they have to struggle to do so. Although it may be difficult on others such as younger family members to watch the oldster completing tasks in a slow determined way, the aging need this sense of accomplishment. Children will often notice that the aging father and mother with diminishing vision cannot keep their kitchen as clean as formerly. The aging father and mother likewise may be slower and less meticulous in carpentry tasks or gardening. To maintain the elderly's sense of self-respect, nurses and family members need to encourage them to do as much as possible for themselves

independently. Many young people err in thinking that they are helpful to older people when they take over for them and do the job much faster and more efficiently.

Some older people who are ill appear to enjoy the dependent role of being waited on and attended to. Nurses in this instance need to show an interest in these people as persons and set realistic, achievable goals. Praise and recognition for each accomplishment, no matter how small, is important. Success at getting out of bed independently or feeding oneself, if recognized by the nurse, can encourage people to achieve more and more. Some people may be afraid that they are not going to get better; others may feel that the dependency role brings them more recognition and importance. The nurse needs to understand each person's feelings and concerns before helping the older person toward independence. Patients should know, for example, that an increasing level of wellness is possible and that as much attention by the nurse will be offered when they attempt tasks independently as when they are dependent; they probably will feel better about progressing on the road to independence.

Respect.   Aging people need to be recognized for their unique individual characteristics. It can be more difficult to recognize these differences sometimes, since the elderly have less energy than young folks to show how they are different. Perhaps this is one reason the elderly tend to talk about past accomplishments, jobs, deeds, and experiences.

The ability to think, to reason, and to make decisions is important to recognize. Most elderly are willing to listen to suggestions and advice, but few if any need to be ordered around. Decisions made should be supported even if eventually a reversal of a decision needs to be made because of failing health.

Thoughtfulness, consideration, and acceptance of one's waning abilities is appreciated by old people. For example, having dinner out in a well-lighted restaurant or not expecting grandmother to baby sit for too many hours, if at all, are actions that recognize the diminishing vision and energy level of older people.

The values and standards held by older people need to be accepted, whether they are related to ethical, religious, or household matters. For example, the fact that an older person prefers to use a washboard rather than an automatic washing machine, prefers to hang up the laundry outside rather than use a dryer, or prefers to cook on an old wood stove needs to be respected.

SUMMARY

Adolescence is a critical period of development in which people become physically and psychologically mature. In America, adolescence extends to 18 years for girls and to 20 years for boys. Because the skeleton grows more rapidly than muscles at this stage of development, many young adolescents appear poorly coordinated. Often they feel tired until the heart and lungs develop sufficiently to service the body's increased growth needs. Major physical changes noted in boys are the appearance of facial hair (14–15 years), voice changes shortly thereafter, and gradual enlargement of the penis and testes. In girls the menarche occurs at about 12 to 13 years of age, the breasts mature gradually, and maximum heights are reached by 16. Physical growth during adolescence is influenced by heredity, nutrition, and physical health. Thus the major needs of this group include nutrition (increased calories, protein, calcium, and vitamin D), rest, and sleep up to 10 hours a day. Sexual education is also needed and should include information about venereal diseases, the reproductive process and pregnancy, birth control measures, and sexual codes of conduct.

Seven major psychologic tasks face adolescents. These include relating with their parents at a time when they are gaining independence and yet need guidance; development of a stable self-concept that recognizes both strengths and weaknesses; adjusting to sexual roles; establishing appropriate life value systems; selecting a vocation or career; developing cognitively; and relating effectively with the peer group. Common health problems affecting adolescents include obesity, acne, accidents, pregnancy, venereal disease, gastric indigestion and acidity, and drug abuse.

Adulthood encompasses the years from the end of adolescence to retirement. *The young adult* refers to people between 20 and 40 years of age and includes the pregnant female; *the middle-aged adult* refers to people between 40 and 65 years of age. Young adults are at peak efficiency physically, and physical changes are minimal throughout this period with the exception of pregnant women. Psychologic development offers several new experiences. Selecting educational pursuits or employment, choosing a mate, and getting engaged or married are some major experiences. After marriage, if this is chosen, newlyweds also face many adjustments. Learning to live together as a couple, delineating household tasks and financial matters, developing effective sexual relations, planning for children, and promoting relationships with family and friends are essential tasks.

The experience of pregnancy produces additional adjustments for couples. The parental role is now necessitated, and both partners need to share responsibilities required in preparing for an expected baby, adjusting living conditions, and learning to care for a baby.

Physical changes induced by pregnancy not only involve the reproductive organs but many other bodily systems. Cessation of menses occurs due to the maintenance of high levels of progesterone and estrogen after fertilization occurs. The uterus becomes enlarged and anteflexed and softens at the cervix (Goodell's sign) and at the isthmus (Hegar's sign). Braxton Hicks contractions occur thoughout pregnancy. Vaginal changes include Chadwick's sign, increased acidity, and profuse, thick vaginal secretions. Tingling and throbbing sensations occur in the breasts as they enlarge. Pigmentation of the nipples and areola increases, Montgomery's glands appear, and blood vessels increase in prominence. Striae gravidarum frequently show on the abdomen, breasts, buttocks, and thighs.

Other changes include blood volume and red blood cell increases, alterations in gastrointestinal functioning, increased urinary elimination, decreased fasting blood sugar levels, the secretion of HCG and human placental lactogen by the placenta, and adrenal enlargement with increased production of aldosterone. A total weight gain of up to 12.7 kg (28 lb) occurs during pregnancy.

Emotional changes parallel the physiologic changes. Included are feelings of ambivalence in the early stages of pregnancy, rapid mood swings due to hormonal changes, discomfort about body image changes, passive and introverted behavior, and changes in sexual desire.

The major needs of pregnant women are nutrition, rest, and exercise. Common discomforts include nausea and vomiting, breast soreness, fatigue, urinary frequency, constipation, heartburn, food cravings, backache, muscle cramps, and edema. Specific suggestions for the relief of each discomfort are listed.

During the puerperium, the uterus undergoes involution, the endometrium regenerates, and lochia is discharged, progressing through three stages of color (rubra, serosa, and alba). The breasts become engorged about the third day under the influence of prolactin. Emotional changes include a taking-in phase and a taking-hold phase. Postpartum depression is not uncommon. The major physical needs of women during this period are nutrition and protection from infection, which includes breast care and perineal care. The common problems are painful perineal sutures, constipation, and hemorrhoids.

The middle-aged adult undergoes a number of physical changes. Gray hair, facial crease lines, and fat deposits on the abdomen appear. Energy is quickly expended, and metabolic activity decreases. Hearing acuity may diminish, and visual changes often require the use of bifocals. The menopause and the climacteric are the major endocrine changes. Psychologic changes accompany these physical changes, such as anxiety about aging and fears of sexual

changes. Nutrition, rest and sleep, psychosocial adjustments, and acceptance of a changing self-image are the major needs of middle-aged people. Common health problems include obesity, osteoarthritis, excessive use of alcohol, cardiovascular disease, neoplasms, and depressive disorders.

The elderly person is faced with progressive physical deterioration but can also enjoy an enriched lifestyle. Obvious physical changes include skin inelasticity and thinness, muscle weakness, joint stiffness, flexed posture, shortened stature, reduction of sight, hearing, taste, and smell, poor coordination

Table 11-3.   Physical Development Summary

	Intrauterine	Birth to 2 yr	2–8 yr	Puberty and Adolescence (9–16 yr)	Adulthood	Old Age
Bones and muscles	70% of head growth is prior to birth	Most rapid growth during first year; posterior fontanelle closes at 2–3 mo; holds head up at 3 mo; crawls at 9 mo; walks at 12 to 14 mo	Slow growth; anterior fontanelle closes 12–18 mo	Rapid growth; strength is greater in boys (muscle growth is stimulated by testosterone)	Maximum height is reached in early twenties, maximum strength in early adulthood; gradual loss of skeletal integrity	Decreased mass; calcification of some cartilage and ligaments; thinning of intravertebral discs; decrease in muscle bulk and muscle strength
Teeth	None	Teething starts at 6 mo; has 6 teeth by 1 yr	Permanent teeth start at 6–7 yr	Has 27 or 28 permanent teeth by 13 yr	Wisdom teeth (4) by 17–25 yr; full development of teeth complete	Loss of teeth; need for dentures
Fat	Begins to develop at 7 mo; 16% adipose tissue at birth	Increase in adipose tissue to 9 mo followed by decrease to 2½ yr	Slower decrease to 5½, then unchanged	Unchanged to 11 yr; increases rapidly 11 to 13 yr; decrease in latter part of puberty	Tends to increase at middle age; weight gain may be steady in fifties and sixties	Fat stores are generally lost starting in seventies
Nervous system and senses	Rapid	Rapid growth; brain reaches 90% of total size by 2 yr	Rapid growth to 4 yr and continues throughout childhood; brain almost reaches full size by 8 yr	Slowly grows to maturity	Weight of brain decreases with age	Failing hearing, eyesight, and taste

and balance, slowed speech, and delayed reaction times. Other measurable changes include increased blood pressure, reduced respiratory efficiency, and lowered body temperature.

Several psychologic adjustments are required of the elderly. Changes in housing are usually necessitated because of reduced income, widowhood, or limited independence, and are influenced by proximity of family and friends, transportation, health, and other services. Housing for the elderly needs to be equipped to provide adequate heating, lighting, and safety handrails. Retirement years offer many pleasures but also require many adjustments. Establishing ways to keep active, adjusting to being home all day, and maintaining social relationships are some of these. Many communities offer socializing activities and lodging facilities for the elderly. Facing bereavement, solitude, and dying are major adjustments of this period.

The major needs of elderly people correlate with the physical changes that occur with aging and with the psychologic adjustments required for the last years of life. Included are protection from accidents, adequate nutrition, balanced rest and exercise, attention to elimination, independence, and self-respect.

Human physical development from the intrauterine stage to old age is summarized in Table 11-3.

SUGGESTED ACTIVITIES

1. Select a patient whose age comes in the stage of life considered elderly. Assess his or her health and living problems. Compare these with the needs common to that stage of development.

2. With reference to Erikson's or Duvall's stages of development, briefly analyze your own development.

3. Interview an adolescent. Assess his or her developmental needs and problems.

SUGGESTED READINGS

The Adolescent

Brown, Mary Agnes. February 1973. Adolescents and VD. *Nursing Outlook* 21(2):99–103.

The attitudes of nurses toward teenagers, the present sex education programs, the lack of services, and specifically how a nurse can assist teenagers in regard to prevention and treatment are described.

Curtis, Frances L. S. January 1974. Observations of unwed pregnant adolescents. *American Journal of Nursing* 74(1):100–102.

This article compares the differences between interpersonal relationships and interests (hobbies and recreation) of unwed pregnant adolescents and a nonpregnant group. The attitudes about pregnancy are also included.

Giuffra, Mary J. October 1975. Demystifying adolescent behavior. *American Journal of Nursing* 75(10):1724–1727.

A maternal-child specialist and consultant discusses some specific techniques she has found effective in helping adolescents to develop "putting his/her act together".

Lore, Ann. July 1973. Adolescents: people, not problems. *American Journal of Nursing* 73(7):1232–1234.

This article discusses the freedom adolescents want and the security they need and emphasizes that the way nursing care is given to hospitalized adolescents is just as important as what care is given.

The Adult

David, Miriam L., and Doyle, Elaine W. December 1976. First trimester pregnancy. *American Journal of Nursing* 76(12):1945–1948.

This article discusses the reasons for the changes in the pregnant woman's body and what can be done to make her pregnancy easier. Included is a table of commonly used antiemetics for pregnant women.

Diekelmann, Nancy L. August 1976. The young adult: the choice is health or illness. *American Journal of Nursing* 76(8):1272–1277.

Nurses can help young adults to recognize the importance of health maintenance and promotion by encouraging them to develop proper sleeping, eating, and exercising habits and fulfilling emotional tasks. Many problems can occur in later life if attention to health is lacking between the ages of 20 and 35.

———. June 1975. Emotional tasks of the middle adult. *American Journal of Nursing* 75(6):997–1001.

This article outlines four areas in which middle-aged adults become more self-oriented. Specific examples of how several couples and singles view these years enhance the content.

Diekelmann, Nancy L., and Galloway, Karen. June 1975. A time of change. *American Journal of Nursing* 75(6):994–996.

Psychologic, physical, environmental, value, and social changes occur in the middle-aged adult. The nurse's role in teaching and preparing families for these changes is outlined.

Dresen, Sheila E. August 1976. The young adult adjusting to single parenting. *American Journal of Nursing* 76(8):1286–1289.

The nature of the crisis of single parenting is discussed; some available resources that can provide counseling services and help are included. From several people who have been through this crisis, advice is offered.

———. June 1975. The full life, *American Journal of Nursing* 75(6):1008–1011.

This article focuses upon the experiences of one woman during the menopause and the middle adult years.

———. June 1975. The sexually active middle adult. *American Journal of Nursing* 75(6):1001–1005.

This article includes sexual patterns in middle age and some associated problems. It discusses the relationship between a good marriage and satisfactory sexual activity. An emphasis is that the nurse gain self-awareness about his or her own attitudes and feelings before attempting to counsel or help people with sexual problems.

Galloway, Karen. June 1975. The change of life. *American Journal of Nursing* 75(6):1006–1011.

The problems and concerns of both men and women at the change of life are outlined as well as the nurse's role in helping people cope with these changes.

Graber, Edward A., and Barber, Hugh R. October 1975. The case for and against estrogen therapy. *American Journal of Nursing* 75(10):1766–1771.

These obstetric and gynecologic specialists caution that more scientific facts are needed to support the estrogen therapy that is frequently prescribed for postmenopausal women.

Hammons, Chloe. February 1976. The adoptive family. *American Journal of Nursing* 76(2):251–257.

This article discusses some of the stresses inherent in adoption and stresses to the adoptive family. Successful adoption depends upon how well the parents perform their special tasks of telling the child that he or she is adopted and how well they assist the child in identity formation.

Hott, Jacqueline Rose. September 1976. The crisis of expectant fatherhood. *American Journal of Nursing* 76(9):1436–1440.

This article emphasizes that pregnancy is a crisis for the man as well as the woman.

Hargreaves, Anne G. October 1975. Making the most of the middle years. *American Journal of Nursing* 75(10):1772–1776.

This article discusses some of the reactions to middle age. The outcomes of crises in midlife are influenced by the kind of help offered to a person from family, friends, and care-givers.

Johnson, Linda. June 1975. Living sensibly. *American Journal of Nursing* 75(6):1012–1016.

Changes in patterns of diet and exercise are required of the middle-aged adult. Routine preventive care, in addition, can promote healthier and happier people.

Obrzut, Lee Ann Joy. September 1976. Expectant fathers' perception of fathering. *American Journal of Nursing* 76(9):1440–1442.

Increasingly, fathers are becoming more involved in childbearing and childrearing. However, how fathers describe the role of fathering is not always aligned with the way nurses do so.

Owen, Bernice Doyle. June 1975. Coping with chronic illness. *American Journal of Nursing* 75(6):1016–1018.

Increased adjustments are required of the middle-aged adult when he or she is ill.

Peplau, Hildegard E. October 1975. Mid-life crises. *American Journal of Nursing* 75(10):1761–1765.

The role changes, physical changes, and new social needs are potential stressors in the middle years. Nurses can help people recognize some of these stressors and help them to resolve these and enjoy what can be a productive period of life.

Prock, Valencia N. June 1975. The mid-stage woman. *American Journal of Nursing* 75(6):1019–1022.

The middle years may be more stressful for women, resulting in lowered self-esteem.

Wuerger, Mardelle K. August 1976. The young adult: stepping into parenthood. *American Journal of Nursing* 76(8):1283–1285.

Five goals are suggested for parental growth by which the nurse can assess the status of the family. The skills of parenting are not always easily learned.

The Elderly

Alfano, Genrose J. October 1975. There are no routine patients. *American Journal of Nursing* 75(10):1804–1807.

Adaptation to the aging process results in diminished capacity and, for some, chronic illness; however, aging need not result in helplessness. This article presents several patient examples to support the content.

Anderson, Edna G., and Andrew, Avery A. September 1973. Senior citizens health conferences. *Nursing Outlook* 21(9):580–582.

A visiting nurse association provided health maintenance services to elderly suburbanites. Their experience revealed that the elderly living in suburban, middle-class communities are confronted with the same financial, physical, and emotional problems as those elderly living in low-income urban areas.

Armacost, Betty Lou. August 1970. Organizing a visiting service for the isolated elderly. *Nursing Outlook* 18(8):20–23.

This nurse tells how she organized visiting services by community residents for some elderly. She recounts the experiences of six people prior to and after receiving the visiting service and how the project became recognized and expanded.

Burnside, Irene Mortenson. October 1975. Listen to the aged. *American Journal of Nursing* 75(10):1801–1803.

Much can be learned from the aged about living and dying; about problem-solving, grief, sensory deprivation, and survival; and how to be courageous, loving, and generous.

Burnside, Irene Mortenson. March 1977. Recognizing & reducing emotional problems in the aged. *Nursing 77* 7(3):56–59.

General, verbal, and physical signs of emotional problems in the aged are offered. Specific nursing measures to reduce the effects of anxiety, grief, loneliness, and paranoia are given.

Conti, Mary Louise. August 1970. The loneliness of old age. *Nursing Outlook* 18(8):28–30.

This article reveals some interesting insights about loneliness. Inclusion in a group is not the answer to everyone's loneliness.

Davis, Robert W. April 1968. Psychologic aspects of geriatric nursing. *American Journal of Nursing* 68(4):802–804.

This article considers the psychodynamic needs of the older patient and ways in which the nurse can contribute to his or her total welfare. The author says older people are good dissemblers; they quickly tend to adopt whatever role is expected of them.

Greenberg, Barbara. December 1973. Reaction time in the elderly. *American Journal of Nursing* 73(12):2056–2058.

Practical suggestions are offered by this author, a nurse, about the nursing care of the elderly and how it relates to studies concerning reaction times.

Hahn, Aloyse. August 1970. It's tough to be old. *American Journal of Nursing* 70(8):1698–1699.

This is the true story, according to the author, of her grandmother's thoughts and feelings while in a nursing home. Security, understanding, and hope are needed but most of all, love, says this grandmother.

Harmon, Verna C. February 1975. Rx for RN retirement: speaking out. *Nursing '75* 5(2):22–23.

Like everyone else nurses are subject to birthdays, and recurring birthdays eventually lead to retirement. Six basic prescriptions are offered for nurses in their retirement that can help maintain a healthy perspective.

Horn, Mildred. October 1975. Hospital-based home care. *American Journal of Nursing* 75(10):1811.

Expensive in-hospital residence is reduced by bringing the therapeutic resources of the hospital to the patient.

Macdonald, Myrtle I. April 1977. Practical concerns for nursing the elderly in an institutional setting. *The Canadian Nurse* 73(4):25–30.

Physical and psychosocial needs of the elderly are closely intertwined. The author itemizes the physical and psychosocial care goals by first listing the changes that occur with aging; then she discusses related nursing care measures.

Morlok, M. Ann. April 1977. Community resources for the elderly: day therapy centre: the role of the primary care nurse. *The Canadian Nurse* 73(4):50–51.

This article describes some services in Hamilton, Ontario, that help the elderly to delay the need for institutionalized care and the role of a primary nurse as a nursing team leader and patient advocate.

Schattschneider, Hazel. April 1977. Community resources

for the elderly: day hospital. *The Canadian Nurse* 73(4):47–49.

This article describes some services in Edmonton, Alberta, that help maintain people in their own homes and communities.

Schwab, Sister Marilyn. October 1975. Nursing care in nursing homes. *American Journal of Nursing* 75(10):1812–1815.

This author discusses the many meanings of quality care to different people. She emphasizes that in long-term care institutions there are times when human needs should take precedence over medical needs.

———. December 1973. Caring for the aged. *American Journal of Nursing* 73(12):2049–2053.

This article includes knowledge needed by the nurse to care for the older patient such as accepting a cluttered atmosphere as therapeutic, and cardiovascular changes such as asymptomatic hypertension.

Schwartz, Doris. December 1966. Problems of self-care and travel among elderly ambulatory patients. *American Journal of Nursing* 66(12):2678–2681.

One problem, such as difficulty in ambulating, can lead to a number of other problems, such as inadequate nutrition and financial embarrassment.

Stone, Virginia. October 1969. Give the older person time. *American Journal of Nursing* 69(10):2124–2127.

Timing is very important in the care of the elderly. Nurses need to adjust their pace to the elderly as they need time to perceive, time to learn, time to respond, and time to move and act.

SELECTED REFERENCES

Babcock, Dorothy Ellen, 1972. *Introduction to growth, development and family life*, 3rd ed. Philadelphia: F. A. Davis Co.

Birchenall, Joan, and Streight, Mary Eileen. 1973. *Care of the older adult*. Philadelphia: J. B. Lippincott Co.

Broadribb, Violet, and Corliss, Charlotte. 1973. *Maternal-child nursing*. Philadelphia: J. B. Lippincott Co.

Bromley, D. B. 1966. *The psychology of human aging*. Baltimore: Penguin Books Ltd.

Duvall, Evelyn Millis. 1977. *Marriage and family development*, 5th ed. Philadelphia: J. B. Lippincott Co.

Gedan, Sharon. October 1974. Abortion counselling with adolescents. *American Journal of Nursing* 74:1856–1858.

Hellman, L. M., and Pritchard, J. 1975. *Williams obstetrics*, 15th ed. New York: Appleton-Century-Crofts.

Hurlock, Elizabeth B. 1972. *Child development*, 5th ed. New York: McGraw-Hill Book Co.

Hymovich, Debra, and Barnard, Martha. 1973. *Family health care*. New York: McGraw-Hill Book Co.

Inman, Merilee. 1975. What teen-agers want in sex education. Reprinted in *Nursing of Children and Adolescents.* New York: The American Journal of Nursing Co.

Kaluger, George, and Kaluger, Meriem Fair. 1974. *Human Development: the span of life.* St. Louis: The C. V. Mosby Co.

Kleinman, Carol S. 1977. Psychological processes during pregnancy. *Perspectives in psychiatric care.* 15(4):175–178.

Mitchell, Helen S., et al. 1976. *Nutrition in health and disease,* 16th ed. Philadelphia: J. B. Lippincott Co.

Murray, R., et al. 1975. *Nursing assessment and health promotion through the life span.* Englewood Cliffs, New Jersey: Prentice-Hall, Inc.

Reeder, Sharon R., et al. 1976. *Maternity nursing,* 13th ed. Philadelphia: J. B. Lippincott Co.

Robinson, Corinne H., and Lawler, Marilyn R. 1977. *Normal and therapeutic nutrition,* 15th ed. New York: Macmillan Publishing Co. Inc.

Rubin, R. December 1961. Puerperal change. *Nursing Outlook* 9(12):753–755.

Scipien, Gladys M., et al. 1975. *Comprehensive pediatric nursing.* New York: McGraw-Hill Book Co.

Smith, David W., and Bierman, Edwin L., eds. 1973. *The biologic ages of man: from conception through old age.* Philadelphia: W. B. Saunders Co.

Sutterley, Doris Cook, and Donnelly, Gloria Ferraro. 1973. *Perspectives in human development: nursing throughout the life cycle.* Philadelphia: J. B. Lippincott Co.

Vaughan, Victor C. III, and McKay, James R., eds. 1975. *Nelson textbook of pediatrics,* 10th ed. Philadelphia: W. B. Saunders Co.

Williams, Sue R. 1977. *Nutrition and diet therapy,* 3rd ed. St. Louis: The C. V. Mosby Co.

UNIT III

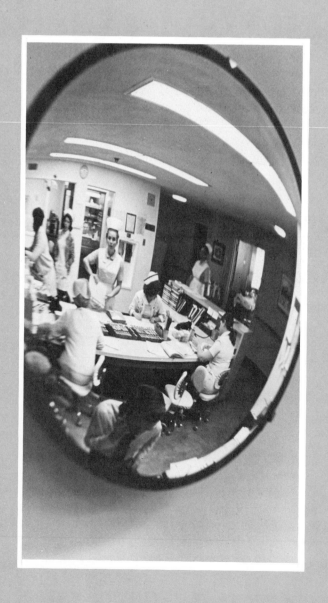

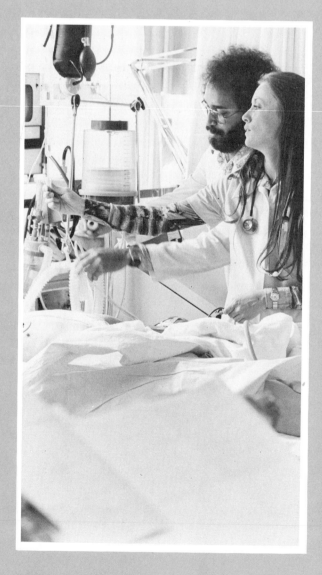

INTEGRATING SKILLS

CHAPTER 12

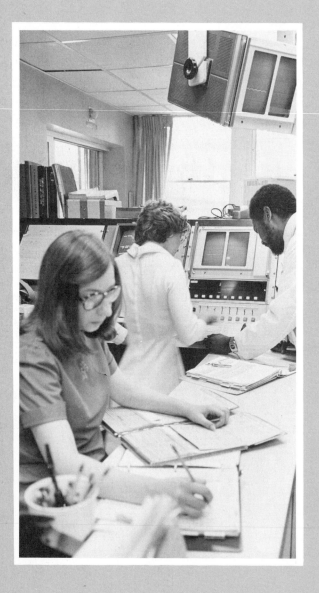

THE FOUR PARTS OF THE NURSING PROCESS

Need and Problem Defined

ASSESSMENT

Objective and Subjective Data

The Collection of Data

Sources of Data

Methods of Data Collection

The Nursing History

Problem Statement

THE NURSING PROCESS

PLANNING NURSING CARE

Setting Priorities

Determining Resource Personnel

Establishing Goals

Writing a Plan of Action

IMPLEMENTATION OF THE PLAN

EVALUATION

OBJECTIVES

Describe the four steps of the nursing process.

Outline data that are necessary to acquire a complete data base.

- List four sources of data.

- Outline specific data that are obtained from various health records.

- Compare the medical history and the nursing history.

- Discuss five basic methods nurses use when collecting data.

- Describe how problems are stated.

- Discuss four factors to consider in planning nursing care.

- Describe three components of nursing objectives (goals).

- Describe five components of nursing orders.

- Discuss the purposes and process of evaluation.

The term *nursing process* emerged in the mid-1960s and has become widely accepted to describe the series of steps that a nurse takes when planning and implementing care. It is similar to the scientific method and to the problem-solving process (see Table 12–1). The nursing process, in contrast to the other methods, emphasizes the solution of immediate problems presented by patients and their families using knowledge and skills that are already available.

The nursing process has four essential elements:

1. It is planned.
2. It is patient, family, or community centered.
3. It is problem oriented.
4. It is goal directed.

The *nursing process* is a systematic method used to identify patients' health problems, to specify plans to solve them, to implement these plans or delegate· others to implement the plans, and, finally, to evaluate the effectiveness of the plans in resolving the problems that were identified. Implicit in the nursing process is the need to involve the patient and her family and the need to individualize the approach for each patient's particular needs.

THE FOUR PARTS OF THE NURSING PROCESS

The nursing literature reveals a variance of from three to six steps in the nursing process. Common to all is the inclusion of four specific parts: assessment, planning, nursing intervention, and evaluation.

The four-step nursing process recommended in this textbook outlines the different skills and concepts that are required when using this process. The steps are as follows:

1. Assessment
    a. Data collection
        (1) By observation
        (2) By interviewing
        (3) By physical examination
    b. Problem statement (nursing diagnosis)
        (1) Analysis of data
        (2) Writing the nursing diagnosis
2. Planning
    a. Setting priorities
    b. Determining necessary resource personnel
    c. Establishing goals
    d. Writing a plan of action (nursing orders)
3. Implementing the plan
4. Evaluating the effectiveness of the plan

Need and Problem Defined

The two terms *need* and *problem* are used within the context of the nursing process. A *need* is a requisite for living, something required by people in order to maintain homeostasis (see pages 100 to 108). A *problem* is an unmet need or anything that interferes with a person's ability to meet her needs. For example, a patient has a need for nourishment, but the ability to meet this need may be threatened by a number of problems such as difficulty in swallowing, vomiting, or excessive intake of carbohydrate.

ASSESSMENT

Assessment is the deliberate, systematic, and logical collection of data from presenting situations and then the assignment of a meaning to the data. During the assessment phase the nurse must first collect data about the patient from all sources available. The nurse then assigns meaning to the data by writing a statement of the patient's problems. The latter can be called the *nursing diagnosis.*

All other steps in the nursing process depend upon the collection of the data, which need to be complete, relevant, and descriptive. An item of *data* is factual information, not information that is interpretive. It is a common error of some nurses to offer opinions, generalizations, and interpretations rather than to describe facts. For example, a patient may be described as "uncooperative." The behavior that resulted in this interpretive label may be his refusal to take a deep breath and to cough after surgery. However, the actual description of the behavior is more useful and provides specific data that can be explored

Table 12-1.   Comparisons of Three Processes

Scientific Method	Problem-Solving Method	Nursing Process
1. Define the problem	1. Gather data in a situation	1. Assessment: data collection, problem statement
2. Collect data from observation and experimentation	2. Analyze data and state the problem	2. Planning or goal setting
3. Formulate and implement solution	3. Decide a plan of action	3. Intervention
4. Evaluate the solution	4. Carry out the plan	4. Evaluation
	5. Evaluate the plan and its results	

as to cause. Perhaps the patient is afraid of rupturing his suture line, or perhaps he is experiencing severe pain when he coughs.

Patients also can generalize or be nonspecific in verbalizing their concerns. They may describe their reasons for coming to the hospital as a "spell" or as "chest pain." It is important that the nurse clarify specifically what the patient has actually experienced. For example, the chest pain needs to be described as to its nature, location, how it was relieved, when it occurred, and whether it was a new experience.

Objective and Subjective Data

Objective data are detectable by an observer or can be tested by using an accepted standard. For example, discoloration of the skin, a blood pressure reading, or the act of crying are objective data. *Subjective data,* on the other hand, are apparent only to the person affected and can be described or verified only by the person involved. Itchiness of the skin, pain, and feeling worried are examples of subjective data.

Some nurses may use terms other than objective and subjective data. A *sign* or *overt data* refers to something observed, whereas a *symptom* or *covert data* is hidden from the observer.

The term *data* has a broader meaning than signs or symptoms. It also includes other information about the patient that is not related to the specific disease process. In the context of the problem-oriented record the terms *data base* and *baseline data* are also used (see page 309).

The Collection of Data

The systematic collection of data is called *data gathering*. The purpose in gathering data from a patient is to

provide information that determines the areas where the patient requires nursing intervention. Sometimes the data that are gathered by the nurse may reflect problems that indicate intervention by other members of the health team. All data collected are combined with the data obtained by other team members in order that an overall plan can be designed to assist the patient. The information that is necessary to collect in order to have a complete data base should include:

1. The patient's lifestyle, something about the person as an individual.

2. Usual patterns and practices for coping with activities of daily living.

3. Problems with which the patient can no longer cope.

4. Current health status, current abilities, and resources.

5. The plan of care prescribed by the physician.

Sources of Data

There are four resources that are usually available to the nurse when making an assessment: the patient, family members or a friend, health team members, and medical and related records. The chief source is usually the patient, unless the patient is unable to communicate because of illness or in the case of the very young or the confused person. The patient can usually provide subjective data, which no one else can offer. However, a stoical patient may understate symptoms while another patient may exaggerate.

Family members or significant others can also be of some assistance. They may supplement information or verify information provided by the patient. They can often convey information about the stresses the patient may have had prior to illness, the family background in relation to illness and health, and the patient's home environment.

Other members of the health team also can provide information about the patient and the patient's health. The physician may have known the patient before, or a social worker may have already helped the patient as may community workers such as the public health nurse.

The hospital admissions record in many settings provides the following data:

Name

Address

Age and birthdate

Sex

Occupation, employer, and length of employment

Religious preference

Attending physician

Legal next of kin

Person to notify in case of serious illness and relationship

Admitting diagnosis

Medical and nursing histories also provide considerable data about the health of patients. The medical history usually includes:

1. Findings of the physician's examination.
2. Past illnesses and therapies.
3. Presenting complaints of the patient.
4. A differential diagnosis about possible disease processes.

The nursing history is discussed later in this chapter.

Other clinical records such as laboratory records, radiologic reports, and special neurologic or vital signs records offer other pertinent data about the patient. The nurse may find from a laboratory record, for example, that the patient's hemoglobin is low or from a radiologic report that an obstructive lesion exists.

Methods of Data Collection

There are five basic methods used by nurses when collecting data: interview, observation, examination, consultation with other team members, and review of records and reports.

Interview

Nurses are increasingly using a nursing history as a tool in initial contact interviews. The patient largely

influences both the time taken for the interview and the assessment itself. When patients are very ill the data gathering may be limited to observation and examination only. On the other hand, when patients are conscious, their willingness to reveal information other than their immediate health problems can facilitate or impede data collection.

During any initial assessment interview, the purpose on the nurse's part is to obtain information and on the patient's part, to convey information. For the nurse this requires thinking, observing, and verbal and nonverbal activity. At the same time nurses, by their behavior, are initiating relationships that will become therapeutic (helpful) for patients.

The nurse is largely responsible for the physical arrangements for the assessment interview. It is best carried out in a setting where the patient and the nurse can be uninterrupted. Privacy is important in that the patient is more likely to feel comfortable and provide highly personal information. The assessment interview has four parts:

1. The introduction.
2. The body.
3. The recapitulation.
4. The plans for continuity in the patient/nurse planning.

The introduction should include a number of points:

1. The name of the nurse and the position of the nurse in the agency.
2. The kinds of information required and what use is to be made of the data.
3. Where the data will be recorded and who will be able to see it.
4. How long the interview will take.
5. The right of the patient to refuse or consent to provide the data.
6. The right of the patient to privileged communication with the nurse.

An example of an introduction might be as follows:

Nurse: Hello, Ms. Goodwin, I'm Ms. Fellows. I'm a student nurse, and I'll be assisting with your care here on this unit.
Patient: Hi. Are you a student from the college?
Nurse: Yes, I'm in my final year and I'd like to sit down with you here for about 10 minutes to talk about how I can help you while you're here.
Patient: I'd be glad to talk with you. What do you want to know?
Nurse: Well, in order to plan your care after your operation, I'd like to obtain some information about your normal daily activities

and what you expect here in the hospital. I'd like to make notes while we talk in order to get the important points and have them available to the other staff who will also look after you.
Patient: Okay. . . . I guess that's all right with me.
Nurse: If there is anything you don't want to say, please feel free to say so, and if there is anything you would rather I didn't write down, just tell me and it will remain confidential. Shall we start now?
Patient: Sure, now is as good a time as any.

In the body of the assessment interview the patient communicates what she thinks, feels, and is experiencing. The information that the nurse requires may well be outlined in the nursing history tool. At this time the nurse has several responsibilities:

1. To listen carefully (see Chapter 18).

2. To clarify points that are not understood.

3. To select the communication technique with which the nurse is comfortable and which elicits the data.

4. To be aware of building a relationship of respect, trust, concern, and interest.

5. To refocus the patient if he or she wanders from the subject.

There are basically three types of questions that the nurse can use in order to elicit information: (a) open-ended questions or suggestions, (b) closed questions, and (c) biased or leading questions.

An *open-ended question* or suggestion is designed to obtain an answer that is longer than one or two words. It can often obtain descriptive or comparative responses. It also allows the patient to divulge information the patient is ready to disclose. The response to this type of question may also convey to the nurse some attitudes and beliefs held by the patient. The chief disadvantage of the open-ended question is that the patient may spend time conveying irrelevant information.

Examples of open-ended questions and suggestions are: "How have you been feeling lately?" "Tell me how you feel about that." "How do you feel about coming to the hospital?"

Closed questions require only one or two words for the answer. The response may be "Yes" or "No," or it may involve giving one's age or marital status. Closed questions are more easily answered by the highly stressed person and the person who has difficulty communicating. The amount of information gained is generally limited. Examples of closed questions are: "What medication did you take?" "Are you having pain now?" "How long have you lived in the United States?"

Biased or *leading questions* contain in them some information as to what the questioner expects in the answer. This type of question can present a problem in that the patient may want to argue with the nurse and hence not give accurate information. Examples of biased questions are: "You haven't had any emotional problems?" "You haven't ever had a venereal disease, have you?"

The use of words about which the patient has many emotions can also bias a question. For example, masturbation and incest have a connotation of being bad to some people, and hence their mention can bias a question.

The recapitulation follows once the required data have been obtained. The recapitulation serves to help the nurse organize, set priorities for, and verbalize the main points that were identified. It also conveys to the patient what the nurse heard and gives the patient an opportunity to validate or revise the nurse's data.

The plans for continuity in the patient/nurse planning then serve to conclude the interview. At this time the patient should obtain some idea of how he or she will be expected to participate in care planning, who will be seeing the patient in this regard, and when. For example, the nurse might say:

> Ms. Goodwin, I will be responsible for giving you care three days per week while you are here. I will be in to see you each Monday, Tuesday, and Wednesday between 8 o'clock and 12 o'clock noon. At those times we can adjust your care if it is needed. When I am not here, Ms. Brown will be looking after you.

Additional information relative to communicating is provided in Chapter 18.

Observation

To *observe* is to gather data by the use of any of the four senses of sight, smell, hearing, and touch, with an understanding of what has been detected. When nurses observe, they must realize the significance of their observations and then interpret them. For example, when a nurse observes that a patient's face is flushed, it is important to then interpret what the flushing means in relation to other data. Some related data might be an elevated blood pressure or an elevated body temperature.

Observation is a highly developed skill that uses knowledge from the physical and social sciences as its basis. When nurses have an understanding of normal

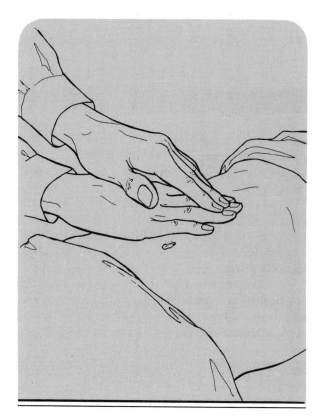

Figure 12-1.   Deep palpation of the abdomen using the pads of the fingers to examine the internal organs.

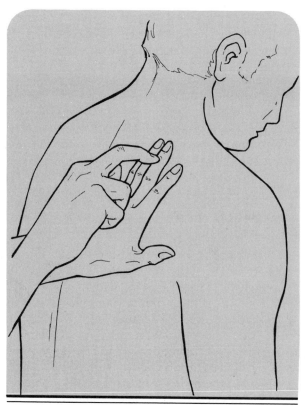

Figure 12-2.   Percussion of the chest is done by striking the middle finger sharply just proximal to the distal interphalangeal joint.

behavior, they are then able to recognize abnormal behavior. Likewise knowledge of normal human physiology is necessary before abnormal physiology can be recognized.

Examination

Visual examination of a person is called *inspection.* The observations are carried out in an orderly manner focusing upon one area of the body at a time. A patient's body can also be examined by touch, that is, by use of the fingers. This is called *palpation* (Figure 12–1). Through palpation the nurse is able to assess hardness, size, texture, movability of an internal organ or part, swelling, and texture. In palpation the pads of the fingers, the most sensitive area of the fingers, are used. *Percussion* (Figure 12–2) is the examination of the body by tapping it with the fingers. The technique most commonly used today is to place one hand on the body surface with the middle finger,

called the *pleximeter,* over the area to be percussed. With the other hand the middle finger strikes rapidly and sharply just proximal to the distal interphalangeal joint. The sound that results comes from the vibration of the body structures adjacent to the pleximeter. Specific percussion sounds of body parts are discussed in Chapter 14.

Auscultation is the process of listening for sounds produced from within the body. The particular sounds that are most frequently listened for are those of (a) the abdominal and thoracic viscera and (b) the movement of the blood within the cardiovascular system. Direct auscultation by using the ear only is seldom done. Indirect auscultation is generally carried out with the use of a stethoscope. The diaphragm of the stethoscope picks up the sounds which are then conveyed to the ear pieces and hence to the listener's ears. The assessment of the body using auscultation is described in detail in Chapters 13 and 14.

Physical examination of the patient is increasingly becoming a nursing responsibility. It incorporates the methods of interviewing and observation. Thirteen functional areas of the patient have been identified that require assessment. These are social, mental, emotional, body temperature, respiratory, circulatory, nutritional, elimination, and reproductive status; state of rest and comfort; state of skin and appendages; sensory perception; and motor ability (McCain 1965:135). The student is referred to the section in this chapter, "The Nursing History," and to Chapters 13 and 14 for assessment skills.

Consultation with Other Health Team Members

Through consultation the nurse is often able to supplement the data about a patient. Other health personnel may have had contact with the patient and family previously or currently. Often their data can verify the nurse's information and augment it or, in some situations, indicate conflicting information, which will need clarification. Which members of the health team need to be consulted will depend to some degree upon the patient and the patient's problems. Usually a physician will be able to offer some information in regard to a patient, particularly if the physician has been involved with the patient's health problems for some period of time. Some of the other members of the health team who may have pertinent information are the social worker, laboratory technologist, dietitian, and community nurse.

Records and Reports

The various data supplied by records and reports from other health workers have already been discussed in this chapter. It is important for the nurse to use all available resources to obtain a complete data base about each individual patient. Once the nurse has gathered the data, they need to be classified into categories. There are a number of classifications suggested in the literature. One of these suggests (a) personal characteristics, (b) social data, (c) medical data, and (d) goals and expectations (Bower 1972:66).

The Nursing History

The *nursing history* is a systematic way of collecting information about a patient. It focuses upon the meaning of the illness to the patient and family, and as such, it is a basis for planning nursing care. See Figure 12–3 for a sample nursing history.

The nursing history is usually completed when the patient initially comes to the health agency, for example, when the patient is admitted to a hospital. Generally, a nursing history includes the following areas:

1. The patient's understanding of the illness.
2. Some indications of the patient's expectations.
3. Significant data in terms of daily living patterns.
4. A brief social and cultural history.
5. Some indications of the patient's expectations.
6. The patient's concerns.
7. A statement of what contributes to the patient's feelings of safety and being cared for.
8. Information about a patient's allergies, current medications, and present contact with other health team personnel. Some nursing histories also include information regarding sexuality and a section for the impressions of the nurse.

The formats for nursing histories vary. Some are interview guides, others are check lists or have objective formats. Nursing histories are adjusted for the age of the patient. See Figure 12–4 for a nursing history of an infant.

Vital Statistics

Vital statistics include name, address, age, marital status, birthplace, citizenship, employment, education, and religious preference. Much of this information can be obtained from an admission record if the patient has been admitted to a hospital. From these data the nurse can learn much about the patient. The address may indicate some information about socioeconomic status. The patient's birthplace may reflect a cultural preference and the languages the patient speaks. Knowledge of the patient's age, sex and marital status help the nurse to understand how the patient perceives the illness and some of the problems it presents. It is also important to know about the patient's next of kin or other significant persons who may or may not be perceived as a support system. For example, a young woman who has three small children and an unemployed husband will probably be anxious to get well to help with the children and return to her job.

Knowledge about a person's education and employment is sometimes helpful in anticipating the patient's ability to understand health problems and participate in planning care. Religious preference may be reflected in some of the patient's attitudes and beliefs relative to health. For example, a young

INITIAL DATA

ADMITTED: WALKING ✓	WHEELCHAIR —	STRETCHER —

PHYSICAL DATA	PROSTHESES —	GLASSES *Bifocals Required*

DENTURES *Uppers Only*   HEARING AID —

OTHER SENSORY OF MOTOR DEFICITS — *N/L*

T-P-R *36·6°C/78/16*   BP *132/60*   HEIGHT *6'1"*   WEIGHT *105 Kg.*

NUTRITION *Likes Italian food*   ELIMINATION: BOWELS *Daily p·c· breakfast*

SKIN INTEGRITY *Intact*   BLADDER

CHRONIC CONDITIONS — *None Reported*

PSYCHO-SOCIAL DATA:

FAMILY and/or SIGNIFICANT OTHER — *Wife: Margareta*   PHONE No. *922-5743*

WHO WILL VISIT — *Wife; 4 daughters; 2 sons*   WHEN? *Wife daytime; others evenings*

TYPE OF RESIDENCE *Not applicable to present illness.*

EMPLOYMENT *Self employed. Pizza Parlor. Family managing during hospitalization*

FINANCIAL STATUS *Not affected by illness.*

COMMUNICATION *Italian first language but speaks English*

BELIEFS OR PRACTICES *None that affect nursing care*

UNDERSTANDING OF ILLNESS *States "Has to pass water often". "The Dr. says he'll fix it with an operation". "I have a big gland."*

EXPECTATIONS OF HOSPITALIZATION *"My operation is tomorrow. I'll be home Saturday."*

HOBBIES and/or SPECIAL INTERESTS — —

SIGNATURE *Janice Reed R.N.*   DATE *Sept. 22/78*

BATH *Partial bed bath post-op.*   SAFETY MEASURES —

DISCHARGE & REHAB PLANS

SPECIAL CONSIDERATIONS *Wife will visit patient pre-op.*

	SURG/DEL/TESTS
ALLERGIES *None known*	
NEXT OF KIN *Wife, Margareta* PHONE *922-5743*	*TUPR Sept 23 - 0800*
ADDRESS *1123 Carnavelli Drive* DIAGNOSIS *Prostatic*	*CBC + Hb Sept 22*

AGE *62*	RELIGION *R.C.*	MAR. STATUS *M*	ADM. DATE *Sept. 22/78*	*Enlargement*	*Urine for C&S Sept.22*

NAME *CROSSETI, MIKE*   ROOM *423 B*   DOCTOR *S. L. SKINNER*

Figure 12-3.   A concise initial data base that is part of the patient care Kardex. (Courtesy St. Paul's Hospital, Vancouver B.C.)

THE HOSPITAL FOR SICK CHILDREN

NURSING HISTORY — INFANT

Damian Fields
7 mos.
Persistent Vomiting and
Failure to Thrive

INFORMATION ABOUT INTERVIEW: INFORMANT: **Mother**

LANGUAGE OF PARENTS: **English**   OF CHILD: **—**

INTERPRETER?   (NAME & PHONE)   **—**

UNUSUAL CIRCUMSTANCES INFLUENCING INTERVIEW: **Admission not planned; sent from Doctor's office**

CIRCUMSTANCES LEADING TO THIS HOSPITALIZATION

WHY DID YOU BRING YOUR CHILD TO HOSPITAL? **Damian has not been gaining adequate weight and has been vomiting small amounts several times a day.**

WHAT HAS THE DOCTOR TOLD YOU ABOUT YOUR CHILD'S ILLNESS?   TESTS, SURGERY, ETC. PLANNED. **Damian will have an X-ray of his digestive system and blood and urine tests will be done**

HAS THE PATIENT BEEN RECEIVING ANY MEDICATIONS AT HOME?   ALLERGIES:

WHAT?	DOSE & FREQUENCY	WHEN LAST GIVEN?	FOOD	DRUGS	OTHER
—	—	—	orange juice	—	—

PREVIOUS HOSPITALIZATIONS   NO **✓**   YES   HOSPITAL:

WHAT WAS THE CHILD ADMITTED FOR:

WHAT WAS HIS AND PARENTS' REACTION TO HOSPITAL?

FAMILY BACKGROUND	OTHER IMPORTANT FAMILY MEMBERS	VISITING PLANS
SIBLINGS (NAMES & AGES)	Grandma and Grampa Fields (maternal grandparents live out west)	Mother - daily
Michael — died at eight months of age of Sudden Infant Death Syndrome (2 years ago)		Father - after work
	HOUSEHOLD PETS	WAYS PARENTS WOULD LIKE
	Cocker Spaniel — "Floppy"	TO PARTICIPATE IN CARE
		bath
		feeding (lunch and supper)

HABITS OF DAILY LIVING	FOOD & FLUIDS:	TEMPERATURE OF FLUIDS: **warm**
LIKES: oatmeal pablum, peaches, pears, carrots, green beans, veal and beef	TYPE OF FORMULA: SMA	CONSISTENCY OF SOLIDS **strained**
	AMOUNT/ FEEDING: 4-5 oz.	(STRAINED, MINCED, CHOPPED)
	FREQUENCY OF FEEDS: every four hours	# MEALS & SNACKS three meals;
DISLIKES: peas, apricots	CUP (BOTTLE) 5 bottles each day	Breakfast: Supper - Pab: Fruit
	2 oz. apple juice mid-morning	Lunch: Meat and vegetables
SLEEP: BEDTIME: 8:30pm	SOOTHER OR SPECIAL TOY: Soother	
NAPTIMES: afternoon only 1-4pm	BEDCLIMBER? —	
SLEEPS THROUGH NIGHT — very rarely	SPECIAL SLEEP HABITS: likes to sleep on tummy	

33385

POMR (27)

Figure 12-4.   A sample nursing history for an infant (continued on p. 228). (Courtesy The Hospital for Sick Children, Toronto, Ontario.)

ELIMINATION:	TOILET-TRAINED? —	BLADDER EXPRESSION, ENEMA
USUAL BOWEL HABITS: 3-4 each day	TERMS USED-URINE: —	ROUTINE, LAXATIVE —
FREQUENCY: every day	STOOL: —	
TIMES: usually after feedings	POTTY OR TOILET —	
	DIAPERS AT NIGHT? Yes	

RECREATION AND SOCIABILITY	SPECIAL BELONGINGS: ARE THEY WITH CHILD?
FAVOURITE TOYS & ACTIVITIES musical clown mobile, small blue elephant rattle	soother and rattle
	USED TO BABY SITTERS? Grandparents only
PLAY WITH OTHERS OR ALONE? likes to watch children play	PREVIOUS EXPERIENCE AWAY FROM HOME
LANAGUAGE SKILLS (SPECIAL WORDS) makes gurgling sounds only	DAY CARE, VISITS, ETC. No

CAPABILITIES OF PHYSICALLY &/OR MENTALLY HANDICAPPED CHILD:	
RESTRICTIONS —	MOBILITY —
	FEEDING —
SELF-HELP. —	
	SPEECH —

QUESTIONS ASKED BY PARENT &/OR PATIENT: Will the radiation from the X-ray harm Damian? Will the nurses check him often during the night? Do many babies come into hospital because of vomiting?

PERTINENT OBSERVATIONS MADE DURING INTERVIEW: (PARENTS' REACTIONS AND CONCERNS, PARENT-CHILD INTERACTION)

Mother appeared extremely anxious and looked very tired. She was tearful when talking about her first child's death and expressed a fear that Damian may also die. Through out the interview Mrs. Fields held Damian on the edge of her knee and watched him constantly.

NURSING OBSERVATIONS OF PATIENT ON ADMISSION: (PHYSICAL APPEARANCE, ADJUSTMENT TO HOSPITAL)

Damian is a small pale infant who smiles frequently and is alert and interested in his surroundings. He seemed hungry and kept putting his fingers in his mouth. He regurgitated three times during my interview with mother.

PROBLEMS IDENTIFIED FOR THE PATIENT CARE PLAN:

Note frequency, amount and pattern of vomiting.
Observe appetite and response to food.
Observe interaction between mother and child.
Allow for consistency and continuity in assigning nurses to Damian.

DATE: July 27 _____ SIGNATURE J. A. Henderson RN.

Figure 12-4.   Cont'd

woman who is Roman Catholic might be expected to be very anxious about the threatened loss of a fetus during pregnancy. The following is a sample of obtained information which will assist in planning a patient's care:

Name	Robert Skimski
Address	6943 Mountain View Drive, Albany
Sex	Male
Birthdate	December 6, 1930
Marital status	Married
Birthplace	Bucuresti (Bucharest), Romania
Religion	Roman Catholic
Citizenship	U.S.
Language spoken	English, Romanian, Russian
Education	University graduate in engineering, Bucharest University
Employment status	Lumber grader in a mill

The Patient's Understanding of the Illness

In this area the nurse assesses in three main areas:

(a) the patient/ perceptions of the illness,

(b) the goals related to health, and

(c) whether these goals are realistic.

Patients' perceptions regarding illness may be accurate or very inaccurate. Even if patients know their health problem, they may not understand fully its implications. Sometimes patients are not ready to accept reality and will deny they are ill or that anything is really wrong. Questions such as "Why did you go to your doctor?" or "Why do you think you became ill?" will elicit some information in regard to patients' perceptions of their health. An example of a nurse's assessment of this information is as follows:

PERCEPTIONS OF ILLNESS. States he went to the doctor because he felt "tired all the time." Says he does not know what is wrong.

GOALS. Says he wants to return to his job in 2 weeks when his sick time is used up.

IMPRESSION RE: GOALS. Unable to assess at this time until medical diagnosis and therapeutic regimen have been established.

The Patient's Expectations

These include what patients expect will happen to them in the hospital or the clinic, how long they expect to be in the hospital or attend the clinic, how they expect to manage when they go home, and what they expect from the nursing staff.

Patients' previous contact with some area of the health care system may affect their expectations. By asking which nursing activities were helpful and which ones were not helpful during a previous hospital admission, a nurse can often obtain information as to the patient's perception of the nurse's role. A sample of the patient's information is:

EXPECTATIONS. Mr. Skimski expects nurses to be very busy and states he will need very little care; he says, "I just need to rest and then I'll feel better."

Patterns of Daily Living

A knowledge of the patient's daily living practices can also assist in planning care. The areas of usual concern are nutrition, rest and sleep, elimination, hygiene, smoking, and alcohol.

Nutrition. The usual pattern of eating, the patients' appetite, and foods they usually eat, or food from which they have indigestion need to be noted. How is the patient's appetite? Is he or she on a special diet? Does he or she follow the diet? If the patient is a young child, it is very important to know the foods the child is accustomed to and whether he or she sits in a highchair or has other individualized habits.

Rest and sleep. The number of hours of sleep the patient usually needs and the hour at which the patient goes to bed need to be learned. What habits or aids to sleep does the patient usually follow, such as an evening snack or reading in bed? This information is particularly helpful for the patient who is admitted to a hospital and will be remaining overnight. A young child may be accustomed to a nap between noon and 2 o'clock.

229

Elimination.   Habits in regard to bowel and bladder elimination are also assessed. How often does the patient defecate and are there any problems? Does the patient take laxatives? Often elderly patients find it necessary to take laxatives or to follow particular practices such as taking hot lemonade to defecate regularly. Does the small child use a toilet? What words does the child know to indicate the need to defecate and urinate? Is the urinary elimination normal? Does the patient need to urinate during the night? Does the patient experience frequency or urgency at any time?

Hygiene.   The habits of daily hygiene are also important. Does the patient shower or have a tub bath? Does the patient take it in the morning or evening? Is a tub bath part of the before-sleep ritual? Does the small child bathe in a small tub, or does the child use the family bathtub? How often and when does the male patient shave?

Smoking and Alcohol.   Increasingly a person's habits about smoking and alcohol are being assessed. Whether a person smokes and, if so, how often are investigated. For some people who do not smoke, it is equally important that they do not share a room in a hospital with a person who does smoke. The amount and frequency with which a person drinks alcohol and smokes can be helpful in detecting potential problems and current health problems. A sample of this patient information is:

NUTRITION. Eats three meals per day and has a large snack before going to bed. Likes cabbage and all meats and fish. Has indigestion from curry. Eats well when on shift.

REST AND SLEEP. Sleeps 8 hours per day. Sleeps well even when on shift rotation. Takes no sedatives.

ELIMINATION. Has one bowel movement every other day. Never takes laxatives. No problems with urination except gets up once during sleep.

HYGIENE. Showers after a shift of work. Shaves upon arising and after work. Washes hair in shower daily.

SMOKING AND ALCOHOL. Stopped smoking 2 years ago. Used to smoke two packs per day. Likes beer and drinks about six bottles per week, usually with friends.

Social and Cultural History

This area needs to include those aspects of particular concern for the individual patient. For example, a patient who was born and lived in another country most of his life may have attitudes and beliefs that differ from those of many other citizens in the United States. Beliefs that people only go to the hospital to die may be highly relevant to a patient's anxiety and related to cultural background.

It is often important also to know whether the patient lives with the family. For the hospitalized patient who will be discharged, information in regard to living accommodations, stairs to be climbed and the nearness of stores can be helpful in anticipating problems and making realistic plans. This is of particular concern for elderly and disabled patients. A sample of this information is:

SOCIAL HISTORY. Mr. Skimski lives with his wife and one daughter (age 19 years) in a house. The neighborhood has stores nearby. House has bedrooms upstairs and one bathroom upstairs.
Parents are dead and one brother is still in Romania. He has two sons and three daughters, all married and living in the city.
Has lived in the United States for the past 15 years.

The Patient's Concerns

It is important for the nurse to appreciate what the patient is concerned about if a supportive, helping relationship is to be established. There are three aspects in this assessment: those matters about which the patient expresses concern, those matters which are of importance to the patient, and the concerns that the nurse might have but that the patient does not verbalize.

Patients may well express concern about a business, children at home, or a possible diagnosis. Nurses are not always able to help with concerns, but sometimes the suggestion of a homemaker, for example, may assist the patient who is worried about her children. People vary in what is of particular concern to them. One person may be especially concerned about her pain, another his wife, while another her business. Sometimes matters such as being able to talk to a family member on the telephone mean a great deal. If the nurse assists the patient with this, the patient may feel that the nurse understands and may feel more comfortable and secure.

Sometimes a nurse might be concerned about matters that the patient does not discuss, such as the meaning of a diagnosis. In these situations there are a number of possible reasons why the patient does not voice concerns:

1. The patient is unaware of the matter.
2. The patient is not ready to accept or discuss it.
3. Because of the patient's particular value system the patient is not concerned.
4. The patient does not want to discuss this with the nurse.

Discussion with the patient or other members of the health team can often clarify the reasons. It is important that the nurse accepts the patient's behavior and that the nurse's values are not imposed upon the patient. A patient sample is:

```
CONCERNS. Mr. Skimski states
that, "I miss my garden and
working in it and I hope I can get
back to work before my sick leave
runs out."
```

The Patient's Feeling of Comfort and Well-being

There is a wide variety of behaviors that contribute to different people's feelings of comfort and well-being. For one person it may be a joke, for another a cup of tea, and for another, an interested listener. By asking the patient who has been previously ill about how the nurses were helpful, the nurse can get an idea as to what the patient finds comforting. An example of this is:

```
COMFORT. Mr. Skimski finds it
comforting when his wife and
daughter visit. He also likes to
talk about his family and his
garden.
```

Allergies and Medications

Increasingly patients are aware of allergies and some will even wear a wrist band or tag stating allergies. It is important to note these in order that any medical therapy and nursing measures will consider these. Some patients take medications that may affect other medications they can safely take. With the incompatibilities of drugs, this information needs to be known before additional medicines are prescribed or administered.

Problem Statement

Once the nurse has gathered all the information about the patient, the next step in the assessment process is to identify the patient's problems. The problem statement is also referred to in some settings as the *nursing diagnosis* or *data analysis*. A *problem* was defined earlier in this chapter ("Need and Problem Defined"). It can also be described as "any condition or situation in which a patient requires help to maintain or regain a state of health, or to achieve a peaceful death" (Becknell and Smith 1975:4).

Problems arise when a patient, family, or community:

1. Cannot meet a need.
2. Need(s) help to meet a need.
3. Is not aware of an unmet need.
4. Has conflict of apparently equally important needs.
5. Must choose from several alternative ways of meeting needs (Bower 1972:68).

It is important when identifying problems to assess persons in their environment and to assess the resources they may possess internally and externally. Problems may be either actual or potential. An *actual problem* is one that is causing a patient difficulty at present such as painful urination. A *potential problem* is one that may occur in the future, perhaps as a result of a disease process, diagnostic tests, or a plan of therapy. An example of a potential problem is a decubitus ulcer or foot-drop if appropriate preventive measures are not implemented.

Problems need to be stated in clear, precise terms that every member of the health team will understand. There are various ways of stating problems. One way is simple description: Mr. Roach "cannot chew solid food," Mrs. Johnson has "edema of her lower extremities," Mr. Skimski says he is "tired all the time." Another way is to relate data in a kind of cause-effect manner. Using the above examples: Mr. Roach is "edentulous and cannot chew solid food," Mrs. Johnson has "edema of the lower extremities due to lack of understanding and inconsistent use of 'water pill' (diuretic)," Mr. Skimski is "anemic and feels tired all the time." In the problem-oriented method, each of the patient's problems are listed separately but are then related in terms of reference. For example, the patient's problems may be listed as:

1. Pernicious anemia.
2. Feels tired all the time (see problem no. 1).
3. Sick time expires in 2 weeks.
4. Worried about finances (see problem no. 3).

However problems are written, they must be specific, clear to all concerned and written in terms of what the problems are for that particular patient (see Figure 15–1, for a Patient's Problem Sheet).

PLANNING NURSING CARE

Planning nursing actions involves setting priorities, determining resource personnel who can best handle the patient's problems, establishing goals (objectives) for the nursing care, and writing a plan of action that includes the problems, the intervention, and the expectations of the nursing care.

Setting Priorities

Each of the problems that has been identified is assigned a priority rating: high, medium, or low priority. This is a nursing judgment, but it must also include the patient's views. Maslow's hierarchy of needs as adapted by Kalish are helpful in setting priorities (see Chapter 7). In sum, these are as follows:

1. Physiologic needs—food, air, water, temperature, elimination, rest, and pain avoidance.
2. Need for knowledge—sex, activity, exploration, manipulation, novelty.
3. Need for safety—safety, security, protection (Kalish 1966).
4. Need for love and belonging—love, belonging, closeness.
5. Need for esteem and self-worth.
6. Need for self-actualization.

From these, it can be seen that physiologic needs take precedence and that even within a category some needs are of greater importance than others. The need for air is essential for the maintenance of life, and people can live longer without water than without air. Once physiologic needs are met, then other needs can assume a higher priority. The priorities of needs are continually changing just as the patient's health status changes.

There are other factors that also affect the priority assigned to problems. These are the availability of other personnel, the cost of needed services, and the patient's point of view in regard to urgency.

Determining Resource Personnel

Once priorities have been set for the patient's problems, it may well be that other personnel may be better able to help the patient with one or more problems. These personnel may be the patient, the family, other health team members, and other personnel such as a family priest. It is important for nurses to recognize that they cannot help the patient with all problems.

The patient and nurse can discuss the alternatives and then decide upon whose assistance is required. The particular resources will depend upon the individual patient and the available resources. In some instances the resources of an urban setting may not be available to people in a rural one.

Establishing Goals

A goal is a hoped-for outcome. A goal or objective is stated in terms of anticipated patient outcomes, not in terms of nursing activities. Goals are of two types, short-term and long-term. A short-term goal might be "the patient will raise right arm to shoulder height once every two hours during the day." A long-term goal in the same context might be "the patient will regain full use of right arm."

Goals must be realistic in terms of patient potential and nursing ability. To set a goal that requires the assistance of a nurse when in fact the nurse cannot help is unrealistic. The goals are worded in a clear concise manner that can be understood by all health team members. They are planned by the patient and the nurse in most situations.

The objectives for a patient have the following characteristics:

1. Written in terms of patient behavior.
2. Realistic.
3. Clear and concise.
4. Exact, rather than general in wording; a specific behavior.

When an objective is written, it needs to contain three components: the subject, the behavior, and the conditions under which the behavior can be expected to be demonstrated.

Subject.   This is usually the patient, or it might be a family member or other significant person, or it might be a physiologic part of the body such as the ankle or arm.

Behavior.   Behavior may be one of four types: psychomotor, affective, cognitive, or physiologic (Becknell and Smith 1975:92). *Psychomotor* behavior involves muscle control, such as writing or walking. *Affective* behavior includes feelings and attitudes such as joy or anger. *Cognitive* behavior includes the use of the intellectual processes such as remembering and understanding. *Physiologic* behavior is activity of the body processes such as the skin, respirations, and elimination.

Conditions.   Conditions are those circumstances in which the behavior can be expected to be demonstrated. They are used primarily to make terminal goals more explicit, but they are not necessary for all objectives. Examples are "the patient walks *unassisted,*" or "the patient will walk *using a walker.*"

Specific criteria of acceptable performance can further clarify a goal. Phrases such as "once an hour" or "the length of the hall" specify minimum performance of expected behaviors.

Writing a Plan of Action

Once the goals have been determined, the next step is to determine a plan for nursing action. The nursing action or intervention involves assisting patients to meet their goals.

It is also at this time that the nurse may require additional information from perhaps the patient or from resources such as current literature. The latter data can add to the rationale for the basis for nursing action. *Rationale* refers to an explanation, which includes facts, principles, and knowledge.

The plan of action initially involves a decision about each problem for which there are usually three alternatives open to the patient and the nurse:

1. No action is necessary or perhaps possible at this time.
2. The problem needs to be referred to another member of the health team or perhaps to a member of the family.
3. Nursing intervention is indicated to help the patient resolve the problem.

Previously the problems have been placed in a hierarchical order. It is important now that each problem be considered in this sequence. After the problem has been assessed as to its disposition as just discussed and if nursing intervention is indicated, the nurse considers the alternative nursing actions. For most problems there are a number of alternatives possible, and the ones that are selected need to be realistic. This judgment is generally based upon experience, knowledge, and data from other resources.

For example, if one problem is "edematous legs and stasis ulcer (2.5 cm) on medial aspect of right ankle," the planned nursing interventions (also referred to as *nursing orders, nursing approaches,* or *nursing actions*) may include the following:

1. Footboard and bed cradle continuously.
2. Elevate legs on foot stool with two pillows when up in chair.
3. RN to instruct re: cause of edema.
4. RN to apply sterile dressing to ulcer b.i.d. (0900, 1800).
5. RN to consult Doctor re: method of cleansing ulcer.
6. Administer lasix as ordered every morning (q AM).
7. Measure and record fluid intake and output.
8. Measure and record ankle circumference q 2 days (every two days).

In choosing the most desirable nursing action a number of criteria should be considered:

1. Will it be effective?
2. Is it realistic for the patient and the nurse?
3. Is it acceptable to the patient and perhaps the family?

These nursing interventions are then written in the nursing care plan or on specific nursing order sheets.

The degree of detail included in the nursing orders will depend to some degree upon the health personnel who will carry out the order. It is advisable, however, to be exact in regard to the order. For example, writing "the patient will force fluids" may have different meanings for different people, whereas "the patient will drink 5000 ml each 24 hours" provides a precise guide for the patient and to all the health team personnel.

Nursing orders need to include five components:

1. The date.
2. A precise action verb and possibly a modifier.
3. Content area.
4. Time element.
5. Signature (Little and Carnevali 1976:213).

Date.   Nursing orders are dated when they are written and reviewed regularly depending upon the individual patient's needs. If a patient is acutely ill, in an intensive care unit for example, the plan of care will be continually monitored and revised. In a community clinic, weekly or biweekly reviews may be indicated.

Action Verb.   The verb starts the order and is precise in nature. For example, "Explain (to the patient)

the actions of his insulin" is a more precise statement than "Teach (the patient) about his insulin." Sometimes a modifier for the verb can make the nursing order more precise. For example, "Apply spiral bandage to left lower leg *firmly*" is more precise than "Apply spiral bandage to left leg."

Content Area.   Content involves the where and the what of the order. In the above order, "spiral bandage" and "left leg" state the what and the where of the order. The nurse can also clarify whether the foot or toes should be exposed.

Time Element.   The time element answers when, how long, or how often in regard to the nursing order. Examples are "Assist patient with tub bath at 0700 hr daily"; "Immerse patient's left arm in sterile saline, soak for 1 hr,"; or "Assist patient to change his position every 2 hr, 1200, 1400, etc., between 0700 and 2100 hr."

Signature.   The signature of the nurse prescribing the order shows the nurse's accountability and has legal significance.

IMPLEMENTATION OF THE PLAN

Implementation of the nursing plan is the actual assistance provided the patient and family by nursing personnel in order to help them meet the identified goals. A nurse may carry out the activities, or the actions may be delegated to other nursing personnel. To *delegate* is to authorize another as one's representative or to entrust authority to another. Delegating nursing activities is not a simple function; it requires the following knowledge:

1. The needs of the patient and family.
2. The goals of the patient and the nurse.

3. The nursing activity that can help the patient meet goals.
4. The skills of the various nursing personnel.

It is important in the implementation of nursing that it be carried out competently and skillfully. Implementation involves technical, communicative, and intellectual skills.

During the time of implementation, it is important that the nurse continually assess the patient's needs and revise the plan of care accordingly.

EVALUATION

Evaluation is the process of determining to what extent the goals of the nursing care have been attained. It is an exceedingly important step in the nursing process in that as a result of the evaluation conclusions are drawn and the nursing plan may need to be changed.

If the patient's problem and goals were identified and written in precise terms, then the evaluation process is relatively simple. Did the patient drink 3000 ml of fluid in 24 hours? Did the patient walk unassisted the specified distance per day?

There are a number of possible outcomes of evaluation:

1. The patient has responded as expected.
2. Short-term goals were achieved, but intermediate and long-term goals are not yet met.
3. No goals were achieved.
4. New problems have arisen.

The evaluation is carried out purposefully and in an organized way. It is an intellectual activity in which the patient is assessed in terms of the identified goals. Both the patient and the nurse participate whenever this is possible.

During the evaluation the nurse can reflect on a number of questions. What factors affected the attainment of the goal? Was the problem correctly identified? Why was the problem not resolved? Was the nursing intervention directed toward the stated goals? What other nursing interventions are more likely to assist the patient to attain the stated goals?

SUMMARY

The four basic steps of the nursing process include: assessment (data collection and problem identification), planning nursing care, nursing intervention, and evaluation. Although the terms *needs* and *problems* are often used interchangeably, their meanings are different. A need is a requisite for living, while a problem is something that interferes with a person's ability to meet needs.

The importance of systematic and logical collection of data is stressed in the assessment phase, on which all other phases of the nursing process are dependent. Data collected must be descriptive, relevant, and complete, and both objective and subjective data need to be considered. A complete data base usually includes the patient's lifestyle, usual ways of coping with the activities of daily living and current problems in coping with these, current health status, and the plan of care prescribed by the physician.

Many sources of data are available to the nurse. The major source is the patient, since only the patient can provide subjective data. Other sources include the patient's family or a close friend, other health team members who have had contact with the patient such as a dietitian, and clinical health and associated records. The latter include hospital admission records, medical and nursing histories, and laboratory and radiologic records.

Five basic methods of collecting data need to be employed by nurses: (a) interview, (b) observation, (c) examination, (d) consultation with other health workers, and (e) review of records and reports. During the initial assessment interview, privacy and an appropriate introduction are important in order to put the patient at ease and elicit as much information as possible. The patient needs to know what use will be made of the information, by whom, and for what purpose. The patient's rights to refuse to offer data must be considered. The nurse needs to select appropriate communication techniques. The use of both open-ended questions and closed questions is necessary. Biased or leading questions should be avoided. This initial interview is concluded with a recapitulation of the findings and plans for continuity in patient care planning.

Observation involves the use of all senses with the exception of taste. The use of sight is referred to as *inspection* and is carried out in an orderly way. Touch is referred to as *palpation*, while percussion involves both touch and hearing senses. Auscultation can be direct or indirect, the latter involving the use of a stethoscope. The physical examination that incorporates both interviewing and observational techniques is increasingly becoming a nursing responsibility.

The nursing history is a systematic collection of information about the patient. Taking the history involves both interviewing and some observational methods. Relevant facts are gathered about the patient's vital statistics, the patient's understanding and perceptions of the illness, and the patient's expectations of the health team. Some social and cultural data can influence the manner in which short- and long-term care is planned. The patient's immediate concerns and factors that contribute to the feeling of well-being are also important. Another major part of the nursing history is fact-finding about the patient's usual patterns of daily living and areas in which illness has altered the patient's ability to cope with these. Notations also need to be made about the patient's allergies or current medication therapy.

After the nurse has collected data, the next part of assessment involves identification of the patient's problem or writing the nursing diagnosis. Problems are written and listed in a variety of ways, but the diagnosis needs to be specific, individualized, and clear to all concerned.

Planning nursing care is the second step of the nursing process. Priorities are determined, resource personnel available are considered, and goals are established. Goals, either short term or long term, are best stated in behavioral terms and need to be realistic for a particular person. They should be determined by the patient, the nurse, and family members collectively. Goals are written keeping three components in mind: the subject, the behavior, and the specific conditions in which the behavior will be demonstrated. After goals are determined, the nurse then writes a plan of action (nursing orders) for all nursing personnel to follow in the care of that particular patient.

Implementing the plan of action and evaluation are the final two steps of the nursing process. It is then that the nurse can determine whether the patient's problems are resolved or aided by the specific plan of care outlined.

SUGGESTED ACTIVITIES

1. Compare three nursing history tools and evolve a meaningful one for your own use.

2. Interview a fellow classmate using a selected nursing history tool of your choice. Practice some interviewing techniques, and discuss feelings and reactions about being interviewed.

3. From the data obtained in activity 2, make recommendations about the person's health habits and together devise goals to promote better health habits.

4. In a clinical setting select a patient and:

   a. Take a nursing history.

   b. Write two or three problem statements.

   c. Establish possible goals.

   d. Write some nursing orders to achieve the goals.

   e. List evaluative criteria relative to the above.

SUGGESTED READINGS

Eggland, Ellen Thomas. July 1977. How to take a meaningful nursing history. *Nursing 77* 7(7):22–30.

This article discusses how a nurse can take a good history. Included is a sample of a history format and a list of 15 do's and don'ts in interviewing.

Ryden, Muriel B. 1977. Energy: a crucial consideration in the nursing process. *Nursing Forum* 16(1): 71–82.

This article discusses human energy using assessment, planning, implementation, and evaluation. In particular, some questions are suggested as a means of assessing energy.

Smith, Dorothy M. February 1971. Writing objectives as a nursing practice skill. *American Journal of Nursing* 71:319–320.

Ms. Smith explains that objectives of nursing must be stated in terms of patient behavior. Included are a variety of stated objectives.

Wolff, Helen, and Erickson, Roberta. February 1977. The assessment man. *Nursing Outlook* 25:103–107.

This article describes a simple assessment tool that students can use in the clinical area. The format follows head to toe using the categories of initial impression, patient's body, extremities, and environment.

SELECTED REFERENCES

Aspinall, M. J. September–October 1975. Development of a patient completed admission questionnaire and its comparison with the nursing interview. *Nursing Research* 24:377–381.

Becknell, Eileen P., and Smith, Dorothy M. 1975. *System of nursing practice.* Philadelphia: F. A. Davis Co.

Bloch, Doris. November 1974. Some crucial terms in nursing. What do they really mean? *Nursing Outlook* 22:689–694.

Bloch, Doris. July–August 1975. Evaluation of nursing care in terms of process and outcome: issues in research and quality assurance. *Nursing Research* 24:256–263.

Bower, Fay Louise. 1977. *The process of planning nursing care: a model for practice,* 2nd ed. St. Louis: The C. V. Mosby Co.

Carlson, Sylvia. September 1972. A practical approach to the nursing process. *American Journal of Nursing* 72:1589–1591.

Gebbie, Kristine M., and Lavin, Mary Ann, eds. 1975. *Classification of nursing diagnoses.* St. Louis: The C. V. Mosby Co.

Gebbie, K., et al. February 1974. Classifying nursing diagnoses. *American Journal of Nursing* 74:250–253. Reprinted in *Contemporary Nursing Series: The Nursing Process in Practice.* 1976. New York: The American Journal of Nursing Company, pp. 188–196.

Hagar, Lorraine. October 1977. The nursing process: a tool to individualized care. *The Canadian Nurse* 73(10):38–41.

Hamdi, Mary Evans, and Hutelmyer, Carol M. July–August 1970. A study of the effectiveness of an assessment tool in the identification of nursing care problems. *Nursing Research* 19:354–358.

House, M. J. July 1975. Devising a care plan you can really use. *Nursing 75* 5(7):12–14.

Kalish, Richard A. 1977. *The psychology of human behavior,* 4th ed. Monterey, California: Brooks/Cole Publishing Co.

Krall, Mary Louise. February 1976. Guidelines for writing mental health treatment plans. *American Journal of Nursing* 76:236–237.

Little, Dolores E., and Carnevali, Doris L. 1976. *Nursing care planning,* 2nd ed. Philadelphia: J. B. Lippincott Co.

Manthey, Marie E. October 1967. A guide for interviewing. *American Journal of Nursing* 67:2088–2090.

Mayers, Marlene G. May 1972. A search for assessment criteria. *Nursing Outlook* 20:323–326.

McCain, R. Faye. April 1965. Nursing by assessment—not intuition. *American Journal of Nursing* 65:82–84. Reprinted in *Contemporary Nursing Series: The Nursing Process in Practice,* 1974. New York: The American Journal of Nursing Company, pp. 133–138.

McPhetridge, L. Mae. January 1968. Nursing history: one means to personalize care. *American Journal of Nursing* 68:68–75.

Rajabally, Mohamed H. September 1977. Nursing education: another Tower of Babel? *The Canadian Nurse* 73(9):30–31.

Schaefer, Jeannette. October 1974. The interrelatedness of decision making and the nursing process. *American Journal of Nursing* 74(10):1852–1856.

Simon, J. R., and Chastain, Sally. September 1960. Take a systematic look at your patients. *Nursing Outlook* 8:509–512.

Smith, Dorothy M. November 1968. A clinical nursing tool. *American Journal of Nursing* 68:2384–2388.

Taylor, Deane B., and Johnson, Onalee H. 1974. *Systematic nursing assessment: a step toward automation.* DHEW Publication no. (HRA) 74:17.

Yura, Helen, and Walsh, Mary B. 1973. *The nursing process: assessing, planning, implementing, evaluating,* 2nd ed. New York: Appleton-Century-Crofts.

Zimmerman, Donna Stulgis, and Carol Gohrke. February 1970. The goal-directed nursing approach: it does work. *American Journal of Nursing* 70:306–310.

CHAPTER 13

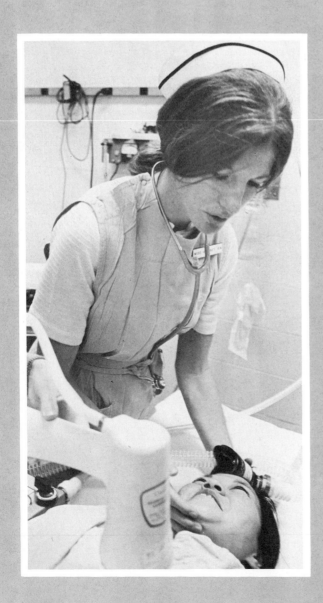

ASSESSMENT OF VITAL SIGNS

RESPIRATIONS

Rate

Depth

Rhythm

Character

BLOOD PRESSURE

Factors that Control Blood Pressure

Factors that Affect Blood Pressure

Measuring Blood Pressure

OBJECTIVES

- Discuss the vital signs as reflecting vital physiologic functions.

- Define the terms used to report these vital functions.

- Explain normal differences according to age.

- Describe the techniques used to measure these vital functions.

- Demonstrate skill in the techniques of measuring temperature, pulse, respirations, and blood pressure.

- Demonstrate beginning skill in observing deviations from the normal related to the vital signs.

Assessment as part of the nursing process has been discussed in Chapter 12. This chapter will deal specifically with assessment skills that are used to assess a person's vital physiologic functions.

Nurses have always assessed their patients' conditions, but increasingly they are employing specific techniques to ascertain health status. In some agencies nurses carry out the complete physical examina-tion and report their findings to the physician by way of the patient's record. Nursing students need to become familiar with the policies and practices in a specific agency before initiating particular assessment techniques.

This chapter is oriented to the assessment of the vital signs of a patient of any age.

VITAL SIGNS

The *vital* or *cardinal signs* are body temperature, pulse, apical rate, respirations, and blood pressure. These signs monitor the functions of the body in a precise manner, reflecting changes in function that otherwise might not be observed.

Within the realm of normalcy there are also variations in an individual person's vital signs. The time of day, amount of exercise, age, emotional status, and even the eating of a meal can affect some of the vital signs. As a basis for assessing changes in a patient's condition the vital signs are usually taken on initial contact with a nurse or physician whether the contact be in a hospital, home, or a physician's office.

BODY TEMPERATURE

The *body temperature* is the balance in the body of the heat that is produced and the heat that is lost from the body. Heat is produced by the metabolism of food, in particular by the cellular activity of the muscles and the secreting glands. Such activities as exercise, shivering, or the unconscious tensing of muscles produce heat. In addition, heat production can be increased or decreased by the presence of disease, an important fact to remember when assessing a person's body temperature.

Heat Production

Food Metabolism and Activity

The metabolism of food produces heat referred to as *obligatory heat*. This rate of metabolism is referred to as the *basal metabolic rate* (BMR). Additional activity such as exercise adds to the BMR, that is, to the heat produced. *Shivering*, which is the contraction of the arrector pili muscles in the skin, can increase heat production of the body as much as five times (Guyton 1976:963).

Increased Thyroxine Production

The hypothalamus, in response to cooling, is stimulated to release the thyrotropin-releasing factor. This factor stimulates the release of thyrotropin from the adenohypophysis, which in turn stimulates the output of thyroxine by the thyroid gland. This thyroxine increases the rate of cellular metabolism throughout the body and hence the increase in heat production.

Chemical Thermogenesis

Chemical thermogenesis is the stimulation of heat production through the circulation of norepinephrine and epinephrine or through sympathetic stimulation.

Heat Loss

Heat is lost from the body through four major methods: radiation, conduction, convection, and vaporization. Through sweating, panting, lowering the environmental temperature, and decreasing the amount of clothing, these avenues of heat loss can be facilitated.

Radiation

Radiation is a method of transfer of heat from the surface of one body to the surface of another without contact between the two objects. In this instance one object will contain more heat than the other; the latter, however, will gain heat through the process of radiation.

Conduction

Conduction is the transfer of heat from one molecule to another. Again a temperature gradient is implied: the heat transfers to a molecule of lower temperature. Conductive transfer necessitates contact between the molecules and normally accounts for minimal heat loss except in situations such as when a body is immersed in ice water for a period of time.

Convection

Convection occurs with the movement of air. As the air near a body becomes warmed it moves away to be replaced by cooler air, which will subsequently be warmed by heat from the body. Convection is employed as a mechanism for heat transfer by the use of fans and open windows. Convection and conduction are less important than radiation and vaporization in heat loss from the body.

Vaporization

Vaporization or evaporation is the fourth method of heat loss. Vaporization occurs continuously through the respiratory tract and through insensible perspiration from the skin. Body sweating will increase heat loss by this method, providing that the surrounding air is not saturated (humid) and is able to assimilate the additional fluid. For further information regarding sweat see Chapter 29.

Body Heat Production and Loss in Balance

In health the body is able to maintain an almost constant temperature despite changing environmental conditions. Temperature control is such that a person's body temperature rarely normally varies more than 0.77° C (1.4° F).

The main thermoregulatory organ is considered to be the hypothalamus. It is believed that the mechanism involves the relative concentrations of sodium and calcium ions within and around the posterior hypothalamus. Body temperature is maintained through a negative feedback system (see Chapter 7, "Homeostasis"). In this instance the temperature of the body is sensed, and specific motor responses are activated to deal with this temperature, for example, by increasing heat production in the case of a sensed lowered body temperature.

Factors that Affect Body Temperature

A number of factors affect the body temperature. Some of these are age, time of day, sex differences, emotions, exercise, and the environment.

Age

The age of a person to some degree affects body temperature (see Table 13–1). When a baby is born, the body temperature mechanism is imperfect. As a result the baby is greatly influenced by the temperature of the environment and must be appropriately protected from extreme changes with clothing and covers. In the newborn the normal body temperature will fluctuate between 36.1° and 37.8° C (97° and 100° F). In fact, a child's temperature will continue to be more labile than an adult's until puberty. By two years body temperature will be around 37.8° C (100° F), by three years it will be about 37.2° C (98.9° F), and by 12 years it will average 37° C (98.6° F), the same as that of an adult. In old age the body temperature tends to be lower and is more greatly affected by cold weather. For example, an 80-year-old man may have a normal temperature of 35° C (95° F) in the early morning.

Table 13-1. Variations of Body Temperature by Age

Age	Average Fahrenheit	Average Centigrade
Newborn	97.0–100.0°	36.1–37.7°
2 years	100.0°	37.8°
3 years	98.9°	37.2°
7 years	98.6°	37.0°
12 years	98.6° (oral)	37.0°
Adult	98.6°	37.0°
Elderly	About 95.0° (oral)	About 35.0°

Note: Rectal temperatures tend to be about 0.4° C and 0.7° F higher than oral temperatures.

Time of Day

The human, like many animals, has variations in vital signs such as temperature and blood pressure, which occur with cyclical rhythm over 24 hours. This cycle is called *circadian rhythm*. It is observable in the body temperature, which can vary as much as 1.1° to 1.6° C (2° to 3° F) between the early morning (4 AM or 0400 hr) and the late afternoon (8 PM or 2000 hr). The point of highest body temperature is usually reached between 8 and 11 PM (2000 and 2300 hr), and the lowest point is reached during sleep between 4 and 6 AM (0400 and 0600 hr).

The variation in rhythm is chiefly accounted for in terms of muscular activity and the digestive processes, which are at a minimum in the early morning while sleeping. For people such as nurses who work at night, an alteration in the temperature rhythm can be noted. Some people change readily during nocturnal employment while others may take longer, thus feeling the difficulty of inverting the cycle.

Sex

Whether a person is male or female can also affect body temperature. At the time of ovulation the increased level of progesterone raises the body temperature of a woman about 0.3° to 0.5° C (0.5° to 1° F). In addition, estrogen and testosterone also increase the basal metabolic rate. Because estrogen causes an increase in the deposition of adipose tissue, women are usually better insulated than men, and thus the internal body temperature of women is better maintained.

Emotions

Extremes in emotional states and behavior can affect the body temperature. Just as heightened emotions can increase the temperature, lowered emotions such as apathetic depression lower the heat production.

Exercise

The body temperature can become considerably elevated as a result of muscular activity. For example, trained athletes after strenuous activity can raise their temperatures as much as 2.7° C (5.0° F). Vigorous chewing of gum for a few minutes can also raise an oral temperature as much as 0.5° C (1.° F). In the same context, taking ice water can lower the oral temperature about 0.9° C (1.6° F).

Environment

The environment can also affect a person's temperature, even that of an adult. Although it is not a major factor of concern, on a hot day a patient in the hospital may register an elevated oral temperature for no reason other than that of the environment.

Body Temperature Measurements

A person's body temperature can be measured by three routes: oral, rectal, and axilla. Each of these measures vary somewhat. A rectal temperature will measure about 0.4° C (0.7° F) higher than an oral temperature. An axillary temperature will on an average be 0.6° C (1° F) lower than an oral one.

Oral (Per Ora)

An *oral temperature,* a temperature taken by mouth, is the one most frequently used in hospitals and health agencies. It is the most convenient and generally the least disruptive to the patient. It is generally contraindicated in the following situations:

1. Babies and very young children, who can be unpredictable; there is a danger of the thermometer breaking in their mouths.

2. Patients who have oral pathology or surgery, or who have difficulty breathing through their noses.

3. Confused and irrational patients, who may also break an oral thermometer.

4. Patients who are receiving oxygen through a mask or nasal cannulae.

For an oral temperature reading, the thermometer is placed under the tongue, where it registers heat largely from the small blood vessels at the surface under the tongue. Critical to the accurate measure of the temperature is the length of time that the thermometer is left in place before it is read. Literature provides differing instructions in regard to oral readings. It has been recommended that the thermometer remain in place eight minutes for men and nine minutes for women where the room temperature is between 18.3° C (65° F) and 23.8° C (75° F) (Nichols and Kucha 1972:6). On the other hand, it is not uncommon for agencies to recommend that the thermometer remain under the tongue for two minutes. Nursing students are advised to check the recommended practices of their own agency.

Rectal (Per Rectum)

Rectal temperatures are taken in the rectum. They are considered to be highly accurate reflections of the body's temperature. A rectal temperature is not affected by the ingestion of hot or cold fluids or by the mouth breathing as is the case in the oral method.

Rectal temperatures are indicated for (a) the very young and (b) the unconscious or irrational and confused patient. They are generally contraindicated for patients who have rectal pathologic conditions or who have had rectal surgery.

The rectal thermometer is usually left in place two or three minutes before the body temperature is observed. In some settings it is a policy to take a rectal temperature for all patients who have elevated temperatures (fevers). In this way the most accurate reading is obtained.

Axilla

An axilla temperature is considered to be a safe way to obtain the body temperature; at least it is generally safer than the oral method. The *axilla temperature* is measured in the axilla of the arm. It is, however, the least accurate of the three methods, although it is more convenient than the rectal method. If the axilla has recently been washed, it is indicated to wait about 10 minutes until the friction effect of drying no longer will influence the temperature reading.

The thermometer is left in place 10 minutes to obtain a reading. It may be necessary in some instances for the nurse to hold the thermometer in place for that time. Temperature by axilla is standard practice in some newborn nurseries after the initial body temperature after birth is taken per rectum.

Equipment

The thermometer is the commonly used tool for measuring body temperature. There are a number of thermometers available. The most common type is the glass tube within which there is a column of mercury. The principle underlying the use of the thermometer is that with heat the mercury expands, thus extending the column along the glass tube where it can be measured against marked calibrations.

Thermometers are calibrated in either one of two scales: centigrade or Fahrenheit degrees. The scale of a centigrade thermometer usually extends from 35.0–43.3° C. A Fahrenheit scale usually extends from 94–110° F. It is unusual for body temperatures to occur above or below these ranges (see figure 13-1).

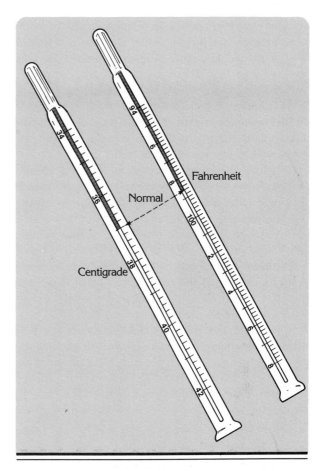

Figure 13-1.   Fahrenheit and centigrade thermometers showing normal adult temperature (98.6°F and 37°C).

It is sometimes necessary for the nurse to convert a Fahrenheit reading to centigrade and vice versa. To convert from Fahrenheit to centigrade, deduct 32 from the Fahrenheit reading and then multiply by (5/9). That is:

$$C = (5/9)(F - 32)$$

To convert from centigrade to Fahrenheit, multiply the centigrade reading by the fraction 9/5 then add 32. That is:

$$F = (9/5)C + 32$$

There are other methods for taking a patient's temperature. An electric thermometer has been developed that registers a body temperature in a few seconds. There are also infrared thermometers, which also provide an almost instant reading. Another device used to measure body temperature is a disposable tape. It is applied to the abdomen, and the tape, which is temperature sensitive, responds to the body temperature by changing color. The tape is removed and discarded after the color has been noted. This method is particularly useful at home and for infants whose temperatures are to be monitored for any reason. There are also disposable thermometers as well as thermometer probes. The latter are used to continuously monitor a patient's temperature in acute settings such as an intensive care unit.

Before inserting a thermometer, one should wipe off any disinfectant solution with a soft tissue. It is wiped from the bulb toward the fingers holding the thermometer. The nurse is then wiping from the cleanest to the least clean area. In the wiping motion, the thermometer is rotated within a piece of tissue while moving toward the bulb when it is contaminated and toward the fingers when disinfectant is being removed. With this motion all sides of the thermometer can be wiped.

A thermometer should also be shaken down so that the mercury is in the bulb end. To do this, the thermometer is held by the thumb and forefinger at the far end from the bulb. The wrist is then flicked sharply, forcing the mercury to descend because of gravity. If the column does not descend below the lowest reading, continue shaking the thermometer.

After the thermometer is inserted for the prescribed length of time, it is removed and the temperature noted. To do this the nurse holds the thermometer at eye level and rotates it between the thumb and forefinger until the calibrations and the column of mercury are in view.

Important also is the removal of any organic material, such as mucus or feces, from the thermometer before it is placed again in disinfectant. These organic materials can inhibit the action of the disinfectant solution if they are still present on the thermometer. Washing the thermometer in warm soapy water, then rinsing it under running cold water will effectively cleanse it. It is then dried with a soft tissue. In a home setting, a thermometer is generally washed in warm soapy water, dried, and stored for reuse. If a person using it is suspected of having an infection that can be transmitted through body secretions, the thermometer will need to be disinfected with an appropriate agent.

Procedure 13-1.   Measuring Body Temperature by Mouth

Action	Explanation
Assemble Equipment	
1. Oral thermometer.	Oral thermometers may have a blunt bulb end or a narrowed bulb. In some agencies oral thermometers have white or silver columns.
2. Soft tissue.	To wipe the thermometer.
3. Pencil or pen.	To record the temperature.
4. Book, record, or work sheet.	Upon which to record the temperature.
To Measure the Temperature	
1. Wash hands.	To remove any microorganism, which should not be transmitted to the patient.
2. Explain to the patient what you plan to do. Adjust the explanation to the patient's need.	To reassure the patient by knowledge of what will happen. To identify the patient. To ascertain that an oral temperature method is appropriate.
3. Wipe the thermometer with a soft tissue or rinse it under cold water. Wipe from the bulb end to fingers in a rotating fashion. Discard the tissue.	The disinfectant may be irritating to mucous membrane and unpleasant to taste. Use cold water because hot water will expand the mercury and can break the thermometer.

4. If using an electric thermometer, assemble the kit and disposable probe covers. Place a cover on the probe. Warm up the machine by switching on the *on* button.

5. Check the level of the mercury in the thermometer. Shake it down by holding it between the thumb and forefinger. Sharply flick the wrist downward. Repeat until the mercury is down.

   It should be below 35° C (95° F)

6. Ask the patient to open his or her mouth, and place the thermometer under the tongue.

   The thermometer will reflect the temperature of the blood in the superficial blood vessels under the tongue.

7. Ask the patient to hold the thermometer with the lips.

   Holding with the teeth can result in biting and breaking the thermometer.

8. Leave the thermometer in place according to agency policy.

   The recommended time is eight minutes for men and nine minutes for women if there is no policy. If using an electric thermometer (oral), hold thermometer under the tongue about 10–20 seconds.

9. Remove the thermometer.

10. Wipe with a tissue starting at end held by the nurse, and wipe in a rotating manner toward the bulb. Discard tissue.

    Wipe from the area of least contamination to that of greatest contamination.

11. Hold the thermometer at eye level and rotate it until the mercury column is clearly visible. Read the temperature.

    The upper end of the mercury column reflects the patient's body temperature. Each long line on the thermometer reflects 1°. Each short line indicates 0.2°.

12. Return the thermometer to its container after shaking it down again.

    Note if thermometer is broken, and replace if necessary.

13. Wash hands.

14. Record temperature in the book or on the record or work sheet.

    Record immediately before it is forgotten.

Procedure 13-2.   Measuring Body Temperature by Rectum

Action	**Explanation**
Assemble Equipment	
1. Rectal thermometer.	In some agencies the rectal thermometers have a round bulb end and a blue liquid column.
2. Soft tissue.	To wipe the thermometer.
3. Lubricant.	To lubricate the thermometer in order to ease insertion into the rectum.
4. Pencil or pen.	To record temperature.
5. Book, record, or work sheet.	Upon which to record temperature.

To Measure the Temperature

1. Wash hands.

    To remove any microorganisms, which should not be transmitted to the patient.

2. Explain to the patient what you plan to do. Adjust the explanation to the patient's need.

    To reassure the patient by knowledge of what will happen. To identify the patient. To ascertain that a rectal temperature method is appropriate.

3. Wipe the thermometer with a soft tissue or rinse it under cold water and dry. Discard the tissue.

    The disinfectant may be irritating to the mucous membrane. Use cold water because hot water will expand the mercury and can break the thermometer. Dry so that water will not interfere with the application of lubricant on the thermometer.

4. Check the level of the mercury in the thermometer. Shake it down by holding it between the thumb and forefinger. Sharply flick the wrist downward. Repeat until the mercury is down.

    The mercury should be below 35° C (95° F).

5. Assist the patient to assume a lateral position. Provide privacy before folding the bedclothes back to expose the buttocks.

    Exposure of the buttocks could be embarrassing to the patient. An infant can remain in a supine position.

6. Place some lubricant on a piece of tissue. Then apply lubricant to the thermometer. For an adult, lubricate 1 to 1½ inches along the thermometer from the bulb end. For an infant, lubricate from ½ to 1 inch.

    The lubricant in the jar or tube will not be contaminated by the thermometer. The lubricant facilitates the easy insertion of the thermometer without irritating the mucous membrane.

7. With one hand raise the upper buttock to expose the anus. For the infant hold both ankles by one hand and raise the legs to expose the anus.

8. Insert the thermometer into the anus anywhere from ½ to 1½ inches, depending upon the age and size of the patient. For example, ½ inch for an infant, 1½ inches for a large adult. Do not force insertion of the thermometer.

    Do not force the thermometer on an infant. Inability to insert the thermometer on a newborn could indicate that the rectum is not patent. Asking the patient to take a deep breath will relax the external sphincter muscle, thus easing insertion. If using an electric thermometer, make sure the end of the probe is not embedded into feces.

9. Hold the thermometer in place according to agency policy.

    The recommended time is two to three minutes. Hold an electric thermometer 10–20 seconds.

10. Remove the thermometer.

11. Wipe it clean with a tissue starting at the end held by the nurse and wipe in a rotating manner toward the bulb. Discard tissue.

    Wipe from the area of least contamination to that of greatest contamination.

12. Hold the thermometer at eye level and rotate it until the mercury column is clearly visible. Read the temperature.

    The upper end of the mercury column reflects the patient's body temperature. Each long line on the thermometer reflects 1°. Each short line indicates 0.2°.

13. Wash the thermometer in warm soapy water. Rinse it in cold water.

    To remove any organic material, which could interfere with the action of an antiseptic.

14. Shake it down.

15. Return the thermometer to its container.

Note if the thermometer is broken, and replace it if necessary.

16. Assist the patient to a comfortable position.

17. Wash hands.

18. Record the temperature in the record book or on work sheet.

Procedure 13—3.   Measuring Body Temperature by Axilla

Action	**Explanation**
Assemble Equipment	
1. Axilla thermometer.	Oral thermometers are usually used in most agencies.
2. Soft tissue.	To wipe the thermometer.
3. Towel.	To wipe the axilla.
4. Pencil or pen.	To record the temperature.
5. Book, record, or work sheet.	Upon which to record the temperature.
To Measure the Temperature	
1. Wash hands.	To remove any microorganism, which should not be transmitted to the patient.
2. Explain to the patient what you plan to do. Adjust the explanation to the patient's need.	To reassure the patient by knowledge of what will happen. To identify the patient. To ascertain that an axilla temperature is appropriate.
3. Wipe the thermometer with a soft tissue or rinse it in cold water and dry. Discard the tissue.	The disinfectant may be irritating to the skin in the axilla. Use cold water because hot water will expand the mercury and could break the thermometer.
4. Check the level of the mercury in the thermometer. Shake it down by holding it between the thumb and forefinger. Sharply flick the wrist downward. Repeat until the mercury is down.	The mercury should be below 35° C (95° F).
5. Expose the patient's axilla. Dry the axilla with a patting motion if it is moist.	Friction can raise the temperature of the axilla.
6. Place the thermometer in the patient's axilla.	
7. Assist the patient to place the arm tightly across the chest.	To maintain the thermometer closely in the axilla.
8. Leave the thermometer in place.	The thermometer should be in place 10 minutes.
9. Remove the thermometer.	

10. Wipe with a tissue starting at the end held by the nurse, and wipe in a rotating manner toward the bulb. Discard the tissue.

    Wipe from the area of least contamination to that of greatest contamination.

11. Hold the thermometer at eye level and rotate it until the mercury is clearly visible. Read the temperature.

    The upper end of the mercury column reflects the patient's body temperature. Each long line represents 1°. Each short line represents 0.2°.

12. Wash the thermometer in warm soapy water. Rinse it in cold water.

    To remove any organic material, which could interfere with the action of the disinfectant.

13. Shake it down.

14. Return the thermometer to its container.

    Note if the thermometer is broken, and replace it if necessary.

15. Assist the patient to a comfortable position and cover the axilla.

16. Wash hands.

17. Record temperature in the book or on the record or work sheet.

Fever

An elevated body temperature is called a *fever* or *pyrexia*. A very high fever is *hyperpyrexia*. An extremely low body temperature is referred to as *hypothermia*. There are three types of fevers: (a) intermittent, (b) remittent, and (c) relapsing.

An *intermittent* or *quotidian fever* is one in which the body temperature is elevated but returns to normal sometime in the 24-hour period. It is not unusual for an intermittent fever to be highest in the late afternoon or evening and lowest in the early morning hours.

A *remittent fever* is one in which there is a wide range of temperatures over the 24-hour period, all of which, however, are above normal.

In a *relapsing fever*, the body temperature is elevated for perhaps several days, and then there will be one or two days of normal temperature. The periods of normal temperature are irregularly spaced.

A fever can also be described according to the type of onset and the type of termination. A fever can start gradually or suddenly, and the temperature can return to normal either suddenly (*crisis*) or gradually (*lysis*).

Fevers are caused by an increase in heat production, a decrease in heat loss, or a combination of both. For every 1° C rise in body temperature, heat produc-

tion increases 13%. The highest temperature at which a person can survive is thought to be about 46° C (114.8° F). However, studies indicate a temperature ceiling in most cases of febrile disease of about 40.6° C (105° F) or 41.1° C (106° F) (MacBryde et al. 1970:456).

The signs of a fever vary depending upon the stage of the fever, that is, the onset, the course, or the termination.

Onset

Symptoms during the onset of a fever are as follows:

1. Shivering or strong muscle contractions result in shaking chills.
2. Body metabolism is increased.
3. Increased cardiac rate is reflected by an increased pulse rate.
4. The skin is pallid due to peripheral vasoconstriction.
5. The arrector pili muscles contract, shown as "goose-flesh" appearance.
6. Sweating is reduced.
7. The patient complains of feeling cold.
8. With extremely high temperatures, convulsions can occur, particularly in children.

Course

Symptoms during the course of a fever are as follows:

1. The skin feels warm to the touch.

2. Peripheral vasodilation results in skin flushing.

3. The patient usually complains of neither heat nor cold.

4. The patient may state that he or she has a headache. The patient is irritable or restless due to irritation to the central nervous system.

5. With extremely high temperatures the patient may be disoriented and confused.

6. There is generalized weakness and aching of body parts.

7. With a prolonged fever, weight loss occurs.

8. Anorexia, nausea, and vomiting occur.

9. Sweating and increased vasodilation can occur when the temperature is falling.

10. Dehydration can occur with a prolonged fever; as a result, the skin and mucous membranes become dry (see section on underhydration, Chapter 30). This is a particular problem for babies and young children.

Termination

Symptoms during the termination of a fever are as follows:

1. Increased diaphoresis and reddening of the skin accelerate heat loss.

2. Dehydration can occur.

PULSE

The *pulse* of a person is the pulse wave of blood that is created by the contraction of the left ventricle of the heart. A pulse can be palpated on certain superficial areas of the body, for example, where an artery passes over or alongside a bone. By slight pressure on the artery the pulse wave can be felt as the blood is pumped around the body.

Pulse Sites

A pulse is commonly taken at a number of sites: temporal, carotid, brachial, radial, femoral, popliteal, posterior tibial, and pedal (dorsalis pedis) (see Figure 13-2). The most commonly used is the radial site. An apical pulse is usually taken on babies and young children under two or three years.

Temporal Pulse

The temporal pulse is taken at a site superior and lateral to the eye. At this site the temporal artery passes over the temporal bone of the head.

Carotid Pulse

The carotid pulse is felt at the side of the neck. If an imaginary line is drawn from the lobe of the ear down along the anterior border of the sternocleidomastoid muscle, the carotid pulse can be felt along this line. It is likely to be felt most clearly near the angle of the jaw.

Brachial Pulse

The brachial pulse can be felt on the inner aspect of the biceps muscle. It is found a few centimeters below the axilla on the inner aspect of the arm or medially in the antecubital space.

Radial Pulse

The radial pulse is found on the inner aspect of the wrist on the radial or thumb side. It is the most commonly used site because it is readily accessible with usually little disturbance to the patient.

Femoral Pulse

The femoral pulse is found in the groin about at the midpoint, that is, the midpoint of the inguinal ligament.

Popliteal Pulse

The popliteal artery can be palpated behind the knee. It is a more difficult pulse to find but the assessment is facilitated if the patient flexes the knee and the nurse's fingers are pressed into the center of the popliteal space.

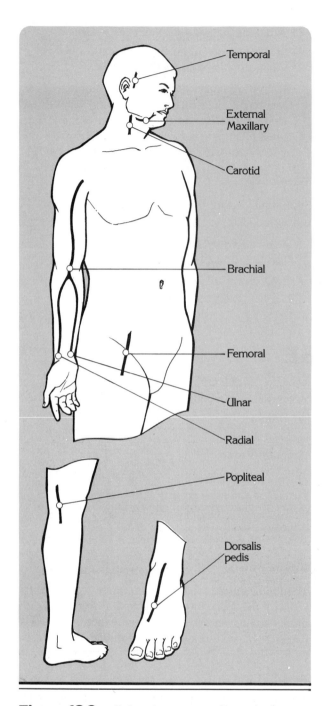

Figure 13-2.   Pulse sites commonly used where an artery passes over or alongside of a bone.

Posterior Tibial Pulse

This pulse can be found by placing the fingers in the groove between the Achilles tendon and the tibia just above the medial malleolus and then pressing toward the tibia.

Pedal (Dorsalis Pedis) Pulse

This pulse in the foot, the dorsalis pedis pulse, can be felt by palpating the instep of the foot on an imaginary line drawn from the middle of the ankle to the interdigital space between the big toe and the second. toe.

Reasons for Taking a Pulse

There are basically two broad reasons for taking a patient's pulse:

1. To assess the adequacy of the blood flow to an area, as for example, taking the dorsalis pedis pulse to assess blood flow to a foot.

2. To assess the rate, rhythm, volume, and tension of a pulse, which may reflect a central problem, such as a slow heart rate.

The peripheral pulses are the ones generally checked to assess the adequacy of blood flow to a particular area. Nurses are expected to do this for a variety of reasons such as taking a dorsalis pedis pulse after the application of a leg cast to assess any restriction of the blood flow to the patient's foot, or assessing the radial pulse after surgical procedures to an elbow.

When assessing the rate, rhythm, volume, and tension of a pulse, it is customary to use the radial pulse because of the convenience for most people. If the radial pulse is not readily available, such as when a patient has both arms bandaged, a temporal or carotid pulse is customarily taken.

Pulse Rate

The rate of the pulse is expressed in beats per minute (beat/min). Usually when a pulse is regular it can be counted for 15 seconds and then multiplied by 4 to obtain a relatively accurate estimate. If a pulse is irregular, however, it is advisable to count it for a longer period (one minute) to obtain a more accurate measure.

A pulse rate varies according to a number of factors: age, sex, exercise, emotions, heat, and body position, for example.

Age

The pulse of a newborn baby will vary from 120–160 beats/min. By two years it will have slowed to 80–140 beats/min and to 110 beats/min at three years. By 12 years a boy's pulse will be between 65 and 105 beats/min and a girl's between 70 and 110 beats/min when resting. In adolescence a boy's pulse will drop to between 60 and 100 beats/min and will be 50–90 beats/min at 18 years of age. A girl's will drop somewhat less; at 14 years it will be between 65 and 105 beats/min, and by 18 years it will have dropped further to between 55 and 95 beats/min.

During adulthood, the pulse tends to remain at the 18-year-old level, generally between 60 and 100 beats/min, until old age, when it tends to increase slightly. The average pulse rate of an elderly person is on the average 70 to 80 beats/min.

Sex

The pulse rate tends to vary somewhat between men and women of similar ages. Reference is made to the previous section in regard to adolescence and adulthood.

Exercise

The pulse rate normally increases with activity. Increased need for oxygen by the muscles during exercise results in an increased heart rate in an effort to deliver that oxygen through the blood stream.

Emotions

The heart rate alters in response to both the sympathetic and parasympathetic divisions of the autonomic nervous system. Emotions such as fear, anger and worry, as well as the perception of pain, stimulate the sympathetic system. As a result, the heart rate as well as the contractility of the heart are increased. The parasympathetic stimulation slows the heart and the contractility of the atria. Digitalis is a frequently used drug that stimulates the parasympathetic system, specifically the vagus nerve.

An excessively fast heart rate is referred to as *tachycardia*. A rate of over 100 beats/min in an adult is considered to be cardiac tachycardia. *Bradycardia* refers to a slow rate of heart contraction, usually any rate below 60 beats/min.

Heat

The prolonged application of external heat as well as the internal occurrence of a fever also can accelerate a heart (pulse) rate. The pulse rate increases in response to the lowered blood pressure, which in turn is a result of a peripheral vasodilation response to the heat.

Body Position

Prolonged assumption of a horizontal position can also result in increased heart and pulse rates. Physiologically the normal blood volume in the extremities is diminished, moving more centrally in the systemic circulation. Therefore the heart is required to beat more rapidly in order to pump out this additional blood volume.

Pulse Rhythm

The *rhythm* of the pulse is the pattern of the beats and the intervals between the beats. A normal pulse has characteristically an equal time period between each beat; this is called *pulsus regularis*. A pulse that has an irregular rhythm is referred to as an *arrhythmia*.

In an irregular rhythm the irregular beats may come at random or they may come at predictable times, thus forming a regular irregularity.

Pulse Volume

A pulse *volume* refers to the force of blood with each beat. Usually a pulse volume is the same with each beat. A normal pulse can be felt with moderate pressure of the fingers, and it can be obliterated with greater pressure. A forceful or full blood volume that is obliterated only with difficulty is called a *full* or *bounding* pulse. A pulse that is readily obliterated with pressure is referred to as *weak, feeble,* or *thready*. It feels weak and less full to the person palpating the artery.

The Arterial Wall

The arterial walls can also be palpated with the fingers. Elderly people often have inelastic arteries, which may feel twisted and irregular. Normally arteries are straight and smooth.

By emptying an artery the nurse is able to more clearly feel any beading or roughness. To do this two fingers are placed over an artery, and the artery is compressed firmly. The finger distal to the heart is then moved along the artery that will be empty. An artery that is very hard may feel gritty to the touch.

Procedure 13-4.   Assessing the Pulse

ACTION	EXPLANATION
Assemble Equipment	
1. Watch with a second hand.	To count the pulse rate.
2. Pencil or pen.	To record pulse data.
3. Book, record, or work sheet.	Upon which to record pulse data.
To Assess the Pulse	
1. Wash hands.	To remove any microorganisms, which should not be transmitted to the patient.
2. Explain to the patient what you plan to do. Adjust the explanation to the patient's need.	To reassure the patient by knowledge of what will happen. To identify the patient.
3. Select the pulse point.	Normally the radial pulse is taken unless it cannot be exposed or circulation to another body area is to be assessed.
4. Place three middle fingertips over the pulse point.	Place fingertips lightly and squarely on the site.
5. Count pulse for 15 seconds and multiply by 4 if pulse is regular. If it is irregular, count for one full minute. Count one full minute for an infant.	For an accurate rate a full minute's count is needed for an irregular pulse.
6. Assess the pulse rhythm by noting the pattern of intervals between the beats.	A normal pulse has an equal time period between each beat.
7. Assess the pulse volume. A normal pulse can be felt with moderate pressure.	Normally the pressure of the blood with each beat is equal, and a forceful pulse volume is referred to as full. A pulse easily obliterated is called weak.
8. Palpate the arterial wall by compressing the artery firmly and running a finger distal to the heart along the artery.	A normal arterial wall will be felt to be smooth and straight.
9. Assist the patient to a comfortable position. Cover him/her if necessary.	
10. Wash hands.	
11. Record pulse rate, rhythm, volume and arterial wall.	

To Take a Pulse

To take a pulse the nurse should first make sure that the patient is in a comfortable position. If the patient has been active, the pulse observation should be deferred for 10–15 minutes until the patient is resting.

The nurse then palpates the pulse using the first, second, or third fingers. Using the thumb is contraindicated because there is a pulse in the thumb, which the nurse could mistake for the patient's pulse.

Once the pulse has been located, the nurse then counts the beats. If the pulse is regular, counting for 15 or 30 seconds is considered to be satisfactory, but if it is irregular, a full minute of counting is advised. If the count is carried out for a fraction of the minute, the count is then multiplied accordingly to obtain a count in beats per minute. The nursing student is advised to check the recommended practice of the agency regarding the length of time to count a pulse. While taking the rate of the pulse, the nurse should

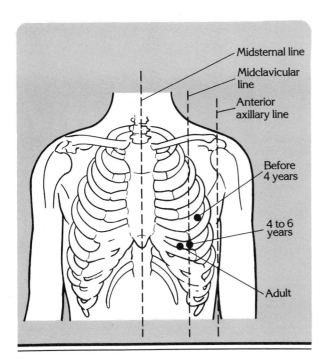

Midsternal line

Midclavicular line

Anterior axillary line

Before 4 years

4 to 6 years

Adult

Figure 13-3. The location of the apical pulse, also called the point of maximum intensity (PMI), for a child under 4 years, a child 4 to 6 years, and an adult.

also assess the rhythm, volume, and the condition of the arterial wall. These observations should also be recorded.

The Apical-Radial Pulse

It may be necessary to take an apical-radial pulse for a patient. This will require two nurses: one takes the radial pulse and the other nurse takes the apical rate. The number of beats of both are counted at the same time.

Each nurse will require a watch with a second hand, and one will require a stethoscope. The stethoscope is placed over the apex of the heart, which in an adult is under the fourth, fifth, or sixth intercostal space, that is, 2–3 inches (no more than 8 cm) to the left of the sternum, just below the left nipple. Another way of locating the apex is to find the midclavicular line or just medial to it at the fourth, fifth, or sixth intercostal space. (See Figure 13-3.) Sometimes it is easier to locate the point of maximum intensity of the heart (PMI) by palpation.

The apical pulse in a child seven to nine years old is generally located between the fourth and fifth intercostal space. Before four years of age it is left of the midclavicular line, between four and six years it is at the midclavicular line, and after seven years it is to the right of the line. (See Figure 13-3.)

To determine the apical rate, the bell of the stethoscope is placed as described above, and the beats are counted for one minute. Each heartbeat will be heard as a *lubb-dubb*. The *lubb* is the closure of the atrioventricular valves (the bicuspid and tricuspid valves), and the *dubb* is the closure of the semilunar valves (pulmonary and aortic valves). Any beats in addition to these should also be counted.

To take the apical-radial pulse, one nurse counts the apical rate at exactly the same time as the other nurse counts the radial pulse. Usually one nurse gives a hand signal to initiate counting, and each person counts for one full minute. The difference between the apical and radial pulse is referred to as the *pulse deficit*. When there is a deficit of this type, it indicates that some contractions of the heart are too feeble to pass along a palpable wave of blood at the radial pulse site.

Frequently the apical pulse alone is taken. For example, for patients who are receiving digitalis therapy, some agencies specify that the apical pulse should be taken in preference to the radial pulse. Other agencies specify that if the radial pulse rate is 60 beats/min or less, then the apical pulse rate should be taken.

Fetal Heart Sounds

Fetal heart sounds are generally first heard sometime between the eighteenth and twentieth weeks of the pregnancy. The fetal rate will usually be between 120 and 160 beats/min. It can be detected during the early months of pregnancy over the symphysis pubis; however, in later months the location varies depending upon the position of the fetus.

There are several positions that the fetus can assume in utero. Therefore in order to obtain the fetal heart rate the position of the fetus must initially be determined by abdominal palpation. The heart sounds are heard most predominantly through the back of the fetus. See Figure 13-4 for five common presentations and positions of the fetus during birth.

In vertex presentations (when the head is nearest the cervical opening and is born first) the fetal heart sounds are heard most audibly between the umbilicus and the anterosuperior spine of the ilium. For LOA (left occipital anterior) and LOP (left occipital posterior) positions, auscultation of the left lower quadrant will usually produce the best sounds. In contrast, for breech presentations the fetal heart sounds are generally heard loudest at the level of the umbilicus.

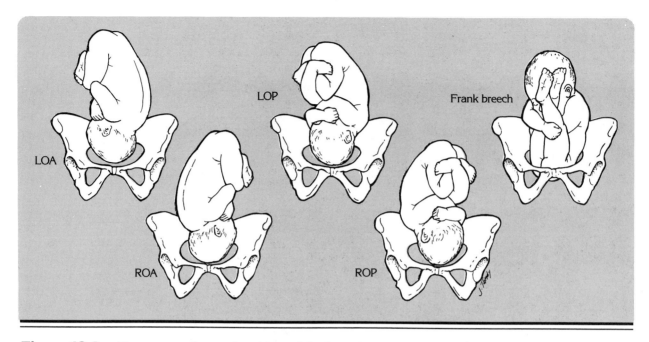

Figure 13-4.   Five presentations and positions of the fetus during childbirth are left occiput anterior (LOA), right occiput anterior (ROA), left occiput posterior (LOP), right occiput posterior (ROP), and frank breech.

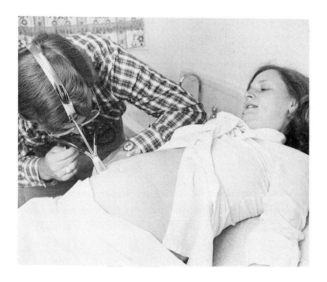

Figure 13-5.   A fetal heart is assessed using a fetal heart stethoscope.

To listen to the fetal heart, an ordinary bell stethoscope can be used if held by the use of rubber bands. A head stethoscope can augment the sounds, however, since sounds are transmitted by bone conduction through the headpiece in addition to the eardrum of the nurse. Special fetal heart stethoscopes are available. These have large weighted bells for fetal heart auscultation, and some are interchangeable in that a smaller bell can be attached to monitor the mother's blood pressure (Figure 13-5).

When counting the fetal heart rate, the nurse listens and counts for one minute. Two other blowing or whizzing sounds referred to as *souffles* may be heard during fetal heart auscultation. One is the funic (umbilical cord) souffle and the other, the uterine souffle. The funic souffle, a sharp hissing sound, is caused by blood rushing through the umbilical cord and is equivalent to the fetal heart, that is, the rate is around 140 per minute. It is not heard in every person (about 15%) and occurs when the umbilical arteries are subjected to pressure, torsion, or tension. The uterine souffle, a softer blowing sound, is due to blood propelled by the maternal heart through large dilated blood vessels of the uterus. Thus it synchronizes with the maternal heart rate, for example, 75 beats/min. It can be heard distinctly when the lower portion of the uterus is auscultated. Later in pregnancy, other sounds also become audible such as the maternal gurgling of gas or fetal sounds produced by its movement.

Assessment of fetal heart sounds is of particular importance in the first and second stages of labor. It is monitored generally every one-half to one hour in the first stage and then every five minutes in the second stage. Fetal distress is indicated when the rate slows to below 100 beats/min for as long as 30 seconds. During labor, the fetal heart rate normally slows (physiologic bradycardia) after the onset of a contraction, but this slowing normally ends by 10 or 15 seconds before the contraction is completed. Because the uterine muscle is tense during a contraction and because lying still during a contraction is difficult for the mother, assessment of the fetal heart rate may be more difficult. Electronic and ultrasound techniques are being used increasingly for high-risk mothers such as those with diabetes or a previous history of stillbirths.

RESPIRATIONS

Respiration is the act of breathing; it includes the intake of oxygen and the output of carbon dioxide. Reference is often made to *external respiration* and internal respiration. The former refers to the interchange of oxygen and carbon dioxide between the alveoli of the lungs and the pulmonary blood. *Internal respiration*, on the other hand, takes place throughout the body; it is the interchange of these same gases between the systemically circulating blood and the cells of the body tissues.

The term *inhalation* or inspiration refers to the intake of air into the lungs. *Exhalation* or expiration refers to breathing out or the movement of gases from the lungs to the atmosphere. *Ventilation* is another word used to refer to the rate of movement of air in and out of the lungs. *Hyperventilation* refers to very deep, rapid respirations; *hypoventilation* refers to very shallow respirations.

There are basically two types of breathing that nurses will observe, *costal* or thoracic breathing and *diaphragmatic* or abdominal breathing. Costal breathing involves chiefly the external intercostal muscles and other accessory muscles such as the sternocleidomastoid muscles. It can be observed by the movement of the chest upward and outward. In contrast, diaphragmatic breathing chiefly involves the contraction and relaxation of the diaphragm, and it is observed by the movement of the abdomen, which occurs as a result of its contraction and downward movement.

Respirations are observed to determine (a) rate, (b) depth, (c) rhythm, and (d) character.

Rate

The respiratory rate varies according to a number of factors. It also varies normally with the age of the person. In the newborn respirations will range anywhere from 35 to 50 respirations per minute, and they will be irregular, quiet and shallow. At 2 years of age they will have slowed to 25–35 breaths per minute. By 12 years they will be further slowed, and this decrease continues throughout adolescence. The normal rate of respirations for an adult will be between 16 to 20 breaths per minute. In the older person the respiratory rate increases, and respirations are generally shallow. These changes are due primarily to two physiologic changes of aging:

1. Decreasing elasticity of the lungs.
2. Impaired gaseous exchange between the alveoli and the pulmonary capillaries.

A number of terms are used in relation to respiratory rate. Normal effortless breathing is referred to as *eupnea*. A respiratory rate greater than 24 breaths per minute is called *tachypnea*. A count of fewer than 10 respirations per minute is described as *bradypnea*. The complete absence of respirations is *apnea*, which is often described in terms of time periods, for example, 30 seconds of apnea. Prolonged apnea results in death.

Depth

The depth of a person's respirations can be established by watching the movement of the chest. It is generally described as either deep or shallow. Deep respirations are those in which a large volume of air is inhaled and exhaled, inflating most of the lungs. Shallow respirations involve the passage of a small volume of air and often the use of minimal lung tissue.

The depth of respirations can also be measured accurately by the use of pulmonary equipment (see pulmonary capacities in Chapter 28).

The capacity of the lungs varies with sex, age, stature, physical development, and body position. Men generally have a greater vital capacity than women of the same age. Variance by age is obvious in that the baby will have a smaller vital capacity than the child and the child less than that of the adolescent and subsequently the adult. However, elderly people usually have a reduced capacity compared to their capacities as young adults.

Stature also effects lung volume in that tall, thin people usually have a greater vital capacity than obese people. The athlete who is physically well developed may well have a vital capacity that is above normal.

Body position also affects the amount of air that can be inhaled. In the supine position two physiologic processes operate: an increase in the volume of the intrathoracic blood and compression of the chest. Consequently, patients lying in a supine position have poorer lung aeration, which can predispose to the stasis of fluids and subsequent infection.

Rhythm

The rhythm of respirations refers to the regularity of both the expirations and the inspirations. Normally respirations are evenly spaced. The terms used to describe rhythm are *regular* or *irregular*.

Character

The character of respiration refers to those aspects of breathing which are different from the normal effortless breathing. Some of these are the amount of effort a patient requires to breathe, the sound of breathing, and skin color.

Usually breathing does not require effort; however, in some instances, increased effort is required to breathe. Difficult breathing is referred to as *dyspnea*. This is usually evidenced by the obvious effort of the accessory muscles, such as the sternocleidomastoid, to maintain respirations.

The sound of breathing is also significant. Normal breathing is silent, but there are a number of abnormal sounds that a nurse will observe. Wheezing occurs when the airway is constricted; the wheezing is usually more apparent on expiration. Acute constriction of the trachea produces a harsh crowing sound on inspiration called *stridor*. This usually reflects respiratory distress. *Rales* or *rhonchi* are bubbling or crackling sounds that are evident with respiration. These sounds occur as a result of the presence of fluid in the lungs and are more clearly heard with a stethoscope.

Procedure 13-5.   Assessing Respirations

ACTION	EXPLANATION
Assemble Equipment	
1. Watch with a second hand.	To count respiratory rate.
2. Pencil or pen.	
3. Book, record, or work sheet.	
To Assess Respirations	
1. Wash hands.	To remove any microorganisms, which should not be transmitted to the patient.
2. Explain to the patient what you plan to do. Adjust the explanation to the patient's need.	To reassure the patient through knowledge of what will happen. To identify the patient.
3. Place a hand against patient's chest and observe chest movements.	This is conveniently done directly after taking the pulse.
4. Count respiratory rate for 30 seconds if they are regular. Count for a full minute if they are irregular.	
5. Observe for depth. Deep respirations will take in a large volume of air. Shallow respirations take in a small volume.	

6. Observe respiratory rhythm. It may be regular or irregular.

7. Observe for character of respirations such as sound and effort.

8. Wash hands.

9. Record respiratory rate, depth, rhythm and character.

BLOOD PRESSURE

Blood pressure is a measure of the pressure of the blood as it pulsates through the arteries. Because the blood moves in waves, there are two blood pressure measures: the *systolic* pressure, which is the pressure of the blood as a result of contraction of the ventricles, that is, the pressure at the height of the blood wave, and the *diastolic* pressure, which is the pressure when the ventricles are at rest. Diastolic pressure, then, is the lowest pressure, and it is present at all times within the arteries. The difference between the diastolic and the systolic pressures is called the *pulse pressure*.

Blood pressure is measured in millimeters of mercury (mm Hg). This is indicated upon a sphygmomanometer, which reflects the pressure of air in a rubber cuff that is wrapped around a patient's extremity, for example, the upper arm.

Factors that Control Blood Pressure

The blood pressure is controlled chiefly by five factors: the cardiac output, the blood volume, the elasticity of the arterial walls, the viscosity of the blood, and the size of the arterioles and capillaries.

Cardiac Output

Cardiac output is the amount of blood ejected from the heart at each ventricular contraction. At rest the left ventricle normally puts out about 70 ml; this is the stroke volume. Cardiac output is normally about 5 liters, that is, 70 ml multiplied by the number of contractions per minute (70) equals 4900 ml or 5 liters/min.

Cardiac output increases with fever and exercise, and the systolic pressure may be increased as a result. On the other hand, cardiac output can be decreased as a result of heart disease, and the systolic blood pressure may then be low.

Blood Volume

An increased or decreased blood volume also affects blood pressure. Normally an adult has about 6 liters of blood in the circulatory system. Loss of blood volume due to hemorrhage or dehydration results in a lowered systolic and diastolic pressure. Excessive blood volume, such as with a quickly administered blood transfusion, can result in an increased blood pressure.

Elasticity of the Arterial Walls

Arterial walls normally have some elasticity, which permits them to yield somewhat during systole and then retract during diastole. With arteriosclerosis the arteries lose much of their elasticity and become more rigid. This condition is frequently seen in elderly people. As a result of this, the systolic pressure is generally elevated because the arteries do not yield to the pressure, and the diastolic pressure is generally lower because the arteries have limited retractability upon ventricular relaxation.

Size of the Arterioles and Capillaries

The size of the arterioles and the capillaries is basic to the peripheral resistance to the blood in the body. A lumen (plural: lumina) is a channel within a tube.

The smaller the lumina the greater the resistance. Normally the arterioles are in a state of partial constriction. Increased vasoconstriction raises the blood pressure, whereas decreased vasoconstriction lowers the blood pressure.

Factors that Affect Blood Pressure

A number of factors affect a person's blood pressure from time to time. Some of these are age, exercise, emotion, and physical stress.

Age

The newborn normally has a systolic pressure of 40–70 mm Hg, and the adult pressure is normally between 110 to 140 systolic, 60 to 80 diastolic. See Table 13-2 for variations in blood pressure by age.

Exercise

Exercise increases the cardiac output and hence the blood pressure. Therefore a patient needs to be resting when her blood pressure is taken to obtain a reliable reading.

Emotional and Physical Stress

Emotions such as anxiety and fear and physical stress such as moderate pain can also increase the blood pressure. Stimulation of the sympathetic nervous system results in increased cardiac output and vasoconstriction of the arterioles. On the other hand, severe pain can cause a fall in the blood pressure and

Table 13-2.   Variations in Blood Pressure by Age

Age	Normal Blood Pressure
Newborn	40–70 systolic
1 month	About 80 systolic, 46 diastolic
2 years	80–90 systolic
3 years	90 systolic, 60 diastolic
11 years (girls)	145 systolic, 90 diastolic
13 years (boys)	145 systolic, 80 diastolic
15 years	119 systolic, 62 diastolic (mean measures)
Adult	110–140 systolic, 60–80 diastolic
Elderly	As for the adult or slightly higher

subsequent shock. In this case the vasomotor center is inhibited, and vasodilatation takes place.

Measuring Blood Pressure

There are two methods of measuring the blood pressure, the direct and the indirect methods. Direct measurement involves the insertion of a catheter into a large vein (the superior vena cava) and taking the measure of the central venous blood pressure (CVP) prior to its entry into the right auricle of the heart. Generally physicians insert the catheters, and nurses are responsible for monitoring the pressure readings. This is a relatively accurate pressure reading.

The indirect method of taking the blood pressure, in this case arterial blood pressure, is commonly carried out by nurses. The equipment required for this is a stethoscope and a sphygmomanometer with a cuff. The cuff is a rubber bag that can be filled with air. It generally is covered with a cloth and it has two rubber tubes attached to it. One serves as the attachment for the rubber bulb that blows up the cuff. The other tube is attached to a manometer indicating the pressure of air within the cuff.

There are two types of manometers commonly used. One is the aneroid manometer. It is a calibrated dial with a needle or pointer that points to the calibrations. The second type of manometer is a tube or cylinder filled with mercury. In this case the nurse reads the pressure by looking at the meniscus of the mercury when it is at eye level. By looking up at the column of mercury or down at it, distortions in the reading can result. See Figure 13-6.

Blood pressure cuffs come in six standard sizes. For the average adult a cuff width of 12–14 cm is generally satisfactory. There are smaller cuffs for babies and small children. Some cuffs hook together; others wrap or snap in place. It is particularly important to use the appropriate size of cuff and cuff length in order to obtain accurate blood pressure readings. Too narrow a cuff can result in erroneously high readings, while too wide a cuff can produce low readings.

In some settings electronic equipment is used, which eliminates the need to use a stethoscope. As the pressure in the cuff decreases, a light flashes on at the systolic and diastolic measures in some models.

When taking a blood pressure by using a stethoscope, the nurse will hear a series of sounds. Initially the cuff is pumped up until no sound is heard, that is, until the blood is stopped from running through the arteries. The pressure is then slowly reduced until the blood can again flow through. At this point a sharp

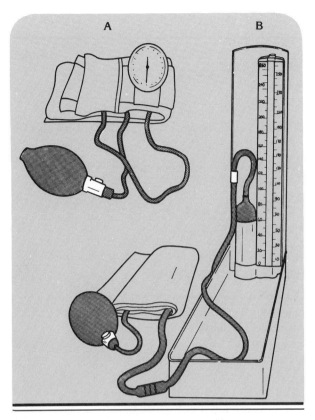

Figure 13-6. Blood pressure equipment. **A,** Aneroid manometer and cuff and **B,** mercury manometer and cuff.

sound will be heard with each ventricular contraction. These sounds are called Korotkoff sounds. The first clear sound heard when the pressure is released is the systolic blood pressure.

As the pressure is further decreased in the cuff, the sounds become muffled, and finally they disappear entirely. It is a matter of debate as to how best to measure the diastolic blood pressure, that is, the pressure in the arteries when the left ventricle of the heart is relaxed. Most authorities believe that neither of the above points, the muffled sound or the cessation of sound, is the true diastolic pressure. In people who have healthy arteries the true diastolic pressure is considered to be about 10 ml below the first muffled sound. This may coincide with the cessation of sounds. For people who have arteriosclerotic arteries, however, the muffled sounds may continue after the true diastolic pressure.

The American Heart Association recommends that three figures be recorded when a blood pressure reading is taken. These are:

1. The systolic pressure: the point when the first sounds are detected.

2. The first diastolic pressure: the point when the muffled sounds are first heard.

3. The second diastolic: the point of cessation of sound.

If this practice of noting three pressures is not followed in an agency, the student is advised to determine whether the first or second diastolic pressure is taken. A second diastolic pressure may be zero; that is, the sounds are heard even when there is no air pressure in the blood pressure cuff. In some instances, also, muffling of the sounds may not be detected, in which case a dash is inserted where the reading would normally be recorded (see Figure 13-7).

Normal blood pressures have been discussed earlier in the chapter (Table 13-2). Pressures of adults that are above 160 mm Hg systolic and/or 100 mm Hg diastolic are referred to as *hypertensive*. Pressures below 100 systolic are considered *hypotensive*.

The frequency with which blood pressure measurements are taken largely depends upon the patient's physical condition. After surgery it may be taken every half hour or even continually monitored electronically. Nurses are expected to use their own judgments in regard to taking or rechecking a blood pressure reading if for any reason a problem in accuracy is suspected.

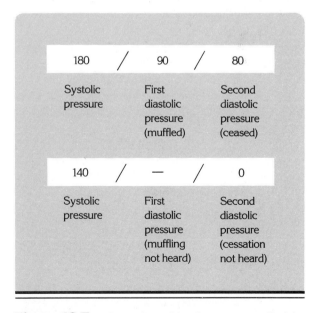

Figure 13-7. Recording a blood pressure reading, including systolic pressure, first diastolic pressure, and second diastolic pressure.

Procedure 13-6.   Measuring Blood Pressure

ACTION	EXPLANATION
Assemble Equipment	
1. One stethoscope.	To listen to pressure changes.
2. Blood pressure cuff of appropriate size.	There are cuffs for adults (12–14 cm) and smaller ones for children and infants.
3. Sphygmomanometer.	An instrument for measuring pressure in the artery.
To Measure Blood Pressure	
1. Wash hands.	To remove any microorganisms, which should not be transmitted to the patient.
2. Explain to the patient what you plan to do. Adjust the explanation to the patient's need.	To reassure the patient through knowledge of what will happen. To identify the patient.
3. Assist the patient to a comfortable position if this is necessary.	Discomfort can elevate the blood pressure. Use a sitting position unless it is otherwise indicated because position also affects the blood pressure.
4. Expose the upper aspect of the arm to be used. Usually an arm is used, although a leg may be used in rare instances.	
5. Wrap the cuff evenly around the upper arm. For an adult the lower edge of the cuff should be about 2 cm (1 inch) above the antecubital space. For infants the lower edge can be nearer the antecubital space.	The bladder of the cuff must be directly over the brachial artery to obtain an accurate reading.
6. Palpate the brachial artery with the finger tips.	The brachial artery is normally found medially in the antecubital space.
7. Place the bell of the stethoscope on the brachial pulse.	The bell can be held with the thumb or first few fingers.
8. Put the ear attachments of the stethoscope in the ears. The ear attachments should be put in the ears in such a way that they direct slightly forward.	In this way they follow the direction of the ear canal, thus facilitating hearing.
9. The stethoscope must hang freely from the ears to the bell.	Any rubbing against an object can obliterate the sounds reflecting the waves of blood.
10. Close the valve on the pump.	To close turn clockwise.
11. Pump up the cuff until the sphygmomanometer registers about 20 mm above the point of the last sound. Palpate until point of obliteration, then pump 20 mm more.	At this point the blood is prevented from flowing through the artery. This point is generally about 180–200 mm for an adult.
12. Open the valve on the pump carefully, permitting the air to escape very slowly.	The manometer should reflect a decrease in pressure of about 2 mm for each heartbeat.
13. Note the point on the manometer where the first sound is heard.	This is the systolic pressure.

14. Continue to release the pressure slowly.

15. Note the point on the manometer where the sound first becomes muffled.

 This is the first diastolic pressure.

16. Continue to release the pressure slowly.

17. Note the point on the manometer where the sounds cease.

 This is the second diastolic pressure. Note agency policy regarding diastolic pressure. In some agencies only one diastolic pressure is measured; it may be either one of the diastolic pressures described.

18. If there is any doubt about any of the pressures, repeat the blood pressure.

 Often blood pressures are taken twice as a routine practice to ensure accuracy.

19. Remove the cuff from the patient's arm and fold.

20. Assist patient to cover the upper arm.

21. Wash hands.

22. Record blood pressures. If three pressures are recorded, for example:

 130/100/80

 130 is the systolic pressure, 100 is the first diastolic pressure, and 80 is the second diastolic pressure. To record two pressures, for example:

 130/80

 130 is the systolic pressure and 80 is the diastolic pressure.

SUMMARY

Although nurses have always assessed their patients' conditions, specific techniques are increasingly being employed to ascertain health status. These techniques include those which assess mental and emotional health as well as those which assess the physical health status. An outline of the physical assessment techniques to determine vital signs as well as influencing factors and points of emphasis follows:

I. Body temperature

 A. Influencing factors

  1. Age

   a. Newborns: fluctuations between 36.1° and 37.7° C

   b. two years: 37.7° C

   c. three years: 37.2° C

   d. twelve years: 37.0° C

   e. Adults: 37.0° C

   f. Elderly: less than 37.0° C

  2. Time of day

   a. Lowest in the morning

   b. Highest in the evening

  3. Sex: Ovulation increases body temperature

  4. Emotions: Heightened emotions increase the temperature

  5. Exercise: Elevates body temperature

  6. Temperature of environment: Direct relationship to body temperature

B. Routes of measurement

   1. Oral

      a. Taken for two to nine minutes

      b. Contraindicated for infants, young children, nose breathers, the confused, and patients receiving oxygen by cannula or mask

   2. Rectal

      a. Indicated for the very young, unconscious, or confused patient

      b. Contraindicated for patients with rectal pathologic conditions or trauma

      c. Taken for two or three minutes

      d. Must be held in place

   3. Axilla

      a. Least accurate of the three methods

      b. Taken for 10 minutes

C. Types of fever

   1. Intermittent (quotidian)

   2. Remittent

   3. Relapsing

D. Symptoms of fever

   1. During fever onset

      a. Shivering and chills

      b. Increased pulse rate

      c. Pallor and skin coldness

      d. Gooseflesh

      e. Convulsions with high temperature

   2. During fever course

      a. Skin feels warm

      b. Flushing

      c. Headache, irritability, restlessness

      d. Disorientation with high temperature

      e. Weakness

      f. Dehydration

   3. During fever termination

      a. Increased diaphoresis

      b. Skin redness

II. Pulse measurement

A. Pulse sites

   1. Temporal

   2. Carotid

   3. Brachial

   4. Radial

   5. Femoral

   6. Popliteal

   7. Posterior tibial

   8. Dorsalis pedis

   9. Apical

B. Factors influencing pulse rates per minute

   1. Age

      a. Newborns: fluctuates between 120 and 160

      b. Two years: 80–140

      c. 12 years: boys, 65–105; girls, 70–110

      d. 18 years: boys, 50–90; girls, 55–95

      e. Adults: 60–100

      f. Elderly: 70–80

   2. Sex: Men tend to have lower pulse rates than women

   3. Exercise: Increases pulse rates

   4. Emotions: Tachycardia with sympathetic nervous system stimulation

   5. Heat: Prolonged external heat elevates pulse rate

   6. Body position: Prolonged horizontal position increases pulse rate

C. The apical-radial pulse

   1. Requires two nurses for assessment

   2. Locations of the apical pulse vary with age

D. Fetal heart sounds

1. Heard by 18 to 20 weeks of pregnancy

2. Normal fetal heart rate is 120 to 160 per minute

3. Sounds are heard predominantly through the back of the fetus

4. Locations of sounds depend upon the fetal position

5. Sounds must be differentiated from souffles (the funic and the uterine)

6. Assessment is of utmost importance during labor

III. Respirations

   A. Variations in respiratory rate by age

      1. Newborns: 35–50, irregular and shallow

      2. Adult: 16–20

      3. Elderly: Increased rate and shallow

   B. Measurements in addition to rate

      1. Depth: Observed by movement of the chest or by the use of pulmonary equipment

      2. Capacity: See Chapter 28, pulmonary volumes

      3. Rhythm: Normally regular

      4. Character: Normally silent and effortless

         a. Note abnormal sounds of breathing (rales or rhonchi)

         b. Notable effort by accessory muscles of respiration and dyspnea

IV. Blood pressure

   A. Measured in mm Hg

      1. Systolic pressure

      2. Diastolic pressure

   B. Factors controlling blood pressure

      1. Cardiac output

      2. Blood volume

      3. Elasticity of arterial walls

      4. Blood viscosity

      5. Size of arterioles and capillaries

   C. Factors influencing blood pressure

      1. Age

         a. Newborn has systolic pressure of 40–70

         b. Adult has systolic pressure of 110–140 and a diastolic pressure of 60–80

      2. Exercise: increases blood pressure

      3. Stress: moderate stress increases blood pressure but severe stress may lower the pressure

   D. Methods of measurement

      1. Direct (CVP)

      2. Indirect by use of stethoscope, cuff, and sphygmomanometers: the aneroid manometer or the mercury manometer

      3. Electronic equipment without a stethoscope

   E. Abnormalities

      1. Hypertension: above 160 systolic (adults)

      2. Hypotension: below 100 systolic (adults)

SUGGESTED ACTIVITIES

1. Select three patients of differing ages. Take their vital signs (temperature, pulse, respirations, and blood pressure) and compare them.

2. At a local health agency determine the policies governing taking vital signs. Compare these with the data obtained by other students at other agencies.

3. At a physician's office listen to fetal heart sounds. Determine the location at which the sounds were most clear and relate this to the position of the fetus.

SUGGESTED READINGS

Blainey, C. G. October 1974. Site selection in taking body temperature. *American Journal of Nursing* 74:1859–1861.

This article discusses rectal temperatures, their advantages and disadvantages, and the sublingual temperature as well as other sites. The author concludes that the sublingual site provides the most accurate reflection of body temperature under normal conditions.

Roberts, Sharon L. April 1975. Skin assessment for color and temperature. *American Journal of Nursing* 75:610–613.

This article describes assessment of the skin, including the significance of changes in color and temperature in different areas of the body.

Warren, Freda M. April 1975. Blood pressure readings: getting them quickly on an infant. *Nursing 75* 5(4):13.

The author describes the flush method of obtaining a blood pressure reading.

SELECTED REFERENCES

Bell, S. April 1969. Early morning temperatures? *American Journal of Nursing* 69: 764–766.

Felton, G. January–February 1970. Effect of time cycle change on blood pressure and temperature in young women. *Nursing Research* 19(1): 48–58.

Guyton, Arthur C. 1976. *Textbook of medical physiology,* 5th ed. Philadelphia: W. B. Saunders Co.

MacBryde, C.M. et al. eds. 1970. *Signs and symptoms applied pathologic physiology and clinical interpretation,* 15th ed. Philadelphia: J. B. Lippincott Co.

Murray, R. et al. 1975. Nursing assessment and health promotion through the life span. Englewood Cliffs, New Jersey: Prentice-Hall Inc.

Nichols, Glennadee A. and Kucha, Delores H. June 1972. Taking adult temperatures: oral measurement. *American Journal of Nursing* 72: 1090–1093.

Nichols, Glennadee A. June 1972. Taking adult temperatures: rectal measurements. *American Journal of Nursing* 72: 1092–1093.

Thompson Laverne R. February 1963. Thermometer disinfection. *American Journal of Nursing* 63:113–115.

Whitner, W. et al. January–February 1970. The influence of bathing on the newborn infant's body temperature. *Nursing Research* 19(1): 30–36.

CHAPTER 14

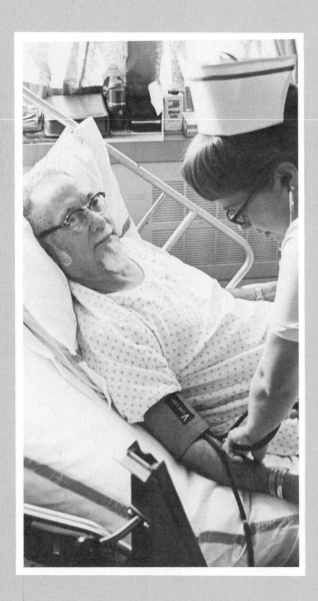

GENERAL ASSESSMENT SKILLS

BREASTS

AXILLAE

ABDOMEN

Observation

Auscultation

Palpation

Percussion

GENITALS AND RECTUM

Adult Female Genitals

Adult Female Rectum and Anus

Adult Male Genitals

Adult Male Rectum and Anus

EXTREMITIES

Reflexes

NEUROLOGIC AND MENTAL-EMOTIONAL ASSESSMENT

The Cranial Nerves

Cerebral Functioning (Mental Status)

The Cerebellum

The Sensory System

The Motor System

OBJECTIVES

- Describe normal height and weight according to age.

- Describe normal skin, hair, and nails.

- Demonstrate beginning skill, measuring an infant's skull circumference.

- Describe the closure of the skull sutures.

- Demonstrate beginning skill palpating an adult's neck for lymph nodes and the thyroid gland.

- Demonstrate beginning skill examining eyes, ears, nose, mouth, and pharynx.

- Explain how to examine the chest.

- Describe how to examine the heart and the fetal heart.

- Demonstrate beginning skill in examining the breasts, axillae, and the abdomen.

- Describe the examination of the genitals and rectum of males and females.

- Demonstrate beginning skill testing body reflexes.

- Explain the various aspects of a neurologic and mental-emotional assessment.

General assessment skills are being used increasingly by nurses. This assessment provides data about the patient and assists all members of the health team in identifying the patient's problems and in evaluating the effectiveness of therapy. Some techniques, such as measuring a person's weight, are carried out frequently; whereas other examinations are performed only when indicated, such as auscultating the abdomen of a surgical patient for bowel sounds. Some assessment skills must be adjusted to the individual's age; for example, an infant's height is measured in the supine position, and a child's vision is tested with a special Snellen chart until the alphabet is learned.

In some agencies, nurses carry out the complete physical examination and report their findings to the physician by way of the patient's record. Nursing students need to be familiar with the policies and practices in a specific agency before initiating particular assessment techniques.

In Chapter 13, general assessment methods such as observation, palpation, and auscultation were discussed. The sources of pertinent data have also been described. This chapter is oriented to the assessment of a patient of any age. Some laboratory tests have been included. The student is referred to Chapter 38 for additional information about tests and examinations.

Because the patient as a total person must be considered, techniques for assessing basic mental-emotional health are also included in this chapter. This aspect of assessment is considered to be as important as the physical assessment.

HEIGHT AND WEIGHT

Height and weight are standard measures of people that are taken frequently in physicians' offices, schools, and hospitals. Height is a measure of growth of a child, and weight is in many ways a measure of health for all people. For more information, refer to Chapter 2 and the incidence of obesity and morbidity statistics of the general population.

The length of a newborn in the United States is usually from 47.5 to 52.5 cm (19 to 21 inches). The average is about 50 cm (20 inches). During the first 6 months the newborn grows another 13.75 cm (5.5 inches); the newborn grows 7.5 cm (3 inches) during the last 6 months of the first year. Each year during the preschool years children add another 5.0–6.4 cm (2.0–2.5 inches) to their height. At six years both boys and girls will be about 115 cm (46 inches). They will usually be 140 cm (56 inches) by age 12 years. For reference to growth cycles see Chapter 10. The growth spurt before puberty often results in girls becoming taller than boys of the same age at this particular stage.

During adolescence the maximum height for boys is generally reached at age 18 or 19 years and for girls at about 15 or 16 years.

In the elderly there is usually some decrease in overall stature due to the atrophy of the intervertebral discs.

To measure the length of a baby who cannot stand, place the baby on a hard surface with the soles of the feet supported in an upright position. The knees are extended, and the measure is taken from the soles of the feet to the vertex of the head. The head should be in such a position that the eyes are facing the ceiling.

After a child can stand, the height can be measured if the child stands with heels, back, and head against a wall. A small flat board from the top of the head to the wall will give an accurate measure of height, that is, the distance from the floor to the board.

The weight of a person is more likely to vary from the norm than is height. Genetic influences, diet, and activity are just a few of the factors that affect a person's weight.

At birth most babies weigh between 2.7–3.8 kg (6.0–8.5 lb). Initially some of this birth weight (about 10%) is lost the first few days due to fluid loss. Children can be expected to double their weights by 4 to 6 months of age and to weigh about 5.4 kg (12 lb) at 1 year and 10.8 kg (24 lb) at 2 years.

At 3 years a toddler will probably weigh 15 kg (33 lb) and by 5 years between 18.0 and 20.4 kg (40 and 45 lb). During school-age years a child averages 3.2 additional kilograms (7 lb) each year. By the time the adolescent reaches maximum height, weight will tend to stabilize until the middle years, when additional weight gain tends to take place. Tables 14-1 and 14-2 refer the student to suggested height and weight for health according to body frame.

The weight of a person who can stand is generally measured by a standing scale. The person stands on a platform, and the weight is transmitted to a dial

Table 14-1.   Weight According to Frame (Indoor Clothing), Women of Ages 25 and Over*

Height†			Small Frame		Medium Frame		Large Frame	
Feet	Inches	cm	Pounds	Kilograms	Pounds	Kilograms	Pounds	Kilograms
4	10	147.3	92–98	41.7–44.5	96–107	43.5–48.5	104–119	47.2–54.0
4	11	149.9	94–101	42.6–45.8	98–110	44.5–49.9	106–122	48.1–55.3
5	0	152.4	96–104	43.5–47.2	101–113	45.8–51.3	109–125	49.4–56.7
5	1	154.9	99–107	44.9–48.5	104–116	47.2–52.6	112–128	50.8–58.1
5	2	157.5	102–110	46.3–50.0	107–119	48.5–54.0	115–131	52.2–59.4
5	3	160.0	105–113	47.6–51.3	110–122	49.9–55.3	118–134	53.5–60.8
5	4	162.6	108–116	49.0–52.6	113–126	51.3–57.2	121–138	54.9–62.6
5	5	165.1	111–119	50.3–54.0	116–130	52.6–59.0	125–142	56.7–64.4
5	6	167.6	114–123	51.7–55.8	120–135	54.4–61.2	129–146	58.5–66.2
5	7	170.2	118–127	53.5–57.6	124–139	56.2–63.0	133–150	60.3–68.0
5	8	172.7	122–131	55.3–59.4	128–143	58.1–64.9	137–154	62.1–69.9
5	9	175.3	126–135	57.2–61.2	132–147	59.9–66.7	141–158	64.0–71.7
5	10	177.8	130–140	69.0–63.5	136–151	61.7–68.5	145–163	65.8–73.9
5	11	180.3	134–144	60.8–65.3	140–155	63.5–70.3	149–168	67.6–76.2
6	0	182.9	138–148	62.6–67.1	144–159	65.3–72.1	153–173	69.4–78.5

For women between 18 and 25, subtract 0.5 kg (1 pound) for each year under 25.
*Courtesy of the Metropolitan Life Insurance Company.
†With shoes on—5.1 cm (2-inch) heels

Table 14-2.   Weight According to Frame (Indoor Clothing), Men of Ages 25 and Over*

Height†			Small Frame		Medium Frame		Large Frame	
Feet	Inches	cm	Pounds	Kilograms	Pounds	Kilograms	Pounds	Kilograms
5	2	157.5	112–120	50.8–54.4	118–129	53.5–58.5	126–141	57.2–64.0
5	3	160.0	115–123	52.2–55.8	121–133	54.9–60.3	129–144	58.5–65.3
5	4	162.6	118–126	53.5–57.2	124–136	56.2–61.7	132–148	59.9–67.1
5	5	165.1	121–129	54.9–58.5	127–139	57.6–63.0	135–152	61.2–68.9
5	6	167.6	124–133	56.2–60.3	130–143	59.0–64.9	138–156	62.6–70.8
5	7	170.2	128–137	58.1–62.1	134–147	60.8–66.7	142–161	64.4–73.0
5	8	172.7	132–141	59.9–64.0	138–152	62.6–68.9	147–166	66.7–75.3
5	9	175.3	136–145	61.7–65.8	142–156	64.4–70.8	151–170	68.5–77.1
5	10	177.8	140–150	63.5–68.0	146–160	66.2–72.6	155–174	70.3–78.9
5	11	180.3	144–154	65.3–69.9	150–165	68.0–74.8	159–179	72.1–81.2
6	0	182.9	148–158	67.1–71.7	154–170	69.9–77.1	164–184	74.4–83.4
6	1	185.4	152–162	68.9–73.5	158–175	71.7–79.4	168–189	76.2–85.7
6	2	188.0	156–167	70.8–75.8	162–180	73.5–81.6	173–194	78.5–88.0
6	3	190.5	160–171	72.6–77.6	167–185	75.8–83.9	178–199	80.7–90.3
6	4	193.0	164–175	74.4–79.4	172–190	78.0–86.2	182–204	82.6–92.5

*Courtesy of Metropolitan Life Insurance Company.
†With shoes on—2.5 cm (1-inch) heels

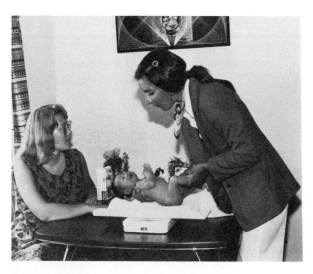

Figure 14-1.   Weighing a baby in the home.
(Courtesy City of Vancouver Health Department.)

on the scale. Usually weight is taken without shoes, in which case a clean paper towel on the platform assists the patient to maintain the cleanliness of feet.

To weigh a patient who is too ill to stand, some agencies have a scale not unlike a jack in principle (see Chapter 22). These have canvas straps that fit around the patient. The patient is mechanically lifted, thus conveying the weight measurement to a scale, which the nurse can read.

There are a number of types of weight scales that can be used to weigh babies. In a hospital there is usually a weigh scale with a container in which the baby can be laid for weighing. Another handy type of scale is portable (Figure 14-1). It is important to weigh a baby unclothed or to weigh the clothes separately and subtract this weight.

SKIN

Observation of the skin includes all skin surfaces of the body and the hair and nails. Usually this observation is done gradually while the nurse is observing parts of the body for other data. The skin is normally observed for (a) color, (b) texture, (c) temperatures, and (d) lesions.

Color

Description of skin color needs to include any deviations from the normal, including any increased pigmentation. The skin may reflect pallor, flushing, jaundice, or cyanosis. *Pallor* appears as a whitish-grayish tinge. *Flushing* is a redness, which may also be generalized or idiosyncratic to a particular area. A *jaundiced* skin is tinged yellow and is often most readily seen in the sclera of the eyes, particularly in people who normally have a yellow tinge to their skins. *Cyanosis* is a bluish color appearing around the mouth and in the nails by pressing them downward. In dark-skinned persons it is important to check the color of the mucous membranes to obtain an accurate assessment.

Color also includes an increased or decreased pigmentation. Some increased pigmentation is perfectly normal and temporary, for example, the brown patches on the forehead and cheeks of some pregnant women commonly called "the mask of pregnancy" (chloasma gravidarum). This particular pigmentation usually disappears spontaneously after childbirth.

The presence of hair on the body can also be observed. Hirsutism is the presence of darker, thicker hair on the body than is usual. It has little significance in men but should be noted in children and women.

Texture

Texture or skin turgor can be assessed by picking up and pinching the skin. Healthy skin springs back into position, whereas a dehydrated person's skin will remain pinched for a short time.

Texture also includes dryness, flaking, wrinkling, or excessive moisture, all of which may reflect more serious problems.

Temperature

Palpation of the skin will reveal to the nurse whether it is normally warm or whether it is unusually hot or cold. Skin temperature may be similar throughout the body or it may be particular to one area, such as the coldness of the skin of a foot due to decreased blood flow to the part.

Lesions

There are many types of lesions that occur on the skin. The nurse's main responsibility is to describe them accurately, including (a) distribution and location, (b) size, (c) contour, and (d) consistency.

The student is referred to Table 14-3, which describes the different types of primary skin lesions.

Hair

The characteristics of the hair as well as its distribution are of importance. Hair that is not usual on any area of the body needs to be reported. If the normal scalp hair has changed in its texture to thinning fine hair, this should also be reported. This change can be indicative of thyroid problems.

Nails

Nails usually grow regularly, but this growth can be stopped at times of severe stress or illness. When the patient's nails begin to grow again, a deep line will become visible. This is called *De Beau's line.*

It is important to observe *clubbing,* which involves the nail and later the terminal phalanx. With clubbing the proximal aspect of the nail is elevated and the nail bed becomes soft. With more advanced clubbing the terminal aspect of the finger becomes wider and rounder and the nail becomes more curved. Clubbing frequently results from a long-term lack of oxygen.

Table 14-3.   Primary Skin Lesions

Type	Description	Size	Example
Macula	Flat circumscribed area of color with no elevation of its surface	1 mm to several cm	Freckles
Papule	Circumscribed solid elevation of skin	Less than 1 cm	Acne
Nodule	Solid mass extending deeper into dermis than does papule	1–2 cm	Pigmented nevi
Tumor	Solid mass larger than nodule	Over 2 cm	Epithelioma
Cyst	Encapsulated fluid-filled mass in dermis or subcutaneous layer	Over 1 cm	Epidermoid cyst
Wheal	A relatively reddened, flat, localized collection of edema fluid	1 mm to several cm	Mosquito bite; hives
Vesicle	Circumscribed elevation containing serous fluid or blood	Less than 1 cm	Herpes; chickenpox
Bulla	Larger fluid-filled vesicle	Over 1 cm	Second-degree burn
Pustule	Vesicle or bulla filled with pus	1 mm to 1 cm	Acne vulgaris

THE HEAD AND NECK

Examination of the head includes assessment of the skull shape, the skull circumference, the fontanelles, the hair and scalp, the face and skin, and the ears, eyes, nose, mouth, and throat. These latter five structures will be discussed subsequently. Examination of the neck includes mobility, pulsation, symmetry, and the presence or absence of enlarged underlying structures. Methods used for assessment are largely those of observation and palpation with the exception of the eyes and the ears. For infants a measuring tape is needed to obtain skull size, and a flashlight may be necessary for transillumination of the skull.

Skull Circumference

The skull is measured at its greatest diameter from above the eyes to the occipital protuberance. Steel, cloth, or disposable paper tapes are available for measurement. If a cloth tape is used, it is recommended that it be checked periodically against a metal standard, since cloth ages and tends to stretch.

Assessment of skull circumference is of particular importance in infants and children in order to determine the rate and appropriate growth of the skull and the brain. An infant's head should be measured at every visit to the physician or nurse until the age of two years. It usually does not need to be done routinely after the age of three years; however, for any initial examinations of young children this measurement always needs to be included (See Figure 14-2).

Normal head circumferences *(normocephaly)* are often related to chest circumferences. At birth the average head circumference is 35 cm (14 inches) and generally only varies 1 or 2 cm (0.5 inches) either way. The chest circumference of the newborn is usually less than the head circumference by about 2.5 cm (1 inch). As age advances, the chest circumference becomes larger than that of the head. See Table 14-4. At about 9 or 10 months the head and chest circumferences are about the same and after one year of age the chest circumference is larger than the head circumference.

Abnormalities in head circumferences are referred to as *macrocephaly* (a large head) or *microcephaly* (a small head). The former is often the result of excessive cerebrospinal fluid within the skull *(hydrocephalus).*

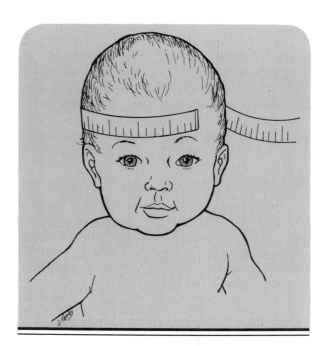

Figure 14-2.   An infant's head circumference is measured around the skull above the eyebrows.

Skull Shape and Fontanelles

Most newborn babies have misshapen heads. This is due to the molding of the head that occurs during vaginal deliveries. Molding of the head is made possible by fontanelles (unossified membranous gaps) in the bone structure of the skull and by overriding of the sutures (junction lines of the skull bones). Within a week the newborn's head usually will regain its symmetry, a fact that reassures parents.

The cranium is composed of eight bones, each separated by sutures, which gradually ossify during

Table 14-4.   Average Head, Chest, and Abdominal Circumferences in Centimeters by Age

	Boys			Girls		
Age	**Head**	**Chest**	**Abdomen**	**Head**	**Chest**	**Abdomen**
Newborn	35.3	33.2	—	34.7	32.9	—
3 months	40.9	40.6	38.5	40.0	39.8	38.4
6 months	43.9	43.7	41.4	42.8	43.0	41.4
9 months	46.0	46.0	43.4	44.6	45.4	43.4
12 months	47.3	47.6	44.6	45.8	47.0	44.5
15 months	48.0	48.6	45.1	46.5	47.9	45.0
18 months	48.7	49.5	45.5	47.1	48.8	45.5
2 years	49.7	50.8	46.2	48.1	50.1	46.3
2½ years	50.2	51.7	46.7	48.8	51.2	47.0
3 years	50.4	52.4	47.2	49.3	51.9	47.7

From Vaughan, Victor C., III, and McKay, R. James. 1975. *Nelson textbook of pediatrics*, 10th ed. © 1975 by the W. B. Saunders Co., Philadelphia. pp. 46, 47.

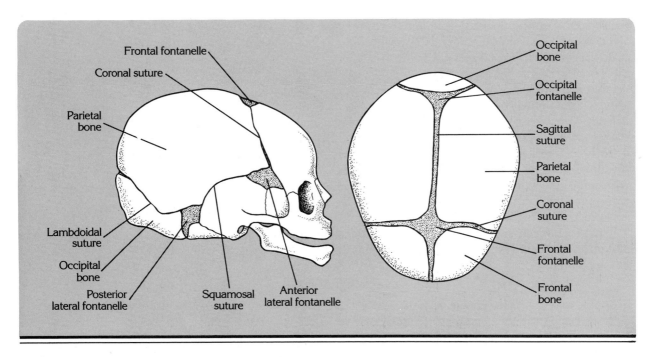

Figure 14-3. The bones of the skull of an infant showing the fontanelles and suture lines.

childhood. These bones are the frontal bone, the occipital bone, two parietal and two temporal bones, and the sphenoid and ethmoid bones (Figure 14-3). Six fontanelles are present at birth, but the two most prominent ones are the frontal (anterior) and the occipital (posterior) ones. The latter is the smaller of the two (1–2 cm in diameter) and is generally closed by two months. At birth the posterior fontanelle may not be palpated for a few hours because of the overriding of the sutures during delivery. The larger anterior fontanelle (4–6 cm in diameter and diamond shaped) can increase in size for several months after birth. After six months, the size gradually decreases until closure occurs between 10 and 18 months.

Examination of the head of infants for symmetry of shape and for palpation of the fontanelles is best achieved while the infant is sitting comfortably in the mother's lap. Normally during crying, coughing, or vomiting, the anterior fontanelle has a certain tenseness, fullness, and bulging. This is indicative of increased intracranial pressure. Continual bulging is abnormal and associated with tumors or infections of the brain or hydrocephalus due to obstruction of the cerebrospinal fluid circulation of the ventricles. Depression of the anterior fontanelle is generally indicative of dehydration.

Asymmetry of the scalp can be caused by a number of factors. Frequently a newborn will have disfiguring localized swellings over a portion of the scalp at birth or shortly after birth. *Caput succedaneum* is an edematous swelling of the soft tissues of a part of the scalp that was encircled by the cervix before the latter became fully dilated. This condition commonly occurs over the occipitoparietal region (the presenting part of the fetus) and disappears spontaneously within a few days of birth. Bilateral symmetrical swellings of the scalp can also occur in difficult deliveries that require the use of forceps.

Another type of swelling of the scalp in the newborn is called *cephalhematoma*. This differs from caput succedaneum in that the swelling occurs directly over a bone or portion of it and is not visible until several hours after delivery. The cause is an effusion of blood between the periosteum and the bone (subperiosteal); it most commonly occurs over the parietal bones. This hematoma increases gradually in size for about a week and then slowly disappears. Misshape of the head can also occur because of premature closure of the cranial sutures. Flattening of a part of the scalp frequently occurs in infants who sleep in one predominant position.

The Scalp

The scalp is observed and palpated for sutures, hair condition, scaliness, and infections. Sutures in the newborn can be felt as ridges, since overriding of the bones occurs during delivery. Flattening occurs by about six months, and some infants normally have wide spaces. After six months any other ridges or breaks in the cranial bones usually indicate fractures.

Normal hair has a resilient texture and color and is evenly distributed People with severe protein deficiency *(kwashiorkor)* have faded hair colors that appear reddish or bleached. This hair is also coarse and dry. Some therapies for cancer can cause alopecia (baldness), and the coarseness of hair can also vary with some disease conditions. The presence of ringworm, pediculi (lice), or nits (eggs) should also be assessed.

The scalp itself should be free from infections and scaliness. To observe the scalp, the hair needs to be well parted.

The Neck

Observation of the neck commences by noting the skin. Then the range of motion is assessed by asking the patient to flex, extend, hyperextend, and rotate the head. For young children and people who cannot do this themselves, the nurse can passively move the patient's head and neck through these motions. Older children can be asked to follow a bright light moved up and down and sideways to assess ease of

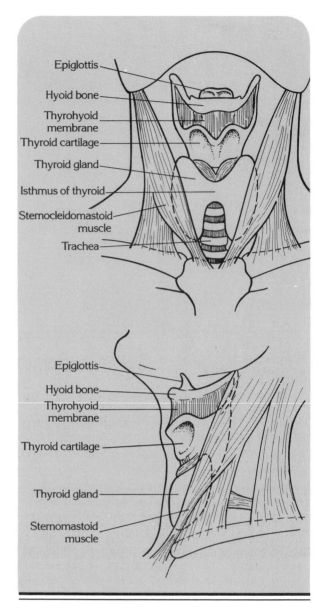

Figure 14-5.   The thyroid gland is located lateral to the trachea.

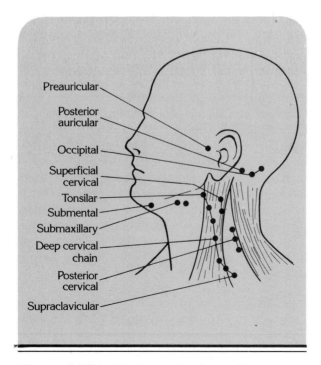

Figure 14-4.   The four major chains of lymph nodes in the neck.

neck motion. Control of the head must also be assessed in young children. Normally, infants will show some head lag when pulled from a sitting to a lying position up to three months of age. After this age, head lag suggests a neuromuscular defect such as cerebral palsy.

The neck needs also to be palpated for lymph nodes, which may be enlarged. Lymph nodes occur in chains. One of these lies behind and below the angle of the jaw. An anterior chain of nodes lies downward behind the muscle that starts behind the ear and goes forward toward the clavicle. The third chain, the posterior chain, lies further behind the anterior chain. The fourth group of nodes is above and below the clavicles (see Figure 14-4).

A further observation pertaining to the neck is of the larynx or voice box. Any abnormality in the person's voice such as hoarseness needs to be noted.

The size of the thyroid gland also needs to be assessed (Figure 14-5). A grossly enlarged gland is obvious visually. The gland can also be palpated with the fingers. The patient is asked to swallow, and the gland will move past the nurse's fingers. In this way the gland's size can be assessed and any nodules felt.

EYES

An examination of the eyes needs to include an assessment of the external structures: the eyebrows and eyelashes, eyelids, eyeballs, conjunctivae, sclera, cornea and iris, pupils, and fundus. It should also roughly test the visual acuity of the person, which can be done either by having the patient read an eye chart or less accurately by having the patient read a newspaper.

Eyebrows

The eyebrows are normally present over both eyes. Tweezing eyebrows is a normal practice today for men and women; the complete absence of eyebrows, however, is abnormal and needs to be noted.

Eyelashes

Eyelash follicles need to be observed for infection, which produces a red stye that the patient will usually say is painful.

Eyelids

Eyelids need to be observed primarily for discoloration, edema, any lesions, and positional faults. Edema is readily seen on the eyelids because this skin is thin and loosely attached to the underlying tissues. Positional faults include *ectropion* (a rolling out of the lids) and *entropion* (an inturned lid). The former usually requires surgical intervention; the latter is normally present in Oriental children and is generally harmless unless the cornea becomes abraded by the eyelashes.

Eyeballs

The eyeballs are observed to see whether they are situated deeply in the eye socket or whether they protrude abnormally from the socket. Patients who are dehydrated or emaciated often appear to have sunken eyeballs, while a patient who has hyperthyroidism may have protruding eyeballs. The latter is called *exophthalmos*.

By palpating the eyeball with the finger when the eye is closed, the relative hardness or softness of the eyeball can be noted. In glaucoma the eyeball is abnormally hard due to the increased pressure of the aqueous humor. The exact pressure can be assessed by a physician using a *tonometer*. Particularly soft eyeballs can often be detected in a patient who is dehydrated.

Conjunctivae

The conjunctivae of the eye are observed for inflammation and for paleness and cyanosis in darkskinned people. The lower portion of the conjunctiva can be observed by pulling down gently on the skin just below the eye. The upper conjunctiva is observed by everting the upper eyelid. This is done by gently pulling the eyelid down when holding the eyelashes. Then an applicator is placed against the upper border of the eyelid and the lid everted by moving the eyelashes toward the eyebrow.

The conjunctivae of the newborn may have small hemorrhages, which normally disappear relatively soon after birth. See Figure 14-6 for parts of the eye.

Sclera

The sclera of the eyes should be white and clear and are observed chiefly for their color. Jaundice will be reflected in a yellow tinge to the sclera. Newborns usually reveal a slightly bluish tinge, and the sclera of black races is frequently slightly brownish. A bluish sclera can indicate glaucoma.

Cornea and Iris

These structures are chiefly observed for irregularities and abrasions. By shining a flashlight from the side these defects can generally be detected.

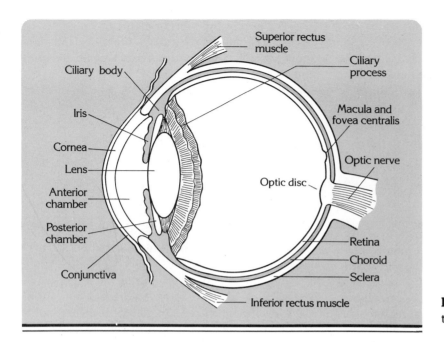

Figure 14-6. The external anatomical structures of the right eye.

Pupils

Testing the reaction of the pupils and the size of the pupils is of particular importance. Pupils normally dilate in a darkened environment and constrict in a bright light. They are normally of the same size. Pressure on the brain from, for example, a cerebral hemorrhage can result in uneven pupils, and certain drugs make the pupils pinpoint regardless of the light.

To test the reaction of the pupils the room is darkened and a flashlight beam is then shone from the side into the pupil. Normally the pupil will have dilated in the darkened room, and with the sudden light it will contract quickly.

Fundus

To examine the interior of the eye, an ophthalmoscope (Figure 14-7) is used. This is a lighted instrument that can focus a beam of light into the eye. It also has a series of lenses by which the nurse can focus on various parts of the eye.

The patient can assume either a supine or sitting position and is asked to look straight ahead and not to move the eye. The nurse holds the ophthalmoscope with the right hand and looks into the right eye of the patient with the right eye. The left eye is then used to look into the patient's left eye. Normally when the light enters the eye the nurse will see through the

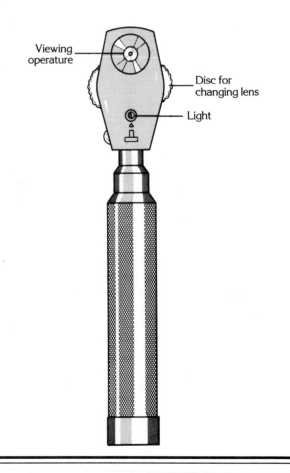

Figure 14-7. The ophthalmoscope is a lighted instrument used to examine the interior of the eye.

ophthalmoscope a reddish orange reflected light. Each structure in the eye should be clearly seen by changing focus of the ophthalmoscope. If there is a pathologic condition present that interferes with the passage of the light, for example, a cataract (an opacity of the eye lens), then dark lines will appear.

Fundoscopic examinations in infants may be done at two to six months of age unless other assessments such as the neurologic examination suggest pathologic conditions. For proper visualization a mydriatic is required. Generally the drops are instilled three times before the test at 15-minute intervals. The baby can be positioned in the supine position on the examining table or held by the mother, either on her lap or held upright over one shoulder. The optic disc of infants is paler than that of adults, and edema of the optic disc is rarely seen in situations of increased intracranial pressure, since the sutures and fontanelles are open.

Retina.   The retina of the eye has certain landmarks, which need to be identified. The optic disc is the central point on the retina. The sensor organs come together at this point, forming the optic nerve, which goes to the brain. The optic disc is normally a flat, white, or grayish round area. In conditions in which there is increased intracranial pressure, the disc may appear to bulge or push forward into the eye.

The blood vessels of the retina can also be seen on the retina. The arterioles appear red, while the venules are reddish purple. They are normally distributed over the retina forming wide curves. In some pathologic conditions they may appear narrowed in places and tortuous. See Figure 14-8 for a normal ocular fundus.

The macula of the eye will also be seen lateral to the disc. It is yellow and most readily seen in brunettes, whose retina is normally darker red than that of a fair person. It is at the macula that the cones are most greatly concentrated; thus it is the point of maximum visual acuity and the point of central vision.

Usually the structures of the eye and any abnormalities are described as to their placement by the clock. For example, a hemorrhage of the right eye might be described as at "7 o'clock," that is, below the disc, and "out one disc diameter."

Lens and Chambers.   If the lens is opaque, it will appear as a grayish white opacity, often impairing visualization of the retina. Bleeding into the posterior eye chamber may also give a reddish haze to the structures in the eye.

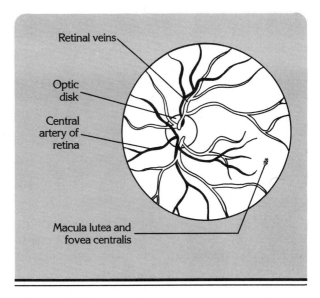

Figure 14-8.   The fundus of a left eye.

Labels on figure: Retinal veins · Optic disk · Central artery of retina · Macula lutea and fovea centralis

Visual Acuity

The ability of the person to see can be tested with the use of the Snellen chart. In children who are three years or older a Snellen E chart can be used. After children know the alphabet the regular Snellen chart can be used. Each eye is tested separately.

Visual acuity is stated in terms of the test distance of 20 feet. Normal vision is stated as 20/20. Vision of 20/40 means that the person can only read at 20 feet what a normal person can read at 40 feet. A child's visual acuity changes with age; at three years vision is 20/40, at four and five years it changes to 30/40, and by six years it is usually 20/20. During adolescence, myopia tends to increase, often requiring corrections by glasses.

In the middle-aged and elderly, eyesight often deteriorates. This is frequently due to an opacity of the lens, called a *cataract. Presbyopia* (ineffective powers of accommodation) occurs as a result of hardening of the lens. *Hyperopia* (farsightedness) commonly occurs in middle age.

Eye Movement

The eyes normally move synchronously to the right and left, upward and downward, and diagonally. All children over six months of age require screening tests to detect *strabismus*, a condition commonly referred to by lay people as a squint or crossed eyes. In strabismus the eye movements are not coordinated and deviate from the normal visual axis. Some deviations are readily apparent; others are very subtle and are seen only when the child's eyes are fatigued.

One screening test that can be carried out to assess for the subtle strabismus is referred to as the *cover test*. The child is asked to focus the eyes on an object about one foot away and to keep the eyes very still for the duration of the test. The nurse then holds a card in front of one eye for several seconds, removes it quickly, and observes the eye that was covered. This test is repeated for the other eye and can be repeated for both eyes focused on a more distant object. If the eye jerks after the cover is removed, some strabismus is indicated.

EARS

There are two major aspects to an assessment of the ears: first, observation of the external ear structures, ear canal, and tympanic membrane, and second, a test of hearing acuity.

External Ear

The external structures of the ear can be observed for skin lesions, pus, and blood. The external canal is vis-

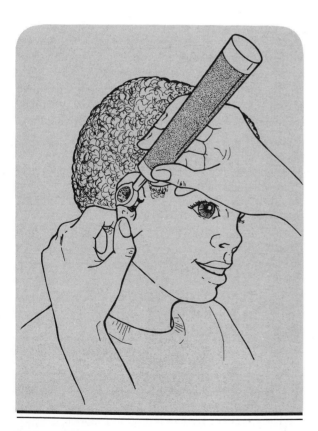

Figure 14-9.   In inserting an otoscope into the external auditory canal of a child, the auricle is pulled backward and downward to straighten the canal.

ualized with the use of an otoscope. This is a lighted instrument with a funnel-shaped part that is inserted into the external auditory canal (Figure 14-9).

To insert the otoscope, one must straighten the ear canal. In an adult the auricle is pulled upward and backward. The auricle is pulled backward and downward for infants and backward and upward for older children.

With the otoscope any cerumen in the canal can be observed as well as the tympanic membrane. The latter appears as a light gray, translucent membrane. Any abnormalities of the tympanic membrane such as perforations, scars, bulging, and discharges need to be reported. See Figure 14-10 for a normal tympanic membrane.

A child needs to be carefully restrained for this procedure. Infants under one year of age can be laid on their backs on the examining table with their heads turned to one side and their arms placed over their heads. The arms can be held securely at the elbows by the mother. The nurse then leans her body on the infant's chest and examines the ear with both hands. Young children sit on their mother's lap with their legs restrained between the mother's knees and their arms restrained against their chest. The mother can then with her free hand hold the child's head against her chest. Older children generally cooperate when standing or sitting.

Hearing

Hearing acuity can be roughly tested by using a watch. The nurse's hearing is compared to the patient's if the nurse's hearing is normal. A watch is held to the patient's ear and slowly withdrawn until the patient can no longer hear the ticking. This distance is then compared with the distance at which the nurse can no longer hear the watch tick.

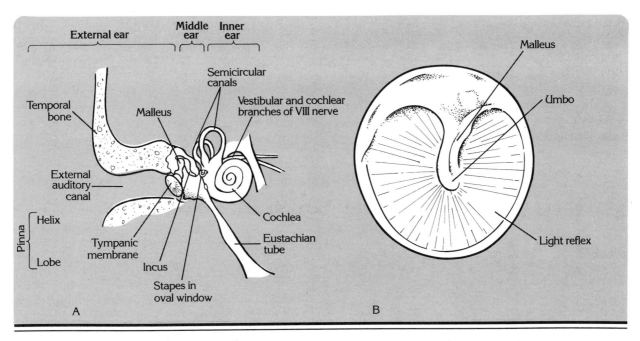

Figure 14-10.   **A,** External anatomical structures of the ear and, **B,** Right tympanic membrane.

NOSE

The nose can be examined very simply with a flashlight, but before doing this the external nares should be observed for any crusts or discharge that might be present. The nose itself needs also to be examined as to its size, shape, and the symmetry of the two sides. Observation of the nasal passages can then be carried out. The patient tips the head back, and the flashlight is shone up each nostril. In some cases the otoscope is also used. It is inserted carefully up each nostril. The otoscope should never be forced if an obstruction is encountered, but this fact needs to be noted. Any discharge in the nostrils also needs to be noted. The mucous membrane is normally pink. Any variations such as the redness of inflammation or the grayness of an allergy need to be noted.

Normally the nasal septum lies in the midline dividing the two nasal passages. Any deviation or protuberance needs also to be noted. After this, the openness of the passage can be assessed by pressing one side of the nose so that one nostril is closed and then asking the patient to breathe out through the other nostril, that is, with the mouth closed, to assess any obstruction. This is then repeated using the other nostril.

MOUTH AND PHARYNX

The external portion of the mouth, the lips, are first observed for color and moisture. Abnormalities such as undue redness, swelling, and crusts, for example, are also observed.

A tongue depressor and a flashlight or otoscope are used for detailed observation. Dentures need to be removed by the patient. The mucous membranes need to be observed for ulceration, bleeding, swelling, redness, and, in some instances, pus. The teeth also need to be observed for discoloration and caries. The odor of the patient's mouth can also in some instances be a clue to an infective process.

The tongue should be situated in the midline of the mouth, and when the patient sticks it out it should remain on the midline and it should not have a tremor. The tongue also needs to be assessed for color, moisture, and any lesions. Normally the top of the tongue has a velvety appearance due to the presence of the tastebuds and small furrows. A person who is dehydrated may have deep furrows on the tongue that run anterior to posterior.

The throat or pharynx is also observed. Often this is best done by viewing one side at a time in order to avoid initiating the gag reflex. The tongue depressor is placed to the back and side of the tongue while the patient sticks the tongue out. The mucous membranes should normally be pink and smooth. The uvula should be in the midline. Behind the fauces on each side is a tonsil. The presence of pus or large amounts of mucus needs to be noted. This might be evidence of an infection in the nasopharynx or sinuses.

THE CHEST

The thorax, lungs, heart, breasts, and axilla are included in the assessment of the total chest in this chapter. The techniques of observation (inspection), auscultation, palpation, and percussion are utilized in total chest examination.

The Thorax

For examination of the thorax the patient removes all clothing to the waist and assumes a sitting or standing position. The chest is first observed for posture, shape, symmetry, and motion.

Posture

The patient's posture is important to note. Some people with chronic respiratory problems tend to bend forward or even prop their arms on a desk in order to elevate their clavicles. This is an attempt to get more chest expansion and thus breathe with less effort.

Shape and Symmetry

In the infant the thorax is rounded in shape, that is, the diameter from the front to the back (anteroposterior, A-P) is equal to the transverse diameter. It is also cylindrical, having a nearly equal diameter at the top and the base. By six years of age the anteroposterior diameter has decreased in proportion to the transverse one. In adults the anteroposterior diameter is smaller than the transverse diameter, and the overall shape of the thorax is elliptical, that is, it has a smaller diameter at the top than at the base.

Assessment of the shape of the chest is done by inspection of all sides of the chest, front, sides, and back. Several deformities of the chest can occur. *Pigeon chest*, a permanent deformity, is caused by rickets. It is one in which the transverse diameter is narrowed, the A-P diameter is increased, and the sternum protrudes. A *funnel breast* is the opposite of pigeon breast in that the sternum is depressed, thereby causing a narrow A-P diameter. Spinal deformities such as kyphosis or scoliosis can also be seen during examination of the thorax. Some changes in the chest wall such as a bulge can be caused by cardiac enlargement or neoplasms. Conversely, depressions in the chest may be seen as a result of the surgical removal of some ribs, for example.

The thorax also needs to be inspected for symmetry of expansion. This assessment is assisted by palpation. Both hands are placed on the lower part of the posterior chest with the thumbs adjacent to the spine and the fingers stretched laterally (see Figure 14-11).

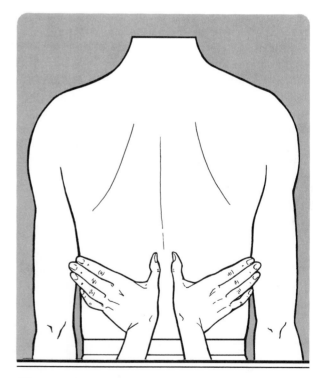

Figure 14-11.   The position of the hands on the posterior chest to test for symmetry of chest expansion.

During a deep inspiration the thumbs normally move an equal distance apart from the spine at the same time. This process is repeated for the upper thorax and for the anterior thorax. In the latter instances the fingers are placed along the rib cage laterally and the thumbs along each costal margin. Wide variations between the upper and lower chest expansions also need to be noted. A symmetry of expansion can be due to many factors such as atelectasis (collapse of a lung), fractured ribs, or acute pleurisy. During chest expansion the nurse also needs to note bulging or retraction of intercostal spaces.

Lung Percussion

The percussion technique was described in Chapter 12. It was noted that the more solid the underlying tissue the less it vibrated with percussion. Therefore the lung that is filled with air vibrates more than a lung without air. Two normal percussion sounds over the thorax are resonance and dullness. *Resonance,* the lower pitched sound, is found over normal lung tissue, while *dullness,* a higher pitched sound, is found over the heart or liver.

Abnormal percussion sounds that can occur are hyperresonance and flatness. *Hyperresonance* is a lower pitched sound than resonance and occurs over a lung portion that is abnormally filled with air such as may occur in severe emphysema or with a pneumothorax. *Flatness* is an extreme amount of dullness and therefore is higher pitched. This sound can be simulated by percussing the thigh, which is a totally nonaerated tissue. Some authorities use the term *flatness* to describe the normal sound over the heart or liver. Many, however, consider flatness an abnormality and prefer the term *dullness* to describe the normal percussion sound over the heart or liver.

Any dullness found over areas that are normally resonant is also considered abnormal. When large amounts of fluid, pus, or blood collect in the lung (alveolar spaces or pleural spaces), percussion will reveal dullness rather than resonance. This occurs in such conditions as pneumonia, pulmonary edema, or tumors, to name a few.

When percussing the thorax, a systematic method is used starting superiorly and progressing inferiorly (Figure 14-12). Parallel areas of each side of the chest are percussed at each level, anteriorly and posteriorly. For posterior percussion the patient can cross the forearms at the waist to separate the scapulae. The top of each shoulder is percussed as well to assess the resonance over each lung apex. The scapular areas and sternum need to be avoided, since the skeleton obscures the normal sounds.

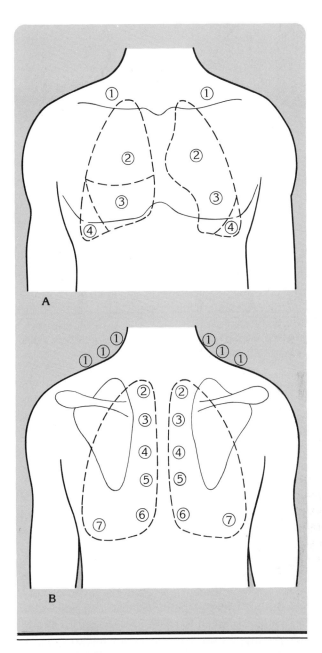

Figure 14-12. Chest percussion sequence on the, **A,** anterior and, **B,** posterior chest.

Identifying the location of the heart and the liver is important. The upper border of the liver is normally found at the right fourth or fifth intercostal space and will be found readily by percussing down from the right midclavicular line. The heart location is discussed later in this chapter in the section "The Heart."

Lung Sounds

Lung sounds include breath sounds, voice sounds, and adventitious sounds (abnormal sounds). Lung

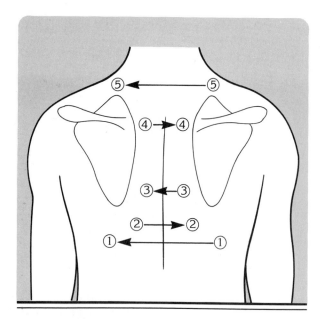

Figure 14-13. Auscultation of the posterior chest using a stethoscope.

sounds can be heard with or without the use of a stethoscope. Normal breathing is a quiet process, but with the use of a stethoscope breath sounds can be heard as soft air vibrations. Some sounds can be heard only with a stethoscope. (See Figure 14-13.)

When auscultating the chest, a quiet room is advised, particularly for a beginning student. The character and quality of the breath sounds and of the whispered voice as well as the presence of adventitious sounds need to be determined.

The excursion of the diaphragm can also be percussed on the posterior chest. Normal excursion is 3–5 cm in females and 5–6 cm in males. This is done by noting the difference between the levels of dullness during a deep inspiration and a deep expiration. The patient is asked to take in a deep breath and to hold it while the nurse percusses downward until the quality of the percussion tone changes noticeably. This area is then marked on the chest. The patient is then asked to exhale and to hold it while the nurse repeats the percussion procedure and marks the place where the tone changes. See Figure 14-14 for levels.

Breath Sounds

Normal breath sounds are of three major types: vesicular, bronchial, and a combination of the two, bronchovesicular.

The vesicular sounds can be likened to a sigh and/or a soft, quiet rustle or swish. These sounds are produced in the alveoli and the terminal bronchioles. They are heard over most lung areas during respira-

tion but are louder during inspirations. This is because during inspiration the flow rate is more rapid, and the air is transported into smaller and smaller channels. Expiration is more passive and one and one-half times longer than inspiration, thus creating less air turbulence and less sound.

The bronchial sounds are loud tubular sounds that are louder during expiration. They are heard normally over the trachea and major bronchi, that is, in the vertical line below the neck over the sternum.

The bronchovesicular sounds, which are a combination of the two, are heard over parts of the chest where a bronchus is situated near the lung parenchyma, in the upper anterior chest lateral to the sternum or posteriorly between the scapula. To auscultate for breath sounds the diaphragm of the stethoscope needs to be warmed in the palms of the nurse's hands if it is cold and then placed firmly against the chest wall. Ask the patient to breathe quietly with the mouth open. (Deep breathing converts vesicular sounds into bronchovesicular.) The latter prevents the interference of sounds produced in the nares and nasopharynx. The chest is systematically auscultated similar to chest percussion (see Figure 14-13 for the auscultation sequence).

Adventitious Breath Sounds

Descriptions of the adventitious breath sounds vary to some degree in the literature. Some of the common sounds, however, are discussed.

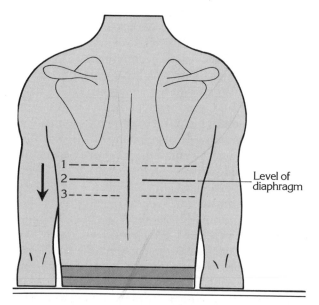

Figure 14-14. To determine chest excursion, a posterior view.

Rhonchi. Rhonchi is a Greek term meaning "a wheezing sound" and is a sound generally heard more prominently during expiration when the air passages are normally contracted. Rhonchi are described as continuous, coarse, wheezy, whistling sounds that are produced in the large bronchi by air passing through mucus and/or a narrowed air passage. The pitch varies in accordance with the size of the bronchus. Larger bronchi produce a lower pitch than smaller ones. Any disease process that narrows the lumen of a bronchus such as asthma, tumors, accumulation of mucus, or edema will create rhonchi.

Rales. Rale is a French term meaning "a rattle" and is a sound generally heard during inspiration. Rales are sounds produced by the bubbling of air through fluid in the alveoli or air passages. They can be described as a shower of bubbling sounds, short and interrupted. The pitch of rales also varies with the location. Those produced in the alveoli are high pitched and sound close to the ear. Those produced in the bronchioles are crackling and lower pitched and are not unlike a carbonated beverage that fizzes when the bottle is opened. When rales are heard the patient should be asked to cough. If the rales are accentuated or do not disappear, fluid accumulation due to congestive heart failure or inflammatory disease such as pneumonia can be suspected.

Sometimes rales are also referred to as *creps* or *crepitations.* Some people use the term solely to describe the rales produced in the terminal airways and liken it to the sound of cellophane being crumpled.

Pleural Rub. The pleural rub is a coarse leathery or grating sound produced by the rubbing together of the surfaces of the pleura, and thus it is often referred to as a *friction rub.* It occurs when these surfaces are inflamed and is generally heard over the lower lateral areas of the thorax, particularly the anterior portion where there is greater chest expansion. It is important that the nurse hold the diaphragm of the stethoscope firmly when auscultating. Sliding the bell can produce artificial sounds similar to a rub. A pleural rub can be simulated by placing the palm of one's hand tightly over the ear and then rubbing the back of the hand with one finger of the other hand.

Voice Sounds

Talking produces vibrations in the larynx, which are transmitted through the respiratory system to the chest wall. These vibrations are referred to as *vocal fremitus* and can be heard with a stethoscope or felt by the palms of the hands during palpation (tactile fremitus). Fremitus is best heard or felt in the superior portion of the chest wall rather than at the base. It varies among individuals, being more pronounced in males and people with thin chest walls. Normally when a person is asked to whisper a few numbers, the examiner will hear the sounds as muffled and the words will not be clearly differentiated or distinguished. When the words are heard more loudly and the words are distinguishable, it is suggestive of consolidation of the lung tissue, that is, the lung tissue has become more solid. This can be due to an infectious process such as pneumonia. Consolidation facilitates the transmission of the voice sounds.

To determine tactile fremitus, the nurse places the palms of the hands symmetrically against the chest wall. The patient is asked to say (not whisper) a few words such as "ninety-nine" or to count "one, two, three." A mild vibration can be felt. Fremitus should be felt equally on each side. Any increase, decrease, or absence needs to be noted. Consolidated lung tissue conducts voice vibrations better than the normal lung containing air, and therefore fremitus is increased where it occurs. Absence of fremitus can be noted when air is not conducted, for example, when a bronchus is obstructed. Fremitus is decreased when the pleural space is thickened or enlarged with fluid or air such as occurs in a pneumothorax or fibrosis of the pleura.

In infants tactile fremitus can be assessed when the baby cries. The nurse places the palm of the hand and fingers over the anterior, lateral, or posterior chest wall.

THE HEART

The state of the heart's function can be obtained to a large degree by findings in the history such as symptoms of shortness of breath or by the patient's general appearance, which may reveal some cyanosis or edema of the legs. Direct examination of the heart, however, offers more specific information, including the heart sounds, the heart size, and other phenomena such as lifts, heaves, or murmurs. The techniques used for examination of the thorax are also used to examine the heart that is, observations (inspection), palpation, percussion, and auscultation, in this same sequence. Auscultation can be more meaningful when data from the previous methods are obtained first. Examination of the heart in infants and children is generally carried out in the same manner as for the adult.

Heart Size and Location

The area of the chest overlying the heart is referred to as the *precordium*. In the average adult the base of the heart (both atria) lies slightly to the right of the sternum and toward the back, while the apex of the left ventricle lies to the left of the sternum and points forward. The apex touches the anterior chest wall at or medial to the left midclavicular line (MCL) and at or near the fifth left intercostal space (LICS) (see section on apical-radial pulse, Chapter 13. An apical impulse, also referred to as *point of maximum impulse* or point of maximum intensity (PMI) can be seen in about 50% of the adult population. The apical impulse is a good index of cardiac size. If the heart is enlarged, this impulse is found lateral to the MCL. The distance between the apex and the MCL should be noted in centimeters. In people in whom the apical beat is not observed, the apex may be located by palpation, but not always. The apex of a newborn lies in a more horizontal position than the adult's and can be palpated in the third or fourth intercostal space. The apex may normally be lateral to the midclavicular line (See Figure 13-3 for apical pulse locations).

An abnormal *lift* or heave may be noticed in some people. These refer to a lift of the sternum or ribs with each heartbeat. It occurs when cardiac action is very forceful and should be confirmed by palpation using the palm of the hand. A *heave* is more forceful than a lift. Enlargement or overactivity of the left ventricle produces a heave lateral to the apex, while enlargement of the right ventricle will produce a heave at or near the sternum.

Locating the left cardiac border is achieved by percussing the patient's chest while the patient is in a standing or sitting position. The heart falls away from the chest wall in a supine position, reducing the area of normal dullness, and therefore this position is not recommended. Percussion should start from the anterior axillary line toward the midline in the fourth LICS, and this is then repeated in the fifth and sixth LICS. The LICS at which the cardiac border is furthest laterally is noted. The right cardiac border cannot be percussed appropriately, since it lies beneath lung tissue and the sternum.

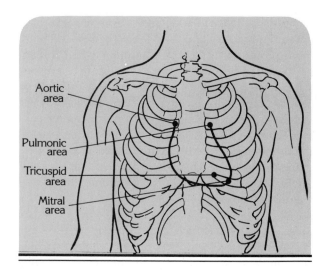

Figure 14-15.   The placement of the bell of the stethoscope to hear heart sounds.

Heart Sounds

Several heart sounds can be heard by the use of auscultation techniques. Only the first and second heart sounds will be emphasized in this text. The normal first two heart sounds are produced by closure of the valves of the heart.

The first heart sound (S_1) occurs when the atrioventricular (A-V) valves close. These valves close when the ventricles have been sufficiently filled. Although the right and left A-V valves do not close simultaneously, the closures occur closely enough that they are heard as one sound (S_1), a dull, low-pitched sound.

After the ventricles empty their blood into the aorta and pulmonary arteries, the semilunar valves close, producing the second heart sound (S_2). S_2 has a higher pitch than S_1 and is also shorter. These two sounds, S_1 and S_2, occur within one second or less, depending upon the heart rate.

Associated with these sounds are systole and diastole. *Diastole* is the period in which the ventricles are relaxed. It starts with the second sound and ends at the subsequent first sound. *Systole* is the period in which the ventricles are contracted. It begins with the first heart sound and ends at the second heart sound. Systole is usually shorter than diastole. Normally no sounds are audible in these periods.

When auscultating the heart, the nurse stands at the patient's right side and the patient is examined in two positions, the upright position and the recumbent position. Certain sounds are more audible in certain positions. The nurse then places the stethoscope on the patient's chest and auscultates the entire precordium.

Although the two heart sounds are audible anywhere on the precordial area, they are heard best over specific valve areas (see Figure 14-15). These areas are the tricuspid valve area, which is near the lower sternum, the mitral valve area, which is located at the cardiac apex, the aortic valve area, and the pulmonic valve areas. The aortic area is located in the second right intercostal space (RICS) near the sternal border, and the pulmonic area is in the second LICS at the sternal border.

Auscultation should not be limited to these areas. The nurse needs to locate these areas and then move the stethoscope around to find the most audible sounds for each particular patient. Both sounds need to be distinguished in every area of auscultation. It is also necessary when auscultating to concentrate on one particular sound at a time in each area: the first heart sound, then the second heart sound, followed by systole, and then diastole.

Normally both cardiac sounds are heard loudest in the aortic area, with S_2 being distinctly louder. The intensity or loudness of the sounds is described as normal, absent, diminished, or accentuated as contrasted to normal sounds. The quality of sounds can be described as sharp, full, booming, or snapping.

A systematic method of auscultating these areas is recommended, starting at the aortic area, then the pulmonic, followed by the tricuspid area, and last the mitral area. A stethoscope with a bell and a diaphragm attachment are needed for adequate auscultation. The bell attachment transmits lower pitched sounds best, while the diaphragm transmits the higher pitched sounds best. The bell attachment should be used for the tricuspid and mitral valve areas. The heart sounds are described and compared in accordance with the valve areas in Table 14-5. In infants the first heart sound is usually louder than the second heart sound at the apex. Murmurs are frequently heard at the left sternal border because of the newborn's changing circulatory system. Repeated follow-up is required to assess abnormalities. Other cardiovascular signs such as respirations, color, and pulses will usually confirm any abnormality. Note in Table 14-5 that S_2 is usually louder in the pulmonic area in children and young adults and that by about

Table 14-5. Heart Sounds

| Sound | Description | Area | | | |
		Aortic	Pulmonary	Tricuspid	Mitral
S_1	Dull, low-pitched and longer than S_2	Less intensity than S_2	Less intensity than S_2	Louder than S_2 or equal	Louder than S_2 or equal
S_2	High-pitched, snappy, and shorter than S_1	Louder than S_1	Louder than S_1 in children and young adults; if louder in adults over 40 it is abnormal	Less intensity than S_1 or equal	Less intensity than S_1 or equal
Systole	Normal silent interval between S_1 and S_2				
Diastole	Normally no sounds; interval between S_2 and next S_1				

Table 14-6. Grade System Describing the Intensity of Cardiac Murmurs

Six-grade system	Four-grade system
Grade 1: Faintest murmur audible; may not be heard at first	Grade 1: Faintest murmur audible
Grade 2: Faint murmur audible without difficulty	Grade 2: Soft murmur
Grade 3: Soft murmur louder than Grade 2	Grade 3: Loud murmur
Grade 4: Loud murmur	Grade 4: Very loud murmur
Grade 5: Louder murmur, but if stethoscope is removed slightly off chest, not audible	
Grade 6: Maximum loudness; audible if stethoscope is lifted from chest	

age 30 most adults have a louder S_2 in the aortic and pulmonic areas. As part of the auscultation procedure, therefore, the loudness of S_2 should be compared between the aortic and pulmonic areas. When the pulmonic S_2 is found to be louder than the aortic S_2 in adults over age 40 years, the finding is abnormal. The loudness of S_2 in the pulmonary area relates to the blood pressure in the pulmonary artery, while the loudness of S_2 in the aortic area is related to the arterial blood pressure in the systemic circulation. Thus when the pulmonary artery pressure increases, as in some chronic obstructive lung diseases, the loudness of S_2 pulmonic also increases. In contrast, the S_2 aortic sound will be augmented above normal in hypertensive disease.

Cardiac Murmurs

Murmurs result when blood flow becomes turbulent within the heart due to valvular defects or abnormal openings between the compartments of the heart. Not all murmurs indicate cardiac disease. Murmurs are described in relation to their location of maximum intensity, loudness, pitch, and any change that occurs during movement or exercise of the patient or during respiration. The intensity of murmurs is often described by a four- or six-grade system (Table 14-6). Murmurs are generally also described as systolic or diastolic. Diastolic murmurs are usually considered to be abnormal. Systolic murmurs occur during systole; diastolic murmurs occur during diastole.

BREASTS

The breasts of men, women, and children need to be examined. Men and children will have some glandular tissue beneath each nipple, while a mature woman will have glandular tissue throughout the breast. In the newborn the breasts may be slightly enlarged due to maternal hormones. This usually disappears in a few days. During adolescence, asymmetrical development is not unusual, and boys may have some breast development in early adolescence.

During pregnancy both breasts become enlarged. In the second month the areola of the breast normally becomes raised, pigmented, and edematous. About the third month it is not unusual for some colostrum to be expressed from the breast. This is best done in a sitting position. The nipples are observed for any discharge, crusting, and edema. There should also be noted any retraction and disease. Although the former may not be indicative of any disease process, it needs to be noted.

The breasts also need to be observed for their size, shape, and position, and then each breast should be compared according to these criteria. The normal size varies according to age, heredity, endocrine functions, and the amount of adipose tissue that is present.

Breasts must also be palpated for any masses that may be present. Women today are being encouraged to palpate their own breasts regularly for this reason.

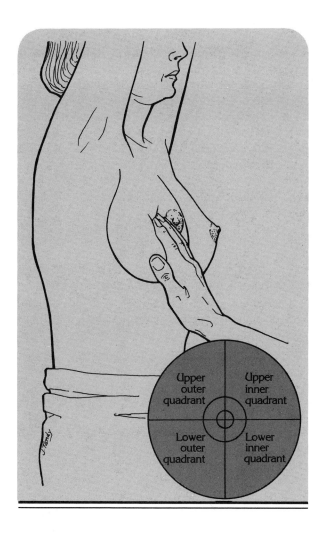

One technique is to press the palmar surfaces of the first, second, third, and fourth fingers down on the breast, moving them in a slightly rotary motion, pressing the tissue against the chest wall. By dividing the breast into four imaginary quadrants such as the upper outer quadrant (left), the nurse has a reference point for recording any palpated masses. This palpation is repeated completely around one breast and then around the other (See Figure 14-16). Sometimes the second hand can be used to support the tissue to get a better estimate of the size of any nodules. Masses need to be described in terms of the following criteria.

1. Location in the breast, such as right inner quadrant, right breast.
2. Shape, for example, nodules, round and smooth.
3. Mobility: moves freely or is fixed.
4. Discomfort, for example, appears painful to touch.
5. Consistency, such as hard, soft, rubbery.

The second breast is then palpated in the same manner.

Figure 14-16.   Palpating the right breast using the palmar surfaces of the first, second, third, and fourth fingers.

AXILLAE

The axillae are most usually palpated for enlarged lymph nodes as well as for the condition of the skin, the latter of which has already been discussed.

To palpate the axillae, assist the patient to relax the arm, perhaps by resting it on a table. The nurse's fingers are then pressed as far up toward the apex of the axilla as possible and brought downward, pressing against the chest wall. Nodes in the central area of the axilla and toward the thorax may be palpated in this manner. The central nodes are the most readily palpable. If the thoracic nodes are palpable and/or either group of nodes feels enlarged, this needs to be reported. The procedure is then repeated on the other axilla.

ABDOMEN

There are a number of organs in the abdominal cavity, some of which extend beyond the normal landmarks of the abdomen. There are two methods by which the abdomen is imaginarily divided in order to aid in description: one is by quadrants, and the other divides the abdomen into nine areas. To di-

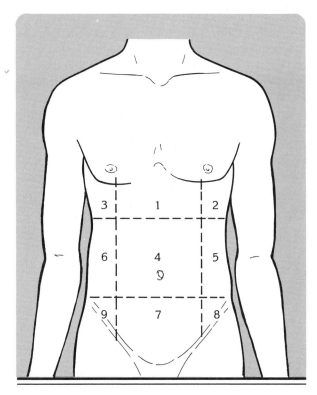

Figure 14-17. Nine abdominal areas. *1*, Epigastrium; *2,3*, left and right hypochondriac; *4*, umbilical; *5,6*, left and right lumbar; *7*, suprapubic or hypogastric; and *8,9*, left and right inguinal or iliac.

vide the abdomen into quadrants, a vertical line is made from the xiphoid process to the symphysis pubis, and a horizontal line is drawn across the abdomen at the level of the umbilicus. These quadrants are labeled upper left quadrant, upper right quadrant, lower right quadrant, and lower left quadrant (Figure 14-18). The second method, division into nine areas, requires two vertical lines, which extend superiorly from the midpoints of the inguinal ligaments, and two lines drawn horizontally, one at the level of the edge of the lower ribs and the other at the level of the iliac crests. See Figure 14-17.

Generally the following structures lie in the quadrants:

> Right upper quadrant: liver, gall bladder, kidney at the back, part of the colon and small intestine
>
> Left upper quadrant: stomach, pancreas, spleen, kidney at the back, part of the colon and small intestine
>
> Left lower quadrant: colon, rectum, and urinary bladder
>
> Right lower quadrant: colon, appendix, rectum, and urinary bladder

To examine the abdomen four methods are used: observation, auscultation, palpation, and percussion. The patient needs to be in a supine position, with a pillow for the head.

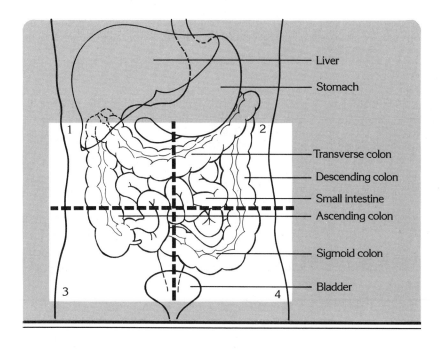

Figure 14-18. The four abdominal regions and the underlying organs. *1*, Right upper quadrant; *2*, left upper quadrant; *3*, right lower quadrant; and *4*, left lower quadrant.

Observation

The abdomen is observed for skin rashes, lesions, and scars. Also observe for any generalized or localized swelling.

In the newborn it is normal for the abdomen to protrude slightly due to the undeveloped abdominal muscles. In childhood the abdomen protrudes in standing, but the protuberance disappears when the child lies down.

Normally the abdomen is flat; in the obese adult, however, the abdomen may assume a more rounded appearance. Localized swellings may indicate a hernia. These are most likely to occur above and below the inguinal ligaments, along the midline, and near any scars from previous operations.

Normally peristalsis of the intestines cannot be observed through the abdominal wall; however, in acute intestinal obstruction, waves may be seen. This is abnormal and needs to be reported.

In a woman who is pregnant it may be possible to see the fetus move during the later stages of the pregnancy.

Auscultation

There are two particular sounds for which the nurse must listen: bowel sounds and vascular bruits. In the pregnant woman fetal sounds are also assessed. A *bruit* is a murmur or sound, which is frequently abnormal.

Bowel sounds are heard with the use of the stethoscope, and they can be heard in all four quadrants. They are caused by the gas and food products moving along the intestines. When the intestine is not functioning correctly, the bowel sounds may be heard at a slow rate, for example, one per minute. This occurs in the situation of paralytic ileus, an occasional after-effect of surgery.

In situations in which the patient has diarrhea, the bowel sounds occur at a very fast rate, perhaps as frequently as every three seconds. This is referred to as *hypermotility*.

Bruits

Bruits are listened for in each quadrant and along the midline, where a problem of the abdominal aorta may be heard. These may sound like a blowing or swishing sound.

Fetal Heart Sounds

About the fifth month of pregnancy fetal heart sounds can usually be heard. This is done using a fetoscope, an instrument like a stethoscope. See Chapter 13 for additional information.

Palpation

Palpation can be either superficial or deep. In *superficial* palpation the abdominal wall is pressed, but no effort is made to feel more deeply. With the palmar surface of the four fingers the muscle layer can be palpated. It will normally be firm, but it will also yield to pressure. Observed protuberances can also be palpated in this manner for size, hardness, mobility, and tenderness.

Deep palpation is also carried out on the entire abdomen. This is done in order to detect tenderness and any masses that may be present. In this instance the fingers are pressed more deeply, often using both hands. Each quadrant is deeply palpated, and certain structures are identified. The liver edge can frequently be detected about 5 cm (2 inches) below the costal margin in the right upper quadrant at the midclavicular lines. When the patient takes a deep inspiration, the fingers are pressed firmly down. If the liver edge is not detected, ask the patient to take in another breath; this may be repeated several times. This activity should not be painful, although it is normal for the liver edge to be tender to pressure. If the patient experiences pain, then there may be an inflammatory condition or infection present in the liver or the gall bladder or both.

The nurse also examines the liver edge in order to assess whether it is smooth or nodular as well as its position in the abdominal cavity.

The spleen should also be checked in the left upper quadrant. It is found in the same manner as the liver; however, a normal spleen is rarely palpable. In disease it may be sufficiently enlarged to be felt.

In the newborn the tip of the spleen can be felt beneath the left costal margin, and the liver edge is felt about 2 cm below the right costal margin.

In children the examination is carried out much as for an adult. Special attention needs to be paid to any tenderness in the right lower quadrant (appendicitis) and for protuberances indicative of inguinal hernias.

The kidneys are also not normally palpable except in very thin people. The nurse should first try to locate the lower aspect of the right kidney, which is easier to find than the left because it lies in a lower position. The nurse's left hand is placed in the lumbar curvature, and the right hand is pressed toward it palm down at the level of the umbilicus. As the patient inhales, the nurse's hands are pressed together, and the lower, rounded end of the kidney will be felt. This is repeated for the left kidney, which lies a little higher.

The kidneys are generally palpated in newborns while supporting them at about a 45° angle with the knees slightly flexed. The other hand then palpates for each kidney, which can normally be felt.

Tenderness of an abdominal area needs to be carefully assessed and accurately described. It is im-portant to find the point where the tenderness is greatest (point of maximum tenderness).

Percussion

Percussion is used in order to help establish the presence of gas, fluid, and/or masses. The method is similar to that used for the chest. If the urinary bladder is distended, the percussion will sound dull rather than normally resonant. On the other hand, percussion of the colon when gas is present will produce a tympanic sound in contrast to the usually dull sound around the umbilicus. Tympany over the gastric area is also normal.

GENITALS AND RECTUM

In the newborn the genitals need to be examined for normalcy, for example, that a urinary meatus is on the glans penis in a boy and that it is patent. The testes are also palpated within the scrotum. If both testes have not descended, this needs to be noted. Normally the testes have descended at birth.

In the female newborn the vaginal orifice needs to be inspected. Any discharge should be noted and recorded, although a reddish tinged discharge may be perfectly normal.

The first rectal temperature is taken with particular care in case the anus is closed over (imperforate anus).

During childhood, particular reference is made to any problems involving the genitals. Bed wetting may result from a urinary infection or because of a child's anxiety. Young boys' scrotums also need to be palpated to check for descended testicles.

The external genitals of the female child are usually inspected, but a pelvic examination is normally not carried out.

In male adolescents it is most important to establish the presence of the testicles in the scrotum as previously mentioned; undescended testes need to be noted.

For girls during adolescence the examination is limited to an inspection of the external genitalia unless the girl is sexually active. In this instance it is advocated that a Papanicolaou smear (Pap smear) be taken once a year to detect cancer of the cervix and uterus. To do this a uterine speculum is carefully inserted into the vagina and opened. The spatula or applicator provided is rotated against the cervix, then withdrawn and smeared on a glass slide or inserted in a tube as the case might be.

If the adolescent is sexually active and has an increased or abnormal vaginal discharge, specimens should be taken for the presence of sexually transmitted (venereal) disease.

Pelvic examination of the woman may also provide evidence indicative of pregnancy. Three of these signs are (a) Goodell's sign, (b) Chadwick's sign, and (c) Hegar's sign. See Chapter 11 for information about these signs.

Adult Female Genitals

To examine the genitals of the adult female the patient is best assisted to a lithotomy position either in bed or on an examining table where she can place her feet in stirrups. The patient can be assisted for comfort with appropriate draping and with a pillow for her head. Some women also prefer to have the head of the bed elevated to 35°.

The external genitalia are first examined for lesions, rashes, inflammation, and swelling. Any discharge such as pus or blood needs to be noted.

A vaginal speculum is required for a thorough assessment of the vagina and cervix. The size of the speculum will depend upon the size of the vagina. Women who have had children will probably need a large speculum, the elderly and children require a very small speculum, and women who have not had children need an average size. Usually children do

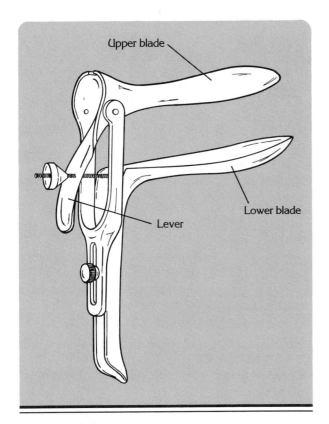

Figure 14-19. A vaginal speculum used to examine the cervix and vagina.

not have pelvic examinations unless it is specifically ordered. The speculum is then lubricated and inserted sidewise with the blades closed and pointing upwards. When the blades are in the vagina, the speculum is turned so that the handle is down, and then the blades are opened. (See Figure 14-19 for the parts of a vaginal speculum.)

With a flashlight the cervix can be observed for color, shape, and firmness. Normally it is pale pink, round, smooth, and firm to touch. It is at this time that a specimen is usually taken for a Papanicolaou smear.

The speculum is then removed and the internal organs are examined manually. Note that in some settings the manual examination is carried out before the speculum is inserted. Usually the nurse puts gloves on one or both hands, then the tips of the first and middle fingers are lubricated with the designated lubricant. With the fourth and fifth fingers curled into the palm and the thumb stretched out, the two lubricated fingers are inserted into the vagina. The nurse's arm needs to be raised in order that the fingers will follow the vagina, which angles backward.

The cervix can be palpated readily. It normally feels relatively firm, smooth, and rounded in the non-

pregnant woman. Usually one's finger cannot enter the cervical canal, therefore if it does enter, this needs to be noted and recorded.

With the other hand upon the abdomen (bimanual examination or two-handed examination) and pressing by starting below the umbilicus and working downward, the fundus of the uterus can be felt by the fingers in the vagina. The fundus is generally anterior to the cervix. It is normally mobile and has a smooth, regular surface. Its size should also be noted.

The fallopian tubes and ovaries can also be palpated. The hand on the abdomen presses about midway on the inguinal ligament, and the hand in the vagina presses to the right or left and toward the abdominal wall to detect each ovary. The size of the ovary, its firmness, and the regularity of the surface of the ovary need also to be assessed. If the ovary feels tender to the patient, this needs to be noted.

Usually a fallopian tube cannot be palpated; however, any enlargement needs to be reported. The nurse's hand is then removed from the vagina, the glove removed, and the patient assisted to a comfortable position.

Adult Female Rectum and Anus

To examine the female's rectum and anus the patient can remain in a supine position with her knees flexed, (Figure 14-20).

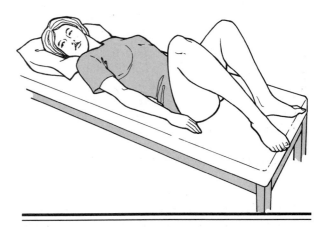

Figure 14-20. A dorsal recumbent position with legs flexed.

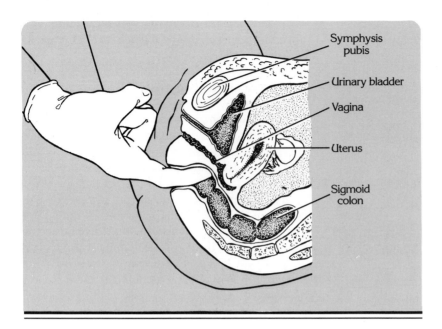

Figure   14-21. Anatomical structures of the female reproductive tract with index finger inserted for examination of the rectum.

Initially the anus is observed for any protruding hemorrhoids (distended veins, which appear as red bodies), fissures, and cracks. When the patient bears down as if to defecate, other hemorrhoids may become visible.

To palpate the anus and rectum the nurse puts on a glove and lubricates the index finger. The patient is asked to bear down, and then the lubricated finger of the nurse slips through the anus into the anal canal. The muscle around the anus will tighten, but this should not be painful to the patient. As the finger moves up the rectum it needs to palpate both the anterior and the posterior walls, being sensitive to any masses (see Figure 14-21). If a mass is encountered it needs to be described as to its location, size, firmness, mobility, smoothness, tenderness, and regularity. On the anterior wall of the rectum the cervix will be palpated. It will feel smooth, round, firm, and movable, and it will not be tender to palpation. During pregnancy it has already been mentioned that the cervix becomes larger and softer. During labor the opening of the cervix will increase in size (dilate) in readiness for the passage of the baby. After the completion of the rectal examination the glove is removed, the hands washed, and the observations recorded.

Adult Male Genitals

It is not unusual to wear gloves when examining the male genitalia because of the danger of acquiring an infection. If gloves are worn, the reason needs to be explained to the patient in a manner that will be unoffensive to him.

The male pubic area needs to be examined for the absence or thinness of the pubic hair. In some instances missing hair can be indicative of a problem such as cirrhosis of the liver. Normally hair of the genital region does not grow on the penis, except at the base or on the scrotum.

The penis is then examined for lesions, swellings, and any discharges. In the uncircumcised male the foreskin (prepuce) is drawn back to expose the glans, which is normally reddish. Ulcers need to be noted particularly on the glans or just inside the urinary meatus. The latter can be opened usually with slight pressure near the tip of the glans.

The scrotum usually has loose skin, and it appears wrinkled. By palpation each testis can be felt. They are normally oval, firm, smooth, and freely movable within the scrotum. The testes are usually 4 cm in length and about 2.0–2.5 cm in width, varying from one end to the other, like a chicken egg. The epididymis can be felt at the lower aspect of the testis and extending along the posterior surface. The spermatic cord can also be palpated where it extends from the superior pole of the testis upward entering the inguinal canal and subsequently the abdominal wall.

The scrotum is observed for lesions and the testes for swelling, masses, and inflammation. Any mass needs to be described as for size, mobility, position, firmness, and regularity of its surface.

The inguinal region is then palpated for enlarged lymph nodes. This is done by pressing one's

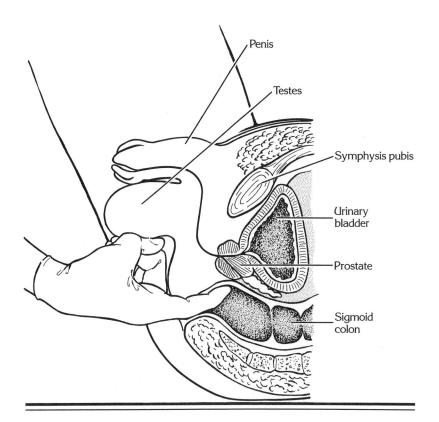

Figure 14-22. Anatomical structures of the male reproductive and urinary tracts with the index finger inserted for examination of the rectum.

Labels on figure: Penis; Testes; Symphysis pubis; Urinary bladder; Prostate; Sigmoid colon

fingers along a line from the base of the penis up toward the crest of the ilium. Any weakness should also be noted at this time as a sign of a possible inguinal hernia.

Adult Male Rectum and Anus

For this examination the patient can assume one of several positions. The most comfortable is probably the lateral lying position with the upper leg acutely flexed. The anus is inspected just as it is done for the female, and the gloved finger is similarly inserted into the rectum for the rectal palpation. In the male rectum the prostate gland can be palpated on the anterior wall (see Figure 14-22). Each lobe of this gland then is felt for masses, consistency of size of the two lobes, firmness, and tenderness. As with the female it is important to examine the rectal wall for any nodules or masses.

EXTREMITIES

The extremities (the arms and legs) are palpated, inspected, and moved. First the skin is observed as it was on other parts of the body. The limb itself is assessed for any unusual joint angle, which could well indicate a current or old bone fracture. The joints are next moved in order to assess range of motion. See Chapter 23, "Movement of the Joints." The joints are also observed for their size, complaints of pain, and redness.

Finally the muscles are observed for any tremor or unsteadiness. A fine tremor can sometimes be observed by asking the patient to hold the arms out in front of him or her for a few minutes. These observations are made for each extremity.

The feet and legs need also to be observed for color and edema (excess fluid). The swelling may be tense and hard, stretching the skin, or it may be possible to press the skin and produce an indentation that disappears in a few minutes. The latter is called *pitting edema.*

Another observation of particular importance for the legs is the appearance of distended bluish veins, which may be tortuous and lumpy. These are varicose veins and may well be tender to the touch.

Until about two years of age a child will appear somewhat bowlegged.

Reflexes

A *reflex* is an automatic response of the body to a stimulus. In Chapter 10, reflexes normally present at various ages were discussed.

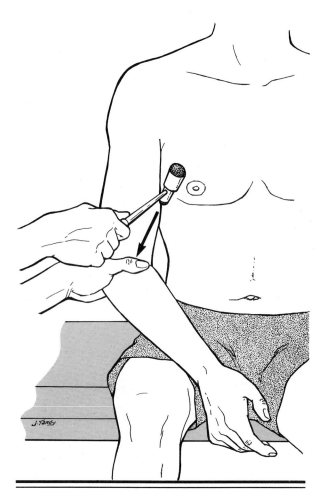

Figure 14-23. The biceps reflex. Note placement of the nurse's thumb.

Reflexes are tested using a percussion hammer. They are described on a scale as 0, +, ++, +++, and ++++. 0 means no reflex, + is minimal activity (hypoactive), ++ normal reflex, +++ more active, and ++++ maximum activity (hyperactive). In assessing reflexes it is important to compare one side of the body with the other.

Several reflexes are normally tested during a physical examination. These are (a) the biceps and triceps reflex, (b) the patellar reflex, (c) the Achilles reflex, and (d) the plantar reflex.

Biceps and Triceps Reflexes

This reflex is tested with the nurse's thumb on the biceps tendon while the patient's arm is supported. The nurse's thumb is then tapped with the hammer, and normally the biceps muscle can be seen to contract (see Figure 14-23).

In the triceps reflex test the patient's arm is again supported in a relaxed fashion and the patient's arm

is tapped with the hammer just above the olecranon process. Normally the forearm will straighten (see Figure 14-24).

Patellar Reflex

To test this reflex the patient sits on the edge of a table, for example, with the legs hanging freely. The hammer is used to strike the area just below the patella, and normally the lower leg will kick forward (see Figure 14-25).

Achilles Reflex

Again in the same position as for the patellar reflex the toes are slightly supported and the Achilles tendon is tapped. The normal response is a downward jerk of the foot (see Figure 14-26).

Plantar Reflex

This reflex is also referred to as the *Babinski reflex.* The sole of the foot is stroked with a thumb nail or the sharper end of some percussion hammers (see Figure 14-27). Normally all five toes bend downward; this is called *negative Babinski.* In an abnormal response, *positive Babinski,* the toes spread outward and the big toe moves upward.

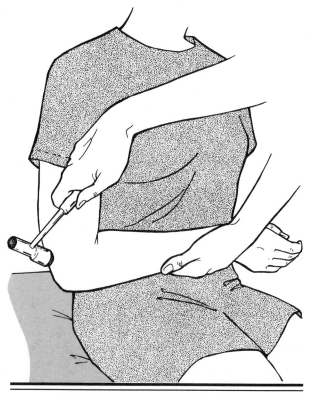

Figure 14-24. The triceps reflex.

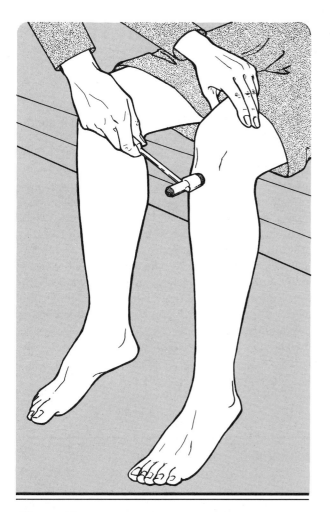

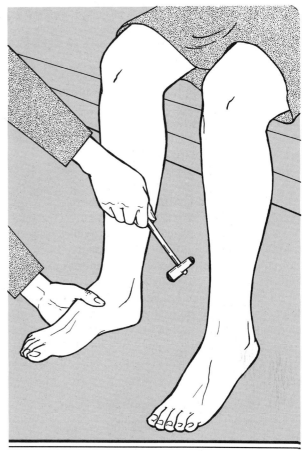

Figure 14-26.   The achilles reflex.

Figure 14-25.   The patellar reflex.

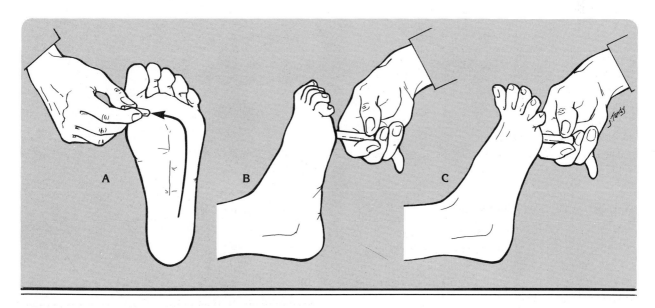

Figure 14-27.   The plantar reflex. **A,** The line of stroking; **B,** negative Babinski (normal); and **C,** positive Babinski (abnormal).

NEUROLOGIC AND MENTAL-EMOTIONAL ASSESSMENT

Neurologic assessment includes examination of the reflexes, the cranial nerves, and the functions of the cerebrum, the cerebellum, and the sensory and motor systems. The reflexes have been previously described in the assessment of the extremities.

The Cranial Nerves

Assessment of the functions of the twelve pairs of cranial nerves is included to a large degree in an examination of the head and neck. Specific examination of these nerves is usually conducted by a neurologist as the situation warrants. However, the routine neurologic assessment portion of a basic physical examination includes some of these cranial nerves. For the

specific functions of each cranial nerve see Table 14-7. The nurse needs to be aware of these to relate abnormalities.

The sense of smell (cranial nerve I) and the sense of taste (cranial nerves VII and IX) are not routinely tested. Vision and eye movements have been previously discussed. These activities involve cranial nerves II, III, IV, and VI. The cranial nerves V (trigeminal) and VII (facial) are not routinely tested other than by observing facial expression and asymmetry for the latter nerve. Any weakness of the face is made more obvious by having the patient close the eyes tightly, wrinkle the forehead, and show the teeth. For the eighth cranial (vestibulocochlear) nerve, only the cochlear branch is routinely tested, that is, hearing ability. The vestibular branch con-

Table 14-7.   Functions of the Cranial Nerves

Nerve	Name	Type of Nerve	Function
I	Olfactory	Sensory	Smell
II	Optic	Sensory	Vision and visual fields
III	Oculomotor	Motor	Extraocular eye movement (EOM) and movement of sphincter of pupil and ciliary muscles of lens
IV	Trochlear	Motor	EOM, specifically moves eyeball downward and laterally
V	Trigeminal	Motor and sensory	
	Ophthalmic branch	Sensory	Sensation of cornea, skin of face, and nasal mucosa
	Maxillary branch	Sensory	Sensation of skin of face and anterior oral cavity (tongue and teeth)
	Mandibular branch	Motor and sensory	Muscles of mastication; sensation of skin of face
VI	Abducens	Motor	Moves eyeball laterally
VII	Facial	Motor and sensory	Facial expression; taste (anterior tongue)
VIII	Vestibulocochlear (acoustic)		
	Vestibular branch	Sensory	Equilibrium
	Cochlear branch	Sensory	Hearing
IX	Glossopharyngeal	Motor and sensory	Gag reflex, tongue movement, taste (posterior tongue)
X	Vagus	Motor and sensory	Sensation of pharynx and larynx; swallowing and phonation
XI	Accessory	Motor	Head movement; shrugging of shoulders
XII	Hypoglossal	Motor	Protrusion of tongue

cerned with balance is not routinely tested but will be subsequently discussed with assessment of cerebellar functions. Swallowing, the gag reflex, tongue movement, and phonation, involving cranial nerves IX, X, and XII, are routinely included in examination of the mouth. The former two nerves (IX and X) are tested at the same time. Each side of the pharynx is touched with a tongue blade, and normally, when the pharyngeal muscles contract, the patient gags. Another test is to have the patient say "ah." The soft palate normally moves. Imperfect movement suggests difficulty with these nerves (IX and X). The latter nerve (hypoglossal) can be readily examined by having the patient protrude the tongue as far as possible. Deviation of the tongue toward one side or the other suggests paralysis. The accessory nerve (cranial nerve XI), which is the motor nerve of the sternocleidomastoid muscle, can be tested by asking the patient to shrug the shoulders while the nurse's hands are pressed down upon them. Any weakness is noted.

Cerebral Functioning (Mental Status)

The highest functions of the nervous system are carried out in the brain. These functions include intellectual (cognitive) ones as well as emotional (affective) functions. A large part of the mental status assessment is included in the history taking. If disorders of speech, behavior, memory, or thought are detected then a more extensive examination is required. Various classifications are available for mental status assessment. Some of the major areas follow:

Behavior and Appearance

The patient's style of dress and hygiene, the appropriateness of gestures and facial expression, ability to relax and relate to persons and things in the environment and the patient's attentiveness to the nurse can all provide clues about a person's mental status. The posture a person assumes and the quality and quantity of speech also provide significant clues. For example, is the patient's posture tense, slumped, or relaxed? Does the patient speak quickly, loudly, clearly, coherently? Speech is a complex act involving the tongue, mouth, palate, larynx, respiratory system, and the cerebrum and cerebellum. Thus, disturbances of speech may or may not relate to the nervous system.

In newborns and infants the overall appearance, activity, alertness, and the cry need to be assessed. Some postural deviations such as marked hyperextension of the head, continual turning of the head to

one side, stiffness of the neck, or extension of the extremities can indicate severe intracranial problems.

Consciousness

The state of consciousness or level of alertness is often determined at the beginning of the physical examination. It varies from a state of hyperalertness to alertness, drowsiness, stupor, and coma. These levels are assessed by describing the patient's response to various verbal and physical stimuli (see "Stages of Consciousness," Table 34-1).

Emotional State

Evaluation of the emotional state, mood, or affect is made by observation and by questioning. Appropriate or inappropriate responses throughout the interview can be observed. For example, being overly cheerful in response to bad news, laughing while discussing a serious topic, or crying when talking about a pleasant topic are suggestive of inappropriate affect. The patient's approachability and openness should be noted. Is the patient overly active (euphoric, agitated, or hostile) or underactive, (flat or unresponsive)?

Questioning the patient about mood may also be necessary. Asking about how well the patient sleeps at night or if the patient gets discouraged and feels down or cries frequently can help to determine whether the patient is depressed. Other questions then may determine the depth of a depression. For example, ask whether the patient ever feels life is not worth living or whether things are getting too bad for the patient to cope. Affirmative answers to these questions warrant other questions such as, "Have you ever thought of killing yourself or tried to kill yourself?" and "How did you do it or how do you plan to do it?" By gradually leading up to questions of suicide the depth of a depression can be estimated.

Intellect

Intellectual or cognitive functions include the areas of orientation, memory, concentration, calculations, knowledge, judgment, and thought processes.

Orientation.   The patient's orientation to time, place, and person is determined by tactful questioning. These orientations are easily obtained by inquiring about the patient's place of residence (city and state), by inquiring about the time of the day, date of the month, day of the week, or duration of illness, and by asking the names of family members. More

297

direct questioning may be necessary for some people, such as, "Where are you now?" or "What day is it today?" or "What is your name?" These questions are readily accepted by most people when initially the nurse asks, "Do you get confused at times?"

Memory.   Three categories of memory are tested: immediate recall, recent memory, and remote memory. *Immediate recall* can be tested by having the person repeat a series of digits that have been given slowly, such as 7-4-3-5-6-7-2. Most people readily recall the seven digits. *Recent memory* refers to the events that occurred in the same day, such as how the patient got to the clinic. This information should be validated against other sources, however. A series of words can also be given early in the interview, such as an address, and then the patient can be asked to recall it. *Remote memory* refers to events that occurred several years in the past such as an anniversary, birthday, or surgical procedure.

Concentration and Calculation.   The ability to concentrate or attention span can be tested by asking the patient to repeat a series of digits forward and backward. Normally most adults are able to recall correctly five to eight digits forward and four to six digits backwards. The use of consecutive digits or those that form easily recognized dates such as 1980 should be avoided in this test. Concentration can also be tested by other tests of varying difficulty. Some of these include reciting the alphabet or counting backward from 100.

The ability to calculate can be tested by having the patient subtract a seven or a three progressively from 100, that is, 100, 93, 86, 79, or 100, 97, 94, 91. This standard test is often referred to as the *serial sevens* or *serial threes* test. Normally one adult can complete the serial sevens test in about one and one-half minutes with three or fewer errors. Because calculating ability is affected by educational level and by language or cultural differences, this test may be too difficult for some. These patients can be asked to add or to subtract small numbers.

Knowledge.   The knowledge or the information a person has is also influenced by cultural background and education. In addition, it is closely related to memory. A series of questions may be asked, such as "What are the five largest cities in America?" "When are potatoes planted?" or "What are the four seasons of the year?" Vocabulary can also be assessed by asking the patient the meaning of various words such as *extract, imitate, microscope,* and *multiple.*

Judgment.   To test judgment the questions need to be relatively simple and take into consideration the person's cultural background. Direct questions can be asked about what a person would do in certain situations such as being stopped for failing to stop at a stop sign, or after breaking a piece of borrowed equipment. Another test is to have the person pick out a word in a series that does not relate to the other two. For example: large, small, and red, or up, left, and down.

Thought Processes.   The relevance and organization of thought processes is noted throughout the history the patient describes. The patient may reveal bizarre behavior in which the patient appears to be looking or listening to stimuli undetected by you. In this situation it is necessary to ask additional questions in order to determine whether the patient is hallucinating or having illusions or delusions.

Some patients have insight or recognize that they see or hear things or are aware that their delusions are not justified. Others do not reveal insight, and the examiner can ask whether the patient actually believes the delusions or ever questions the reality of the hallucinations. These questions can arouse anger and elicit responses about whether you think the patient is crazy. It is important in these situations to acknowledge truthfully that you find some responses unusual, but avoid telling the patient that he or she is normal or abnormal until it can be verified.

The Cerebellum

The center for balance and muscle coordination is in the cerebellum. There are many tests that can be used to assess normal functioning of this center. A few are outlined below.

Coordination Tests

These tests are familiar to most and are referred to as the finger-to-nose test, the alternating motion test, and the heel-to-shin test. For the *finger-to-nose test* the patient is asked to abduct and extend the arms at shoulder height and to rapidly touch the nose alternately with one index finger and then the other. The test is repeated with the eyes closed if the test is first performed easily. In abnormal responses the patient will miss the nose and may bring the finger beyond the nose (past-pointing).

Alternating motions are coordinated by the normal person but are slow and incorrect in persons with cerebellar dysfunction. For this test the patient can be asked to rub his abdomen in a circular fashion with one hand while patting the top of the head with the other hand. Another way of examining alternating motion is to have the patient tap the floor with the toes and at the same time rapidly promote and supinate the hands.

The *heel-to-shin test* is carried out while the patient is lying in a supine position on the examining table. The patient is asked to rapidly move the right heel down the shin bone to the ankle of the opposite leg. The test is repeated for the left heel and the right leg.

Balance Tests

Balance or equilibrium tests are conducted while the patient walks or stands. Abnormalities of gait such as a staggering or unsteady gait not unlike that seen in intoxicated people should be noted. When the patient is standing with the eyes open and the feet together, disequilibrium of stance or posture can be observed. If the patient does not lose balance or does not begin to fall with eyes open, the test is repeated with the eyes closed. It is important to be prepared to assist patients should they begin to fall. The test conducted with the eyes closed is referred to as *Romberg's sign.* If disequilibrium is noted, the Romberg test is recorded as positive.

The Sensory System

The sensory functions include those of touch, pain, vibration, position, temperature, and discrimination. The first three are routinely tested in a few locations. Generally the face, arms, legs, hands, and feet are tested for touch and pain, although all parts of the body can be tested. For any areas that the patient states are numb or where peculiar sensations occur or paralysis exists, sensation should be checked more carefully over flexor and extensor surfaces of limbs. Abnormality of touch or pain should then be mapped out clearly by examining responses in the area about every 2 cm or one inch. This is a lengthy procedure. A more detailed neurologic examination includes position sense, temperature sense, and discrimination.

Superficial Touch

The sensation of touch is tested with a wisp of cotton. Because sensitivity to touch varies normally with specific skin areas, it is important to compare the sensa-

tion in symmetrical areas of the body such as the cheeks. The patient is asked to close the eyes and to respond whenever the cotton touches the skin.

Pain

By using the point and the blunt end of a safety pin the sharpness or dullness of pain can be tested. Again the patient is asked to close the eyes and to respond to which end of the safety pin is touching. Areas of reduced or heightened sensations should be noted, although responses can be somewhat subjective and difficult to assess. Where deficits to pain exist, the temperature sense is usually also impaired, since distribution of these nerves over the body is similar. Thus testing the temperature may prove more reliable. Distal and proximal areas should be compared.

Vibration

The vibratory sense is tested by the use of a tuning fork, which is held firmly against a bone. Bones commonly used are at the thumb side of the wrist, the outside of the elbow, the ankle on either side, or the knee. Routinely the distal bones of an extremity are tested first, and then if some impairment is noted the more proximal bones are also tested. Other bones may also be checked such as the sternum or the iliac crests.

To perform the vibratory test, a tuning fork is struck fairly hard and held against the patient's chin. He can then feel the vibration or buzz. Then the wrists and ankles are tested while the patient states whether the buzz can be felt. The patient is asked also to state when the buzz stops. This test can be compared to your own response. If there is any doubt about the patient's reliability to differentiate between the buzz from the vibration and the pressure of the tuning fork, the tuning fork can be struck but placed on the patient after you stop the vibration.

Position

Testing the sense of position is conducted when the patient has the eyes closed. Commonly the middle fingers and the large toes are tested. To test the fingers, the arm is supported and the palm held in the palm of your free hand. To test the toes the heels must be supported on the examining table.

It is important for the examiner to grasp the finger or toe on either side firmly between the thumb and index finger and to exert the same pressure while moving the part. The finger or toe is then moved up, down, and straight out and the patient is asked to respond with the appropriate "Up," "Down," or "Straight" position. A series of brisk up-and-down movements can also be done until suddenly the toe or finger is stopped in one of the three positions. Normal persons can easily determine the position of their fingers and toes.

Temperature

Temperature sense is determined by touching the skin with test tubes filled with hot and cold water. The patient then identifies which one feels hot or cold. If the pain sensation test is normal, it is not necessary to conduct this test.

Discrimination

The ability to discriminate can be tested in several ways. One way is to have the patient discriminate between one- and two-point stimuli. The skin is stimulated alternately with two pins simultaneously and then one pin. Since the fingertips are particularly sensitive, the normal person can differentiate between a one- and two-point stimulus within 2–3 mm, while on the chest differentiation occurs at about 75 mm apart.

Another test for discrimination assesses the ability to recognize objects by touching them. This ability is referred to as *stereognosis*. Familiar objects such as a key, paper clip, or coin are placed in a person's hand and the patient asked to identify them. If the patient has a motor impairment of the hand and is unable to voluntarily manipulate an object, the examiner can write a number or letter on the patient's palm and then ask for identification.

Two other tests of discrimination are referred to as *point localization* and *the extinction phenomenon*. The former involves having the patient close the eyes and stimulating a point on the skin with a pin. The patient is then asked with her eyes opened to point to the place touched. The latter (extinction phenomenon) involves the simultaneous stimulation of two corresponding symmetrical areas of the body such as the thighs, the cheeks, or the hands. Normally both points of stimulus are felt.

The Motor System

The motor system is assessed by determining the function of the voluntary skeletal muscles. This includes tonus, size, strength, and any involuntary movements.

Tonus

Normally the muscles feel firm and are maintained in a state of slight contraction, that is, they have a normal tone. This tone is maintained by the central nervous system acting through the peripheral nerves. When muscle tone is lacking, the muscles become relaxed, flabby, and weak, and eventually they atrophy, resulting in what is referred to as a *flaccid paralysis*. Involuntary movements such as a localized twitching are often associated with atrophy and flaccidity. These are referred to as *fibrillations* or *fasciculations*. Normal persons also experience fibrillations periodically such as the quivering of an arm or the twitching of an eyelid.

Rigidity and *spastic paralysis* refer to muscles that have increased tone; the latter is more severe. The muscles feel firmer and harder than normal. A spastic muscle is difficult to move, springing back sometimes when the examiner lets go of the muscle. A rigid muscle usually offers increased resistance but can be moved relatively easily by the nurse. Sometimes a cogwheel rigidity occurs. This means that the muscle vacillates between periods of increased tone and normal tone.

When assessing muscle tone, the nurse can palpate muscles for firmness and in addition note any restrictions in active movement. Various joints of the body can also be passively moved through their ranges of motion. For example, to test the arm muscles, the wrist is firmly grasped with one hand while the arm is bent and straightened at the elbow with the other hand. Slight resistance to movement is normal. This procedure is repeated for other joints such as the fingers, wrist, shoulder, knee, or ankle.

Muscle Size

Slight asymmetry in muscle size can be normal. Any deviations in symmetry of one muscle group as contrasted to the same group on the opposite side should be noted. These should be observed in the assessment of the neck and extremities.

Muscle Strength

Muscle power can be tested against the examiner's resistance or against gravity. The former is commonly used. By having the patient move each joint in every direction the nurse can oppose the motions with his or her hands. For example, ask the patient to extend the wrist while you oppose this movement. Muscle strength varies among individuals, for example, between an elderly woman and a young athlete. Therefore, judgment by the examiner is required in determining relative weakness. Both extensor and flexor muscle groups should be checked as warranted. See Chapter 23 for normal range of joint movements.

Involuntary Movements

Abnormal muscle movements can be readily observed in adults. Some terms used to describe abnormal movements are *fasciculation, tics, tremors,* and *athetosis.* Fasciculations have been previously described. Tics are also twitching of muscles but are repetitive and often occur in the face or upper trunk. Tremors are involuntary rhythmic movements, some of which may become noticeably more pronounced on movement or activity, others at rest. The former is referred to as an *intention tremor,* the latter as a *resting tremor. Athetosis* refers to involuntary twisting and writhing movements such as occur in cerebral palsy.

SUMMARY

I.   Height and weight

   A.   Average heights by age

      1.   Newborns: about 50 cm (20 inches)

      2.   One year: about 70 cm (28.5 inches)

      3.   Preschool years: add 5–6 cm (2–2.5 inches) for each year

      4.   Six years: about 115 cm (46 inches)

      5.   Adolescence

         a.   Maximum height for boys at about 18 years

         b.   Maximum height for girls at about 15 years

      6.   Elderly: decrease in height due to atrophy of intervertebral discs

   B.   Average weights by age

      1.   Newborns: 2.7–3.8 kg (6.0–8.5 lb)

      2.   Six months: double the birth weight

      3.   One year: 5.4 kg (12 lb)

      4.   Two years: double the first-year weight

      5.   Three years: 15 kg (33 lb)

      6.   Five years: about 20 kg (45 lb)

      7.   School-age years: add 3.2 kg (7 lb) per year

II.   Skin

   A.   Skin color

      1.   Pallor

      2.   Flushing

      3.   Jaundice

      4.   Cyanosis

   B.   Skin texture

      1.   Turgor

      2.   Dryness, flaking, excessive moisture, or wrinkling

   C.   Skin temperature

   D.   Skin lesions: Note distribution, location, size, contour, and consistency

      1.   Macules

      2.   Papules

      3.   Nodules

      4.   Tumors

      5.   Cysts

      6.   Wheals

      7.   Vesicles

III.   Nails: Note Beau's lines and clubbing

IV.   Head and neck

   A.   The head

      1.   Measurement of skull circumference

         a.   The greatest diameter above the eyes to the occipital protuberance is measured

         b.   Measurements are taken until the age of two years

c. Newborn average circumference is 35 cm (14 inches)

d. Normocephaly relates to chest circumferences

(1) At birth the head circumference is larger

(2) At 9 to 10 months the head and chest circumferences are the same

(3) After one year chest circumferences are larger

e. Abnormalities of head circumference are macrocephaly and microcephaly

2. Observation of skull shape and fontanelles

a. Newborn skulls are misshapen

b. By one week of age symmetry is regained

c. Six fontanelles are present at birth

d. At birth the posterior fontanelle may not be palpated

e. The anterior fontanelle increases in size for several months

f. The anterior fontanelle closes between 10 and 18 months

3. Observation of the scalp: Note hair condition, scaliness, and infections

B. The neck

1. Range of motion

2. Head control of infants

3. Palpation of lymph nodes

4. Voice changes

5. Size of the thyroid

V. The eyes

A. External structures

1. Eyelash follicles for styes

2. Eyelids for discoloration, edema, lesions, ectropion, and entropion

3. Eyeballs for sunkenness or exophthalmos or excessive pressure by tonometry

4. Conjunctivae for inflammation

5. Sclera for discolorations

6. Cornea and iris for irregularities and abrasions

7. Pupils for reaction

B. Fundus of the eye by ophthalmoscope: Proper visualization requires the use of a mydriatic.

1. The retina

a. The optic disc (normally flat, round, and white or grayish in color)

b. The blood vessels (arterioles appear red, while venules appear reddish-purple)

c. The macula (normally yellow)

2. The lens and chamber

a. Opacity

b. Bleeding

C. Visual acuity is assessed by use of Snellen charts

D. Eye movements are normally synchronous in all directions

VI. The ears

A. External structures

1. Visually note the presence of skin lesions, pus, or blood

2. With the use of an otoscope note:

a. Excessive cerumen in the ear canal

b. The tympanic membrane (normally light gray and translucent)

B. Hearing Acuity

VII. The nose

A. External structures

1. Observe encrustations or discharges

2. Observe symmetry

B. Internal structures by a flashlight or otoscope

1. Observe the color of the mucous membrane

2. Observe the position of the nasal septum

3. Observe the patency of the nasal passages

VIII. The mouth and pharynx

   A. The mouth

      1. The color, moisture, and character of the lips

      2. The status of the oral mucous membrane

      3. The condition of the teeth and gums

      4. The presence of malodor

      5. The tongue movement and appearance

   B. The pharynx

      1. The condition of the mucous membranes

      2. The position of the uvula

      3. The appearance of the tonsils

IX. The chest

   A. The thorax and lungs

      1. The state of posture

      2. The chest shape and symmetry in accordance with age variations

      3. The symmetry of expansion by palpation

      4. The lung percussion sounds

      5. The location of the heart and liver by percussion

      6. The lung sounds by auscultation

      7. The excursion of the diaphragm by percussion

   B. The heart

      1. Heart size and location by percussion

      2. Heart sounds by auscultation over specific valve areas

      3. The presence of cardiac murmurs

   C. The breasts

      1. Symmetry of size, shape and positions (asymmetry is not unusual in adolescence)

2. The presence of abnormal discharges

3. Palpation for tumors

   D. The axillae: Palpation for enlarged lymph nodes

X. The abdomen

   A. The external appearance

      1. Observation for skin rashes, lesions, scars, and edema

      2. Observation for localized swellings or generalized protuberances

      3. Observations for contractions during labor or peristalsis during acute bowel obstructions

      4. Auscultation for bowel sounds, vascular bruits, and fetal heart sounds

      5. Palpations to detect tenderness, masses, and the position of the liver and spleen

      6. Percussion to determine the presence of gas, fluid, and/or masses

XI. The genitals and rectum

   A. The genitals

      1. Observation for patency of the urinary meatus in newborns

      2. Palpation of the scrotum to check for descent of testes in newborns and boys

      3. Observation for abnormal vaginal discharge

      4. Observation for imperforate anus prior to rectal temperature assessment in newborns

      5. Papanicolaou smear in mature females

      6. Inspections for veneral disease for all adults

      7. Pelvic examination for females

      8. Palpation of scrotum for masses and swelling

      9. Palpation of inguinal canal for lymph node enlargement or hernia in males

   B. The rectum

      1. Inspection of the anus for protruding hemorrhoids or fissures

2. Palpation of anterior wall to assess the prostate gland or the cervix

3. Palpation of rectal walls for nodules or masses

XII. The extremities

1. Inspection of the skin for color and edema

2. Range of joint motions

3. Observation for muscle tremors

4. Observation for varicosities

5. Status of reflexes using a percussion hammer

   a. Biceps and triceps reflex

   b. Patellar reflex

   c. Achilles reflex

   d. Plantar reflex

XIII. Neurologic and mental-emotional assessment

1. Examination of the reflexes

2. Tests for cranial nerve function

3. Observations of mental status during history taking. Includes:

   a. Behavior and appearance

   b. Level of alertness

   c. Emotional state

   d. Intellect, including orientation, memory, concentration, calculations, knowledge, judgment, and thought processes

4. Coordination tests

   a. Finger-to-nose

   b. Alternating motion test

   c. Heel-to-shin test

5. Balance tests

6. Sensory function tests

   a. Superficial touch

   b. Pain

   c. Vibration

   d. Position

   e. Temperature

   f. Discrimination

7. Motor function tests

   a. Tonus

   b. Muscle size

   c. Muscle strength

   d. Observation of involuntary movements

SUGGESTED ACTIVITIES

1. In a laboratory setting, practice auscultation and percussion of a classmate's chest.

2. Choose a patient, and, using a stethoscope, assess lung and heart sounds.

3. Using an ophthalmoscope, examine the interior of a classmate's eyes. Make a diagram of your findings.

4. Visit a public health nurse in a school. Observe or note the assessment tests used in this setting.

5. Visit a nursing home. Select an elderly patient and assess his or her emotional and intellectual status.

SUGGESTED READINGS

Derbes, Vincent J. March 1978. Rashes: recognition and management. *Nursing 78* 8(3):54–59.

The author has updated his March 1973 article. He discusses rashes which nurses may encounter, how to recognize them, and the nurse's role in treatment.

McVan, Barbara, ed. April 1977. What the nose knows odors. *Nursing 77* 7(4):46–49.

This article includes the physiology of the sense of smell, different odors, and their sources. Deodorants are also discussed as well as measures to reduce body odors.

Sloboda, Sharon. September 1977. Understanding patient behavior. *Nursing 77* 7(9):74–77

A psychological assessment is described including self-concept, perception, stress, and loss. Listening attentatively, being objective, and using open-ended statements are advised.

SELECTED REFERENCES

Alexander, Mary M., and Brown, Marie Scott. Physical examination series parts 1 to 18. *Nursing '73, '74, '75, '76.*

Bates, Barbara. 1974. *A guide to physical examination.* Philadelphia: J. B. Lippincott Co.

Derbes, Vincent J. March 1973. Rashes: recognition and management. *Nursing '73* (3):44–49.

Hobson, Lawrence B. 1975. *Examination of the patient: a text for nursing and allied health personnel.* New York: McGraw-Hill Book Co.

Jarvis, Carolyn Mueller. May 1977. Perfecting physical assessment: Part 1. *Nursing 77* 7(5):28–37.

———. June 1977. Perfecting physical assessment: Part 2. *Nursing 77* 7(6):38–45.

———. July 1977. Perfecting physical assessment: Part 3. *Nursing 77* 7(7):44–53.

Kahn, Howard. October 1974. Visual dysfunctions. Some easy tests for detecting them in children. *Nursing 74* 4(10):26–27.

Macbryde, Cyril Mitchell, and Blacklow, Robert Stanley.

eds. 1970. *Signs and symptoms. Applied pathologic physiology and clinical interpretation,* 5th ed. Philadelphia: J. B. Lippincott Co.

McFarlane, Judith. December 1974. Pediatric assessment and intervention. Some simple how-to's for ambulatory settings. *Nursing 74* 4(12):66–68.

Murray, Ruth, and Zenter, Judith. 1975. *Nursing assessment and health promotion through the life span.* Englewood Cliffs, New Jersey: Prentice-Hall, Inc.

Roach, Lora B. November 1972. Color changes in dark skins. *Nursing '72* 2(11):19–22.

Sherman, Jacques L., and Fields, Sylvia Kleiman. 1976. *Guide to patient evaluation,* 2nd ed. Flushing, New York: Medical Examination Publishing Co., Inc.

Slessor, Gail. April 1973. Auscultation of the chest—a clinical nursing skill. *The Canadian Nurse* 69(4): 40–43.

CHAPTER 15

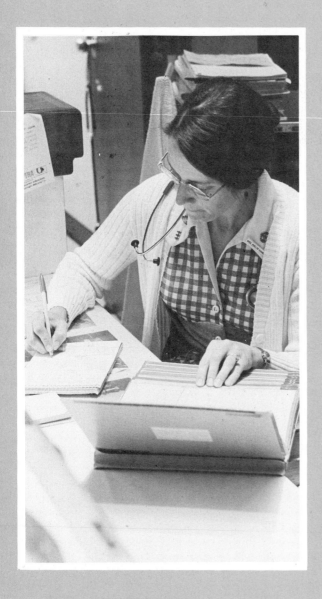

REASONS FOR RECORDS

THE PROBLEM-ORIENTED MEDICAL RECORD

Defined Data Base

Problem List

Plans

Progress Notes

TYPES OF PROGRESS RECORDING

RECORDING AND REPORTING

TRADITIONAL PATIENT RECORDS

The Kardex Record

GUIDELINES FOR RECORDING

LEGAL CONSIDERATIONS FOR RECORDING

Terms, Abbreviations, and Symbols

REPORTING

Guidelines for Reporting about Patients

OBJECTIVES

- Explain four purposes for communication about patients between health team members.

- Describe six purposes of the patient's record.

- Name four basic components of the Problem-Oriented Medical Record (POMR).

- Discuss the values of the four basic components of POMR for the patient and for involved health personnel.

- Describe the systematic format for writing SOAP progress notes.

- Discuss three kinds of progress notes related to POMR.

- Describe six parts of the traditional patient record.

- List the kinds of information included on the traditional patient record.

- Discuss the advantages of the Kardex record.

- Outline guidelines for the nurse when recording.

- Discuss some legal factors to consider when recording.

- Interpret commonly accepted terms, symbols, and abbreviations used in charting.

- Outline some guidelines for reporting about patients.

Reporting and recording are two methods of communication used extensively by health personnel. A *record* is written communication; a report is one type of verbal or written communication. Discussion is another type of verbal communication used by nurses and other members of the health team. A *discussion* is the verbal consideration of a specific subject by two or more persons, often resulting in a decision. To *report* is to give a verbal or written accounting to one or more people, such as when a nurse in a hospital finishes a shift and reports to others about the patients.

Communication between members of the health team is an important aspect of patient care. Accurate, complete communication serves several purposes:

1. It facilitates the coordination of care by several people.

2. It prevents the patient from having to repeat information to each health team member.

3. It assists in accuracy in the provision of care and hence the avoidance of error.

4. It helps health personnel make the best use of their time by preventing overlapping of activities.

REASONS FOR RECORDS

Written records have traditionally been considered an important aspect of care. All types of health agencies have written records, although the form of the record may vary considerably from place to place.

A patient's record or chart is a written record about health status and health care. It specifies the patient's individual health, the diagnostic and therapeutic measures that are employed, and the patient's response to these measures. The record is usually kept current while the patient is attending the health agency.

The patient's record has a number of purposes: communication, legal documentation, research, education, statistics, and audit.

Communication

The record serves as the vehicle by which different members of the health team communicate with each other. Although health team members will communicate verbally, the record serves as an efficient and effective method of communication. An accurate record can prevent errors such as duplication of a medication. It also allows health team members on different shifts to convey meaningful information about the patient to one another.

Legal Documentation

The patient's record is a legal document and is admissible in court as evidence. In some jurisdictions the record is considered inadmissible as evidence when the patient objects because of the confidentiality of the information given to the physician by the patient.

A record is usually considered to be the property of the agency, although increasingly it is believed that the patient upon request has a right to the information in the record (Berni and Readey 1974:17). The Patient's Bill of Rights supports this view (see Chapter 5). There have been legal decisions in California recognizing this right (Creighton 1975:309). Some agencies, however, do not permit the patient access to the record; thus the nurse needs to be guided by the policy of each particular agency.

Research

The information contained in a record can be a valuable source of data for research. By studying the treatment plans for a number of patients with the same illness, information can be helpful in treating a particular patient.

A record made years previously may also assist members of the health team with a current problem. A patient's memory of an illness may limit the data the patient can provide, but a record of that illness will generally reveal accurate data perhaps forgotten by the patient. Records are also very important where experimental drugs and treatments are being used.

Statistics

Statistical information from patient records can also help an agency anticipate the future needs of people and plan for these. For example, the number of births or kinds of illnesses can be obtained from these records. Some statistics are required by law, such as the records of births and deaths, which are filed with a government agency and become a part of the local, national, and international statistics.

Education

Students in the various health disciplines can use patient records as tools in education. A record can frequently provide a comprehensive view of the patient, the illness, and the various kinds of assistance provided. In this context the records are used by nursing students, interns, dietitians, and people in most of the health disciplines.

Audit

The patient's record is used also to monitor the care that the patient is receiving and the related compe-

tencies of the people giving that care. Specifically, a nursing audit monitors the nursing care, and it is often a retrospective audit in that the care has already been given. This care is then measured against established standards.

The nursing audit, when carried out by other nurses, is sometimes referred to as the *peer review*. Many agencies have audit committees that monitor individual nurse practice. Audits are also carried out by outside groups in instances where approval and accreditation are being considered.

In nursing audits various aspects of the care are assessed: the data base, the identification of the health problems, the goals of the nursing intervention, the nursing interventions that were chosen, and the evaluation of the goal attainment. Included in this audit are skills of the nurse as well as the judgment and knowledge used in the provision of the care.

THE PROBLEM-ORIENTED MEDICAL RECORD

The *problem-oriented medical record* (POMR) or problem-oriented record (POR) is increasingly becoming the means of communicating information. It is also referred to as the *Weed system* after its originator, L. L. Weed. The Weed system provides a patient-centered problem-solving approach to care, one that all health disciplines contributing care to the patient can use together. The record first lists all of the patient's identified problems at a point in time and then relates the therapy plans for each identified problem. The system integrates the care given by all health-team members in contrast to the traditional patient record, which separated the medical problems, nursing problems, and others into different sections of the record.

The POR has the following basic components: (a) defined data base, (b) complete problem list, (c) initial plan for each identified problem, and (d) progress notes.

Defined Data Base

The *data base* consists of all the information known about the patient when the patient first enters the health-care agency. It includes the nursing history

and assessment, the physician's history, and the physical examination. To this are added social and family data from other sources such as the social worker, and baseline laboratory and radiographic data. Important in the data is the chief complaint of the patient. In most agencies a standardized form is used, which assists people to obtain a complete data base.

Problem List

This is a carefully drawn up list of the problems presented by the patient. Some of the problems will be obvious upon initial contact with the patient; others will be established as additional data are gathered.

The initial problem list is usually made by the physician or the person who assumes primary responsibility for the patient's care. Contributions are made subsequently by other members of the health team.

The problems list, to be complete, includes socioeconomic, demographic, psychologic, and physiologic problems. The list is attached to the front of the patient's record. Each problem is labeled and numbered so that it can be identified throughout the record. This list has been likened to an index or table

UNIVERSITY OF MARYLAND HOSPITAL

PATIENT'S PROBLEM SHEET

PROBLEM NUMBER	DATE OF ONSET	DATE PROBLEM RECORDED	ACTIVE PROBLEMS	INACTIVE/RESOLVED PROBLEMS	DATE RESOLVED
1	Aug. 31 1977	Sept. 1 1977	Suddenly Passed Out / Scalp Laceration		9/1/77 / 9/8/77
2	2 yrs. +	Sept. 2 1977	Diabetes Mellitus — Uncontrolled Long Standing Out of Control		Controlled 10/5/77
3	10 yrs.	Sept. 1 1977	Obesity	March, 1978	
4	Sept. or Oct. 1976	Sept. 1 1977	Pre Tibial Varicose Ulcers / Walked into furniture Sept. & Oct, 1976	Feb, 1978	Feb, 1978
5	1 yr. + or	Sept. 4 1977	Family Problems — Because "he is always sick"	Feb, 1978	Feb, 1978
6	Gradual Onset ?time	Sept. 4 1977	Impotence (complete)		April, 78
7	Nov. 24 1977	Nov. 25 1977	I "don't care" / I am "down in the dumps" / I cannot eat the way I want		April, 78
8	2 wks.	Jan. 3 1978	Toe Nails Get Sore Especially Rt. Big Toe	Feb 15, 1978	
9	June 10 1978	June 10 1978	Congestive Heart Failure. { Dyspnea / Leg Edema / Tender Abdomen	June 24, 1978	
10	3 days	June 10 1978	Cloudy Smokey Urine		
		Current	Summation of Patient's Problems as of July 15, 1978 (over)		

3020

Figure 15-1.   Sample patient's problem sheet. (Courtesy Medical Records Community of the Medical Board of The University of Maryland Hospital, Baltimore, Md.)

of contents (see Figure 15-1). Problems are also usually listed according to their status such as active or inactive.

If a problem is potential rather than actual, it is usually entered on the progress notes rather than on the problem list. Only when the problem actually becomes active is it added to the list.

Plans

The initial list of plans is made with reference to the active problems. Each plan has a number correspond-

ing to the related problem and has three parts: diagnostic workup, therapy, and patient education.

In the *diagnostic workup* the physician indicates what needs to be done first. This indication of priority helps with planning in that it can help prevent duplication and eliminate some distress for the patient, and it is often economical in terms of time and money. Included in the diagnostic workup may be plans to collect further data in order to establish a medical diagnosis or to assist in the therapeutic management of the patient.

The *therapy* aspect of the planning includes the physician's orders, of which drug therapy and specific treatments are often a part. The orders are also numbered according to the problem with which they deal. This type of organization presents to the reader (the nurse) considerable information about the plan, including the reason for a physician's specific order.

The *patient education* aspect of the plan will include the needs of the patient for skills that will assist in the management of the illness as well as the patient's needs for information in this regard.

Progress Notes

Progress notes are the fourth part of the POR. These notes are made by all members of the health team who are involved in a patient's care: nurse, occupational therapist, dietitian, physician, and social worker are examples.

There is a systematic format for writing progress notes known as *SOAP*, which stands for Subjective data, Objective data, Assessment, and Planning. Compiling *subjective data* would include reporting what the patient perceives, and the way the patient expresses it. Entering subjective data initially helps to see the patient as a person and to identify emotional responses such as anger or frustration and hence to use these more therapeutically (Woody and Mallison 1973:1173).

Objective data include the measurements such as the vital signs, observations made using the senses, laboratory and radiographic findings, as well as responses to other diagnostic and therapeutic measures such as medications.

The *assessment stage* is the one in which the observer makes interpretations and conclusions from the subjective and objective data. Again all team members need to make their assessments, using the knowledge in their possession.

In the traditional method of recording, nurses are not usually expected to draw conclusions and make interpretations. Thus for many nurses the assessment stage is a difficult one to learn. It involves the use of a knowledge base as well as logical thinking.

The fourth stage of SOAP, the *plan*, involves a revision of the initial plan. It may include the need for immediate change or for future changes. The plans include what the patient has been taught and what the patient has learned. The plans then have three major aspects to be considered: the educational, diagnostic, and therapeutic. In many settings there is only one narrative progress note for all health team members, thus encouraging communication and coordination. Each plan needs to be signed, dated, and timed by the person writing it.

TYPES OF PROGRESS RECORDING

Three kinds of progress notes are generally recognized: (a) narrative notes, (b) flow sheets, and (c) discharge notes.

Narrative Notes

These record the patient's progress on a day-to-day basis. They are keyed to the related patient problems and are filled out by all members of the health team who are involved. It may only be necessary to enter "as above" if there is no additional information to record.

Flow Sheets

These are used when a patient's progress needs to be recorded accurately in regard to specific or operative variables such as pulse, blood pressure, medications, or progress in learning a new skill. In these cases the

narrative notes would be too long, but the flow sheet, a graphic record, would reflect the patient's condition quickly. See Figure 15-2 for a "Nurses Activity Flow Sheet."

The time parameters for flow sheets can vary from minutes to months. In an intensive care unit of a hospital, a patient's blood pressure may be monitored by the minute, whereas in an ambulatory clinic, a patient's blood sugar may be recorded once a month. Once a problem on a flow sheet is resolved, a narrative note is written.

Discharge Notes

The discharge note may be written by the physician or another member of the health team, depending upon the health care agency. In a home visiting service or community clinic it may be done by the nurse. The discharge note refers to the problems identified

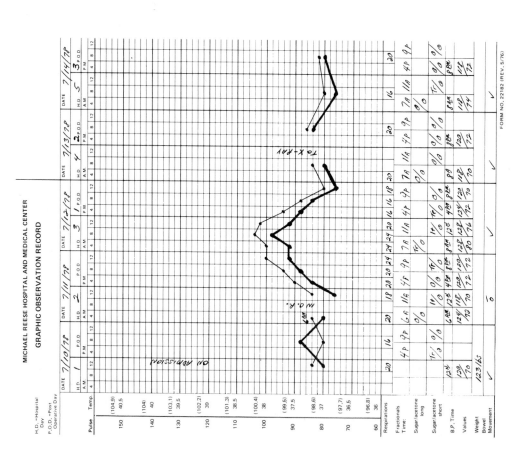

Figure 15-2. Sample graphic observation record. Normally the pulse is shown in red. We have widen the pulse line here so you can distinguish between the two lines. (Courtesy Michael Reese Hospital and Medical Center, Chicago, Ill.)

THE MONTREAL GENERAL HOSPITAL

NURSING DISCHARGE PROFILE
RESUME DU DOSSIER SOINS INFIRMIERS

SMITH, MRS. JANE

PATIENT'S LEVEL OF SELF CARE
HABITUDES QUOTIDIENNES DU PATIENT

	INDEP.	ASSIST(E)	DEPEND.	COMMENTS (COMMENTAIRES/PREFERENCES)
BATH/BAIN	✓			☐ BED BATH / BAIN AU LIT ☑ TUB BATH / BAIN: BAIGNOIRE ☑ SHOWER / DOUCHE
DRESSING/HABILLEMENT	✓			
FEEDING/ALIMENTATION	✓			
AMBULATION/DEPLACEMENT	✓			
STAIRS/ESCALIERS	✓			

NUTRITION/DIETE	BLADDER/VESICALE	BOWELS/INTESTINALE	VISION/VUE
☑ Regular/Régulière	☑ Normal	☑ Normal	☑ Adequate/Suffisante
☐ Diabetic/Diabétique	☐ Incontinent/Incontinence	☐ Incontinent/Incontinence	☐ Impaired/Déficiente
☐ Low Salt/Sel↓	☐ Frequency/Frequence	☐ Diarrhea/Diarrhée	☐ (R) Eye/Oeil droit
☐ Other/Autre AS TOLERATED	☐ Catheter/Sonde	☐ Constipation	☐ (L) Eye/Oeil gauche
	☐ Ostomy/Ostomie	☐ Aids/Moyens	☐ Glasses/Lunettes
			☐ Contact Lens/Verres de contact
HEARING/OUIE	SPEECH/EXPRESSION	LANGUAGE/LANGUE	
☑ Adequate/Suffisante	Difficulty/Difficultés	☑ Eng./Anglais ☑ Fr./Français	
☐ Impaired/Déficiente	☐ Yes/Oui ☑ No/Non	☐ Other/Autre	
☐ Aid/Appareil			

NURSING CONCERNS/PROBLEMES SOINS INFIRMIERS	NURSING APPROACH/APPROCHE SOINS INFIRMIERS
1) WOUND CARE (DRAIN SITE OOZING SMALL AMOUNT SEROUS FLUID)	CLEANSE WITH NORMAL SALINE DAILY. APPLY DRY DRESSING.
2) FATIGUE (TIRES EASILY, HAS FOUR YOUNG CHILDREN TO CARE FOR)	HOMEMAKER x 5 DAYS

ATTITUDES TO PLAN OF CARE/ATTITUDES ENVERS LE PLAN DE SOINS (PATIENT & FAMILY/MALADE & FAMILLE) ANXIOUS TO GO HOME. AWARE THAT SHE WILL NEED LOTS OF REST

TEACHING DONE/ENSEIGNEMENT FAIT UNDERSTANDS & HAS DEMONSTRATED WOUND CARE. KNOWS THAT SHE CAN CALL SOCIAL WORKER FOR EXTENSION OF HOMEMAKER SERVICES

RESOURCES/RESSOURCES (FAMILY/FAMILLE, COMMUNITY/COMMUNAUTE) HOMEMAKER x 5 DAYS. PARENTS LIVE NEARBY - CAN HELP WITH CHILDREN

DISCHARGE DIAGNOSIS/DIAGNOSTIC AU RENVOI DU MALADE CHOLECYSTECTOMY

MEDICATION RECEIVED DAY OF DISCHARGE/MEDICAMENTS RECUS LE JOUR DE RENVOI —

DATE OF DISCHARGE/JOUR DE RENVOI JULY 11/78 TIME/HEURE 10.30 TO/A HOME

FOLLOW-UP APPOINTMENTS/RENDEZ-VOUS JULY 26, 1978 - SURGICAL CLINIC

SIGNATURE (NURSE/INFIRMIER(E)) A. Carpenter, N. DATE July 11, 1978

NURSING DISCHARGE PROFILE

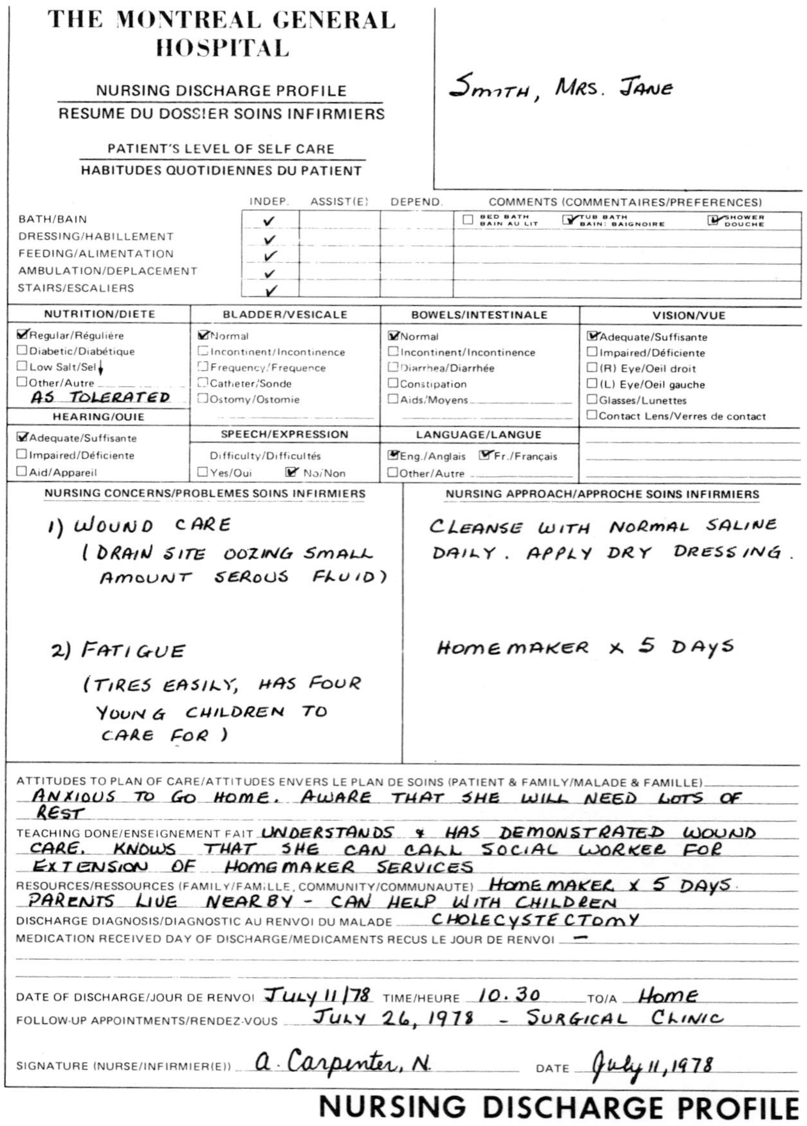

Figure 15-3. Sample nursing discharge profile. (Courtesy Montreal General Hospital, Montreal.)

earlier and describes the degree to which each problem has been resolved. If the patient has been referred to another agency, this is also noted.

Some agencies have a nursing discharge profile which contains significant information about the patient relevant upon discharge (see Figure 15-3).

TRADITIONAL PATIENT RECORDS

The traditional patient record is a source-oriented record, that is, each person or source has his or her own individual record. Information about a particular problem is therefore distributed throughout the record, and some problems that are identified at one time may or may not be followed up by other health team members. For example, a patient who has a fractured femur may have been taking dicumarol (an anticoagulant) at home; however, the physician may not be aware of this and thus deal only with the fracture.

Traditional patient charts generally have six parts: the admission sheet, the face sheet, the physician's order sheet, the history sheet, the nurses' notes, and other special reports and records.

The *admission sheet* is a part of the record in most agencies. It generally contains specific data about the patient, including an identification number. In hospitals most admission sheets contain the following information: the patient's full name, address, date of birth, name of attending physician, sex and marital status, nearest relative, occupation and employer, financial status for hospital payments, religious preference, date and hour of admission to the hospital, hospital unit or agency of admission, previous hospital admission or call, admitting diagnosis or problem, and identification number.

The *face sheet* is the front sheet of the chart. It has a number of uses, one of the most frequent of which is a list of the allergies presented by the patient.

The *doctor's order sheet* is a written record of the physician's orders. The physician is expected to write the date with the order and to sign each order or to sign once for several orders written at the same time. Often agencies have a method of flagging a patient's chart to indicate to the nurse that there is a new order.

When physicians phone in orders about a patient, these are written on the doctor's order sheet by the recipient of the order and signed by that person indicating a telephone order. Often the physician is expected to countersign the telephone order within 24 or 48 hours of giving the order.

The *history sheet* is a record of the patient's health history written by the physician. Often the physician

also uses this sheet to record progress notes on the patient and any future plans for the patient.

The *nurses' notes* are a record of the nursing intervention carried out by the nurse(s) as well as an assessment of the patient and evaluation of the effectiveness of the intervention. In summary, nurses' notes record the following kinds of information:

1. The assessment of the patient by various nursing personnel, for example, assessment of skin color or the aroma of urine.

2. Nursing intervention ordered by the physician such as medications or treatment.

3. Nursing intervention carried out in the nurses' judgment, for example, special skin care or health teaching.

4. Evaluation of the effectiveness of nursing intervention.

5. Specific measures carried out by the physician, for example, shortening a drain in an incision.

6. Visits by members of the health team such as a consulting physician.

Special reports and records also become a part of a patient's chart. These often include radiographic reports, laboratory findings, reports of surgery, and anesthesia records. Often nurses can obtain significant data from these reports that will contribute to a plan of nursing care. See Figure 15-4 for a sample.

The Kardex Record

The Kardex is a widely used, concise method of recording significant data about a patient, which is quickly accessible to members of the health team. The system is a series of cards, which are usually kept in a portable index file. The card for a particular patient can be quickly turned up to reveal significant data about the patient. Often Kardex data are written in pencil and changed frequently to be up to date (see Figure 15-5).

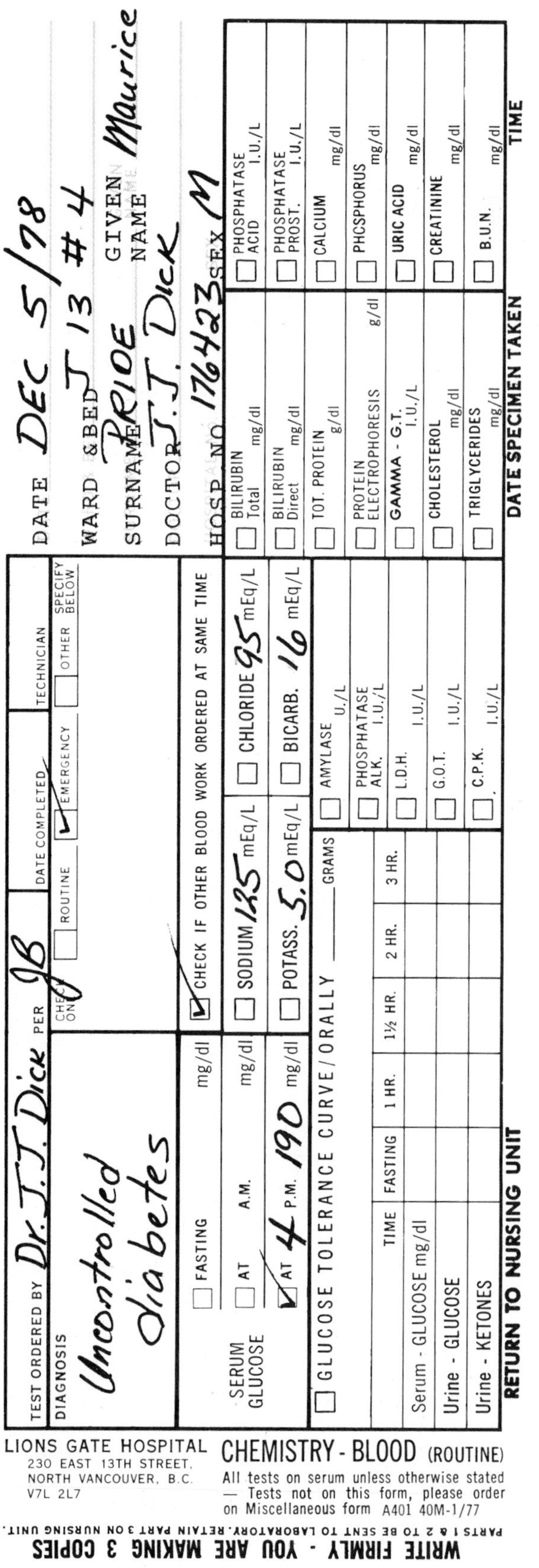

LIONS GATE HOSPITAL
230 EAST 13TH STREET,
NORTH VANCOUVER, B.C.
V7L 2L7

CHEMISTRY - BLOOD (ROUTINE)

All tests on serum unless otherwise stated — Tests not on this form, please order on Miscellaneous form A401 40M-1/77

TEST ORDERED BY Dr. J.J. Dick PER JB | DATE COMPLETED | TECHNICIAN

DIAGNOSIS Uncontrolled diabetes | CHECK ONE: ☐ ROUTINE ☑ EMERGENCY ☐ OTHER SPECIFY BELOW

DATE DEC 5/78
WARD & BED J 13 #4
SURNAME PRIDE GIVEN NAME Maurice
DOCTOR J.J. Dick
HOSP. NO 176423 SEX M

SERUM GLUCOSE: ☐ FASTING mg/dl; ☐ AT A.M. mg/dl; ☑ AT 4 P.M. 190 mg/dl

☑ CHECK IF OTHER BLOOD WORK ORDERED AT SAME TIME

☐ SODIUM 125 mEq/L ☐ CHLORIDE 95 mEq/L
☐ POTASS. 5.0 mEq/L ☐ BICARB. 16 mEq/L

☐ GLUCOSE TOLERANCE CURVE/ORALLY ______ GRAMS

TIME	FASTING	1 HR.	1½ HR.	2 HR.	3 HR.
Serum - GLUCOSE mg/dl					
Urine - GLUCOSE					
Urine - KETONES					

☐ AMYLASE U./L
☐ PHOSPHATASE ALK. I.U./L
☐ L.D.H. I.U./L
☐ G.O.T. I.U./L
☐ C.P.K. I.U./L

☐ BILIRUBIN Total mg/dl
☐ BILIRUBIN Direct mg/dl
☐ TOT. PROTEIN g/dl
☐ PROTEIN ELECTROPHORESIS g/dl
☐ GAMMA - G.T. I.U./L
☐ CHOLESTEROL mg/dl
☐ TRIGLYCERIDES mg/dl

☐ PHOSPHATASE ACID I.U./L
☐ PHOSPHATASE PROST. I.U./L
☐ CALCIUM mg/dl
☐ PHCSPHORUS mg/dl
☐ URIC ACID mg/dl
☐ CREATININE mg/dl
☐ B.U.N. mg/dl

RETURN TO NURSING UNIT | DATE SPECIMEN TAKEN | TIME

WRITE FIRMLY - YOU ARE MAKING 3 COPIES
PARTS 1 & 2 TO BE SENT TO LABORATORY. RETAIN PART 3 ON NURSING UNIT.

Figure 15-4. Sample laboratory report. (Courtesy Lions Gate Hospital, North Vancouver, B.C.)

Figure 15-5. Nursing Kardex information. (Courtesy Mount Saint Joseph's Hospital, Vancouver, B.C.)

X-MATCH

DATE	MEDICATIONS	TIME	DATE	I.V.'s
JULY 4	MYLANTA 15cc q.2.h.	06-0870 12-14-16		
"	HALDOL 1mgm. T.I.D.	08-14-20		
"	FROSST 292 -CRUSHED FOR PAIN	P.R.N.		
"	BIONETS TO SUCK	P.R.N.		
"	SLIDING SCALE TORONTO INSULIN			
	5% GIVE 12 UNITS.			
	3% " 10 "			
	2% " 8 "			
	2%-0 " 0 "			TREATMENTS/PROCEDURES
JULY 11	AZOGANTRISIN T̄ Q.I.D.	06-11 16-22	JULY 4 CLINITEST T.I.D ¥ H.S ~ 07-11 17-H.S.
			JULY 8 IRRIGATE FOLEY CATH. DAILY ⨍c NS
JULY 4 H.S. MED. DALMANE 30 mgm.		H.S.		
JULY 14 Amitriptyline (ELAVIL) 25 mgm		H.S		

NAME	ROOM	DOCTOR	015
FOO MUI SENG	306·A	T·Y· TUNG.	

DATE	No.	PROBLEM LIST	RESOLVED	DATE	OTHER RELEVANT DATA (Include x-rays and tests)
JULY 17	#1	PT. STILL VERY DEPRESSED			DATE OF BIRTH
	#2	L-SIDED WEAKNESS		JULY 17	CHEST PHYSIO.
	#3	COMMUNICATION PROBLEMS		JULY 14	BARIUM MEAL ✓

HEALTH CARE CONSULTANTS

DATE REVIEWED

DIET
☒ Regular CHINESE
☐ Soft
☐ Fluid
☐ Clear Fluid
☐ N.P.O.
☐ Other

FEEDING
☒ Self ⨍c SOME ASSISTANCE
☐ Assist

FLUIDS
☐ I. & O.
  Am't Daily
☐ I.V.
☐ Preferred Fluids

ELIMINATION
☐ B.R.
☒ Commode
☐ Ostomy
☐ Incontinent
☐ Condom
☐ Catheter
  Size #16 Date JULY 30cc BALOON
☐ Other Specify:

ACTIVITY
☐ Up ad lib
☐ B.R.P.
☐ Amb c asst
☐ Walker
☒ Chair T.I.D 08-12-16
☐ Dangle
☐ Bed rest

HYGIENE
☒ Self ⨍c SOME ASSISTANCE
☐ Partial
☐ Bed
☐ Tub
☐ Shower
☐ Mouth Care

SAFETY
Side Rails
☒ Constant
☐ Night Only
Other

PROSTHESIS
☐ Glasses
☐ Hearing Aid
☐ Dentures
☐ Other - Specify

V.S. FREQUENCY
☒ B.P. ⎰O.D
☒ T.P.R. ⎱@ 0800

☐ Other - Specify

SPECIAL CONSIDERATIONS:
Ⓛ-SIDED WEAKNESS

ALLERGIES

DISCHARGE AND REHAB. PLANS: DATE REVIEWED

DATE	PROBLEM AND SHORT TERM GOAL	APPROACH
JULY 17 #1	PT. WILL BE LESS DEPRESSED, PARTICIPATE MORE IN A.D.L.-↑ HER SELF-ESTEEM	① SHOW CARING BY BEING PATIENT AND UNDERSTANDING. ② BE CONSISTENT IN INVOLVING HER AS MUCH AS POSSIBLE IN A.D.L - AND PRAISE HER WHEN SHE ACCOMPLISHES THEM. ③ MAINTAIN A ROUTINE OF CARE ¥ EXPECT HER TO DO HER SHARE.
JULY 17 #2	PT. WILL BE ABLE TO PARTICIPATE AS MUCH AS POSS. IN A.D.L AND BE AWARE OF POSITIONING OF Ⓛ LIMBS	① ASSIST PT. WHENEVER NECESSARY ② EXPECT PARTICIPATION IN A.D.L. ③ KEEP PT. AWARE OF LEFT LIMB POSITIONS.
JULY 17 #3	PT. WILL UNDERSTAND PROCEDURES ETC.	① GET INTERPRETER WHEN NEC. ② SPEAK SLOWLY

Next of Kin: HUSBAND - FOO YUNG TOY   S.I.   Isolation:

Occupation: HOUSEWIFE   Surgery: JULY 4 - ESOPHAGOSCOPY.

Age	Religion	Mar. Status	Adm. Date	Diagnosis
61	NIL	M.	JUNE 21/78	① ACID INGESTION ② DIABETES ③ OLD Ⓛ C.V.A.

Name	Hosp. No.	Accom.	Doctor	016
FOO MUI SENG		Ⓦ P SP	T·Y· TUNG	

GUIDELINES FOR RECORDING

The following guidelines will assist the nurse in recording on the patient's chart in either recording system, the traditional or the problem-oriented.

1. *Brevity.* The recording needs to be brief, yet all pertinent data must be included. Extra words such as the patient's name and the word *patient* should be omitted. Reference to *patient* is not needed because it is obvious about whom the nurse is recording. Correct terms and acceptable abbreviations and symbols are to be used. See the appendix, "Terms, Abbreviations, and Symbols."

2. *Accuracy.* All data recorded must be accurate and specific. For example, the exact time that a patient takes a medication is charted, not the approximate time, that is, "1425 hours," not "about 1400 hours." It is also important that all pertinent information is included on the record, since the omission of significant data is also regarded as an inaccuracy.

3. *Legibility.* All recording must be legible to the reader. Recording is normally done in ink because pencil does not provide a permanent record. Print or script writing is acceptable. Correcting an error in charting is discussed subsequently in this chapter.

4. *Correct spelling.* Spelling is important in terms of accuracy. Two medications may have similar spelling, for example, Digoxin and Digitoxin, and yet be decidedly different drugs.

5. *Differentiating between observation and interpretation.* The nurse must relate observations of the patient accurately and indicate when an interpretation is made. For example, to state that a patient "is crying" is an observation, but to write that he is "depressed because of his illness" is an interpretation of the crying. If, on the other hand, the patient states that he is worried about his diagnosis, this should be quoted directly on the chart: "I am worried about my gut." Record what is seen and heard.

6. *Consecutive lines.* Recording is done chronologically and on consecutive lines. When a statement does not fill the entire line, a straight line is drawn through to the end of the line to prevent inserts. Capital letters are used to begin each thought, and periods are used to complete each thought, for example, "Is dyspneic on exertion." or, "Appetite is poor."

7. *Signature.* The nurse's signature must include the first initial, complete surname, and status, such as registered nurse, for example, "J. Brown, RN" The signature follows each entry of recording and is entered at the far right of the nurse's notes.

8. *Where and when to chart.* Information is recorded in accordance with agency policies. Some specific data are recorded on clinical flow sheets, such as vital signs, medications, or appetite. Any abnormal data recorded on these records are often then repeated on the nurse's notes with additional relevant details. All medications and treatments are recorded after administration to the patient rather than before. The time that is recorded is the time the treatment is performed, not the time that the recorder does the recording. In many agencies, the nurse makes an initial entry on the record indicating the nurse's tour of duty, for example, 0900 to 1600 hours. Subsequent recording then designates the specific time of data.

Frequency of recording is primarily dependent upon the patient's degree of illness and therapies administered. General guidelines include:

a. Record immediately after initial or other assessments such as when the patient is admitted to the agency or after transfer from the operating room, anesthetic recovery room, or other area.

b. Record analgesics immediately after administration.

c. Record immediately prior to leaving the patient for any extended period of time such as for lunch or coffee breaks, particularly for those patients whose condition is critical.

LEGAL CONSIDERATIONS FOR RECORDING

Reference has already been made to the use of the patient's record as evidence in a court of law. In recording there are a number of practices that need to be followed in regard to the legal status of the record. If a nurse makes an error in recording, a line is placed through the error and the correct material is added. In some settings the nurse also writes "error" and signs initials or name nearby. Erasures on a legal document can be cause for suspicion and are generally avoided.

The nurse is required to sign his or her *legal name*. This may or may not be the name the nurse uses in day-to-day life. Another precaution for nurses is to chart nursing intervention as a record of what has been done for the patient. However, in settings where problem-oriented recording is used, nursing intervention has been added to the progress notes (Creighton 1975:309).

It is also important that all health-team members use the abbreviations that are recognized and accepted by their particular agency; otherwise a particular abbreviation may mean one thing to one person and something else to another.

Problem-oriented charting has brought up the question of the legality of nursing practice and related charting. This has arisen from nurses' diagnosing and providing initial assistance (therapy) to patients in regard to their problems. Nurses are advised to consult the definitions of nursing in their respective states and provinces. It is important that nurses practice within these dimensions in order that their activities are considered legal.

Terms, Abbreviations, and Symbols

In most health agencies there are terms, abbreviations, and symbols that are considered acceptable and are understood by all members of the health team. These may differ somewhat from one agency to another, and often a hospital will have an official list to be used in recording.

In some specialty areas, terms, abbreviations, and symbols may also be used that are common only to that particular specialty. The student is advised to be familiar with the terms used in a particular agency before charting, writing, or interpreting reports. The student is referred to the Appendix for abbreviations, terms, and symbols in common use.

REPORTING

Reporting can be either verbal or written. Its purpose is generally to communicate specific information to a person or group of people. A report should be short and concise. It needs to include pertinent information but not extraneous detail.

Guidelines for Reporting about Patients

These guidelines can assist nurses in the preparation and presentation of reports about patients:

1. Start with the patient's name in order that the thinking of the listeners or readers can immediately relate the subsequent information to the particular patient. For example, "Ms. Jessie Jones has a reddened area on her left hip," *not* "There is a reddened area on the left hip of Ms. Jessie Jones."

2. Report only pertinent information; do not include other data that are not relevant for the patient care.

3. Provide exact information, such as "Ms. Jessie Jones received Demerol 100 mg intramuscularly at 2000 hours (8 PM)," *not* "Ms. Jessie Jones received some Demerol during the evening."

4. When reporting about a series of patients, follow a particular order, for example, by room number in a hospital or by time of appointment in a community clinic.

5. When reporting about one patient, select the pertinent information in order of: assessment, planning, intervention, and evaluation. For example, "Mr. Ronald Oakes states he has an aching pain in his left calf. Inspection revealed no other signs. Rest and elevation of his legs on a footstool provided relief."

SUMMARY

Accurate communication about patients between health-team members is important in facilitating coordination of patient care and accuracy in providing care. Patients are ensured that all health-team members are informed about their needs and that overlapping of activities is avoided.

Written records about patients serve several purposes. Communication that is written ensures transmission of information about patients between all health workers involved. Research, educational, and statistical data are also obtainable from records. In addition, patient care standards can be audited. The patient's record is also admissible as evidence in a court of law.

The POMR (Weed system) is increasingly recognized as a method that provides a patient-centered problem-solving approach to care. All health disciplines cooperate in recording the patient's problems, plans of therapy, and progress in response to the planned therapies on integrated records. The POMR includes four basic components: a defined data base, a complete labeled problem list, an initial plan for each identified active problem, and progress notes. The defined data base incorporates the physician's and nurse's initial assessment as well as those of other health workers. The problem list includes both active and inactive physiologic, psychologic, socioeconomic, and demographic problems. Initial plans include a diagnostic workup, therapy, and patient education. Progress notes incorporate the systematic format of SOAP and involve narrative notes, flow sheets, and discharge notes.

Traditional patient records are source-oriented records in that each health worker has separate records. This kind of record generally includes six parts: the admission sheet, the face sheet, the doctor's order sheet, the physician's history sheet, the nurses' notes, and other special records such as the laboratory record. The Kardex record is widely used as a quick accessible method of current data about patients.

Guidelines for recording include explanations about brevity, accuracy, legibility, chronology, use of consecutive lines, signatures, and where and when to chart. The potential use of the record as a legal document makes accuracy in recording, the use of legal names, and the use of acceptable terms and abbreviations important. Many commonly accepted abbreviations, terms, and symbols are listed alphabetically in the Appendix.

Reports about patients need to be concise and pertinent. Guidelines are included.

SUGGESTED ACTIVITIES

1. Review a traditional patient record, and note the information that is included.

2. Review a problem-oriented record, and compare it with the traditional patient record. Be specific in regard to the content and method of recording.

3. Establish a problem-oriented record for a member of your class who conveys to you a specific health problem.

4. Select a patient, and over a five-day period record the progress notes using the SOAP format.

SUGGESTED READINGS

Kerr, Avice H. February 1975. Nurses' Notes "That's where the goodies are!" *Nursing 75* 5(2):34–41.

This article explains the importance of nurse's notes and provides guides for the nurse in charting. The use of the chart as a means to improve nursing care is indicated throughout the article.

Lambert, Kathryn. 1974. Basic principles of the problem-oriented system. In *The problem-oriented system—a multi-disciplinary approach.* 1974. Pub. No. 20-1546. New York: National League for Nursing.

The POR can be adapted to a variety of settings. Information is provided about the data base, problem list, initial plan, and progress notes (plan of action). Examples of the various records are provided.

SELECTED REFERENCES

Abruzzese, Roberta S. 1974. The nursing process and the problem-oriented system. In *The problem-oriented system—a multi-disciplinary approach.* 1974. Pub. No. 20-1546. New York: National League for Nursing.

Ansley, Betty. August 1975. Patient-oriented recording: a better system for ambulatory settings. *Nursing 75* 5(8):52–53.

Berni, Rosemarian, and Readey, Helen. 1974. *Problem-oriented medical record implementation.* St. Louis: The C. V. Mosby Co.

Bloom, Judith T., et al. November 1971. Problem-oriented charting. *American Journal of Nursing* 71:2144–2148.

Creighton, Helen. 1975. *Law every nurse should know,* 3rd ed. Philadelphia: W. B. Saunders Co.

Larkin, Patricia Dubbert, and Backer, Barbara A. 1977. *Problem-oriented nursing assessment.* New York: McGraw-Hill Book Co.

Weed, Lawrence L. 1971. *Medical records, medical education and patient care: the problem-oriented record as a basic tool.* Cleveland: Case Western Reserve University Press.

Woody, Mary, and Mallison, Mary. July 1973. The problem-oriented system for patient-centered care. *American Journal of Nursing* 73:1168–1175.

Woolley, F. Ross, et al. 1974. *Problem-oriented nursing.* New York: Springer Publishing Co., Inc.

CHAPTER 16

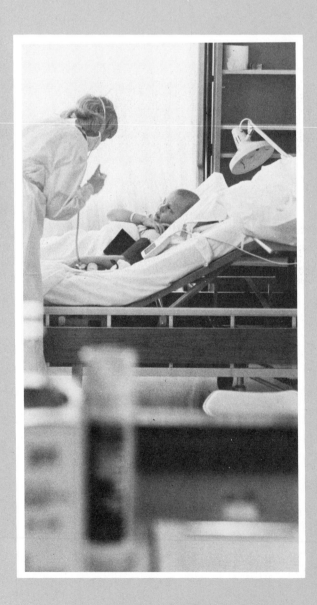

INFECTION CONTROL: MEDICAL ASEPSIS

OBJECTIVES

- Explain medical asepsis and surgical asepsis.

- Define terms used in relation to infection.

- Describe the chain of infection.

- Discuss the various factors that affect a person's susceptibility.

- Identify common sources of infection.

- Describe the course of an infection.

- Identify the symptoms of an infection.

- Explain the types of isolation precautions and the characteristics of each.

- Provide isolation precautions while carrying out nursing functions.

Microorganisms are always present in the environment. Some live on the skin, others are common inhabitants of the intestinal tract, and others are found, among other places, in the air, in the soil, and on our clothes. Most of these microorganisms do not produce disease; those which do are called *pathogens*. The control of the spread of pathogens and the protection of people from the acquisition of infectious diseases are practiced on four levels: international, national, community, and individual.

On the international level, there are regulations regarding the kinds of protection people must have against certain diseases before they can visit a specific country and regulations about the protection needed for American and Canadian citizens returning to their own country.

Nationally there are regulations such as those regarding the interstate and interprovincial transportation of food. These are designed to protect people from receiving contaminated food. There are also regulations regarding pollution of water, air, and, in fact, the entire environment, a subject which is currently receiving a great deal of publicity.

On a community level there are regulations regarding the disposal of sewage and the purity of drinking water, for example, all of which are designed to protect people from disease.

Protection from disease is also very much an individual responsibility. Not only are hygienic practices relevant, such as oral hygiene as a preventive measure for periodontal disease (see Chapter 20, "Personal Hygiene"), but there is also individual responsibility regarding diet and exercise.

An *infection* is the invasion of the body of a person by pathogenic organisms that multiply and overcome the flora normally present and the subsequent physiologic reaction of the body to these organisms. If this infection can be passed on readily to others, such as smallpox or typhoid fever, it is referred to as a *communicable disease*.

Trauma is injury to the body. It can refer not only to physical trauma, such as a cut by a piece of glass, but it also includes injury caused by invading microorganisms. Thus an infectious process can be described as trauma. Sometimes a cut can serve as the place of entry for microorganisms.

Etiology is the study of specific causes; in the case of an infection it is the identification of the invading microorganism. It may be a virus such as the chickenpox virus or a bacteria such as *Staphylococcus aureus*.

ASEPSIS

Asepsis refers to the absence of all disease-producing microorganisms. When hands are washed with a disinfectant, they can be considered to be aseptic; that is, any disease-producing microorganisms have been destroyed. *Sterilization* is the absence of *all* forms of microorganisms: bacteria, viruses, spores, and fungi. Unlike the skin, articles such as forceps can be sterilized, thus destroying all microorganisms.

There are two types of asepsis with which nurses need to be familiar: medical asepsis and surgical asepsis. *Medical asepsis* (clean technique) is concerned with limiting the spread of microorganisms. It includes those practices which are intended to confine a specific microorganism to a specific area. For example, a child at home who has measles is kept in bed in the child's room and is not permitted to have direct contact with brothers and sisters. The measles virus is thus confined to the child's room.

Surgical asepsis (sterile technique), on the other hand, refers to keeping microorganisms from a specific area. For example, after an operation, a patient's incision is cleansed and dressed using surgical aseptic technique in order that microorganisms are unable to gain entrance to the body through the incision.

THE CHAIN OF INFECTION

Six factors or elements are involved in the infectious process:

1. The etiologic agent or pathogen.
2. The source of the pathogen or the reservoir.
3. The exit or method of escape of the pathogen from the source.
4. The method of transmission or the vehicle.
5. The portal or method of entry.

6. The susceptibility of the person (the host) to the pathogen.

The Etiologic Agent

Microorganisms and parasites are the sources of infection. A *parasite* is an animal or plant that lives in or on another and obtains its nourishment from it. Some microorganisms, such as the gonococcus bacillus, are parasites. There are five general categories of microorganisms concerned with infection: protozoa, fungi, bacteria, rickettsiae, and viruses. The extent to which any microorganism is capable of producing a disease depends upon a number of factors such as:

1. The number of organisms.
2. The virulence and potency of the organisms.
3. The source of the organisms.
4. Their ability to enter the body.
5. Their ability to establish themselves within the body.

Some microorganisms such as the smallpox virus have the ability to infect almost anyone upon first contact. On the other hand, other microorganisms such as the tuberculosis bacillus attack a relatively small number of the population, often people who are poorly nourished and living in unsanitary conditions. Some animals and humans are *carriers*, that is, they carry pathogenic organisms in their bodies although they are not ill themselves. They can pass the pathogen along to other people. An example are persons who harbor the typhoid bacillus in the gallbladder, thus excreting it in feces, but do not manifest any symptoms of the disease themselves.

Some bacteria form spores; that is, they can assume a round or oval form with a tough resistant capsule. They assume this form in response to adverse conditions, and as such they are difficult to destroy.

Sources and Source Characteristics

There are many sources or reservoirs of pathogens. They may be other humans, plants, animals, or the environment generally. Quite commonly people serve as the source of infection for others. The person who has a virus such as the influenza virus may frequently spread this infection to others. Sometimes people carry a pathogen themselves and yet are not ill. Only when other conditions such as fatigue are present does an infection emerge.

Commonly animals and birds can be the sources of infection. The *Anopheles* mosquito is known to serve as the source of the malaria parasite. Food, water, milk, and feces also can be reservoirs for pathogens, for example, contaminated chicken at a club luncheon.

The reservoir for a pathogen must have certain characteristics so that the organisms can live and grow. Some of these follow.

Food

All living microorganisms require nourishment of one sort or another. Some require organic matter, whereas others can make use of carbon dioxide and simple inorganic compounds.

Water

Most living organisms require water, although their needs vary widely. For example, in the spore form some bacteria can live without water for years.

Oxygen

Some microorganisms (obligate aerobes) require oxygen to live, for example, the *Staphylococcus aureus* bacillus, while others, such as the tetanus bacillus (*Clostridium tetani*) cannot live with oxygen. These are referred to as obligate anaerobes. *Obligate* means "obliged."

Temperature

Organisms have their own temperatures, at which they thrive, and low and high temperatures, at which they are destroyed. This is an important factor when destroying organisms in asepsis.

pH

Microorganisms are sensitive to changes in pH. Most grow best somewhere between pH 5 and 8.

Light

Microorganisms are either inhibited or killed by ultraviolet rays, which are used as a method for disinfecting instruments in hospitals.

Antibiosis

An *antibiotic* is a chemical agent produced by one microbe that inhibits or kills other microbes. Antibiotics are used frequently to combat infections, such as penicillin, which is used to treat syphilis.

Exit from the Source

For an infectious process to be established, the pathogen must leave the reservoir (the source). In a person there are a number of exits from the body, depending upon the pathogen and the site of the reservoir.

Respiratory Tract

The *respiratory tract* is one of the most common exit routes for pathogens. While one is sneezing, coughing, breathing, and even talking, pathogens can leave the tract through the nose and the mouth.

Gastrointestinal Tract

The *gastrointestinal tract* is another site of exit. Pathogens can be expelled in feces, through drainage, such as gallbladder drainage, and even in vomitus. One example is the typhoid bacillus, which in some patients is carried in the gallbladder and/or the large intestine and expelled in the feces.

Urinary Tract

Reservoirs in the *urinary tract* (the kidneys, the bladder, and the urethra) can be sources for pathogens that exit in the urine.

Reproductive Tract

Pathogens in the *reproductive tract* of women exit by way of the vagina. In men, they exit through the urinary meatus. Thus in males they may also be in the urine, while in females they exit in a vaginal discharge.

Blood

In some people there may be a reservoir for pathogens in the circulating *blood*, such as the virus of serum hepatitis. In these instances, any situation that permits blood to leave the circulatory system provides a portal of exit for the pathogen.

Tissues

The *tissues* of the body can also be a reservoir for pathogens, and thus any opening into the tissues can serve as the portal of exit. For example, wounds can become infected and produce drainage that contains a high concentration of pathogens.

Method of Transmission

Once a pathogen has escaped its reservoir, then it must have a means of transmission to another person or host. There are various vehicles to carry the organisms to a person. Some of these are (a) direct contact, (b) air, (c) fomites, (d) food and water, and (e) animals and insects.

Direct Contact

By coming in contact with a person who has an infection, the pathogen can transfer directly to the second person. For example, kissing, sexual intercourse, or touching provide direct contacts and can permit direct transmission of pathogens.

Air

The air can readily serve as a vehicle for transmission of some pathogens. By sneezing, for example, pathogens are sprayed into the air where they can be inhaled by others. Pathogens can attach themselves to dust particles in the air and be carried quickly to other people even over some distance.

Fomites

A *fomite* is an object other than food that can harbor microorganisms. For example, dishes, silverware, forceps, and dressings can serve to transfer organisms from one person to another. The use of disposable equipment in hospitals and the modern methods for disinfection have reduced this method of transmission considerably in recent years.

Food and Water

Food and water are also ways of transmitting pathogens. In cities in the United States and Canada there are laws that protect the public from contaminated food and water. However, in remote areas of the country water can still serve as a vehicle of transmission when it becomes contaminated. An example would be the virus of infectious hepatitis, which is transmitted through water.

Animals and Insects

Both animals and insects can spread pathogens such as the *Salmonella* bacillus, which is a natural pathogen of domestic animals and causes gastroenteritis in humans. Flies carry microorganisms also; thus they contaminate food and fluids with which they come in contact. A fly, for example, may pick up pathogens from the feces of soiled diapers, and then transmit them to various exposed foods.

Portal of Entry

For a person to become infected, the pathogen must be able to enter the body. The skin of a person serves as a barrier to infections; however, any break in the skin can readily serve as a portal of entry. Microorganisms can enter a body through the same routes that they can leave the body. See "Exit from the Reservoir."

A PERSON'S SUSCEPTIBILITY

Whether an organism causes an infection depends upon a number of factors already mentioned. One of the most important factors is the susceptibility of a person, which is affected by (a) stress, (b) nutritional status, (c) fatigue, (d) sex, (e) genetic inheritance, (f) age, and (g) concomitant medical treatment.

Stress

The level of stress experienced by a person can influence susceptibility to infection. The person whose stress level is elevated, who has been exposed to stressors for a long period of time, may have little energy left for coping with infection; the person may be more likely to acquire an infection than if the stressors had been fewer and spaced over a shorter period. For example, a person recovering from a major operation is more likely to develop an infection than a healthy person who has not had surgery.

Nutritional Status

The nutritional status of a person directly affects the health of body tissues and hence susceptibility to infection. Unhealthy tissues are more likely to become infected and are slower to heal. Protein is an essential element in the tissue building and growing process. Some infections, such as tuberculosis, are found more frequently among poorly nourished people.

Fatigue

Fatigue also affects a person's susceptibility to disease. A tired person's coping mechanisms are less effective,

and thus the person is unable to resist stressors as she normally could. A common example is the overworked, overtired person who becomes vulnerable to the cold virus.

Sex

Whether one is a man or woman can also affect one's susceptibility to some infections. For example, pneumonia more frequently occurs in men, whereas scarlet fever is more likely to be seen in women.

Genetic Inheritance

Some people, because of their genetic inheritance, are more likely to acquire infections. For example, some people may be deficient in immunoglobulins, which play a significant role in the internal defense mechanism of the body.

Age

Age is also a major factor in relation to susceptibility to infections. A neonate will have antibodies from the mother which will provide protection for the first two or three months. These gradually provide decreasing protection. Infections are one of the major causes of death of newborn children. Growing children normally develop their own immune globulins. A young child readily acquires colds, common infectious diseases, and intestinal infections. An only child may experience these chiefly when entering nursery school, while a child with older brothers and sisters will acquire these infections earlier. For adults viral diseases are a common reason for intermittent illness. The immune responses become poorer with age, so that again the elderly person, like the young child, more readily acquires infections.

Concomitant Medical Treatment

Some forms of medical treatment, because of their effects, can predispose a person to infection. For example, treatments by radiation destroy tissue, thereby rendering it more vulnerable to infections. Treatment for leukemia lowers the white blood cell count, thereby having a similar effect.

THE COURSE OF AN INFECTION

The course of an infection can be divided into three stages: the incubation period, the period of illness, and the convalescent period.

The Incubation Period

The incubation period is the time between the entrance of the pathogen into the body and the onset of the symptoms of the infection. It is during this time that the causative organism adapts to the person and multiplies sufficiently to produce disease. The length of an incubation period varies greatly, depending upon the pathogen. For example, rubella (measles) takes from 10 to 14 days, whereas tetanus (lockjaw) takes from 4 to 21 days to develop.

The Period of Illness

The period of illness can be divided into two stages: the prodromal stage and the full illness stage. During the *prodromal stage* the patients have some early manifestations of illness. The signs are usually nonspecific but will indicate to persons that they are not well; patients may have fever, feel tired and irritable, and may complain of malaise. It is during this stage that persons are most infectious and are most likely to spread the disease. A prodromal stage usually lasts a short time, hours or days at the most. Following this is the full illness stage, in which more specific signs and symptoms develop. The severity of the symptoms and the length of the illness vary from pathogen to pathogen and from one person to another.

Systemic Symptoms

Systemic symptoms are symptoms relating to the whole body. These symptoms can be:

1. Fever (one of the most constant symptoms associated with most infections).
2. Lassitude, malaise.
3. Anorexia, nausea.
4. Headache.
5. Lymph node enlargement and tenderness.

Symptoms of Localized Infections

Localized infections are infections relating to a particular body area or part. Symptoms include the following:

1. Swelling.
2. Redness.
3. Pain or tenderness.
4. Heat at the infected area.
5. Loss of function of the involved body part.

See Chapter 8, "The Inflammatory Adaptive Response."

Symptoms of Generalized Infections

These infections affect a general body part or area. The symptoms are:

1. Sneezing or discharge from the nose.
2. Skin rash and lesions of the mucous membranes.
3. Vomiting or diarrhea.
4. Enlargement of body lymph glands.

The Convalescent Period

During the convalescent period, the symptoms disappear and there is a return to health. Depending upon the severity of the illness and the patient's general condition, the length of convalescence can vary greatly from a few days to months.

PRINCIPLES RELATED TO INFECTIONS

Principles related to infections are as follows:

1. Microorganisms are always present in the environment. When the conditions are appropriate, some microorganisms can cause infection.

2. The body has various barriers to infections, such as the skin, mucous membranes, and certain body secretions (such as lacrimal and vaginal secretions). When these barriers are altered for any reason, the person is more susceptible to infections.

3. Pathogens can be killed by exposure to moist heat at 121° C (250° F) for 15 to 20 minutes. Such moist heat also destroys spore-forming bacteria.

4. Cleanliness inhibits the growth of microorganisms.

5. Disinfection destroys most pathogenic non-spore-forming microorganisms.

6. Pathogenic organisms are usually transmitted to others unless some precautions are taken. Patients tend to be more vulnerable to infections while in hospitals than in their own homes because of their own health problems, such as a surgical procedure which depletes resistance, and their lack of immunity to the organisms present there.

PREVENTION OF INFECTIONS IN HEALTH

Environmental Measures

In the United States and Canada, the responsibility for establishing and maintaining a safe environment in regard to health is delegated to state, provincial, and local health departments. These departments maintain four broad categories of service relative to environmental health.

Preventive Services

Preventive services provide programs for immunizations (see Chapter 21), the investigation of sources of disease, and case finding for such diseases as tuberculosis and venereal diseases. Most centers will offer diagnostic and treatment services as well as follow-up care.

Special Health Services

This group includes such specialized services as laboratories, statistics, and record keeping. In many instances, the laboratory service related to infection and communicable disease control is available to physicians in a community in order to assist them with diagnoses.

Health Centers

Health centers provide both community and home services. School nurses advise parents in regard to children's health, and they assist with the identification of infectious health problems in a school or community. For example, a school nurse may identify ringworm on a child and assist parents to obtain adequate treatment before the child returns to school.

Sanitation Services

These services involve the practices concerned with the disposal of garbage, the sale of food, water purification, and the control of rodents, to mention just a few. States and provinces have laws governing the preparation and distribution of food, especially dairy products and meat. These laws are intended to protect the public from infections that could be spread by these vehicles.

Public concern about the natural environment, especially about pollution of water and air, has been growing. People are becoming aware of the many dangers that a polluted environment can have for health.

Individual Measures

There are a number of personal practices that individuals can carry out to help prevent infections. They can be generally placed in two major groups: those which strengthen the body's barriers against infection and those clean practices which minimize the number of microorganisms and decrease the chances of developing an infection.

Strengthening the Body's Barriers Against Infection

A number of measures can be taken to strengthen the body's infection barriers:

1. *Immunization.* The immunologic system is the body's major defense against infections. Not only does the body gradually build up defenses against pathogens with which it comes in contact, but it can also be assisted artificially by immunizations (see Chapter 21, "Immunizations").

2. *Nutrition.* A balanced diet enhances the health of all body tissues. Thus it assists the skin to remain intact and to be able to repel microorganisms. An adequate nutritional status also enables tissues to maintain and rebuild themselves. One of the body's defenses that requires nourishment is the reticuloendothelial system. This is the system of connective tissue cells (phagocytes) that combat and prevent infections by ingesting microorganisms, other cells, or foreign matter. There are three types of phagocytes: reticuloendothelial cells, which line the liver, spleen, and bone marrow; macrophages, which wander in the tissues; and microglia, which are located in the central nervous system.

3. *Adequate rest and sleep.* Rest and sleep are necessary to restore the body; they are essential elements in the health of a person and in the ability to perform one's usual activities. See Chapter 24, "Comfort, Rest, and Sleep," for additional information.

4. *Normal stress level.* Elevated stress predisposes a person to infection. A balanced life, for example, between work and recreation is important. See Chapter 7, "Psychological Homeostasis."

Minimizing the Number of Microorganisms

There are a number of personal hygienic practices that, if carried out in daily living, will decrease the likelihood of acquiring an infection:

1. *Hand washing.* Washing one's hands after urination and fecal excretion will prevent the transfer of microorganisms to other objects and food. Hand washing before handling food will also prevent contamination of the food and subsequent ingestion of the organisms.

2. *Perineal Care.* Cleansing a female's rectum and the perineum after elimination by wiping from the area of least contamination (the urinary meatus) to the area of greatest contamination (the anus) helps to prevent genitourinary infections. See Chapter 20, "Perineal and Genital Care."

3. *Regular Bathing.* Bathing serves to remove the microorganisms from the skin surface, thus helping to prevent infections. See Chapter 20.

4. *Brushing Teeth Regularly.* See Chapter 20, "Oral Hygiene."

5. *Blowing One's Nose.* Blowing the nose and sneezing clear microorganisms from the upper respiratory tract. They also assist in the removal of organisms and dust that have been caught in the cilia (tiny hairlike processes inside the nose). Children need to be taught not to pick their noses. This is an unclean practice resulting in contamination of the hands and possible damage to the mucous membrane that lines the nose.

6. *Coughing.* Coughing assists in the removal of organisms and dust from the lower portions of the respiratory tract. When coughing, one should cover one's mouth with a tissue, thus preventing spraying of organisms into the air for someone else to breathe.

7. *Nail Care.* Carefully cutting the nails and not the side tissue will maintain the integrity of the nail-skin barrier to organisms. The tissues around nails may also need to be lubricated regularly with an oil in order to prevent drying and cracking.

PREVENTION OF INFECTIONS IN ILLNESS

Medical Aseptic Practices

When a person is ill, the usual measures that are taken in health continue to apply. In addition, there are specific measures that can be employed to restrict the spread of microorganisms. If a person has an infection, whether at home or in a hospital, it is necessary to restrict the spread of the pathogens to others. The problem of confining the organisms and subsequently killing them or inactivating them involves a number of practices referred to earlier in the chapter as *medical asepsis.*

Medical aseptic practices include those practices carried out to prevent the transfer of organisms by any person or object that has come in contact with the infected person. A nurse who is caring for a patient needs to take precautions not to acquire the patient's pathogens. Care should be taken that dishes, equipment, and body discharges do not serve as means of transmission of the pathogens to others. This can be accomplished by the destruction of organisms after they leave the body.

Hospital-Acquired Infections

Hospital-acquired infections continue to pose a problem. Prior to the introduction of antisepsis and aseptic practices in hospitals in the late nineteenth century, hospital-acquired (nosocomial) infections were uncontrolled. Aseptic techniques are responsible for some measure of control. However, since 1947, the incidence is again on the rise. There are a number of reasons for this increase, such as the development of strains of organisms that are resistant to antimicrobial agents and laxity in aseptic technique practices. A survey in 1970 indicated that at any one time, 15.5% of hospital patients had an active infection, but 98% of those patients with infections did not require special precautions (Garner and Kaiser 1972: 734).

Cleaning

An article is considered *clean* when it is free of pathogenic organisms. An article that has pathogens on it is considered dirty or *contaminated*. Most articles, whether artery forceps or drawsheets, can be cleaned by rinsing them in cold water to remove any organic material, washing them with hot soapy water, then rinsing them again to remove the soap. The following steps should be considered when cleaning in a hospital or home setting where pathogens exist.

1. Rinse the article with cold water in order to remove organic material. Hot water coagulates the protein of organic material and tends to make it stick to the article. Examples of organic material are blood or wound drainage such as pus.

2. Wash the article in hot water and soap. Soap has an emulsifying action and reduces surface tension, which facilitates the removal of dirt. Rinsing with water assists in washing the dirt away.

3. Use an abrasive such as a stiff-bristled brush to clean various types of equipment that have grooves and corners.

4. Rinse the article well with hot water.

5. Dry.

6. Disinfect or sterilize if indicated.

Disinfection and Sterilization

Disinfection is a process by which most microorganisms are destroyed, with the exception of spores. Spore-forming organisms such as *Bacillus anthracis* (which causes anthrax) and *Clostridium tetani* (which causes tetanus) are killed by sterilization processes. It is therefore important, when arranging precautions, to know the type of pathogen and how it is destroyed.

Methods of Disinfection and Sterilization

Various methods exist for disinfecting and sterilizing hospital objects:

1. *Hot-air oven.* Hot-air ovens are used to sterilize glassware and some metal objects in hospitals. By means of dry air at a temperature of 180° C for two hours, all microorganisms and spores are destroyed.

2. *Steam.* Steam under pressure and free steam can be used to sterilize. The autoclave uses steam at 17 pounds pressure, 121° C for 30 minutes. When microorganisms are exposed to this pressure and temperature for 30 minutes, all of them, including spores, are destroyed. Autoclaving is used to sterilize surgical dressings, surgical linens, parenteral solutions, and metal and glass objects.

Free steam (100° C) is used for objects that would be destroyed at the higher temperature of the autoclave. Usually it is necessary to steam the article for 30 minutes on three consecutive days. The spacing is required so that the spores not killed at that temperature will return to their vegetative state during the intervals, thus becoming vulnerable to the heat.

3. *Radiation.* Ultraviolet light rays are also used for disinfection and sterilization. They are used in some hospitals and in industry. They provide a relatively safe and quick method for killing microorganisms.

4. *Ultrasonic waves.* In this method sound waves above the hearing level, that is, above 20,000 cycles per second are used. They break up microorganisms and provide sterilization of objects.

5. *Chemical methods.* There are several chemicals that work either by interfering with the metabolism of microorganisms or by destroying the protoplasm of the organisms. There are basically two types of anti-infectives: (a) those which are applied for local action, such as disinfectants and antiseptics in the skin, or to a body excretion such as the feces, and (b) those with a systemic action, such as antibiotics and specialized agents, such as para-aminosalicylic acid, which is effective against the tuberculosis bacillus.

6. *Pasteurization.* Pasteurization is the disinfection of milk and similar substances. They are heated to a moderate temperature for a specific time. One method heats the product at 71° C for 15 seconds. The milk is then cooled and placed in the containers.

7. *Ethylene oxide gas.* Ethylene oxide gas sterilization is also used in some institutions. Microorganisms subjected to a temperature of 43.3° C (110° F) in a concentration of ethylene oxide of 440 mg/liter are destroyed (Shull 1962: 603–607). This type of sterilization is generally used for delicate plastic or rubber objects that can be harmed by higher temperatures. Examples of articles sterilized by gas are oxygen or suction gauges, blood pressure apparatus, stethoscopes, sheepskins, motors, plastic drinking glasses, and catheters.

ISOLATION TECHNIQUES AND PRECAUTIONS

The purpose of isolation techniques and related precautions is to keep pathogens within a defined area by establishing mechanical barriers to their escape. The boundaries for pathogens may be the patient's room or a bed unit. A whole room provides better isolation of pathogens than a part of a room because airborne spread is more easily restricted, and there is decreased danger of inadvertent contamination by another patient who may unknowingly touch a part of the isolated unit.

Types of Isolation

Isolation techniques and precautions are intended to confine pathogenic microorganisms within a given and recognized area. There are a number of kinds of isolation techniques and precautions.

Respiratory Isolation

Respiratory isolation is indicated in situations in which the pathogens are spread on droplets from the respiratory tract. In this type of isolation, masks are generally worn by the nurses, and in the case of small infants, gowns are also worn because of the possibility of drooling by the infant. When possible, patients should be taught proper tissue techniques in order to prevent the transmission of infection. For example, they should always hold several layers of tissue in front of their noses and mouths when they sneeze and cough, and they should dispose of these directly in the appropriate receptacle provided.

Visitors also need instruction. They need to learn the reasons for the use of masks and appropriate application and disposal of them.

In some agencies patients also wear masks when they are transported and where there are a number of people. When the patient is masked, the nurse need not mask.

Respiratory isolation is indicated for patients who have respiratory illnesses such as active pulmonary tuberculosis, pertussis (whooping cough), and pneumonia due to *Staphylococcus aureus*. Precautions must be taken when acquiring sputum specimens. Specimen containers should have close-fitting lids and be double-bagged prior to sending them to the laboratory.

Enteric Isolation

Enteric isolation is indicated in situations in which the pathogens are transmitted in the feces. Transmission depends upon oral ingestion of the pathogen. In some instances throat secretions or vomitus may be indirectly contacted; these also require special precautions in handling. In most settings it is appropriate for the patient to use the usual toilet and bedpan units where feces and urine are normally treated for any microorganisms. However, the bathroom is not used by other patients. Usually, leftover food and fluids are also disposed of in the toilet.

For this type of isolation it is not necessary to wear a mask, but it is recommended that gloves and gowns be worn when handling feces and urine containers and soiled linen. If it is necessary to destroy pathogens before disposing of excreta, this is usually done by adding 0.5–1.0% chloride of lime solution to the excreta and permitting it to stand for one hour. This type of isolation practice is indicated for patients who have diseases such as typhoid fever, salmonellosis, hepatitis, and dysentery (amebiasis).

Some patients who are carriers of the typhoid bacillus can live safely and comfortably at home. Their only precaution is to put the chloride of lime solution with their feces before emptying the toilet. For patients with hepatitis, special precautions are required when needles and syringes are used. See "Blood Isolation."

Wound and Skin Isolation

This type of isolation is for pathogens that are found in wounds and that can be directly transmitted by contact with the wound or by contact with articles heavily contaminated from the wound, such as dressings or linen. The isolation involves retaining the pathogens in a wound area and preventing transmission to other parts of the patient or to another patient. The pathogen in this instance is confined in the wound drainage of the skin, mucous membrane, or any body orifice or tract.

Usually gowns are worn for this type of isolation, and in some cases gloves are also worn. Masks (respiratory precautions) are recommended for some specific pathogens, such as staphylococcus coagulase positive and streptococcus, beta-hemolytic group A. Important in this type of isolation is the safe disposal of dressings, clothes, and equipment that was used to treat the wound. Examples of indications for wound and skin isolation are abscesses, boils, or infected burns. Precautions for gas gangrene require strict isolation measures.

Blood Isolation

This isolation is intended to prevent transmission of pathogens that are found in the blood. Therefore, any equipment that comes in contact with the patient's blood will need to be carefully disinfected before touching another object or person. Examples of infections that indicate this type of isolation are malaria and serum hepatitis.

Strict Isolation

Strict isolation is indicated where the pathogen can be spread by contact and by air. It is used for all highly communicable diseases that can produce serious disease in other susceptible persons. Techniques usually involve the use of gowns, masks, gloves, and a single room for the patient. Strict isolation is indicated for diseases such as diphtheria, smallpox, and rabies.

Protective Isolation

This isolation is also referred to as *reverse barrier technique*. Its objective is to protect an uninfected patient with lowered resistance from potential pathogens in the environment. In this instance, the pathogens are kept *out* of a designated area. One way of accomplishing this is to enclose the patient in a large plastic bubble into which purified air is circulated.

This technique is indicated for patients who are particularly susceptible to infections, for example, pa-tients with defective immunologic reactions, those taking immunosuppressive drugs for cancer therapy, or patients who have leukemia.

Suspect Isolation

Suspect isolation is an interim one used only for short durations. It is used when an infection is suspected but confirmation is needed by laboratory tests. Isolation precautions are initiated to alert and protect others from possible transfer of organisms. Examples of indications for this type of isolation are fevers of unknown origin, draining wounds that seem to be infected, and undiagnosed diarrhea and jaundice with a suspicion of hepatitis.

When tests confirm that a communicable disease or infection is present, the appropriate category of isolation is initiated. If the tests indicate that the patient is not infectious, the suspect isolation precautions are discontinued, and routine care is established. Table 16-1 presents a summary of types of isolation and precautions.

Guidelines for Isolation Techniques

Nurses are faced with a number of problems when helping a patient who is on isolation techniques or using some isolation practices. There are a number of guidelines that can assist in providing safe care for patients.

1. Floors are contaminated; therefore when any object falls on the floor it will need to be disinfected or sterilized before use. The dust on the floors is contaminated; thus the floors need to be wet-mopped with a disinfecting solution so that dust is not stirred up.

2. Paper towels can be used to handle some contaminated objects so that the nurse's hands can remain clean.

3. Drafts can carry airborne organisms from one patient to another.

4. Two nurses can often effectively maintain good isolation technique more easily than one, as in double bagging materials to be removed from the unit or obtaining a throat culture.

5. When anything is removed from an isolation unit, it must be adequately bagged and labeled for sterilization or disinfected at the unit.

6. Always be aware of your hands when in an isolation unit. Once they are contaminated, they should not touch any clean objects such as the nurse's hair, watch, or medication tray.

Table 16-1.   Recommended Types of Isolation and Precautions

Type of Isolation	Precautions					
	Mask	Gown	Gloves	Articles	Indications	Duration of Isolation
Respiratory	For all personnel entering room; for patient when transported out of room; usually not required for patients with pneumonia	Only when holding infant in arms; not needed for care of adults	Not needed	Disinfect articles contaminated by respiratory secretions	Chicken pox	7 days after eruption disappears
					Diphtheria	After two negative nose and throat cultures once off antibiotics
					Meningitis (meningococcal)	24 hours after therapy is started
					Mumps	7 days after onset of swelling
					Pneumonia	Duration of iilness
					Rubella	5–7 days after rash appears
					Smallpox	Until all crusts are shed
					Tuberculosis	Until therapy begins and swab is negative
					Whooping cough	Duration of illness
Enteric	Not needed	When handling soiled linen or feces and urine receptacles or any article contaminated by feces and urine	Same as for gown	Disinfect articles contaminated by feces, urine, or vomitus; for hepatitis, special precautions are needed with needles and syringes	Cholera	Duration of illness
					Hepatitis (infectious)	Duration of hospitalization
					Salmonellosis	Duration of illness
					Typhoid fever	After three daily negative cultures
Wound and skin	Only for specific pathogens, e.g., *Staphylococcus* coagulase positive, *Streptococcus* (beta hemolytic Group A)	For all personnel having contact with patient's linen or dressings	Same as for gown	Precautions needed for linens, dressings, and instruments used in dressing changes	Abscesses and boils Purulent wounds	Duration of illness Healing, or one negative culture
					Venereal disease	24–48 hours after therapy is started

					Gas gangrene Conjunctivitus	Negative culture 24–48 hours after therapy is started
Blood	Not needed	Possible enteric precautions	Possible enteric precautions	Disinfect any articles contacting the patient's blood such as syringes and needles	Malaria Hepatitis	Duration of hospitalization Duration of hospitalization
Strict	For all persons entering room	For all persons entering room; for smallpox, cap and shoe covering is also recommended	For all persons entering room	Usual isolation disposal of all articles	Rabies Diphtheria Smallpox Pneumonia (a) *Streptococcus* (beta hemolytic Group A), (b) *Staphylococcus* (coagulase positive)	Duration of illness See Respiratory See Respiratory See Respiratory
Protective (reverse barrier)	For all persons entering room; for patient when transported out of room	For all persons entering room; sterile gown for burn patients; for patients when transported out of room	For direct contact with patient; sterile gloves for burn patients	Sterile linen for burn patients; linen hamper in room not necessary; terminal disinfectant not necessary	Defective immune responses Receiving immunosuppressives Leukemia Leukopenia Burns	Duration of illness Duration of illness Duration of illness Duration of illness Duration of illness
Suspect	When required for suspect respiratory problems	For all persons entering room	As required to protect self and others	Precautions with tissues, etc., for respiratory problems; precautions with linen, feces, and urine for enteric problems; precautions with linen, dressings, and instruments for wound problems	Fever of unknown origin; undiagnosed diarrhea; draining wounds; jaundice; suspicion of hepatitis; possible tuberculosis or meningitis or any communicable disease	Until diagnosis is confirmed for all infections

7. Contaminated gowns should not be worn outside the isolation unit because of the chance of contaminating other people or objects and spreading microorganisms.

8. If a nurse acquires a cut or scratch, this should be reported since it may be a portal of entry for microorganisms. Thus the nurse may be unable to care for a patient on isolation until the wound is healed.

9. When hands are contaminated, wash them using the prescribed technique.

Equipment for Isolation Precautions

A unit that is set up for isolation technique (barrier technique) needs to have the following equipment:

1. Sink with soap dispenser.

2. Paper towels.

3. Laundry hamper.

4. Table on which to place supplies, such as stethoscope and dressing supplies.

5. Toilet, which can also be used as a garbage disposal.

6. Tub or shower.

7. Garbage receptacle with plastic liner.

8. Rack for hanging gown, if gown is reused.

9. Bedside necessities for the patient, such as tissues, paper bags, water pitcher, disposable cup, back rub lotion, and mouth wash.

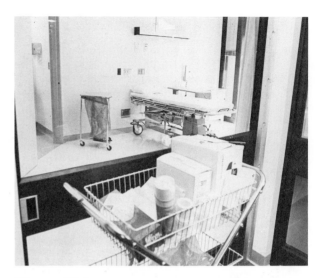

Figure 16-1. An especially designed isolation unit in a modern hospital.

10. A designated area out of the patient's room or an isolation cart for clean supplies such as gowns, paper towels, plastic garbage bags, isolation tags or tape to mark contaminated items, and disinfectant solutions as required. In some agencies, a paper bag containing masks is taped onto the door. This obvious place alerts staff to the need for masking before entering the room.

11. Door cards stating "Isolation" and "Visitors Inquire at Desk."

See Figure 16-1 for a unit in a hospital which is designed for isolation practices.

MEDICAL ASEPSIS TECHNIQUES

Hand Washing

Hand washing is carried out in order to prevent the transfer of microorganisms by the hands to another person, either directly or by way of an object such as a glass or a bottle of back rub solution. Hand washing is carried out with a soap. In hospitals the soaps often contain a germicide because of the presence of pathogenic organisms. A number of detergents are used, such as benzalkonium chloride (Zephiran), which acts as both a detergent and a disinfectant. Another is povidone-iodine (Betadine), which is also a detergent and *germicide* (a substance that kills microorganisms).

Hand washing involves both mechanical and chemical action. The running water and friction of rubbing supply the mechanical cleansing, while the soaps emulsify and lower surface tension and thus facilitate the removal of microorganisms, dirt, and oils. The time required to cleanse the hands adequately is usually one to two minutes.

General Technique for Hand Washing

1. The nails must be filed and short.

2. Turn on the water so that it is warm and comfortable to the touch. Excessively hot water opens pores and can irritate the skin.

3. Hold hands below the level of the elbows and wet thoroughly. The hands will be more contaminated than the elbows, hence the water

should run from the area of least contamination (the elbows) to the area of greatest contamination (the hands) (Figure 16-2).

4. Apply soap or detergent. (Soap may be in a liquid form or in a bar.) A bar of soap needs to be rinsed before it is returned to the container.

5. Wash each hand thoroughly, using a rotary motion. Wash each finger separately, and make sure the interdigital spaces are well cleansed. Continue for one to two minutes.

6. Cleanse nails with a brush or an orange stick.

7. Rinse hands so that water flows from the arms to the hands.

8. Repeat steps 3–6.

9. Dry the arms and hands, starting at the elbows and working toward the hands. Discard the towel after it has reached the hands. In some places warm-air driers are used.

10. Turn off the faucet, using a paper towel if it has a hand control, because the handle is contaminated. Foot and leg controls are frequently used for sinks, and in these situations a towel is not required to turn off the water.

If while washing the hands they accidentally touch a contaminated object, such as the sink or the faucet handle, the handwashing procedure needs to be repeated from the beginning. If the nurse's hands are becoming dry and cracked from frequent washings, it is advisable to use a lubricating lotion or cream.

Gowning Technique

Gowning technique is used for two main reasons: (a) to cover clothes so that they will not become contaminated by pathogens that are around a patient, and (b) to cover clothes so that microorganisms on the clothing will not be transferred to a patient; for example, a mother wears a gown when she visits her sick newborn baby in the nursery.

The gown needs to be large enough to cover entirely the clothing under it. It should have sleeves with tightly fitting cuffs and a belt or tie for the waist. Gowns used in hospitals open down the back and usually have a tie at the neck and perhaps one or two other ties at the back. The most effective method for using gowns is to put on a clean one each time and discard the used one before leaving the patient's room. When taking the gown off, care needs to be taken that the nurse's hands, which are contami-

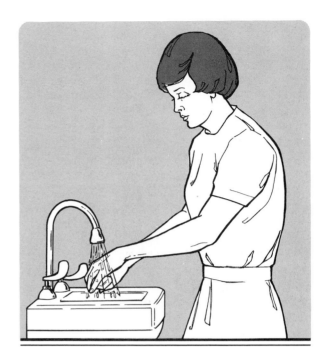

Figure 16-2. Hand washing for medical asepsis. Note the hands below the elbows.

nated, do not touch anything but the gown until they are washed. The outside of the gown (the contaminated side) should not touch the nurse's clothing or any clean, uncontaminated objects. The hands are then washed (see "General Technique for Hand Washing").

In some hospitals, gowns are reused rather than discarded after use. To put on a used gown, it is necessary to remember that the inside of the gown is clean and the outside is contaminated. The neck band and the fasteners at the neck are also considered clean. The gown is usually hanging on a stand designated for that purpose; the nurse picks it up from the inside and then slides hands and arms down the sleeves. If the hands will not move easily through the cuffs, the nurse can pull the sleeve over the hand with the opposite hand, which is still in the sleeve. The second hand may then be pushed through, or the sleeve can be pulled on by taking a clean paper towel and grasping that second sleeve on the outside. However, it is important that both hands remain clean and do not touch the outside of the gown. If the hands do become contaminated, they need to be washed before the neck of the gown is secured. The gown is then fastened at the neck; the gown is overlapped, left over right side, as much as possible at the back, and then the waist tie or belt is secured (see Figure 16-3).

To remove a gown that is to be kept for reuse, the nurse first unties the waist ties, then washes the

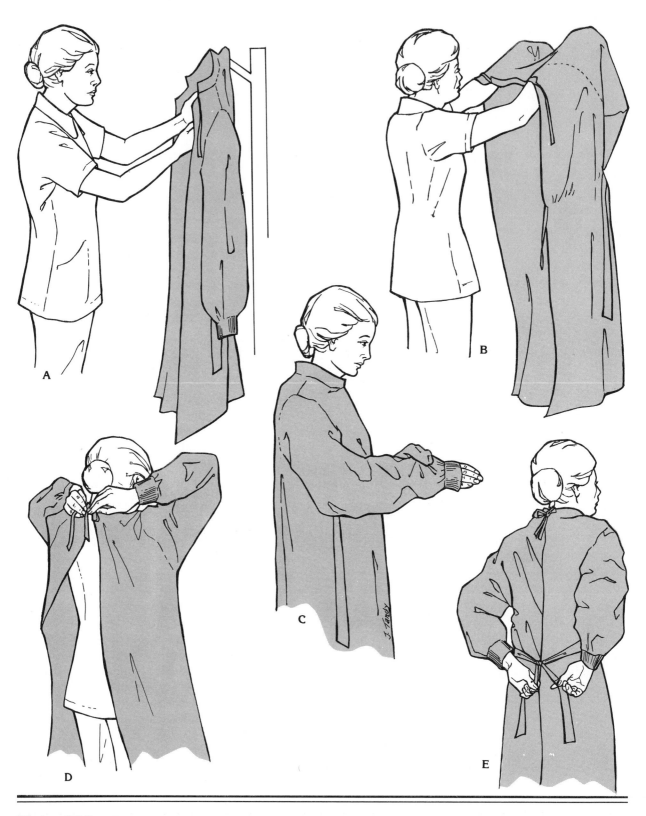

Figure 16-3.   Donning a gown for medical asepsis. **A,** Reaching to the inside at the shoulders; **B,** sliding arms down the sleeves; **C,** pulling hands through the cuffs; **D,** tying gown at the neck; and **E,** fastening gown at the back by placing left side under right side.

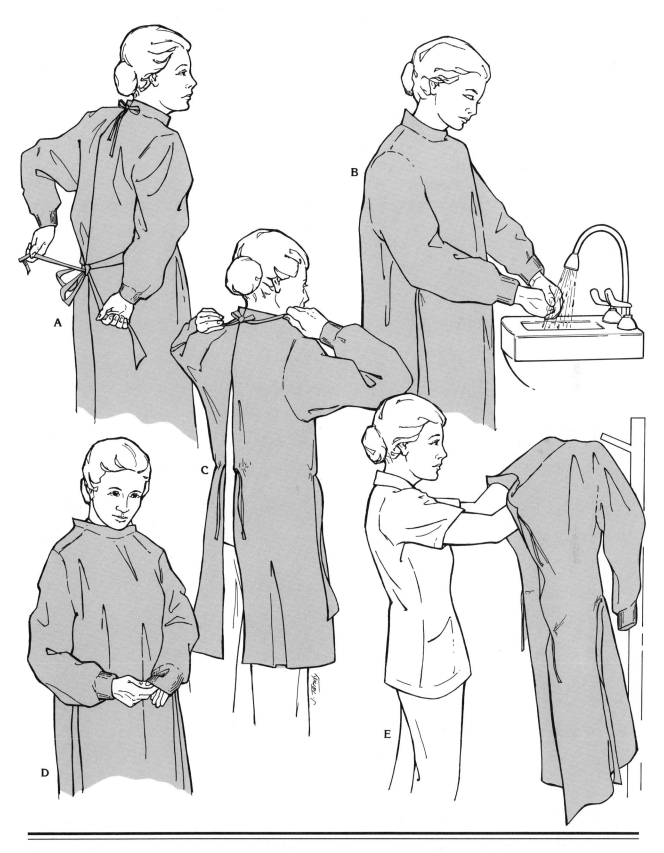

Figure 16-4. Removing isolation gown. **A,** Untie the waist ties; **B,** wash hands; **C,** untie neck ties; **D,** remove arms from sleeves touching only the inside of the gown; and **E,** hang gown on rack or dispose of appropriately.

hands before untying the neck and taking off the gown, being careful to touch only the inside of the gown. It is then hung on the rack by holding it on the inside. The neck ties are clean and are permitted to fall down on the inside of the gown. By holding the gown with both hands inside the shoulders at the shoulder seams, the hands can be brought together and then one shoulder of the gown inverted over the other. This ensures that the clean part of the gown is on the outside. The gown is then hung outside the isolation unit on a rack ready for reuse.

Some agencies are now using disposable gowns, which are used once and then destroyed. These are usually disposed of in a covered garbage can. See Figure 16-4 for removing a gown.

Procedure 16-1.   Gowning Technique

Action	Explanation
Assemble Equipment	
1. Clean isolation gown.	
To put on a clean isolation gown:	
1. Remove watch and rings. A plain wedding ring can remain.	Jewelry can harbor microorganisms.
2. Wash hands.	To remove any microorganisms that should not be transmitted to the patient.
3. Explain to the patient what you plan to do. Adjust the explanation to the patient's needs.	To reassure the patient by knowledge of what will happen. To identify the patient.
4. Hold the gown at the neck on the inside, permitting it to unfold. The open part of the gown is toward the nurse.	
5. Slide hands and arms down the sleeves.	If putting on a gown that is contaminated on the outside, be careful not to touch the outside. If there is difficulty sliding hand through the cuff, the hand still in the sleeve can pull the other cuff over the other hand. The second hand can be pushed through by using a clean paper towel to grasp the sleeve.
6. Fasten ties at the neck.	
7. Overlap the gown at the back as much as possible, left side under right side.	
8. Secure waist band or belt.	
Removing a contaminated gown	
1. Untie the waist belt or ties.	These are considered contaminated.
2. Wash hands.	To remove microorganisms that contaminate them.
3. Untie the neck ties. Be sure not to touch the outside of the gown.	These are considered clean. Allow them to fall inside the gown, which is clean.
4. Slide the gown down arms and over hands.	If the cuffs will not slide easily over the hands, use a clean paper towel to pull first cuff over hand, and then pull second cuff over by using first hand, which is inside the sleeve.

5. Hold the gown with both hands inside the shoulders at the shoulder seams. The hands are then brought together, and the gown is rolled and discarded in the container provided.

6. The gown is then hung on the isolation rack.

7. Wash hands.

Make sure that the gown does not touch the uniform. If the gown is to be reused, one shoulder of the gown is inverted over the other shoulder; now the clean part of the gown is outermost.

Use a towel to turn off the tap after washing because it will be contaminated.
Open the door using a paper towel because the inside handle will be contaminated.

Face Masks

Masks are generally used to prevent the spread of microorganisms to and from the respiratory tract. Nurses wear masks basically in two situations: either to prevent the passage of organisms from their own respiratory tracts to the patient or to prevent inhaling pathogenic microorganisms.

Masks are made of a variety of materials, for example, cotton or glass fiber; disposable masks are being used increasingly. Masks should be worn only once and then discarded to ensure effective filtering of microorganisms. Masks that become wet are less effective and should also be discarded. It is advised that masks be worn no more than one hour at a time.

Masks need to cover both the mouth and the nose and fit tightly around the face to prevent escape of microorganisms around the sides. If a person wears glasses, the upper edge of the mask should fit under the glasses to help prevent the glasses from steaming. A mask is put on with clean hands prior to donning a gown.

To Remove a Mask

In medical asepsis, where a mask is used to protect the nurse from the patient's pathogens, it is removed with clean hands. If the gown is to be discarded, the mask is removed after the gown is removed and after the hands have been washed. The nurse should not touch the mask proper, only the ties or ear loops. If the gown is to be retained for reuse, the mask is removed after the hands are washed, and the hands are washed again before the gown is removed.

If a mask needs to be changed, the hands are washed, the mask is discarded, hands are rewashed, and a clean mask is put on. Masks should not be al-lowed to dangle around the neck, and they should not be carried in pockets for reuse. This is neither a clean nor a safe practice.

Gloves

Gloves are used in medical asepsis to protect the nurse from pathogens. They serve as a barrier to infection when a nurse is handling feces or wound drainage, which may contain highly virulent microorganisms.

The gloves used for this purpose are usually clean but not sterile and are often of the disposable variety. Generally the gloves are removed in the patient's unit after handling the contaminated articles, and the patient's care is completed without the use of them.

Linen

Clothes, linens, blood pressure cuff covers, and similar items are usually sent to the hospital laundry for disinfection. The linen is double bagged; that is, the bag with the linen is placed in another bag, the outside surface of which is kept free of the pathogenic organisms. The bag is labeled to indicate that it contains contaminated linens and taken to a laundry isolation storage area or chute.

Most hospital laundries have standard laundering techniques that safely disinfect the linens from most microorganisms. The spore-forming organisms will require special treatment, usually with steam at a high temperature, to ensure their destruction.

The double bagging of linen requires an assistant, who stays outside the room and holds the outside bag. The nurse inside the room puts on her gown

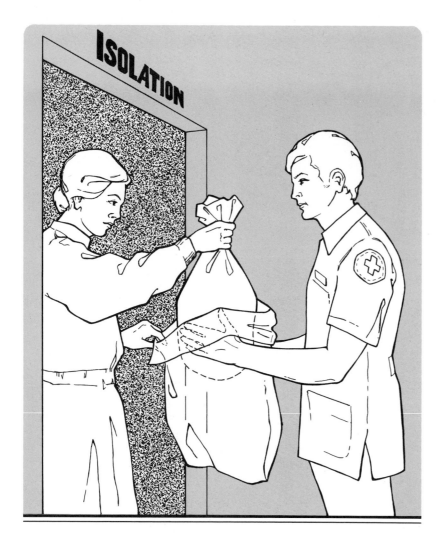

Figure 16-5. Double bagging is used to safely dispose of contaminated linen and supplies.

(and mask if indicated), closes the top of the linen bag securely, and takes the bag to the doorway to be placed in the outer bag. The nurse outside the room cuffs the upper part of the bag so that the hands are well covered and receives the soiled bag from the nurse in the room. Care is taken not to contaminate the outside of the outer bag. The nurse outside the room then closes the bag securely and tags it appropriately, according to agency policy. Some agencies use colored bags for the outer bag. A clean bag is then given to the nurse to place in the linen hamper in the patient's room (see Figure 16-5).

Garbage

Disposal of garbage is handled in a fashion similar to linen bags, that is, it requires an assistant outside the room and the double bagging technique. Once double bagged, the garbage is then transported directly to the incinerator by a chute or special area provided.

Food and Dishes

Food left on a tray is normally put down the patient's toilet or into the patient's plastic-lined garbage receptacle. Dishes are rinsed with cold water and then either soaked in disinfectant for a prescribed period of time or are dried and placed in a bag, sealed, and sterilized. Some hospitals use disposable plastic or paper dishes. Silver cutlery may be washed, dried, folded in a paper towel, and left in the patient's room.

A patient who is isolated usually keeps his or her own tray, and the dishes are transferred to it from the tray on which the food is delivered. In this way, the tray does not have to be disinfected after each meal.

Equipment

When isolation precautions are being carried out for a patient, it is usual to leave the equipment that is used regularly, such as a thermometer, blood pressure cuff, stethoscope, and tourniquet, in the patient's room until the patient is discharged or until the isolation practices are considered to be no longer necessary.

A good deal of equipment used in most hospitals today is disposable, thereby lessening the need for *concurrent disinfection* (disinfection of equipment used while the patient is ill). With disposable equipment, it is only necessary, in most instances, to bag it safely and have it destroyed. Most hospitals have incinerators that can be used for this purpose.

Equipment that cannot be disposed of, such as special instruments, is washed, double bagged, and sealed. The outside of the outer bag is kept clean. It can then be autoclaved to kill any present pathogens or soaked in a disinfectant for the prescribed time.

Used Dressings

Used dressings are disposed of in a bag in the patient's room, which is then double bagged in another garbage disposal bag and labeled "Isolation." The garbage is then sent to the incinerator for burning.

Taking Vital Signs

The sphygmomanometer, thermometer, and stethoscope are kept in the patient's room for the duration of isolation. A thermometer can be stored in a test tube that is taped to the mirror over the sink. The test tube is filled with a cotton fluff, to preserve the tip of the thermometer, and disinfectant solution, which is changed daily. Some agencies advocate the use of a clean thermometer each time a temperature is taken. Agency practices need to be checked in this regard.

To take the patient's pulse and respiration, the nurse must place the watch on a paper towel on the patient's overbed table. The nurse gowns if necessary and takes the vital signs. The nurse then removes the gown and washes both hands. The watch is then picked up, being careful to touch only the top or clean surface of the paper towel. The towel is discarded before leaving the room, but it can first be used to open the door of the isolation room.

If a separate blood pressure cuff is not supplied for the patient, it is necessary to have the patient put on a clean, long-sleeved gown. Thus the cuff touches only the clean gown. After determining the blood pressure, the apparatus is placed on clean paper towels. Any surfaces that have contacted the patient, for example, the bell of the stethoscope, are then sprayed with disinfectant after the nurse has degowned and washed both hands. The apparatus is not used again until the appropriate time has elapsed for disinfection, which is usually 20 minutes. Notations of the vital signs are done on a piece of paper left on the isolation cart outside the room. The paper then remains clean.

Procedure 16-2. Taking Vital Signs

Action	Explanation
Assemble Equipment	
1. Thermometer.	This equipment usually remains in the isolation unit while the patient is on isolation.
2. Sphygmomanometer.	
3. Blood pressure cuff.	
4. Stethoscope.	
5. Watch.	The watch is placed on a clean towel in a position so that the nurse can see it when taking the patient's pulse and respirations.
6. Book, record, or work sheet, pencil.	These are left outside the area and remain uncontaminated.
To take the vital signs	
1. Wash hands.	To remove any microorganisms that should not be transmitted to the patient.
2. Explain to the patient what you plan to do. Adjust the explanation to the patient's needs.	To reassure the patient by knowledge of what will happen. To identify the patient. To ascertain the appropriate route for the temperature measurement.

3. Gown if there is any danger of the uniform becoming contaminated.

Gown for children and confused patients.

4. Take the vital signs.

See vital sign techniques, Chapter 13.

5. Wash hands.

6. Remove the gown if one has been put on and wash hands again.

7. Pick up the watch and discard the paper towel.

Touch only the clean surface of paper towel.

8. Record vital signs.

Giving Medications

All medications are prepared according to agency practices and taken to the isolation unit. The medication tray and card are left outside the room, and the medication taken into the room. For oral medications, it may not be necessary to put on a gown if the patient is rational and cooperative. The medicine cup is discarded in the wastebasket or patient's bedside paper bag. The nurse hand washes prior to leaving the room and then charts the medications.

For injectable drugs, the nurse must don a gown. Only the prepared syringe and needle are taken into the room. Most agencies now use disposable needles and syringes. These are not put into wastebaskets in the patient's room but are usually placed in specially provided isolation containers at the nursing station. They may be wrapped in clean paper towels to transport them from the patient's room as required. Some agencies put a can in the room labeled to receive used needles. In this instance the isolation needles are placed in this can, and the disposable syringes are placed in the garbage receptacle.

Collecting Urine and Stool Specimens

The outside of the specimen container is kept clean. The lid is placed on the isolation cart outside the room, and the container is taken into the patient's bathroom and placed on clean paper towels. The nurse then puts on a gown and acquires the specimen of urine or feces. Urine is poured from the bedpan into a graduate pitcher and then some is poured into the specimen container, care being taken not to contaminate the outside of the container. Tongue blades are used to transfer stool specimens into the appropriate container; the blades then are wrapped in paper

towels and disposed of in the waste basket. The bedpan is cleaned and returned to the bedside unit. The nurse then hand washes, removes the gown, and repeats the hand washing. The specimen is then taken out of the room, covered, and labeled twice to denote the type of specimen and that it is an isolation specimen. Some agencies swab the outside of the bottle with a disinfectant; others place it in a paper bag prior to sending it to the laboratory.

Transporting Isolation Patients

Sometimes it is necessary to transport patients who are on isolation technique to other places such as the radiography department. Prior to transport, the patient is given a clean gown and robe. If the patient is on respiratory isolation, a mask or tissues and bag also may be provided so that proper tissue technique may be utilized. A clean sheet is then placed over the stretcher or wheelchair, making sure that all areas to be touched by the patient are covered. Stretcher straps can be fastened over the clean sheets, and the patient is instructed to keep the hands under the sheet. When transportation of the patient is finished, the linen is placed in the patient's hamper, and the transport vehicle is sprayed with disinfectant if necessary.

Handling Patients' Money, Letters, and Documents

Money collected from an isolation area does not usually require special precautions but may be sprayed with disinfectant to alleviate any apprehension on the part of personnel. If desired, the coins are placed on clean paper towels on the isolation cart outside the room, sprayed, and allowed to stand for a period of time. Outgoing mail likewise does not require disinfectant measures, except in cases of smallpox. The patient may need reminding that the letters should be kept free from expectorations or secretions. Thus, a mask may need to be worn while writing the note. Some agencies advocate that envelopes be sealed and stamped at the nurse's station.

Signing of documents by the patient is sometimes required. The document can be placed on the patient's overbed table on clean paper towels and can be read by the patient without the patient touching it, or it may be touched if the patient washed hands. Prior to signing the document, a paper towel can be placed over it, leaving just the exposed space required for signature. The patient can use his or her own pen or the nurse's pen, which can then be sprayed or wiped with disinfectant. The document is then taken outside with one hand, the paper towels are discarded, and the hands washed.

SUMMARY

Medical aseptic practices are involved in all nursing activities, since microorganisms are always present in the environment. A knowledge of medical asepsis and an awareness of how microorganisms are transmitted are essential for safe nursing practice. The chain of an infection involves the etiologic agent, the source, the exit, the method of transmission, the portal of entry, and the susceptibility of the person.

Many factors affect a person's susceptibility to infection. Included in the chapter are stress, nutritional status, fatigue, sex, genetic inheritance, age, and concomitant medical treatment.

There are three stages during the course of an infection: the incubation period, the period of illness, and the convalescent period. During the period of illness, signs and symptoms are evident. Localized infections are noted by the signs of inflammation, that is, swelling, redness, heat, pain, and loss of function. Systemic symptoms include fever, malaise, anorexia, headache, and lymph node enlargement.

Many measures are employed to prevent infections and to maintain health. These are categorized as environmental measures and individual measures. The environmental measures include preventive programs for immunization, communicable disease laboratory services, health centers that educate people about health, and sanitation services. Individual preventive measures are employed to strengthen the body's barrier against infections and to minimize the number of microorganisms present. Examples that strengthen the body's barriers are adequate nutrition, immunization, and adequate rest. Personal hygienic practices minimize the numbers of microorganisms.

The prevention of infections for ill persons requires the use of medical aseptic practices such as cleaning, disinfection, and sterilization. Methods of disinfection include hot-air ovens, steam, radiation, ultrasonic waves, chemical methods, and pasteurization.

Various types of isolation techniques are employed in accordance with the way in which specific pathogens are transmitted. Seven types of isolation are discussed: respiratory, enteric, wound and skin, blood, strict, protective, and suspect. The purpose of each of these types is to keep pathogens within a defined area. General guidelines that apply to all types of isolation and the equipment necessary for setting up an isolation unit are included.

Specific isolation nursing techniques are outlined such as hand washing, gowning, applying and removing face masks, and gloving. The way in which other general nursing measures are handled for the isolation patient are also outlined. These include the handling of linen, disposal of food and garbage, disinfection of dishes and other equipment, the taking of vital signs, administration of medications, and collecting specimens.

SUGGESTED ACTIVITIES

1. In the nursing laboratory set up an isolation unit. With a classmate as a patient in the unit take his/her pulse and blood pressure. Serve the patient a tray as for a meal.

2. Interview a patient who is or has been on isolation in a hospital. Find out how that person viewed the isolation precautions.

SUGGESTED READINGS

Castle, Mary. May 1975. Isolation: precise procedures for better protection. *Nursing 75* 5(5):50–57.

Photographs and step-by-step techniques are used to outline procedures in isolation care.

Garner, Julia S., and Kaiser, Allen B. April 1972. How often is isolation needed? *American Journal of Nursing* 72:733–737.

    A survey of infections in hospitals and the types of isolation practices indicated for communicable disease are discussed.

SELECTED REFERENCES

Dubay, Elaine C., and Grubb, Reba D. 1973. *Infection: prevention and control.* St. Louis: The C. V. Mosby Co.

Greene, V. W. November 1969. Microbial contamination: control in hospitals. *Hospitals* 43(11):78.

Hardy, C. S. August 1973. Infection control: what can one nurse do? *Nursing 73* 3(8):18–21.

Jenny, J. November 1976. What you should be doing about infection control. *Nursing 76* 6(11):78–79.

Lee, R. V. December 1973. Antimicrobial therapy. *American Journal of Nursing* 73:2044–2048.

Litsky, Bertha Yanis. 1973. *Hospital sanitation, an administrative program.* Chicago: Modern Hospital Press, McGraw-Hill Publications Co.

McInnes, Mary Elizabeth. 1975. *Essentials of communicable disease,* 2nd ed. St. Louis: The C. V. Mosby Co.

National League for Nursing. 1975. *Infection control.* Pub. No. 20-1582. New York: National League for Nursing.

Nordmark, Madelyn T., and Rohweder, Anne W. 1975. *Scientific foundations of nursing,* 3rd ed. Philadelphia: J. B. Lippincott Co.

Streeter, S., et al. March 1967. Hospital infection—a necessary risk? *American Journal of Nursing* 67:526–533.

US, Department of Health, Education, and Welfare. 1975. *Isolation techniques for use in hospitals,* 2nd ed. DHEW Publication No. (CDC) 76-8314.

CHAPTER 17

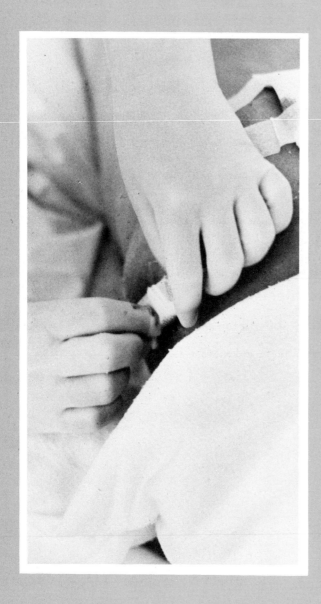

WOUND CARE AND SURGICAL ASEPSIS

Open and Closed Methods of Wound Care

Dressings

Dressing Materials

Changing Dressings

DRAINS

Cleansing the Drain Site

REMOVING SKIN CLIPS AND SUTURES

Common Methods of Suturing

Guidelines for Removing Sutures

Removing Sutures

Retention Sutures

IRRIGATIONS

Wound Irrigation

Eye Irrigation

Ear Irrigation (External Auditory Canal)

Gargling

Throat Irrigation

Vaginal Irrigation (Douche)

SUPPORTING AND IMMOBILIZING WOUNDS

Materials

Principles Related to the Use of Binders and Bandages

Guidelines for Bandaging

Basic Turns in Bandaging

Common Types of Binders

HEAT AND COLD THERAPY

Physiologic Responses to Heat and Cold

Perception of Heat and Cold

Tolerance to Heat and Cold

HEAT APPLICATIONS

Reasons for Applying Heat

Factors of Concern in Regard to Applications of Heat

Contraindications to the Application of Heat

Moist Applications of Heat

Compresses and Hot Wet Packs

Dry Applications of Heat

COLD APPLICATIONS

Reasons for Applying Cold

Factors of Concern in Regard to Cold Applications

Contraindications to the Application of Cold

Moist Applications of Cold

Dry Applications of Cold

OBJECTIVES

- Describe the appearance of a clean wound.

- List the principles of surgical asepsis.

- Define the terms commonly used to classify wounds.

- Demonstrate safe handling of sterile supplies.

- Demonstrate gowning technique.

- Explain the technique for preoperative skin preparation.

- Change a dressing using good sterile technique.

- Describe how to shorten a drain.

- Demonstrate beginning skill in irrigation techniques.

- Explain the factors that affect and promote wound healing.

- Demonstrate the five basic turns used in bandaging.

- Demonstrate beginning skill in applying binders.

- Explain the body's physiologic responses to heat and cold.

- Apply relevant principles in nursing intervention involving the application of heat and cold.

- Describe the contraindications in the application of heat and cold.

Although the body is remarkably protected from trauma (injury) by the skin and by the subcutaneous and adipose tissues, trauma does occur intentionally and unintentionally. *Intentional* trauma is that which occurs during therapy, such as an operation, venipuncture, or radiation. Though it is therapeutic to remove a tumor, the surgeon must cut into the body tissues, thus traumatizing them.

Unintentional wounds are acquired by accident, for example, a fractured arm from an automobile accident. If the tissues are traumatized without a break in the skin, the result is a closed wound. A blow from a hard instrument that causes bruising is called a *contusion,* which is considered to be a closed wound. An open wound occurs when the skin or mucous membrane surface is broken.

Wounds are further described according to the presence or absence of infection. A *clean* wound is one in which there are no pathogenic organisms. An *infected* or contaminated wound is one in which pathogens are present. Wounds that are produced intentionally are generally clean, while those that are unintentional and open are considered contaminated.

One of the functions of the nurse is to promote wound healing, which may involve changing dressings, shortening and maintaining drains, applying heat and cold, and applying bandages and binders. Surgical asepsis is implemented for most of these measures to prevent the introduction of pathogens to vulnerable wounds.

TYPES OF WOUNDS

Wounds are frequently described according to the manner in which the wound is acquired. There are six categories of wounds by this classification: (a) incised, (b) contused, (c) abraded, (d) puncture, (e) lacerated, and (f) penetrating.

An *incised wound* is an incision made with a sharp instrument. It can be intentional, such as a wound made with a surgeon's scalpel, or accidental, such as a wound made from a sharp knife.

A *contused wound* is a closed wound that occurs as the result of a blow from a blunt instrument. As a result, the skin appears bruised (ecchymotic) because of the release of blood into the tissues from the damaged blood vessels. Contused wounds are usually unintentional, although contusions of some tissues may occur because of surgical manipulation.

An *abraded wound* is a type of open wound that occurs as a result of friction; for example, a scraped knee from a fall on the road surface. Abraded wounds can also be intentional, such as a dermal abrasion of the skin in which the superficial layers of the skin are removed either by sandpapering or by an abrasive machine, in order to remove scars and pock marks.

A *puncture wound* is also called a *stab wound.* It is an open wound made by a sharp instrument that penetrates the skin and the underlying tissues. Puncture wounds can be accidental, such as a wound made by stepping on a nail, or they can be intentional, such as a stab wound made by a surgeon for the insertion of a drain for drainage of an area. Venipuncture and intramuscular injections are common puncture wounds induced intentionally.

Lacerated wounds or lacerations occur when the tissues are torn apart, resulting in irregular edges. Lacerations are accidental and can be seen often as the result of an automobile accident or from accidents involving machinery.

A *penetrating wound* is one in which an instru- ment penetrates deeply into the tissues through the skin or mucous membrane. Usually penetrating wounds are accidental, as from a bullet or the pen- etration of metal fragments. In a penetrating wound, a bullet, for example, may lodge in an internal organ.

WOUND HEALING

Measures that Promote Wound Healing

Factors that affect tissue healing were discussed in Chapter 8. In addition to these, there are a number of measures that can promote wound healing.

1. Protection against infection of the wound by the use of sterile technique and appropriate immuniza- tions; for example, tetanus antitoxin for a wound in which there is soil and in which the tetanus bacillus may be present.

2. Protecting a wound from additional injury and stress, such as additional stretching and pulling of tissues.

3. If a wound has draining exudate, the patient needs to assume a position that will encourage the drainage. For example, if a patient has a wound on his or her side, a side-lying position on the wound side will encourage the drainage to flow.

4. If a wound is infected, the process of localizing the infection is promoted by the local application of heat and by restricting movement of the part. Heat brings additional blood to the area, thus increasing the antibody supply to the area and nourishment to the tissues. Restricting movement discourages the spread of the inflammatory process to adjacent areas.

5. Elevating an inflamed body part above the level of the heart facilitates the return venous flow and lymphatic drainage. As a result, swelling is fre- quently reduced, and circulation within the affected area is improved.

6. The application of cold to a recent contusion can assist in localized constriction of the arterioles and consequently assist in preventing the leakage of blood into the tissues. Cold applications decrease swelling (edema). Resting the part can also help to reduce the swelling and to decrease the bleeding.

Principles of Wound Healing

1. Healing can occur in two basic ways: by repair of the injured cells and by regeneration of tissue. If the wound is not large and if cells are not completely destroyed, they can often repair themselves with ade- quate nourishment and rest. Some tissues of the body can regenerate, that is, new cells can be produced and appropriately organized as specific tissue. Nervous tissue, elastic tissue, and muscle tissue have very lit- tle, if any, ability to regenerate.

2. The protective covering of the body, the skin and mucous membrane, normally have microorganisms present on them. Therefore the use of a disinfectant on tissues surrounding a wound decreases the num- ber of organisms in the area and thus decreases the chances of an infection developing in the wound.

3. The presence of lysozyme, an enzyme present in skin secretions, nasal secretions, and saliva, is bac- teriostatic to many bacteria. It is therefore a natural barrier to infections of intact skin and mucous mem- branes.

4. Normal skin is relatively dry. Excessive and con- tinuous moisture, however, can cause skin macera- tion. Excessive dryness of the skin, on the other hand, results in scaling and cracking. Mucous membranes are normally moist. Excessive dryness of the mucous membranes results in limited cleansing of the area, which is normally performed by the mucous secre- tions.

5. The circulatory system, specifically the blood, supplies a wound with the nourishment it requires in order to heal. Therefore, any factors that affect the circulation to an area affect the healing process. In addition, any factor that limits the flow of debris and toxins from the area also inhibits the wound healing process.

6. Normal healing of a wound occurs from the deepest point to the surface. Any foreign materials,

such as glass, metal, or a surgical wound drain, prevent healing of that area. If the skin of a wound heals over, leaving foreign material and allowing the subsequent formation of pus, an abscess forms.

Factors Inhibiting Wound Healing

The progress of wound healing can be halted by a number of problems.

1. *Infection.* Infection not only halts the healing process but also damages additional tissue cells, thus increasing the size of a wound, both in width and depth.

2. *Hematoma.* A *hematoma* is a blood clot. Usually blood in a wound is gradually absorbed back into the systemic circulation as debris from the wound. However, a large clot may take weeks to dissolve and absorb, thus inhibiting the healing process. These hematomas can be removed if they are inhibiting healing for a prolonged period.

3. *Foreign objects.* Foreign objects, such as a piece of wood, or microorganisms, can also inhibit healing. The object may well form an abscess before it is removed. This abscess is made up of serum, fibrin, dead tissue cells, and *leukocytes* (white blood cells), which form a thick liquid called *pus.* This stage in the inflammatory process is known as *suppuration.*

If the foreign object is left in the wound, pus will continue to be formed and will either drain by breaking through the skin surface or by being absorbed into the lymphatic system. Microorganisms that cause pus to be formed are called *pyogenic,* but not all microorganisms are pyogenic.

4. *Localized ischemia. Ischemia* is defined as localized anemia due to the obstruction of the flow of blood to a part. Dressings, bandages, and casts that are applied too tightly can cause ischemia of an area, as can the internal obstruction of the blood vessels by a blood clot.

Appearance of a Clean Healing Wound

Wound healing by primary union (first intention) occurs usually when the tissue surfaces have been approximated by sutures. A healing wound has a characteristic appearance.

1. The area around the wound will appear reddened (natural inflammatory response).

2. There will be some serous drainage. *Serous* refers to the clear portion of the blood. The amount varies with the location of the wound. Perineal wounds usually have a large amount of drainage; wounds of the face have less.

The serous drainage will appear clear or slightly brown because of the presence of some old blood, and it is watery. New wounds usually have some sanguineous (bloody) drainage for a few days. When both serous and sanguineous drainage occur, the drainage is referred to as *serosanguineous.*

3. A blood clot may appear in the wound. This provides the framework for the growth of new tissue in some wounds.

4. Pink-white tissue (granulation tissue) appears at the skin edges and grows in to fill the wound.

5. Often drains are placed in deep wounds to keep them open until the underlying tissues have healed. Deep wounds need to heal from the bottom so that fluid is not trapped in the wound. Skin regenerates more rapidly and can seal over deep tissues first.

6. By the seventh to eighth day, granulation (pink) tissue will have covered most wounds.

Wound healing by secondary union (second intention) requires the formation of considerably more granulation tissue. These wounds are usually large, and the skin edges cannot be approximated; they take much longer to heal, and there is usually extensive scar tissue. Second intention healing also can occur subsequent to a wound infection.

PRINCIPLES OF SURGICAL ASEPSIS

Surgical asepsis has been defined as those measures which render and maintain objects free from microorganisms (pathogens and nonpathogens). It is also referred to as *sterile technique.* Sterile technique is employed in many situations, such as the operating room and delivery rooms, and for many techniques such as dressing changes, catheterizations, administering injections, and intravenous solutions. Whenever the skin barrier is broken or whenever a body cavity that is considered free from organisms is entered, sterile technique is employed. In all situations basic principles apply.

1. *Sterile objects become contaminated unless touched only by other sterile objects.* In other words:

Sterile to sterile = Sterile

Sterile to clean = Contaminated

Sterile to contaminated = Contaminated

Sterile to questionable = Contaminated

2. *Sterile items that are out of vision or below the waist level of the nurse are considered contaminated.* Sterile objects can be accidentally touched by unsterile objects if not in view. Thus nurses should never leave a sterile field unattended. They also need to hold objects in view and above waist level, and not to turn their backs on a sterile field.

3. *Sterile objects are contaminated by airborne sources.* The environment in which sterile technique is carried out must be as clean as possible. Such areas are usually damp cleansed with detergent germicides to reduce the number of contaminants in the area and to reduce the transfer of them by air currents. Most institutions provide a room designed to be used for only clean and sterile techniques. Clothing worn by personnel must also be clean. Headgear, when worn, needs to cover the hair completely in order to prevent particles and organisms dropping from the hair strands.

Airborne contaminants can be dispersed by droplets from the mouth and nose, especially when talking, laughing, sneezing, or coughing. Therefore nurses are advised to minimize talking over sterile fields or to wear masks in order not to contaminate the field. Any nurse who has a mild upper respiratory infection should refrain from performing sterile measures or should double-mask while performing such tasks.

Air currents can be produced by moving objects. Therefore traffic must be kept to a minimum, and items should not be moved over a sterile field. Sterile bundles or packages are opened in such a manner that the nurse does not reach over the sterile field, since particles can drop from the nurse's arm. Once a sterile item is exposed, the nurse needs to refrain from reaching over it and must work efficiently to minimize air contact with the sterile objects. Moving sterile objects as little as possible also minimizes chances of their becoming contaminated.

4. *Moist or damp sterile fields are considered contaminated if the surface below is not sterile or if the surface is exposed to the air.* Once moisture penetrates through a sterile object such as a drape, capillary action (a drawing action) brings microorganisms from the unclean surface through to the sterile surface. To prevent this, sterile metal trays are often used beneath sterile objects so that if liquids such as disinfectants need to be added to the sterile field, they are confined to the sterile area. Thus capillary action from an unclean surface is impossible. However, sterile covers that become moistened need to be considered contaminated because of the capillary action with airborne contaminants. Therefore care should be taken when pouring solutions to avoid contamination.

5. *Objects are rendered sterile by the processes of dry and moist heat, chemicals, and radiation.* Sterility is maintained by storing sterile articles in double wrappers for prescribed periods of time. Storage areas need to be clean and dry.

6. *Fluids flow in the direction of gravity.* Wet forceps are held with the tips down. If the tips are held up, the fluid will flow to the handle, become contaminated by the hands, and then flow back down and contaminate the tips when the forceps are pointed downward. The surgical hand scrub also applies this principle. The hands are held higher than the elbows when scrubbing to prevent contaminants from the forearms reaching the hands. Hands are dried from the fingertips toward the elbows (from the cleanest to the least clean area).

7. *The edges of a sterile field are considered contaminated.* Because opened drape edges are in contact with an unsterile surface, a one-inch margin around a drape is considered contaminated. When opening disposable packages or removing lifting forceps from a container of disinfectant, the edges of the container are not touched with the forceps because they are also considered contaminated.

8. *Wound exudates are considered contaminated, and dry wounds are considered clean.* Sterile swabs that are used to cleanse a wound become contaminated and are therefore discarded away from the sterile field in a separate receptacle such as a paper bag. When cleansing wounds, each swab is used only once. The wound is cleansed from the center outward toward the skin and from incisions to drain sites (from the cleanest to the least clean area).

9. *Conscientiousness, alertness, and honesty are necessary qualities in maintaining surgical asepsis.* When an object is contaminated its appearance is unchanged. Only the person who saw it become contaminated would know that it was, and only that person can correct the situation.

HANDLING STERILE SUPPLIES

Sterile supplies are handled by using sterile forceps, by wearing sterile gloves, or by enveloping the hands in a sterile drape, but never by the naked hand. Prior to handling sterile equipment, the nurse in all instances needs to scrub hands and forearms thoroughly, and, in some situations, needs to wear a mask, a sterile gown, and sterile gloves. The methods for hand washing, gloving, and gowning are different from methods practiced for medical asepsis because the purposes are different. In surgical asepsis, the goal is to prevent the transfer of any microorganisms, pathogens, and nonpathogens, to the patient or to an area on the patient.

Hand Washing in Surgical Asepsis

In surgical asepsis, hands should be thoroughly cleansed for about three minutes. When washing hands, they are held above the level of the elbows, since the elbows are considered more contaminated after scrubbing than the hands. Water then runs from the area of least contamination to the area of greatest contamination. It is essential that rings and watches are first removed and that the nails are short. The hands are cleansed progressively and thoroughly from the fingertips to the elbows. A nail cleanser or brush can be used to cleanse the nails early in the scrub. It is important to lather well and rinse frequently. Chemical cleansing alone is no substitute for mechanical cleansing done conscientiously. Chemical action, however, is also important, and antiseptic detergents are often used. Rinsing and drying are done in the same manner, from the fingertips to the elbows. The water faucet is then closed by using a paper towel or by a knee gatch or foot pedal.

The Surgical Hand Scrub

Longer hand scrubs of up to ten minutes are employed in the operating room and delivery rooms, particularly at the beginning of the day. Shorter scrubs of three minutes are sufficient between operations but are essential, since bacterial growth is facilitated on warm, moist hands enclosed in surgical gloves. After the scrub, the hands are maintained above the elbows and are held away from the body (see Figure 17-1). If bar soap is used, it is discarded after the scrub. A sterile cloth towel may be supplied for drying in the operating room. One half is used to dry one hand and arm, and the other half is used for

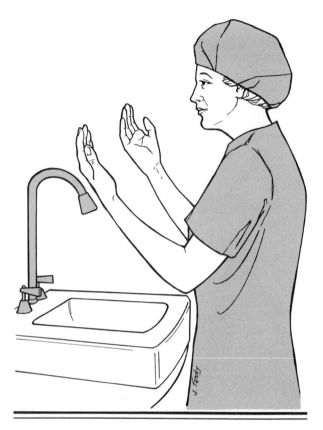

Figure 17-1.   A surgical hand scrub. Note the hands above the elbows.

the other hand and arm. Prior to surgical scrubs, head gear and masks must be applied.

Opening Sterile Wrapped Packages

Sterile packages of such items as dressing gauzes, catheterization trays, or dressing sets are commercially prepared in paper or plastic containers. In hospitals, a double-thickness linen or special paper may be used to wrap nondisposable items. Sterile equipment is stored in clean, dry areas to preserve its sterility. If the equipment is moist or damp, it is considered contaminated and should not be used. The sterilization dates should also be checked to ensure that the wrapped item has not been kept beyond the sterilization period. Frequently, chemical indicator tape is used to fasten sterile packages. These indicator strips change color during the sterilization process, indicating that the contents are sterilized. If the color change is not evident, the package is considered unsterile.

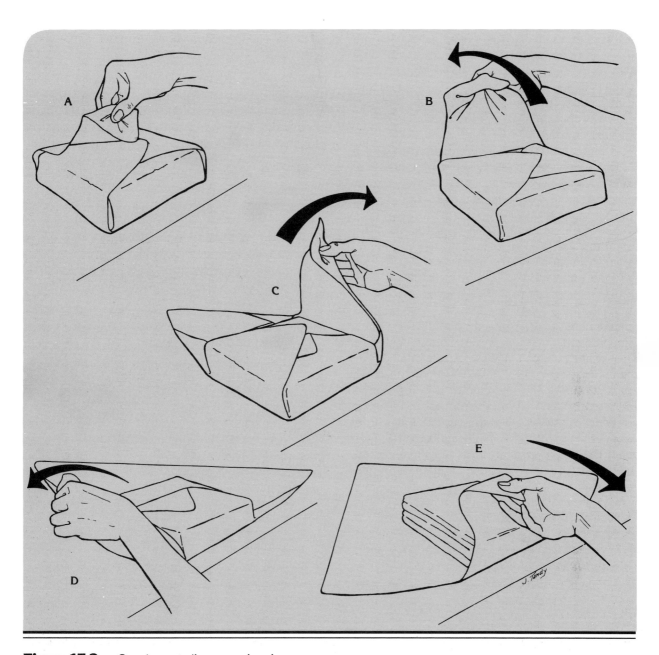

Figure 17-2. Opening a sterile wrapped package.

Sterile packages may be opened by (a) placing them on a table and unwrapping them in such a way that the sterility of the contents, including the inside of the wrapper, is maintained or (b) by holding the outside of the package with one hand and unwrapping it with the other hand. Prior to opening any sterile item, the nurse's hands must be thoroughly washed.

Sterile items are packaged in such a way that the package can be opened without contaminating the contents. A large, clean working area above waist level must be used. The indicator tape on the package is removed rather than torn and is discarded. Tape that is not removed from the linen wrapper later creates problems in the laundry process.

Place the package in such a way that it can be opened away from the body. The flap farthest away is opened first, with care not to reach over the sterile field. The nurse needs to hold his arm out at the side or lateral to the package. Then the side flaps are opened, and the flap nearest the nurse is opened last. When opening the flaps, care must be taken not to touch the inside of the wrapper. Usually the corners are turned outward, so that the nurse can grasp these easily and avoid touching the inside (see Figure 17–2). When opening the last flap, it is important to stand well back from the package—6–12 inches—in order to avoid contamination from the nurse's uniform. If space on the table is limited, it may be necessary to fan fold this flap so that it remains above the waist level of the nurse. Some sterile trays have an additional inner wrapping. This is opened in similar fashion, but sterile forceps must be used.

In some situations, it is also necessary to close or loosely wrap a sterile package. For example, after solutions have been added to a dressing tray, the tray may need to be rewrapped for transport to the bedside. A sterile package is wrapped in the *reverse* order to that of unwrapping. The proximal flap is closed first to prevent reaching across the sterile field, the side flaps next, and the distal flap last.

Smaller or Light Items

Smaller items can be opened by holding them in one hand and opening them with the other hand in the same manner described above. The sterile item can then be transferred to a sterile field or handed to another person. Before the transfer, it is important to enclose the hand holding the package in the sterile wrapper. This is done by grasping all corners of the wrapper with the other hand and securing them above the level wrist of the first hand, thus enclosing the hand completely. The item can then be dropped safely onto a sterile field or, with arm extended, handed to another person who is wearing sterile gloves (see Figure 17–3).

Commercially Prepared Packages

Many disposable items, such as syringes and some dressings, are prepared in sterile paper packages. Usually one end of this package has some unsealed edges, which the nurse grasps (one in each thumb and index finger) and peels apart, taking care not touch the inside of the wrapper. This wrapper can be laid on a table surface and used as a sterile area, or it may be discarded, depending upon the needs of the situation (see Figure 17–4).

Using Sterile Forceps

There are many styles of forceps used for handling sterile supplies. Some of the forceps used most commonly by nurses are:

1. The Kelly or hemostatic forceps with a straight or curved tip (Figure 17-5).
2. The thumb or tissue forceps with or without teeth (Figure 17-5).
3. The handling or sponge forceps, also referred to as a transfer or pickup forceps (Figure 17-5).
4. The Bard-Parker transfer forceps.

Regardless of the type of forceps used, the following principles apply in their use. Forceps are useful in many situations that require the transfer of sterile items from one place to another, for example,

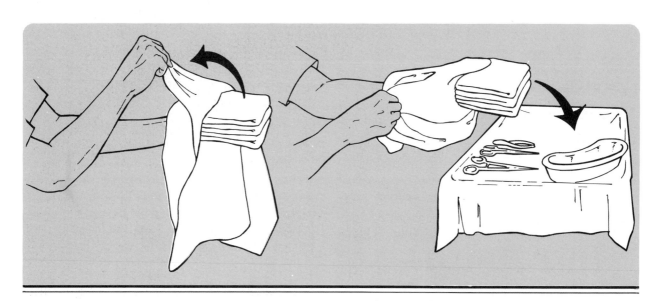

Figure 17-3.   Placing sterile wrapped supplies on a sterile tray. Note that the hand is covered by the wrapper.

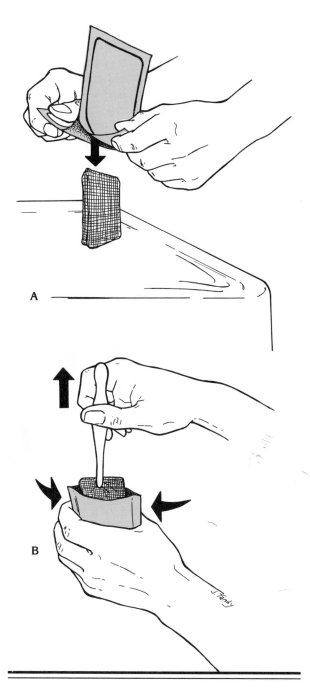

Figure 17-4. Removing contents from sterile commercially prepared packages. Note how package is cupped in **B**.

placing sterile cotton balls or gauzes from a large sterile stock container onto a dressing or catheterization tray.

The practice of storing lifting forceps in germicidal solution and storing sponges and gauzes in large metal containers is decreasing, since the sterility of these is questionable. If these practices are utilized,

the nurse needs to ascertain that the containers are sterilized and the solutions changed at least daily.

1. *Sterile forceps are always held above and in front of the waist* to prevent inadvertent contamination out of the nurse's range of vision.

2. *The tips of the forceps are always considered sterile and need to be held down,* particularly when they become wet. This prevents liquids from flowing from the sterile tips to unsterile hands, becoming contaminated, and then flowing back by gravity to the tips

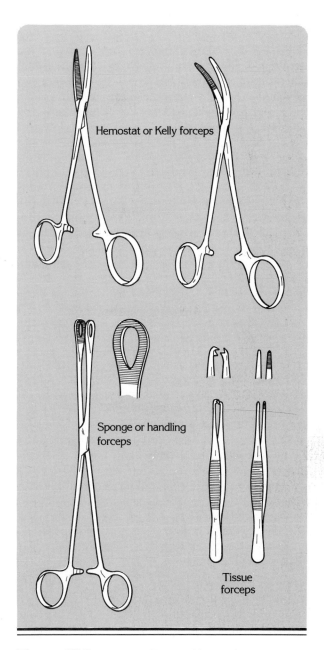

Figure 17-5. Types of surgical forceps.

when they are down again. The nurse needs to learn to abduct her elbows when handling forceps. This abduction facilitates keeping forceps tips in the downward position.

3. *The handles of forceps are considered contaminated except when handled by sterile gloves.* Forceps are placed onto sterile trays with the tips inside the sterile field and the handles outside or at the edge of the sterile field when handled by the naked hand. The entire forceps is placed inside the sterile field when the nurse is wearing sterile gloves.

4. When removing sterile items from a container, *the forceps tips and/or the item should be kept away from the edges of the container or disposable paper package.* The edges are exposed to air and are considered contaminated. Thus, when lifting forceps from a germicidal solution container, the sides and top edges are not touched. When removing gauzes from commercially prepared paper packages, the flaps must be pulled well apart or the package cupped.

5. *Forceps tips that are moistened with germicidal solution should not touch a sterile field when transferring objects.* Sterile articles are dropped gently onto a sterile field. Excess moisture on the forceps tips can first be removed by gently tapping the tips while holding them in the downward position over the solution container. Caution is needed to avoid touching the top edges of the container, which are contaminated.

Pouring Sterile Solutions

The need to handle sterile solutions is frequently encountered by the nurse. Many solutions are contained in sterilized solution bottles, such as those for intravenous fluids, and in vials or ampules, which are used for parenteral medications. The methods of handling these are discussed in Chapters 30 and 36, respectively. Often the need arises to pour a sterile solution from a large or small bottle into another container, such as a solution basin.

Flasks or bottles containing sterile solutions are considered sterile on the inside and contaminated on the outside. Thus, when removing the cap of a bottle, only the outer unsterile surface must be touched. Because the inner part of the cap, including the inner rim, is sterile, the cap, once removed, is placed on the table with the top of the cap against the table or held in one's hand with the inner side pointed downward. This principle also applies to lids of large containers that hold other sterile materials, such as gauzes or cotton fluffs.

Prior to pouring the sterile solutions, it is recommended that a small amount of solution be poured into a sink or waste container in order to cleanse the lip of the bottle opening. The bottle should be held with its label on the upward side to avoid the possibility of wetting it. When pouring the solution, care must be taken not to contaminate the receiving solution basin from contact with the outside of the bottle or the underlying sterile drapes from undue splashing of solution. It is important also to avoid reaching over the sterile field. Therefore the bottle should be held outside the sterile field as much as possible and the top of the bottle kept at a reasonable distance from the solution container. This distance will vary with the size of the bottle. A distance of 4–6 inches is recommended for large bottles, but the distance can be decreased for smaller bottles. The solution flask is then recapped, using the technique described, touching only the outside of the cap.

The Use of Drapes

Sterile drapes are often used in settings to expand a sterile field. These are particularly useful when sterile gloves are worn. Extensive draping procedures are used in the operating rooms, and the student is referred to agency policies for these techniques.

Many sterile trays such as dressing, catheterization, or special diagnostic trays (lumbar puncture) are equipped with sterile drapes. Sizes of drapes vary, but commonly they are approximately 30 cm by 45–60 cm (1 ft by 1½–2 ft). Some drapes are plain pieces of cloth or paper; others have holes in the center. Placement of drapes depends upon the number of drapes present and the procedure involved.

Many drapes are placed in sterile packages in such a way that the nurse can pick up the drape with the naked hand by one corner without contaminating the rest of it (Figure 17–6, *A*). Care must be taken not to contaminate it with the nurse's uniform (Figure 17–6, *B*). By lifting the drape with one hand, the opposite corner of the drape can be grasped with the other hand (Figure 17-6, *C*). The drape is then placed in such a way that the farthest side from the nurse is placed first and then the near side last (Figure 17-6, *D*). This prevents the nurse from reaching across the sterile field. If gloves are used to handle drapes, care must be taken to avoid contamination of fingertips on the bedclothes. This is done by enclosing the fingertips in the corners of the drape prior to placing the drape.

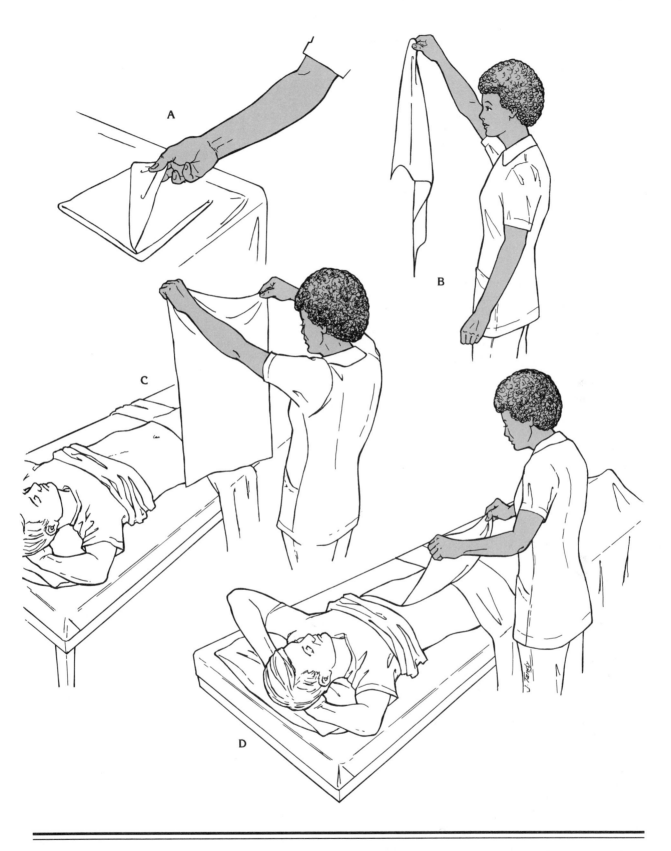

Figure 17-6.   Placing a sterile drape. **A,** Pick up drape at one corner; **B,** hold drape above waist level and away from the nurse's uniform; **C,** hold drape at both corners; and **D,** hang drape down far side first.

DONNING STERILE GLOVES

Sterile gloves are packaged with a cuff of about 2 inches. A surgical scrub must precede gloving. There are two methods for donning sterile gloves: the open method and the closed method. The former method is most frequently employed in areas of nursing practice other than the operating room, since the latter method is dependent upon wearing a sterile gown.

Open Method

To put on the first glove, the nurse grasps the glove by its cuff (on the palmar side) with the thumb and first finger of one hand, being careful to touch only the inside of the glove (Figure 17-7, *A*). The sterility of the outside of the glove must be maintained. Remember that the nurse's hand is considered contaminated. The other hand is then inserted into the glove, and the glove is pulled in place by the hand grasping the cuff (Figure 17-7, *B*). The cuff is left turned down, and care is taken not to touch the wrist.

To put on the second glove, the sterile gloved hand must be used. The second glove is picked up by inserting the gloved fingers under its cuff (Figure 17-7, *C*). This retains the sterility of the outside of both gloves. The second glove is then pulled on (Fig. 17-7, *D*), paying particular attention to the gloved thumb, so that it does not touch the palmar skin or wrist of the second hand. The thumb can be held up and back, or it can exert a pull on the cuff away from the skin. The cuffs of both gloves may then be unfolded by touching only the sterile sides.

If a sterile gown is also being worn, this same technique can be used, but the cuffs are pulled well up over the cuffs of the sleeves. See the section on gowning technique in this chapter.

Closed Method

This method can be used only when a sterile gown is worn, as in the operating room. The gown is first put on so that the hands are in only as far as the cuff seam of the sleeve, and the gown is tied by another person. To put on the gloves, the nurse first grasps the inside of one sleeve cuff with the thumb and index finger. One glove is then picked up and placed palm side down on the palm of the other hand, with the fingers pointing toward the elbow. The cuff of the glove and the gown cuff lie together. The glove is then put on. For a right glove, the left hand (still covered by the

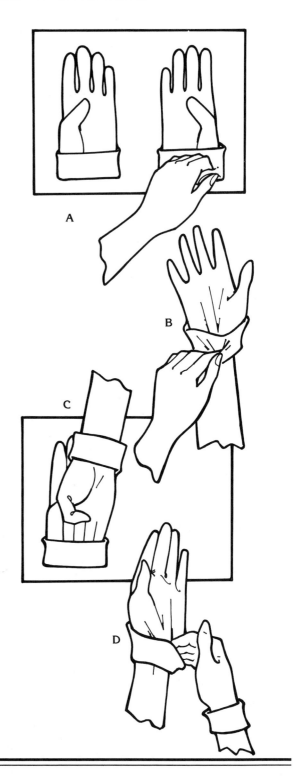

Figure 17-7.   Donning sterile gloves (open method). **A,** Pick up first glove by its cuff; **B,** put on first glove; **C,** pick up second glove under the cuff; and **D,** put on second glove.

sterile gown) grasps the top edge of the glove cuff, and the right hand (also covered by the sterile gown) grasps the bottom edge of the glove cuff. The glove is then pulled on by the left hand, while the right hand directs its fingers into the glove. Care must be taken not to expose the fingers. The left glove is put on in the same manner, except that the gloved right hand can now handle the glove.

DONNING A STERILE GOWN

Sterile gowns are worn in the operating room and the delivery room and when open wound technique is used, as for the burned patient. The gown may be picked up from a sterile pack, or it may be handed to the nurse by someone who is already gowned and gloved. To keep the gowns sterile they are folded inside out and are touched only on the inside. The outside must be kept sterile, and when donned, the part of the gown that is considered sterile is that above the anterior waist and the anterior aspect of the sleeves. Parts of the gown that are considered unsterile are the back of the sleeves, below the waist, the collar area, and under the arms. The gown is put on after the head turban, mask, and surgical scrub.

Procedure 17-1.   Technique for Donning a Sterile Gown

ACTION	EXPLANATION
Assemble equipment	
1. Sterile gown.	
To don gown	
1. Remove watch and rings.	Jewelry can harbor microorganisms.
2. Wash hands.	To remove microorganisms.
3. Pick up the gown by grasping the folded gown at the neck band. Stand well back (1 foot) from the sterile bundle (see Figure 17-8, A).	The neck area and the inside of the gown are considered contaminated.
4. Hold the gown out at arm's length and allow it to unfold naturally (Figure 17-8, B). The inside of the gown (the armholes) must face the wearer.	Do not shake the gown, since this creates air currents or the gown may accidentally touch unsterile objects.

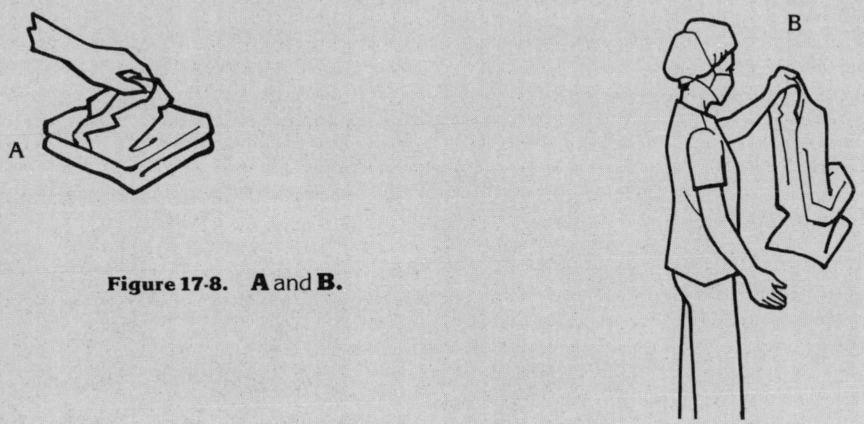

Figure 17-8.   A and B.

Procedure 17-1. Cont'd.

5. Hold the gown by the open inside shoulder seams and put each hand alternately into the armholes (Figure 17-8, *C*).

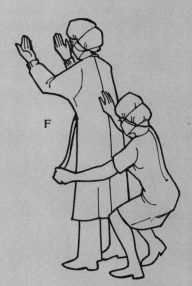

Figure 17-8.   C and **D.**

6. Extend the arms and hold the hands upward at shoulder height when putting them through the armholes.

This holds the gown in place and lessens the chance of contaminating the gown.

7. An unsterile person (circulating nurse) will then assist in pulling the sleeves onto your arms by working from behind and inside the gown. The sleeves may be pulled over the hands, or they may be pulled so that the seams of the cuff are at the fingertips (see Figure 17-8, *D*).

See open and closed methods for gloving.

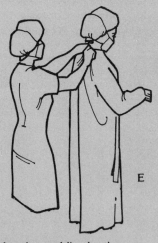

Figure 17-8.   E and **F.**

8. The gown is then fastened at the neckline by the circulating nurse, and the open edges folded or held together (Figure 17-8, *E*).

9. The waist ties are then fastened by the unsterile nurse from behind. These ties are grasped at the tip after the gown wearer bends at the waist (Figure 17-8, *F*).

Bending allows the ties to fall free and away from the sterile gown.

CARE OF WOUNDS

The types of wounds have been previously described in this chapter. Just as there are many types of wounds, there are also many ways of caring for wounds. In general, the care varies in accordance with the type of wound, the size of the wound, the amount of exudate present, whether it is an open or closed wound, the location, the personal preference of the physician, and the presence of complicating factors.

Goals of Wound Care

The goals of wound care are as follows:

1. *To prevent infection* from the entrance of microorganisms through the broken protective barriers of the skin and mucous membranes. This is accomplished by using sterile technique when caring for wounds, by using antiseptic on the skin, and, on occasion, by using antibiotics.

2. *To prevent further tissue damage* of fragile healing wounds from friction or injury. This is done by protecting the wound with dressings and by immobilizing the part with slings or binders.

3. *To encourage measures that promote healing.* This is accomplished by approximating wound edges with sutures, ensuring a good blood supply, supplying essential nutrients, and keeping the area dry.

4. *To cleanse wounds of foreign debris,* such as a piece of glass or excessive exudates. The former can act as an irritant, and the latter can harbor microorganisms. *Debridement* is the cleaning of an injured area to remove debris, and it is usually performed by the physician. Wound irrigations with water or cleansers such as hydrogen peroxide may be used to clear away organic material prior to cleansing wounds with antiseptics.

5. *To provide a means for absorbing inflammatory exudate and to promote drainage.* Rubber or plastic tubes or drains are frequently put into wounds or ducts during surgery to promote drainage. Some of these drains, commonly referred to as *Penrose drains,* are shortened progressively throughout the healing process. They ensure removal of inflammatory exudates or blood prior to the closure of overlying skin. Other drains are placed in ducts, such as the ureter or common bile duct, to ensure patency of the duct and to prevent adhesion or closure of ducts. Drains or tubes may be attached to suction apparatuses, which facilitate drainage. A vacuum suction is sometimes used to drain blood and serous exudate from deep surgical wounds, such as for orthopedic surgery.

6. *To prevent hemorrhage.* Occlusive pressure dressings are commonly applied to surgical incisions. These are left on for the first few days until a dressing change is ordered by the physician. In certain body areas, such as the rectum or vagina, long threads of gauze in varying widths are packed into these orifices to provide pressure to small blood capillaries and prevent bleeding. The packing is usually removed 2–3 days after surgery.

7. *To prevent skin excoriation* around draining wounds. This is accomplished by changing saturated dressings as required and by cleaning and drying wounds and surrounding skin areas. When drainage is excessive, as seen with some bowel surgery (colostomy) or urinary surgery, protective ointments or pastes may be applied to surrounding skin areas to prevent irritation and excoriation. The frequent removal of adhesive tape can also be irritating, and thus Montgomery straps or tie tapes are frequently used.

Open and Closed Methods of Wound Care

The closed method refers to wounds that have a dressing applied, the open method to wounds that do not. The application of dressings to a wound can be advantageous in that they do the following:

1. Help absorb drainage.
2. Protect the wound from microorganisms.
3. Cover unpleasant disfigurements.
4. Can assist in approximating wound edges.
5. Provide emotional rest to some people by the protective covering.

In some situations, the physician may apply a protective covering, such as collodion spray, in lieu of a gauze dressing. This spray hardens like nail polish and can often be peeled from the skin when the wound is healed, or it can be removed with special solutions. This method is often preferred, since the friction effects of a dressing are eliminated and the wound is always observable because the covering is clear and translucent. The wound is kept dry because the spray is moisture-proof. For children, who are active and heal quickly, this spray is frequently used. It is not advised for wounds that have drainage.

361

The open method is used to avoid the disadvantages that dressings may provide, such as (a) dark, warm, moist environments for resident and nonresident microorganisms to multiply; and/or (b) irritation of wounds by friction.

By exposing wounds to the air, a drying effect results. The open method is frequently employed for the burn victim.

Dressings

The order for dressings and the frequency of dressing changes are generally prescribed by the physician. Any special ointments to be applied may also be ordered. For example, the physician may order "Elase ointment to varicose ulcers and dry dressings twice a day." For a surgical incision, the order may read simply, "Change dressing on the third day postoperatively," and the nurse will then apply skin cleansers and/or antiseptics according to agency policy. Some patients are taught to change their own dressings. In this instance the nurse offers assistance and supervision as required.

Dressing Materials

Various types of materials are available for dressing and cleansing wounds.

Materials to Cleanse Wounds

Some people prefer the use of cotton balls because of their absorbent qualities, while others prefer the use of gauze squares, claiming that threads of cotton can stick to sutures. Cleansing agents vary considerably. Some of the common cleansers are:

Alcohol 70%

Aqueous and tincture of chlorhexidine hydrochloride (Hibitane)

Aqueous and tincture of benzalkonium chloride (Zephiran Chloride)

Hydrogen peroxide

Materials to Cover Wounds

Several sizes of gauze are available to cover wounds. The standard sizes are 4 × 4 inches and 8 × 4 inches. The size and the numbers used are dependent upon the nature of the wound, the amount of exudate, and the location of the wound. This is left to the nurse's judgment. Sometimes the gauze is cut halfway

through one side to make it fit around a drain, or it is folded in a special way.

Telfa gauze is a special type of gauze with a shiny, nonadherent surface on one side. It is applied so that the shiny surface is placed directly on the wound. Exudate then seeps through this surface and collects on the absorbent side. This kind of dressing is advantageous for wounds with a sticky exudate or newly formed granulation tissue. When it is removed, it does not adhere and therefore does not cause injury to the wound.

Larger and thicker gauze dressings, called *surgipads* or *abdominal pads,* are used to cover these small gauzes. They hold the other gauzes in place but are also absorbent and thus collect excessive drainage. Surgipads are more absorbent on one side, therefore this absorbent side is placed toward the wound; the less absorbent and protective side is placed outward. The outer side is often indicated with a blue stripe.

Materials to Secure Dressings

Dressings are secured by adhesive tapes, bandages, and binders. Bandages and binders are discussed later in this chapter.

Adhesive Tapes.   After abdominal or other types of surgery, an elastic adhesive tape is commonly applied over wounds because of its ability to compress, thereby controlling hemorrhage. This original tape is removed during the initial dressing change and a lighter dressing applied. Ordinary adhesive tape can be applied in strips across the dressing. It is important to secure the dressing at both ends and across the middle and to use tape of a sufficient width for the dressing and the wound.

Montgomery straps or tie tapes are commonly used for patients who require frequent dressing changes. These straps prevent skin irritation and discomfort to patients by eliminating the need to remove the adhesive strapping each time the dressing is changed. Nonallergenic tape is used for people who have sensitive skin. If this is not available, the application of tincture of benzoin to the skin where the adhesive is to be applied serves as a skin protective.

Changing Dressings

Dressing changes are prescribed by the physician. Some physicians may prefer that a dressing be reinforced with surgipads for excessive drainage rather than removing the existing dressing and applying a new one. It is important for the nurse to review the physician's orders and nurses' notes prior to changing a dressing. The physician may prescribe a specific solution for cleansing. The notes on the Kardex nursing care plan can offer information about the amount of drainage, the quantity of dressing materials required, allergy to adhesive tape, and scheduled times for dressing change. It is mandatory that the nurse determine the existence and location of drains prior to removing dressings to prevent drain dislodgment. This information can be acquired from the patient's chart and is often on the surgical or anesthetic record or on the nursing Kardex. The patient needs a simple explanation about the procedure. Any specific questions the patient has can be asked at this time. It is important that the patient is comfortable and free from pain.

The patient may require assistance with positioning. The linen is fan-folded away from the site, and gowns or pajamas may need to be opened or removed. A bath blanket can be used for draping if necessary. Only the wound site should be exposed. Privacy is also provided to minimize air currents and for the patient's peace of mind.

Preparing the Equipment

Prior to assembling the equipment, the nurse completes a hand wash as described for surgical asepsis and dons a mask as required. Necessary supplies include a dressing tray with a sterile drape, cotton balls or gauzes for cleansing, a metal or plastic basin for cleansing solution, and at least one hemostat, one thumb forceps, and one pair of scissors. In addition to this, a waterproof bag is needed in which to dispose of dressing materials, and a cleansing agent must be added, plus necessary dressing materials such as 4 × 4-inch gauzes, surgipads, and adhesive tape. Some disposable trays also include dressing materials.

The dressing tray may be opened to add solutions or other necessary items in the clean utility room or at the patient's bedside on the overbed table. The tray is opened in the manner described for sterile wrapped packages. Lifting forceps can be used to position instruments appropriately on the tray so that the sterile tips lie inside the sterile field and the handles lie outside. Some dressing sets are prepared in such a way that one hemostat can be removed without touching the sterile field. This hemostat can then be used as a pickup forceps to reposition other instruments or supplies.

The waterproof bag can be taped to the patient's bedside table or to the drawsheet, which prevents the nurse from having to reach across the sterile field or the wound when putting articles in the bag. Other

equipment may be needed, for example, suture scissors to remove sutures and a sterile safety pin when shortening a drain. These procedures are discussed subsequently.

Changing the Dressing

In some agencies, the sterile forceps are used to change the dressing. In other agencies, sterile gloves are used with or without sterile forceps. The gloving procedure has been described previously. If only sterile forceps are used, the tips are considered sterile, while the handles, which contact the naked hand, are considered contaminated. Thus the handles are placed outside the sterile field. If sterile gloves are used with sterile forceps, both the tips and the handles of the forceps are sterile and must remain *within* the sterile field.

Removing the Dressing.   Binders are removed and tie tapes (Montgomery straps) are untied and placed aside. If adhesive tape is present, it should be removed by holding down the skin and pulling toward the wound. By moistening the tape with acetone or similar products, the discomfort of removal can be lessened, particularly from hairy surfaces. The outer abdominal dressing or surgipad is removed first with the naked hand, since its outer surface is contaminated by the patient's clothing and linen. These should be removed in such a way that any drainage present is turned away from the patient's vision.

Underlying gauze is then removed by the use of a sterile forceps and are deposited into the disposable paper bag. Care must be taken, when dropping soiled dressings into the bag, not to contaminate forceps tips or sterile gloves on the edges of the paper bag. The dressings are held about 6 inches above the bag and dropped into it. A cuff made at the top of the bag ensures a wide opening of the bag. It is essential for the nurse to note the type of drainage present, the number of gauzes saturated, and the appearance of the wound for recording purposes. Care must also be taken to avoid dislodging any drains present in or near the incision. In some instances the use of two forceps may be necessary to remove gauzes from around drainage sites. They may stick together because of the drainage. When using forceps, remember that they must be held with the tips down.

Cleansing the Wound.   The wound is cleansed from the cleanest area to the less clean area. Although some agencies have policies prohibiting the direct cleansing of incisions, many advocate that the incision is cleansed. First swab it from top to bottom and progressively outward, or laterally in vertical lines parallel to the incision on each side. A new cotton ball or pledget is used for each stroke and discarded into the waxed paper bag. The process is repeated until all drainage has been removed. (See Figure 17–9.) When sponges are dipped into cleansing solution, excess solution can be removed by pressing the sponge against the inside of the container. This prevents dripping solution on the sterile field.

Dry pledgets are used to dry the skin as required. If a drain is present, it is recommended that it is cleansed *after* cleansing the wound, since more drainage is present in this area and therefore it is considered more contaminated than the incision site. For irregular wounds, such as a decubitus ulcer, the cleansing process is started from the center of the wound outward. Circular motions of the swab may be required, and one swab should be used for one wipe.

Applying the Dressing.   Powders or ointments may be ordered by the physician to apply to specific wounds. Sterile applicators or tongue blades may be used to apply ointments. Powders are shaken directly onto the wound.

Dressings are applied one at a time, starting at the wound center and moving progressively upward and outward from the wound site. Care must be taken when applying dressings not to contaminate gloves or forceps tips. For some incisions, such as flank incisions, it may be necessary to hold one end of the gauze with a forceps on the incision to keep the gauze from slipping. When changing dressings on drain sites, it may be necessary to cut the dressings to fit around the site. When sufficient layers of gauze are applied, as determined by the amount of drainage that was present, the abdominal pads or surgipads are applied. These are applied by touching only the outside of them with the bare hands. The outside is frequently marked with an indicator such as a blue line. Tie tapes and binders are then refastened or clean ones applied as required. Gloves, if used, will need to be removed prior to handling adhesive tape. These are removed by turning the gloves inside out and

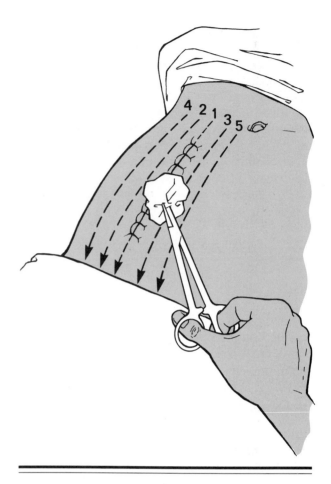

Figure 17-9.   Cleansing a surgical incision starting at the midline.

handling them only from the inside. Equipment is then disposed of appropriately, and the appearance of the wound is recorded. For example:

0930. Abdominal dressing changed. Six 4 × 4 gauzes saturated with serosanguineous drainage. Incision edges well approximated. No apparent inflammation. No complaints of tenderness.

_____RN
(Signature)

Procedure 17-2.   Changing a Surgical Dressing

ACTION	EXPLANATION
Prior to assembling equipment, wash hands and mask.	To remove microorganisms present on the hands, which could contaminate the wound. Some agencies require that a mask be worn in order to prevent contamination from microorganisms in the respiratory tract.

Assemble Equipment

1. Dressing tray, which includes:

    Sterile drape   To cleanse the wound.
    Cotton or gauze balls   For cleansing solution.
    Basin
    1 hemostat
    1 thumb forceps
    1 pair scissors

2. Waterproof bag.   For disposal of the dressing.

3. Add dressing materials to tray.   4 × 4-inch gauze and surgipads are frequently used.

4. Adhesive tape.

5. Add cleansing solution to basin.   It may be necessary to check the patient's dressing to assess what supplies are needed.

6. In some settings sterile gloves are used instead of forceps.

To Change a Dressing

1. Explain to the patient what you plan to do. Adjust the explanation to the needs of the patient.   To reassure the patient by knowledge of what will happen. To identify the patient.

2. For an infant or young child assistance may be required.   An infant or young child might move and contaminate the sterile field.

3. Provide the patient with privacy and expose the area of dressing.

4. Wash hands.   To remove microorganisms present, which could contaminate the wound.

5. Open the sterile tray.   See ''Opening Sterile Wrapped Packages.''

6. Place a bag for the old dressing nearby.   It should be in a position so that the nurse does not reach over the sterile field to get it.

7. Don sterile gloves if used.

8. Remove any large outside dressing by hand.

9. Remove under dressings with tissue forceps.   Note the type and amount of drainage present. If sterile gloves are used, maintain sterility of one glove by not touching old dressings.

10. Discard soiled dressings in the disposal bag.

11. Place the forceps back on the tray without touching other equipment.   These forceps will be contaminated by the old dressing.

12. Cleanse the wound using artery forceps and gauze. Cleanse from the center of the wound to the outside. Use a gauze swab, then discard.   Cleanse from the cleanest area to the least clean, such as toward a drain.

13. Dry the wound in the same manner using gauze.

14. Apply powders and ointments as required.   These will be ordered by the physician. Where there is profuse drainage, ointment will protect the skin from excoriation.

Procedure 17-2. Cont'd.

15. Apply sterile dressings one at a time over the wound.	Start at the wound center.
16. The outside dressing can be applied by hand.	Care must be taken to touch only the outside surface.
17. Retain the dressing with tie tapes.	
18. Assemble equipment on tray.	
19. Assist the patient to a comfortable position.	
20. Remove the tray and disposal bag.	
21. Wash hands.	
22. Chart dressing change and observations.	

DRAINS

Frequently, flexible rubber drains, called *Penrose drains,* are inserted during abdominal surgery to provide drainage and healing of underlying tissues. These drains may be inserted and sutured through the incision line, but they are most commonly inserted through stab wounds a few inches away from the incision line. The latter site allows for the incision to be kept dry. Drains vary in length and width. The length inserted can be 25–35 cm (10–14 inches), and the width, 2.5–4.0 cm (0.5–1.5 inches). In order to facilitate healing and drainage of tissues from the inside to the outside, or from the bottom to the top, the physician commonly orders that the drain be pulled out or shortened 2–5 cm (1–2 inches) from day to day until it falls out on its own. When a drain falls out or is removed, the remaining stab wound usually seals over (heals) within one to two days. In some agencies this shortening procedure is performed only by physicians; in others, it is performed by nurses.

The shortening of the drain is done in conjunction with a dressing change. The preparation of the patient and equipment is the same as for a dressing change. A sterile safety pin or special drain clamp needs to be added to the dressing tray. This is used to hold the drain end in place above the skin. Straight scissors may be needed to cut gauzes that are placed around the drain site and to cut the suture holding the drain in place if it is the first time the drain is to be shortened. It is essential that the doctor's order be confirmed prior to this procedure.

Cleansing the Drain Site

The drain site is cleansed after the incision has been cleansed in accord with the principle of cleansing from the cleanest area to the most contaminated area. Because moist drainage facilitates the growth of resident bacteria, the drain site is considered the most contaminated. If the drain is situated in the center of the incision, the incision can be cleansed from the top toward the drain and from the bottom toward the drain, using separate swabs. The skin around the drain is cleansed with an antiseptic swab held with a hemostat by swabbing in half or full circles around the drain site outward. A tissue forceps may be used in one hand to hold the drain erect for proper cleansing while using the other to cleanse.

Procedure 17-3.   To Shorten a Drain

ACTION	EXPLANATION
Wash hands and mask before assembling equipment.	
Assemble Equipment	
1. Dressing tray.	Set up as for dressing.

2. One sterile safety pin.

3. Sterile gloves can be used instead of forceps.

Add to sterile tray, maintaining asepsis.

To Shorten the Drain

1. Explain to the patient what you plan to do. Adjust the explanation to the patient's needs.

To reassure by knowledge of what you plan to do. To identify the patient.

2. Provide privacy, and assist the patient to a comfortable position.

3. Proceed as for dressing change up to and including cleansing the incision and drain site.

Cleanse from the cleanest to the least clean area. The incision is considered to be cleaner than the drain because of the drainage.

4. With hemostat grasp drain by its full width firmly and gently. Pull out the required length.

To pull evenly.
Usually 2–5 cm (1–2 inches).

5. Using two forceps, insert the sterile safety pin through the drain as closely to the skin as possible.

The pin keeps the drain from falling back into the incision. Insert over a forceps that is holding the drain near the skin.

6. Fasten the safety pin.

7. Cut off the excess drain.

Leave about 2.5 cm (1 inch) above the skin.

8. Complete the procedure as for sterile dressing.

Because of the drainage, additional gauze dressings need to be placed around the drain.

9. Chart technique, including amount and type of drainage present and the amount the drain was shortened.

REMOVING SKIN CLIPS AND SUTURES

Policies vary in relation to the personnel who may remove skin sutures. In some agencies, only physicians remove sutures; in others, registered nurses and student nurses with appropriate supervision may do so. Various suture materials are used, such as silk, cotton, linen, or wire threads, and some synthetics such as nylon or dacron (polyester fiber). Silver wire clips are also available. The physician prescribes the removal of sutures. Usually skin sutures are removed 7–10 days after surgery. Sterile technique and special suture scissors are used. The scissors have a short, curved cutting tip that is readily slid under the suture.

Common Methods of Suturing

Sutures can be broadly categorized as either (a) interrupted (each stitch is tied and knotted separately) or (b) continuous (one thread runs in a series of stitches and is tied only at the beginning and end of the run).

Common sutures of the skin include (a) plain interrupted (Figure 17-10, *A*), (b) mattress interrupted (Figure 17-10, *B*), (c) plain continuous (Figure 17-10, *C*), (d) mattress continuous, and (e) blanket continuous (Figure 17-10, *D*).

Guidelines for Removing Sutures

1. The physician's orders must be carefully confirmed. Many times alternate interrupted sutures are removed one day, and the remaining sutures are removed a day or two later.

2. The suture line is usually cleansed with antiseptic solution before and after suture removal.

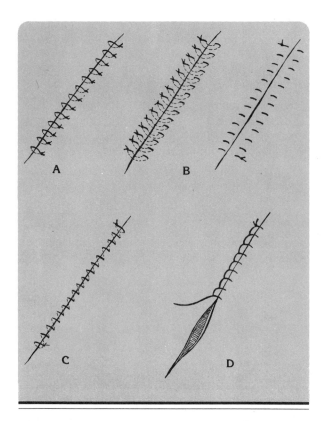

Figure 17-10. Common methods of suturing. **A,** Plain interrupted; **B,** mattress interrupted and continuous; **C,** plain continuous; and **D,** blanket continuous.

3. When removing interrupted sutures, alternate ones are removed first. If gaping (dehiscence) of the wound occurs, the remaining sutures may then be left in place.

4. Because suture material that is visible to the eye is in contact with resident bacteria of the skin, this part of the suture is never pulled beneath the skin during removal. Suture material that is beneath the skin is considered free from bacteria. Therefore, when removing sutures, they are cut at the skin edge on one side of the visible part (Figure 17-11). Suture material that is left beneath the skin acts as a foreign body and elicits the inflammatory response.

5. If wound *dehiscence* (splitting or separating) occurs during the removal of sutures, sterile butterfly tapes should be applied to approximate the wound edges as closely as possible.

6. After suture removal, a small dry dressing is applied. Instruction is given to the patient about follow-up wound care. Generally, if the wound is dry and healing well, showers can be taken in a day or two. If wound discharge occurs, the patient should be instructed to contact the physician.

Removing Sutures

For *plain interrupted* sutures, grasp the suture at the knot with a tissue forceps, cut the suture at the skin edge either below the knot or opposite the knot, and pull the thread out in one piece.

Mattress interrupted sutures do not cross the incision line and have two threads underlying the skin. When possible, the visible part of the suture opposite the knot should be cut at either side and this small visible piece removed. Then the remainder of the suture beneath the skin can be removed by pulling the suture out in the direction of the knot. In some situations, the visible part of the suture opposite the knot is very small, and it may only be possible to cut it once.

Plain continuous sutures can be removed by cutting the thread opposite the knot of the first suture and the thread below on the same side of the second suture. This enables removal of the first stitch and the piece of thread beneath the skin, which is attached to the second stitch. The remaining sutures are then removed by cutting off the visible part of the thread, pulling the underlying loop up by the next stitch, and again cutting the visible part. This process is repeated until the last knot is reached and removed. After the first stitch is removed, the thread is cut all down the same side below the original knot.

Blanket continuous sutures are readily removed by cutting the threads that are opposite the looped blanket edge.

Mattress continuous sutures can be removed in the same manner described for plain continuous su-

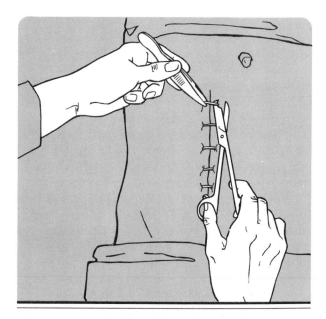

Figure 17-11. Removing plain sutures. Note suture scissors close to skin on side opposite to the knot.

tures. If large pieces of suture material are visible on either side of the incision, removal can be done by cutting and working from side to side of the incision so that visible material is not pulled underneath the skin.

Retention Sutures

Retention sutures, sometimes referred to as *Stay sutures*, are very large plain sutures that are seen in some incisions in addition to skin sutures. These large sutures attach underlying tissues of fat and muscle in additon to the skin and are used to support incisions in obese individuals or in situations in which healing may be prolonged. They are frequently left in place longer than skin sutures (14–21 days) but may be removed at the same time as the skin sutures. Retention sutures may have rubber tubing over them or may be placed over a roll of gauze extending down the incision line. Both measures prevent these large sutures from irritating the incision. Because there are other forms of retention sutures, the nurse should make inquiries whenever in doubt about their removal.

IRRIGATIONS

An *irrigation* is the washing or flushing out of an area. It is done for one or more of the following reasons:

1. To cleanse the area.
2. To apply heat.
3. To apply a medication, such as an antiseptic solution.

Irrigations necessitate the use of sterile technique whenever there is a break in the continuity of the skin. Some irrigations are safely conducted using clean technique, such as eye irrigations, which may be done in order to remove foreign material from an eye.

Wound Irrigation

Open wounds are frequently irrigated to cleanse and to remove excess drainage and sloughing tissue. Sometimes the intent of the irrigation is also to apply heat or an antiseptic solution.

Procedure 17-4.   Wound Irrigation

ACTION	EXPLANATION
Assemble Equipment	
1. Dressing tray.	Set up as for dressing changes.
2. Sterile irrigating syringe.	Bulb syringes are frequently used.
3. Sterile straight catheter.	If the wound is deep and the opening is small.
4. Sterile basin.	For the irrigating solution.
5. Sterile basin.	To receive the solution during the irrigation.
6. Sterile gloves.	For the nurse.
7. Waterproof sterile drape.	To protect the patient and the bed.
8. Irrigating solution, usually 200 ml. of solution at 32.2–35.0°C (90–95° F).	The agency or physician's choice. Dakin's solution or hydrogen peroxide are frequently used.
9. Sterile petrolatum jelly and sterile tongue blade.	To protect skin if it is irritated by drainage.
To Irrigate Wound	
1. Explain to the patient what you plan to do. Adjust the explanation to the patient's needs.	To reassure by knowledge of what you plan to do. To identify the patient.

Procedure 17-4. Cont'd.

2. Assist the patient to a position so that the solution will flow from the wound to a basin below it.

Solution should also flow from the upper end of wound to the lower end before flowing into the basin.

3. Wash hands.

4. Proceed as for changing a sterile dressing up to and including cleansing the wound.

5. Place the sterile basin below wound, and place the waterproof drape over the patient and bed.

To catch irrigating solution.

6. If an irritating solution such as Dakin's is used, protect the skin with the sterile petrolatum.

This can be applied to the skin with a sterile tongue blade.

7. Using syringe and solution, irrigate the wound.

Continue irrigating until the solution becomes clear (no exudate present) or until all solution is used.

8. Dry the area around the wound with sterile gauze.

9. Complete as for sterile dressing.

10. Assist patient to a comfortable position.

11. Collect equipment.

12. Wash hands.

13. Record the irrigation, the solution used, appearance of the wound, and appearance of any exudate and sloughing tissue.

Eye Irrigation

An eye irrigation is administered in order to wash out the conjunctival sac of the eye. It is specifically done for any of the following reasons:

1. To treat an inflammatory process of the conjunctiva.

2. To apply an antiseptic solution.

3. To remove a foreign object or an irritating chemical.

4. To apply heat or cold to the eye.

5. To prepare an eye preoperatively.

For an eye irrigation in the home, an eye cup is frequently used. Ascertain that the eye cup is clean and that it has no chips along the edge, which could injure the skin.

Procedure 17-5.   Eye Irrigation

ACTION	EXPLANATION
Assemble equipment	
1. Sterile container for irrigating solution.	
2. Irrigating solution.	2–8 ounces is generally sufficient at 37.7° C (100° F).
3. Sterile eye syringe or eye irrigator.	An eye dropper can be used where small amounts of solution are required.
4. Sterile cotton balls.	To dry around the eye after irrigation.

5. Sterile kidney basin.	To catch solution.
6. Waterproof drape.	To protect the patient.

To Irrigate the Eye

1. Explain to the patient what you plan to do. Adjust the explanation to the patient's needs.

   To reassure the patient by knowledge of what you plan to do. To identify the patient.

2. Assist the patient to a comfortable position either sitting or lying. Tilt the head toward the affected eye.

   Light should not shine into patient's eyes. The solution will run from the eye to the basin at the side, *not* to the other eye.

3. Place the drape to protect the patient, and place the basin against the patient's cheek.

4. Wash hands.

5. Wipe the eyelid and lashes with irrigating solution and cotton balls.

   To remove any material on the eyelid and lashes so that it will not be washed into the eye.

6. Wipe from the inner canthus to the outer canthus.

   The material will not be wiped into the lacrimal duct.

7. Hold the eye open by separating both lids with the thumb and forefinger.

   Another way is to hold the lower lid down by pressing down on the cheekbone and irrigate, then hold the upper lid up and irrigate (Figure 17-12).

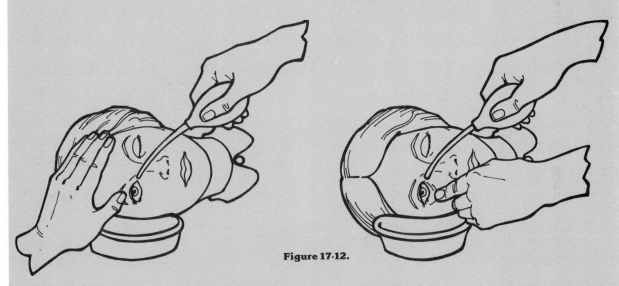

Figure 17-12.

8. Hold the eye irrigator about 2 cm above the eye.

   At this height the pressure of the solution will not damage the tissues.

9. Wash from the inner canthus to the outer canthus.

   Do not touch the eye with the irrigator.

10. Irrigate until the solution leaving the eye is clear (no discharge present) or until all the solution has been used.

11. Dry around the eye with cotton balls.

12. Gather up equipment.

13. Assist the patient to a comfortable position.

14. Wash hands.

Procedure 17-5. Cont'd.

15. Record irrigation, solution used, and appearance of the eye, the pupils, and any discharge. Also include whether the returned solution was cloudy, clear, yellow, etc. Report any pain and other mannerisms such as squinting or rubbing the eyes.

Ear Irrigation (External Auditory Canal)

Irrigations of the external auditory canal are generally carried out for cleansing purposes, although the application of heat and of antiseptic solutions is sometimes prescribed.

Procedure 17-6.   Irrigation of the External Ear Canal

ACTION	EXPLANATION
Assemble equipment	
1. Sterile container for irrigating solution.	
2. Irrigating solution.	About 500 ml. of required solution. Normal saline is frequently used. The temperature is body temperature: for an adult, 37.0° C (98.6° F).
3. Sterile irrigating ear syringe (metal or rubber) or irrigating nozzle.	
4. Basin.	To receive the solution during irrigation.
5. Waterproof towel.	To protect the patient (and bed if required).
6. Applicator swabs.	
7. Towel.	
8. Cotton balls.	To absorb the remainder of the solution at completion of the irrigation.
To Irrigate the External Ear Canal	
1. Explain to the patient what you plan to do. Adjust the explanation to the patient's needs.	
2. Assist the patient to a sitting position or lying position with head turned to the affected ear.	The solution can flow from the ear canal to a basin.
3. Wash hands.	
4. Place the waterproof towel around the patient's ear and shoulder.	To protect the patient from the irrigating solution.
5. Place the basin under the ear to be irrigated.	
6. Cleanse the pinna of the ear and the meatus of the ear canal with the applicator swab and solution.	Any discharge will not be washed into the ear canal.

7. Straighten the ear canal. For infants pull the ear downward and backward. For adults pull upward and backward. (See Figure 17-13, *A*, *B*.) Permit the solution to return freely.

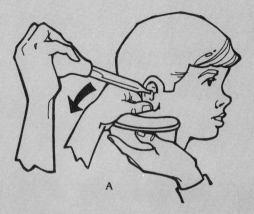

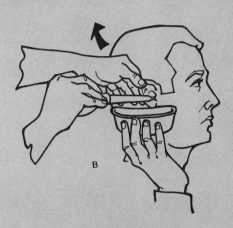

Figure 17-13.

8. Direct the irrigating solution into the auditory canal.

9. Use all the irrigating solution.

10. Dry the outside of the ear.

11. Assist the patient to lie on affected side. Place a cotton ball in the meatus to absorb fluid.

12. Assist the patient to a comfortable position.

13. Collect equipment and dispose of it appropriately.

14. Wash hands.

15. Record irrigation, solution used, appearance of any discharge and returning solution, appearance of the ear, and complaints of pain or discomfort.

To drain out the remaining fluid by gravity.

Gargling

Throat gargling is often performed for the same purposes as a throat irrigation. Gargling has the disadvantages of being fatiguing and painful to irritated, swollen tissues. Gargles do not always reach all tissues of the throat; however, they are generally satisfactory for cleansing the oral pharynx and the mouth.

If gargling with full-strength antiseptic solutions is done for a long period of time, the normal microorganisms present in the mouth are destroyed, and infections are more likely to occur.

Throat Irrigation

Throat irrigations are generally used to cleanse the throat by removing secretions, to apply heat, and to apply an antiseptic. Throat irrigations replace gargling when the latter is painful or when a prolonged effect is desired.

Procedure 17-7.   Irrigating The Throat

ACTION	EXPLANATION
Assemble equipment	
1. Irrigating can and nozzle.	
2. Irrigating solution (about 500 ml). Temperature of solution not above 46.1° C (115.0° F).	Above this temperature the solution could damage tissue.
3. Waterproof drape.	To protect patient.
4. Kidney basin.	To receive irrigation returns.
5. Standard.	Upon which to hang can.
Throat Irrigation	
1. Explain to the patient what you plan to do. Adjust your explanation to the patient's needs.	To reassure the patient by knowledge of what you will do. To identify the patient.
2. Assist the patient to a sitting position with the head tilted forward or a sidelying position with the head over the edge of the bed.	So that the solution will flow freely out of the mouth.
3. Wash hands.	
4. Hang irrigating can on standard about 30 cm (12 inches) above patient's head.	At this height the force of the solution will not injure the tissues.
5. Place basin under mouth.	To catch returning solution.
6. Irrigate the back and sides of the patient's throat. Ask the patient to hold his/her breath while irrigating.	Some patients prefer to do this themselves, thus controlling the flow of the solution. To prevent aspiration of fluid.
7. The nozzle should not touch the back of the tongue or uvula. The uvula is a small mass hanging down from the soft palate.	Touching these areas will stimulate the gag reflex.
8. Use all of the irrigating solution.	
9. Assist the patient to a comfortable position.	
10. Collect equipment and dispose of it appropriately.	
11. Wash hands.	
12. Record the irrigation and solution used, the appearance of the throat and the returning solution, and any perceptions of pain or discomfort by the patient.	

Vaginal Irrigation (Douche)

A vaginal irrigation is the washing of the vagina by a liquid at a low pressure. It is similar to the irrigation of the external auditory canal in that the fluid immediately returns after being inserted.

A vaginal irrigation is done for a variety of reasons.

1. To apply an antiseptic solution that discourages the growth of microorganisms.

2. To cleanse, removing an offensive or irritating discharge.

3. To apply heat or cold as in the treatment of inflammation or hemorrhage.

4. To cleanse preoperatively.

Procedure 17-8.   Vaginal Irrigation

ACTION	EXPLANATION
Assemble Equipment	Sterile equipment is normally used in a hospital and clean equipment at home. Disposable equipment is available.
1. Irrigating solution, 1000–2000 ml at 40.5° C (105.0° F).	Solutions commonly used: Normal saline, tap water, sodium bicarbonate (8 ml in 1000 ml of water) or vinegar (8 ml in 1000 ml of water).
2. Container for solution.	
3. Container with solution to cleanse the perineum and five cotton balls.	Zephiran chloride 1:1000 is commonly used.
4. Nozzle and tubing.	
5. Waterproof drape.	To protect bed.
6. Bedpan.	To collect irrigation returns.
7. Drape.	To cover the patient's legs.
8. Sterile gloves or forceps.	For cleansing the perineum.
9. Standard.	To hang irrigation can.
Vaginal Irrigation	
1. Explain to the patient what you plan to do. Adjust the explanation to the patient's needs.	To reassure the patient by knowledge of what is being done. To identify the patient.
2. Provide privacy.	
3. Ask the patient to void.	To empty the bladder, thus reducing discomfort or trauma during the irrigation because of a distended bladder.
4. Place the waterproof drape under the bedpan.	
5. Assist the patient to a dorsal recumbent position on the bedpan. The hips should be higher than the shoulders.	To facilitate the flow of the irrigation solution into the vagina back to the posterior fornix.
6. Hang the irrigating can on the standard. The base should be about 30 cm (12 inches) above the vagina. Make sure the clamp is tightly on the tubing.	At this height the pressure of the solution should not damage the tissues.
7. Wash hands.	
8. Wash perineum.	
9. Run some irrigating solution through the tubing, then insert the nozzle carefully into the vagina.	Direct the nozzle toward the sacrum, thus following the direction of the vagina.
10. Insert 7–10 cm (3–4 inches) and rotate two or three times to cleanse all areas of the vagina.	For patients who have had vaginal surgery or who have carcinoma of the cervix, do not rotate the nozzle.
11. Use all the irrigating solution.	
12. Dry the perineal area and remove the bedpan.	

Procedure 17-8. Cont'd.

13. Apply a dressing if it is indicated.

14. Assist the patient to a comfortable position.

15. Gather equipment and dispose of it appropriately.

16. Wash hands.

17. Record the irrigation solution used, description of returned fluid, and any discomfort experienced by the patient.

SUPPORTING AND IMMOBILIZING WOUNDS

Bandages and binders are used for a variety of purposes, although support and immobilization are the most common reasons. The purposes of binders and bandages are as follows:

1. To support a wound, for example, a fractured bone.

2. To immobilize a wound, for example, a strained shoulder.

3. To apply pressure, for example, elastic bandages to the lower extremities to improve venous blood flow.

4. To secure a dressing, for example, for an extensive abdominal surgical wound.

5. To retain splints (this applies chiefly to bandages).

6. To retain warmth, for example, a flannel bandage on a rheumatoid joint.

Bandages are available in various widths; the most common widths are 1.5–7.5 cm (0.5–3.0 inches). They are usually supplied in rolls for easy application to a body part.

A binder is a type of bandage. It is a piece of material designed for a specific body part; for example, the triangular binder (sling) fits the arm of a patient. Binders are used to support large areas of the body, such as the abdomen, arm, or chest.

Materials

The materials used in bandaging vary widely, according to the purpose of the bandage.

Gauze is one of the most frequently used materials. It is light and porous, and it readily molds to the body. It is also relatively inexpensive and is generally discarded once it becomes soiled. Gauze is used frequently to retain dressings on wounds and for the fingers, hands, toes, and feet. Gauze can be impregnated with petroleum jelly for application to some wounds. Gauze supports dressings well and at the same time permits air to circulate through them.

Flannel is a soft, pliable material that provides warmth to a body part. It is a strong, fairly heavy material, and it can be washed and reused.

Muslin (factory cotton) is another strong material. It is lighter than flannel, but it also supplies good support. Many binders are made of muslin. It can also be washed and reused.

Crinoline and Kling are types of woven gauze. Crinoline is loosely woven, yet strong. It is impregnated with plaster of Paris as the base for casts. Kling is woven in such a manner that it will stretch and thus mold to the body.

There are a variety of elasticized bandages, which are generally applied in order to provide pressure to an area. They are commonly used as tensor bandages or designed as partial stockings in order to provide support to the legs and improve the venous circulation. Some elasticized bandages have an adhesive backing and can be secured to the skin. These are most frequently used to retain dressings and at the same time provide some support to a wound.

A plastic adhesive bandage is also used to retain dressings. It is waterproof and thus retains wound drainage or keeps an area dry. It has some elastic properties and therefore provides some pressure.

Principles Related to the Use of Binders and Bandages

1. Bandages and binders need to be applied to the body in a way that promotes circulation and does not restrict it. They should be applied so that there is even

pressure over the area and they are tight enough to promote circulation. If possible, the distal end of an extremity should be left uncovered in order that the adequacy of the circulation can be readily determined.

2. Symptoms at a distal part of an extremity, such as coldness, bluish discoloration, and a perception of tingling or numbness, usually indicate that circulation is restricted. The latter needs to be reported and the bandage loosened.

3. When a body part is supported, it should be in a position as close to good body alignment as possible (see Chapter 22).

4. Rubbing can cause the skin to become abraded. Therefore skin surfaces should be separated with gauze before bandaging and bony prominences padded.

5. Warmth and moisture facilitate the growth of microorganisms. Therefore binders and bandages need to be changed regularly unless specifically contraindicated, and the associated skin areas need to be washed and dried. Dirt also promotes the growth of organisms, and its presence indicates that a bandage needs to be changed.

Guidelines for Bandaging

When it is necessary to apply a bandage to a patient, a number of guidelines apply in most situations.

1. Select the material for the bandage according to the purpose of the bandage as well as cost and availability.

2. Select the width of the bandage according to the size of the body part. For example, use a 5 cm (2-inch) bandage for an arm, a 2.5 cm (1-inch) for a finger, and a 7.5–10.0 cm (3- or 4-inch) for a leg.

3. Assist the patient to a comfortable position with the part to be bandaged supported in an aligned position, with slight flexion of the joints unless this is specifically contraindicated.

4. Face the patient who is being bandaged unless specifically instructed otherwise, as for a skull bandage, which is done from behind the patient.

5. Hold the roller bandage with the roll facing upward in one hand and the initial part of the bandage in the other hand.

6. Initiate the bandage by placing it on the limb so that the bandage direction will be from distal to proximal and from medial to lateral. Do not initiate a ban-

dage over a wound or in an area where pressure is contraindicated, such as the sole of the foot.

7. Overlap each bandage turn by two-thirds the width of the bandage and apply the bandage with firm, even pressure.

8. Cover underlying dressings with bandages at least 5 cm (2 inches) beyond the edge of the dressing.

9. Pad bony prominences and separate two skin surfaces in order to prevent friction and subsequent abrasion.

10. Leave a distal aspect of a limb exposed if at all possible in order to check adequacy of the blood circulation.

Basic Turns in Bandaging

Five basic turns are used in bandaging. These turns are spiral, circular, spiral reverse, recurrent, and figure-of-eight. They are often used in different combinations to bandage different parts of the body.

Spiral turns are used to bandage a part of the body that is of about the same circumference throughout, for example, the upper arms, and part of the legs. The turns are carried at a slight angle, about 30°, and each turn overlaps the preceding one by two-thirds the width of the bandage (Figure 17-14, A).

Circular turns are used chiefly to anchor a bandage or to terminate it. They are also used to cover a cylindrical part of the body such as the proximal aspect of the fifth finger. The bandage is wrapped around the body part so that each turn exactly covers the previous turn (Figure 17-14, C). Two circular turns are used to anchor and complete a bandage. These are usually not applied directly over a wound because of the discomfort they may cause.

Spiral reverse turns are used to bandage cylindrical body parts that are not of uniform circumference, for example, the lower leg of a muscular person. To make a spiral reverse, bring the bandage upward at a 30° angle, then place the thumb of the free hand on the upper edge of the bandage. The bandage is unrolled about 14 cm (6 inches), then the hand is pronated so that the bandage folds over on itself and finally continues around the limb. Successive spiral reverses are made at the same point in the turn, each overlapping the previous turn by two-thirds the width of the bandage and at the same angle. (See Figure 17-14, B.)

Recurrent turns are used to cover the distal portions of the body such as the hand, the finger, or the stump after an amputation. The bandage is first anchored by two circular turns around the proximal

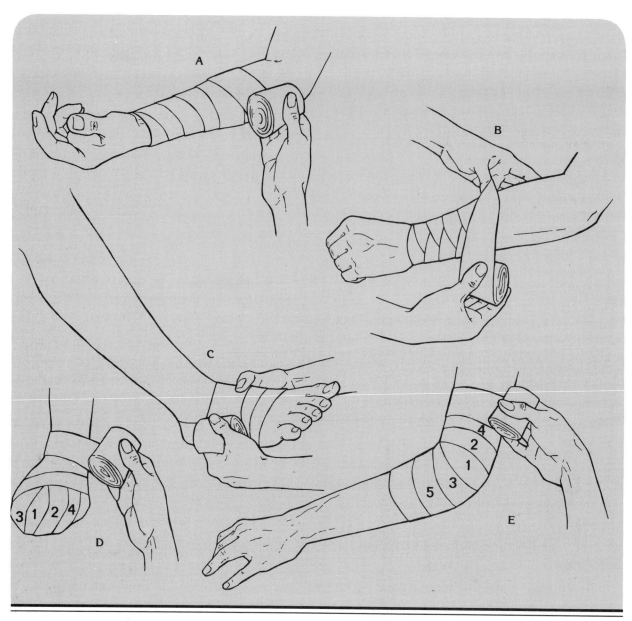

Figure 17-14.   Bandages. **A,** Spiral; **B,** spiral reverse; **C,** circular turns; **D,** recurrent; and **E,** figure-of-eight.

body part, and then the bandage is folded back on itself and brought centrally over the distal end to be covered. It is then taken to the inferior aspect, where it is held with the other hand and brought back over the end but this time to the right of the center bandage, overlapping one-third the width of the bandage. The bandage then is repeated to the left of the center bandage. This pattern of alternate right and left is continued, overlapping all but the first turn by two-thirds the width of the bandage. The bandage is finally secured by two circular turns, which gather in the sides of the bandage (see Figure 17-14, *D*).

The *figure-of-eight* turn is usually used to ban-

dage an elbow, a knee, or an ankle. The bandage is anchored with two circular turns over the center of the joint, then the bandage is carried above the joint, around it and then below the joint, making figure-of-eight turns. Each turn works upward and downward from the joint by overlapping the previous turn by two-thirds the width of the bandage. It is anchored by two circular turns above the joint. (See Figure 17-14, *E*.)

In addition to these basic turns, which are used to bandage most areas of the body, there are special bandages for various parts of the body such as skull, ear, and eye bandages.

Common Types of Binders

There are five commonly used types of binders: the triangular binder (sling), breast binder, many-tailed (scultetus) binder, T-binder (single or double T), and the abdominal binder.

The Triangular Binder (Sling)

The triangular binder is usually of muslin cloth. It can be applied in a number of ways, but it is usually applied as a full triangle to make a large arm sling that supports the arm, elbow, and forearm of a person, (see Figure 17-15).

To make a large arm sling:

1. Place one end of the unfolded triangle over the shoulder of the uninjured side.

2. The binder falls down the front of the patient with the point directed toward the elbow of the injured side (behind the elbow).

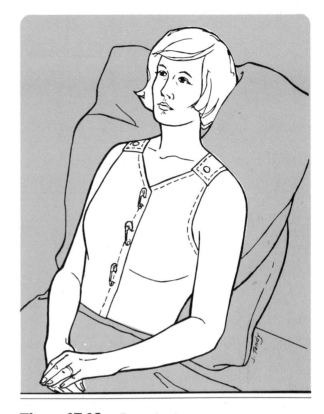

Figure 17-16.   Breast binder.

3. Take the upper corner and carry it around the neck until it hangs over the shoulder on the injured side.

4. Assist the patient to flex the elbow with the thumb upward until it is at right angles to the upper arm.

5. Take the lower corner of the binder and bring it up over the arm to the shoulder of the uninjured side.

6. Secure this corner to the other end with a reef knot.

7. Bring the point of the bandage at the elbow forward and secure it neatly with safety pins. The tips of the fingers should be visible.

Breast Binder

Breast binders are used to promote pressure to breasts, for example, when drying up the breasts after birth, or to support the breasts, as after surgery.

The binder is pinned in front. The pins are placed vertically except for the lower one, which is placed horizontally for the patient's comfort. Breast binders usually have straps that fit over the shoulders and are pinned in front (see Figure 17-16).

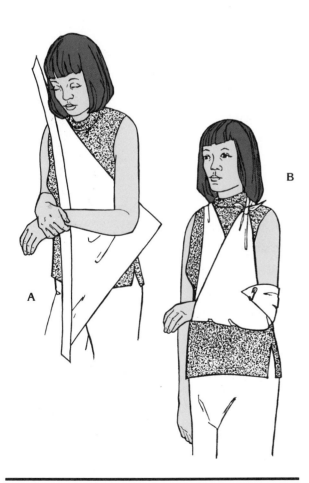

Figure 17-15.   Large arm sling.

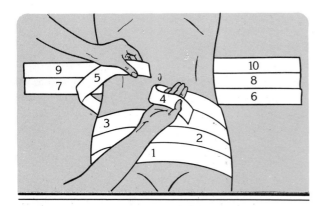

Figure 17-17.   Scultetus' (many-tailed) binder. Each tail overlaps the preceding one by about one-half the width of the tail.

The Many-Tailed (Scultetus) Binder

The many-tailed binder is used to provide support to the abdomen and, in some instances, to retain dressings. The binder is usually made of flannel or cotton. The center of the binder is placed under the patient so that the lower edge is at the gluteal fold (over the buttocks). The tails are then brought over to the center from alternate sides, starting at the bottom. Each tail should overlap the preceding one by about half the width of the tail. In thin people the ends of the tail may extend beyond the other side and require fold-

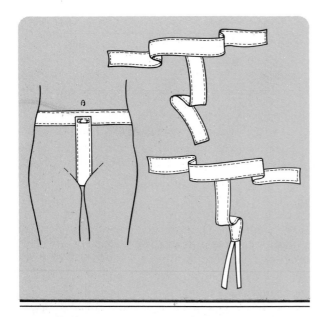

Figure 17-18.   T-binders: single T and double T.

ing back. The last tail is secured with a safety pin. (See Figure 17-17.)

The T-Binder (Single or Double T)

T-binders are usually made of cotton fabric. They are usually used to retain perineal dressings. The bar (top) of the T serves to go around the patient's waist. The stem of the T passes between the patient's legs, posterior to anterior. In the single T, also referred to as the *female T-binder*, the stem is brought upward and attached to the waist band. The double T binder has two tails, that is, the stem of the T splits into two for male patients. These two tails are brought up on either side of the penis to the waist band. Double T-binders may be used for female patients if greater support to the perineum is required. (See Figure 17-18.)

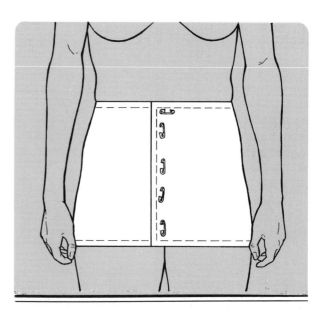

Figure 17-19.   Straight abdominal binder used to support the abdomen.

The Abdominal Binder

The abdominal binder is a rectangular piece of cotton that is long enough to encircle a patient's abdomen with about a 5.0–7.5 cm (2–3-inch overlap for an adult, 2.5 cm overlap for an infant). It should also be wide enough to reach from the gluteal fold to the patient's waist. It is pinned down the center securely and then molded to the patient's body by pinning on the lateral aspects (see Figure 17-19).

HEAT AND COLD THERAPY

Both heat and cold are applied to the body in order to support processes involved in the repair and healing of tissues. Hot and cold applications can be applied in either dry or moist forms. The form of choice generally depends upon the exact purpose of the application and the type of wound. For example, an open wound usually indicates the need for sterile, moist compresses or heat by radiation (dry) in order to maintain the sterility of the area.

When a hot application is applied to a body part, it adds heat to that part; a cold application withdraws heat from the part. Heat to a closed wound is generally applied by a hot pack (hot moist) or an electric pad (hot dry).

Heat is transferred by the processes of conduction, convection, and radiation. *Conduction* means the transfer of heat by molecular interaction; it implies contact between the source of the heat and the body part. An example would be the application of a hot water bottle to an abdomen. A substance that inhibits conduction is known as an *insulator*. *Convection* is the transfer of heat by movement of a liquid or gas. An example of transfer by convection is the sitz bath in which the water continues to run. *Radiation* is the transfer of heat in the form of electromagnetic waves through the air. An example of heat applied in this manner is the ultraviolet lamp.

Heat applications are usually classified as *radiant, conductive,* or *conversive.* The infrared part of the electromagnetic spectrum produces radiant heat; the infrared lamp produces such heat. Penetration of infrared rays is from 1–3 mm, depending upon whether the wavelengths are near or far. Near wavelengths are 7700–14,000 Å, and far wavelengths are 14,000–120,000 Å. (The Å [angstrom] is a unit of wavelength of electromagnetic radiation.) Near infrared radiation penetrates about 3 mm and far infrared about 1 mm. Luminous bulbs produce more near infrared and thus have greater penetration than nonluminous filaments, which also produce far infrared radiation.

Conductive heat is provided by the direct application of heat, such as by a hot water bag or heated air to the body. This heat is relatively superficial; it penetrates 1–2 cm, and it requires about 20–30 minutes in order to produce the desired effect.

Conversive heat involves the conversion of a primary form of energy to heat. An example is medical diathermy. Short-wave diathermy, using wavelengths of 3–30 meters, is used to provide heat to deep tissues. With this method, the greatest increase in temperature is in the subcutaneous fatty tissue; the depth of temperature rise is from 2–3 cm. Short-wave diathermy and other forms of deep heat treatment are usually carried out by a physiotherapist or a specially trained rehabilitation therapist.

Physiologic Responses to Heat and Cold

Heat and cold have different effects upon the body, and their effects are further dependent upon the duration of the application.

External Heat of Short Duration

An application of heat of short duration (15–30 minutes) has the following effects:

1. Increases the temperature of the tissues.
2. Causes vasodilatation.
3. Increases the capillary blood pressure.
4. Increases the amount of capillary surface available for exchange of fluids and electrolytes by relaxing the capillaries.
5. Decreases blood viscosity.
6. Increases tissue metabolism.
7. Causes sedation with the relief of pain and muscle tension.

Increasing the temperature of the tissues increases the metabolic activity of the cells involved, and this adds to further temperature increase and more vasodilatation as more capillaries become patent. Some of this heat is conducted to underlying tissues. Excessive heat is carried to other body parts by blood flow.

Vasodilatation results in a reddening and warming of the skin. The blood flows to the area, which becomes *hyperemic* (has excessive blood). The increase in blood volume facilitates the exchange of nutrients and waste products between the tissues and the blood. The increase in capillary blood pressure also facilitates the movement of nutrients and oxygen from the arterial blood to the tissues. Because the capillaries relax, the surface area of the capillary bed increases, thus increasing the exchange of nutrients and wastes.

When the capillaries of the skin are fully distended, they are capable of holding one-half to two-thirds of the total blood volume. For this reason a person who gets in a hot bath can faint as a result of the blood moving from the vital centers such as the brain to the skin. With heat the blood becomes less viscid (thick). This permits it to circulate more readily and to deliver nutrients more efficiently. Because of this, the tissue cell metabolism is accelerated. The analgesic effects of heat are thought to be due to the equalization of temperature from superficial to deep tissues, but the exact mechanism is not understood.

External Heat of Long Duration

The prolonged application of heat to an area decreases the blood flow to the area. This usually occurs after one hour of application. By removing the heat for 15–30 minutes and then reapplying it, vasodilatation is reestablished.

Extreme Heat Application

The application of extreme heat has the following effects (Table 17-1):

1. Cell metabolism is increased more than the local circulation.
2. Surface arterioles tend to constrict.
3. Muscles tend to remain tense and fail to relax.
4. Cells can be damaged and blisters appear.

External Cold of Short Duration

The application of cold to an area has varying effects, depending upon the degree of cold and the length of time of the application. However, cold applications usually have these effects:

1. Vasoconstriction.
2. Increased venous congestion.
3. Decreased local tissue metabolism.
4. Contraction of the arrector pili muscles.
5. Decreasing sensitivity with a numbing sensation.

Vasoconstriction is the first obvious sign after the application of cold. The arterioles of the circulatory system constrict, thereby limiting the blood supply to the affected part (ischemia). Vasoconstriction results in a pallor to the skin with a coolness that can be observed by touch. The slower circulation and the constriction of the blood vessels result in increased venous congestion, which can be observed as the bluish appearance of the skin. This venous congestion also reduces the amount of fluid entering the tissues, thereby assisting to reduce edema. The decrease in blood flow means that less oxygen and fewer nutrients are available to the tissue cells, which results in decreased tissue metabolism. For this reason, prolonged exposure to cold can result in cell deprivation and subsequent damage.

With an application of cold, particularly over a large area of the body, the body reacts by contracting the arrector pili muscles. This is a normal reaction of the body to produce heat by muscle contraction, and it can be seen as goose flesh on the patient.

Another important effect of a cold application is the decreasing sensitivity of tissue, leading to numb-

Table 17-1.   Effects of Heat and Cold Applications

Heat	Cold
1. Arteriole vasodilatation (reddened skin)	Arteriole vasoconstriction (pale bluish skin)
2. Decreased stroke volume*	Increased stroke volume*
3. Increased respiratory rate	Decreased respiratory rate
4. Increased temperature of local tissues	Decreased temperature of local tissues
5. Increased amount of capillary surface	Decreased amount of capillary surface
6. Decreased blood viscosity	Increased blood viscosity
7. Increased tissue metabolism	Decreased tissue metabolism
8. Increased capillary blood pressure	Decreased capillary blood pressure
9. Muscular relaxation	Muscular contraction
10. Increase in number of leukocytes and inflammation	Reduced inflammation

*Stroke volume is the volume of blood ejected from the ventricle of the heart with each contraction.

ness of the area. This effect is evident with the administration of a local anesthetic, such as ethyl chloride, used for minor local surgery.

External Cold of Long Duration

For long periods of exposure to a cold application, it is generally considered unsafe to employ temperatures that would produce skin temperatures below 4.4° C (40° F) for any length of time. The one exception to this general rule is the use of cold in anesthesia.

Cold for a prolonged period can interfere with the circulation, healing, cell function, and cell resistance to a point where permanent damage to the tissues results. Prolonged exposure to cold results in vasodilatation, as opposed to vasoconstriction. This explains the ruddiness of the skin of a person who has been for a walk in the cold weather.

The symptoms of damaged tissues due to cold are a bluish-purplish mottled appearance of the skin, numbness, stiffness, pallor, and sometimes blisters and pain.

Extreme Cold Application

Extreme cold can damage the cells in the area to which the cold is applied. The fluid in the tissues can freeze, forming crystals, and the cells can die as a result of the lowered temperature and lack of oxygen and nourishment.

Perception of Heat and Cold

The skin of the body is well supplied with nerves, blood vessels, and lymph vessels. The temperature receptors (heat and cold) in the skin are sensitive to temperatures that are either greater or lesser than that of the skin surface itself, which is 33.9° C (93.0° F). With repeated exposure to either heat or cold the person becomes less sensitive. Therefore a person can inadvertently damage tissues by not taking adequate precautions when having hot and cold applications. For example, a patient who is soaking a hand repeatedly in hot water at home would be wise to take the temperature of the water before putting the hand in it.

Heat and cold are perceived as cold, cool, indifferent, warm, and hot. The pain receptors are stimulated by extremes in temperature, that is, 45° C (113° F) and above or 15° C (59° F) and below. A person perceives the temperature of hot or cold applica-

tions most when the temperature of the skin is changing. That is why a hot-water hand soak will feel hottest when the hand is first immersed, not later. Temperatures that are 8.3° C (15.0° F) above the skin temperature, which is normally 33.9° C (93.0° F), and 11.1° C (20.0° F) below the skin temperature, stimulate the temperature receptors in the skin. Temperatures around the temperature of the skin (between 33° and 34° C; 91.4° and 93.2° F) are normally undifferentiated.

The cold temperature receptors lie closer to the skin surface than do the heat receptors. The cold receptors are more plentiful than heat receptors, and both types vary in density on different parts of the body. For example, there are more cold receptors on the forehead, making it more responsive to cold than to heat. Thermal signals are picked up by the heat or cold receptors and transmitted along the sensory nerves to the central nervous system. The impulses then travel by the lateral spinothalamic tract to the thalamus. Some stimuli will continue to the somatesthetic cortex and others to the cerebral cortex. It is as a result of the impulses in the cerebral cortex that the person becomes aware of the sensation of heat or cold.

Tolerance to Heat and Cold

The tolerance of the body physiologically to heat and cold varies according to a number of the following factors:

1. The part of the body. For example, the back of the hand is not very sensitive to temperatures, while the inner aspect of the wrist is more sensitive.

2. The size of the part of the body exposed to the heat or cold. The larger the area exposed, the less the tolerance.

3. The tolerance of the individual person, which to some degree is affected by age and the condition of the skin, the nervous system, and the circulatory system. The very young and the very old generally have the least tolerance.

4. The length of time of exposure to the heat or cold. People feel heat and cold applications most as the skin temperature is changing. After a period of time, tolerance is improved.

See Table 17-2 for recommended temperatures for hot and cold applications.

Table 17-2.   Recommended Temperatures for Hot and Cold Applications

	Fahrenheit	Centigrade	Application
Very Cold	Below 59°	Below 15°	Ice bags
Cold	59°–65°	15°–18°	
Cool	65°–80°	18°–27°	
Tepid	80°–98°	27°–37°	Alcohol and tepid sponges
Warm	98°–105°	37°–40°	
Hot	105°–115°	40°–46°	Aquathermia
			Soaks
			Sitz baths
			Irrigations
			Moist sterile compresses
			Hot-water bag for debilitated or young
Very hot	Above 115°	Above 46°	Hot-water bag for adults
			Heat cradle

HEAT APPLICATIONS

Reasons for Applying Heat

Heat can be applied in a dry form, such as a hot water bottle, or in a moist form, such as a hot compress. Heat is applied for its local effect or its systemic effect. A local effect is one in which the action is confined to a specific area of the body, for example, a finger or a wound. A generalized effect is one in which the body as a whole reacts to the heat; for example, a hot bath warms the entire body.

Heat is applied for any one or more of the following reasons:

1. To relieve muscle spasm.
2. To soften exudates.
3. To hasten the suppurative process.
4. To hasten healing.
5. To warm a part of the body.
6. To reduce the congestion of an underlying organ.
7. To reduce pressure of accumulated fluid.
8. To increase peristalsis.
9. For comfort and relaxation.

To Relieve Muscle Spasm

Contraction of muscles can be painful, as many people know when they get the so-called Charley horse in a leg or a wry neck. The application of heat to the area can serve to relax the muscle that is in spasm and thus dissipate the pain. The underlying mechanism is unknown.

To Soften Exudates

An exudate is a discharge produced by the inflammatory response of body tissues. This exudate, when it dries, hardens and can form a crust, which adheres to the skin, mucous membrane, or wound, as the case may be. Moist heat in the form of a hot compress softens the exudate, thus permitting it to be readily removed.

To Hasten the Suppuration Process

Suppuration means the formation of pus. When heat is applied to an area, the increased circulation brings additional defenders against infection, that is, leukocytes and phagocytes (white blood cells), and takes away toxins that have been produced in the area. The pus will consolidate in an area and may subsequently be absorbed into the circulation or drain to the outside of the body. If localization does not occur, the microorganisms may spread to other cells, causing cellulitis; they may be absorbed into the lymphatic system through the tissue fluid and cause an inflammatory process of the lymph vessels (lymphangitis); or they may reach the lymph nodes, where they may be destroyed or cause a localized inflammation, such as tonsillitis or lymphadenitis.

To Hasten Healing

When heat is applied to the body it causes vasodilatation of the arterioles in the area, which remain dilated. This results in an increased blood supply to the area, which brings additional nutrients for the tissue healing. The arterioles remain dilated for about an hour, after which a vasoconstriction takes place. If the heat is removed for about an hour, it can be reapplied with subsequent vasodilatation again. This is why hot compresses are sometimes given alternated with cold compresses.

To Warm a Part of the Body

Heat (often dry heat) is applied to warm a particularly cold part of the body. For example, a person with a leg cast may find that his foot is cold because of lack of exercise and the fact that he cannot wear a sock and shoe. A hot-water bottle will warm the foot and provide comfort to the patient. Care must be taken to make sure that the coldness of an extremity is not due to impaired circulation, a situation which should be reported immediately for corrective measures.

To Reduce the Congestion of an Underlying Organ

Heat increases blood circulation to the body surface upon which the heat is applied, redirecting the blood from deeper congested areas. The heat itself penetrates no more than 2 mm, but a reflex action is set up. The heat in this instance acts much like an irritant. The cutaneous nerve endings are stimulated, and the stimuli are carried to the spinal cord by the sensory fibers. From there the impulses enter the sympathetic nervous system and hence go to the internal organs. Thus the blood is redirected away from the organ to the body surface.

To Reduce Pressure of Accumulated Fluid

The removal of accumulated fluid in a tissue or joint can also be facilitated by heat. The heat increases the supply of blood to the area, and the capillaries are available for absorption of fluid. Hence, accumulated fluid is more easily absorbed into the circulation from the tissues.

To Increase Peristalsis

A hot drink or hot food increases the strength of peristaltic waves. Peristalsis is the wavelike contractions of the muscles of the digestive tract. It propels the digested products along the tract. This particular increase in peristalsis due to the heat of ingested liquids or food can be used to assist patients to establish regular defecation habits. After hot cereal and coffee at breakfast, a patient can learn to use the resulting peristaltic waves for defecation.

Comfort and Relaxation

Heat applied to the body is also comforting and relaxing to many people. A warm tub bath relaxes the skeletal muscles and is often used to promote sleep.

Very hot applications, that is, those above 46.1° C (115.0° F) produce a reaction of the body similar to that of a cold application. The superficial blood vessels tend to constrict rather than relax, and the muscles fail to relax.

Factors of Concern in Regard to Applications of Heat

The following factors affect the use of heat applications to a body area and the degree of heat to be applied:

1. The size of the body area. The greater the area of the body, the lower the temperature of the application.
2. The use of moist or dry heat. Moist heat penetrates better than dry heat and is less likely to burn. Therefore moist heat is usually tolerated better than dry.
3. The individual tolerance. There is a wide variation in the degree of tolerance of heat between individual people.
4. The particular skin area involved. In any individual person there are a variety of tolerances, depending upon the number of heat receptors present.
5. The age and condition of the patient. Heat is less well tolerated in the very young, the elderly, and in people with circulatory problems.

Contraindications to the Application of Heat

Heat applications are ordered by a physician. However, nurses need to be aware of symptoms that usually contraindicate heat applications. Thus, even though an order has been written, it is a nursing responsibility to question the order in the following circumstances:

1. When vasodilatation will increase a patient's discomfort, for example, by increasing circulation to a swollen joint or by increasing the expansion of gases, as in an infected tooth.

2. When vasodilatation of the blood vessels inside the cranium will increase discomfort. Therefore, heat is rarely applied for headaches.

3. When an inflammatory process is present, for example, in appendicitis.

4. When the possibility of hemorrhage exists, since vasodilatation will increase the bleeding.

Moist Applications of Heat

Moist applications of heat have the following advantages over dry applications. Moist applications:

1. Soften crusts and exudates.

2. Penetrate more deeply than dry heat.

3. Are less likely to burn the skin.

4. Do not dry the skin.

5. Tend to have a more localized effect, thereby reducing the amount of body fluid that can be lost through diaphoresis (perspiration).

Sitz Bath

A sitz bath, or hip bath, is intended to supply moist heat to the patient's pelvic area. The patient is usually immersed from the midthighs to the iliac crests (Figure 17-20). The temperature of the water should be from 43.3°–46.1° C (110°–115° F) unless otherwise ordered by the physician, or unless the patient is unable to tolerate the heat. If the purpose of the bath is to assist the patient to relax, the temperature is usually 36.1–37.7° C (97–100° F). The duration of the bath is generally from 15 to 30 minutes, depending upon the patient's condition.

Special tubs and chairs, as well as disposable basins, are available for sitz baths. The latter are often used in the home. These tubs are perferred to the regular bathtub, which, when it is used, usually involves immersing the entire leg, thus less effectively directing the circulation to the perineum or pelvic area.

When a patient takes a sitz bath, care needs to be taken so that undue pressure is not placed on any body part, such as the sacrum or the posterior aspects

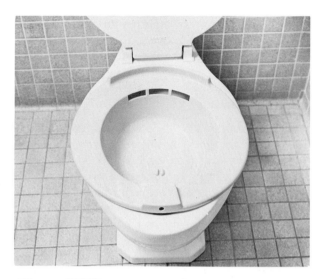

Figure 17-20.   A portable Sitz bath used in hospitals and homes.

of the thighs. A stool for the patient's feet can often assist to support the legs, thus preventing pressure on the thighs. (Some sitz baths are installed at floor level, thus negating the need for a foot stool.) Further precautions also need to be taken to prevent chilling and to guard against burning and fainting. Often a bath blanket over the patient's shoulders will prevent chilling, as will eliminating drafts during the bath. Maintaining the temperature of the bath is also important. The water should be tested every 10 minutes and additional hot water added as necessary. At such time care is taken to prevent burning the patient.

Sometimes patients feel faint and dizzy during a sitz bath. This is particularly true of patients who have just had surgery or when the water temperature is 43.3–46.1° C. A cold cloth on the back of the patient's neck will often prevent fainting; however, close observation is necessary, and the bath should be terminated if the feeling of faintness persists.

Before taking a sitz bath, patients should understand that they are not to touch any wound areas and that they are to ring for a nurse with the signal provided if they feel weak. After rectal surgery, patients need to take a sitz bath after each defecation. Sitz baths may feel uncomfortable initially; however, after the first 3–5 minutes, most patients find them comforting.

The nurse will need to make the following observations:

1. Color of the patient's face. Extreme pallor may precede fainting or vomiting.

2. Pulse rate. An accelerated pulse rate may precede fainting.

3. Sensation of faintness, nausea, or extreme pain.

4. Temperature of the water.

5. Appearance of the perineal area.

Soaks

A soak refers to either immersing a body part, for example, an arm (Figure 17-21), in a solution, or to wrapping a part in gauze dressings and then saturating the dressing with a solution. Soaks may employ either clean technique or sterile technique. The latter is generally indicated for any open wounds, such as a burn or an operative area. Dry dressings are usually applied in between the soaks.

Soaks are usually indicated for any of the following reasons:

1. To apply heat, thus hastening suppuration and softening exudates.

2. To apply medications.

3. To cleanse areas such as wounds in which there is sloughing tissue.

A physician usually will specify in the order the site for the soak, the type of solution, the temperature of the solution, the length of time for the soak, the frequency, and the purpose. Whether sterile technique is indicated is usually a nursing judgment; if there is a break in the skin, sterile technique is indicated.

The equipment required for a soak is as follows:

1. The specified solution. If a temperature is not ordered, 40.5–43.3° C (105–110° F) is usually indicated.

2. The container, such as a basin or special arm bath. This should be sterile if there is a break in the skin.

3. Thermometer to test the temperature of solution.

4. Towels.

5. Sterile drape if sterile technique is used, in order to cover the part and the solution during the soak.

6. Gauze, if indicated.

For the soak, any dressings are removed and discarded. The part is then slowly immersed in the solution. If it is a sterile soak, the affected part is covered with a sterile towel. Ideally the temperature of the solution should be checked frequently, every five minutes, and additional solution added or provided to replace discarded solution in order to maintain the appropriate temperature. Normally a soak lasts from 15 to 20 minutes. Therefore the patient will require

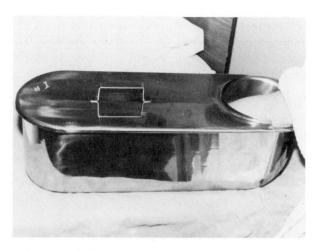

Figure 17-21. An arm soak being used by a patient in hospital. (Courtesy Lions Gate Hospital, North Vancouver, B.C.)

support in order to be comfortable and avoid muscle strain. For example, if a hand is to be soaked, the arm can be supported by a pillow.

The nurse will need to make the following observations:

1. Appearance of the area being soaked. Some erythema (redness) is to be expected from the heat of the solution.

2. Pain in the area.

3. Any untoward reactions, such as numbness in the area.

Compresses and Hot Wet Packs

A *compress* is a moist gauze dressing that is applied frequently to an open wound. Sometimes compresses are ordered to be hot, in which case the solution is heated to a temperature ordered by the physician, such as 40.5° C (105° F). Compresses are usually applied using sterile technique when there is a break in the skin; therefore sterile gloves or sterile forceps are necessary for their application.

A *hot pack* or fomentation is the application of hot moist cloth to an area of the body. Usually it is applied to an area where there is not an open wound and frequently to a larger area than could be covered by a compress. Frequently wool flannel is used for hot packs because it holds heat well.

After a compress or a hot pack has been applied, it is advisable to apply external heat, such as a hot water bottle or heating pad, to help maintain the heat of the application.

Procedure 17-9.   Application of Hot Moist (Sterile) Compresses

ACTION	EXPLANATION
Assemble Equipment	
1. Solution as ordered.	For a sterile compress.
2. Sterile container for solution.	
3. Gauze squares.	
4. Plastic.	For insulation.
5. Sterile gloves or forceps	To wring out gauze.
6. Hot-water bottle or specially insulated electric pad.	To provide additional heat to maintain the heat of the compress.
7. Insulating towel.	

Note: A hot soak (pack) is the unsterile application of moist heat, usually to a large body area. In order to prepare hot packs, special hot-pack machines are available in which pieces of flannel are heated. In this instance a thermometer, gauze, and gloves or forceps are normally not required. The pack is usually applied at as hot a temperature as the patient can tolerate.

ACTION	EXPLANATION
To apply a hot compress	
1. Explain to the patient what you plan to do. Adjust the explanation to the patient's needs.	To reassure the patient by knowledge of what will be done. To identify the patient.
2. Provide the patient with privacy.	
3. Assist the patient to a comfortable position and expose the area of the body that will have the compress.	
4. Wash hands.	
5. Heat the solution.	
6. Remove the dressing if one is on the wound.	Proceed as for a sterile dressing.
7. Cleanse the wound.	See sterile dressing technique.
8. Immerse the gauze square in the solution and wring it out.	
9. Apply it to the designated area.	
10. Cover the gauze with the plastic and the insulating towel.	Mold the compress closely to the body in order to reduce heat loss by evaporation.
11. Apply external heat.	Use a hot-water bottle at 40.5–43.3° C (105–110° F).
12. Assist the patient to a comfortable position.	
13. Gather the equipment and dispose of it appropriately.	
14. Wash hands.	

15. Record the application of compress, solution used, appearance of wound and any exudate, and any statements of discomfort from the patient.

Note: Compresses are usually changed every 1–2 hours. If changes are required less often, the wet compress should be replaced with a dry sterile dressing when it becomes cool (about 30 minutes to 1 hour).

The following equipment is needed for hot wet packs:

1. Flannel pieces or commercial packs
2. Hot-pack machine
3. Petroleum jelly
4. Plastic material for insulation
5. Insulation materials—flannel, towel, etc.
6. Hot-water bottle or heating pad

The hot wet pack is prepared either by boiling or steaming pieces of flannel or by heating commercially prepared packs in hot-pack machines. After heating the pack, it is applied directly to the area to be treated. It is applied as quickly as the patient can tolerate, then covered with plastic and insulating materials, which assist in the retention of heat. Hot-water bottles and especially insulated electric pads are also applied to provide additional heat.

If a patient's skin tends to be irritated by the hot pack, the application of petroleum jelly to surrounding skin areas before the pack is applied will serve to protect it. Hot packs provide heat for a short period of time (about 15 minutes), and they need to be removed after they cool. Sometimes continuous hot packs are ordered to reduce severe muscle spasm.

Dry Applications of Heat

Dry heat is frequently applied to the body for one or more of the following reasons:

1. Comfort.
2. To dry skin areas or a newly applied plaster of Paris cast.
3. To increase blood circulation to an area, such as the application of infrared heat to a decubitus ulcer.

Hot-water Bottles (Bags)

Hot-water bottles, sometimes referred to as hot-water bags, are frequently used as a source of dry heat in the home. They are being used less often in hospitals because of the burns that can result from injudicious use. The following temperatures of the water in the bags are considered safe in most situations and provide the desired effect:

Normal adult	51.6° C	(125° F)
Debilitated, unconscious adult	40.5–46.1° C	(105–115° F)
Child under 2 years of age	40.5–46.1° C	(105–115° F)

In agencies where hot-water bags and heating pads are used, it is not unusual for the patient to be required to sign a release before their use. The release absolves the agency and its employees from any responsibility as a result of any injury incurred in their use.

Hot-water bags are usually filled about two-thirds of their volume. The remaining air is then expelled and the top secured. In this way the hot water bag is light, and it can be readily molded to a body part. After the bag is dried, it is held upside down and tested for leakage. If it is secure, it is then wrapped in a towel or cover and placed on the appropriate body site. Hot-water bags retain their heat for about an hour.

Electric Pads

Electric pads and blankets have become increasingly popular in recent years. They have the advantage of providing a constant, even heat and of being light and easily molded to a body part. Some electric pads have waterproof covers, and these are highly desirable for use in situations were moisture exists. Heating pads used in agencies are frequently set to a specific temperature, while those found in homes usually have a control for the temperature.

Caution needs to be taken, when using electric pads, that pins are not inserted into the pad. A pin can hit a wire inside the pad, thereby damaging the pad and causing a shock to the person holding the pin.

Infrared Lamps and Heat Lamps

Infrared lamps are also used to apply dry heat, usually to a small body area with an open wound. They are also used to promote healing of decubitus ulcers. Heat lamps and infrared lamps are similar in their use and their action. The chief difference is that an infrared lamp has an infrared element, while a heat lamp uses a special bulb or a 60-watt bulb.

Infrared rays penetrate only 3 mm of body tissue, and thus they provide heat chiefly to the surface of the skin or mucous membranes. Two sizes of infrared lamps are commonly available. The larger lamp is placed further from the patient than the smaller one.

Before an infrared lamp is used, the area to be heated should be clean and dry. This lessens the likelihood of burning. A small lamp should be placed 45–60 cm (18–24 inches) from the patient, while the larger lamp is placed 60–75 cm (24–30 inches) away. The treatment usually lasts 15 to 20 minutes, provided the patient is tolerating the heat satisfactorily. The patient should be checked after five minutes for any discomfort, burning, or untoward reaction. Important also in the use of infrared lamps is the need to caution the patient not to touch the lamp, and the lamp should not be draped or placed under any bedclothes because of the chance of initiating a fire. At the first sign of skin redness or discomfort, the treatment should be terminated and the reaction reported and recorded.

Heat Cradles

Heat cradles, sometimes referred to as *bakers*, are also used to provide dry heat to an area. They are usually used to supply heat to large body areas such as the abdomen, legs, or chest. Heat cradles are made of metal and contain a series of bulbs, often 25 watts. The cradle is placed over the patient and usually covered with a bath blanket or sheet. The temperature inside the cradle should not normally exceed 51.6° C (125° F), and the treatment normally lasts 10 to 15 minutes. The heat source inside the cradle should be 45–60 cm (18–24 inches) away from the patient.

K-Matic Pads (Aquathermia Pads)

The K-Matic pad is a device in which warm distilled water circulates, providing heat to a body part. The reservoir of the pad is filled two-thirds full, and air bubbles are removed. The pad is then covered and placed on the body part after the desired temperature is set. Normal temperature is 40.5° C (105° F) and the treatment is usually continued for 10 to 15 minutes. In the event of any unusual redness or pain, the treatment should be discontinued and the patient's reaction reported and recorded.

COLD APPLICATIONS

Reasons for Applying Cold

Cold can also be applied in either moist or dry forms. It is used for both systemic and local purposes. Systemically, cold is applied to lower the body's metabolic rate in preparation for certain types of surgery and to lower the body's temperature in situations where it is persistently elevated.

Locally, cold is applied for any of the following reasons:

1. To decrease and terminate bleeding, for example, after a tonsillectomy.
2. To anesthetize body areas and reduce pain.
3. To reduce inflammation.
4. To control the accumulation of fluid.

To Decrease and Terminate Bleeding

Cold constricts the arterioles and increases the viscosity of the blood. It therefore can act to control bleeding and to prevent the occurrence of a hemorrhage.

To Anesthetize and Reduce Pain

Cold applications also decrease the sensitivity of tissues and create a sensation of numbness. Thus cold can be used as a local anesthetic for a short period of time. This is important to remember when applying cold. However, the patient may be unaware, because of the numbness, that the tissues are being damaged.

To Reduce Inflammation

Cold reduces the inflammatory process and slows the suppurative process by causing vasoconstriction and decreasing local tissue metabolism.

To Control the Accumulation of Fluid

Because of the vasoconstriction of the arterioles, fluid accumulation in body tissues is delayed. Therefore cold is applied in order to prevent swelling due to sprains or to tissue trauma.

The temperature used for cold applications depends upon the purpose of the application, the size of the area to which it is to be applied, and the length of time of the treatment. Applications are usually described as very cold, cold, cool, or tepid. See Table 17-2 for temperature ranges.

Factors of Concern in Regard to Cold Applications

The following factors affect the use of cold applications to an area of the body and the degree of cold to be applied:

1. The size of the body area. The greater the area of the body, the higher the temperature of the cold application.
2. The use of moist or dry cold. Moist cold penetrates better than dry cold; therefore moist applications do not require as low a temperature as dry applications.
3. The age and condition of the patient. Elderly patients and people with impaired circulation tolerate cold less well than younger people with good circulation.

Contraindications to the Application of Cold

Cold applications are normally ordered by a physician. Nurses need to be aware, however, of symptoms that can contraindicate cold applications. When any of these are observed, they need to be reported:

1. Bluish, purplish appearance to the skin or mucous membrane.
2. Cold feeling to the skin or mucous membrane.
3. A feeling of numbness.

4. Pain due to contracted muscles.
5. Shivering and a lowered body temperature.

Moist Applications of Cold

Moist cold is commonly applied in two ways: by moist, cold compresses and by an alcohol or cold sponge bath. Moist, cold compresses can be applied to both closed and open wounds. Where open wounds are involved, sterile technique is indicated. The technique is similar to that for hot compresses, and the student is referred to Procedure 17-9.

Alcohol or Sponge Bath (Tepid Sponge Bath)

The alcohol or sponge bath is used in order to reduce a patient's systemic temperature. Usually it will reduce a fever rapidly. Alcohol and sponge baths are generally ordered by a physician. An alcohol bath is a combination of alcohol and water; a sponge bath uses cool water. Alcohol is less frequently used due to its drying effect. The temperature of both solutions is generally 29.4–37.7° C (85–100° F). The following equipment is required:

1. Basin for the solution
2. Bath thermometer
3. Solution as ordered
4. Washcloths and towel
5. Bath blanket
6. Patient thermometer

Initially the patient's temperature, pulse, and respiration are taken and recorded. If the sponge bath is effective, these vital signs should change when taken after the bath (temperature is reduced).

As with other baths, the patient's privacy is ensured, and the bath blanket is used to cover the patient. Large areas are sponged at one time, permitting the heat of the body to transfer to the cooler solution on the body surface. Often wet cloths are applied to the wrists, groin, and ankles, where the blood circulation is close to the skin surface. Each area is dried by patting rather than rubbing, since rubbing will increase the cell metabolism and thus the rate of heat production.

The temperature, pulse, and respiration are taken 15 to 20 minutes after the bath. A physician may order a sponge bath to be repeated until the temperature reaches a certain point. Sponge baths are generally terminated before the temperature reaches normal because a further drop can be anticipated.

391

If during a sponge bath the patient demonstrates any of the following symptoms, the bath should be terminated and the symptoms reported and recorded:

1. Bluishness (cyanosis) of the lips or nails.

2. Shivering.

3. Accelerated weak pulse.

Dry Application of Cold

A number of dry cold applications are used for both systemic and local effects.

Systemic Cold: Hypothermia

Hypothermia is used in order to decrease a patient's metabolism and to maintain a low body temperature, often for prolonged periods. It is indicated in some instances of cerebral injury and cerebral surgery.

A number of methods are employed in therapeutic hypothermia. Nurses are most likely to be involved in the method in which the hypothermia is induced by cooling the body surface. Another method, the extracorporeal, includes the use of a heart-lung machine (usually during surgery). In this method the blood can be cooled, thereby reducing the patient's body temperature.

In therapeutic hypothermia by surface cooling, the patient lies between two cooling blankets, which are attached to a machine. Within the blanket, coolant circulates, which serves to provide the cooling to the body surface. The following nursing measures are important in caring for patients who are undergoing hypothermia:

1. Monitoring vital signs: temperature, pulse, respirations, and blood pressure.

2. Maintaining skin cleanliness and protecting it with oil as required.

3. Observing any signs of tissue damage and frostbite.

4. Assisting patients to meet their basic needs, such as nutrition, elimination, and hygiene.

Surface hypothermia can also be induced in the following ways:

1. Covering the patient with a wet sheet over which a fan is directed.

2. Covering the patient's body surface with ice bags or plastic bags filled with ice.

3. Immersing the patient in a tub of icy water. This is sometimes done for children in the home.

After a period of hypothermia, a patient's vital signs need to be monitored regularly and frequently until these signs have remained constant for 72 hours.

Local Cold: The Ice Bag

Ice bags are commonly used in both homes and hospitals. They are made commercially of plastic or rubber material. Small pieces of ice are placed in the bag until it is two-thirds full, excess air is expelled, and the top is secured in order to prevent leaking. The bag is then covered with a piece of flannel or towel and placed on the patient so that it molds to the body part. The cover serves to absorb the moisture from condensation and will need to be changed when it becomes wet. Ice bags should usually be removed an hour after application and then reapplied an hour later for maximum effectiveness.

SUMMARY

A common function of the nurse is to care for wounds. This may involve changing dressings, shortening and maintaining drains, administering heat and cold applications, applying bandages and binders, and irrigating body parts. Surgical asepsis is employed for many of these measures.

Wounds may be intentional or unintentional. Six categories are classified and include incisions, contusions, abrasions, lacerations, puncture wounds, and penetrating wounds. Wound healing can be promoted by measures that prevent an infection (use of sterile technique), prevent further injury (immobil-ization by binders), reduce inflammatory swelling (application of cold), and improve blood circulation (application of heat). Factors that inhibit wound healing include the presence of foreign hematomas, infections, and localized ischemia. The appearance of a clean healing wound is described for appropriate assessment of healing.

Surgical asepsis involves the application of several principles, which are outlined in the chapter. Especially important is conscientiousness, alertness, and honesty on the part of the nurse in adhering to standards. All sterile supplies are handled by using sterile forceps, by wearing sterile gloves, or by enveloping the hands in a sterile drape. Each of these techniques is described in detail. In all of these instances the nurse first needs to scrub the hands and forearms thoroughly.

Sterile wrapped packages need to be opened in such a way that the sterile contents are not contaminated. This is done by first opening the flap of the package that is farthest away, then the side flaps, and last the flap nearest the nurse. Many small items are commercially prepared in paper or plastic containers. These, too, require sterile precautions when they are opened.

The care of wounds varies considerably in accordance with the type of wound, its size and location, the amount of exudate, the presence of complicating factors, and sometimes the personal preference of the physician. Advantages and disadvantages of the open and closed methods of wound care are discussed. The types of dressing materials and their indications for use are also outlined.

Prior to changing dressings the nurse needs to ascertain the physician's orders, the presence of drains, the amount of wound drainage, and specific cleansing solutions to be used. The specific techniques involved in preparing necessary equipment, removing soiled dressings, cleansing wounds, and applying clean dressings are described. The technique for cleansing and shortening Penrose drains is also outlined.

Agency policies vary in relation to personnel who may remove skin sutures. Because registered nurses may be responsible for this procedure, five common types of sutures are described, and guidelines for removing them are included.

Irrigations of wounds are often prescribed to cleanse wounds, to administer heat, or to apply medications in solution form. The techniques for wound irrigation and for irrigating the eye, the ear, the throat, and the vagina are outlined in a step-by-step format.

Bandages and binders serve several purposes in the care of wounds, but support and immobilization are the two most common ones. Materials used vary widely and relate to the purpose of the bandage. Examples are flannel, muslin, gauze, and elastic adhesive. Principles and general guidelines for bandaging are outlined as well as the five basic turns required for specific body parts. The five turns are the spiral, circular, spiral reverse, recurrent, and figure-of-eight. Five commonly used types of binders are the triangular binder, the breast binder, the scultetus (many-tailed) binder, the single and double T-binder, and the abdominal binder.

Heat and cold can be applied in either dry or moist forms. Heat therapy is usually classified as radiant (infrared lamp), conductive (hot-water bag), or conversive (medical diathermy). Physiologic responses to heat and cold are outlined. Each thermal effect is further described in accordance with the duration of the application. External applications of short duration and of long duration produce different physiologic responses; however the extremes of both hot and cold applications can damage cells. When administering heat or cold applications, the nurse needs to consider the following factors: size of the body area, type of application (moist or dry), individual tolerances, specific skin area involved, and the age and condition of the patient.

Nine reasons for heat applications are outlined. Included are the relief of muscle spasm, the reduction of congestion, comfort and relaxation, and the hastening of the suppurative process. Hot moist applications include sitz baths, soaks, compresses, and wet packs. Hot dry applications include the hot-water bottle, electric pads, heat lamps, heat cradles, and K-Matic pads.

Cold applications are used to decrease and terminate bleeding, to anesthetize body areas, to reduce inflammation, and to control the accumulation of fluid. The moist application of cold includes the tepid sponge bath. Dry cold applications include hypothermia and the ice bag. Prior to administering any hot or cold application, the nurse needs to recognize symptoms that contraindicate its use.

SUGGESTED ACTIVITIES

1. In a clinical area, identify patients who are receiving heat or cold applications. Determine the reasons for these applications and their effects.

2. Observe several surgical incisions or other open wounds and compare their appearance with the characteristics of clean healing wounds described in this chapter.

3. Observe several irrigations in a home or agency setting. Describe the return irrigation in terms of color, clarity, and odor.

4. In a laboratory setting, mark an incision on the abdomen of a classmate, cleanse the incision, and apply an abdominal dressing using sterile technique.

5. Stitch three different types of sutures into a piece of cloth or tape, and then remove them using sterile technique.

The article describes bandaging techniques that are useful in an emergency situation in the community. Photographs provide step-by-step action for some bandage techniques.

SUGGESTED READINGS

Auld, Margaret E., et al. October, 1972. Wound healing. *Nursing 72* 2:36–40.

This article describes how nurses can assist wounds to heal and how nurses can hinder the healing process.

Castle, Mary. August, 1975. Wound care. *Nursing 75* 5 (8):40–44.

Using many photographs, the author describes wound care with particular reference to the practical problems encountered by nurses.

Devney, Ann Marie, and Kingsbury, Barbara A. August, 1972. Hypothermia in fact and fantasy. *American Journal of Nursing* 72:1424–1425.

This article provides an overview of the methods of hypothermia and the complications significant to nurses that can ensue.

Rinear, Charles E., and Rinear, Eileen E. January, 1975. Emergency bandaging. *Nursing 75* 5(1):29–35.

SELECTED REFERENCES

Dyer, Elaine D., and Bagnell, Howard K. January–February, 1970. Local tissue and general temperature changes in dogs, produced by temperature applications. *Nursing Research* 19:37–41.

Glor, Beverly A. K., and Estes, Zane E. September–October, 1970. Moist soaks: a survey of clinical practices. *Nursing Research* 19:463–465.

Hickey, Mary Catherine. January, 1965. Hypothermia. *American Journal of Nursing* 65:116–122.

Myers, M. Bert. September, 1971. Sutures and wound healing. *American Journal of Nursing* 71:1725–1727.

Nursing 75. October, 1975. Wound suction: better drainage with fewer problems. *Nursing 75* 5(10):52–55.

Powell, Mary. October, 1972. An environment for wound healing. *American Journal of Nursing* 72:1862–1865.

Weinstock, Frank J. October, 1971. Emergency treatment of eye injuries. *American Journal of Nursing* 71:1928–1931.

UNIT IV

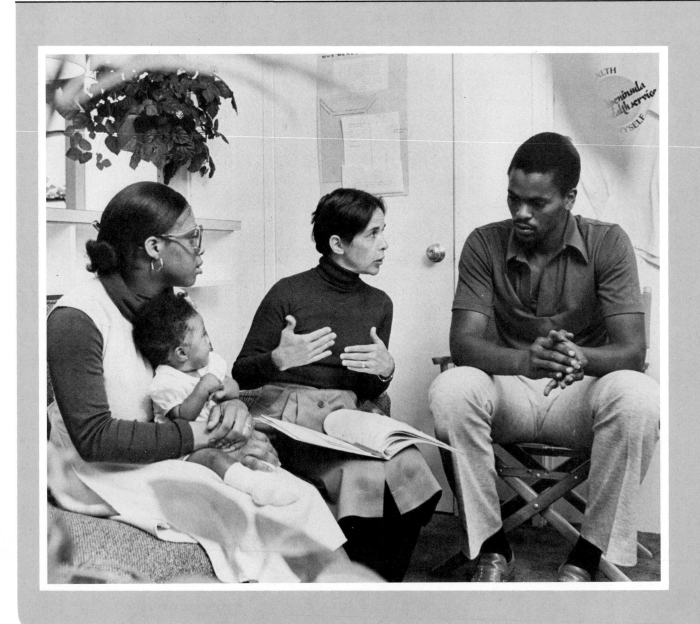

THERAPEUTIC COMMUNICATION

CHAPTER 18

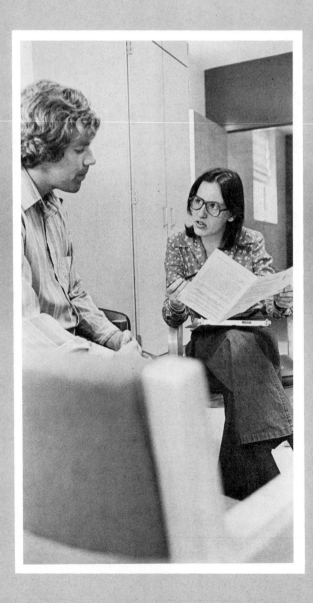

COMMUNICATING EFFECTIVELY

OBJECTIVES

- Define communication and describe the two basic kinds of communication.
- Discuss five characteristics of effective verbal messages.
- Discuss various attributes and limitations of nonverbal communication.
- Describe aspects of nonverbal behavior that need to be observed.
- Explain the four elements of the communication process.
- Describe some techniques that facilitate communication.
- Describe some techniques that inhibit communication.
- Discuss several factors that influence the communication process.
- Outline aspects of the process of communication (language) development.
- Discuss factors that influence language development and ways in which it can be stimulated.
- Outline guidelines for ways of helping patients.
- Describe the four phases of effective nurse-patient relationships.

The term *communication* has various meanings depending upon the context in which it is used. To some, communication is the interchange of information between two or more people; in other words, the exchange of ideas or thoughts. This kind of communication uses methods such as talking and listening or writing and reading. However, communication can also include painting, dancing, and story-telling. Thoughts are not only conveyed to others by spoken or written words but also by gestures or body actions. These will be discussed in the section on kinds of communication.

Communication may have a more personal connotation. In contrast to the interchange of ideas or thoughts, communication can be a transmission of feelings, or a more personal and social interaction between people. In this context communication often is synonymous with relating. Frequently we hear the comment from a wife or husband that the spouse is not communicating. The same holds true for some teenagers who complain about a generation gap—being unable to communicate with understanding or feeling to a parent or authority figure. Sometimes one hears it said about a nurse that she or he is efficient' but lacks something called *bedside manner*. For the purpose of this text, communication is any means of exchanging information or feelings between two or more people and will be regarded as a basic component of human relationships. The intent of any communication is to elicit a response. To communicate effectively with patients and their families, nurses need to become skilled in communication techniques and in developing therapeutic (helping) relationships. Communication by nurses with other health workers was discussed in Chapter 15, Recording and Reporting.

KINDS OF COMMUNICATION

Communication is generally categorized into two basic kinds, *verbal* and *nonverbal. Verbal communication* is that which uses the spoken word; *nonverbal communication* uses forms other than the spoken word, such as gestures. Although both kinds of communication occur concurrently, the majority of communication is nonverbal. This may be surprising to those who associate communication with only the verbal forms of expression such as talking or writing. Learning about nonverbal communication is thus an important consideration for nurses in developing effective communication patterns and relationships with patients.

Verbal Communication

Verbal communication is largely a conscious effort in that the person chooses the words he or she uses. The words used vary among individuals according to the person's culture, socioeconomic background, age, and education. As a result, countless possibilities exist in the way ideas are exchanged. An abundance of words can be used to form messages. In addition, a wide variety of feelings can be conveyed when talking. The intonation of one's voice can express animation, enthusiasm, sadness, annoyance, or amusement, to name some examples. Consider the number of different intonations you have heard when people say "hello" or "good morning." The pacing or rhythm of a person's communication is another variance. Monotonous rhythms or very rapid rhythms can be products of anxiety or fear or lack of energy or interest.

Characteristics of Giving Effective Verbal Messages

When choosing words to say or to write, several criteria need to be considered in order to provide effective communication. These include (a) simplicity, (b) clarity, (c) timing and relevancy, (d) adaptability, and (e) credibility.

Simplicity   The best teachers can state complex ideas in simple words. The same holds true for persons communicating everyday concerns. Simplicity includes the use of commonly understood words, brevity, and completeness.

Many people have a tendency to over-communicate. Their messages tend to be wordy, to contain too many explanations that are extraneous, or to involve words that are highly academic, technical, or are considered to be slang. In the world of nursing, many complex technical terms become natural to nurses. However, these terms can often be misunderstood even by informed laymen. Words such as "discombobulate" or "cholecystectomy" may be meaningful to the speaker and easy to use but are ill-advised when communicating with patients. Nurses need to learn to intentionally select simple words even though effort is required in doing so. For example, instead of saying to a patient, "The nurse will be catheterizing you tomorrow for a urine specimen," it is better to say, "Tomorrow the doctor needs a sample of your urine, and it will be necessary to collect it by putting a tube into your bladder." The latter statement is likely to produce a response from the patient about why it is needed and whether it will hurt or be uncomfortable rather than make the patient wonder what the nurse means.

Another consideration related to simplicity is brevity. Most people have heard lengthy explanations of events by others to which they respond, "Get to the point." By using short sentences and avoiding unnecessary material, brevity can be achieved. This is of particular importance in writing. Busy people do not have the time to read several pages of concerns before discovering the main issue or the recommendations that have been put forth. Reports or memos need to be concise and condensed into a single paragraph or page.

The opposite of over-communicating is under-communicating. Short cuts at the cost of simplicity or brevity can lead to incomplete communication. An example is the use of initials or abbreviations such as b.i.d. (twice a day) or ICU (Intensive Care Unit). Unless the nurse is certain that the initials will be readily understood, they should be avoided. Because clarification is required, abbreviations can waste the listener's or reader's time. Initially names should be expressed in full; later they can be shortened when the nurse is sure that the patient or reader knows the meanings.

Clarity   *Clarity* refers to saying exactly what is meant. It also is aligned with meaning what you say. The latter involves a blending of the speaker's behavior (nonverbal communication) with the words that are spoken. When the words and the behavior of the speaker blend together or are unified, the communication is regarded as consistent or congruent.

The goal of clarity is to communicate so that people know the what, the how, the why if necessary, and the time, person, and place of any specific event. Without consideration to these, people are left in a position to make assumptions. To ensure clarity in communication the nurse also needs to speak slowly and enunciate words well. It is helpful as well to repeat the message and to reduce distractions such as surrounding noises.

Some common pitfalls that can produce unclear communications are the use of ambiguous statements, generalizations, or opinions. For example,

"Men are stronger than women," "Women are better cooks than men," "All of Doctor X's patients hemorrhage postoperatively." Another pitfall is to ask several questions at once. For example, a nurse enters a patient's room and says in one breath, "Good morning, Mrs. Broadbeat. How are you this morning? Did you sleep well last night? Your husband is coming to see you before your surgery, isn't he?" The patient no doubt feels bombarded and confused and wonders which question to answer first, if any.

Another pitfall is to ask a question and then not wait for an answer before making another comment. An example is the husband who asks his wife when she returns from work: "How did the job go today, honey? I must show you my new shoes." In this instance the husband conveys the feeling that he is not really interested in the wife's day at work. Nurses also commit this error. To Mr. Snowball the nurse says, "How is that swollen leg this morning? I'm going to get your bath water now before the doctor comes."

Timing and Relevancy.   No matter how clearly or simply words are stated or written, the timing needs to be appropriate to ensure that words are heard. Moreover, the messages need to relate to the person or to the person's interests and concerns. Consider the problem of the harrassed woman with children crying, the telephone ringing, and the doorbell sounding all at the same time. This is not the best time for the person on the telephone to discuss what to wear to dinner or for the person at the door to try to make a sale, even if the woman is interested.

Nurses need to be aware of both relevancy and timing when communicating with patients. This involves being sensitive to the patient's needs and concerns. These are not always as obvious as in the situation just described. For example, explanations to a female patient about the expected procedures before and after her gallbladder surgery may not be heard if the woman is enmeshed in her fear of cancer. In this situation it is better for the nurse first to encourage the patient to express her concern and at another time to provide the necessary explanations.

Adaptability.   Spoken messages need to be altered in accordance with behavioral cues from the receiver. This adjustment is referred to as *adaptability*. Moods and behavior may change hour by hour or from day to day. In this sense the nurse needs to avoid routine or automatic speech. What the nurse says and how it is said must be individualistic and carefully considered. This requires astute observation and sensitivity on the part of the nurse.

Credibility.   *Credibility* refers to being worthy of belief, to being trustworthy and reliable. It can be regarded as the most important criterion of communication. Being credible to patients depends in part upon the opinion of others. If other health workers and patients regard the nurse as trustworthy, then the patient will. More will be discussed about developing trust later in this chapter in the section "Phases of the Helping Relationship."

To become credible the nurse needs to be knowledgeable about the subject matter being discussed. The information needs to be accurate. The nurse also needs to convey confidence and certainty in what he or she is saying. This is often referred to as *positivism.* People tend to perceive confidence, which is more dynamic and emphatic, as more credible than hesitancy or uncertainty, which is less forceful and less active. However, caution needs to be taken to not sound over-confident or authoritarian. This can be prevented by stating messages in a constructive way that is helpful to patients.

Reliability, the third aspect of credibility, is developed by being consistent, dependable, and honest. People value the nurse who acknowledges limitations and can say, "I do not know the answer to that, but will find someone who does and to whom you can talk."

Nonverbal Communication

Nonverbal communication is sometimes referred to as *body language.* It includes gestures, all body movements, and physical appearance, including adornment. The majority of a person's communication is nonverbal. Nonverbal communication often tells people more about what is felt than what is actually said. The reason for this is that nonverbal behavior is controlled less consciously than verbal behavior. As a result, listeners tend to rely upon body language more than upon words. Nonverbal communication either reinforces or contradicts what is said verbally. For example, the teacher or counselor may say, "I have lots of time to see you (a student)" and yet glance nervously at her watch during the visit. Her actions are contradicting the verbal message. The nonverbal behavior, suggesting "I am very busy," is more likely to be believed.

Certain limitations exist in nonverbal communication. One cannot always be sure of the feelings being expressed by nonverbal behavior. The same feeling can be expressed nonverbally in more than one way. For example, anger may be communicated by aggressive or excessive body motion, or it may be communicated by a frozen stillness. In addition, a variety of feelings such as embarrassment, pleasure, or anger can be expressed by one single nonverbal cue such as blushing (Johnson 1972:104).

Observing and interpreting the patient's nonverbal behavior is an essential skill for nurses. Observational skills using the senses of seeing, hearing, touching, and smelling are required. Interpreting the observations requires validation with the patient, using specific communication techniques discussed subsequently.

The nurse also needs to remember that his or her own nonverbal behavior is under constant scrutiny by patients. It is therefore necessary for nurses to gain awareness of their own actions and to learn to convey understanding, respect, and acceptance to patients.

Observing and Interpreting Nonverbal Behavior

In order to observe nonverbal behavior efficiently, a systematic approach needs to be used. Generally the nurse notes the person's overall physical appearance, including adornment, posture, and gait, and then specific parts of the body such as the face and the hands.

Physical Appearance.   The person's appearance includes physical characteristics and manner of dress. Physical characteristics can denote the person's state of health. Skin color and texture, length of fingernails, weight, or deformities causing physical limitations are a few examples. The skin may appear dry or mottled or pale. Weight may indicate malnourishment. Nails may be well manicured or short. Whatever is observed by the nurse needs caution in interpretation. For example, skin color may appear pale, but it may be normal for that particular person. Nails may be short because they were chewed or because they were broken with hard manual labor.

Clothing and adornment are sometimes rich sources of information about a person. The choice of apparel is highly personal. Clothing may convey a person's social and financial status, culture, religion, group association, and self-concept. Other adornments such as jewelry, perfume, or cosmetics reveal additional information.

How a person dresses is often an indicator of how the person feels. People who are tired or ill may not have the energy or the desire to maintain their normal grooming. The nurse also needs to be alert to sudden changes in a person's dress. A person who is known for immaculate grooming may become lazy about appearance and stay in a nightgown all day, suggesting a loss of self-esteem or perhaps physical illness. Hair care or nail care may be lacking. Appropriateness of dress is also dependent upon context. A swimsuit worn to a beach party is regarded as appropriate, whereas a swimsuit worn to a dinner party usually is not.

In acute general hospital settings, indications that a patient is feeling better often relate to dress, particularly personal adornment. A male patient may request a shave or a female patient may request a mirror and her lipstick.

Posture and Gait. The way people walk and carry themselves is often a reliable indicator of self-concept, current mood, and health. An erect posture and an active, purposeful stride suggest a feeling of well-being. A slouched posture and slow, shuffling gait suggest dejection or physical discomfort. A tense posture and rapid, determined gait suggest anxiety or anger. Likewise the sitting or lying postures of patients can communicate similar feelings.

Facial Expressions. No part of the body is as expressive as the face. Feelings of joy, sadness, fear, surprise, anger, and disgust can be conveyed by facial expressions. The muscles around the eye and the mouth are particularly expressive. Although actors learn to control these muscles to convey emotions to audiences, facial expressions are not generally consciously controlled.

Patients are quick to notice the nurse's facial expression, particularly in situations where patients feel unsure or uncomfortable. The patient who questions the nurse about a feared diagnostic result will watch the nurse's face to see if the nurse looks at him to answer or looks away. The patient who has disfigurement will examine the nurse's face for signs of disgust. Nurses, like actors, need to be aware of their facial expressions and what they are communicating to patients. Although it is impossible to control all facial expressions, the nurse must learn to control some feelings such as fear and disgust in certain situations.

Many facial expressions convey a universal meaning. The smile conveys happiness. Contempt is conveyed by the mouth turned down, the head tilted back, and the eyes directed down the nose. No single expression can be interpreted accurately, however, without considering (a) other reinforcing physical cues, (b) the setting in which it occurs, and (c) the expression of others in the same setting. Consider the person who is smiling among others who are intently watching an accident victim on the street. In this instance the smiling could convey contempt.

Eye contact is another essential element of facial communication. Mutual eye contact acknowledges recognition of the other person and a willingness to maintain communication. Often the eye initiates contact with another person with a glance, thus capturing the person's attention prior to communicating. Eye contact is generally averted or avoided when a person feels weak or defenseless. The communication received may be too embarrassing or too dominating. Animals are also known to succumb to dominance by averting their eyes and then their presence.

Hand Movements and Gestures. Like faces, the hands are another expressive body part. Hands can communicate feelings at any given moment. Envision the person in an interview for a new job. Anxious people may wring their hands or pick their nails; relaxed persons may interlock their hands over their laps or allow their hands to fall over the end of an armrest. Hands also communicate by touch. Hitting someone in the face or caressing another communicates obvious feelings.

Hands are frequently involved in the use of gestures. The handshake, the victory sign, the wave goodbye, the welcome sign as you ask a visitor to sit down are gestures that have relatively universal meanings. Some gestures, however, are socially accepted in one culture while not in another. European women walk together holding hands as a sign of friendship. In contrast, in North American society two women holding hands is usually regarded as socially unacceptable. Even the same gesture can have different meanings in different cultures. The "shoo away" or "go away" gesture of the hands in North America means "come here" or "come back" in some Japanese cultures.

Hands are also very expressive in illustrating or stylizing verbal communication. The French and Italian cultures are noted for using their hands in this manner. Instead of describing the attractive shape and contour of a movie star by words alone, the hands are manipulated to reinforce the verbal message.

For people who have special communication problems, such as deaf mutes, the hands are invaluable in communication. Many of these people learn to speak sign language. For some ill persons who are unable to reply verbally, the nurse and patient can devise a unique communication system using the hands. The patient may be able to raise an index finger once for "yes" and twice for "no." Other signals can often be devised to denote other meanings.

Gestures often involve body parts other than the hands. In some cultures a gentleman may bow before a lady; two European men greet each other by embracing and touching opposite cheeks alternately; men and women kiss to say hello or goodbye.

Elements of the Communication Process

In its simplest form communication has been described as a two-way process involving the sending and the receiving of a message. Since the intent of communication is to elicit a response, the process is ongoing in that the receiver of the message then becomes the sender of a message while the original sender then becomes the receiver. Several sequential models have been proposed for the communication process, incorporating from four to six elements. Essential to all are four elements: (a) the sender, (b) the message, (c) the receiver, and (d) the response (feedback).

The Sender

The sender or person who wishes to convey a message to another is referred to by some as the *source-encoder*. The term *source-encoder* includes the concept that the person sending the message must first have an idea or reason for communicating (source) and second must put the idea or feeling into a form that can be transmitted (encoded). *Encoding* involves the selection of specific signs or symbols (codes) to transmit the message such as the use of English or French words, the specific arrangement of the words, and the tone of voice and gestures to use. For example, if the receiver is Canadian or American, English words will usually be selected. If the message is "No, Johnny, you may not have any more cookies before dinner!" the tone of voice selected will be one of firmness, and a shake of the head or a pointing index finger can reinforce it.

The Message

The second component is the message itself—what is actually said or written (body language accompanies the former) and how it is transmitted. Various channels can be used to convey messages, and frequently these are used in combinations. It is important that the channel chosen is appropriate for the message and is one which will make the intent of the message clear.

Talking directly with a person face-to-face may be more effective in some instances than telephoning or writing a message. Recording messages on tape or

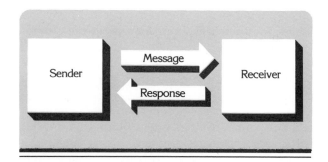

Figure 18-1.   Elements of the communication process.

communicating by radio or television may be more appropriate for larger audiences. Written communication is often appropriate for long lists of explanations or for communication that needs to be recorded. The nonverbal channel of touch is often highly effective.

The Receiver

The receiver, the third component, is the listener. This person must perceive what the sender intended (sensation) and then analyze the information received (interpretation). Perception involves use of all the senses to receive all the verbal and the nonverbal messages. Another term for the receiver is the *decoder*. This means that the receiver must relate the message perceived to his or her storehouse of knowledge and experience and sort out the meaning of the message. How accurately the message is decoded by the receiver in accordance to what the sender intended depends to a large extent upon their similarities in knowledge and experience. For example, Johnny may interpret the message accurately—"No more cookies for me right now." However, if his past experience has taught him that he can help himself to the cookie jar without punishment, he will interpret the message differently.

The Response

The fourth component, the response, is the message that the receiver returns to the sender. It is also called *feedback*. Feedback can be either positive or negative. Nonverbal examples are a nod of the head or a yawn. Either way, feedback allows the sender to correct or reword a message. In the case of Johnny he may cry or move away from the cookie jar or say, "Well, Judy had three cookies and I only had two." The sender then knows the message was interpreted accurately. However, now the original sender becomes the receiver, who is required to decode and respond.

The receiver is not the sole source of feedback. Communicators constantly receive *internal feedback* or that from the self. Internal feedback is often used for written messages. For example, after composing a letter the person will read the letter silently or out loud to see how it sounds. Another example of internal feedback is the social blunder (faux pas) recognized instantly by the sender. In this case, as soon as the speaker has said something, he or she realizes the mistake and says, "That isn't really what I meant" or "I didn't mean it that way."

SOME TECHNIQUES TO FACILITATE COMMUNICATION

Communication, whether it is verbal or nonverbal, can be described as helpful (therapeutic) or unhelpful (nontherapeutic). The former encourages a sharing of information, thoughts, or feelings between two or more people. The latter hinders or blocks the transfer of information.

Several techniques can be used to facilitate communication that will promote understanding on the part of the sender and on the part of the receiver. These techniques can also assist in the formation of a constructive relationship between the nurse and the patient. On the other hand, use of the techniques is no guarantee to effective communication. So many factors are involved in communication that the nurse would be ill-advised to rely solely upon any one or even several specific techniques. Not all people feel comfortable with all techniques, and skill is essential in using them appropriately.

Listening Attentively

Attentive listening is listening actively using all the senses as opposed to listening passively with just the ear. It is probably the most important technique of all. It is an active process that requires energy and concentration. It involves attention to the person's total message. This includes both the spoken verbal messages and the nonverbal messages that modify what is spoken. It also involves noting whether verbal and nonverbal communication are congruent. Attentive listening also yields to both the content and the feeling of the person without selectivity. This means that the listener does not select or listen to solely what he wants to hear and does not focus upon his needs but rather upon the patient's needs. Attentive listening conveys an attitude of caring and interest, thereby encouraging the patient to talk. In summary, attentive listening is a highly developed skill, but fortunately one that can be learned with practice.

How attentive a nurse is in listening to patients can be conveyed in various ways. Commonly used responses are a nod of the head, uttering "uh huh" or "mmm," repeating the same words that the patient says, or responding "I see what you mean." Each nurse will have his or her own characteristic ways of responding in this manner. Caution needs to be taken, however, in not sounding insincere or phony.

Five specific ways that convey physical attending have been outlined (Egan 1975:65–67). Egan defines physical attending as the manner of being present to another or being with another. Listening, in his frame of reference, is what one does while attending. The five ways of physical attending, which convey a "posture of involvement," are as follows:

1. *Face the other person squarely.* This position says, "I am available to you." Moving to the side lessens the degree of involvement.

2. *Maintain good eye contact.* This was discussed in the "Facial Expressions" section. Mutual eye contact, preferably at the same level, recognizes the other person and denotes a willingness to maintain communication. Eye contact should neither glare at nor stare down another but should be natural.

3. *Lean toward the other.* We all move naturally toward another when we want to say or hear something—by moving to the front of a class, by moving a chair nearer a friend, or by leaning across a table with arms propped in front. Whispering a secret into someone's ear is an extreme example. Likewise when sitting, the nurse conveys involvement when he or she leans forward, closer to the patient.

4. *Maintain an open posture.* This posture is regarded as the nondefensive position. It is one in which neither arms nor legs are crossed. It conveys that you wish to encourage the passage of communication as does the open door of a home or an office.

5. *Remain relatively relaxed.* Total relaxation is not feasible when the nurse must listen with intensity. The term *relative* acknowledges that the nurse can appear comfortable by taking time in responding, allowing pauses as needed, balancing periods of tension with relaxation, and using gestures that are natural. The nurse who feels tight and tense will generally offer responses too quickly to the patient and prevent a free flow of thoughts and feelings.

These five attending postures need to be adapted to the specific needs of patients in any given situation. For example, leaning forward may not be appropriate at the beginning of an interview. It may be reserved until a closer relationship grows between the nurse and the patient. The same applies to eye contact. This is generally uninterrupted when the communicators are very involved in the interaction. At times, however, eye contact may need to be interrupted.

Nurses can learn much by examining and becoming aware of their own reactions (feelings) and responses. Although it is difficult to see one's nonverbal communication other than by a videotape feedback, much can be learned by reflecting on what was heard, what was said by the nurse, and when and how it was said. Various methods can be employed such as role-playing, process recordings, and audio tapes.

Paraphrasing

Paraphrasing is also referred to as *restating*. It involves listening for the patient's basic message and then repeating the message (thoughts and/or feelings) in similar words. Usually fewer words are used. Paraphrasing conveys that the nurse has listened and understood the patient's basic message. It may also offer the patient a clearer idea of what he or she said. After the paraphrase the nurse can learn from the patient's response (it may be necessary to ask for a response) whether the paraphrase was accurate or helpful.

STUDENT: Who does he [boyfriend] think he is anyway? He expects me to just jump when the phone rings and to go out with him without any notice. It doesn't matter to him if I have an exam the next day or the flu or anything.

LISTENER: You feel angry because you think he doesn't care about how you feel.

STUDENT: Yeah, I sure do feel angry!

Clarifying

Clarifying is a method of making the patient's message more understandable. It is used when paraphrasing is difficult, when the communication has been rambling or garbled. To clarify the message the nurse can (a) attempt a guess by restating the basic message, or (b) confess confusion and ask the patient to repeat or restate the message (Brammer 1973:85). In the latter instance the nurse might say, "I'm puzzled" or "I'm not sure I understand that and I'd like to," "Would you please say that again?" or "Would you tell me more?"

If the reason for not understanding the message was the nurse's inattention, it is best to admit it and apologize. "I'm sorry, I was distracted by . . ." or "I was thinking about . . ." When possible, the nurse should discuss the distraction with the patient.

The nurse will sometimes need to clarify the message to the patient. This need is generally discovered by the patient's nonverbal feedback. In this instance the nurse might ask a question or say, "It seems to me I didn't make that clear" and then repeat or rephrase the message. Sometimes only one word or phrase in a message will need clarifying.

Open-ended Questions and Statements

An *open-ended question* is one that leads or invites patients to *explore* (elaborate, clarify, or illustrate) their thoughts or feeling. It allows patients the freedom to talk about what they wish. It also places responsibility on patients to explore themselves and to understand in contrast to receiving advice from another (Brammer 1973:87–89). Examples of open-ended questions are "How did you feel in that situation?"; "What do you think she meant by that remark?"; "Would you describe more about how you relate to your child?"

These questions require more than a "yes" or "no" or other short response such as "yesterday" or "I don't know." They encourage patients to discover what their thoughts and feelings truly are. Such questions usually begin with "what" or "how." Questions that begin with "when," "where," "who," "do (did, does)" or "is (are, was)" tend to produce short answers that impede self-exploration. However, in the course of communicating with the patient, the nurse will need to use this latter type of question in certain situations that require information gathering, such as the nursing history.

Indirect questions are often useful at the beginning of an interview or to keep one going. These kinds of questions are commonplace, such as "What would you like to talk about?" or "You were saying?" Sometimes a question can be implied by the use of statements such as "I'd like to hear more about that" or "Tell me more about . . ."

Focusing

Focusing is used when the patient's communication is vague, when the patient is rambling or seemingly talking about numerous things. *Focusing* can be compared to a telephoto lens. The camera lens focuses sharply upon a certain aspect of the view; similarly the nurse assists or leads the patient to focus on one specific aspect of communication. It is important for the nurse to wait until the patient thinks he or she has talked about the main concerns before attempting to focus. The focus can be an idea or a feeling; however the latter is often emphasized to help the patient recognize feelings that have been disguised behind words.

Being Specific, Tentative, and Informative

When responding to another person's comments, it is helpful to make statements that are (a) specific rather than general, (b) tentative rather than absolute, and (c) informative rather than authoritarian. Examples are:

> "You're as clumsy as an ox" (general statement)
> "You stepped on my foot" (specific statement)
> "You seemed unconcerned about Mary"
> (tentative statement)
> "You don't give a damn about Mary and you never will" (absolute statement)
> "I haven't finished yet" (informative statement)
> "Stop interrupting!" (authoritarian statement)

Using Touch

Certain forms of touching behaviors indicate affection. For example, cheek patting, hand patting, and chucking under the chin are valued forms of affection in North America. The "laying on of hands" is a common expression indicating curative and comfort actions. This expression is often attributed to individuals in the healing professions such as religion, medicine, or nursing. Tactile contacts vary considerably among individuals, families, and cultures. Some families have a great deal of tactile contact between all members of the family. Other families, even within the same culture, have minimal contact. Appropriate forms of touch can be helpful in reinforcing caring feelings by the nurse. The use of touch alone often says much more than words for many patients such as those who are terminally ill or who are unable to speak for whatever reason. It is important, however, for the nurse to be sensitive to the differences in attitudes and practices related to touch among individuals, including the nurse's own attitudes.

Using Silence

In everyday conversations natural pauses or silences are often accepted without thought. The listener attentively waits until the talker resumes conversation. These natural pauses are generally taken to recall a name or event or to put thoughts or feelings into the most accurate words possible. Pauses or silences that extend for several seconds or minutes, however, make some listeners extremely uncomfortable. The listener in these instances often interjects with thoughts, questions, or explanations to reduce this discomfort. This listener puts words into the other person's mouth, so to speak. The unfortunate result is that self-expression is blocked for the initial communicator.

When people are ill, communication about how they feel is often difficult for them. Many prefer to remain stoically silent until they are sure that the nurse is interested or to be trusted. Once communication is initiated, it may be expressed awkwardly with many pauses. The nurse needs to learn to be patient and silent in these situations and to wait until the patient is able to put thoughts and feelings into words.

Perception Checking

Perception checking verifies the accuracy of listening skills by the giving and receiving of feedback about what was communicated. It involves paraphrasing what the nurse thinks he or she heard and asking the patient for comfirmation. It is important to allow the patient to correct inaccurate perceptions. The advantage of frequent perception checking is that inaccurate perceptions are corrected before communications become confused and misunderstandings arise. Examples of perception checking are: "You seem to be annoyed with me—is that correct?" or "You seem to have some doubts about the decision you made, and I'd like to see if what I'm hearing is accurate."

Summarizing

Summarizing the main points of a discussion is a useful technique near the end of an interview, after a significant discussion, or as a review of a health teaching session. It clarifies for both the nurse and the patient the relevant points discussed and often acts as an introduction to future care planning. For example, the nurse might say, "During the past half hour we have talked about . . . Tomorrow afternoon we may explore this further" or "In a few days, I'll review what you have learned about the actions and effects of your insulin." A word of caution about summarizing: no new material should be added.

SOME TECHNIQUES THAT INHIBIT COMMUNICATION

Nurses need to recognize nontherapeutic techniques that interfere with effective communication. Often these techniques are used when nurses need to protect themselves from getting too close and having to deal with uncomfortable feelings. Because listening is the most effective technique to facilitate communication, the opposite, *failure to listen,* is the primary inhibitor to communication. It says to the patient, "I'm not interested" or "I'm bored" or "You are not important." It suggests that the nurse needs to be entertained or that the nurse's needs require attention. The nurse may prefer to discuss topics that concern the nurse. Other nontherapeutic techniques are (a) offering reassurance, (b) using judgmental responses, and (c) being defensive (Sundeen 1976:89–90).

Offering Reassurance

Statements such as "You'll feel better soon," "I'm sure everything will turn out all right," "Don't worry," and "You're looking better each day" are futuristic and intended to provide hope for the patient. However, they disregard the patient's feelings of the moment and in many instances are said when there is no hope of improvement. The patient who fears death, for example, needs to express these concerns rather than have them dismissed with false reassurance. The nurse who offers reassurance in this manner needs to examine his or her own feelings and recognize that this type of response is of more help to the nurse than to the patient.

Using Judgmental Responses

Passing judgment on the patient implies that the patient *must* think as the nurse thinks: the patient's values must be the same as the nurse's if the patient is to be accepted. Several responses fall into this category, including the following:

Approval and Disapproval

Approving or disapproving responses such as "That's good (bad)," "You shouldn't do that," or "That's not good enough" tell patients they must measure up to the nurse's standards rather than to their own goals. Perhaps what the nurse considers "bad" the patient considers "good."

Approving or disapproving responses can also be nonverbal. For example, a patient may have managed to bathe herself completely without the nurse's assistance for the first time. Although this activity took time and effort, she is feeling pleased. The nurse, however, thinks she took too long so says nothing and hurriedly makes her bed.

Common Advice

Giving common advice removes decision-making control from the patient to the nurse. It suggests that the patient is inferior and less wise than the nurse. Moreover, it fosters dependency and often is not followed. Note that the adjective *common* is used, not *expert.* This differentiation is significant, since the giving of expert advice can be therapeutic. Brammer (1973:108) writes:

> Advice can be helpful if it is given by trusted persons with expert opinions based on solid knowledge of a supporting field such as law, medicine, or child rearing. Sometimes . . . patients need a recommended course of action supported by wide experience and hopefully, facts.

Common advice, on the other hand, refers to matters dealing with individual choice. Examples are: "Should I move from my home to a nursing home?"

"I'm separated from my husband; do you think I should have sexual relations with another man?" "Do you think I should have an abortion?" or "Should I give up my baby to an adoption agency?" In these situations offering advice such as "If I were you . . ." is unwise for the nurse. The patient needs support to make decisions.

Stereotypes

Stereotyping responses place the patient into categories that negate uniqueness as an individual. *"Stereotypes* are generalized and oversimplified beliefs we hold about various groups of people, which are based upon experiences too limited to be valid . . . (Hein 1973:81). The less one knows about a person, the more the tendency to stereotype. Some examples are "Two-year-olds are brats," "Women are complainers," or "Men don't cry." Depending upon how emotionally charged the stereotype is for the nurse, communication between nurse and patient can be affected. For example, if the nurse discovers that the two-year-old is cooperative, the communication pattern may be only temporarily affected. On the other hand, if the nurse has marked feelings about men who cry, the patient's individualism will probably be ignored.

Another common error is to offer meaningless stereotyped responses to patients:

PATIENT: "I'm sure having a lot of pain."

NURSE: "Really? Most people don't have pain after this type of surgery."

PATIENT: "I don't have the energy I'd like to have."

NURSE: "Rome wasn't built in one day."

Being Defensive

Many times patients will offer opinions or comments about their care. These comments may be directed toward the nurse, the nurse's colleagues, or the institution. Feeling threatened, the nurse may become defensive and prevent the patient from expression of feelings. Following are two examples:

PATIENT: "The food here is lousy."

NURSE: "It's a lot better here than in ——— hospital. You should consider yourself lucky."

PATIENT: "Those night nurses must just sit around and talk all night. They didn't answer my light for over an hour."

NURSE: "I'll have you know we literally run around on nights. You're not the only patient, you know."

These responses prevent the patient from expressing true concerns. The nurse is saying, "You have no right to complain." Defensive responses protect the nurse from admitting weaknesses in the health-care services, including personal weaknesses.

FACTORS INFLUENCING THE COMMUNICATION PROCESS

Some of the factors that affect the communication process have been mentioned previously such as variations in the person's sociocultural background, language, age, and education. The limitations and attributes of nonverbal communication were also mentioned. Other factors of importance are (a) capacity of the communicator, (b) perceptions, (c) personal space, (d) roles and relationships and purpose, (e) time, (f) attitudes, and (g) self-esteem and emotions.

Capacity of the Communicator

The patient's ability to speak, to hear, to see, and to comprehend stimuli influences the communication process. People who are hard of hearing may require messages that are short, loud, and clear. Others who are unable to read or write will be unable to comprehend written information. Some, because of disease processes, are unable to see or to speak. Individualized methods for communication therefore need to be devised.

The receiver of a message also needs to be able to interpret the message. Mental faculties can be impaired for many reasons such as brain damage, use of sedative drugs, alcohol, or age.

Even in the absence of physical impairments the nurse needs to determine how much stimuli the person is capable of receiving in a given time frame. Frequently the receiver is expected to assimilate too much information. The nurse may be talking too fast or presenting too many ideas all at once. This is of particular importance when offering health instruction.

Perceptions

Because each person has unique personality traits, values, and life experiences, each one will perceive and interpret messages differently. For example, the nurse may draw the curtains around a crying woman and leave her alone. The woman may interpret this as "The nurse thinks I shouldn't cry and will upset the other patients" or "The nurse doesn't like crying" or "The nurse respects my need to be alone." It is important in many situations to validate the perceptions of the receiver.

Personal Space

Personal space is the distance people prefer in interaction with others. Middle-class North Americans use definite distances in various interpersonal relationships along with specific voice tones and body language. Communication thus alters in accordance with four distances that have been described as follows (Hall, 1969:45). All distances have a close and a far phase.

1. Intimate (7.5–45.0 cm or 3–18 inches)
2. Personal (0.4–1.2 meters or 1.5–4.0 ft)
3. Social (1.2–3.7 meters or 4–12 ft)
4. Public (beyond 3.7 meters or beyond 12 ft)

Intimate distance communication is characterized by body contact, heightened sensations of body heat and smell, and vocalizations that are low. Vision is intense, restricted to a small body part, and may be distorted. Intimate distance is frequently used by nurses in hospitals and homes. Examples are cuddling a baby, touching the sightless patient, moving patients to position them, observing an incision, and restraining a toddler for an injection. It is a natural protective instinct for people to maintain a certain amount of space immediately around them. The amount of space varies with individuals. It can be noted when someone wanting to communicate steps too close and the receiver automatically steps back a pace or two. Nurses often in their therapeutic roles are required to violate this personal distance. However, it is important to be aware of when it will occur and to forewarn the patient if possible. In many in-

stances the nurse can respect a person's intimate distance. In other instances the nurse may select to use this distance to communicate warmth and caring.

Personal distance is less overwhelming than intimate distance. Voice tones are moderate at this distance, and body heat and smell are less noticed. Physical contact is possible, such as a handshake or touching a shoulder. More of the person is perceived at a personal distance so that nonverbal behaviors such as body stance or the entire face are seen with less distortion. Much communication occurs at this distance between nurses and patients. Examples are sitting with a patient, giving medications, or establishing an intravenous infusion. Communication at a close personal distance can convey involvement by facilitating the sharing of thoughts and feelings. At the outer extreme of 1.2 meters (4 ft), however, less involvement is conveyed. Bantering and some social conversation are usual at this distance.

Social distance is characterized by a clear visual perception of the whole person; body heat and odor are imperceptible, eye contact is increased, and vocalizations are loud enough to be overheard by others. Communication is therefore more formal and is limited to seeing and hearing. The person is protected and out of reach for touch or personal sharing of thoughts or feelings. Social distances allow for more activity and movement back and forth. It is expedient in communicating to several people at the same time or within a short time. Examples are nursing rounds or waving a greeting to someone. Social distance is important in that the business of the day can be accomplished. However, it is also frequently misused. For example, the nurse who stands in the doorway and asks "How are you today?" will receive a more noncommittal reply than if the nurse were to move into the personal distance space.

Public distance involves loud, clear vocalizations with careful enunciation. Although the faces and forms of people are seen within public distance, the individuality of each person is lost. Instead, a general notion is devised about a group of people or a community.

Roles, Relationships, and Purpose

The roles and the relationship between the sender and the receiver are other factors that affect the communication process. Roles such as those of the nursing student and instructor, patient and doctor, or parent and child will affect the content and responses in the communication process. Choice of words, sentence structure, and tone of voice will vary considerably. In addition, the specific relationship between the communicators is significant. The nurse who meets with the patient for the first time will communicate differently than the nurse who has previously developed a relationship with that patient.

The intended purpose of communication also alters interactions with others. For example, if the purpose is to acknowledge another's presence the nurse may say, "Hello, how goes it today?" but if the purpose is to assess the person's pain and the effect of an analgesic, several questions and responses are necessary.

Time

Time includes what precedes and follows the interaction and the setting of the interaction. The patient in a hospital who is anticipating surgery or who has just received news that a spouse has lost a job will not be very receptive to information. If the patient has had to wait for some time to express needs, the patient may respond quite differently than if there had been no waiting period. The setting also influences communication. If the room lacks privacy or is hot, noisy, or crowded, the communication process can break down.

How the nurse uses time can facilitate or inhibit a patient's communication. The nurse whose response to a patient is "I'll be back in a moment" while delivering medications is likely to convey "I haven't time now" or "I've got work to do." Because nurses appear busy, some patients learn that requests need to be made as soon as the nurse appears. Often their request is accompanied with an apology for taking the nurse's time.

The concept of time also has cultural connotations. White people, for example, tend to emphasize punctuality and think in terms of the hour, the day, the week, or the month. American Indians, on the other hand, are governed more by events of nature. In terms of health care, appointments for child care or health screening programs will inevitably be kept by the former group. The latter group, however, may well defer appointments when nature beckons regardless of how well the communication was offered in advance. Priority for them may be that "the salmon are running" or "the geese are flying."

Attitudes

Attitudes convey our beliefs, thoughts, and feelings about people and events. They are communicated convincingly and rapidly to others. Attitudes such as caring, warmth, respect, and acceptance facilitate communication, whereas attitudes such as condescension, disinterest, and coldness inhibit communication.

Caring and *warmth* are terms frequently used to describe the attitudes of people. They convey a feeling of emotional closeness as contrasted to impersonal distance. Caring is more enduring and intense than warmth. It conveys deep and genuine concern for the person. Warmth, on the other hand, conveys friendliness and consideration by acts of smiling and attention to physical comforts (Brammer 1973:31). Caring involves the giving of one's feelings, thoughts, skill, and knowledge. It involves psychologic energy and the risk of little in return yet usually reaps the benefits of greater communication and understanding.

Respect is an attitude that emphasizes a person's worth and individuality. It conveys that a person's hopes and feelings are special and unique even though similar to others in many ways. People have a need to be different from others and at the same time to be similar to others. Being too different can be isolating and threatening.

Acceptance emphasizes neither approval nor disapproval. The nurse willingly receives patients' honest feelings and actions without judgment. An accepting attitude allows patients to express personal feelings freely and to be themselves. The nurse may find that the act of acceptance may need to be restricted, however, in certain situations when patients' actions are personally harmful or harmful to others.

In contrast, attitudes of condescension inhibit communication. *Condescension* is an attitude that conveys one's superiority over the other person. It magnifies the patient's differences and inequality. Nurses are often perceived by patients who feel helpless to be in an elevated position with their knowledge and skill as helpers. In these instances the nurse may convey condescension by an air of superiority and intellectualism. One common condescending act by nurses is to refer to all patients as "honey" or "dear" whether they are male or female, young or old. This makes the nurse a superior mother and the patient an inferior child.

An attitude of *disinterest* also inhibits communication by saying "I'm not interested" or "What you say is not important." This attitude is conveyed when the nurse forgets part of the patient's conversation or does not concentrate sufficiently on it to remember. The nurse may be tired after a long day's work or in a hurry to complete tasks.

Self-esteem and Emotions

All kinds of emotions can influence a person's ability to communicate. Most people have experienced overwhelming joy or sorrow that is difficult to express in words. Anger may produce loud, profane vocalizations or controlled speechlessness. Fright may produce screams of terror or paralyzed silence.

Emotions also affect the person's ability to interpret messages. Large parts of a message may not be heard, or the message may be misinterpreted. This situation occurs frequently in nursing. For example, the patient may not hear the doctor's message that the illness is terminal. Or the patient may not remember all the preoperative instructions offered by the nurse.

Self-esteem also influences communication patterns. Those people whose self-esteem is high communicate honestly, with confidence, and with congruence between verbal and nonverbal messages. Those with low self-esteem or high stress tend to give double messages, that is, the verbal and nonverbal messages are incongruent. Many patterns of communication are used to alleviate feelings of low self-esteem.

DEVELOPMENT OF COMMUNICATION

The development of communication from the cries of the infant to the verbal capacity of the adult is a complex process. The art of language is learned by sharing ideas and feelings with others. The precise ways by which children learn socialized speech are not fully understood. Various theories of language development have been proposed. The learner is referred to other sources for these theories. This section will describe the various sounds and phases of children's language.

The first sound of a newborn is the birth cry as air moves across the vocal cords. This is a reflexive response associated with the air pressure and the temperature changes of extrauterine life. Although infants are speechless for almost one year, they do communicate their needs. Within two to three weeks after birth a mother can describe notable differences in the cries of her infant. Babies cry in one way when they are hungry and in a different way when they are in pain, wet, tired, or wanting attention. The hunger cry may start out in a plaintive way and become increasingly demanding. The cry of pain is usually a sudden yell because the baby is startled about what is happening. The cry of discomfort or the need for attention may sound like complaining because it goes on and on. Some babies will cry when they are put down to sleep. They cry jerkily; some become loudly demanding, and when mother does not appear, they settle down with progressively fading crying spurts. Each mother and infant soon learn to communicate in response to the child's own unique sounds. In contrast, infants also make comfort sounds. Smiling is noted in a number of infants as early as the second week of life. Soon after, some will begin small throaty cooing sounds while feeding or bathing. Babies usually make these comfort sounds when they are contented such as when they are cuddled or when others talk to them.

The Prelinguistic Phase

Until about the age of 10 months or a year the infant's sounds are not related to language and therefore are considered *prelinguistic*. These early sounds are actually exercise for the vocal chords. The first sounds are vowel-like sounds or gurglings from the throat. When the mouth is opened, air is exhaled, resulting in various happy noises such as "uuuuuuu" or "eeeeeeeee." To produce consonant sounds such as "b" or "k," infants need sufficient motor development to manipulate their lips, tongue, throat, and voice at the same time. These sounds therefore appear less frequently and later than vowel sounds. The consonants are then combined into syllables with the vowel sounds. Such sounds as "da" and "ge" are then heard.

The prelinguistic phase includes reflexive vocalization, babbling, and echolalia. *Reflexive vocalization* refers to the nondescriptive sounds infants make in response to various stimuli and environmental conditions. These are the discomfort cries and the comfort coos.

The *babbling phase* begins when infants become aware that they are making noises. They delight in producing and repeating sounds, particularly when they are enjoying themselves. They spend more time making noises and will talk to themselves when alone. Babbling often occurs just after waking up or before going to sleep. It is as if they are practicing self-produced sounds. By about seven months babbling will include some sounds they have picked up from their environment. Now hearing and the sounds they produce are associated. This is referred to as *lalling*: infants are repeating sounds they have heard.

Echolalia is the repetition or echoing of sounds just spoken by another. This involves definite acoustic awareness. Whole sequences of the sound may be strung together such as "dadadadada." At this point there is no meaning associated with the infants' sounds, but they have learned to manipulate their tongue, lips, and throat and to imitate sounds spoken by others. Language and speech development proceed at a faster pace if the parent at this time repeats the baby's sounds. The baby in turn echoes the parent's sounds.

The First Word

The first word of the infant is a notable event for proud parents. By about 10 to 12 months of age children develop a *passive* understanding of the language. They will respond to a few familiar words such as "No" and familiar names—their own and those of their family and household pets. Even when family members are not present, children will turn to look for them when their names are mentioned.

Active use of language follows. The first words that children use may be unrecognized by parents. Children often invent their own first words. A word such as "nenene" may mean many things to a child. It may mean comfort when spoken softly, or it may mean a scolding or wrongdoing when spoken sharply. The word *mama* may mean food, comfort, warmth, and love. To understand this early language it is necessary to listen to what children say in relation to what they are doing and their situation. Whole messages can be involved in one word based on the tone or manner of voice. This is not surprising when one considers that babies respond to their mother's tone of voice as young as four or five weeks when they are comforted by the soothing soft tones. Although the words are not understood, it is known that babies respond differently to the same word said with different intonations at the age of four to five months.

True speech begins between 12 and 18 months of age. This occurs when the child correctly uses a conventional word or facsimile of the word. It is used with intent, and a response is anticipated; a child may bang a cup on the highchair and say "wawa" (water). This type of speech is referred to as *holophrastic speech* (one word expresses a whole sentence). "Wawa" means "I want some water." "Bath" means "I want to take a bath now." Generally children can say about four words at 15 months, about ten words at 18 months, and about 50 words by two years. The vocabulary that children understand is much larger. They can respond to commands such as "Give that to me" and "Touch your nose."

The First Sentence

By two years of age children learn to put words together. This period is considered the beginning of complete speech. Complete speech occurs when a child uses different word combinations in grammatical form.

In the beginning only two words are combined; later three-word and four-word sentences appear until full adultlike sentences are constructed. As with the first words the child's sentences have personalized meanings and do not follow the rules of grammar. Examples are: "See plane," "Kitty sleep," "Byebye Dada." Some peculiar combinations can be made up, such as: "Byebye shoe." Regardless of the combinations, a certain order exists in the child's language. Some words will always appear at the beginning of a phrase and others at the end. "See" is usually at the beginning and "it" is usually at the end.

Learning to use the past tense and to create questions is more complex. Most of the early phrases spoken use the present tense. When learning the past tense children provide much amusement for adults. They initially put an "ed" on every verb so that we hear things like "Dolly eated" or "Mummy boughted it." As the child grows older, questions are formulated. Three stages are involved in transferring a statement into a question (Bee 1975:147–149). These can be exemplified using the statement "Daddy is driving a blue car." Although dozens of words can be used to phrase a question, the word "why" will be used to illustrate the three changes.

1. The word "why" must be added: "Daddy is driving a blue car why?"
2. The word "why" then needs to be moved to the beginning of the statement: "Why daddy is driving a blue car?"
3. Then the verb "is" needs to be moved to follow the word "why": "Why is daddy driving a blue car?"

The earliest questions of a child do not change the sentence structure. Instead inflections are used at the end of a phrase, such as "See tree?," raising the voice as the child says "tree." Then questions will occur without verbs such as "Where my coat?" followed by ones with verbs such as "Why can't do it?"

Children also have various ways of dealing with some consonants. One child who could not pronounce "f" to say her uncle Fred's name constructed the name "Pete" to avoid her difficulty. Another child pronounced Valerie as "Bralerie."

Egocentric and Socialized Speech

The French psychologist Jean Piaget (1952) categorized the conversation of children from ages four to 11 into egocentric and socialized speech. *Egocentric speech* is self-centered noncommunicative speech. Children talk merely to please themselves or to please anyone who happens to be there to hear. Although the conversation is not directed to anyone in particular, the talking is about the child's thoughts and activity of the moment. The child is thinking out loud. Three categories of egocentric speech are repetition, monologue, and collective monologue. An example of repetitive speech is provided by four-year-olds in a nursery school.

JUDY: "I've got a red block."

TRACEY: "I've got a red block."

JUDY: "I've got a red block."

TRACEY: "I've got a red block."

The *monologue* refers to a long speech that occurs when there is no listener. For example, the preschooler who is building a castle with blocks will mutter, "This big red block goes here . . . that's good . . . and now this green block goes there . . . uh . . . let's see, I'll put it this way . . . now where's the bridge? That will keep the bad guys out." In contrast, the *collective monologue* involves the presence of others. Children speak with awareness of another child's presence, but they are indifferent to what others are saying.

In contrast to Piaget, the work of the Russian psychologist Lev Vygotsky (1962:16–17) proposes that egocentric speech is a form of self-guidance and assists the child in problem solving situations. He believes that egocentric speech is both goal oriented and communicative. It is the state between external speech and what he refers to as "silent inner speech" (1962:149). Egocentric or external speech goes underground and becomes internalized as thought processes.

Socialized speech refers to the exchange of thoughts with others and includes questions, answers, commands, and criticism of others. In school-age children the use of egocentric speech gradually diminishes. They predominantly communicate their thoughts to other people.

Semantic Development

Semantics is the study of the meanings of words in a given language. Increasing attention has been given to semantic development in recent years. The words children use do not always indicate their meaning to the adult. A young preschooler said before his birthday that he did not want his birthday in January. After exploring what bothered him about having his birthday in January, his response was, "I want my birthday here at home on the farm." Although the child had the vocabulary, his personalized meaning referred to a place.

Children first learn the meaning of concrete words and their categories; later the abstract words and their categories are understood. The child will learn concrete words such as "chair" or "table" before learning the meaning of the category of furniture, or "apple" and "orange" before learning the category of fruit. Abstract words such as "quality" or "relation" are learned primarily after the preschool years.

Other words in the English language that have double meanings are also difficult for preschoolers. Such words as "sweet" or "crooked" can have either a physical or psychologic meaning. They are not fully comprehended until about the age of 10 years.

FACTORS INFLUENCING LANGUAGE DEVELOPMENT

Growth in language development is affected by a number of factors: (a) intelligence, (b) sex, (c) bilingualism, (d) single child or twin, (e) parental stimulation, and (f) socioeconomic factors.

Intelligence
Brighter children begin to talk earlier. Vocabulary development of intelligent children occurs more rapidly, and they articulate better and use sentences

that are longer and more grammatically correct. Mentally defective children show notable lags in vocabulary growth.

Sex

During the first year there is not much difference in the sounds produced by boys or girls. After this time girls tend to be superior in both the rate of vocabulary development and in articulation. In later school years boys tend to be equal to girls in reading abilities and even superior with certain words. Females on the whole exceed in grammatical word usage and spelling tests.

Bilingualism

Research has contradicted the belief that a child of a bilingual home is hindered in language development. Lambert and Tucker (1972) found that language development was not retarded in bilingual children over a seven-year period. The bilingual children also scored high on tests of creativity.

Single Child or Twin

Recent evidence suggests that twins and triplets exhibit certain aspects of retarded language development, particularly during the preschool years. It is thought that (a) twins may receive less verbal stimulation from parents, (b) they grow up so close together that they understand each other's speech patterns early, (c) they lack the motivation to verbalize with others. The school years are apparently instrumental in resolving these problems (Howard 1946:181–188).

Parental Stimulation

Vocabulary growth occurs at a more rapid pace in children who are spoken to more frequently. A less rapid growth has been noted in children who spend most of their time with other children and who watch a great deal of television. The kind of stimulation offered by parents is significant. Children who have mothers described as "object oriented and noncritical" acquire language more rapidly. These mothers tend to talk and to ask questions about the child's toys rather than criticizing what the child is doing with the toys. In contrast, children who have mothers described as "critical and intrusive" have inhibited language development. These mothers focus on giving their children directions (commands and demands) about what to do with their toys. Vocabulary is enhanced in children who travel away from their homes and who have contact with several different adults.

Socioeconomic Factors

The family setting in which the child is reared affects language development. Children from upper-class families, such as those whose parents are lawyers and doctors, use many more words even by age three than children from lower social classes where parents are unskilled workers. The caliber of conversation overheard by youngsters is an influencing factor. Middle-class and upper-class families tend to discourage the use of profane language or slang; instead, proper word usage and grammar are encouraged and often rewarded by praise. Homes that expose their children to a variety of educational aids also enhance the child's development. The effects of lack of development are noted in homes without magazines, books, newspapers, encyclopedias, radios, or television.

Although differences exist in language development among social classes, lower-class children should not be regarded as inferior. These children possess a fully developed language that is similar to a dialect. They are able to articulate well in their own cultural setting but not as well with the middle-class or upper-class children. The converse also applies. Upper-class or middle-class children have difficulty articulating dialects outside of their own cultural settings.

STIMULATING CHILDREN'S LANGUAGE DEVELOPMENT

Nurses can be instrumental in assisting parents to become active stimulants in the language development of their children:

1. *Improve the parental model.* Parents should try to provide the best possible instruction and to become good models. Some parents may need to attend En-

glish classes; others may need encouragement to acquire educational aids such as storybooks.

2. *Encourage verbal and nonverbal means of communication.* Children need different verbal experiences such as rhyming games, reading aloud, and songs with accompanying nonverbal gestures of smiling and laughing. Expanding upon the child's remarks, drawing, painting, and musical endeavors also are vital parts of learning the communication process.

3. *Provide experiences to talk about.* Children talk when they have something to talk about. Parents need to provide field excursions, pets, toys, picture books, numbers, and colors that the child can experiment with and talk about.

4. *Encourage listening.* Articulation skills of children can be enhanced by teaching them to pay attention and to listen to sounds. Parents can encourage

these by having children listen to and repeat nursery rhymes or jingles or asking questions such as "What was that sound?"

5. *Encourage speech as a substitute for action.* Children's ability to express themselves verbally can be enhanced when parents direct them to say what they want rather than respond to physical action. The child who tugs at a playmate's tricycle can be instructed by the parent to express wants verbally by the remark "Tell him what you want; perhaps he will let you have it."

6. *Use exact terms.* Children learn to distinguish color, size, shape, position, and ownership of objects when exact terms are used. Parents should refrain from using words such as "it" or "thing" or saying "You know what I mean." Asking a child to "Put away your toys" instead of "the toys" can clarify property problems.

THE EFFECTIVE NURSE-PATIENT RELATIONSHIP

An effective nurse-patient relationship is referred to by some as a *therapeutic relationship* and by others as a *helping relationship. Helping* is described as a growth-facilitating process in which one person assists another person to grow in the direction the person chooses (Brammer 1973:3). Several terms are used to describe the persons involved in a helping relationship. Examples are the *helper,* the *helpee;* the *giver,* the *receiver;* the *client,* the *clientee;* and the *counselor,* the *counselee.* For purposes of consistency in this textbook, the term *nurse* or *helper* will refer to the person who gives the help, and the term *patient* will denote the person receiving the help. However, we recognize that various people in all walks of life act as helpers and receivers of help.

Guidelines for Ways of Helping Patients

Although special training in counseling techniques and psychiatry is advantageous for nurses to become effective helpers, there are many guidelines that the nurse can employ to help patients that do not require specialized training. Eleven of these guidelines are outlined as follows (Shanken and Shanken 1976:24–27):

1. Actively listen.
2. Help to identify what the person is feeling.

3. Put yourself in the other person's shoes.
4. Be honest.
5. Do not tell a person not to feel.
6. Do not tell the person what the person should feel.
7. Do not make excuses for the other person.
8. Be personal.
9. Use your ingenuity.
10. Try to summarize to the person at the end of the interview.
11. Know your role: know your limitations.

Active listening was discussed previously. It involves being attentive, clarifying, paraphasing, and asking questions to accurately understand the other person.

Helping patients to identify their feelings requires feedback from the nurse to the patient about how he or she appears. Often patients who are troubled are unable to identify or to label their feelings and consequently have difficulty working them out or talking about them. Responses by the nurse such as "You are angry about taking orders from your boss" or "You're lonely since your wife died" can assist patients to recognize what they are feeling and to talk about it.

Putting oneself into the other person's shoes is referred to as *empathy.* According to Egan (1975:76) empathy involves the ability to:

(1) *discriminate*: get inside the other person, look at the world through the frame of reference of the other person and get a feeling for what the other's world is like; and (2) *communicate* to the other this understanding in a way that shows the other that the helper has picked up both his *feelings*, and the *behavior and experience* underlying these feelings.

Empathy therefore requires more than the sharing of past similar feelings and events that we have all experienced such as fright or depression. The nurse needs to understand the patient's world as if the nurse were inside it; the nurse should see it through the patient's eyes, and feel as the patient feels. Empathy is valuable in supporting patients to explore their situation and to move toward resolution of their problems. Feelings of closeness and understanding gradually evolve between the patient and nurse. Neither person, however, loses a sense of self.

Four steps are outlined by Katz in the process of empathy (Ehmann 1971:77–78). All steps occur rapidly and tend to overlap.

1. *Identification.* To understand the feelings and situation of another, the helper must first lose consciousness of self and become engrossed in the personality and situation of the other person (identification). The nurse needs to relinquish a certain amount of self-control to achieve this.

2. *Incorporation.* This is a step beyond identification in that the experiences of the other person are taken into the helper's self (incorporation). The experience, however, is still recognized as belonging to the patient.

3. *Reverberation.* This is the step that involves understanding the feelings of the other. There is interaction between the nurse's feelings from past experience and the experience incorporated from the patient. Because humans have the same potential for feelings, the experiences people share need not be identical to understand associated feelings.

4. *Detachment.* This refers to the step in which the nurse returns to his or her own identity. The results of the three preceding steps are then combined with other knowledge about the patient. All information is then used collectively as a basis for responding to the patient.

The value of *honesty* was previously mentioned as an aspect of credibility. In effective relationships the nurse honestly recognizes limitations of knowledge by saying, "I don't know the answer to that right now"; openly discusses feelings of discomfort by saying, for example, "I feel uncomfortable about this discussion"; and admits tactfully that problems do exist when a patient expresses such things as "I'm a mess, aren't I?"

Do not tell a person not to feel. Feelings expressed by patients often create discomfort in the nurse. Common examples are the patient who expresses anger or worry or who cries. When the nurse is uncomfortable, common responses are often made such as "Don't worry about it, everything will be fine" or "Please don't cry." These responses inhibit the expression of feelings. Unless feelings are extremely inappropriate, it is best to encourage ventilation (voicing) of them. This allows them to be expressed in words and examined objectively. Indirectly it says also, "My feelings are not that awful if that nurse is not bothered by them."

Do not tell a person what he or she should feel. Statements that indicate to patients how they should feel rather than how they actually do feel need to be avoided. These statements in essence deny patients' true feelings and suggest that they are inapprorpiate. Examples are "You shouldn't complain about pain"; "Many others have gone through this same experience stoically"; "You should be glad that you are alive and not worry about the loss of your arm."

Do not make excuses for the other person. When a person reacts with intense feeling such as anger or tears and assumedly has lost control of behavior to the astonishment or discomfort of others, a common error is to explain the behavior by offering excuses. Examples of such excuses are: "Well, John, you're upset about your bad report but your teacher is unrealistic" or "I guess you've had a tough day at the office." These responses discourage and divert the person from discussing feelings such as anger or inadequacy. With such responses the helper has made *assumptions* about the reasons for the patient's behavior and therefore inhibits exploration of what is really being experienced and felt by the patient.

Be personal. Not all people feel comfortable about offering personal statements about themselves to strangers or to those they do not know well. Used with discretion, however, personal statements can be helpful in solidifying the rapport between the nurse and the patient. Such comments as "I recall when I was in (a similar situation) and I felt angry about being put down." Egan states that the helper "must be spontaneous, open. He can't hide behind the role of counselor. He must be a human being to the human being before him" (1975:35).

Egan refers to this as *genuineness* and outlines five behaviors that it constitutes (1975:90–94):

1. The genuine helper does not take refuge in the role of counselor.

2. The genuine person is spontaneous.

3. The genuine person is nondefensive.

4. The genuine person has few discrepancies, that is, the person does not think or feel one thing but say another.

5. The genuine person is capable of deep self-disclosure (self-sharing) when it is appropriate.

Caution needs to be exerted by nurses when making personal references about themselves. They must be used with discretion. The extreme of matching each of the patient's problems with a better story of one's own is of little value to the patient.

Use your ingenuity to help identify alternatives. There are always many alternative courses of action to consider in handling problems. Whatever course of action is chosen needs to effectively achieve the patient's goals, be compatible with the patient's value system, and offer the probability of success. These actions are not explored until the relationship is well established (see "Phases of the Helping Relationship," this chapter) and is done conjointly by the patient and the nurse. The patient needs to choose the ways to achieve goals; however, the nurse can assist in identifying alternatives. An example is the widower who comes for help because he is depressed and anxious about retirement. The nurse could suggest the following courses of action:

1. Read books and articles on retirement.

2. Consider working part-time at his former employment.

3. Talk to other senior citizens about retirement.

4. Move in to live with a child and grandchildren.

5. Join a senior citizens club.

6. Renew old hobbies such as gardening or golf.

7. Join a counseling group.

8. Move from his house to an apartment.

9. Remarry.

10. Move into a senior citizen's lodge.

11. Join a volunteer service group.

12. Increase church activities.

13. Get involved in politics.

14. Write articles for the local newspaper.

15. Make plans to travel more extensively.

The ingenious nurse will help the patient to select acceptable alternatives. For example, if this gentleman loves animals, young children, and storytelling, the nurse might direct his thoughts toward associated activities such as acquiring a puppy or writing children's stories.

Try to summarize to the person at the end of the interview. Summarizing is the process of tying together several thoughts and feelings into one or two statements at the end of a discussion or interview. It is broader than paraphrasing and includes what was said and how it was said. Several purposes are achieved by summarizing: (a) it helps to terminate the interview, (b) it reassures the patient that you have listened, (c) it checks the accuracy of your perceptions, (d) it clears the way for new ideas, and (e) it assists the patient to note progress and forward direction (Brammer 1973:94). Sometimes patients may spontaneously offer a summary; other times the nurse must initiate it or ask the patient to do so. The nurse may say, "Let's look at what has happened in this interview; what do you think has been accomplished?"

Know your role; know your limitations. Every person has unique strengths and problems. It is important for the nurse to recognize limitations and to be as open about them as necessary. When the nurse feels unable to handle some problems, the patient should be informed and referred to the apppropriate health · professional.

Phases of the Helping Relationship

The relationship process can be described in terms of four sequential phases, each of which is characterized by identifiable tasks and skills. Progression through the stages must occur in succession as each one builds onto the next. Nurses can therefore identify the progress of a relationship by understanding these phases. These four phases are (a) the preinteraction phase, (b) the introductory phase, (c) the working (maintaining) phase, and (d) the termination phase (Sundeen 1976:108–119).

The Preinteraction Phase

In most situations the nurse has information about the patient before the first face-to-face meeting. Such information may include the patient's name, address, age, past medical history, and/or social history. Tasks of this phase for the nurse include reviewing pertinent knowledge, considering some potential areas of concern, and developing plans for the initial interaction. For example, prior to meeting a young pregnant woman in her home, a student nurse may need to review the normal physical changes that occur with pregnancy and the related needs and discomforts. If the woman is in the first trimester of pregnancy, the nurse may anticipate some areas of concern from the mother-to-be such as urinary frequency, nausea, fatigue, or feelings of ambivalence, which are common discomforts during this period. Planning for the initial visit may generate some anxious feelings in the nurse. By recognizing these feelings and by identifying specific information to be discussed, positive outcomes will evolve. It is wise for the nurse to recognize limitations at this stage and to seek assistance as required.

The Introductory Phase

This phase is also referred to as the *orientation phase* or the *prehelping phase*. The tone is set during this phase for the rest of the relationship phases. Some of the tasks of this phase were discussed in Chapter 12 for the nursing assessment interview. Three stages of this introductory phase include:

1. Entry: Preparing the patient and opening the relationship.
2. Clarification: Stating the problem or concern and reasons for seeking help.
3. Structure: Formulating the contract and the structure (Brammer 1973:55).

Opening the Relationship.   Initially the nurse and the patient need to identify each other by name as a friendly gesture and to open the relationship. When the nurse initiates the relationship, it is important to explain the nurse's role to give the patient an idea of what can be expected. When the patient initiates the relationship process, the nurse needs to help the patient express concerns and reasons for seeking help. Vague, open-ended questions are helpful at this stage, such as "What's on your mind today?" The nurse needs to be aware that it is not easy for the patient to receive help. Thus a relaxed, attending attitude is important on the part of the nurse. Providing a setting with minimal distractions and disturbances is also helpful.

Clarifying the Problem.   Initially the patient will not see the problem clearly. To clarify the problems, the nurse needs to employ such techniques as attentive listening, paraphrasing, and clarifying. These techniques were discussed previously in this chapter. A common error at this stage is to ask too many questions of the patient.

Structuring and Formulating the Contract.   A *contract* includes the obligations that are to be met by both the nurse and the patient. These commitments are agreed upon verbally and need to evolve naturally. Contracts need to include:

1. The location, frequency, and length of meetings.
2. The overall purpose of the relationship.
3. The way in which confidential material will be handled.
4. The duration and indications for termination of the relationship (Sundeen 1976:110).

The first three points have been mentioned previously in Chapter 12. Determining the duration of the relationship and indications for termination depends in part upon conditions outside of the relationship process. For example, many relationships are terminated when the patient is discharged from the hospital or when the nursing student ends clinical rotation. In these situations the nurse and the patient need to discuss these limits. When outside controls do not exist, both participants need to agree upon indications for termination. These are largely determined by the purpose of the relationship. An example is the nurse who terminates a relationship after the patient has learned how to care for his colostomy and is able to resume a lifestyle acceptable to himself.

Other important tasks of this introductory phase include getting to know each other and developing a degree of trust. During the initial parts of this phase the patient may display some resistive behaviors and some testing behaviors. *Resistive behaviors* are those which inhibit involvement, cooperation, or change. Three major reasons for their occurrence are (a) difficulty in acknowledging the need for help and thus a dependency role, (b) fear of exposing and facing one's feelings, and (c) anxiety about the discomfort involved in changing problematic behavior patterns. *Testing behaviors* are those which examine the nurse's interest and sincerity. For example, a patient may refuse to talk to test whether the nurse will stay with her for the prescribed period of time.

By the end of the introductory phase, the patient begins to develop trust in the nurse. Both participants also begin to view each other as unique individuals. Characteristics of trusting individuals include (a) a feeling of comfort with growth in self-awareness, (b) an ability to share this awareness with others, (c) acceptance of others as they are without needing to change them, (d) openness to new experiences, (e) consistency between words and actions, and (f) the ability to delay gratification (Thomas 1970:118).

The Working Phase

When the nurse and the patient begin to view each other as unique individuals, they begin to appreciate this uniqueness and *care* about each other. *Caring* is sharing deep and genuine concern about the welfare of another person. Once caring develops, the potential for *empathy* increases. The purpose of the working phase is to accomplish the tasks that have been outlined in the introductory phase.

The working phase has three successive stages: (a) responding and exploring, (b) integrative understanding and dynamic self-understanding, and (c) facilitating action and action (Egan 1975:34–40). A summary of these stages and the specific skills required by both participants follows (Egan 1975:34–40). Each stage builds upon the other, and therefore they must occur in succession.

Responding and Exploring.   During the introductory phase, emphasis was placed upon the listening or attending skills of the nurse. These skills must be continued in the working phase of the relationship, but in addition the nurse now must *respond* to the patient in ways that assist the patient to *explore* thoughts, feelings, and actions.

The nurse requires four skills for this first stage:

1. First level empathy. The nurse must communicate (respond) in ways that indicate the nurse has listened to what was said and understands how the patient feels. The nurse responds to the content or to the feelings or both of these as appropriate.

2. Respect. The nurse must show the patient that he or she respects the patient, is available, and wants to work with the patient.

3. Genuineness (previously discussed in this chapter).

4. Concreteness. The nurse must assist the patient to be concrete and specific rather than speaking in generalities; when the patient says, "I'm stupid and clumsy," the nurse assists him to be specific by pointing out, "You tripped on that scatter rug."

Self-exploration enables the patient to explore the feelings and actions associated with problems. This is also referred to as *self-disclosure.*

During this first working phase, trust and rapport are enhanced. The intensity of interaction increases, and many feelings may be expressed such as anger, shame, or self-consciousness. If the nurse is skilled in this stage and if the patient is willing to explore himself or herself, the outcome is a beginning understanding on the part of the patient about behavior and feelings.

Integrative Understanding and Dynamic Self-understanding.   In this second working stage patients achieve an objective understanding of themselves' and their world (dynamic self-understanding). This ultimately enables patients to change and to take action. More self-exploration occurs, and more information is produced. As a result of this, isolated pieces of information can now be integrated into larger contexts that reveal behavioral patterns or themes.

To acquire this integrative understanding about the patient, the nurse requires additional skills to those of stage 1. Some of these are as follows:

1. Advanced level empathy. The nurse must respond in ways that indicate an understanding not only of what is said but also of what is hinted at or implied nonverbally. Isolated statements become connected.

2. Self-disclosure. The nurse willingly shares personal experiences with discretion.

3. Confrontation. The nurse challenges discrepancies between thoughts, feelings, and actions that inhibit the patient's self-understanding or exploration of specific areas. This is done with empathy, not with a clout.

The skills required by the patient include the following:

1. Nondefensive listening. The patient, with support from the nurse, develops the skill of listening.

2. Dynamic self-understanding. The patient gains insight into personal behavior, and this understanding forms the basis for changing behavior.

Facilitating Action and Action.   Ultimately the patient must make decisions and take action to become more effective. The responsibility for action belongs to the patient. The nurse, however, collaborates in these decisions and may offer alternatives or advice.

When planning action programs, the patient needs to learn to take risks, that is, to accept that either failure or success may be the outcome. Whatever action is taken needs to fall within the person's capabilities.

Short-term and long-term goals are considered, and it is essential that the nurse offer support at this time. Successes need to be reinforced, and failures need to be recognized realistically. The fact that new problems may arise during this period also needs consideration. Often by solving one problem, new problems evolve. Each new problem then needs to be dealt with by beginning again at stage 1 of the working phase.

The Termination Phase

Terminating the relationship is often anticipated as being difficult and filled with ambivalence. However, if the previous phases have evolved effectively, the patient can accept this phase of the relationship without feelings of anxiety or dependency. The patient generally feels positive and able to handle problems independently. However, because caring attitudes have developed, it is natural to expect some feelings relative to any loss, and each person needs to develop a way of saying goodbye.

Many methods can be used to terminate relationships. By summarizing or reviewing the process, a sense of accomplishment can be achieved. This may include a sharing of reminiscences of how things were at the beginning of the relationship as compared to now. It is also helpful for both the nurse and the patient to openly and honestly express their feelings about termination. Thus termination discussions need to start in advance of the termination interview. This allows time for the patient to adjust to independence. In some situations referrals may be necessary, or it may be appropriate to offer an occasional standby relationship to give support as needed.

SUMMARY

Communication incorporates all means of exchanging information between two or more people and is a basic component of human relationships. It is usually categorized as verbal and nonverbal. Verbal communication is effective when the criteria of simplicity, clarity, timing, relevancy, adaptability, and credibility are met. Nonverbal communication, however, often reveals more about a person's thoughts and feelings than verbal communication. It includes physical appearance, posture and gait, facial expressions, hand movements, and gestures. When interpreting nonverbal behaviors, the nurse needs to consider cultural influences and be cognizant of the fact that a variety of feelings can be expressed by only one nonverbal expression. The significant emphasis in communication, however, is that the verbal and the nonverbal expressions are congruent.

The communication process is two-way and involves the sender of the message and the receiver of the message. Because the sender must encode the message and then determine the appropriate channels for conveying the message and because the receiver of the message must perceive, decode the message, and then respond, the communication process includes four elements: (a) the sender, (b) the message, (c) the receiver, and (d) the feedback.

There are many techniques that facilitate communication. These include attentive listening, paraphrasing, clarifying, using open-ended questions and statements, focusing, being specific, using touch and silence, and perception checking. In contrast, there are several techniques that inhibit communication. Examples are offering unvalidated reassurance, providing approving or disapproving statements, stereotyping, and being defensive.

Many factors influence the communication process. Included are the capacity of the communicator, perceptions, personal space (intimate, personal, social, and public distance), roles and relationships, time, attitudes, and self-esteem.

The development of communication is a complex process. Normal descriptions of the sounds and phases of children's language are outlined for the nurse to use when assessing individuals. Sounds of the newborn, the prelinguistic phase, passive and active use of language, true speech, and sentence construction are outlined. Egocentric speech, which includes the monologue and collective monologue, and socialized speech are defined. Semantic development starts with concrete words such as "table" and is then followed by abstract words such as "quality." The factors that influence language development are intelligence, sex, bilingualism, single child or twin status, parental stimulation, and socioeconomic factors. Suggestions for stimulating the language development of children are outlined.

The effective nurse-patient relationship is described as a growth-facilitating process. Eleven guidelines for ways of helping patients are outlined. Four phases of the helping relationship include the preinteraction phase, the introductory phase, the working phase, and the termination phase. Each phase has a specific purpose or goal and requires specific skills of the nurse.

SUGGESTED ACTIVITIES

1. In a clinical situation, analyze your abilities to provide information to a patient using the crite-

ria for giving effective verbal messages outlined in this chapter.

2. Visit an ethnic family or restaurant and observe cultural differences in the use of nonverbal expressions.

3. Analyze a recent interaction with a patient, and identify techniques used that facilitated or inhibited communication. Indicate your own feelings regarding the use of specific techniques, emphasizing those with which you feel comfortable and those which you tend to avoid.

4. In a clinical situation, observe the frequency, purpose, and effectiveness of touch used by several staff members. Discuss and compare your findings with a group of classmates.

5. Assess the language development of an infant and preschool child.

6. In a laboratory setting select a classmate and over a period of weeks alternate roles of being the patient and the nurse. Select some real-life problems for discussion, such as difficulty relating with older patients or anxiety about starting a new clinical experience. Throughout these interactions, analyze the course of your relationship. Emphasize listening skills and empathizing.

SUGGESTED READINGS

Forrest, Jean W. July 1972. Student termination: saying goodbye. *Nursing Papers* 4(1):23–28. Montreal: School for Graduate Nurses, McGill University.

This article outlines the process of termination and the feelings that student nurses experience when saying goodbye to patients. The role of the faculty adviser as an integral part of this experience is also included.

Kelly, Holly Skodol. November 1969. The sense of an ending. *American Journal of Nursing* 69:2378–2381.

In this article the author likens the ending of a relationship to that of grief after bereavement. Devices such as substitution, rationalization, and fantasy, which are used to avoid the pain of separation, are included.

Kron, Thora. November 1972. How we communicate nonverbally with patients. *Canadian Nurse* 68(11):21–23.

This article emphasizes the importance of the nurse's nonverbal communication in conveying self-confidence, interest, respect, and approval to patients. Pertinent examples are given.

MacDonald, Malcolm R. June 1977. How do men and women students rate in empathy? *American Journal of Nursing* 77:998.

This article reveals the empathy ratings of men and women in nursing as contrasted to men and women who are not in nursing. The results are contrary to what many would think.

Travelbee, Joyce. February 1963. What do we mean by rapport? *American Journal of Nursing* 63(2):70–72.

The basic ingredients of rapport are outlined in this article. Nurses are constantly reminded that they need to develop rapport with patients but often are unable to explain its meaning.

SELECTED REFERENCES

Bee, Helen. 1975. *The developing child.* New York: Harper and Row, Publishers, Inc.

Brammer, Lawrence M. 1973. *The helping relationship: process and skills.* Englewood Cliffs, N. J.: Prentice-Hall, Inc.

Brown, Barbara G. July, 1972. The language of space: a silent component of the therapeutic process. *Nursing Papers* 4(1):29–34. Montreal: School for Graduate Nurses, McGill University.

Clark, Carolyn Chambers. 1977. Psychotherapy with the resistant child. *Perspectives in Psychiatric Care* 15(3):123–125.

Edinburg, Golda M., et al. 1975. *Clinical interviewing and counseling: principles and techniques.* New York: Appleton-Century Crofts.

Egan, Gerard, 1975. *The skilled helper: a model for systematic helping and interpersonal relating.* Monterey, Calif.: Brooks/Cole Publishing Co.

Ehmann, V. 1971. Empathy: its origin, characteristics and process. *Perspectives in Psychiatric Care* 9(2):72–80.

Hall, Edward T. 1969. *The hidden dimension.* Garden City, N.Y.:Doubleday and Co., Inc.

Hein, Eleanor C. 1973. *Communication in nursing practice.* Boston: Little, Brown and Co.

Helms, Donald B., and Turner, Jeffrey S. 1976. *Exploring Child Behavior.* Philadelphia: W. B. Saunders Co.

Howard, R. W. 1946. The language development of a group of triplets. *Journal of Genetic Psychology* 69:181–188.

Johnson, David W. 1972. *Reaching out: interpersonal effectiveness and self-actualization.* Englewood Cliffs, N. J.: Prentice-Hall, Inc.

Kesler, Arlene Riley. September, 1977. Pitfalls to avoid in interviewing patients. *Nursing 77* 7(9):70–73.

Landreth, C. 1967. *Early childhood.* New York: Alfred A. Knopf, Inc.

Lambert, W. E., and Tucker, G. R. 1972. *Bilingual education of children: the St. Lambert experiment.* Boston: Newbury House.

Meadow, Lloyd, and Gass, Gertrude Zemon. February, 1963. Problems of the novice interviewer. *American Journal of Nursing* 63(2):97–99.

Montagu, Ashley. 1971. *Touching: the human significance of the skin.* New York: Harper and Row, Publishers.

Nelson, K. 1973. *Structure and strategy in learning to talk.* Monographs of the Society For Research in Child Development, 38 (1–2, Whole No. 149).

Piaget, J. 1952. *The language and thought of the child.* London: Routledge and Kegan Paul, Ltd.

Shanken, J., and Shanken, P. February, 1976. How to be a helping person. *Journal of Psychiatric Nursing and Mental Health Services* 14(2):24–28.

Sundeen, Sandra J., et al. 1976. *Nurse-client interaction: im-plementing the nursing process.* St. Louis: The C. V. Mosby Co.

Thomas, M. 1970. Trust in the nurse-patient relationship. In Carlson, Carolyn E., ed. *Behavioral concepts and nursing intervention.* Philadelphia: J. B. Lippincott Co.

Van Dersal, William R. December, 1974. How to be a good communicator—and a better nurse. *Nursing 74* 4(12):57–64.

Vygotsky, L. S. 1962. *Thought and language.* Cambridge, Mass.: M.I.T. Press.

Wright, Joan. May 1976. Deaf but not mute. *American Journal of Nursing* 76:795–799.

CHAPTER 19

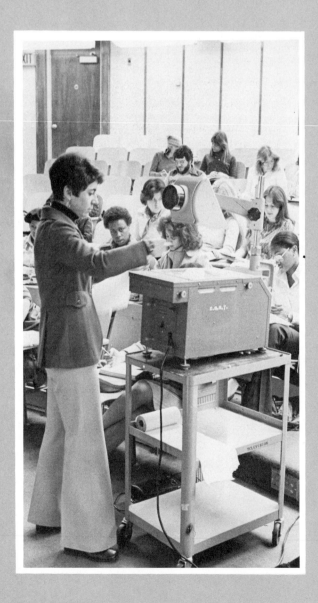

TEACHING AND LEARNING

OBJECTIVES

- Define the terms commonly used in this teaching and learning context.

- Discuss the factors that affect learning.

- Explain the developmental learning needs of persons of various ages.

- Describe the teaching process.

- Demonstrate beginning skill in assessing learning needs of individual people.

- Demonstrate beginning skill in identifying the readiness of a person to learn.

- Develop a plan for learning with a patient.

- Demonstrate beginning skill in implementing a teaching plan.

- Describe methods of evaluating learning.

One of the nurse's functions is to assist patients and their families with their learning needs. This teaching function applies to needs that are related to both health and illness. *A learning need* is a need to change behavior. In this context the behavior is an observable activity such as taking a medication, administering insulin by hypodermic syringe, or following a diet. The areas of learning with which nurses are concerned are:

1. Developmental learning needs.
2. Learning needs related to promoting health.
3. Learning needs related to restoring health.
4. Learning needs related to gaining new skills and knowledge as a result of impaired functioning.
5. Learning ways of coping with a terminal illness.

People continually acquire knowledge and learn new skills. This is most apparent during childhood, when so much is learned in a relatively short time. Consequently nurses are frequently involved in developmental learning such as assisting the parent of a 2-year-old with toilet training. For an adult the learning may be related to new experiences such as illness or to a change of environment, as happens when a person enters the hospital.

Promoting health is an area of nursing function that frequently involves learning on the part of patients and/or their families. This type of teaching may involve the acquisition of knowledge and, in some instances, the acquisition of skills. An example of the former is learning about calories and the caloric values of specific foods by an obese person. Related skills would be cooking attractive meals for a low-calorie diet or learning a program of exercises to assist weight loss.

Learning needs related to restoring health are frequently seen in hospitalized patients. The man who has had surgery may need to learn to look after his incision; the woman who has a paralyzed arm will need to learn exercises to regain the muscular functioning in her arm. This type of learning need is generally readily identified by nurses, since it usually relates directly to the patient's illness.

For patients who have impaired functioning of some type it may be necessary to learn new skills in daily living. Patients who have diabetes may need to learn to give themselves insulin by hypodermic injection, to test their urine for glucose, and to cut their nails in such a way as to avoid cutting the skin and consequently incurring an infection. The patient who has had one leg amputated needs to learn to strap on an artificial leg and to walk with it. Learning of this type is important in that it assists people to resume their daily activities with as few limitations as possible.

The teaching function of the nurse is important in assisting patients and their families with their health problems. Often if the teaching is well done, the patient will be able to function without the nurse. This independence can be one measure of the patient's learning.

THE PROCESS OF LEARNING

Learning is a permanent change in behavior. It is a process that involves active participation by the person; it requires energy. Nurses are concerned with four kinds of learning: psychomotor skills, understandings, attitudes, and social skills. The acquisition of each of these is the first step in learning. The second step is making the material meaningful to the person.

Psychomotor skills such as walking, talking, and eating are learning tasks for some patients. Often exercises and training programs are designed to assist the patient in reeducating muscles. Learning and relearning these skills usually takes both practice and time. Two-year-old children who are learning to walk will fall many times before they walk steadily.

Understanding involves thinking. A patient may need to understand what diabetic coma is, how to identify it, and what to do about it. Another example is a new mother who needs to understand when and how to feed her baby.

Attitudes also need to be learned in many situations. A patient may need to change attitudes toward an illness or toward people. Attitudes are often reflected in behavior and may need to be changed before the behavior can change. Patients who have a colostomy may need to develop healthy attitudes toward it before they can learn to effectively care for it. Attitudes can often be learned from others. Thus colostomy patients may learn attitudes from others who have colostomies.

Social learning is a different type of learning. It involves acquiring sound skills that are needed in social settings. Patients who have had some kinds of brain damage may need to relearn social skills such as eating at a table to function daily. Children learn social skills continually.

FACTORS THAT AFFECT LEARNING

Internal Factors

There are a number of internal factors for patients and their families that can affect learning. Some of these are (a) anxiety, (b) physical status, (c) age, (d) motivation, (e) communication skills, (f) senses, and (g) education and experience.

Anxiety

A greatly elevated anxiety level can impede learning. Patients or families who are very worried may not hear spoken words or may only retain part of the communication. Mild anxiety, however, can often increase learning by focusing attention.

If a patient is very anxious, this might be reduced by certain medications or by information to relieve uncertainty. On the other hand, patients who appear to be disinterested and who have no concern may need to hear about possible problems to increase their anxiety slightly and thus facilitate learning.

Physical Status

Impaired physical status such as fatigue, weakness, and hunger can affect a person's ability to learn. Patients who have just had an operation may need to devote all their energy just to breathing or moving themselves and thus have no inclination to learn about next week's diet. Learning needs to be timed for when patients are ready and when some of their physical energies can be devoted to the learning task. By providing rest periods and comfort, physical stamina can frequently be conserved to meet other needs. It is important to recognize that secondary needs such as learning can be met only after meeting primary needs such as breathing, eating, or resting.

Age

The age of a person is a primary consideration in relation to learning. The very young have obvious limitations as to what and how they learn. A child's nervous system and musculoskeletal system must be sufficiently developed for learning to take place. Therefore parents need to learn skills and knowledge for a child's care. The parents of a newborn baby may need to learn how to bathe the baby safely, or parents of a three-year-old may need to learn to change a dressing on an incision.

Older children can often learn skills and acquire knowledge in regard to their health. Teenagers may need and want help dealing with facial acne; they can learn to follow a diet, wash with a special soap, and avoid squeezing any blackheads and pimples. Adults can also learn to look after their health if they perceive the need. Elderly people, however, may have difficulty learning new skills or new ways of doing things. It may be difficult for older persons to remember to take a medicine every 4 hours, and they may need to have the times written down as a reminder. Often it is helpful to write down the date and the time in especially large letters. Then after taking the medicine they can cross out the time to serve as a reminder that they have taken the medicine. Aids of this type are often needed by elderly patients.

Motivation

Motivation is desire; in the case of learning, it is the desire to learn. The motivation experienced by a person is generally greatest when the person recognizes a need and believes that through learning this need will be met. It is not adequate for the nurse to see and express the need; it must be experienced by the patient. Often this involves assisting the patient to work through a problem and then identify the need for him or herself. Sometimes patients or families need help identifying elements in the situation before they can see a need. Patients who have heart disease may need to know the problems of smoking and being overweight before they recognize a need to stop smoking or know about a weight reducing diet. Adolescents may need to know the consequences of an untreated venereal disease before they see the need to obtain treatment. The readiness of the person is critical to learning.

Communication Skills

Communication skills involve the person's ability to perceive, understand, and convey thoughts and feelings to others. People vary in their abilities in this regard. One patient may have a large vocabulary; another may know only simple words. The ability to understand health needs is also affected to a large degree by the person's value system in regard to health. People who do not want to keep their teeth intact probably will not learn to brush them regularly.

Senses

The acuity of the senses also affects a person's ability to learn. The elderly person who is blind will be unable to learn from a brochure; the deaf person may be unable to hear a recording or the spoken word.

Education and Experience

The ability to learn is also affected by education and experience. Learners' vocabulary may relate to their background. Words such as *feces* or *emesis* may be familiar to some people and strange to others. Parents who have four children will have different needs in learning to care for a handicapped baby than parents learning to care for their first child. Familiarity with the language can also be an important factor. A patient who was born in Korea may have difficulty with the English language. People born in the United States or Canada may be more familiar with another language such as Spanish, Chinese, or French. It is not reasonable to assume that people born in the United States or Canada are comfortable with the nurse's language.

External Factors

There are also factors external to a person that can affect learning. Some of these are (a) physical environment, (b) timing, (c) teaching methods and aids, and (d) content.

Physical Environment

This includes heat, light, temperature, ventilation, noise, and supports such as chairs and tables. For optimum learning a room needs to provide adequate lighting free from glare, a comfortable room temperature, and good ventilation. Perhaps students know what it is like to try to learn in a hot, stuffy room; the subsequent drowsiness interferes with concentration. Noise can also be a distractor. Loud voices, interruptions by others, and outside traffic can interfere with listening and thinking. For the best learning it may be advisable to choose a time in a hospital when visitors are not present and interruptions are unlikely. For some learning, privacy is essential, for example, when a patient is learning to irrigate a colostomy. The presence of other people can serve to embarrass the patient and thus interfere with learning.

It is equally important that the patient be comfortable while learning. Pain and fatigue can also be distractors hindering the patient from concentrating on the subject to be learned. If a group of patients are attending a class such as a baby bath demonstration, each person needs to have a chair that provides good support and comfort.

Timing

The time for learning, the length of the learning period, and the intervals between learning are of great importance. The time chosen needs to be that which is best for the patient. If a patient is rested in the morning, this may well be the best time to learn. For another person it may be the evening or half an hour after an analgesic has been taken. Nurses need to recognize the best time for the patient or family and use that time. If repeated learning sessions are scheduled, it is often helpful if they are at the same time each day. The patient can anticipate the lesson in this way and often prepare for it.

The length of learning periods is also of great importance. If they are too long, patients lose their ability to concentrate; if they are too short, patients may not have enough time to master a skill or to understand the information.

The interval between learning periods should depend upon the patient's needs. For a patient who wants to learn quickly, a learning session in the morning, afternoon, and evening may be appropriate; for another person once a day or every other day may suffice. The intervals should not be so long that patients forget from one session to another, neither should they be so close together that patients do not have time to assimilate what they are learning.

The timing needs also to be considered relative to the need. For example, a patient who is being discharged from the hospital and who will need to be able to irrigate his own colostomy at home will need to learn these skills sufficiently ahead of discharge in order that he can practice the irrigation in the nurse's presence and be able to ask any questions in regard to his care. However, the learning will be less effective if it is done too soon before the patient is aware of his needs upon discharge and before he can even think of going home.

Teaching Methods and Aids

The method the teacher uses to convey knowledge and skills will depend to a large extent upon how the patient best learns. Usually a combination of hearing and seeing on the patient's part is best. Handling equipment and practicing with the nurse present will assist in gaining skill and confidence. Most people are helped in their learning if they have feedback as to how they are doing. *Feedback* is relating the person's performance to the desired goal. Praise when it is deserved also serves to encourage the person and sustain the urge to learn. Praise may be verbal or otherwise. For example, it may take the form of allowing a child an extra five minutes in the playroom or reading him a favorite story.

Content

The content for learning should be related to the learner's needs, not the nurse's. A patient may want and need to know only simple anatomy regarding the colostomy, not a detailed knowledge. The vocabulary the nurse uses should also be appropriate for the learner. Words such as *feces* and *void* may not be understood, whereas *bowel movement* and *pass urine* may be better known by adults and *pooh pooh* and *pee pee* by children. It is very important that nurses assess what words children do use in this regard.

The content needs also to follow a logical sequence, starting at the place where the patient has some information and logically progressing toward the objectives for the learning. When learning is planned over a number of sessions, it is best to review what has already been covered and answer any questions that the patient may have. This way the patient is always starting learning from a base, and the nurse is in no doubt as to what the patient already knows.

The content of the learning needs also to be specific. It is not sufficient to say "a few times," which can have different meanings to people. The nurse needs to say "three times" or whatever is appropriate. In regard to medications, the specific hours need to be planned. For example, an antibiotic may be required four times a day; yet the times the medication should be taken may need to be every 6 hours around the clock rather than four times between 8:00 AM and bedtime.

DEVELOPMENTAL LEARNING NEEDS

People learn from the day of birth to the day of death. Some learning is done with conscious effort; other learning is done with minimal effort and awareness. For example, a patient in a hospital may be unaware that she is learning the time for her medications, and only when they do not come does she consciously realize the time that they are normally delivered. The normal learning needs of people change to some degree when they are ill or injured. They often become secondary needs as physiologic needs take priority. The adolescent who is studying hard for a scholarship may well forget the fact when he is in acute pain. Suddenly relief from pain takes precedence over studying.

During the life cycle the nurse needs to be aware of the normal learning needs of patients and their families and to support these needs when it is appropriate.

Infancy (Birth to Two Years)

From birth to two years infants learn voluntary control over movements. They learn to hold a spoon and put it in their mouth. They also learn to control their bladder and bowels, to chatter nonsensically, and to say a few words. They learn to sleep during the entire night and learn to respond to certain objects. By 18 months they imitate their parents. At this age routines are very important.

For children who are in the hospital at this age it is important that the nurse have certain information to help children with their adjustments and learning needs. To know what stage a child is at in his or her developmental tasks is important. See Table 10–3. Maintaining routines when this is possible and using words the child already knows will assist the child in adjustment. With a change in environment an infant may seem to forget some learning as a result of anxiety, but this is usually temporary. It is best dealt with by the nurse's being supportive, understanding, and noncritical of the child.

It is also helpful to know what foods the child is accustomed to eating and the child's likes and dislikes.

The Preschool Child (Two to Five Years)

It is during this period that children become social beings. They usually are toilet trained by the age of 3 years, although they may still have accidents occasionally. They learn to manage their own clothes, and by 5 years of age they probably have learned to be modest about exposing their body to others. This fact in particular will require tactful handling by the nurse caring for the preschool child.

Preschool children learn to brush their teeth and wash themselves alone. In the hospital the nurse should allow them the time to carry out these tasks they have learned if they are well enough. During these years children learn to talk with others, and by 5 years of age they ask the nurse questions to obtain information. It is important that they receive answers to their questions using vocabulary that they understand.

By the age of 3 or 4 years they will want to play with their peers, whereas at two years they prefer solitary play. Children in this age group like to look at picture books and to have stories read to them. For the nurse to know a child's favorite bedtime story can be helpful to the adjustment in the hospital.

Preschool children focus their feelings chiefly on the parent of the opposite sex. Thus in a hospital, a boy will probably look to a female nurse for support, while a girl will look to a male nurse. Children also play with their bodies and want to know the names of the different parts. This interest may be heightened when they are ill because of others' interest in their bodies as well. They will ask the nurse the names of equipment and what the nurse is doing, expecting answers.

Children at this age have learned to like certain foods and may dislike strong or coarse textured foods. This information will help the nurse provide the child with proper nourishment. Some preschool children may have learned that they do not have to do what they are asked. This can usually be corrected by adequate explanations to accompany requests and by following through with a stated alternative. For example, if a child refuses to eat her meat after the nurse has said that she cannot have dessert unless she does

so, then it is important to follow through in this manner. See "Developmental Tasks of Childhood," Table 10–3.

The School-age Child (Six to Ten Years)

Children in this age group have learning needs concerned with skills involved in daily activities, games such as football and baseball, and communication with peers and others in their social sphere.

Physical activity is usually important to children at this time, and any impairment in their ability to participate with their peers will usually require special support and understanding from parents as well as nurses. School-age children will probably not require a nap during the afternoon but will require activity of one sort or another. Physical activity at this age serves to develop fine coordination.

The peer group is very important at this age. It is then that children learn to play and work with others. Through this activity they become less self-centered and more conscious of others in a group. Children at this age are aware of death as a concept; however, they usually do not have a need to have it explained, and they rarely apply it to themselves.

At this age children ask questions, and they like to be busy. For sick children in the hospital, it is often challenging to provide activities that are within their energy tolerance and yet meet their needs to learn and to accomplish some task.

Adolescence

The learning needs of the adolescent that are of concern to nurses largely center around four areas: the sexual roles, learning to care for and use the body effectively, grooming, and achieving emotional independence. Adolescents need to learn role behavior, and often a role model provides much of this information. An adolescent girl may learn a great deal from a female nurse; a boy may learn from a male nurse. Often learning to care for one's body is a major concern. Hair styling, skin problems, and learning to dress become very important. It is also during this period that adolescents learn what they want in a future mate.

It is equally important at this time for adolescents to learn some emotional independence from their parents. They still need guidance, and they may seek this from another adult. Adolescents want to know about sex, including venereal disease and birth control. They also have learning needs in regard to the

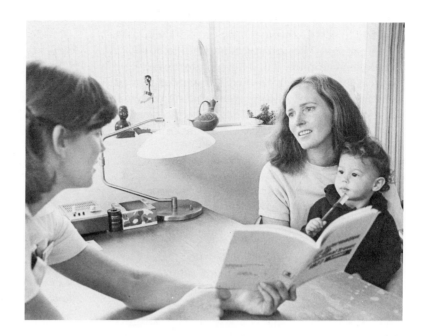

Figure 19-1. A new mother discusses nutrition of her baby with the public health nurse at a community child health clinic.

use of drugs and alcohol. See Table 10–3 on developmental tasks during adolescence.

Adulthood

Adults who become ill will have learning needs largely related to the changes in their health and environment. For the young couple expecting a baby, learning needs are largely related to what is happening, what they can expect, and how they can best prepare for the new baby. The physical and emotional changes associated with pregnancy will need to be understood as well as changes related to body image and sexual desire. They will need to learn about diet (see Chapter 25, "Pregnancy and Lactation") as well as the woman's needs for rest and for exercise. After the birth of the baby the parents have many learning needs in regard to the care of the mother and the child. See Chapter 11, "Needs of the Woman During the Puerperium."

For young adults who become hospitalized, this may be a first experience, not only of being in a hospital but also of being ill. They have learning needs in relation to the expectation of the sick role, the routines of the hospital, and any adjustments they may need to make in life after discharge.

The Middle-aged Adult

During middle age, adults have learning needs primarily in relation to adjustments to their lives as a result of health problems, physiologic changes, and anticipated retirement.

There are a number of common health problems in this age group, which may involve learning a new lifestyle: obesity, excessive use of alcohol, depressive disorders, and cardiovascular disease. The patient who is hospitalized at this time because of a heart condition may need to know about a diet, obtaining adequate rest and exercise, and making adjustments in stress settings, for example, employment. Further learning tasks are related to the developmental tasks of middle age. Refer to Table 10–3 for this material.

The Elderly Person

The special learning needs of the elderly are largely associated with their diminishing physical and mental capacities. With aging, most of the body's tissues are affected, requiring the person to learn to accommodate to these changes. See Chapter 11, "The Elderly Person, Physical Changes." In addition, some elderly people have reduced mental capacities as a result of reduced blood flow to some areas of the brain and increased atherosclerosis. They may think more slowly, have difficulty remembering, and, in some instances, have some difficulty thinking and reasoning.

Elderly people need to learn to take precautions to prevent accidents, such as having adequate lighting, handrails, and a floor area free from clutter. These and other precautions are discussed in Chapter 11, "Needs of Elderly People."

When elderly persons are admitted to the hospital, they need to learn what is expected of them just as other patients. They also probably need to be shown where the bathroom is and how to use the call light, matters nurses sometimes take for granted that patients know or will find out themselves. A change in environment for elderly persons may create some degree of confusion. Thus they require repetitive orientation as to time, place, and person for a while. It is often difficult for an elderly person to change and learn new ways of doing things or learn a new diet. However, most can learn to change with the help of the nurse. Often teaching material needs to be repeated a number of times. Special aids to learning, such as a detailed list of foods to eat, also can be used to help the elderly person learn and remember.

THE TEACHING PROCESS

Teaching can be defined as "activities by which the teacher helps the student to learn" (Redman 1976:9). It involves a special type of communication for which there are specific goals. For example, patients who need to administer their own eye drops or to change an incision dressing share these goals with the nurse. Another aspect of teaching is the relationship between the teacher and the learner. It is essentially one of trust and respect. The learner trusts that the teacher has the knowledge and skill to teach, and the teacher respects the learner's ability to attain the recognized goals. Once a nurse starts to instruct a patient or family, it is important that the teaching process continue until the goals are reached, changed, or considered not to be helping the patient or family meet their learning objectives.

The following principles may be helpful to the nursing student:

1. Teaching activities should help the learner meet individual learning objectives. If certain activities do not assist the learner, then these need to be reassessed; perhaps other activities can replace them. For example, a patient may not be able to learn to handle a syringe by explanation only. The patient may more effectively learn by handling the syringe.

2. Rapport between the teacher and the patient is essential. A relationship that is both accepting and constructive will best assist the patient to learn.

3. The teacher who can use the patient's previous learnings in the present situation encourages the patient and facilitates learning of new skills. For example, a person who already knows how to cook can use this knowledge when learning about special diets.

4. A teacher must be able to communicate clearly and concisely. The words the teacher uses need to have the same meaning to the patient as to the teacher. For example, a patient who is taught not to put water on an area of the skin may think a wet wash cloth is permissible for washing the area. In effect, the nurse needs to explain that no moisture or water should touch the area.

5. The teaching activities are oriented around the learning objectives. Thus information and skills not related to learners' objectives need to be eliminated from the teaching process. If they remain, they may confuse learners or serve as a distraction to effective learning.

ASSESSING LEARNING NEEDS

Assessing learning needs can be divided into three steps: (a) obtaining data, (b) identifying learning needs, and (c) identifying readiness and ability to learn.

Obtaining Data

Data for assessment of learning needs come from two main sources.

1. *The patient and/or the patient's family.* Their perceptions of the needs are highly significant and must be considered initially in any learning plan. Sometimes conveying information can suffice to relieve patients of worry. The hospitalized patient can also tell the nurse about problems in the home that may be of concern. For example, a patient who is to remain in bed except to use the bathroom may have his bedroom on a different floor of the house than the bathroom. Often adjustments in living such as moving to

another room can resolve this problem relatively easily.

2. *The patient's record.* When a patient has been cared for by members of a health team, the health record will provide recent data. It will also probably include information as to the possible eventual outcomes and how the patient is adjusting to illness. The record will also provide information as to financial resources, employment, daily living habits, and other pertinent data (see Chapter 15).

Included in the data will also be information as to how the patient's progress will be evaluated after discharge from a hospital. Often this will involve a plan for visits by a member of the health team and perhaps follow-up teaching if this is indicated.

Identifying Learning Needs

After all the data have been collected, the nurse then identifies the specific learning needs of the patient and/or family. It is important to identify those needs which the patient recognizes and those of which the patient is unaware. Part of the teaching plan can be to make the patient aware at a time when he or she is ready. Therefore these needs need to be noted in order that the learner and the nurse can deal with them at a later time. Sometimes, in the course of gaining some knowledge or skills, patients may become ready to recognize needs that they initially would deny or find impossible to comprehend. Often by questions the patient will reflect the need to learn.

Sometimes a need to learn is reflected in behavior that nurses find difficult. The patient appears angry or orders the nurse around. These behaviors may well reflect a need for the patient to control the environment; but the patient can be taught more acceptable ways of coping with the environment. This type of learning is referred to as *behavior modification*.

Identifying Readiness and the Ability to Learn

The third phase in assessment of learning needs is identifying the patient's or family's readiness and abilities to learn. The following criteria can be used to assess these facts.

Age

Age will provide information as to the person's individual developmental status. Simple questions to school-age children will elicit information as to what they know. Observing children in play also provides information about motor and intellectual development as well as relationships with other children. For the elderly person, conversation and questioning may reveal memory difficulties and learning difficulties often associated with sensory limitations such as deafness.

Education and Socioeconomic Status

These will give the nurse some idea about health beliefs and behavior of the person. Is oral care part of the person's system of health behavior, or does she never brush her teeth? This information will also assist the nurse to evaluate the person's intellectual capacity. For example, a person who has had a university education can be expected to have a larger working vocabulary than a person who has not had this education and does not read. Perhaps an adult patient has had no schooling and can neither read nor write; this will need to be considered in relation to learning needs.

Physical Status

Is the patient physically ready to learn? Does the patient have sufficient strength to learn to walk? Often patients who have been acutely ill may feel stronger than they really are and quickly tire upon slight exertion. Patients may need to try to walk to realize how weak they are and what their limits are at that time.

Emotional Status

Does the patient want to learn, and does the patient have the psychologic energy to do so? When people are ill, they often go through a number of stages from denial and disbelief to acceptance. These stages are described by Kübler-Ross in relation to death and dying (1970:38–137):

1. Denial and isolation—involving disbelief and withdrawal from others.
2. Anger—which is projected into the environment, often at random.
3. Bargaining—including wishing in hope of postponing a future event such as disability.
4. Depression—including a sense of loss.
5. Acceptance—including adaptation to the situation.

The person's ability and desire to learn will be largely related to the stage of the illness. People learn most effectively when they have reached the stage of acceptance and have some sense of their own identity and control.

PLANNING AND IMPLEMENTING LEARNING

Planning

Planning learning involves a number of stages: setting goals, setting priorities, planning learning content, and selecting methods of teaching.

Setting Goals

Setting goals or objectives is done by the patient or family and the nurse. Often the patient can identify the goals that are most meaningful personally and about which the nurse has little information.

Goals can be thought of as immediate and long term. Immediate goals relate to immediate needs of a patient, such as perineal care after birth of a baby. A long-term goal might be related to the need of an obese new mother to lose weight. In this case the goals may relate to a specific weight loss through diet and exercise.

The patient and the nurse should set the learning goals together. If the patient or family is actively involved in planning at this stage, they are more likely to follow through in meeting these goals. In some instances the patient might be grateful to the nurse for doing most of the planning, for example, when the patient is very weak but needs to learn quickly. An example would be a patient who wants and needs to learn responsibility for medications yet has difficulty concentrating upon the subject. A written plan for the patient that is discussed for short periods will often be most helpful at that time.

The goals for learning should be both specific and observable in terms of behavior. A specific goal might be "to take 60 mg Lasix upon identifying ankle edema." For additional information on goals see Chapter 12, "The Nursing Process."

Setting Priorities

The priorities for learning need to be set by the patient or family and the nurse. The final priority list results from a combination of the patient's perceived needs and the nurse's professional judgment.

Planning Learning Content

Learning content needs to be written as a plan. It may consist of a detailed plan, an outline form, or even a few words. However the plan is written, it should be meaningful to all people who are involved. The content is that which needs to be learned, such as how to irrigate a colostomy or how to transfer independently from the wheelchair to the tub. It can often be broken down into elements or steps.

Selecting Methods of Teaching

The methods of teaching selected should be suited to the individual patient's needs. There are many methods of conveying knowledge, feelings, and skills. To the baby the sense of touch and warmth is highly significant. To the child, manipulating objects can be meaningful. For adults, a combination of hearing, seeing, and doing is highly individualistic. Some people can conceptualize from verbal instruction, while others need to see and do for themselves.

Some teaching methods involve group learning where people can learn from each other as well as from the teacher. Other learning involves individual instruction. This permits the nurse to teach at the pace of the learner, and it is particularly appropriate for learning that the patient might find embarrassing, as in the case of learning to do self–urinary catheterization. Often there are special aids that can assist some patients with special learning needs. For example, there are a variety of special syringes to assist a visually impaired person draw up insulin for injection (Boyles 1977:1456–1458).

Demonstration is widely used as a method of teaching for both individual and group instruction. It can be planned or informal; the latter is most often used in one-to-one instruction. During the demonstration it is important for the nurse to follow a step-by-step method. If the patient appears confused, the nurse should stop and clarify the step involved before proceeding.

Audio-visual aids are also helpful to people. Charts, posters, films, and tapes are generally available. The nurse must remember, however, to choose materials that are appropriate to the learner's level. A film that includes many medical terms might serve to confuse rather than assist the viewer.

Implementing

In implementing the teaching plan there are two major concerns, timing and the environment. Both of these factors have been mentioned previously. See "Factors that Affect Learning, External Factors," in this chapter.

EVALUATING LEARNING

Evaluating is an ongoing process in which both the patient and the nurse assess what the patient has learned. There are many ways in which learning can be identified. Some of these are:

1. By the patient's questions and comments, certain knowledge will appear evident.

2. By the answers the patient gives to direct questions.

3. By demonstrating a skill such as giving a baby bath.

4. Through the observations of members of the family and other health team members.

5. By what the patient says he or she does or does not understand.

Evaluation is one means by which the patient can be encouraged in learning. Even the smallest advances are worthy of positive feedback on the part of the nurse, which will encourage the patient. Feedback at frequent intervals is important in order that the patient does not practice incorrectly or retain incorrect information. It is important when evaluating to be objective, that is, to be without personal bias and to focus upon the task, not the person. For example, it is better to say, "You handled the syringe well" rather than, "You are good."

The evaluation needs to be measured against objectives of the learning, and this may necessitate changing the teaching plan if the objectives are not being reached. It may well be that the needs of the patient must be reassessed or that there are factors interfering with learning that have not been considered. It may also be that the teaching methods need to be changed for that particular patient. Often the patient can tell the nurse where there is difficulty and what needs to be changed. The nurse and the patient can then revise the teaching plan accordingly and continue.

SUMMARY

Nurses are concerned with two types of learning in relation to patient care. The first is the developmental learning needs of patients and their families. The second type is learning needs directly related to health. Thus the teaching function of the nurse is important in assisting normal development and in assisting patients to meet needs related to health.

Learning is a permanent change in behavior. Relative to health needs, nurses are concerned with four types of learning: psychomotor skills, understanding, attitudes, and social skills. Learning is affected by many factors, some of which hinder learning and some of which assist learning. It is important to identify these factors in a particular situation and implement learning when it is most likely to be successful.

Developmental learning needs were discussed in Chapters 10 and 11. They vary with each age group and among individual persons in a particular group. Teaching is a process whereby people are assisted to learn. There are a number of principles that can serve as helpful guides to the nurse who is teaching.

Assessing learning needs and readiness to learn are the first steps in teaching. They are followed by drawing up a teaching plan and then implementing that plan. Evaluating the learning subsequently takes place, and the plan is changed if this is indicated. Positive feedback is often important in encouraging the patient about progress, particularly when learning is slow.

SUGGESTED ACTIVITIES

1. Interview a person in the community. Establish the developmental learning tasks of that person. Compare these with the developmental tasks of that age group as described by Havighurst.

2. Interview a patient in a hospital who is convalescing after surgery. Assess the patient's learning needs and develop a plan to assist him or her to meet these needs.

3. Assess the readiness to learn for the patient in activity 2.

4. Implement the plan and evaluate the learning.

SUGGESTED READINGS

Aiken, Linda Harman. September 1970. Patient problems are problems in learning. *American Journal of Nursing* 70:1916–1918.

The teaching function of the nurse begins with the assessment of patient problems. In this way teaching is a continuous process in which the nurse helps patients learn to cope with problems in their environment.

Hitchens, Emily A. March, 1977. Helping psychiatric outpatients accept drug therapy. *American Journal of Nursing* 77:464–466.

Many outpatients require long-term antipsychotic medication. Helping patients accept the need for medications and adjust to the side effects of these is an imperative function of the nurse.

Murray, Ruth, and Zentner, Judith. February, 1976. Guidelines for more effective health teaching. *Nursing 76* 6(2):44–53.

The role of a health teacher is a constant challenge to the nurse. There are a wide variety of factors that affect learning and many teaching techniques that can be used.

SELECTED REFERENCES

Altshuler, Anne, et al. January, 1977. Even children can learn to do clean self-catheterization. *American Journal of Nursing* 77:97–101.

Boyles, Virginia A. September, 1977. Injection aids for blind diabetic patients. *American Journal of Nursing* 77:1456–1458.

Kübler-Ross, Elisabeth. 1970. *On death and dying.* New York: Macmillan Publishing Co., Inc.

Pohl, Margaret L. 1968. *The teaching function of the nursing practitioner.* Dubuque, Iowa: William C. Brown Co., Publishers.

Redman, Barbara Klug. 1976. *The process of patient teaching in nursing.* St. Louis: The C. V. Mosby Co.

Steagall, Barbara. November, 1977. How to prepare your patient for discharge. *Nursing 77* 7(11):6–7.

UNIT V

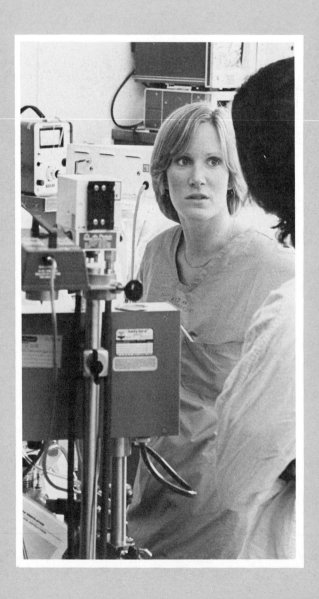
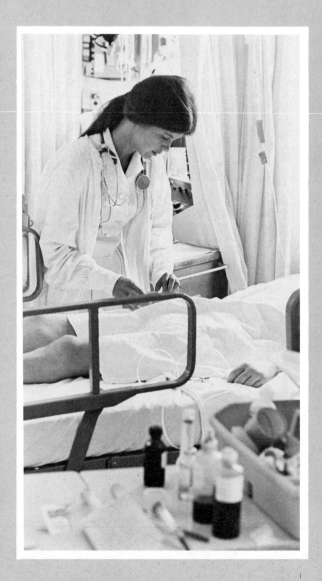

PHYSIOLOGIC NEEDS

CHAPTER 20

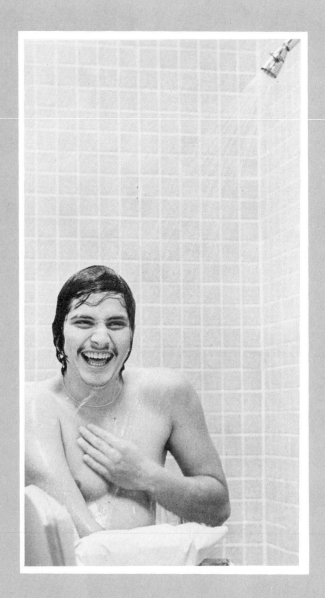

PERSONAL HYGIENE

OBJECTIVES

- Describe some of the factors that affect a person's hygiene practices.

- Identify normal skin, mucous membranes, nails, hair, and teeth.

- Explain the developmental changes of the above organs.

- Discuss the principles related to the care of skin and mucous membranes.

- Describe good oral hygiene.

- Describe good foot and nail care.

- Explain how to care for an artificial eye.

- Recognize symptoms of lice on the body or hairy body areas.

- Identify individual hygienic problems and plan and implement nursing action.

- Describe the purposes of bathing.

- Explain how to bathe a baby and an adult.

- Describe three types of back rubs.

- Explain how to carry out perineal care.

- Describe how to prevent and care for decubitus ulcers.

Hygiene can be defined as a science of health and its maintenance. Personal hygiene is the care that persons themselves take in regard to health. In the literature many types of hygiene are described: mental, oral, sexual, and social are just a few of the subdivisions of the total picture of hygiene.

Hygiene is a highly personal matter and one attached to individual values and practices. The influences in hygiene practices are of four chief sources: cultural, social, familial, and individual. Culture to a large degree influences a person's practices. For example, in some European cultures a full tub bath is normally not taken more than once a week, whereas in North America people generally bathe more frequently. Once a day is not unusual if the water and facilities are available. Social influences also affect a person's hygiene practices. Teenagers who want to be accepted by the members of their peer group will wash frequently and use the latest advertised deodorants and hair creams. If the football hero of the school uses a particular toothpaste, so will other boys who admire him.

The family also plays a large part in the development of hygienic values and practices of a person. Some of these practices will be related to physical conditions such as the availability of hot water, the number of people in the family who need to bathe, as well as their own family customs. Perhaps the father

of a family believes the use of a deodorant is unmanly, and thus his sons may adopt this attitude. Or, on the contrary, they may use deodorants because of other influences. The individual person in the end establishes practices influenced by a number of factors such as those alredy mentioned, as well as knowledge of health and hygiene, and perception of personal comfort and needs. For some people to be in a tub of water is a luxury, an activity to be enjoyed after a day of work; to others it assists in relaxation before going to bed. People also have individual needs about which they may or may not be aware. It is unlikely that a person with particularly odorous feet would not be aware of this problem; however, people with underarm perspiration problems may need assistance, for example, from a nurse, in order to cope effectively with the problem.

When people are ill, hygienic practices frequently become secondary to other body functions such as breathing, which in health is taken for granted. One sign that a formerly ill or depressed patient is feeling better is the interest in shaving or hair care or makeup.

Hygiene practices involve care of the skin, hair, nails, teeth, the oral and nasal cavities in men and women, and the vagina in women. The skin, hair, and nails are referred to commonly as the *integumentary system*.

ANATOMY AND PHYSIOLOGY OF THE INTEGUMENT

Skin and Mucous Membrane

The skin covers the entire surface of the body, and as such it is the largest organ of the body. At body orifices such as the ears, eyes, nose, rectum, and vagina the skin is continuous with the mucous membrane that lines these orifices. Skin varies in thickness from

about 0.5 mm over the ear lobes to 1.5 mm on the palms of the hands and the soles of the feet.

The skin of the body is made up of three major layers: the epidermis, the dermis or corium, and the subcutaneous tissue or hypodermis. The *epidermis* is made up of five layers in most areas of the body, none of which have blood vessels in them. The outermost layer is the stratum corneum or horny layer, which is continually being shed. It is made up of dead cells referred to as *keratized cells,* because they are converted to protein before being shed. The other layers of the epidermis are the stratum lucidum, stratum granulosum, stratum spinosum, and the deepest layer, the stratum germinativum. It is in this last layer that new cells are formed and start to move toward the surface; it is also here that *melanin* is formed, which gives skin its dark pigment. The pink tint of skin is due to blood vessels in the dermis. Exposure to the sunlight stimulates melanocytes to produce melanin, hence the tan some people obtain. Certain races have more active melanocytes and hence darker pigmentation to the skin. The distribution of pigmentation in dark-skinned people varies considerably. People from the Mediterranean area tend to have very blue lips. Blacks usually have a bluish pigmentation to their gums either evenly distributed or in patches. The observable portion of the sclera may also have melanin deposits.

The *dermis* is situated under the epidermis. It is a tough, elastic, flexible tissue, which is highly vascular and contains nerves and nerve endings. Hair follicles, the sweat glands, and oil-supplying glands *(sebaceous glands)* are situated in this layer of the skin.

Below the dermis is the *hypodermis.* It is a loosely knit connective tissue containing blood and lymph vessels, nerves, and fat globules. It serves to anchor the other skin layers and provides the springy base for the skin.

The normal skin of a healthy person has present on it microorganisms that are not harmful. Adults will usually have present some resident micrococci, bacteria of the genera *Corynebacterium* and *Propionibacterium,* and a genus of fungi, *Pityrosporum.* Children also have gram-positive, spore-forming rods and *Neisseria sp.* bacteria.

Transient microorganisms vary considerably from one person to another. They do not maintain themselves on the skin. Normally the skin can rid itself of pathogenic microorganisms in *three* general ways: the drying and the chemical effects of the fatty acids in the sebum, and the normal skin pH of 5–6 (acid medium), which is unsupportive of many microorganisms (Cahn, 1960:994).

Mucous membrane, which is continuous with the skin, lines the digestive, urinary, reproductive, and respiratory tracts and the conjunctiva of the eyes. It is an epithelial tissue, and it forms mucus, concentrates bile, and secretes or excretes enzymes, as for example in the digestive tract.

The skin of the body serves five major purposes:

1. Regulates the body temperature.
2. Protects underlying tissues from drying and injury by preventing the passage of harmful microorganisms.
3. Secretes sebum, which has antibacterial and antifungal qualities.
4. Contains nerve receptors, which are sensitive to pain, temperature, touch, and pressure thus transmitting these sensations.
5. Aids in vitamin D production.

Mucous membranes also serve four major functions. They protect the underlying tissues, provide support for body structures such as the teeth, absorb nutrients into the body, for example, in the small intestine, and they secrete mucus, salts, and enzymes.

Nails

The nails at the dorsal ends of the fingers and the toes are hard flattened keratin cells. They grow at the rate of about 1 mm per week. A lost fingernail takes about 3½ to 5½ months to regenerate, and a toenail takes 6 to 8 months (Jacob and Francone, 1978:78).

Hair

Hair grows on the whole body surface with six exceptions. It does not grow on the palms of the hands, the soles of the feet, the dorsal surfaces of terminal phalanges, and parts of the genitalia (inner surface of the labia and inner surface of the prepuce of the glans penis).

Hair on the body is of two types: the *vellus,* which is the fine nonpigmented hair covering large areas of the body, and *terminal hair,* which is longer, coarser, and pigmented. Hair grows at varying rates and is shed at varying times. The scalp of the average person loses between 20–100 hairs per day. Body hair is shed in 3 to 4 months, whereas hair in beards lasts 3 or 4 years (Brown, M.S. et al. 1973:39).

The visible part of a hair is called the *shaft.* The root of a hair is in a tube known as a *hair follicle.* There are muscles known as *arrector pili muscles,* which are attached to the hair follicles. When these contract, the skin assumes a goose flesh appearance. Sebaceous glands grow from the walls of hair follicles. They secrete *sebum,* an oily substance that lubricates the skin.

Sebum is produced in greater quantities on the scalp and the face.

Sweat Glands

Sweat glands or *sudoriferous glands* are on all body surfaces with the exception of the lips and parts of the genitalia. The body has from two to five million, which are all present at birth. They are most numerous on the palms of the hands and the soles of the feet. Sweat is made up of water, sodium, potassium, chloride, glucose, urea, and lactate. Sweat glands are classified as *apocrine* and *exocrine*. The apocrine glands, located specifically in the axilla and pubic areas, are of little use. Bacteria act upon the sweat produced by these glands, causing odor. The exocrine glands are of utmost importance physiologically. The sweat produced from these glands is responsible for cooling the body through the process of evaporation.

Teeth

A tooth has a number of parts: the crown, the root, and the pulp cavity. The *crown* is the exposed part of the tooth, which is outside of the gum. It is covered with a hard substance called *enamel*. The internal part of the crown below the enamel is ivory colored and is referred to as the *dentin*. See Figure 20-1.

The root of a tooth is embedded in the jaw, and it is covered by a bony tissue called *cementum*. The pulp

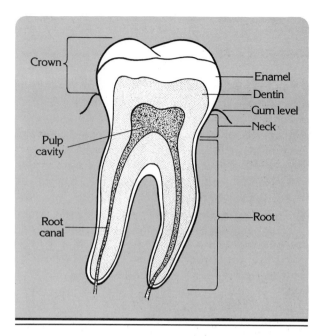

Figure 20-1.   The anatomical parts of a tooth.

cavity in the center of the tooth contains the blood vessels and nerves.

Teeth are used to masticate food in order that it can be digested in the stomach and the intestine.

APPEARANCE OF THE NORMAL INTEGUMENT

Normal Skin

Normal skin has a number of observable characteristics. Normal skin:

1. Has variations in pigment within races.

2. Has good tissue turgor, that is, once the skin is pinched it will quickly fall back into place when released.

3. Is smooth, soft, and flexible.

4. Can have a variety of pigmented spots; for example, mongolian spots are normal in black, Chicano, Oriental, and Mediterranean babies. Freckles in whites are normal.

5. Has no evidence of cyanosis, jaundice, or pallor.

Normal Mucous Membrane

The normal mucous membrane is pink, moist, and smooth.

Normal Nails

Normal nails have pink nail beds; they are convex and smooth. Normal nails blanch when pressed but quickly turn pink when pressure is released.

Normal Hair

Normal hair is soft, fine and shiny; it may be thicker and dryer in blacks.

Normal Teeth

Normal teeth are white and are aligned.

DEVELOPMENTAL CHANGES

Skin

In early embryonic life the skin is a single layer of cells. Other layers develop quickly. The skin of an infant is thinner than an adult's, usually mottled, and in whites it varies from pink to red and becomes ruddy when the baby cries. Babies who are genetically dark-skinned are lightly pigmented at birth. Dark bluish areas are often apparent on the lower back or buttocks of nonwhites. These are referred to as *mongolian spots* (no relation to mongolism) and usually disappear spontaneously during the first year. Skin pigmentation gradually increases until about 6 or 8 weeks. Infants, like adults, show a freckle-like pigmentation of the gums, the oral cavity, the tongue edges, and the nail beds.

Sweat glands of babies begin to function at about one month of age.

In adolescence the sebaceous glands increase in activity as a result of increased hormone levels. As a result, hair follicle openings enlarge to accommodate the increased amount of sebum.

The older person will also experience skin changes. The skin tends to be thinner, drier, with fine wrinkling and some inelasticity. This process appears at various ages, anytime from 40 years and older. The elderly person's skin typically will show wrinkles, sagging, pigmentations, and keratotic spots usually on areas exposed to the sun. The older person's skin will also be less resilient, that is, when it is pinched it will return to place more slowly than the skin of a younger person.

Nails

Nails are normally present at birth. The continue to grow during life, and they change very little until people are old. At that time the nails tend to be tougher, more brittle, and in some cases thicker. The nails of an elderly person will normally grow less quickly than those of a younger person, and they may be ridged and have grooves.

Hair

Newborns may have *lanugo* over the shoulders, the back, and the sacrum. Lanugo is the fine hair on the body of the fetus also referred to as *down* or *woolly hair*. This generally disappears, and the hair distribution becomes noticeable on the eyebrows, head, and eyelashes of young children. Some newborns have some hair on their scalps; others are free of hair at birth but grow hair over the scalp during the first year of life.

Pubic hair usually is formed between the ages of 8 and 12 years followed in about 6 months by the growth of axillary hair. Boys will develop facial hair about 6 months later.

In elderly people the hair is generally thinner, grows more slowly, and loses its color as a result of the tissues aging and circulation diminishing. Men often lose their scalp hair and may become completely bald. This phenomenon may occur even when a man is relatively young. The older person's hair also tends to be drier than normal. With age, axillary and pubic hair becomes finer and more scant in contrast to the eyebrows, which become bristly and coarse. Most women develop hair on their faces, which may be a problem to them.

Teeth

Teeth start to develop in the fetus at the seventh week and appear at about 5 months of fetal age. Temporary or deciduous teeth generally begin to show above the gum at about 5 to 8 months, although some newborns may have teeth partially through when they are born.

By the time children are 2 years old they usually have all 20 of their temporary teeth. About the age of 6 or 7 years permanent teeth start to appear. The first permanent teeth to appear are the first molars just behind the temporary teeth. These are followed by the central and lateral incisors. From 9 to 12 years the cuspids, first bicuspids, and second bicuspids appear.

The second molars appear about age 12 or 13. The third molars, also referred to as the *wisdom teeth*, erupt at any time between 21 and 25 years. This completes the permanent dentition process so that each jaw contains 16 teeth.

By the time adults have reached advanced years, they may well have very few of their permanent teeth left. About 75% of elderly people have lost all their own teeth by age 70 (Anderson 1971:110). This is attributed mostly to periodontal disease rather than to dental caries; the latter are common in the middle-aged adult. Preventive dental care is important.

The actual age when people lose teeth or have them removed is highly individualistic. It is dependent upon many factors, including dental care, diet, and dental hygiene, such as frequency of brushing. Many of the elderly have dentures.

GUIDELINES RELATED TO THE CARE OF THE SKIN AND MUCOUS MEMBRANE

1. *Intact skin and mucous membranes serve as the first barriers of defense for the body against injury and disease.* The skin and mucous membranes are not readily permeable to fluids, chemicals, or microorganisms.

2. *The degree to which the skin protects the underlying tissues from injury depends upon the general health of the cells, the amount of subcutaneous tissue and melanin, and the degree of dryness of the skin.* Skin that is poorly nourished and dry has less ability to protect and is more vulnerable to injury. The greater the amount of subcutaneous tissue the more padding there is, in particular, over bony prominences. Skin in which there are very active melanocytes, which produce melanin, is less likely to react to sunlight and burn than is skin with very little melanin.

3. *Hygienic practices vary between individuals, between people of different economic status, and between cultures.* Just as people learn from their family and from reading about hygienic practices, they are also influenced by the availability of facilities such as hot water and the customs of their culture.

4. *Sensory receptors in the skin are sensitive to heat, pain, touch, and pressure.* These receptors can adapt to repeated stimuli; for example, repeated exposure to hot water can result in adaptation to the heat, and it is then no longer perceived as being as hot as it was originally perceived.

5. *Soaps act by lowering the surface tension of water, which aids in the emulsification of fats.* Glands in the skin secrete sebum, an oily substance that lubricates the skin. The collection of sebum over a period of time can be irritating to the skin; thus washing with soap is a part of basic hygiene.

6. *Excessive moisture in contact with skin for a period of time can result in irritation.* Skin should be dried carefully after it has been cleansed, and diapers on a baby need to be kept dry to avoid irritation.

7. *Excessive dryness of the mucous membrane, for example, in the oral cavity, can result in crusting and infections.*

ORAL HYGIENE

Good oral hygiene includes daily stimulation of the gums (gingiva), mechanical scrubbing of the teeth, and flushing of the mouth. Regular checkups by a dentist every six months are also recommended. The nurse is often in a position to help people, young or old, ill or well, to maintain oral hygiene. He or she may assist by helping or teaching people to carry out their own oral hygiene, by inspecting to see that hygiene has been carried out, particularly with children, or by actually providing hygienic measures for some patients such as the ill or incapacitated. The nurse can also be instrumental in identifying and referring problems that require the services of a dentist.

Brushing Teeth

Thorough brushing of the teeth is important in preventing tooth decay (see Figure 20–2). Teeth should be brushed at least four times a day, after meals and at bedtime. The use of a medium or soft multibristled brush is advised, since it minimizes the chance of the gums being traumatized. The mechanical action of brushing removes food particles that can harbor and incubate bacteria. It also stimulates the gums, thus maintaining their healthy firmness and the circulation.

The technique for brushing the teeth includes placing the bristles of the brush at the junction of the teeth and gums and moving the brush back and forth for the inside and outside surfaces. Use short strokes. For the biting surfaces, brush back and forth. For the inside surfaces of the upper and lower front teeth, place brush vertically (Figure 20-2).

An abundant variety of toothpastes are marketed, any of which can be used to assist in the cleansing process. The advantage of these is that they are flavored and scented to make them pleasant tasting. However, a good dentifrice can be made by combining two parts of table salt to one part of baking soda.

After brushing the teeth, the mouth is rinsed with water to remove the dislodged food particles and excess cleanser. Many antiseptic mouthwashes are also marketed, and some people may prefer these for rinsing. If brushing cannot always be done after meals or the intake of food, vigorous rinsing of the mouth with water is recommended.

Children should be taught the habit of brushing their teeth by the age of 2 when the teeth appear. Because children will not be able to manage this independently for several years, parents are advised to do this for them. A small stool can be provided in the bathroom for the child to reach the sink, and a special place for the child's toothbrush can enhance positive attitudes for this habit.

Dental Flossing

Flossing of the teeth is advised daily. It is especially beneficial in preventing the formation of plaque and removing it from the teeth, particularly at the gumline. A method for flossing is described in Figure 20-3.

The Use of Fluoride

The use of fluoride is known to prevent dental caries, although by itself it does not eliminate tooth decay. Many regions have water supplies that contain fluoride. Children who drink fluoridated water when their teeth are forming can develop a resistance to cavities that carries over to their adult life. Some benefit is also received if a child starts drinking fluoridated water even after the teeth are formed. For children who do not have access to fluoridated water, a fluoride solution can be applied to the teeth at regular intervals by a dentist or dental hygienist. Using a toothpaste that contains fluoride is also helpful in preventing tooth decay.

Fluoride supplements are also recommended as an alternative to fluoridated water, starting in the first month of the baby's life until age 14. Some preparations are made in combination with vitamins, but these are not necessary. Prevention of tooth decay is dependent upon regularity of ingestion of fluoride. Recommended dosages of the supplement are as follows:

2 drops daily	0–1 year
4 drops daily	1–4 years
6 drops daily	4–8 years
8 drops or 1 tablet	over 8 years

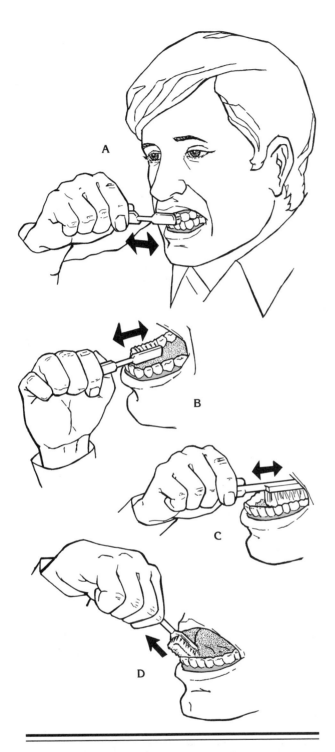

Figure 20-2.   To brush teeth, position the brush as in **A** and use short strokes back and forth for the outer surfaces. **B**, For inside upper and lower front teeth, place brush vertically and gently move it back and forth over the teeth and gum tissue. **C**, For cleansing inner surfaces, place brush horizontally and use short strokes cleansing the teeth surfaces from the gum line to the top of the crown. **D**, To cleanse biting surfaces, move brush back and forth.

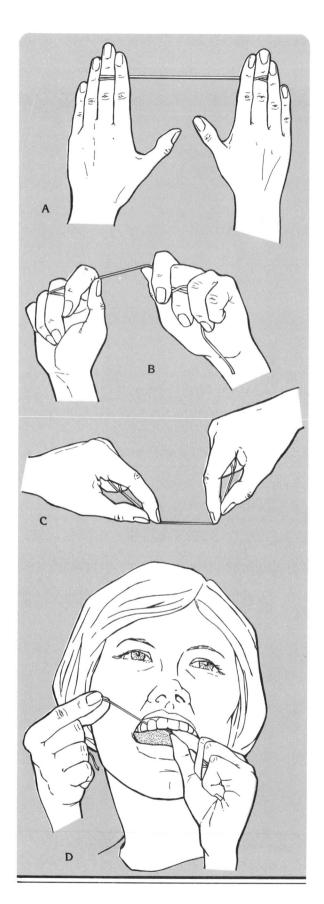

Figure 20-3.   To floss teeth, hold floss between the third fingers of each hand, **A**. To floss upper teeth, use thumbs to stretch floss, **B**. To floss lower teeth, use second fingers to stretch floss, **C**. In flossing, move floss back and forth, inserting gently between teeth, **D**. Do not force floss. Floss to the gum surface but do not damage the gums.

The supplement can be acquired without a prescription and can be taken with water, milk, or juice. It needs to be kept out of the reach of children.

Regular Examinations by a Dentist

It is recommended that children be taken to the family dentist by the age of 2½ or 3. This early age is advised because it helps the child become accustomed to going to a dentist and because the preventive measure of topical fluoride application can be commenced then. By this age 50% of children have tooth decay, and prompt treatment is necessary. Small cavities in primary teeth can progress to large ones within a few months. A cavity is never too small for treatment. Unlike bones that can heal themselves, teeth must be filled. Nothing but a filling will arrest tooth decay. Dentists can at this time also offer helpful advice about the care of the child's teeth and identify any problems concerning the teeth.

Some people hold the illusion that it is not necessary to fill primary teeth, since they will inevitably be replaced. The nurse can be instrumental as a health teacher in this situation. It is important that primary teeth are looked after, since some must last up to 12 years. Primary teeth are needed for proper chewing of food, as guides for permanent tooth eruption, for stimulating natural growth of jaws, and for an attractive appearance. Primary teeth that are decayed can cause dental pain and can be lost earlier than prescribed by nature. Both effects can interfere with proper eating and chewing, and the latter can cause permanent teeth to erupt out of line. Once a tooth is lost, an adjacent tooth drifts over to close in the space, which then interferes with the eruption of the underlying permanent tooth. Because the space for the new permanent tooth to erupt is narrowed, it is forced to grow either in toward the tongue or out toward the cheek. Temporary space maintainers can be inserted by dentists until the permanent tooth erupts to prevent malalignment. Early loss of primary teeth can also lead to poor speech habits. Normal speech development is dependent upon the teeth, which allow the tongue to form certain sounds. In essence, good teeth are needed for a child's health and appearance. The following is a listing of measures to combat tooth decay:

1. Brush teeth thoroughly after meals and at bedtime. Assist children or inspect to be sure teeth are clean.

2. Floss teeth daily.

3. Ensure adequate intake of nutrients, particularly calcium, phosphorus, vitamins A, C, and D, and fluorine.

4. Avoid sweet foods and drinks between meals. Take them in moderation after meals.

5. Eat coarse, fibrous foods (cleansing foods) such as fresh fruits and raw vegetables.

6. Take a fluoride supplement daily until age 14 as an alternative to fluoridated water.

7. Have topical fluoride applications as prescribed by the dentist.

8. Have checkups by a dentist every 6 months.

Oral Hygiene for Hospitalized Patients

When patients are hospitalized, it is the nurse's responsibility to assist them in carrying out oral hygiene. Most patients who are ambulatory can do this independently. Most bedridden patients will require very little assistance other than the provision of a glass of water, dentifrice, a mouthwash as desired, a kidney basin for rinsing the mouth, and a towel to wipe their mouth. Afterward, the nurse will need to clean the patient's toothbrush and kidney basin. For patients who are fasting for surgery or diagnostic tests, oral hygiene is greatly appreciated. Their mouths are dry, and they feel thirsty. Oral hygiene can do much to alleviate their thirst.

Dependent Patients

Patients who are unconscious or who have hemiplegia need oral hygiene provided for them completely or partially. Unconscious patients need to be positioned on their sides with the head of the bed lowered to prevent the danger of aspiration of fluids. A kidney basin or a towel can be placed under the patient's chin. For edentulous patients, the gums, cheeks, roof of the mouth, and tongue should be thoroughly cleansed. The cheeks will need to be retracted with one hand. Commercially prepared applicators soaked with glycerine and lemon juice can be used for cleansing. If these are not available, a gauze square rolled around the index finger and dipped in a glycerine and lemon juice preparation or into an anti-

septic mouthwash is also effective. Only small amounts of solution are needed to moisten the mucous membranes. Large amounts of fluid are to be avoided because they can be aspirated by patients who have swallowing difficulties. Excesses of fluid, however, can be drawn out by gravity if the patient is in an appropriate position. The patient's mouth is then dried, and a lubricant such as petroleum jelly can be applied to the lips.

For dentulous patients, in addition to the above measures, the nurse needs to brush the patient's teeth. Brushing someone else's teeth requires some practice in order to apply sufficient pressure for cleaning the teeth but not too much pressure that could be injurious to gum tissue. Rinsing of the mouth can be accomplished by the use of a rubber-tipped bulb syringe and water if warranted.

Hemiplegic Patients

These patients frequently require assistance from the nurse because food particles tend to collect in the affected side of the mouth. Due to loss of sensation and muscle power on the one side of the mouth, a thorough cleansing is often difficult for these patients.

Care of Dentures

Most patients in a hospital are self-sufficient and will wash their own dentures. However, for the incapacitated or for the bedridden elderly or confused patients, it becomes the nurse's responsibility. In order to remove upper dentures the nurse grasps them at the front with the thumb and index finger. They may need to be moved slightly up and down to overcome the suction effect on the roof of the mouth. Lower dentures are readily removed by retracting the cheek, turning them slightly, and pulling them out through the lips on one side and then the other. Dentures must be handled carefully, since they can break if dropped or knocked against metal water taps. Most agencies supply special containers for patient's dentures, which are labeled with the patient's name and stored at his bedside. Dentures are cleansed with a toothbrush and dentifrice and then well rinsed with water. Replacing dentures in the patient's mouth is facilitated if the dentures are moist. Water, saline, or commercial preparations can be used to soak dentures during the night.

Special Mouth Care

Disease processes and inadequate nutrition can alter the normal moist mucous membranes of the mouth and the tissues of the lips. For example, dehydration can cause halitosis (bad breath), furry tongues, and sordes. *Sordes* is the accumulation of foul matter that collects on the teeth and lips and consists of food, microorganisms, and epithelial elements. In order to remove sordes it is necessary to use solutions containing hydrogen peroxide or brandy. Special mouth care usually means increased frequency of mouth care and increased mechanical cleansing and lubrication.

Symptoms of Oral Problems

The presence of the following symptoms in regard to the mouth can reflect a problem that may require the assistance of a physician or a dentist. Nurses need to be aware of these symptoms as their patients may describe them or as they are observed.

1. Halitosis (bad breath).
2. Inflamed, swollen, receding and/or bleeding gums.
3. Discomfort or pain in a tooth when eating or taking hot or cold fluids.
4. Pain in a part of a jaw.
5. Crusts on the mucous membranes.

Common Problems of the Mouth

Dental disease is common in North America. A study carried out in 1960–62 found that the average American had 20 to 32 teeth either missing, filled, or decayed. It is also estimated that three out of four adults who have their natural teeth show evidence of *periodontal* disease (a disease process around the teeth). It is further estimated that there is a backlog of 800 million unfilled cavities as a result of tooth decay (Milgrom 1975:29–30).

The most common oral problem in younger people is the occurrence of *dental caries* (tooth cavities). Dental caries is a pathologic process in which the enamel and the dentin gradually dissolve with eventual involvement of the pulp of the tooth. The underlying cause of dental caries is thought to be the presence of enzyme-producing bacteria of the lactic acid bacilli group. These bacteria, which are present in saliva, convert carbohydrates to lactic acid, which in turn dissolves tooth enamel, allowing for bacterial invasion and caries formation. The number of lactic acid bacilli can be reduced by the intake of fluoridated water or by topical application of fluoride, thus reducing dental caries.

Periodontal disease is a disease of the tissues that support the tooth. These tissues include the cementum, the periodontal ligament, alveolar bone, and the gingiva (gums). Often periodontitis, the inflammation of the periodontal tissue, occurs as an extension of gingivitis. Initially in the process of periodontal disease plaques form on the teeth, particularly at the gum line. A plaque is made up of mucin, carbohydrates, and the microorganisms normally found in the mouth. Mucin is the chief constituent of mucus and is a glycoprotein substance.

Stomatitis is an inflammatory condition of the mouth. Glossitis and gingivitis are localized forms. *Glossitis* is inflammation of the tongue (glossa), and *gingivitis* is inflammation of the gums (gingiva).

Parotitis is the inflammation of the parotid salivary gland. It can occur in patients who have maintained poor oral hygiene, such as persons who are unable to provide their own care because of paralysis and who have not received assistance.

Many pathogenic organisms can cause these inflammations, such as the streptococcus organism and viruses such as herpes simplex and measles. The inflammatory process can extend to any of the salivary glands, which empty into the oral cavity. Good oral hygiene, which includes brushing teeth and the use of dental floss, will help prevent the occurrence of these inflammations.

When a patient is taking very few or no fluids and little or no food, it is of utmost importance that oral hygiene be maintained as a preventive measure.

Halitosis may be the result of poor oral hygiene, or it may be caused by a systemic condition. If it is the result of bacterial action upon food particles, cleaning the teeth, including between the teeth, and the use of a mouthwash will be helpful. If the cause is systemic, hygiene is of limited help.

BATHING AND SKIN CARE

Purposes of Bathing

Bathing has a number of purposes and functions. The skin is physiologically bathed continuously with sebum and perspiration from the sebaceous and sudoriferous glands, respectively. Sebum and perspiration have protective functions; sebum prevents dryness, and perspiration provides a slightly acid medium, which discourages bacterial growth.

These two processes, however, can be injurious to a person or disadvantageous if bathing is not carried out regularly, that is, when perspiration, sebum, and dead skin cells are permitted to accumulate. Excessive perspiration on the skin interacts with the bacteria present, causing body odor, considered to be offensive. An accumulation of sebum on the skin can be irritating in itself, since it assists the growth of bacteria. Large numbers of bacteria on the skin can cause problems, particularly when the skin integrity is interrupted, for example, from a cut. Dead skin cells also harbor bacteria. Bathing, then, removes accumulated oil, perspiration, dead skin cells, and some of the bacteria. The quantity of oil and dead skin cells that are produced can be more readily appreciated when nurses observe the skin of a person after the removal of a cast that has been on for 6 weeks. The skin will be crusty, flaky, and dry underneath the cast. Applications of oil are usually necessary over several days to remove the debris. Excessive bathing, on the other hand, can interfere with the intended lubricating effect of the sebum, thus causing dryness of the skin. This is an important consideration for people who produce a limited amount of sebum.

In addition to its cleansing value, bathing also stimulates circulation. A warm or hot bath dilates superficial arterioles, bringing more blood and nourishment to the skin. Vigorous rubbing also has the same effect. Rubbing with long smooth strokes from the distal to proximal parts of extremities is particularly effective in facilitating venous blood flow.

Bathing also produces a sense of well-being for people. It is refreshing and relaxing and frequently boosts a person's morale, appearance, and sense of self-respect. A morning shower is often taken by some people for its refreshing, stimulating effect. An evening bath, on the other hand, can be relaxing. These effects are more prominent when a person is ill. For example, it is not uncommon for patients who have had a restless or sleepless night to feel relaxed and comfortable or fall asleep after a morning bath.

The effectiveness of bathing in eliminating some body odors is also important. The apocrine glands, which produce sweat, are situated in the axilla and pubic areas and appear at puberty. Their secretions are decomposed by bacterial action, resulting in a prominent foul odor that is distasteful to others if not to oneself. Apocrine glands are thought to secrete less after menopause and to enlarge and become more active before and after monthly menses. The use of anti-perspirants to control perspiration and odor from the axillae is prevalent in North America. On occasion the nurse may recommend its use to those people who have a problem.

The bathing procedure can serve several advantages for the nurse when caring for ill patients. It gives the nurse an opportunity to observe the condition of the skin and the patient's general physical condition such as sacral edema or rashes. The skin is said to mirror one's health, but it is not always an accurate index. While assisting a patient with a bath the nurse can also assess the patient's mental and emotional states, for example, orientation to time and abilities to cope with the illness. Opportunities to assess learning needs are also provided, such as foot care for the person who has diabetes.

Time and Frequency of Bathing

The time of day and frequency of bathing are highly variable. Some people prefer morning baths, whereas others prefer baths in the evening. The environment and activity of the person dictate the frequency of bathing. If the weather is hot or if a person engages in athletic endeavors, more than one bath may be taken daily. The age of the person also dictates the frequency. Elderly people rarely require bathing more than once or twice a week because of the reduction in the amount of their skin oil and perspiration.

When people are ill, the frequency of bathing may need to be increased. Very ill patients may require at least one bath daily. When people are confined to bed, they are not subjected to the usual air currents that normally help to evaporate perspiration. This is accentuated for patients who have high fevers and are diaphoretic. In other situations the reverse holds true. Body perspiration can be decreased by some illnesses.

Usually a hospital has policies that prescribe the frequency of baths. It is not unusual for full baths and complete bed linen changes to be offered twice a week for patients, and partial baths, that is, of the face, hands, axilla, and pubic areas are offered the rest of the time. This does not preclude the taking of baths as necessitated by illness or in the nurse's judgment. Commonly, too, the time for baths in institutions is in the morning. For patients who are accustomed to bathing in the evening before retiring, this routine may be a source of frustration.

Procedure 20-1.   Bathing a Patient in Bed

ACTION	EXPLANATION
Assemble Equipment	
1. Bath towels.	One for the face and one for the remainder of the body.
2. Washcloth.	
3. Soap.	
4. Basin.	For wash water.
5. Skin lotion.	To massage body prominences, including the patient's back.
6. Bath blanket.	To cover the patient during the bath.
7. Water between 37.7° and 40.5° C (100° and 115° F) for adults. For the newborn the bath water should be between 43.3° and 58.3° C (100° and 105° F).	The water should feel comfortably warm to the patient. The infant's skin is very sensitive. People vary in their sensitivity to heat. Most patients will verify a suitable temperature.
8. Other toiletries desired by the patient.	
To Bathe a Patient	
1. Explain what you plan to do. Adjust the explanation to the patient's needs.	To reassure the patient by knowledge of what will happen. To identify the patient. To assess if any special equipment is needed, such as a razor.
2. Make sure the room is free from drafts by closing windows and doors.	The room temperature should be about 23.9° C (75° F). Air currents increase the loss of heat from the body by convection.
3. Provide privacy.	Draw curtains or close doors. Hygiene is a personal matter.
4. Offer the patient the bed pan or urinal.	
5. Wash hands.	To prevent transmission of microorganisms to the patient.
6. Place bed in high position.	To avoid undue strain upon the nurse's back.
7. The top bed linen is removed and replaced with the bath blanket.	If bed linen is to be reused, it is placed over the chair. If it is to be changed, it is placed in the linen hamper.
8. Assist patient to move near you. Remove gown.	
9. Make a bath mitt with the washcloth (see Figure 20-4). Place a towel across the patient's chest.	
10. Wash the patient's eyes with water only and dry well. Use a separate corner of the washcloth for each eye, and wipe from the inner to outer canthus.	In order to prevent crusts and microorganisms from entering the nasolacrimal ducts.
11. Wash the patient's face, neck, and ears. Some patients may not want soap used on their faces. For infants wash the scalp. Wash and rinse each part well and then dry.	Soap has a drying effect. The face, being exposed to the environment more than other body parts, tends to be drier.

12. Place a towel under the patient's arm, and wash and dry it using long, firm strokes, distal to proximal. Give special attention to the axilla. Repeat for other arm (see Figure 20-5).

To increase venous blood return.

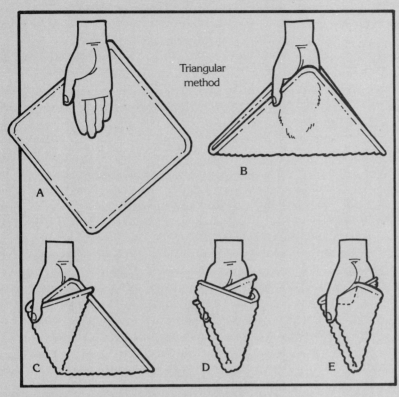

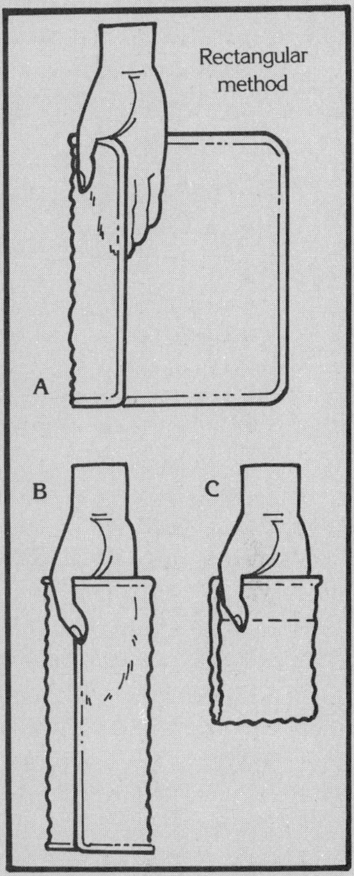

Triangular method

Rectangular method

Figure 20-4.   To make a bath mitt using a wash cloth. Triangular method: **A,** Lay hand on wash cloth; **B,** fold corner away from you over the hand; **C,D,** fold over other two corners; and **E,** tuck second corner under cloth on palmar side to secure. Rectangular method: **A,** Place hand on cloth and fold one side over hand; **B,** bring second side over hand; and **C,** fold top down and under cloth next to the palm of the hand to provide a pad and secure.

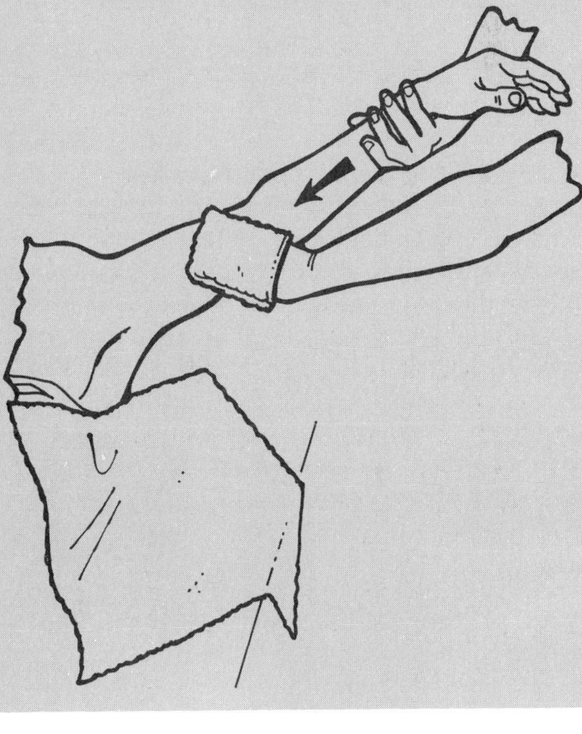

Figure 20-5.   To wash a patient's extremities, use long smooth strokes moving from distal to proximal to promote venous circulation.

Procedure 20-1. Cont'd.

13. Wash the patient's chest and abdomen. For infants wash the entire trunk.

14. Wrap the blanket around the patient's legs and feet. Use long, firm strokes from the ankle to the knee and from the knee to the thigh. Feet can be placed in the basin of water.

    To avoid exposing the perineal area.

    To stimulate venous blood circulation.

15. Obtain fresh bath water.

    Change water more frequently if it becomes cool.

16. Assist the patient to turn on his or her side to wash the back, buttocks, and upper thighs. Then give a back rub (see Procedure 20-2).

17. To give perineal care, assist the patient to the supine position (see "Perineal and Genital Care" later in this chapter).

    Many patients may prefer to cleanse their own perineums if they are able because of embarrassment when it is done by another person.

18. Assist the patient to dress.

19. Comb the patient's hair.

20. Make the bed.

21. Assist the patient to a comfortable position.

22. Return the bed to the low position.

    It is easier for the patient to leave it in this position.

23. Gather equipment and put it away.

24. Wash hands.

25. Record significant observations, such as skin abrasions or complaints of discomfort.

NOTE: Particular attention should be paid to body areas with creases and folds such as behind the ears, beneath the breasts, the axilla, between fingers and toes and gluteal folds.

Hygienic Care of the Newborn

Practices in the hygienic care of the newborn vary from agency to agency. When the baby is first admitted to the nursery, some agencies offer an admission bath, and others remove any blood or vernix from the infant's face for aesthetic reasons only, then diaper and wrap the baby loosely in a blanket. The newborn's temperature-regulating mechanisms are undeveloped, so measures to avoid chilling are important. Hexachlorophene soap was previously used for admission baths to prevent the incidence of staphylococci infections in nurseries. However, its use has been largely discontinued, since it was suggested that central nervous system damage follows repeated use. After the newborn's status is stabilized, the daily hygienic care of the baby includes a sponge bath (optional) until the cord falls off, cleansing the genitals and buttocks with diaper changes, cord care, and, for some male infants, circumcision care. If sponging is done, small soft washcloths or cotton balls should be used. The vernix caseosa usually disappears in about 24 hours. If it does persist in creases and folds, it can become an irritant and needs to be removed with gentle wiping with a cotton ball moistened with warm water.

The cord falls off spontaneously, usually in 5 to 8 days, but it may last up to 2 weeks. Attempts should *not* be made to remove it. In order to encourage drying of the cord and to discourage infection, the base of the cord is wiped once a day with alcohol. In most nurseries the cord is left exposed to the air; however, in some places a small gauze dressing is applied. This needs to be changed periodically when soiled.

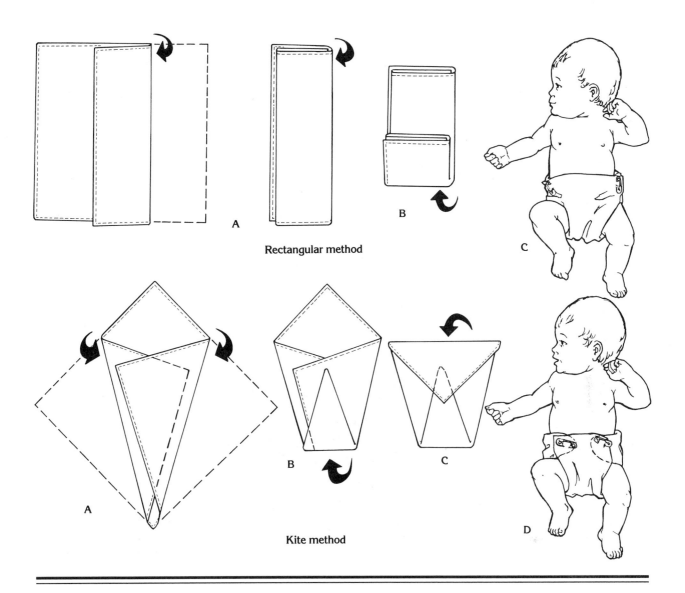

Figure 20-6.   Diaper folding. Rectangular method: **A,** Fold diaper into a rectangle by bringing side over; **B,** fold bottom edge up to provide appropriate size; and **C,** apply to infant, pinning at the sides. Triangular method: **A,** Make a triangle by folding side corners to the center; **B,** bring bottom corner up to center; **C,** fold down top corner; and **D,** apply to infant, pinning at the sides.

For babies who are circumcised, the penis must be inspected for bleeding, although most incisions heal rapidly. By diapering the baby lightly over the penis, bleeding will not go unnoticed if it occurs. Immediately after a circumcision the area is covered with a sterile gauze saturated with petroleum jelly. In some situations this gauze is left on until it falls off spontaneously. In other situations this dressing is removed when the infant voids, the area is cleansed gently with moistened cotton balls, and a new dressing is applied each time the diaper is changed.

Smegma, a curdlike secretion, may collect under the prepuce of the glans in male babies and between the labia in female babies. This can be removed with a moistened cotton ball. For females one swab should be used for each stroke and should be moved from the front of the body toward the back.

Babies are usually clothed in a shirt and a diaper, although the shirt may or may not be necessary depending upon the temperature of the environment. Babies do not perspire for the first month nor do they respond with goose flesh; therefore the nurse must use judgment when clothing babies appropriately. If they are too hot, they develop prickly heat, a pinhead papular rash on the face or neck and/or in places where skin surfaces touch.

Infant Bathing

Sponge baths are given to infants until the cord stump disappears and the umbilicus is well healed. The general measures previously discussed should be employed for the infant's bath, paying particular attention to preventing undue exposure.

The equipment required for sponging the baby will depend upon agency facilities and policies. Generally included are a shirt, diaper, safety pins, soft washcloth, cotton balls, towel, paper bag for soiled cotton balls, facial tissue or toilet tissue to remove feces, and a basin of warm water at 40.6° C (105° F). The water should feel slightly warm to the inside of the wrist or the elbow. Other materials are optional and may include alcohol to apply at the base of the cord stump, mineral oil or petroleum jelly for protection against diaper rash, and mild soap. If soap is used, it should be used sparingly, since it can be drying to a baby's skin. Cotton-tipped applicators are contraindicated for cleansing. The applicators can break when the baby moves, causing injury to the mucous membranes of the nose or to an eardrum. Powders are also to be avoided, since the baby may inhale them while they are shaken from their container. Powders also tend to cake with moisture and cause skin irritation.

Sponging

For a sponge bath the infant's face, neck, ears, and scalp should be cleansed before the baby is undressed. The baby's eyes, behind the ears, and between-the-neck creases can be wiped with a cotton ball. Wipe the eyes from the inner canthus to the outer canthus using one sponge for each stroke. The inside of the ears can be cleansed with a rolled wisp of cotton. Dampen it and rotate it gently in the ear. To cleanse the baby's scalp, pick up the baby securely by sliding your hand under the baby until the baby's head is well supported in your palm. Hold the baby's head over the basin, soap it, rinse it, and then dry it thoroughly.

The infant's shirt is then removed and the trunk, arms, and legs are washed. The infant will need to be turned to wash the back. Alcohol may be applied at the base of the cord stump before applying the shirt. To put on an open-fronted shirt, lay the baby in the shirt and then reach through the sleeve and grasp the arm to pull it through the sleeve. For pullovers it is important to pull the neck opening rapidly over the baby's head and then pull the arms through the sleeve.

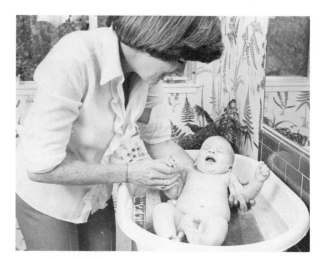

Figure 20-7.   To support an infant in a tub during a bath, the head is supported with the forearm and the infant is held under the axilla.

The buttocks and perineum are finally cleansed. First remove excess feces from the baby with facial tissue or toilet tissue. Cleanse the genital area from front to back. Circumcised areas should not require special care, and the trend is *not* to retract the foreskin of uncircumcised males. The folds between the labia and around the scrotum should receive particular attention and be dried thoroughly. A baby's skin usually does not warrant the need for oil on the perineum. However, if the skin is excessively dry or excoriated, petroleum jelly or mineral oil can offer protection. To apply the diaper see Figure 20-6.

Tub Bath

Infants can be given tub baths when the umbilicus is well healed, usually within the first two weeks of life. In most situations, this can be a pleasurable experience for the baby. Preparation of the environment and of supplies is the same as for the sponge bath. It is important to keep safety pins out of the infant's reach and to have all supplies available. Infants must never be left alone on a bassinette even for a few seconds because they do move and can fall. Before putting the baby in the bath, the face, neck, eyes, and scalp are washed in the manner already described for the infant sponge bath. The baby is then undressed and excess feces wiped away.

The baby must be submerged gradually in the tub and held firmly (see Figure 20-7). The baby is then soaped with the nurse's free hand and rinsed. If the baby appears to be enjoying the experience, the bath can be offered in a leisurly manner. When the baby is removed from the tub, he or she should be wrapped completely in a towel and gently patted dry. Special attention is given to drying body creases. The baby is then dressed.

The Back Rub

The back rub is a massage of the back with two chief objectives: to relax and relieve tension (sedative effect) and to stimulate the blood circulation to the tissues and the muscles. In a back rub the friction from the rubbing produces heat at the skin surface. This causes the peripheral blood vessels in the area to dilate, thus increasing the blood supply to the area. Because tissues are under pressure when a patient is in bed and muscles are usually relaxed, stimulation of the circulation is essential so that these tissues obtain the necessary nutrients and oxygen.

There are four different types of techniques that can be used in a back rub:

1. The *effleurage* is a smooth, long stroke, moving the hands up and down the back. The hands are moved lightly down the sides of the back maintaining contact with the skin but are moved firmly up the back. This rub has a relaxing, sedative effect if slow, light pressure is used.

2. In the *tapotement* the little-finger side of each hand is used in a sharp hacking movement on the back. Care must be taken with this type of rub to not hurt the patient. This motion is not advised for debilitated patients or patients who have pathologic conditions of the back.

3. The *petrissage* is a large pinch of the skin, subcutaneous tissue, and muscle quickly done. The pinches are taken first up the vertebral column and then over the entire back. The tapotement and the petrissage are primarily stimulating, especially if they are done quickly with firm pressure.

4. The *three-handed effleurage* is a smooth stroking motion that gives the patient an impression of three hands. The nurse starts at the base of the patient's neck and moves to the lateral aspect of the shoulder. The other hand then makes the same movement to the other shoulder before the first hand is removed from shoulder to return to the base of the neck. This rub is particularly effective in relieving tension of the neck muscles.

A number of preparations can be used for back rubs. Alcohol preparations are cooling. They are refreshing, and they toughen skin by hardening the skin protein. However, they tend to dry the skin, and very dry skin is likely to crack. Alcohol preparations are particularly undesirable for use on elderly patients, whose skin is usually dry. Patients who are dehydrated and poorly nourished may also find an alcohol backrub disadvantageous because of the drying effects. Emollient creams and lotions are frequently used. These have a lubricating effect upon the skin.

For a patient to receive a back rub the position of choice is the prone position (lying on the stomach). The second preferred position is the side-lying position. The disadvantage of this position is the difficulty of massaging the lateral aspect of the hip on which the patient is lying. This necessitates turning the patient to the other side.

In addition to the rubs just described, circular motions on bony prominences will increase circulation to these areas.

Other pressure points on the body that generally benefit from massage and the application of lotions are the elbows, knees, and heels. Sometimes massage of the anterior aspects of both ilia (iliac crests) of very thin patients is also indicated.

During the back rub nurses need to observe any reddened areas that do not disappear after a few minutes of massage, any breaks in the skin, and any bruising. They should be reported and recorded. Often these conditions predispose to the occurrence of decubitus ulcers. (See "Prevention of Decubiti," later this chapter).

Nurses are advised not to rub tender reddened areas on the lower legs of patients, in particular the calf of the leg. Redness, tenderness, and heat, particularly along the course of a vein, may indicate a thrombus (blood clot) formation in the area. Any massage might dislodge the clot, which could travel to the heart or the lung, causing myocardial or pulmonary emboli. This can present a very serious problem for a patient.

Procedure 20-2. Back Rub Technique

ACTION	EXPLANATION
Assemble Equipment	
1. Back rub solution.	Alcohol is refreshing. Creams and lotions are moistening for dry skin.
Back Rub (For an Adult)	
1. Explain to the patient what you plan to do. Adjust the explanation to the patient's needs.	To reassure the patient by knowledge of what will happen. To identify the patient.
2. Provide privacy.	
3. Wash hands.	Use warm water to warm the hands if they are cold.
4. Warm lotion if the back feels cold.	
5. Assist the patient to the prone or side-lying position.	
6. Fold down top bed clothes to the middle area of the patient's buttocks. Expose the back by separating the gown.	To expose the shoulder areas to the sacral area.
7. With lotion on hands, rub in a circular motion over the sacrum (see Figure 20-8).	To stimulate blood circulation.
8. Move hands up the center of the back and laterally over both scapulae.	
9. Massage in a circular motion over the scapula.	
10. Move hands down the back on the lateral aspects.	

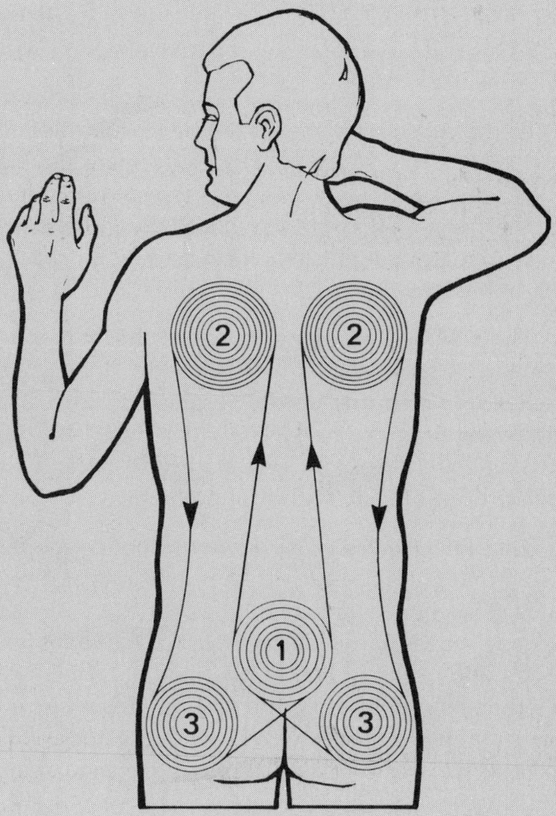

Figure 20-8. Standard back rub technique. 1, Start with circular motion over the sacrum; 2, move both hands up the medial area of the back and provide circular motion over the two scapula; 3, move hands down the lateral aspects of the back and massage the areas over the right and left iliac crests.

11. Repeat for 3 to 5 minutes.

12. Provide extra massage to reddened areas.

13. Observe for abrasions.

14. Assist the patient to a comfortable position.

15. Put away back rub solution.

16. Wash hands.

17. Record any redness, abrasions, or bruises.   These could predispose to decubitus ulcers.

PERINEAL AND GENITAL CARE

Perineal care is an embarrassing procedure for most patients. Nurses also may find it an embarrassment initially, particularly if the patient is of the opposite sex. Most patients who require a bed bath from the nurse are able to cleanse their genital areas with minimal assistance. The nurse may need to hand the moistened washcloth and soap to the patient; rinse the washcloth, and provide a towel. Because many people lack the appropriate terminology for the genitals and genital area, it may be difficult for some nurses to explain to the patient what is expected. Most patients can understand what is meant if the nurse simply says, "I'll give you a washcloth to finish your bath." Many elderly patients are familiar with the term *private parts*. Whatever expression the nurse chooses to use, it should be one that the patient understands and one that is comfortable for the nurse to use.

For Females

When providing perineal care for female patients the nurse places a towel under the patient's hips parallel to the legs and positions the patient with the knees flexed and spread well apart. One end of the towel is used to dry the anterior perineum and the other the posterior perineum. Appropriate draping of the legs with a bath blanket is done to avoid undue exposure. When cleansing the perineum, first wash the area between thighs and the labia. This can be done with a washcloth. The area should be well rinsed and dried. Then the labia are spread, and the folds between the labia major and labia minora are well cleansed. This part can be cleansed with disposable cotton balls or with separate corners of the washcloth, wiping in the direction from the pubis to the rectal area. For menstruating women it is advisable to use cotton balls or gauze. For patients with indwelling catheters it is particularly important to observe the state of the skin around the urethra and to see that the area is dry and clean. Incidents of bladder infection have occurred when perineal care has been neglected for patients with catheters because of the large numbers of microorganisms that grow in this moist, dark area. Some nurses at this point place the patient on the bedpan and rinse the perineum well with a pitcher of warm water. This action ensures the removal of the soap. To cleanse between the buttocks the patient is helped to turn on her side and the area well cleansed, paying particular attention to the anal region. Prior to washing it is important to clean the area with toilet tissue as much as possible if it is soiled. It is poor technique to use a soiled washcloth to cleanse the patient. After drying the area, powder can be applied sparingly. If the skin appears excoriated, zinc oxide or petroleum jelly can offer protection.

For Males

The nurse assists a male patient in the same position as the female for genital care. The penis is washed first with firm strokes. In uncircumcised males the foreskin is retracted and the glans and prepuce washed and dried to prevent the accumulation of

459

smegma. Smegma that accumulates not only causes an offensive odor but facilitates bacterial growth. The outside of the foreskin, scrotum, and medial thighs are washed and dried well. The buttocks are cleansed in the same manner as the female's with the patient lying on his side. In most agencies perineal care is given by male nurses or orderlies; however, in settings where the number of males is limited, the female nurse is responsible for providing this care. Because of the sensitivity of the penis to manipulation there is always the possibility that the patient may have an erection during this procedure. It is recommended that this possibility and ways of dealing with it be discussed beforehand by nursing students.

Some suggestions are to leave the room for a short period and return later to complete the bath, to ignore the erection and complete the bath, or to cleanse the scrotum prior to the penis although the former may be more soiled (Gibbs 1969:125).

The question frequently arises as to whether the nurse should wear gloves when giving perineal care. Those who oppose their use say gloves suggest to the patient that he is dirty and distasteful. Those who wear gloves suggest that bacteriologically the area becomes more soiled without gloves. Each nurse will need to judge which method to employ according to the individual patient. The important point is that perineal care is provided.

COMMON PROBLEMS OF THE SKIN

Nurses will frequently observe common problems of the skin. Some of these problems need to be brought to a physician's attention; others require minimal care, and others will eventually disappear.

In the infant, *milia*, also referred to as *prickly heat rash*, appear as small red irritated lesions due to excess heat. Usually if the baby is kept cooler, often with fewer clothes, they disappear. *Xanthomas* are small yellow fat plaques that can often be identified across the nose of a newborn baby; sometimes they are called milk spots. They will normally disappear in a few weeks with no treatment. *Mongolian spots* were referred to earlier. They are bluish discolorations usually seen in dark-skinned babies and are found in the sacral area. They may well disappear as the baby gets older.

Hemangiomas are vascular lesions that are present at birth. There are a number of types, most of which disappear eventually. However, nurses should refer the child to a physician for accurate diagnosis of the type and treatment if it is indicated. In observing a hemangioma the size, shape, exact color such as pink or port wine color, and whether it is flat or raised from the skin need to be noted and recorded.

Diaper rash is also referred to as *ammonia dermatitis*, since it is caused by skin bacteria reacting with urea, a product related to ammonia and excreted in the urine. This is irritating to the perineum and buttocks, causing them to appear red and sore. In most situations diaper rash can be prevented by keeping the buttocks clean and dry. Protective ointments such as baby oil or petroleum jelly (Vaseline) may be preventive but are not usually needed. Pastes that are difficult to remove should always be avoided. A good treatment for diaper rash is to expose the baby's buttocks to the air and to a 40-watt gooseneck lamp placed a foot away. This can be done several times a day for about a half hour. The lamp provides a drying effect as well as warmth for the baby. Boiling the diapers is helpful to remove the bacteria; however, most detergents now have antibacterial agents in them. Efficient rinsing is a must to remove the detergent.

Erythema or redness is associated with a variety of rashes, infections, and drug reactions. *Petechiae* are tiny pinpoint red areas in the skin, and *ecchymoses* are collections of blood beneath the skin, commonly known as *bruises*. They appear initially as bluish purple, firm, and tender and become yellowish and soften as the blood is absorbed.

Acne is a common problem in adolescence. A number of factors are involved in the development of acne. Some of these are hormone levels, diet, secondary bacterial infection, exercise, nervous tension, and fatigue. The hair follicle becomes obstructed, causing the sebum to accumulate in the follicle and a comedo (blackhead) to form. The sebaceous gland is eventually destroyed, releasing fatty acids into the surrounding tissues, causing an inflammation and the acne nodule. There are a wide variety of theories as to the best treatment for acne. Cleanliness of the skin is important in all treatments in order to prevent secondary infection.

DECUBITUS ULCERS

Decubitus ulcers are also referred to as *pressure sores, bed sores,* or *decubiti.* They are ulcerations of the skin and progressively of the underlying tissue. They are chiefly due to the deprivation of nutrition to the area because of pressure that occludes the blood supply to the tissues. Decubitus ulcers are frequently seen in the elderly who have difficulty moving in bed.

A number of conditions predispose to the development of decubitus ulcers, although pressure is considered to be a primary cause. Some of the predisposing factors are moisture, a break in the skin surface, poor nutrition, impaired circulation to the area, thinness resulting from little subcutaneous tissue and adipose tissue to pad bony prominences, lack of sensation in the area so that the patient cannot feel the tingling and so-called pins and needles of pressure, and the presence of pathogenic microorganisms (see Figure 20-9).

Prevention of Decubiti

There are a number of measures, which, if employed, can prevent the occurrence of decubitus ulcers. These are as follows:

1. Change the patient's position every 2 hours so that another body surface bears the weight. Four body surfaces can usually be used: prone, supine, and right and left side-lying positions.

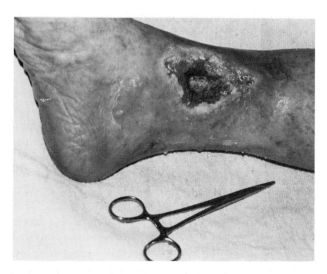

Figure 20-9.   A stasis ulcer of the leg appears similar to a decubitus ulcer. (Courtesy City of Vancouver Health Department.)

2. Encourage joint range of motion exercises to promote circulation (see Chapter 23 for major range of motion exercises).

3. Provide good nutrition for the patient, particularly a diet high in protein.

4. Keep the skin clean and dry, and protect damaged skin. Damaged skin can be further irritated and macerated by urine, feces, sweat, incomplete drying after a bath, soap, and alcohol.

5. Powders on ischemic tissues are preferred to rubbing alcohol and benzoin tincture. Alcohol produces vasoconstriction, thus increasing ischemia, and benzoin tincture can be irritating.

6. Lubricate dry skin areas to prevent cracking. Superfatted soaps and oils act to lubricate skin.

7. Teach patients to be aware of discolored areas or of sensations such as tingling, which can indicate pressure.

8. Provide a smooth, firm, wrinkle-free foundation on which the patient can lie.

9. Provide frequent massage of bony prominences and pressure areas such as the heels, ankles, iliac crests, and sacrum.

10. Use foam rubber pads and sheepskins under pressure areas such as the sacrum and heels.

11. Use special mattresses to decrease pressure on body parts, such as an alternating pressure mattress, eggshell mattress, or flotation mattress. See descriptions in the section on beds in this chapter.

The early symptoms of pressure sores are redness or whiteness of an area, tenderness, an unpleasant sensation frequently described as burning, coldness of the area, and localized edema.

Treatment of Decubiti

Pressure sores are a challenge for nurses to cure. Often they are larger inside than they appear on the outside. In addition to providing preventive measures, the following can also be carried out.:

1. A specimen of the drainage is sent to the laboratory to ascertain the presence of any invading organisms. Subsequent appropriate medications are then provided.

2. A cleansing agent is used on the ulcer, such as hexachlorophene compound, elase ointment, or hydrogen peroxide.

3. Heat is often applied by an electric 100-watt lamp. This is placed from 45–60 cm (18–24 inches) from the ulcer and left in place for 10 minutes. (See Chapter 17, "Application of Dry Heat.")

4. After the ulcer is dry, it can be dusted with cornstarch, and an aeroplast dressing sprayed on. This keeps the ulcer dry and clean, thus promoting healing.

5. Surgical closure may be necessary in some instances.

6. Filling the ulcer cavity with granulated sugar can assist an ulcer to heal (Verhonick 1961:69).

It is wise for nurses to remember that decubitus ulcers are prone to infection. Moist, poorly nourished tissue is a good medium for the growth of pathogenic bacteria. If an ulcer is infected, the techniques of medical asepsis need to be employed in order to prevent spread of the microorganisms.

CARE OF THE FEET

At birth a baby's foot is relatively unformed. The arches are supported by fatty pads and do not take their full shape until 5 or 6 years of age. Feet are not fully grown until about the twentieth year.

During childhood the bony structure of the feet and the small muscles are easily damaged by tight, binding stockings and ill-fitting shoes. In fact, in China, it was customary for a girl baby's feet to be bound in order to limit growth. This practice was outlawed by Chou En-lai in the 1930s. It is important that the arches are supported and that the bony structure and the feet are permitted to grow with no external restrictions.

Common Problems of the Feet

A number of foot problems are commonly observed, which can provide considerable discomfort to people. Among these are calluses, corns, unpleasant odors, plantar warts, fissures between the toes, fungus infections such as athlete's foot, incurvated nails, and paronychia.

A *callus* is a thickened portion of epidermis, a mass of keratotic material. It is flat and usually found on the bottom or the sides of the foot over a bony protuberance. Calluses are usually caused by pressure of the shoes. Calluses can be softened by soaking in warm water with Epsom salts and removed by an abrasive substance such as a pumice stone. Creams with lanolin can also be used to keep the skin soft and prevent the formation of calluses.

A *corn* is a keratosis caused by friction of the shoes and pressure from shoes. It commonly occurs on the toes, usually the fourth and fifth toes, and usu-

ally on a bony prominence such as a joint. Corns are usually conical (circular and raised). The base is the surface of the corn and the apex is in deeper tissues, sometimes even attached to bone. Corns are generally removed surgically and prevented from reforming by relieving the pressure on the area and massaging the tissue to promote circulation.

Unpleasant odors occur as a result of perspiration and its interaction with microorganisms. Regular and frequent washing and wearing clean hosiery will assist to minimize the odor. Foot powders and deodorants will also help prevent this problem.

Plantar warts appear on the sole of the foot. These warts are caused by the virus *papovavirus hominis*. They are moderately contagious. They are frequently painful, often causing the patient to walk with difficulty in order to avoid the pain. The treatment ordered by a physician may be curettage, freezing with the application of solid carbon dioxide several times, or repeated applications of salicylic acid.

Fissures between the toes occur frequently as a result of dryness of the skin and subsequent cracking. The treatment of choice as well as good foot hygiene is the administration of an antiseptic in order to prevent infection. Often a small piece of gauze between the toes will assist in applying the antiseptic and when left in place assists in healing by allowing air to reach the area.

Athlete's foot or tinca pedis (ringworm of the foot) is caused by a fungus. The symptoms are scaling and cracking of the skin, particularly between the toes. Sometimes small blisters form with a thin fluid inside of them. In severe cases the lesions may also appear on other parts of the body, particularly the hands.

Treatment varies from potassium permanganate soaks, 1:8000 solution, to the application of commercial anti-fungal ointments or powders. Preventing such infection is important. Permitting feet to be well ventilated and wearing clean socks or stockings is essential. Avoidance of going barefoot in public showers will help prevent contraction of the infection.

Guidelines to Prevent Foot Problems

Many foot problems can be prevented from occurring by following simple guidelines.

1. Wear correctly fitting shoes that neither restrict the foot nor rub on any area; the latter will prevent corns and calluses.

2. Wash feet regularly and dry them well.

3. For feet that have an unpleasant odor due to excessive perspiration, frequent washing is advised together with changing socks and shoes. Special deodorant sprays are also helpful.

4. Wear only clean stockings and socks.

5. Avoid walking in bare feet in public showers and change areas in order to prevent contracting common infections such as athlete's foot.

6. Avoid excessive drying of the skin of the feet. Use creams or lotions to moisten or soak feet in warm water with Epsom salts. This will soften calluses, which can then be removed with an abrasive such as pumice stone.

PROBLEMS OF NAILS

Incurvated nails are a relatively common condition. The toe nail grows in such a manner that it impinges into the soft tissue. The symptoms are pain on walking and upon pressure on the nail, tenderness, and sometimes redness if an inflammatory process has started in the soft tissues. The treatment usually carried out is to remove that part of the nail which has curved into the tissue and clearing any debris and callus tissue in the area. The nail groove is then packed in such a way that the nail will grow forward rather than into the soft tissue. Any secondary infection is generally treated with an antibiotic ointment or powder.

Paronychia is an inflammation of the tissue surrounding the nail. Acute paronychia is called *thecal whitlow*; it is a painful red swelling which develops quickly. It usually follows a hangnail or injury. This condition occurs most frequently in people who have their hands in water a great deal, and it is three times more common in patients who have diabetes.

Prevention is stressed by careful manicuring in order not to injure the adjacent soft tissue. If a hangnail develops and is not infected, it can be carefully flattened and held in place with collodion. Often, oil rubbed into the tissue around the nail will lubricate the tissue and prevent the development of hangnails.

CARE OF EYES

The eyes of people are extremely important organs, which require no special care in daily living. The lacrimal glands, situated in a depression in the frontal bone at the upper outer angle of the eye orbit, produce lacrimal fluid, which continually washes the eyes. This fluid empties into the lacrimal sac, which is situated in the inner canthus. From the lacrimal sac the fluid drains through the lacrimal duct to the inferior meatus of the nose. The fluid keeps the eyeball moist and helps wash away foreign particles. Excessive lacrimal fluid forms tears.

A common problem of the eyes are secretions that dry on the lashes as crusts. These may need to be softened and wiped away. In hospitals this is usually done with a sterile cotton ball moistened with water sterile water or normal saline. The nurse wipes from the inner canthus of the eye to the outer canthus, thus preventing the particles and fluid from draining into the nasolacrimal duct. In the home it is usually not necessary for the fluid to be sterile in order to remove crusts from the eyes. The excess fluid is then usually wiped away with a soft tissue.

In newborns the eyes are treated soon after the baby is born to prevent ophthalmia neonatorum (gonorrheal conjunctivitis). Penicillin and silver nitrate are the drugs of treatment. A treatment for this disease is mandatory by law in all states in the United States. The method of instilling the drops and wiping eyes is the same for babies as for children and adults. (See Chapter 36, "Instillation of Eye Drops").

Artificial Eyes

Patients who have artificial eyes usually have their own ways to remove the eye and to cleanse them, the sockets, and surrounding tissues. Nurses should ask patients how they wish to do this and what equipment they require.

If a patient is unconscious or for some reason is unable to do this, the nurse will need to assist. To remove the artificial eye from the socket, the lower lid is pulled down and slight pressure is placed just below the eye. This will usually break the suction, and the eye will come out. The nurse must make sure to catch the eye and not scratch it in any way.

Another method to remove the eye is to place the tip of a small rubber bulb (syringe bulb or medicine dropper bulb) directly on the eye. The bulb is first squeezed to create a suction effect. This suction counteracts the pressure holding the eye in place, causing the eye to come away with the bulb.

Artificial eyes are usually washed with warm normal saline, as is the eye socket and the surrounding tissues. Again, cleansing is done from the inner canthus to the outer canthus.

The eye can be replaced by again pulling the lower lid down and slipping the eye gently into its socket. It should fit neatly under the upper lid.

Eyeglasses

Eyeglasses are worn by people of all ages, from children to the elderly. The most common reasons for glasses are: (a) stabismus, (b) myopia (nearsightedness), (c) hyperopia (farsightedness), (d) presbyopia, (e) astigmatism, and (f) cataract.

Strabismus or so-called crossed eyes is seen chiefly in children. The muscles of the two eyes are not coordinated, and thus the child will have one eye directed ahead while the other eye perhaps is directed toward the nose at the same time. Eyeglasses are sometimes worn to correct a strabismus, and surgery is also done in some cases on the eye muscles.

Myopia or nearsightedness occurs when the image of a distant object comes to focus in front of the retina. It can be caused by an abnormally long distance between the cornea of the eye and the lens or the lens and the retina. By employing a concave lens in eyeglasses, the image is brought to focus further back on the retina of the eye. This person needs glasses to see objects at a distance.

Hyperopia or farsightedness occurs when the image of a distant object comes to focus behind the retina. A convex lens is used to bring the object to focus in a more forward position, that is, on the retina. This person needs glasses for close work such as reading.

Presbyopia or oldsightedness occurs with increasing age. The lens loses its elasticity so that it cannot accommodate for close vision or distant vision. This person usually needs glasses for both close and distant vision.

Astigmatism is a defect in the curvature of the cornea of the eye or the lens. As a result there is distortion in the perception of an object. A cylindrical lens placed in the appropriate axial position is used to correct this.

Cataract is opacity of the lens. It occurs frequently in people over the age of 65 years and is corrected in many people by surgery.

Care of Eyeglasses

Most eyeglasses manufactured today are impact resistant. That is, with a forceful blow they will not fragment as glasses did in years past. Plastic is also being used in eyeglasses today. It is a safe material; however, it does have the disadvantage of scratching easily.

Most patients have their own way of washing their glasses and drying them. If nurses are required to clean glasses, this can be done with warm water, then they can be wiped dry with a soft tissue. If the patient has plastic lenses, the use of soft tissue may be contraindicated, and a special cloth or soft paper is used to wipe off the water.

Contact Lenses

A contact lens is a small oval disk that fits directly on the eye. It may be a hard or soft lens. Most people have special small containers for their contact lenses when they are not wearing them. Contact lenses have several advantages over eyeglasses for some people. First, they cannot be seen, thus having a cosmetic value. Second, they can be highly effective in correcting some types of astigmatism when there is a problem in the curvature of the cornea. Third, they can be

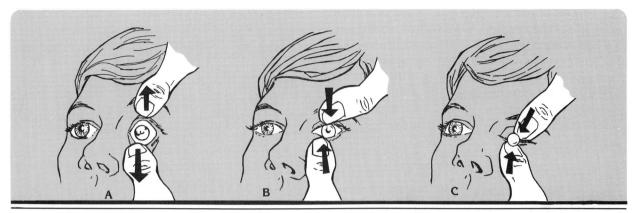

Figure 20-10.   To remove a hard contact lens for a patient **A**, spread the eyelids apart, **B**, bring eyelids to the edge of the lens, and **C**, press the lower lid margin more firmly under the contact lens to tip the lens. By moving both lids closer together, the lens slide off the eye and out.

safer than eyeglasses in activities such as sports and physically active jobs.

Contact lenses should not be worn continually without removal because of irritation to the eyes. They are normally worn for a maximum of 12–15 hours daily and removed when sleeping, swimming, and in very smoky environments. If a patient cannot remove his or her own contact lenses, the nurse assumes this responsibility to prevent resulting damage to the eyes.

Removal of Contact Lenses

Contact lenses are normally worn directly over the cornea of the eye. In order to remove a hard lens for the patient who is unable, the upper and lower eyelids are separated, one with each thumb, until they are beyond the edges of the lens. Pressure is exerted toward the bony orbit above and below the eye, not directly on the eye. The lower eyelid margin is then gently moved up toward the lens, and the upper eyelid margin is moved down to the lens edge. The lower lid margin is then pressed more firmly under the contact lens while the top is held stationary. The lens will tip with this pressure and lift out on the bottom edge. Then by moving both eyelids toward each other the lens will slide off the eye and out. If a lens is misplaced from the cornea, it should be moved back into the proper place prior to removal. This can be done with gentle pressure on the eyelid, moving in the direction indicated (See Figure 20-10).

To remove a soft contact lens ask the patient to look upwards. Retract the lower lid with the middle finger and place the tip of the index finger on the lower edge of the lens. Slide the lens down to the

inferior aspect of the eye. Compress the lens slightly between the thumb and index finger. Rolling the thumb and index finger together causes the lens to double up and air to enter underneath the lens. The lens can be removed from the eye.

Application of Contact Lenses

Lenses are stored in specially designed containers that are dry or contain a solution. Each lens slot is labeled, one for the right eye and one for the left eye. It is essential that the correct lens be applied to the

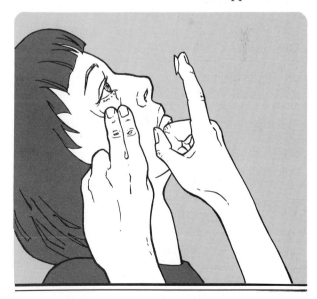

Figure 20-11.   To insert hard contact lens ask patient to look upwards, then separate both lids and with the lens on the tip of the index finger of other hand place it directly over the cornea.

correct eye, since individual lenses are ground to fit the appropriate eye. Prior to inserting a contact lens, the lens should be cleansed with a sterile nonirritating solution. Wetting agents are then applied to the lens prior to insertion. The use of saliva as a wetting agent should be discouraged, since it harbors many pathogens. To insert the contact lens, it is placed directly over the cornea by placing it on the tip of your index finger and separating the eyelids sufficiently to expose the area (see Figure 20-11). This is best done by having patients either lie on their back or bend their head backward. Soft lenses can be inserted by flexing the lens between the thumb and index finger. The edge should be erect and pointing slightly inward for the lens to be in the correct position for application (see Figure 20-12).

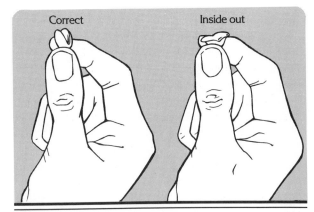

Figure 20-12. Before inserting soft contact lens, cup the lens with thumb and index finger. It is in correct position when edge is erect and pointing inwards.

CARE OF THE NOSE AND EARS

The nose and the ears require minimal care in normal hygiene. For babies and small children a small piece of absorbent cotton moistened with warm water and then twisted between the fingers can be used to cleanse the nostrils and the external ear canals. It is inserted, then rotated inside the body orifice to catch any foreign materials. Neither sticks nor bobby pins should be used because of the danger of abrading the

mucous membrane or, in the case of the ears, puncturing the eardrum.

A common problem of the ears is the collection of cerumen or ear wax in the external auditory canal. This may cause a person some difficulty hearing, and it can cause discomfort when it hardens. The treatment for this is to syringe the ears, and this is generally carried out by a physician.

CARE OF THE HAIR

Relative to hygiene there are three aspects to the care of hair: daily care by brushing and combing, shampooing the hair in order to maintain its cleanliness, and the treatment of hair for infestations such as lice.

matting, it should be combed at least daily. In some instances patients are pleased to have it tied neatly in the back or braided until other assistance is available or until they feel better and can look after it themselves.

Brushing and Combing Hair

Hair needs to be brushed daily in order to be healthy. Brushing has three major functions: it stimulates the circulation of blood in the scalp, it distributes the oil along the hair shaft, and it helps to arrange the hair for the patient, although most people use a comb for this purpose.

Long hair may present a problem to patients when they are unable to obtain the assistance of a hairdresser for a prolonged period. To prevent it from

Shampooing

The cleanliness and grooming of both men's and women's hair is frequently related closely to their sense of well-being. Often after patients have been ill and then begin to feel better, having their hair done is a boost to morale and feelings about their appearance.

The frequency with which a person needs to shampoo is highly individualistic, depending to a large degree upon their activity and the amount of sebum secreted by the scalp. Oily hair tends to appear as stringy, dirty hair and to feel dirty to the person. There are a wide variety of shampoos available on the commercial market, and most patients have their own favorite brands. If a person's hair tends to tangle after it is washed, a cream rinse can be used after the shampoo to prevent this.

A patient who is unable to sit up at a sink for a shampoo may be able to lie on a stretcher with the head at the edge of a water basin. When a nurse assists a patient with a shampoo, it is most important that all the shampoo solution is rinsed from the hair. This is particularly important for dandruff shampoos, which, if they remain in the hair, may damage the hair and irritate the scalp.

A Black Person's Hair

To the white nurse the hair of a black person can present a special challenge. The following are guidelines to the care of a black person's hair.

1. A black person's hair is shampooed just as a white person's hair.

2. Before the hair is dry it needs to be combed to avoid tangling. A wide-toothed comb is best used because of the thickness of the hair. A stiff-bristled brush is also helpful.

3. Often the hair will appear dry. The application of small amounts of mineral oil or petroleum jelly will help lubricate it.

4. For styling, the hair may be rolled on regular curlers or braided in order to prevent matting and tangling (Giles 1972:86–87).

Care of Infestations

Ticks

Ticks take many forms and can adapt themselves to various conditions. The genera *Ornithodoros* and *Dermacentor* are found in North America. They can be attached to human beings and are found frequently in the hair. They can be as large as one-half inch and appear as gray-brown. They attach to a person with the apparatus by which they suck blood. They should not be torn off a person, because the sucking apparatus is left in the skin and becomes infected. If oil is poured on the tick, it loses its hold because it is deprived of oxygen, and it withdraws its sucker.

Ticks transmit several diseases to people, in particular, Rocky Mountain spotted fever and tularemia.

Lice

There are hundreds of varieties of lice that are parasitic to humans. Three types that are particularly common are (a) *Pediculosis capitis,* also called *head lice* or *scabies,* (b) *Pediculosis corporis* or body lice, and (c) *Pediculosis pubis* or crab lice.

Pediculosis capitis is found on the scalp of a person and tends to stay hidden by the hairs as does *pediculosis pubis,* which stays in pubic hair. *Pediculosis corporis* tends to cling to clothing; the lice suck blood from the person and lay their eggs on the clothing. Thus when a patient undresses, the body lice may not be in evidence on the body. However, the nurse will be able to suspect their presence in the clothing by three chief symptoms: (a) the person will habitually scratch, (b) there will be scratches on the skin, and (c) there will be hemorrhagic spots on the skin where the lice have sucked blood.

Head and pubic lice lay their eggs on the hairs; they look like oval particles, like dandruff clinging to the hair. Bites and pustular eruptions may also be noticed at the hair lines and behind the ears.

Lice are very small, grayish white, and difficult to see. The crab louse in the pubic area has red legs. Lice may be contracted from cloak rooms and through direct contact with an infested person.

The treatment now used in most areas is with gamma benzene hexachloride (Kwell). It comes as a cream, a lotion, and a shampoo. For head lice the hair is washed with the shampoo and the bed linen is changed. This treatment may be repeated again from 12 to 24 hours after the first if it is needed. For pubic and body lice, the patient has a bath or shower and after drying applies the lotion or cream to the entire body surface for body lice and to the pubic area and adjacent areas for pubic lice. The lotion is left on 12 to 24 hours, then washed off, and clean clothing and linen is supplied.

Common Problems of the Hair

Problems related to hair with which nurses commonly come in contact are dandruff of the scalp and hirsutism. The latter is the excessive growth of body hair with specific reference to women.

Dandruff appears as a diffuse scaling of the scalp often accompanied by itching. In severe cases it involves the auditory canals and the eyebrows. Mild cases of dandruff can usually be effectively treated with one of the commercial shampoo agents specifically recommended for dandruff. In severe or persistent cases the patient may need the advice of a physician.

Hirsutism is the growth of excessive body hair. The acceptance of body hair in the axilla and on the legs is largely dictated by culture. In North America the well-groomed woman as depicted in magazines has no hair on her legs or under her axillae. This idea is changing. Also, in many European cultures it is not customary to remove this hair in order to be considered well groomed.

However, excessive facial hair on a woman is thought to be unattractive in most Western and Oriental cultures. For example, some Japanese brides follow the custom of shaving their faces the day before the wedding.

The cause of excessive body hair is not always known. Elderly women may have some on their faces, and women during the menopause may also experience facial hair. The causes of these conditions may well involve the endocrine system. It is also thought that a heredity factor may influence the pattern of hair distribution as well as the production of androgens by the adrenal glands.

There are a number of ways of removing hair: waxing, pulling with tweezers, shaving with a razor,

lotions, and electrolysis. In the waxing process, warm wax is poured on the area with hair and allowed to harden. The hairs become embedded in the wax and come away from the skin when the wax is removed. Tweezers are commonly used to remove excess hair from the eyebrows and the face. It can be a time-consuming project if there is a great deal of hair, and it needs to be repeated when the hair grows back, often in 2 to 3 weeks. Shaving with a razor is used frequently for leg and axilla hair. It is an inexpensive and effective method, but it must be repeatedly carried out.

Depilatory creams and lotions are used also for excessive hair. Through a chemical action the hair shaft is destroyed so that the hair comes away easily. This method of hair removal is relatively expensive compared to shaving. Care needs to be taken in the initial use of a product in order to assess the amount of irritation it can cause the skin. People need to be advised to put it on a small area initially and observe for any signs of irritation.

Electrolysis is the only permanent way of removing hair. By means of an electric current the hair follicle is destroyed. Usually, repeated treatments on a follicle are needed before it is completely destroyed. This method of treatment is relatively expensive.

BEDS

Ill persons are frequently confined to a bed, sometimes for weeks or months. A bed then becomes an important piece of furniture, and the patient's ability to rest and sleep are often directly related to it.

There are a number of different types of beds, and patients who are ill at home may find their own beds quite satisfactory as long as the periods of illness are not long. A hospital bed has certain characteristics that are particularly suited to people who are in bed continuously or for a long time. Some of the chief characteristics are as follows:

1.   It is adapted to save a patient energy. Many hospital beds are motorized so that by pushing a button the patient can raise or lower the head or the foot.

2.   It is adapted to so that a nurse can easily reach a patient in bed. Most hospital beds are 66 cm (26 inches) from the floor or can be raised to that level by a motor or lever. A nurse then does not need to bend

over as is necessary for most beds in the home. It is 0.9 meters wide and 1.8 meters long (3 ft wide and 6.5 ft long). Thus the hospital bed is narrower than a normal bed.

3.   The mattress is generally firm to permit good body support. Special mattresses are also available, including sponge rubber, alternating pressure, eggshell, and water mattresses. Hospital mattresses are generally covered with a water repellent material so that they do not soil readily.

4.   A rubber or plastic drawsheet can be used over the middle area of the bed in order to protect the mattress and bottom bed sheet from drainages.

5.   Linen is generally long and wide enough so that the bed will stay in a comfortable, neat condition for a period of time.

6.   Linen and blankets are of a durable quality in order to withstand many washings.

7. Hospital beds are easily moved. Each leg has a caster, usually made of hard rubber. These casters turn easily, making it possible to move the bed readily without jarring the patient.

Hospital beds can be adjusted to a number of positions. The most common are the following:

1. For the *Fowler's and semi-Fowler's positions*, see Chapter 22, "Bed Positions for Patients."

2. In the *Trendelenberg position* the head of the bed is lowered, the foot of the bed is elevated, and the mattress remains unbent. Sometimes this position is provided by placing the blocks, often referred to as *shock blocks,* under the legs at the foot of the bed (see Figure 20-13, *A*). This position is contraindicated in shock, head injury, chest injury, and respiratory problems.

3. The *reverse Trendelenberg position* is the opposite of the Trendelenberg position. The head section is elevated, and the foot is lowered. In this case the legs at the head of the bed may be placed on blocks (see Figure 20-13, *B*).

4. Another position in which a hospital bed can be placed is the *contour position.* The head and foot sections of the mattress are lowered, permitting a break of about 15° (see Figure 20-13, *C*).

Hospital beds usually have a bedside table and an overbed table for the patient's use. A bedside table will have a drawer and a cupboard. The drawer is used for the patient's personal possessions. The cupboard usually contains a wash basin and kidney basin. There is usually a rod situated on the back of the table for the patient's towels and washcloths. The overbed table is, as its name states, a table that fits over the bed. It will permit a patient to sit in bed and eat from the table in relative comfort. Most overbed tables can be raised or lowered, whichever the patient needs.

There are also one or two chairs as part of the hospital bed unit together with a closet or locker, lights, and a signal light at each bed. When the switch is pulled or the button is pressed, the signal turns on a light outside the patient's room and in other places on the hospital unit, for example, the nursing office, to indicate to the nursing staff that a patient requires assistance.

Nurses need to be able to make hospital beds in different ways in order to suit specific purposes. For example, it is necessary in many instances to make a bed while the patient remains in it (occupied bed), or to make a bed for a patient who is having surgery (anaesthetic bed). Although in most instances nurses will delegate bed making to other personnel, a nurse

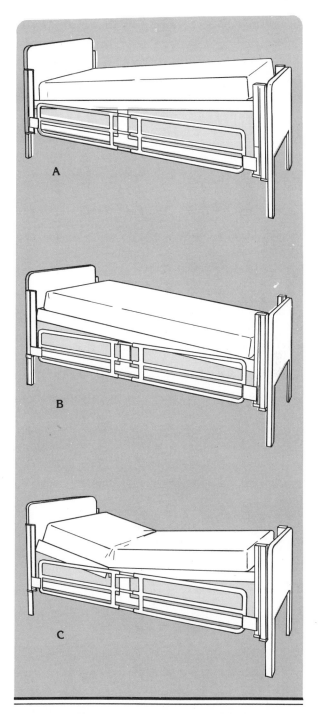

Figure 20-13.   Bed positions. **A,** Trendelenberg position; **B,** reverse Trendelenberg; and **C,** contour position.

should know how to make beds quickly and expediently in order to disturb a patient as little as possible.

Hospital beds are either open or closed. An *open* bed is one currently being used by a patient; generally the top covers are folded back to make it easier to get in. A *closed* bed has the top covers under the pillows; it is generally not being used.

'

Procedure 20-3.   Making an Unoccupied Bed (Open or Closed)

ACTION	EXPLANATION
Assemble Equipment	
Wash hands. Obtain linen required; for a complete change this includes:	
1. Mattress pad	
2. 2 large sheets	
3. 1 cloth drawsheet	
4. 1 plastic or rubber drawsheet	
5. 1 blanket	
6. 1 bedspread	
7. 2 pillow cases	Obtain additional cases if extra pillows are used
8. 1 bath towel	For patient's use
9. 2 wash cloths	For patient's use
10. 1 hospital gown or pajamas	If required
11. linen hamper	For soiled linen
To Strip the Bed	
1. Place fresh linen on the bedside chair, not on another patient's bed.	This prevents cross contamination (movement of microorganisms on the linen).
2. Screen the bed if it is in a room with other patients.	To decrease the spread of microorganisms when moving the linen.
3. Raise bed to its highest level.	This is a working height at which the nurse will not need to bend to reach, reducing or preventing back strain.
4. Moving from the head of the bed on the side on which you are working, loosen the foundation of the bed around to the head of the bed on the other side.	
5. Starting at the head of the bed, remove the linen and deposit it in linen hamper.	Place any linen to be reused over the bedside chair.
To Make a Bed	
1. Move the mattress up to the head of the bed before making the foundation.	Mattresses move toward the bottom of the bed when the bed is in Fowler's position.
2. Moving from the bottom to the top of the bed, put on the bottom sheet.	
3. Tuck in the head of the bed and the side on which you are working.	Extend the bottom sheet just over the bottom end of the mattress; do not miter the corner, thus the sheet is readily changed without taking off the top covers.
4. Miter the top corners.	See section "Mitering the Corner of a Bed."

5. Place the plastic and cloth drawsheets on the bed; tuck them in on the side on which you are working.

6. Tuck in all bottom linen on the other side of the bed.

Pull linens tightly so that they are free of wrinkles.

7. Returning to the first side, place the top sheet on the bed; tuck it in, making a toe pleat at the bottom. The top of the sheet should be even with the top edge of the mattress.

See Figure 20-14.

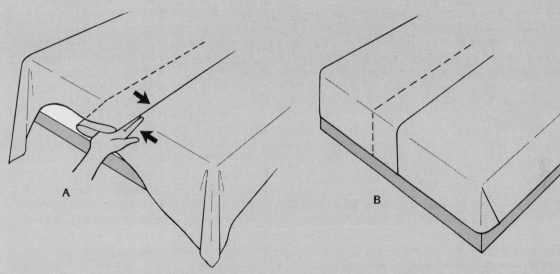

Figure 20-14. A vertical toe pleat is made by making a 2 inch fold in the sheet, **A**, and blankets perpendicular to the foot of the bed before the end is tucked in, **B**.

8. Place the blankets and spread on the bed.

A toe pleat may be indicated for the blankets and spread.

9. Fold the spread under the top blanket, and fold the top sheet over the spread at least 14 cm (6 inches).

The blanket will not come in contact with the patient's face and irritate it.

10. Put clean pillow cases on the pillows.

If there is a soft and a firm pillow, place the soft pillow on top for comfort.

11. Attach the signal light and reading light to the bed.

They should be within easy reach of the patient.

12. Place clean towels and the patient's gown in an appropriate place.

If the unit is unoccupied, place them in the bedside table drawer. If the unit is occupied, give the gown to the patient to put on and put the towels on the rack.

13. Place dirty linen in linen disposal bag, not on the floor or another patient's bed.

Hold linen away from your uniform to limit contamination. Do not wave linen in the air, to prevent airborne spread of contaminants.

14. Remove any other excess equipment no longer used.

For example, dishes usually go to the kitchen.

15. Wash hands.

In order not to spread microorganisms to another patient.

Mitering the Corner of a Bed

1. Tuck the sheet in firmly under the mattress at either the top or the bottom of the bed.

2. Lift the sheet at point A (see Figure 20-15) and bring it to a position along the upper edge of the mattress.

3. Then grasp the sheet at point B and bring it up onto the surface of the bed.

4. Tuck in under the mattress the part of the sheet that is hanging down below the mattress.

5. Bring point B down and tuck it under the mattress. One hand can hold the underfolded sheet (C) so that it remains even with the upper edge of the mattress.

Fitted sheets are being used increasingly, and with these, corners are not necessary.

Making an Occupied Bed

When making an occupied bed, it is important that the nurse works quickly, disturbs the patient as little as possible, and assists the patient to keep body alignment and comfort. It is easier to make a bed when it is flat; however, this may not always be possible if the patient needs to maintain another position. For example, a patient who is having difficulty breathing may not tolerate a supine position. In this instance the bed must be made with the head elevated because of the patient's safety and comfort.

To make an occupied bed the following steps describe one widely used method: Loosen the top covers at the foot of the bed. Remove the top bedding with the exception of the sheet. Fold the top edge to the bottom edge and then across the bed in quarters. Put the bath blanket over the top sheet and, with the patient holding it or after tucking it under the shoulders, remove the sheet by pulling it out from under the bath blanket. Soiled linen can be placed on the seat of the chair or in the linen hamper. Bath blankets provide warmth needed by most patients.

Move the mattress up to the top of the bed. Some patients can assist by grasping the head of the bed and pulling themselves up. If the patient is unable to help, then a second person is usually needed to assist by grasping the lugs of the mattress on the other side of the bed, and both people slide the mattress upward. A nurse might be able to do this alone by going from one side to another, sliding the mattress a little each time. It is usually not possible for one person to move a mattress under a heavy, helpless patient. As-

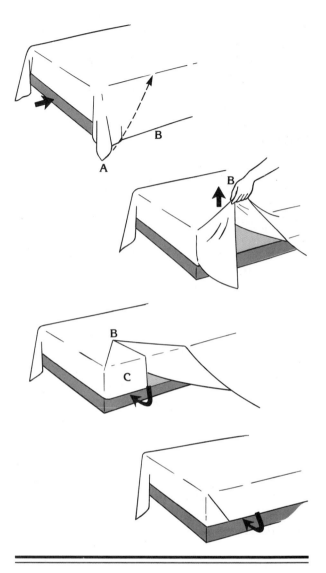

Figure 20-15.   To miter a corner of the foot of a bed, **A**, tuck in bottom of bed; **B**, lift point and bring to position along upper edge; **C**, grasp lower edge where the sheet folds and release point; **D**, fold sheet under at the side; and **E**, bring point down and tuck under. The underfold should be even with the edge of the mattress.

sist the patient to the far side of the bed. A side-lying position is considered best in that it frees a considerable portion of the bed.

Loosen the foundation of the bed on the near side and near half at the head of the bed. Fold the linen at the center of the bed against the patient's back. Place the clean linen on the bed with the excess for the other half of the bed fan folded in the center. Place the bottom sheet with the bottom edge in line with the end of the mattress and the top tucked under the mattress. There should be about 18–42 cm (12–18 inches) of sheet under the top of the mattress in order to keep the sheet secure when the head of the bed is elevated. Miter the top corner and tuck in the side of the bottom sheet. Tuck in the plastic drawsheet and the linen drawsheet under the mattress. Have the patient turn to the clean side of the bed. Complete the far side as the first side. Pull the sheets tightly to make them wrinkle free.

Place the top sheet on the bed and remove the bath blanket. Place the blankets and spread on the top of the bed and miter the bottom corners. A toe pleat is usually put in the top bed clothes. Lift the sheet and blankets and make a 5 cm (2-inch) fold perpendicular to the foot of the bottom edge before tucking them in. The top sheet should be able to fold at least 14 cm (6 inches) over the blankets and spread at the head of the bed.

Put clean pillow cases on the pillows. If there is a soft and firm pillow, the soft pillow should be on top of the firm pillow. Complete making the bed as for an unoccupied bed. Assist the patient to a comfortable position.

A Crib for an Infant or Child

Cribs are made in a similar fashion to a bed. The major differences are that no drawsheets are used because most crib mattresses have plastic covers, and the crib sides are always in the up position when the nurse is not actually working at that side.

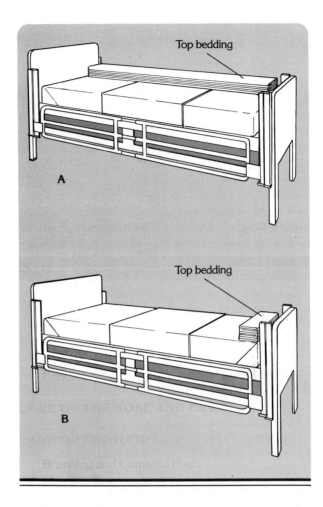

Figure 20-16.   Two types of surgical beds. **A,** Top bed clothes are folded to the side, and **B,** top bed clothes are folded to the foot of the bed.

Surgical Bed (Recovery, Anesthetic, or Operative Bed)

A surgical bed is made specifically for a patient who has had an operation or, in some hospitals, for any patient who has received an anesthetic, for example, during a bronchoscopy. The objectives of this type of bed are as follows:

1. To provide as clean an environment as possible, usually for an operative patient.
2. To provide a bed into which a patient can easily move or be transferred.
3. To provide a bed that can be readily changed with minimal disturbance to the patient if it becomes soiled, for example, with vomitus.

These beds are made in various ways in different settings. Generally the following practices are used in most places:

1. All clean linen is used for the bed.
2. The foundation of the bed is made as for other beds.
3. A plastic sheet and an additional linen drawsheet may be put on the top of the bed where pillows are usually placed. In some places a disposable pad is used.
4. The top covers are not tucked under the mattress. They are generally folded up on the sides and the end, making a 14 cm (6-inch) cuff, and fan folded lengthwise either to the side of the bed or to the center. They may also be fan folded widthwise to the bottom of the bed (see Figure 20-16).
5. Pillows are usually placed on the bedside chair.
6. The bed is left in a high position to meet the level of the stretcher and facilitate transference of the patient.

Special Beds

There are a number of special beds, which are designed to meet the specific needs of some patients. The *water bed* or flotation bed has already been mentioned in the care of decubitus ulcers. This bed has a mattress that is really a plastic bag filled with water. The principle behind the use of this type of bed is that of displacement. The body loses the amount of weight of the liquid displaced; therefore the body weight is lightened, and there is less pressure upon weight-bearing areas (Pfaudler, 1968:2352). A similar bed is the alternating pressure bed or the *air bed*. In this the mattress is filled with air, and as the patient moves the pressure changes on the different body areas.

A *Stryker frame* or Foster frame is another specialized bed. It is used for patients who are unable to move, for example, as a result of fractured vertebral column. The patient lies on a series of canvas pieces attached to a metal frame. When the patient needs to turn, a similar frame is placed on top of him or her and attached to the lower frame. Then the frame is unlocked and turned so that the patient's position is reversed. The upper frame over the patient is then removed.

Another type of bed is fastened to a circular frame. It functions electrically and can be operated by the patient. One of its major advantages is that it permits a patient to assume a standing position without exertion (see Figure 20-17).

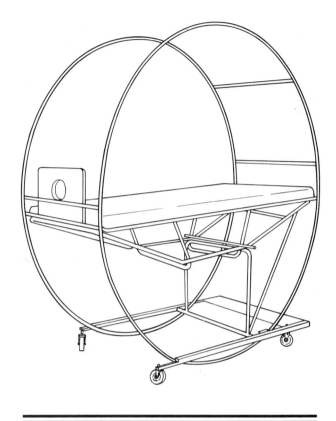

Figure 20-17.   An electric circular bed permits a patient to assume a variety of positions such as prone, vertical, and supine.

SUMMARY

The total picture of hygiene includes mental, sexual, social, oral, and personal aspects. Hygiene practices are influenced to a large degree by family influences. When people become ill, hygienic practices often assume a secondary role to other vital body needs such as rest or breathing. In such instances the nurse then assumes responsibility for the hygienic care of patients.

A review of the physiology of the integument includes the four major purposes of the skin and mucous membranes. The appearance of the normal integument is emphasized as a baseline for assessment purposes, but the developmental differences outlined in the chapter must also be considered. Aspects of the apocrine glands, the hair, nails, and teeth are included that are applicable to hygiene and the maintenance of health. Seven principles related to the care of the skin and mucous membrane serve as a guide for the nurse when providing or assisting with the hygienic care of patients.

Good oral hygiene includes daily dental flossing, mechanical scrubbing of the teeth, and flushing of the mouth four times a day. Dental checkups are recommended every 6 months starting at 2 ½ to 3 years of age. Fluoride supplements are recommended as an alternative to fluoridated water from 1 month to 14 years. Hospitalized patients often require assistance from the nurse to maintain oral hygiene. Various techniques are described, which include the positioning of the unconscious patient, the care of dentures, and the use of commercially prepared cleansing applications. Halitosis and sordes require special mouth-care measures. The common oral problems are dental caries, periodontal disease, glossitis, gingivitis, stomatitis, parotiditis, and halitosis.

The major purposes of regular bathing and skin care are the removal of dead skin cells, excessive perspiration, and sebum, which, if left to accumulate, harbor bacteria. Other benefits of bathing are the stimulation of circulation and a sense of well-being. From the nurse's point of view, assisting patients with bathing can provide an opportunity to assess the patient's state of health. The frequency of bathing patients is largely determined by their preferences, age, degree of illness, and agency policies. The technique for bathing patients in bed is outlined as well as the specific needs of newborns and infants.

The back rub is an essential part of hygiene care for patients confined to bed. Four techniques can be used when massaging backs: effleurage, tapotement, pétrissage, and three-handed effleurage. A number of preparations can be used depending upon the nature of the patient's skin. For example, alcohol is cooling and refreshing, and it toughens the skin protein, but it is usually contraindicated for elderly persons who do not require the drying effects.

For patients who are incapacitated, the nurse needs to provide perineal care. Because this procedure can create embarrassment for both the patient and the nurse, it needs to be handled matter-of-factly. Techniques for providing this care are described for female and male patients. Emphasized is the need to thoroughly cleanse and dry the perineal area because of the large number of microorganisms present.

Many problems of the skin are frequently observed by nurses. Some need to be brought to the attention of the physician; others require nursing intervention, and still others spontaneously disappear. Milia, xanthomas, mongolian spots, hemangiomas, and diaper rash are common among infants. Acne is prevalent amongst adolescents, and erythema, petechiae, ecchymoses, and skin ulcers are common in adults. Decubitus ulcers are a constant threat among hospitalized patients on prolonged bedrest. Several preventive nursing measures are listed and specific treatment measures outlined should ulcers occur.

Common problems of the feet are calluses, corns, plantar warts, unpleasant odors, fissures between the toes, and fungus infections. For each, the causes and treatment measures are outlined. Six guidelines are emphasized that are designed to prevent these problems. The nails also require regular attention to prevent incurvation and paronychia.

Eye care is normally minimal in health. Dried secretions on the lashes or the inner canthus need softening and removal. Newborns initially require eye medications to prevent ophthalmia neonatorum. The nurse also needs to be cognizant of measures related to artificial eyes, eyeglasses, and contact lenses. Common problems of the eyes include strabismus, myopia, hyperopia, presbyopia, astigmatism, and cataracts. The nose and ears also require minimal care. For infants these orifices are cleansed with moistened absorbent wisps of cotton.

Hair care includes daily combing, brushing, and regular shampooing. The black person's hair may also require lubrication. Dandruff, hirsutism, ticks, and lice are problems frequently encountered by the nurse.

Bed-making techniques are included as part of hygiene practices for hospitalized patients. It is important that beds are clean, warm, dry, and comfortable for ill patients. Surgical beds and other special beds such as the Stryker frame are mentioned.

SUGGESTED ACTIVITIES

1. In a health agency, explore the specific oral hygienic practices that are recommended.

2. When caring for a patient in a hospital, explore what hygienic practices the patient carries out. Explain how these differ from your own practices, and consider why.

3. Identify a situation with a patient of any age in which you, the nurse, can offer health guidance about a hygienic matter.

4. In a long-term care setting, identify the special arrangements that are made to assist patients to meet their hygienic and grooming needs. Compare your findings with the practices in an acute hospital setting.

5. Visit a local school nurse and determine the specific hygienic practices the children are taught.

6. In a hospital setting make an occupied bed and provide needed skin care. Discuss in a group what problems you encountered.

SUGGESTED READINGS

Block, Philip Lloyd. July, 1976. Dental health in hospitalized patients. *American Journal of Nursing* 76(7):1162–1164.

   This article emphasizes the need for active hospital oral care programs. Practical guides are offered along with specific oral care devices and their use.

Gruis, Marcia L., and Innes, Barbara. November, 1976. Assessment: essential to prevent pressure sores. *American Journal of Nursing* 76(11):1762–1764.

This author specifies characteristics of the skin that indicate pressure as well as environmental factors contributing to pressure sores. Assessment of relevant factors such as the circulatory status and medication therapy are also included.

Simko, Michael V. September, 1967. Foot welfare. *American Journal of Nursing* 67(9):1895–1897.

This article, written by a podiatrist, includes practical suggestions for corns, calluses, athlete's foot, ingrown toenails, and bunions. Nurses are often in a position to provide temporary relief measures.

Temple, Kathleen D. October, 1967. The back rub. *American Journal of Nursing* 67(10):2102–2103.

This article outlines the different purposes and types of back rubs. The author likens the back rub to a telephone wire, which conducts a message and is well constructed and properly insulated.

Zucnick, Martha. May, 1975. Care of an artificial eye. *American Journal of Nursing* 75(5):835.

This article lists the steps involved in removing, cleaning, and inserting an artificial eye. Five photographs support the steps.

SELECTED REFERENCES

Anderson, Helen C. 1971. *Newton's geriatric nursing,* 5th ed. St. Louis: The C. V. Mosby Co.

Bardsley, Christine, et al. May, 1964. Pressure sores: a regimen for preventing and treating them. *American Journal of Nursing* 64(5):82–84.

Barnhill, Sue Ellen, and Chenoweth, Elizabeth Emery. March, 1966. Cleansing the perineum. *American Journal of Nursing* (66):566.

Brown, Marie Scott, et al. September, 1973. Physical examination. Part 3. Examining the skin. *Nursing 73* (3)39–43.

Cahn, Milton M. July, 1960. The skin from infancy to old age. *American Journal of Nursing.* 60(7):993–996.

Carney, Robert G. June, 1963. The aging skin. *American Journal of Nursing* 63(6):110–112.

Davis, Ellen D. November, 1970. Give a bath? *American Journal of Nursing* 70:2366–2367.

Derbes, Vincent J. March, 1973. Rashes: recognition. *Nursing 73* (3):44–49.

Dyer, Elaine D., et al. July, 1976. Dental Health in adults. *American Journal of Nursing* 76:1156–1158.

Gibbs, Gertrude E. January, 1969. Perineal care of the incapacitated patient. *American Journal of Nursing* 69:124–125.

Giles, Sarah Fisher. 1972. Hair, the nursing process and the black patient. *Nursing Forum* 11(1):78–88.

Jacob, Stanley W., and Francone, Clarice Ashworth. 1978. *Structure and function in man,* 4th ed. Philadelphia: W. B. Saunders Co.

Metropolitan Life Insurance Company. 1969. *Looking for health.* Ottawa.

Milgrom, Peter. The quality of general medical services by dentists. In Leininger, Madeline, ed. 1975. *Barriers and facilitators to quality health care.* Philadelphia: F. A. Davis Co.

Miller, Marian E., and Sachs, Marvin L. 1974. *About bedsores. What you need to know to help prevent and treat them.* Philadelphia: J. B. Lippincott Co.

Nursing 77. (Prepared in consultation with M. A. Kauchak-Keyes). September 1977. Four proven steps for preventing decubitus ulcers. *Nursing 77:*58–61.

Pfaudler, Marjorie. November, 1968. Flotation, displacement, and decubitus ulcers. *American Journal of Nursing* 68:2351–2355.

Piper, Doris A. November, 1968. Weightless ward. *American Journal of Nursing* 68:2360–2361.

Roach, Lora B. March, 1974. Assessing skin changes: the subtle and the obvious. *Nursing 74.* (3):64–67.

Roach, Lora B. November, 1972. Assessment of color changes in dark skins. *Nursing 72:*19–22.

Rogers, Helen M. November, 1968. A water pillow, too. *American Journal of Nursing* 68:2359–2360.

Slattery, Jill. July, 1976. Dental health in children. *American Journal of Nursing* 76:1159–1161.

Stilwell, Elizabeth Jones. November, 1961. Pressure sores—one method of care. *American Journal of Nursing* 61(11):109–110.

Verhonick, Phyllis J. August, 1961. A preliminary report of a study of decubitus ulcer care. *American Journal of Nursing* 61(8):68–69.

CHAPTER 21

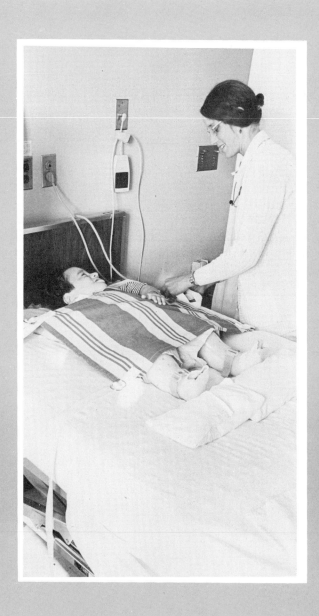

THE SAFE ENVIRONMENT

FACTORS THAT AFFECT PEOPLE'S ABILITY TO PROTECT THEMSELVES

THE INCIDENCE AND CAUSES OF ACCIDENTS

SAFETY PRECAUTIONS IN HEALTH

Infants

Toddlers

Preschoolers

School-Age Children

Adolescents

Adults

The Elderly

PROTECTION

SAFETY PRECAUTIONS IN ILLNESS

Falls and Other Mechanical Traumas

Burns

Chemical Trauma

HEALTH PRACTICES IN THE COMMUNITY RELATED TO DISEASE PREVENTION

Immunizations

Environmental Sanitation

SPECIAL HAZARDS

Radiation

Fire

OBJECTIVES

- Describe a safe home and community environment.

- Identify those aspects of a specific environment which are unsafe.

- Identify those mechanisms needed by people in order to protect themselves.

- Understand the measures to be implemented to assist patients to protect themselves.

- Advise patients on recommended immunizations.

- Be aware of some health practices in the community that are designed to prevent disease.

- Be aware of special precautions to take in relation to radiation and fire.

The need of people to protect themselves and in some instances to be protected is always present. The environment around us contains many hazards, both seen and unseen. The automobile, which may run down a pedestrian, is obvious as a seen hazard. Microorganisms and radiation are unseen hazards.

The need for a safe environment relates to national concerns as well as to the community and to the immediate environment of a person. Nurses are voicing their thoughts as individuals and collectively about such issues as air pollution, the pollution of lakes and rivers, and the safety of foods, cosmetics, and medications. Safety in travel on the highways is always before us as the newspapers report morbidity and mortality from automobile accidents. Increasingly governments are being pressed to take action and legislate in these areas in order to make the environment safer. In addition, people are also becoming aware of safety hazards in their local communities. Regulations to control the speed of boats on lakes used for swimming and local ordinances in regard to burning refuse and the release of smoke by industry are all indications of how people are seeing the importance of a safe environment.

Nurses have traditionally thought of safety in relation to a patient's immediate environment, and this is no less important today in spite of the broader focus on human protection. The need to be aware of what constitutes a safe environment for a particular person and how this environment can be made as safe as possible is a primary concern. The blind person may need railings, the crawling baby and toddler a protective gate at the head of the stairs, and the elderly person secure footing and an uncluttered floor. Nurses are thus focusing their attention upon preventing accidents and injury as well as upon assisting people who have been injured.

The word *environment* usually refers not only to factors external to the person but also to internal influences. In this chapter, however, the word is used with reference to the external influences.

THE SAFE ENVIRONMENT

A *safe environment* is one where the likelihood of a person becoming ill or injured because of factors in the environment is reduced to the lowest degree of possibility. The environment in this context refers to all factors, both physical and psychologic, that impinge upon a person. Physical factors may include heat, light, or furniture. Psychologic factors include, for example, the worry experienced by the parents of a sick child.

A safe environment is one in which people can function safely and one in which they obtain a sense of security. Maslow wrote that the safety and security needs of people were second in priority of needs, preceded only by physiologic needs such as food, air, and water. (See Chapter 7.)

A safe environment has a number of general characteristics; it means freedom from injury: thermal, mechanical, radiational, electrical, microbiologic, chemical, and psychologic. It also means the freedom from any unpleasant stimuli to the senses of odor, touch, sight, or hearing as well as comfortable environmental conditions.

Temperature

The temperature of the environment affects the comfort of people and in extremes the safety of people. What is considered a comfortable temperature varies from one person to another and from one cultural setting to another. In North America a room temperature between 18.3 and 25° C (65° and 77° F) is generally considered comfortable. However, in Great Britain, for example, a comfortable temperature is more likely to be lower. Wide variations in the external temperature can affect people's behavior; people are more likely to be impatient and lose their temper, to work less efficiently, and to become ill more quickly (Hillman 1973:692).

The temperature a person finds comfortable also varies according to a person's age (the very young and the elderly usually prefer a warmer temperature), activity, and illness. The inactive and ill person frequently prefers a warmer temperature.

Humidity

Humidity is the degree of moisture in the air; it is expressed as a percentage. Most people are comfortable when the humidity is between 30% and 60%. When the humidity is high, the rate of evaporation of perspiration is decreased; conversely, when the humidity is low, evaporation of perspiration is accelerated. In some situations a high-humidity environment is provided as a therapeutic measure. For example, steam inhalations increase the humidity of the air inhaled and thus facilitate breathing.

People who live and work in air-conditioned settings often encounter a low humidity. As a result they often experience dry mucous membranes of their noses and throats, resulting in an increased incidence of irritation and infection.

Light

Adequate lighting is important for people so that they can accomplish given tasks with minimum eye strain. Adequate light is one that is neither dim nor glaring and one in which there are no deep shadows. Some people are more sensitive to bright light than others. For comfort a patient may prefer a soft light, whereas the nurse may need a brighter light to perform nursing tasks safely.

Children and elderly people often find a night light helpful. It assists them to orient themselves to strange surroundings at night and even in familiar home settings to get to a bathroom safely. A night light needs to be situated so that it does not shine on the person's eyes, and yet it needs to give good lighting to the floor where a person will walk.

Noise

Noise is another factor in the environment that at certain levels can be considered to be unsafe. Sound levels above 120 decibels (units of loudness) are not only painful, but they are also damaging to people's ears. What a person considers noisy is to a large degree individualistic. The person who lives in a rural community may find the city sounds noisy, whereas the person who lives in the city may not even notice these sounds. Teenagers enjoy playing music at a sound level that parents often consider to be very loud.

Noise pollution is a concern of modern industrial society. It is considered that much of the hearing loss experienced by the elderly is due to the noise of the urban environment.

People who are ill are frequently sensitive to noises that normally would not disturb them. Loud voices, the clatter of dishes, and even a nearby television can be disturbing and produce angry reactions.

There are a number of ways by which noise can be minimized. Acoustic tile on ceilings, walls, and floors as well as drapes and carpeting all absorb sound. Background music has also been found to minimize noise and have a comforting effect upon people.

Smog, Smoke, and Dust

Pollution of the atmosphere has received considerable publicity in recent years. Smog, smoke, and dust are all threats to people's health and are of particular concern in industrialized centers.

Smoking is also generally recognized as a health hazard. The incidence of lung cancer and heart disease are higher in smokers than nonsmokers. Increasingly nonsmokers are asking for seats in theaters, restaurants, and transport vehicles that are segregated from smokers.

Microorganisms

Microorganisms in the environment are a continual source of injury to people. These include *pathogens* (microorganisms that are capable of producing disease), which can affect people who are not protected or who are ill and hence particularly vulnerable. See the section in this chapter, "Immunizations." See also Table 21-1.

Table 21-1.   A Safe Environment

1. Adequate lighting	Adequate lighting eliminates shadows, which may be confusing. A night light may be indicated.
2. Neat and clean	Clutter and litter are removed. Spilled food and liquids are cleaned up. Furniture is in its accustomed place.
3. Safe equipment	Furniture and equipment are regularly maintained. Electrical equipment is in good repair.
4. Noise level is "comfortable"	This is an individual matter; however, sound above 120 decibels is considered painful and damaging to the ears.
5. Cleanliness	Excessive dirt and microorganisms can endanger health by causing infections.
6. Medications and poisons are labeled and kept separately in cupboards out of reach of children.	Accidental ingestion can cause illness and even death.

FACTORS THAT AFFECT PEOPLE'S ABILITY TO PROTECT THEMSELVES

The ability of people to protect themselves from injury is affected by a number of factors. Each of these factors needs to be considered by nurses when they are assisting patients and when they are teaching patients to protect themselves.

Age

Age is an important factor that affects people's ability to protect themselves. Through knowledge and through accurate assessment of the environment, people can learn to protect themselves from many injuries. Children walking to school learn to stop before crossing the street and to wait for oncoming traffic. They also learn not to put their hand on a hot stove, thus avoiding a burn. For the very young, learning about the environment is important. It is only with knowledge and experience that children learn what is potentially harmful. Acquiring this knowledge in a manner that does not include serious accidents is an important aspect of living. Parents normally attach a great deal of importance to teaching children what is potentially dangerous and at the same time arranging the home environment in order to prevent them from having accidents. The safety precautions that may be adequate for an older child or an adult are not adequate for a young child. For example, children's inability to read means that they cannot read the poison label on a drain cleanser bottle or the prescription label for their mother's medicine. It is only through the experience of living that young children can perceive the dangers in the environment.

Elderly people also can have special problems protecting themselves from injury. Often balance is impaired, and once lost it is not readily regained. Thus an elderly person may need to learn to stand up slowly, thus preventing the loss of balance that can result from a quick, sudden movement. Slowness of movement and decreasing sensual acuity also contribute to the likelihood of injury. Elderly persons may neither see nor hear an oncoming car. They may not see a foot stool. They may also be too weak to pull themselves out of a bathtub safely.

Orientation and Level of Consciousness

The ability of persons to orient themselves to their surroundings and to respond to environmental stim-uli are important factors in their ability to protect themselves. Some of the common situations encountered by nurses are:

1. Unconscious or semiconscious persons. Such persons may be completely comatose or may arouse from the coma for brief periods and then lapse back. See Chapter 34, "States of Awareness."

2. Persons with neurologic impairments who may not perceive stimuli such as heat or pain.

3. Persons whose communication is affected so that they cannot convey their perceptions to another person.

4. Paralyzed persons who are unable to move even though they perceive discomfort.

5. Confused patients who may not understand where they are or what to do to help themselves.

6. Patients who perceive stimuli that do not exist, such as the person who is withdrawing from alcohol intoxication and thinks he sees worms crawling on his bed.

For people to protect themselves, they must be able to perceive environmental stimuli accurately. These stimuli, which are received by sensory receptors of the body, travel by way of the sensory pathways of the nerves to the central nervous system. For a reflex action such as occurs when one's hand touches a hot object, some of the impulses travel directly to motor neurons, which then convey the impulses to the muscles necessary to effect the sudden, quick withdrawing of the hand. At the same time other sensory impulses travel to the brain where in the cerebral cortex the person becomes aware of the stimulus and initiates further impulses to the muscles to provide voluntary movement of the body. Impairment of any of these areas—the sensory receptors, sensory pathways, the internuncial neurons which transmit the impulse from the sensory pathways to the motor pathways, the motor pathways, or the cerebral cortex—can impair a person's ability to respond normally to environmental stimuli.

A state of *unconsciousness* is a state in which a person is not aware of the environment. There are varying levels of unconsciousness, that is, levels of lack of response to the environment. One unconscious patient may respond to painful stimuli, for example, whereas another may not.

Consciousness is a state of awareness of oneself and the environment (perceptual and physical stimuli) (Mitchell 1973:168). A number of terms are used to describe these levels (see also Table 34-1).

1. Alertness. The person is in full possession of his senses.

2. Drowsiness (lethargy). Similar to continual sleep; the person can be aroused but returns to sleep when left alone.

3. Stupor. A loss of consciousness. The person can be aroused with difficulty. Usually the person's thinking will be confused, awareness is limited, and perception is distorted.

4. Coma. The person cannot be aroused, and no voluntary movements occur. Breath rate changes in response to painful stimuli. Corneal reflexes may or may not be present. Cough reflex is absent, and swallowing will be impaired.

Emotions

Some emotions experienced by people can also alter their abilities to perceive environmental hazards. Acute anxiety in a person results in reduced perceptual awareness. The person who is depressed may think and react more slowly than normal in response to environmental stimuli. In addition a person can only take in and respond to a certain number of stimuli at one time. A person who is barraged with questions and talks with many people at work may well not remember a telephone call from his wife during that day. A patient in the hospital may be preoccupied with her illness and pain and thus fail to hear a nurse's teaching about her diet.

Injury and Illness

Persons who are ill are especially prone to accidents. They are often weak and less able to carry out their normal physical activities. Often they are not fully aware of their weakened condition; for example, a patient may think he is able to walk to a chair but may fall while trying.

As a result of some illnesses patients become helpless or semihelpless. They may be unable to move or to even help themselves with the simplest function. At these times they will need to depend upon others for their safety. In some instances the therapy for a disease process may in itself make patients more vulnerable to illness and injury. Some medications have side effects such as drowsiness, which make it more difficult for patients to protect themselves. Other medications, such as Mercap-topurine, deplete the white blood cell count, thus making patients more prone to infections.

In addition, worry about illness in regard to oneself and to others can preoccupy people's minds, thus making them less perceptive of potentially harmful stimuli such as an oncoming automobile or a street curb.

Senses

Impaired body senses are a major factor involved in injuries. Not only do hearing, taste, smell, and visual acuity often decrease in the elderly, but they can also be impaired as a result of disease and accident. The person with impaired vision often develops other senses to help compensate for this problem; however, in some situations the person needs the assistance of others for protection. The person may not see a toy and may trip over it or may not see a signal cord at a hospital bed unit. The deaf person may not hear a warning call in regard to traffic, and the person with impaired olfactory sense may not smell burning food or escaping gas. The person who cannot feel may not be aware of the burning of a hot-water bottle, and the person whose sense of taste is impaired may not detect contaminated food.

Lack of sleep can also affect a person's sensual acuity. With fatigue, acuity usually decreases, as is evidenced by the driver who fails to see a sign on the side of the highway or the parent who does not hear a teenager's verbal request for help with a school problem.

In addition to impaired senses is the problem of adaptation of the senses to stimuli that might prove dangerous or embarrassing. The homeowner does not notice the gradual escape of gas; a patient may not notice an offensive odor which is apparent to someone coming in from the fresh air.

Information

Information is a critical factor related to a person's safety. In new situations such as a hospital, patients frequently need specific information to protect themselves. A great deal of equipment is strange to them: oxygen tanks, intravenous tubing, and surgical drains are just a few. Often simple explanations to children and adults can prevent them from having accidents and incurring additional illness. Just to know that a steam kettle is hot is sufficient explanation for most people who are able to protect themselves. For others, special precautions need to be taken by nurses to help the patients protect themselves.

Accident Proneness

For some time it has been recognized that some people are *accident prone*. These are people who have accidents more frequently than the average person. Some children frequently cut themselves and fracture bones more often than their peers. Some adults drive a car for 15 years without an accident, while others have at least one accident each year.

Accident proneness is thought to have an emotional basis. There are a number of theories accounting for its causes. One theory is that emotional tension impairs a person's perceptions and judgments, thus making that person more likely to have an accident. It is also proposed that accidents may serve a person's masochistic and hostile needs. Some people may find it easier to be cared for by others than to be responsible for themselves.

THE INCIDENCE AND CAUSES OF ACCIDENTS

Accidents, rather than disease, are the major cause of death among children over 1 year of age. In Canada more than 2000 children between the ages of 1 and 15 die annually from accidents, and 8000 others suffer permanent disabilities (Canada 1972). Countless other children are involved in accidents of a less serious nature. Of all home accidents to preschoolers, 75% were due to negligence (Canada 1972:2, 3).

In the United States, 12,500 children from the age of 1 to 14 die annually from accidents (US DHEW 1974:33, 34). In fact, throughout the life span of humans, accidents remain among the ten leading causes of death of people. From the age of 15 to 44, accidents are still the leading cause of death. From the age of 45 to 64, accidents rank fourth as a leading cause of death, and above the age of 65, accidents rank sixth. See Table 21-2 for death rates in the United States according to age.

There are seven major external causes of accidents among children and adults. These include, in order of prevalence: motor vehicles, falls, fires and flames, drowning, poisoning (by solid and liquid substances), suffocation by inhalation and ingestion of objects (including food causing obstruction), and firearms. See Figure 21-1 and Table 21-3 for statistics.

Table 21-2.   Deaths and Death Rates from Accidents According to Age in the United States, 1970

Age	Number	Rate*
1–4	4,300†	31.5
5–14	8,203†	20.1
15–24	24,336†	68.7
25–44	23,979†	50.0
45–64	24,164	57.8
65 and over	27,268	135.9

*Per 100,000 population.
†Leading cause of death in specified age group.
From US, Department of Health, Education, and Welfare, Public Health Service, Health Resources Administration, National Center for Health Statistics, 1974, *Facts of life and death*, Rockville, Md., pp. 33–38.

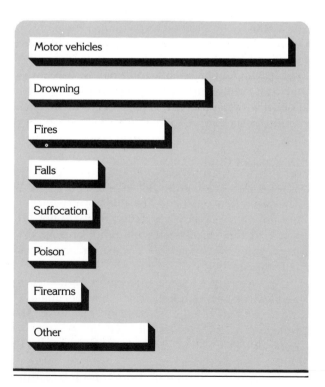

Figure 21-1.   Seven major causes of accidental death in the 1 to 15 age group in Canada. (From Department of Health and Welfare, 1972. Keep Them Safe, Ottawa, p. 2.)

Table 21-3.   Major Causes of Accidental Death, United States, 1970*

	Number	Rate
Motor vehicles	54,633	26.9
Falls	16,926	8.3
Fires and flames	6,718	3.3
Drowning*	6,391	3.1
Poisoning	3,679	1.8
Suffocation	2,753	1.4
Firearms	2,406	1.2

*Drowning may supersede falls, fires and flames as a cause of death in children age one to 15.
From US, Department of Health, Education, and Welfare, 1974, *Facts of life and death*, Rockville, Md., p. 44.

SAFETY PRECAUTIONS IN HEALTH

Most accidents are due to negligence and are preventable, and most communicable diseases are preventable. This section will deal specifically with accidental hazards to life and health. Age as a factor governing a person's protective mechanisms has been previously mentioned. The fact that protection and education are essential commodities throughout life's stages of growth and development is obvious; however, the development of safe living habits varies in accordance with age.

Infants

Although infants are completely dependent upon others for personal care, they soon learn to roll from side to side, to put anything within reach into their mouth, and to creep and walk. They are oblivious to such environmental hazards as falling or ingesting harmful substances. The need for constant surveillance of the infant on the part of the parent is essential. Parents or surrogates must also ensure the provision of protective measures.

Some of the special precautions to be observed in the care of infants are as follows:

1. Provide only toys that are soft and large and that do not have parts that can be removed and swallowed.
2. Always have the sides of the crib up when the baby is not being handled. The rungs of the cribsides need to be close enough together so that the baby cannot get his or her head between them.
3. At feeding time, hold the baby. There is danger of choking if he or she is propped up with a bottle.
4. Put pins, needles, buttons, and nails out of reach of the baby because infants like to put things in their mouth.
5. Use guard rails at the top and bottom of the stairs when the baby starts to crawl.
6. Cover electric outlets, and install safety outlets if possible. Babies like to explore by putting their fingers in holes.
7. Do not leave a baby alone in the bath or on a bed or a table because the baby may roll off.

Toddlers

Toddlers are curious and like to feel and taste everything they can reach. They walk during their second year although they will be unsteady on their feet. Toddlers like to climb and explore, and many things such as garden pools and a busy street fascinate them. As a result toddlers need constant supervision and protection. It is at this age that training in safety can begin.

Some special precautions for toddlers include the following:

1. Knives and other sharp tools and matches need to be kept safely away from the toddler's reach.
2. Pots on the stove need to be kept on the back burners away from the toddler's reach.

3. Cleaning solutions and insecticides need to be kept in locked cupboards.

4. All medicines need to be stored in a locked cupboard.

5. The play area outside should be free of deep ditches, wells, and pools.

6. Teach the toddler what "no" and "don't" mean and that these words are meant when they are spoken at times of risk for the toddler or for others.

Preschoolers

Accident prevention for preschoolers includes teaching them to observe and to act safely. This is particularly important at this age as they become increasingly independent. Preschoolers are very active; they run, climb, and often act before they think. They like to imitate their parents, and it is through example that many safe ways of behaving can be taught.

1. Preschoolers need to learn to cross streets safely and to obey traffic lights.

2. They need to learn to play on a sidewalk or the grass rather than in the road.

3. In their play they need to learn to expect to fall and thus be relaxed when falling.

4. They need to learn to swim and to understand that water can be dangerous.

5. Preschoolers should not run with sharp utensils or with hard objects in their mouth because if they fall they may well injure themselves.

6. They can learn to put their toys away so that they and others will not trip over them.

School-age Children

By the time children are attending school they are learning to think before they act. They like doing things with grown-up equipment rather than with toys. They want to be active with other children in activities such as bicycling, hiking, swimming, and boating.

School-age children have the following needs to protect themselves from accidents:

1. School-age children need to learn to use equipment such as the stove and garden equipment safely.

2. They will need to understand traffic rules before bicycling. See Figure 21-2.

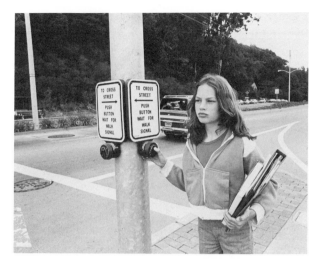

Figure 21-2.   A school-age child knows safety rules as a pedestrian.

3. They will still need help and supervision with much equipment, and if they live in the country, they will need to learn to handle farm animals.

Adolescents

Adolescents spend much of their time away from home with their peer groups. However, they still need guidance from parents. The accident rate involving adolescents is high, and the major cause involves automobiles. In addition, adolescents are likely to become injured while riding motorcycles, snowmobiles, and minibikes. Firearms and drowning are other causes of deaths among adolescents.

Some safety measures that adolescents require in order to prevent these accidents are the following:

1. Developing an inner discipline, which is necessary to be a safe driver.

2. Wearing safety helmets when riding motorcycles and similar vehicles.

3. Learning to swim and understanding water safety.

4. If using firearms, learning how to use these competently.

5. Understanding the dangers involved in the use of drugs and alcohol.

Adults

In middle age, accidents rank fourth as the cause of death. Alcohol is a significant factor in many of these accidents. Consequently adults need to learn not to drink if they are driving motor vehicles or boating.

The Elderly

Elderly people are particularly prone to accidents. They require a safe home environment. Toys need to be out of the way, rugs need to be fastened so that they will not slip. Hand railings in bathrooms and the placement of dishes and frequently used supplies within easy reach are a few of the precautions which can assist in the prevention of accidents. See Chapter 11 about safe housing for the elderly.

SAFETY PRECAUTIONS IN ILLNESS

There are a number of dangers that are of particular significance for people when they are ill or injured. Three of these are falls and similar mechanical traumas, burns, and various chemical traumas such as the overdose of medication.

Falls and Other Mechanical Traumas

Falls are not only common for the very young and the very old, but they also occur frequently to those people who are ill or who have been injured in some way. The latter groups generally have less strength than they are accustomed to having and frequently lose their balance readily.

In hospitals and homes nurses need to be very much aware of patients who may fall. A number of safeguards are generally taken to try to prevent these accidents.

1. Bedside tables and overbed tables are placed near the bed or chair so that patients do not need to overreach and consequently lose their balance.

2. Patients who have had surgery or have been in bed for some time are advised to have assistance when first getting out of bed.

3. Footstools are supplied with rubber feet, which do not slip, and wheelchairs with locks for the wheels.

4. Floors have nonslip surfaces; rugs and carpeting are fixed securely in place so that they will not slip. In some hospitals special nonskid flooring is used in the halls and stairs, and special mats are placed in bathtubs.

5. The environment is kept tidy so that people do not trip over light cords, toys, or misplaced furniture.

6. Some hospitals provide ambulating patients with railings along the corridors and in the bathrooms.

In addition to the above measures there are also specific safety devices that can be employed to assist patients to protect themselves or to be protected. These measures are discussed subsequently.

In some agencies the use of these devices is dependent upon a physician's order or an agency policy, and in others their use is at the nurse's discretion. It is of utmost importance that patients understand why these devices are being employed and what is expected of them at this time. Many nurses can recall patients who did not understand the need to call for assistance when they wanted to use a toilet. Consequently they climbed over siderails on their beds with surprising agility, resulting in unfortunate falls.

Side Rails

Sometimes referred to as *cribsides,* side rails are attached to the side of the bed, and when elevated, they can help prevent a patient from falling out of bed (Figure 21-3). If an adult patient wants to get out of bed, side rails are unlikely to stop him or her.

Side rails are frequently used on beds when the patients are unconscious, confused, or sedated. In ad-

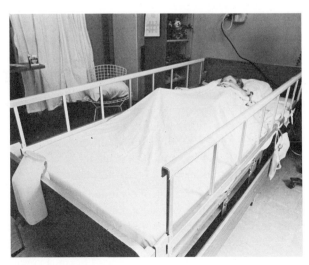

Figure 21-3. Side-rails on a hospital bed provide a sense of security as well as protection from falling.

dition, in some hospitals side rails are applied to the beds of all patients over 70 years of age, particularly at night. In other settings side rails are used for all patients at night regardless of age.

It is usual for nurses to take down the side rail at the side of the bed at which they are working. It is important, however, to elevate the rail when leaving the bedside. Although an unconscious patient or child may appear quiet and unlikely to move, he or she may suddenly move and fall out of bed when the side rail is not in place.

Although some patients may state that a side rail is embarrassing, many others find that they provide a sense of security. This is particularly true with hospital beds, which are at a fixed height, higher from the floor than the normal bed at home, and narrower.

Restraints

In recent times there has been a desire to use means other than restraints to offer protective measures to patients. Restraining can result in increased restlessness and anxiety with the resultant loss of self-control. In many instances, however, restraints are necessary to prevent injury or interruption of therapy. Envision the patient who tries to pull out a urinary or intravenous catheter or the infant who wants to scratch eczematous skin lesions. When the nurse finds it necessary to apply a restraint, there are a number of guidelines to be borne in mind:

1. Allow the patient as much freedom to move as possible and at the same time serve the purpose of the restraint.

2. The patient's circulation must not be occluded by the restraint.

3. Pad bony prominences under a restraint in order to avoid skin abrasions.

4. The restraint needs to permit the body to assume its normal position, for example, slight flexion of the arms.

5. Use the least conspicuous type of restraint possible. Even if the patient is not aware of the restraint, visitors often find them disturbing. For example, a crossover jacket restraint is less noticeable than arm and leg restraints.

6. At the first indication of occluded peripheral circulation (pallor, blueness, cold, tingling, or pain) the restraint needs to be loosened and the limb exercised.

7. Remove restraints at least every 4 hours. Exercise the limb and provide skin care to prevent skin abrasions.

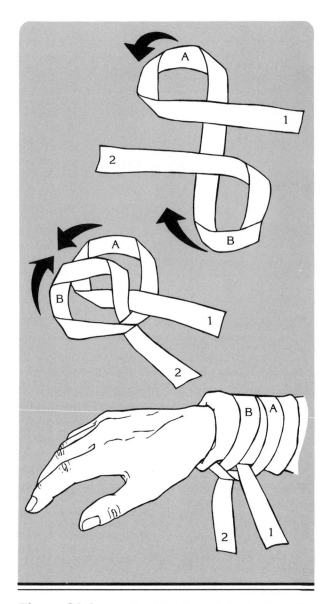

Figure 21-4.   A clove hitch is made by forming a figure eight and then gathering up the two loops.

Hand and foot restraints are used to keep a limb relatively immobilized as in the case of an intravenous infusion or to prevent the confused patient from removing a urinary catheter or nasal tube.

The wrist or ankle is padded with a thick gauze dressing or special felt pads. The cloth restraint is then tied on the body using a clove hitch (which will not tighten upon pulling) (Figure 21-4), and the ends are tied to the bed frame under the mattress.

Jacket restraints are used for both children and adults. The jacket is usually put on with the ties at the back, but in some situations it is put on with the ties at the front (Figure 21-5). The straps from the jacket are then tied to the bed frame under the mattress or to the legs of a chair.

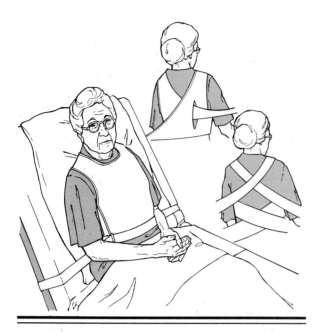

Figure 21-5.   A jacket restraint (note various styles).

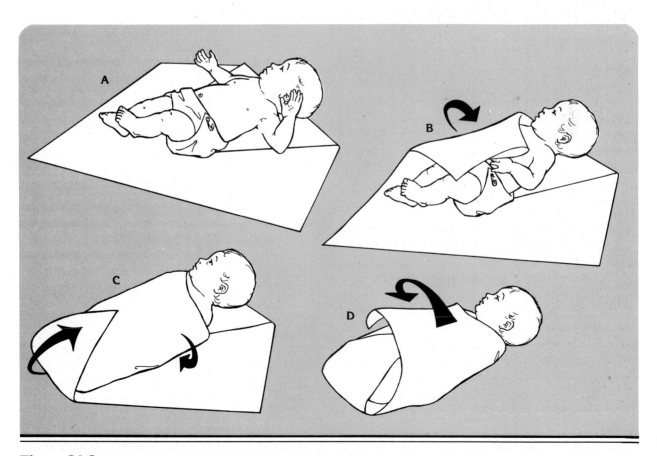

Figure 21-6.   A mummy restraint is used to restrain infants during treatments and examinations.

For small children the mummy restraint and the papoose board are frequently used. The *mummy restraint* (Figure 21-6) is a special folding of a blanket or sheet around the child in order to prevent him or her from moving during a procedure such as a gastric washing, an eye irrigation, or when obtaining a blood specimen. The child lies in a supine position on a blanket with the upper edge of the blanket slightly above the shoulders and the lower edge at least 10 to 12 inches below the feet. The child's right arm is placed at his or her side, then the blanket is brought from that side over the body and between the left arm and body and tucked under the body. Then the left arm is placed in anatomical position, and that side of the blanket is brought over the length of the body and tucked under the child. The long end of the sheet is then brought over the child and tucked in beneath him or her.

A papoose board (Figure 21-7) is used to restrain children for periods of time varying from 15 minutes to several hours. It can be used when intravenous infusions are being administered, for circumcisions, and for other minor local surgical procedures. The

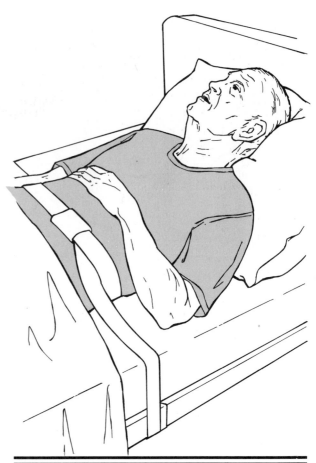

Figure 21-8.   Safety belts are commonly used to secure patients to beds and to stretchers.

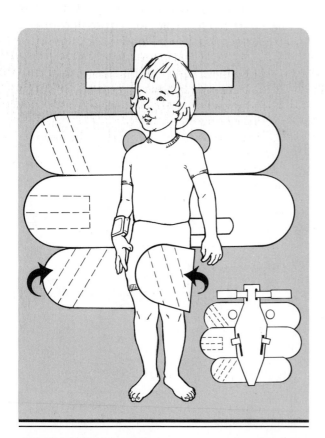

Figure 21-7.   A papoose board can be used to restrain infants and small children.

child lies face up on the board. The board flaps are extended, and a blanket can be used for padding under the child. The child's wrists are placed through the loops on the board. The center strap is brought over the arms and body and fastened securely. This is then repeated with the chest strap, and last, the leg strap is brought over the thighs and lower legs.

Safety belts (Figure 21-8) are used on older children and adults. They come in locked and unlocked models. The belt, which goes around the patient's waist, is attached to a longer belt, which is fastened in turn at each end to the bed frame under the mattress. If a locked safety belt is used, the key is kept by the nurse.

An *elbow restraint* (Figure 21-9) is also used on occasion for small children. This is a piece of cloth into which there are either rigid supports or slots into which tongue blades will fit. The restraint is wrapped around the elbow and tied at the ends. The ties on the upper edge are then pinned to the baby's shirt in order to prevent the restraint from sliding down the arm. Elbow restraints are commonly used for small children to prevent them from bending their elbows and touching an incision or scratching their skin.

Mitt restraints (Figure 21-10) are used for confused patients in order to prevent them from using their hands or fingers to injure themselves. With mitts on, patients are unable to remove a urinary catheter or pull off surgical dressings yet are able to move their arms freely. Mitts are highly advantageous for ambulatory patients, since other types of restraints confine them to bed or to a chair.

Commercially prepared mitts are available, or the nurse can make them using large dressings and stockinette. The patient's hand assumes a natural position, and he is given a soft pad to grasp. The patient's wrist is padded with large dressings to prevent skin abrasions, and all skin surfaces are carefully separated to also prevent abrasions.

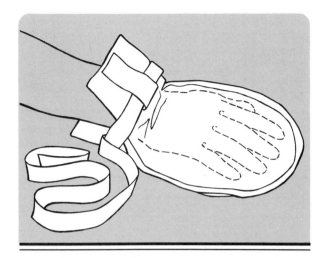

Figure 21-10.   A mitt permits freedom of movement of a limb.

Two large dressings are then placed over the hand, one from side to side, the other from the ventral surface to a dorsal surface. These are then secured with gauze bandage in a recurrent pattern (see Chapter 17, "Basic Turns in Bandaging") and with adhesive tape.

Stockinette is then put over the hand and secured just above the wrist pad with adhesive tape.

Mittens need to be removed at least once in 24 hours to permit the patient to wash and to exercise the hands. If the patient indicates any discomfort, the mitten needs to be taken off and circulation checked.

Burns

The possibility of burns to patients is a continual problem. Patients who are ill may be unaware that they are being burned. People can be accustomed to heat that in fact is injurious to tissues. The use of heat as a therapeutic measure is discussed in Chapter 17. It is important to assess the degree to which patients can protect themselves and what if any special precautions need to be taken by the nurse.

Equipment used for patients who are ill is often strange to them, and they will usually require an explanation as to which areas are hot or dangerous to touch. For small children this kind of equipment needs to be placed out of their reach. Explanations to 2-year-olds often just make them more curious, and children learn by touching things.

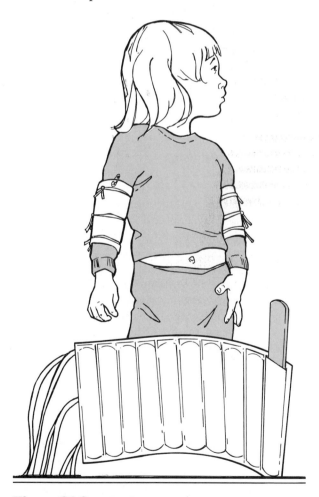

Figure 21-9.   An elbow restraint for a young child.

Burns due to fire are another important area of potential injury. These are discussed later in this chapter.

Chemical Trauma

Accidents do occur as a result of the use of chemicals. In health this is exemplified by toddlers who ingest their parents' tranquilizers. In illness, medication errors account for many of the injuries of this nature. Some of these are as follows:

1. The physician orders the incorrect medication or the incorrect dosage.
2. The nurse administers or the patient takes the incorrect medication or the incorrect dosage.
3. The patient receives a medication intended for another patient.

The provision of medication by nurses is discussed in Chapter 36. There guidelines for nursing actions are provided.

It is important that patients who will be taking their own medications be provided with the assistance necessary to prevent accidents. Some of these follow:

1. Label medications in large enough print so that the patient can read it, and write the directions in understandable words.
2. Parents with young children may need cautioning to place the medicine out of reach of the children.
3. Patients who take their own medication while in the hospital will need to have this recorded on their charts and have the physician's permission. This may prevent a double dose of a medication from being taken by a patient.

HEALTH PRACTICES IN THE COMMUNITY RELATED TO DISEASE PREVENTION

The health practices learned by a person are determined to a large degree by the cultural and social groups (community) in which the person lives. Generally if a community places a high value on medical care or recreational facilities, for example, it will have these to use. Thus if a community places a high value on the prevention of disease, it will generally ascribe to those practices that it believes will prevent disease. Unfortunately, those practices which prevent disease are not always known, and superstitious beliefs or ignorance can prevail. An example of a superstitious belief is wearing a piece of garlic on a string around one's neck in order to cure a cold. Practices in regard to immunizations may be unknown to people, or it may be believed that diphtheria, for example, no longer exists because people have not seen anyone with that disease.

Some aspects of disease prevention in a community are carried out by government agencies, others by voluntary or unofficial agencies. Some services are also controlled by law, but the acquisition of others is left up to the individual person.

Immunizations

Immunity is the body's resistance to disease; the body possesses specific antibodies that resist disease. Im-

munizations are directed toward protecting a person from contracting communicable diseases. *A communicable disease* is one that can spread from one person to another. Infections, on the other hand, are the establishment of pathogens in the person that multiply and cause a disease. The pathogens in the latter case may come from other people, from the air, from animals, or from food. Infection and infection control were discussed in Chapter 16. See Table 21-4.

Epidemiology is the study of the occurrence and distribution of disease as it occurs in humans. *Epidemic* refers to the occurrence of disease in many people at the same time or in rapid succession in an area. *Pandemic* refers to the occurrence of a disease in many parts of the world at the same time.

The process of acquiring immunity involves antigens and antibodies. An *antigen* is a protein or protein-polysaccharide substance that is capable of producing antibodies in the body. Most antigens are considered to be foreign to the body and when taken into the body stimulate the production of antibodies. However, there is some recent evidence that some antigenic substances are not immune to the body.

An *antibody* is a specific chemical substance (an adapted serum globulin) formed by the cells of a person; the antibody has the capacity of neutralizing an antigen or reacting with it.

Table 21-4. Incidence (Reported Cases) of Selected Communicable Diseases in the United States, 1963 and 1970

Disease	1963	1970
Botulism	47	12
Diphtheria	314	435
Infectious encephalitis	1,993	1,580
Infectious hepatitis (includes serum hepatitis)	42,974	56,797
Malaria	99	3,051
Measles	385,156	47,351
Rubella (German measles)	—	56,552
Tuberculosis	54,062	37,137
Typhoid fever	566	346
Gonorrhea	278,289	600,072
Syphilis	124,137	91,382

From US Department of Health, Education, and Welfare, 1974. *Facts of life and death*, DHEW Pub. No. (H.R.A.) 74-1222. Rockville, Md.

Resistance

The resistance of a person to disease is both specific and nonspecific. *Specific resistance* refers to such barriers as an intact skin, body secretions, which normally can kill many pathogens, and the cilia of the respiratory tract, which can trap microorganisms. *Nonspecific resistance* is less well understood. It is thought that the blood and body fluids offer some resistance and that the environmental factors such as temperature and humidity also have an effect upon individual resistance.

Immunity

There are different types of immunity: natural or acquired; the latter is further broken down into active and passive. See Chapter 8 for discussion of "The Immunologic Adaptive Response."

Immunization Process

The process of immunization to communicable diseases is a preventive health measure advocated by government agencies in the United States and Canada.

At birth newborn infants have limited ability to produce antibodies. It is only at about 3 months that they protect themselves in this way. During the last few months of the pregnancy certain antibodies in the mother pass through the placenta to the infant, thus providing the baby with some passive immunity. This immunity is temporary and needs to be supplemented with other practices such as good hygiene, sterilized formula, and separation from people who have infections.

Tables 21-5 and 21-6 indicate immunizations advised in the United States and Canada. In addition it is recommended that boys and girls prior to puberty are immunized against rubella if this has not already been done. Contraction of rubella during the first trimester of pregnancy may result in a baby born with defects which are likely to affect the eyes, heart, and brain.

Table 21-5. Immunization Schedule—United States*

Age	Agents	
2 months	DTP (combined diphtheria toxoid, tetanus toxoid, pertussis vaccine)	TOPV (trivalent oral polio vaccine)
4 months	DTP	TOVP
6 months	DTP	TOVP (optional)
12 months	Tuberculin test; repeated tests depend upon exposure and incidence in reference population	
15 months	MMR (combined measles, mumps, rubella vaccine)	
18 months	DTP	TOPV
4 to 6 years	DTP	TOPV
14 to 16 years	TD (tetanus and diphtheria toxoid, combined adult type)	
After 16 years	TD every 10 years; tetanus toxoid at time of injury	

* Revised schedule for active immunization and Tuberculin testing of normal infants and children in the United States. Approved by the Committee on Infectious Diseases, American Academy of Pediatrics, 1977.

Table 21-6. Recommended Routine Immunization Schedules—Canada*

Age	Agents
3 months	DTP, 1.0 cc (combined diphtheria toxoid, tetanus toxoid, pertussis vaccine)
	OPV (Sabin), 0.2 cc (oral polio vaccine)
4 months	DPT, 1.0 cc
5 months	DPT, 1.0 cc
	OPV (Sabin), 0.2 cc
7 months	OPV (Sabin), 0.2 cc
12 months	Rubeola (MMRor), 0.5 cc (MR)
	MMR (combined measles, mumps, rubella vaccine)
	Rubella vaccine may be deferred until 11 years for girls
13 months	Rubella, 0.5 cc
15 months	DPT, 1.0 cc
5 or 6 years	DPT or DT, 1.0 cc (diphtheria and tetanus toxoid)
	Rubella (both sexes if never given previously), 0.5 cc
	Rubeola (if never given previously), 0.5 cc
	OPV (Sabin), 0.2 cc
10 years	Diphtheria toxoid (40/50 LF), 0.2 cc
	OPV (Sabin), 0.2 cc
11 years (girls)	Rubella, 0.5 cc (if never given previously)
15 years	DT, 0.5 cc
	OPV (Sabin), 0.2 cc
16 years or over	DT, 0.5 cc

*From Canada, Department of Health and Welfare. September 24, 1977. *Canada Diseases Weekly Report*, Ottawa, p. 154.

Immunity Tests

It is advisable in some situations to test the individual for susceptibility to a specific disease before giving the toxoid or vaccine. Diphtheria toxin, 0.1 ml, can be given intracutaneously to test for the presence of the antitoxin in the blood. This is called the *Schick test*. If the antitoxin is present, the site of the injection will become red with some infiltration in 24 to 48 hours (See "Intradermal Injections," Chapter 36).

Another test carried out is the intracutaneous administration of Old Tuberculin as a test for the presence of tuberculosis antibodies. The usual initial dose

is 0.1 ml of a 1:1000 dilution of Old Tuberculin. A positive reaction is indicated by an area of redness at the site of the injection, often with a papule at the point of insertion of the tuberculin.

Immunizations are normally not given if the person has a fever, but mild infections such as a cold without a fever do not contraindicate immunizations. The most frequent reaction to an immunization is a slight fever; occasionally a reaction can be more severe, consisting of a high fever, sleepiness, even convulsions. Physicians need to be consulted if there is a severe reaction or if the person persists in feeling ill after 48 hours.

Environmental Sanitation

The sanitation of the environment has a direct effect upon people's health. Food or water that is contaminated with pathogenic microorganisms can cause widespread disease and in some cases severe illness and even death.

Issues in regard to the environment are popular topics for newspaper and magazine articles. The community in which people live directly affects their lives.

Measures involving environmental sanitation are also necessary to prevent communicable disease and other illnesses such as Q fever, caused by a rickettsia that can infect cattle and be passed on to people through milk that has not been pasteurized. Some specific areas of concern in environmental sanitation follow.

Water

Nearly all water used by people has been polluted while falling as rain or running over the surface of the ground or through the soil. The pollution by wastes has further contaminated many water supplies. The most important diseases conveyed by water are diseases of the intestinal tract: typhoid fever, dysentery, paratyphoids, infectious hepatitis, and cholera. The incidence of these diseases has declined in recent years, primarily due to (a) water treatment including filtration and chlorination, (b) protection of water supply areas, (c) improved waste disposal methods, and (d) immunizations during times of epidemics.

The presence of fluoride in the water in minute quantities (0.6–1.7 mg/liter) has been found to reduce the incidence of dental caries as much as 65% in children (Ehlers and Steel 1965:53).

The US Public Health Service has established standards in regard to drinking water; these are enforced by the state departments of health.

Air Pollution

Air pollution is the presence in the outdoor atmosphere of one or more contaminants such as dust, fumes, gas, mist, odor, smoke, or vapor in sufficient quantities and of sufficient duration as to be harmful to humans, plants, or animals. Air pollution is an increasing problem in all countries where urban growth is accompanied by industrial development and where automobiles are used extensively.

Health problems incurred because of air pollution include respiratory disease and eye, nose, and throat irritations.

Disposal of Human Wastes

One of the most important aspects of environmental sanitation is disposal of human wastes. Sewage normally contains microorganisms such as *Escherichia coli* (E coli), which normally inhabits the intestines of humans, and *Aerobacter aerogenes* and *A. cloacae*, which are also found in feces and in soils. Some of the diseases that can be communicated through sewage are typhoid, paratyphoid, poliomyelitis, and hepatitis.

Some individual sewage disposal systems for people in rural areas are cesspools and septic tanks. Treatment of sewage in an urban area can be carried out by a number of methods: filtration, dilution, or activated sludge, just to mention three. The purposes of sewage treatment are (a) to make the sewage inoffensive, (b) to eliminate the danger of contaminating water and bathing areas, and (c) to prevent the destruction of fish and wildlife.

Milk

Milk can be a vehicle for the spread of diseases such as tuberculosis, diphtheria, dysentery, and streptococcal infections. Not only does milk need to be free of disease, it must also be clean, with a small number of bacteria. In order to produce safe, clean milk the following are necessary:

1. Healthy cows.
2. Clean and healthy dairymen.
3. Clean barn and surroundings.
4. Separate milk room.
5. Clean utensils.

6. Pasteurization, which is the application of heat to milk in order to destroy any disease-producing microorganisms that may be present.

Food Sanitation

Contaminated food can cause serious illness and even death in humans. The five types of contaminants are as follows:

1. Animal parasites such as tapeworms in meat or fish.
2. Microorganisms such as the bacteria that cause typhoid fever and dysentery.
3. Toxins, which are produced by certain bacteria in food, for example, *Clostridium botulinum*.
4. Poisonous plants such as toadstools.
5. Poisonous sprays, which adulterate foods.

There are laws that govern the preparation, storage, transportation, and sale of food, including the sanitation of eating and drinking establishments.

Insects, Vectors, and Rodents

Insects are important in disease transmission. A *vector* is animate (often an animal) and transmits disease. Some of the more important are mosquitoes, which pass on malaria, encephalitis, and yellow fever; flies, which transmit human disease by conveying bacteria from excreta to food; cockroaches; and bedbugs. Cockroaches are found in crevices of houses and in sewers. They can contaminate food with bacteria they bring with them from the sewers. Bedbugs do not transmit any communicable diseases, but they do bite and feed upon humans and animals. Fleas are another type of insect that also can transmit disease such as typhus and some bacteria.

Insects are controlled in various ways. There has been a worldwide effort to control the mosquito responsible for the transmission of malaria. The incidence of malaria in the United States is exceedingly small because of better protection of rural homes from mosquitoes, drainage of swamp waters where mosquitoes breed, mass medication, and spraying. Other insects are also controlled by sprays.

Rodents such as rats are also a potential source of disease such as typhoid fever, hemorrhagic jaundice, and amebic dysentery. It is estimated that the rat population in the United States equals the human population (Ehlers and Steel 1965:340).

The rat population can be controlled in two ways: using adequate garbage disposal so that garbage is not available to the rats and the use of poisons such as warfarin, an anticoagulant.

SPECIAL HAZARDS

Radiation

Radiation has become a more recently recognized cause of injury to people. There are forty elements in earth's soil that are radioactive. These are used in a variety of settings. Specifically, nurses are concerned with those radioactive materials which are used in diagnostic and therapeutic practices. Injury from radiation can occur as a result of overexposure to radiation or as a result of exposure to radiation that treats specific tissues and at the same time injures other tissues.

Radioactive materials are used in diagnostic procedures such as radiography, fluoroscopy, and nuclear medicine. In the last situation, specific radioactive materials that have an affinity for specific tissues are taken into the body, usually by ingestion or intravenous routes. Some of these elements are calcium, which has an affinity for bones; iodine, which is attracted to the thyroid gland; and phosphorus, which is attracted to blood.

Radioactive materials are provided in sealed sources and unsealed liquid sources. An example of the former is cobalt implants; iodine 131 and phosphorus 32 are examples of liquid unsealed sources.

Factors that directly affect the degree of exposure to radiation are as follows:

1. The longer the time that a person is in the presence of radiation the greater the exposure.

2. The closer a person is to the source of the radiation the greater the exposure.

3. Substances such as lead can be used to shield a person from radiation.

Assisting Patients who Are Receiving Radioactive Materials

Often nurses will be involved in helping patients who are being treated by radiation or who are receiving radioactive materials concerned with diagnostic measures.

When a patient is receiving radiography or fluoroscopy, the exposure is generally minimal, and few precautions are necessary for the patient. For the nurse who may need to assist a small child to remain still, shielding by use of a lead apron is advised.

If a patient has received radioactive materials such as implants, these will be a source of radiation to the immediate environment. If a nurse needs to be in close contact with such a patient, lead-shielded aprons are indicated.

It is important to deal with any radioactive body discharges in a safe manner. Nurses need to wear rubber gloves and in some instances may need to place specific excreta in special containers for special disposal. It is also important that the nurse's gloved hands are washed well before the gloves are removed and that any contaminated materials are placed in a special container for disposal.

A hospital that uses radioactive materials will usually have a radioisotope committee. This committee establishes policies and procedures to be used in the care of patients who receive radioactive materials. It is important for nurses to be aware of these and to familiarize themselves with them when the need arises.

One important aspect in the nursing care of such patients is their understanding about the treatment and the precautions they need to take. Often such patients are restricted to bed or to a confined area to protect others. Like patients who are on isolation precautions, it is important that they have an understanding of what is happening and that they receive the required emotional support to deal with the problem.

Fire

Fire is a constant danger in any environment, inside and outside of a hospital. Statistics show that electrical fires are the most common type of fire in homes and hospitals. They are usually due to faulty electrical equipment. The second most common cause of fire in a hospital is smoking in bed. Here patients are often incapacitated and unable to leave the building without assistance.

There are simple guidelines, which, if followed, can assist a nurse at the time of an emergency.

1. Know where the fire exits are in the building.

2. Know where the fire extinguishers are and how to operate them.

3. Be familiar with the practices of the hospital and with the alarm system.

Most hospitals have their own practices in case of a fire. Nurses should carry these out regardless of how small the fire is initially. A small fire in a wastebasket can quickly become a large fire. Some of the practices that are carried out in many hospitals are as follows:

1. Initiate the fire alarm if there is one nearby.

2. Notify the switchboard of the hospital as to the location of the fire.

3. Remove any patients who are in immediate danger.

4. Use the fire extinguisher on the fire.

5. Close windows and doors to reduce ventilation.

6. Turn off oxygen and any electrical appliances in the vicinity of the fire.

7. Clear fire exits if necessary so that they are unobstructed.

If the fire is outside a door, it is advisable to place damp cloths or blankets around the edges of the door to prevent the entry of smoke.

Kinds of Fires

There are generally three kinds of fires: paper and wood fires (class A); flammable liquid fires, such as grease and anesthetics (class B); and electrical fires (class C).

All fires require three elements: sufficient heat to start the fire, a combustible material (a material that will burn), and sufficient oxygen to support the fire.

Types of Fire Extinguishers

There are a number of fire extinguishers available today. Five types are generally used.

1. *Carbon dioxide extinguisher.* This is used for both class B and C fires. It is effective for grease fires as well as for electrical fires. The nurse pulls the trigger of the extinguisher, thereby releasing carbon dioxide, which, when directed to the cause of the fire, excludes oxygen.

2. *Soda and acid extinguisher.* This is a water extinguisher, which can be used to put out paper and rubbish fires. The extinguisher is turned upside down, thus mixing the acid and the soda. These produce carbon dioxide, which permits the water to be released under pressure. When it is necessary to stop the flow from the extinguisher, the can is returned to its original position.

This type of extinguisher is not used for either electrical or grease fires because electricity is conducted by water and the grease is splattered by the water, thus possibly spreading the fire.

3. *Dry chemical extinguisher.* This type of extinguisher is used to blanket a fire with a foamlike material, which excludes oxygen from the fire. It contains chemicals, sodium bicarbonate, and carbon dioxide. It is used for both electrical and rubbish fires. To operate, a pin is pulled and either a valve is opened or a lever on the extinguisher is pressed. The nozzle valve is then squeezed.

4. *Water pump extinguisher.* This extinguisher uses water, which is pumped out by hand. It is used for class A and C fires. To operate, the handle is pumped, and the nozzle is directed toward the fire.

5. *Antifreeze or water extinguisher.* In this extinguisher, water or antifreeze is stored under pressure. There is a pressure gauge on the outside of the can indicating the pressure and its readiness for use. To use this type of extinguisher, it is necessary to pull the pin and then the handle of the extinguisher. It is also used for class A and B fires.

Removing Helpless Patients

There are four methods of carrying persons from the scene of a fire. Generally they are used for patients who are unable to walk themselves and when it is not possible to wheel the patient's bed or to remove the patient by a stretcher.

1. *Swing carry.* This carry involves two nurses. The patient in a sitting position places his or her arms around each nurse's shoulders. Each nurse holds the patient's wrists, which are over the nurse's shoulders to support the patient. Each nurse then reaches behind the patient and grasps the other nurse's shoulder or upper arm. The nurses then release the patient's wrists, reach under the patient's thighs, and grasp each other's wrists. The patient is then lifted in this sitting position and moved as is necessary.

2. *Pack strap carry.* This carry can be done by one nurse. The nurse faces the seated patient and grasps the wrists. The nurse's right hand grasps the patient's left wrist, the left hand the right wrist. The nurse then pivots and slips under one of the patient's arms so that the nurse's back is to the patient and the patient's arms are crossed in front of the nurse. With a broad stance by the nurse, one leg in front of the other, the patient is rolled on the nurse's back.

3. *Hip carry.* For this carry the patient lies laterally at the side of the bed facing the nurse. The nurse is facing the head of the bed. The nurse's arm that is closest to the patient is placed over the patient's back and under the lower axilla. The nurse then turns

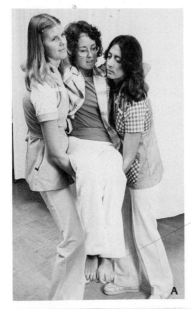

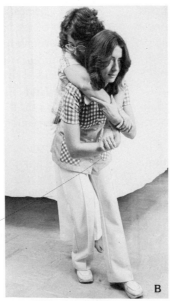

Figure 21-11. Three carries that can be used in an emergency. **A,** Swing carry; **B,** pack strap carry; and **C,** hip carry.

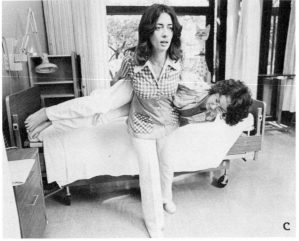

away from the patient and places the second arm around and under the thighs. The nurse with a broad stance for balance then draws the patient on to the nurse's hips so that the patient's abdomen is over the nurse's hips. See Figure 21-11.

4. *Three person carry.* See "Lifting a patient between a Bed and a Stretcher," Chapter 22.

SUMMARY

The provision of a safe external environment is a constant focus of the nurse. Physical factors in the environment and psychologic and physiologic abilities of the individual person need to be considered. General characteristics of a safe environment include a comfortable temperature, which varies with the age of individuals, adequate humidity, appropriate lighting, noise levels below 120 decibels, freedom from pollution, and protection from disease-producing microorganisms.

Many factors affect people's ability to protect themselves. Age determines the capacities with which people are able to protect themelves. For example, the young lack the knowledge and experience of hazards in the environment, and the elderly often lack the sensory acuity necessary to perceive hazards. One's orientation and level of consciousness is another factor. Unconscious patients cannot respond to normal stimuli, and confused patients may be unaware of surrounding stimuli. Acute emotions can also alter a person's ability to perceive or to judge hazards accurately. In many situations injury and illness interfere with the physical strength and abilities required for self-protection.

Accidents are emphasized as the major cause of death among children over 1 year of age. Seven major external causes of accidents for people of all ages include motor vehicles, falls, fire and flames, drowning, poisoning, suffocation, and firearms. Most accidents are due to negligence and are preventable.

Safe living habits and precautions vary in accordance with age. Infants require constant surveillance and protection by adults. Protective measures for infants include guard rails at the top and bottom of stairs, covered electrical wall outlets, large soft toys that do not have parts that can be removed and swallowed, crib sides with rungs close together, and constant observation during feeding or when on the bath table. Toddlers, because of their curiosity and explorative nature, need to have dangerous items such as medicines, sharp tools, and cleaning solutions out of reach. Fences should enclose pools or ditches and the play area. Teaching toddlers that "no" and "don't" are spoken at times of risk is essential. Preschoolers can be taught to observe and to act safely. Lessons such as traffic safety, playing in safe areas, swimming, and keeping toys away from walking areas are important. Safe ways of behaving are imitated from the parents. School-age children prefer using grown-up equipment to toys. They therefore need safety instruction about their use. Adolescents need additional safety guidance from parents about the use of motorized vehicles, firearms, drugs and alcohol, and water safety. The elderly need home safety devices that counteract their diminished sensory acuity and balance.

During illness people are prone to a number of hazards. The major ones are falls, burns, and chemical traumas such as medication overdoses. Nurses need to anticipate persons who are particularly prone to falls and to initiate protective measures. Some of these include side rails on the bed, placement of objects within easy reach, and assistance with ambulation. In some situations restraints are necessary to prevent injury or the interruption of therapy. The use of various restraints is described. Included are hand and foot, jacket and mummy restraints, the papoose board, safety belts, and mitts.

Community disease prevention programs are another important aspect of a safe environment. Communicable diseases and epidemics are minimized. Immunization schedules advised in the United States and Canada are provided in table form starting at 2 or 3 months of age.

Environmental sanitation is important for health maintenance. Food sanitation, protection of water supplies, safe sewage disposal, reduction of air pollution, milk pasteurization, and control of insects, vectors, and rodents are essential.

Special hazards in hospitals and the community include radiation and fire. Preventive measures are emphasized.

SUGGESTED ACTIVITIES

1. Assess your own living environment and determine which aspects of it meet the characteristics of a safe environment.

2. Visit a home of a family with growing children or an elderly couple and assess what safety education is required.

3. Visit a school nurse and identify the safety education programs offered to children in grades 1 to 6, 7 to 10, and for adolescents.

4. Determine the immunization schedules recommended in your locality.

5. Invite a public health worker to your school to discuss the specific environmental sanitation measures conducted in your community.

SUGGESTED READINGS

Feycock, M. W. January, 1975. A do-it-yourself restraint that works. *Nursing 75* 5(1):18.

This article describes how to make a restraint that can be used to elevate a limb.

Mylrea, K. C., and O'Neal, L. B. January, 1976. Electricity and electrical safety in the hospital. *Nursing 76* 6(1):52–59.

This article describes the basics of electricity, electrical hazards, and points on how to prevent problems. Explanations about voltage, current, resistance, alternating current, and capacitance are also included.

SELECTED REFERENCES

Boeker, Elizabeth H. April, 1965. Radiation safety. *American Journal of Nursing* 65(4):111–115. Reprinted in Myers, M. E., ed. 1967. *Nursing fundamentals.* Dubuque, Iowa: William C. Brown Co., Publishers.

Breeding, Mary Anne, and Wollin, Myron. May 1976. Working safely around implanted radiation sources. *Nursing 76* 6(5):58–63.

Canada, Department of Health and Welfare. 1972. Keep them safe. Ottawa.

Ehlers, V. M., and Steel, E. W. 1965. *Municipal and rural sanitation.* New York: McGraw-Hill Book Co.

Hillman, H. May, 1973. The optimum human environment. *Nursing Times* 69(22):692–695.

Kukuk, Helen M. May 1976. Safety precautions: protecting your patients and yourself. Part 1. *Nursing 76* 6(5):45–51. June 1976. Part 2. *Nursing 76* 6(6):49–52.

Kummer, Sylvia B., and Kummer, Jerome M. February, 1963. Pointers to preventing accidents. *American Journal of Nursing* 63:118–119.

Long, Barbara C., and Buergin, Patricia S. June 1977. The pivot transfer. *American Journal of Nursing* 77:980–982.

Morris, Ena M. July, 1968. In case of fire emergencies. *American Journal of Nursing* 68:1496–1499.

O'Grady, R., and Dolan, T. January 1976. Whooping cough in infancy. *American Journal of Nursing* 76:114–117.

Phegley, Diane, and Obst, Jerry. July, 1976. Improving fire safety with posted procedures. *Nursing 76* 6(7):18–19.

Scheffler, Gustav L. October, 1962. The nurse's role in hospital safety. *Nursing Outlook.* 10:680–682. Reprinted in Meyers, Mary E., ed. 1967. *Nursing fundamentals.* Dubuque, Iowa: William C. Brown Co., Publishers.

US Department of Health, Education, and Welfare. 1974. *Facts of life and death.* Rockville, Maryland.

CHAPTER 22

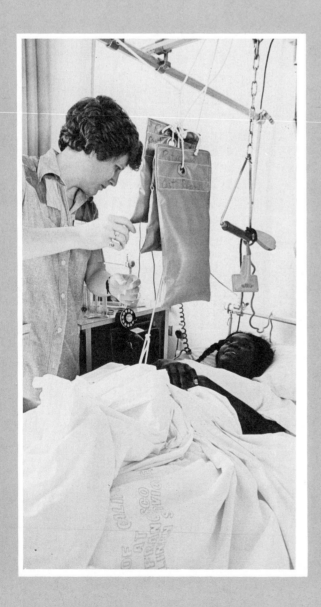

BODY ALIGNMENT AND POSITIONS

OBJECTIVES

- Define body mechanics.
- Describe the well-aligned person standing and sitting.
- Describe postural variations that occur with age.
- Assess body posture of persons of all ages
- Assist patients to assume good body alignment if it is incorrect.
- Explain the physiology of body movement.
- Apply guidelines in assisting patients to move in bed and between a bed and a chair or stretcher.
- Describe the various bed positions.
- Assist patients to assume these positions.
- Assess body positions for alignment.

Many people who are ill are able to move relatively easily, much as they would when well. They may move a little more slowly than usual and perhaps less steadily; however, with the presence of a nurse and the consequent reassurance that help is present if it is required, walking and turning over in bed, for example, are not major problems to many patients.

There are patients, however, for whom even moving in bed can be a major problem. For these patients who have difficulty in moving or a complete inability, skillful nursing assistance is extremely important. There are a number of situations in which nurses can anticipate that assistance to move will be required. Some of these are the following:

1. Patients who are unconscious or paralyzed.
2. Patients who are in weakened states, for example, because of surgery, prolonged periods in bed, or recent injury.
3. Patients who are very young or who are elderly.

4. Patients who have certain disease conditions, such as multiple sclerosis.
5. Patients who require rest and who must not exert themselves, such as, a patient who has recently had a myocardial infarction.

The degree of assistance that patients require from nurses will depend upon their own ability to move and the amount of exertion they can safely expend. In most instances, the nurse needs to be sensitive to the needs of patients to function independently and at the same time sensitive to patients' needs for assistance to move. Frequently, explanations from the nurse as to the reason for the assistance at the particular time, together with reassurance regarding future independent functioning if this is possible, will assist people to accept assistance.

This chapter will include the principles and techniques that can be employed by both patients and nurses to assist patients to move in bed, to move between a bed and a stretcher or chair, and to ambulate.

BODY MECHANICS

Body mechanics refers to the movement and coordination of the body in response to stimuli and to the body's coordinated efforts to maintain its balance while responding to these stimuli. The coordinated body movement of a barefoot person who steps on a piece of jagged glass on a beach in an effort to maintain balance can be described as body mechanics.

In a restricted sense, the term *body mechanics* is commonly used to describe body movements used by people when they move other persons or objects. However, body mechanics are operant in periods of rest in addition to activity, such as when standing, sitting, or lying. Good posture while standing, for example, involves the synergistic action of muscle

groups enabling balance and stability. The major purpose of good body mechanics is to facilitate safe and efficient use of appropriate groups of muscles to support physiologic function at a minimum level.

The use of good body mechanics is not restricted to the health-illness environment. Good posture is one criterion of beauty and enhances health. Conversely, poor posture detracts from beauty and can affect normal body functioning. In this context, *body alignment* and *good body posture* are used as synonymous terms. *Alignment* refers to the position of the body that facilitates body function as does good body posture.

BODY ALIGNMENT

Normal body alignment or good body posture is essential to the effective functioning of the body. When the body is well-aligned, undue strain is not placed upon the joints, muscles, tendons, or ligaments of the body so that the person can maintain balance. Muscles are usually in a state of slight flexion, referred to as *tonus*, when the body is healthy and well-aligned.

This state requires minimal muscular force and yet assists in maintaining adequate support for the body's internal framework and organs. The terms *posture* and *body alignment* are often considered in reference to the standing and sitting positions of the healthy human. However, when a person is ill and confined to bed, body alignment in several sitting and lying positions is of extreme importance. Following are some criteria of the well-aligned person in a standing position and a sitting position.

The Well-Aligned Adult in a Standing Position

1. Has a vertical line falling from the body's center of gravity (located on the midline halfway between the umbilicus and the symphysis pubis) between the feet (the body's base of support).

2. Has toes pointed forward.

3. Has ankles flexed to maintain the feet at right angles to the lower leg.

4. Has knees slightly flexed. A line drawn through the patella and the middle of the ankle ends at the second or third toe.

5. Has hips straight.

6. Has hands positioned midway between pronation and supination with fingers slightly flexed. The wrists are neither flexed nor extended.

7. Has arms falling at the sides with elbows slightly flexed.

8. Has the head erect, neither flexed forward nor extended backward nor flexed laterally with the chin held in.

9. Has normal vertebral curves. In the infant, the primary vertebral curve is posteriorly convex. After children can hold up their heads, stand, and walk, the following three vertebral curves are present:

    a. The lumbar curve is anteriorly convex.

    b. The thoracic curve is posteriorly convex.

    c. The cervical curve is anteriorly convex.

The above normal curves may differ among individuals as a result of variations in walking, prolonged changes in posture, and pregnancy.

10. Has the main body weight borne well forward on the outer sides of the feet.

11. Has the lower abdomen pulled in and up.

12. Has an appearance of being stretched full but is relaxed and poised with minimal muscle strain (see Figure 22–1).

Anatomical position is a term used to describe a position of normal alignment and also serves as a reference for the three body planes: transverse, frontal,

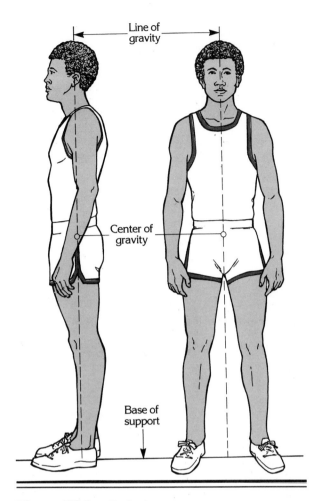

Figure 22-1.   Body alignment.

and sagittal. In anatomical position, a person stands as follows:

1. The arms are at the side.

2. The thumbs are adducted, the hands are pronated, and the fingers are slightly flexed.

3. The head is erect, neither flexed nor hyperextended.

4. The feet are directed ahead with ankles in normal flexion.

5. The knees are slightly flexed.

6. The hips are straight.

The Well-Aligned Adult in a Sitting Position

1. Has head erect, neither flexed forward nor extended backward.

2. Has normal alignment of the vertebral column.

3. Has the weight of the body from the head to the buttocks centered upon the buttocks and thighs.

4. Has both feet on the floor with normal flexion of the ankle joints as in the standing body alignment position. One foot may be placed slightly ahead of the other for comfort.

5. Has the popliteal spaces at least one inch away from the edge of the chair to avoid pressure upon the blood circulation and the nerves of the legs.

6. The thighs are in a horizontal position.

7. Forearms are supported on the lap or arm rests or a table in front.

POSTURAL VARIATIONS WITH AGE

Body alignment or posture changes significantly during growth and with age. An understanding of the normal variations is helpful for the nurse in promoting good posture and in identifying and assisting people to correct postural faults. The following are descriptions of normal developmental postural variations.

The Newborn and Infant

In the newborn, the neck is short and straight. The head moves freely from side to side and flexes and extends easily. The spine is straight, but it can be flexed. Shoulders, scapula, and iliac crests are on the same plane. All extremities are generally flexed, but they can be passively moved through a full range of motion. For example, in the upper extremities, the fists are clenched; the wrists flex more than 90° and extend slightly less than 90°; the arms can be extended, but they promptly return to a state of flexion. In the lower extremities, the feet of the newborn appear flat due to a fat pad in the position of the transverse arch. They may normally turn inward (*inversion*); they can be passively turned outward (*eversion*). The lower legs flex onto the thigh and the knees extend but do not hyperextend. The range of motion of the hip joint is normally about 160°–170° in flexion and extension, and the thighs, when they are flexed at the hip, abduct to an angle of approximately 160° between the thighs. The abdomen is rounded and prominent but not overly extended.

Toeing-in or pigeon-toeing is normal in early infancy. This is due to internal tibial torsion or inward rotation of the lower legs. However, if the lower legs are straight and toeing-in occurs in early infancy, it can be due to an abnormal congenital condition called *metatarsus adductus*, which warrants treatment. Toeing-in can also be caused by an internal rotation of the hip, in which case the entire limb is internally rotated. When the internal hip rotation extends beyond the normal position of the hip, it is called femoral anteversion.

The appearance of flat footedness normally exists in infants and may appear as a fat pad in the instep of toddlers with a mild degree of knock-kneedness. In most cases tibial torsion, femoral anteversion, and mild metatarsus adductus tend to disappear without treatment as the child grows.

When babies learn to stand at about one year of age, they stand with the feet far apart, the toes turned outward, and the knees locked. The head and upper part of the trunk are carried forward. Their balance is rather precarious, and when they fall, they usually fall backwards.

The Toddler

Posture of the toddler reveals a marked lumbar lordosis with an abdomen that protrudes. The pelvis tilts forward, and there is only a slight convex curvature of the thoracic spine. Some toeing-out and a wide stance may occur in 2-year-olds due to a normally slight outward rotation of the hips. Feet are typically everted. Growth with its functional stresses eventually produces an inward rotation of the hips, which results in the disappearance of the foot eversion.

Childhood

In early childhood all children become slimmer, taller, and more solid looking. They assume the so-called little adult appearance as the protrusion of the abdomen decreases and the length of arms and legs increases. By the time children are 3 years old, they are more steady and evenly balanced on their feet. They walk erect, can stand on one foot, and can go upstairs alternating their feet. They begin to swing their arms in an alternating pattern similar to the adult and no longer widely abduct their arms for balance.

Five-year-olds are even more closely knit and in greater control. Their arms are held near the body, and their stance is even more narrow. In late childhood, from ages 9 to 11, all body parts increase in size and function. Muscles and ligaments become firmer and stronger, and thus body posture is improved over that of the young child. Both body stance and balance are efficient for erectness.

Adolescence

Significant changes in body proportions and contours occur during adolescence. In early adolescence, a boy's form is characterized by straight leg lines, narrow hips, wide shoulders, broad chest, and noticeable muscular development in shoulders, arms, and thighs. In contrast, a young adolescent girl has curved leg lines; her hips become wider, and her breasts develop. In the buttocks, thighs, and upper arms, fat is deposited.

Motor awkwardness is of great concern at this age because of the rapid and uneven growth of the muscles and bones. For example, when the bones grow more quickly than the muscles, the muscles become tight and respond in quick, jerky motions. If, on the other hand, the muscles grow more quickly than the bones, the muscles are loose and sluggish, resulting in a clumsy performance. This awkwardness of leg and arm movements disappears once the growth of the bones and muscles is stabilized.

Postural problems at this age often occur because of the physical discrepancies in weight and height

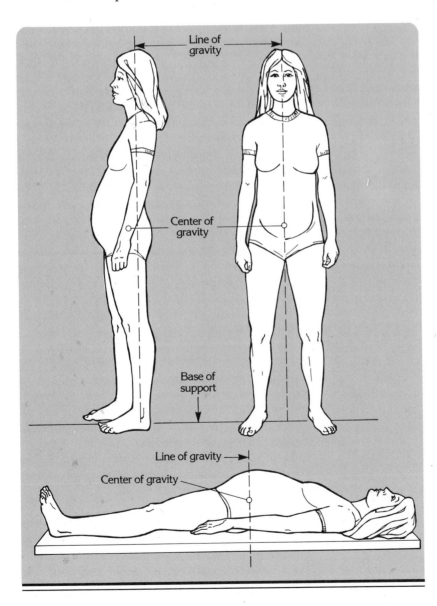

Figure 22-2. Body alignment during pregnancy.

between girls and boys. Because the growth spurt in girls occurs between 8½ and 11½ years of age as contrasted to 10½ to 14½ years of age for boys, it is not uncommon for girls to hover above their male partners on a dance floor. Postures may suffer as a consequence. By late adolescence, the gawky look and awkwardness of early adolescence disappears.

Adult

Body alignment and posture of the adult have been described in this chapter.

During Pregnancy

During pregnancy, both gait and posture change due to the increasing weight of the growing uterus, a changing center of gravity, stretching of the abdominal muscles, and relaxation of pelvic muscles and ligaments as a result of hormonal influences. In the typical pregnant stance a woman leans backward to counterbalance the weight of the enlarging uterus. This produces a progressive spinal lordosis and the common complaint of backache. Improper shoes with high heels can aggravate this balance, adding increased strain on the lower back and pelvic muscles.

Back discomfort and body alignment in pregnancy can be significantly improved by emphasizing good posture and body mechanics in daily activities. The woman needs to learn to pull her abdomen up and in, and to line her head, shoulders, and spine against a wall as much as possible (Figure 22–2). She may also need a reminder to stand as tall as possible without being rigid and to distribute her weight on the outer borders of her feet. Better balance can be achieved by encouraging the pregnant woman to broaden her base of support, standing with feet separated and one leg slightly forward.

Abdominal, pelvic, and back exercises such as abdominal contraction, pelvic floor contraction, and pelvic tilting are advised (Chapter 23). The use of firm, supporting, low-heeled shoes, the avoidance of stooping, and the use of the leg muscles to spare the back such as when lifting objects or when climbing stairs are recommended. For example, when climbing stairs she needs to avoid leaning forward by placing the entire sole of the foot on the stairs and use her leg muscles to raise herself from step to step. All activities during pregnancy may need to be of shorter duration than usual. Periods of standing, walking, and sitting should be varied frequently. Rest periods need to be interspersed with the feet elevated.

The Aged

The typical posture of elderly people is one of flexion. The head and neck are flexed slightly forward with eyes turned downward. The spinal column is flexed in the thoracic and lumbar areas producing a mild dorsal kyphosis and loss of the normal lumbar lordosis. Slight flexion exists at the hips and the knees. During ambulation, the speed of gait is therefore slowed in response to this flexed posture. Small shuffling steps are taken, and the ability to balance without the strength of the hip and knee extensor muscles is reduced.

PHYSIOLOGY OF BODY MOVEMENT

Body movement involves the function of the bony skeleton, the muscles, and the nervous system. The *skeleton* is made up of bones, which are joined together by ligaments, cartilage, and muscles. The skeleton serves three main purposes. The skeleton:

1. Protects the soft tissues of the body that lie under the skeleton.
2. Provides a lever system for movement. A *lever* is a rigid bar that revolves around a fixed point.
3. Provides a structural framework for the body.

In the body, bone is continually being formed and torn down. In a state of homeostasis, a balance is maintained between these two processes. Bone is composed of organic substances, which provide it with pliability, and inorganic substances such as calcium salts, which give it hardness. The amount of inorganic substances increases with age; thus the bones of a 2-year-old child are normally more pliable than those of an adult, and the bones of an elderly person are less pliable than those of a middle-aged person.

Body movements are brought about through the action of muscles. As a result of neuroelectrical factors and complex chemical processes within the muscle fibers involving glucose and phosphocreatine, the muscles contract, and thus the fibers shorten and thicken. In short, chemical energy is converted to mechanical energy in muscles.

Muscular activity is controlled by the nervous system, with centers chiefly in the cerebral cortex, the brainstem, the cerebellum, and the spinal cord. Skeletal muscles are normally in a state of slight contraction or tonus.

In movement of the body, the bones act as levers. As such, these levers vary both in size and in rigidity. These bones are attached to the body muscles. The *origin* of a muscle is the fixed or least movable attachment to a bone. The *insertion* is the point of attachment of the muscle that is the most movable. When a person wants to lift a book, a stimulus originates in the cerebral cortex and is transmitted by the motor pathways to the medulla. There the majority of the nerve tracts cross over and enter the spinal cord. The stimuli then pass along the motor fibers in several tracts of the cord. They synapse with lower motor neurons in the anterior horns, and the individual muscles are innervated by the spinal nerves, which leave the anterior horns and travel to the muscles. To *synapse* is to join as between two neurons.

GUIDELINES FOR MOVING PATIENTS

There are specific concepts and principles basic to body mechanics, which can be applied to effective and safe movement of patients.

1. Use major muscle groups

The major muscle groups should be used rather than smaller muscles. For example, to lift a heavy object, the gluteal and femoral muscles should be used rather than the sacrospinal muscles of the back. The former are employed by flexing the knees and the hips to grasp an object to lift it rather than by bending from the waist. The major muscle groups used in lifting and moving patients are the following:

a. Flexors, extensors, and abductors of the thighs.

b. Flexors and extensors of the knees.

c. Flexors and extensors of the upper and lower arms.

d. Flexors of the abdominal cavity and the pelvic floor.

A *flexor muscle* acts to bend at a joint, decreasing the angle between two bones. An *extensor muscle* acts to straighten a joint, increasing the angle between two bones. An *abductor muscle* draws away from a center or median. An *adductor muscle* draws toward a center or median line. (See Chapter 23, "Synovial Joint Movements," for further information.)

For major muscle groups used in movement, see Table 22–1.

2. Use a wide base of support with center of gravity in the middle

The body should be balanced on a wide base of support (a wide stance). By using a wide stance and maintaining the body's center of gravity in the middle, the stance balance is maintained. *Gravity* (weight) is the tendency toward the center of the earth. The center of gravity of a person is considered to be on the midline halfway between the umbilicus and the symphysis pubis.

3. Prepare pelvic muscles

Muscles in the pelvic area need to be prepared before being brought into action. This has two aspects: putting on the internal girdle and making a long midriff.

The internal girdle is made by contracting the abdominal muscles upward and the gluteal muscles (buttocks) downward. The long midriff is made by stretching the muscles at the waist. By preparation of these muscles the pelvis is stabilized and the abdominal muscles support the abdomen. As a result, all of these involved muscles can assist the muscles of the arms and legs in their activities such as lifting and pushing.

4. Use your own weight to push or pull

A person's own weight can be used to counteract an object or patient's weight, thereby requiring less energy. Nurses can use their own weight to push or pull a patient, thus minimizing the muscle energy required.

5. Avoid working against gravity

Because of the gravitational pull, more force is required to lift an object (overcoming the gravitational pull) than is required to push or pull an object. The latter does not involve the necessity of directly overcoming the gravitational pull.

6. Use the least amount of effort

In good body mechanics, the least amount of muscular effort that is required should be used. To accomplish this the following should be noted:

a. The body movements need to be smooth and rhythmical.

b. When lifting or carrying heavy objects, they should be held as close to the body as possible.

c. Objects should be pushed or pulled along a surface rather than lifted if possible. In many instances, patients can assist by pushing or pulling themselves.

d. When moving a heavy object, the person should directly face the direction of the force. For example, when a nurse assists a patient toward the head of the bed, the nurse's body should face the head of the bed.

e. A work level should be such as to avoid muscle strain; for example, when a nurse assists a patient with a bath in bed, the bed itself should be elevated and side rails lowered so that the nurse does not need to stoop or stretch unnecessarily.

7. Reduce friction

Friction can increase the amount of effort required to move an object. *Friction* is that force which opposes motion. Friction can be reduced by a smooth surface as contrasted to a rough surface. Nurses can apply this principle by ensuring a firm smooth foundation for a bed before moving a patient in the bed.

8. Prevent muscle fatigue

To prevent muscle fatigue, rest periods need to be interspersed with periods of use. Continuous muscular exertion can result in muscular strain. *Muscular strain* is the overstretching or overexertion of muscles.

9. Use others or mechanical aids as required

Some objects are too heavy to be moved without assistance. There are mechanical devices that can assist nurses to move patients, thereby avoiding muscle strain. These are discussed later in this chapter.

Table 22-1.   Major Muscles Used in Moving Patients

Body part	Muscles	Function	Body part	Muscles	Function
Forearm	Biceps brachii	Flexes the forearm	Lower Leg	*Quadriceps Femoris group*	
	Triceps brachii	Extends the forearm		1. Rectus femoris	Flexes thigh and extends the leg
Upper arm	Deltoid	Abducts upper arm Assists in flexion and extension of upper arm		2. Vastus lateralis	Extends the leg
				3. Vastus medialis	Extends the leg
	Pectoralis major	Flexes upper arm upward		4. Vastus intermedius	Extends the leg
	Latissimus dorsi	Extends upper arm downward		*Hamstring group*	
				Biceps femoris	Flexes leg and extends the thigh
Thigh	*Gluteal group*		Abdomen	External oblique	Compresses abdomen, pulls front of pelvis upward, and flattens lumbar curvature
	1. Gluteus maximus	Extends and rotates the thigh outward		Internal oblique	
	2. Gluteus medius	Abducts the thigh and rotates it outward		Transversalis abdominis	
	3. Gluteus minimus	Abducts the thigh and rotates it inward		Rectus abdominis	
	Iliopsoas	Flexes the thigh	Pelvic floor	Levator ani	Supports floor of pelvic cavity
	Rectus femoris	Flexes the thigh and extends the lower leg		Coccygeus	

ASSISTING PATIENTS TO MOVE IN BED

Patients require varying degrees of assistance to move while they are in bed. Some are completely helpless and require the assistance of nurses to make the smallest change in position. Other patients who are weak or very ill frequently require assistance from a nurse, although they may be able to help themselves a little.

Before nurses assist any patients to move, they need to be aware of the following information:

1. The degree to which the patients can exert themselves, specifically considering their physical condition. For example, it may be that patients who have cardiac pathologic conditions should not exert themselves in the slightest even though they feel well enough to help. Although a patient wants to be helpful, it may be contraindicated at that particular time.

2. The position that the patient needs to assume and the degree of tolerance of the patient in another position. The patient who has a respiratory patho-logic condition may require a Fowler's sitting position while in bed to be able to breathe satisfactorily. This patient may or may not be able to tolerate lying flat on the back even for a few minutes.

3. Any discomfort a patient experiences when moving or assuming a particular position. An example would be a patient with an advanced malignancy who finds any movement painful. Nurses can help move such a patient at a time when the analgesic is most effective, for example, half an hour after an injection of morphine, to minimize discomfort.

4. Any special problems a patient might have, such as particularly fragile skin, bones, or blood vessels. Patients with some diseases may have specific problems in that even normal, gentle handling by a nurse can cause a bone to fracture or blood vessels to break. In these instances, soft pads can be used by the nurse to provide less pressure on a specific area of the skin and to provide broader support when helping the patient turn in bed.

Procedure 22-1.   Assisting a Patient to Move up in Bed

Moving a patient up toward the head of the bed is facilitated if the patient can safely tolerate having the head of the bed down and the removal of the head pillow for a few minutes. If this is not possible, the nurse would be wise to obtain the assistance of a second person who could help from the other side of the bed. In this way, with the additional assistance, the patient will experience less exertion and less discomfort. The following steps are followed by either one nurse or two nurses.

Action	Explanation
1. Explain to the patient what you plan to do.	To reassure the patient and gain the patient's assistance if possible.
2. Wash hands.	To transmit no microorganisms to the patient.
3. The head of the bed is lowered, if already elevated, to the degree suitable for the individual patient.	To avoid working against gravity.
4. If the head pillow can be removed, it is placed against the head of the bed.	The pillow serves as a pad to prevent the patient's head from hitting the headboard when moving up.
5. The nurse stands at the side of the patient's bed facing the point at the head of the bed toward which the patient will move. A broad stance is assumed with the foot closest to the bed head in front of the other foot.	Use a wide base of support.
6. The nurse's knees and hips are flexed to bring the forearms to the height of the bed surface.	Use major muscle groups and work close to the patient.

Procedure 22-1. Cont'd

7. The nurse places one arm under the patient's shoulders and the other arm under the patient's thighs (Figure 22-3, *A*).

Figure 22-3.

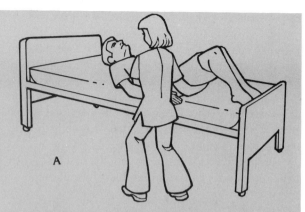

A

8. The patient flexes the knees, thus bringing the heels up toward the buttocks, and places the chin on the chest. If the patient can grasp the bed head, this will also assist in moving, or the patient may be able to push with the hands on the bed surface by flexing the elbows and hyperextending the shoulder joints.

9. The nurse's weight shifts from the rear leg to the forward leg as the patient pushes with feet or arms (Figure 22-3, *B*).

Use the least amount of effort. Have the patient assist by pushing or pulling and reducing friction.

Use your own body weight to push.

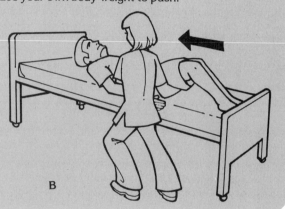

B

Procedure 22-2.   Assisting a Patient to Move up in Bed (Two Nurses)

This second method of assisting a patient to move up in bed requires two nurses. It requires use of the body muscles, particularly the femoral and gluteal muscles.

Action	Explanation
1. Explain to the patient what you plan to do.	To reassure the patient and gain the patient's assistance if possible.
2. Wash hands.	To transmit no microorganisms to the patient.
3. The head of the bed is lowered to the degree suitable for the patient.	So that the patient is not being lifted against the force of gravity.
4. Remove the pillow and place against the head of the bed if the patient can tolerate this.	The pillow serves as a pad for the patient's head against the headboard.

5. Each nurse stands on an opposite side of the bed facing the patient. They stand opposite the patient's waist with knees flexed.

This is opposite the heaviest portion of the patient. Knees are flexed to bring the nurse to a working level using the femoral muscles, thus avoiding back strain.

6. A broad stance is assumed.

To provide balance by placing the center of gravity between the nurse's feet.

7. The feet are turned toward the head of the bed. The leg nearest the patient's head is in front of the other leg.

To move in the direction being faced.

8. Each nurse places one arm under the patient's shoulders and the other under the buttocks.

9. The nurses then grasp each other's forearm (see Figure 22-4).

Figure 22-4.

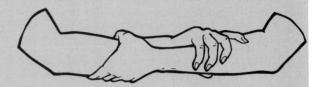

10. The patient lifts the head to the chest.

The neck will not be injured by hyperextension during the move.

11. The patient flexes his or her knees, bringing them as close as possible to the buttocks.

To provide push by using femoral muscles.

12. The nurses extend their knees.

This lifts the patient slightly.

13. The weight is shifted from the foot nearest the foot of the bed to the other foot. At the same time the nurses' bodies pivot toward the head of the bed. The patient pushes with his feet.

The nurses' weight and major gluteal and femoral muscles move the patient. The nurses' arms function to hold the patient.

14. The patient moves up toward the head of the bed.

15. Repeat if it is necessary to move the patient up further.

16. Place pillow under the patient's head and assist the patient to a comfortable position.

17. Wash hands.

Procedure 22-3.   Assisting the Back-Lying Patient to the Side of the Bed

Occasionally the nurse will need to assist a patient who must remain on his or her back to the side of the bed. This may be necessary when changing a bed or carrying out some treatment for the patient within easy reach. In this movement, the nurse's weight is used to counteract the patient's weight; the nurse's arms serve as connecting bars between the patient and the nurse.

Action

Explanation

1. Explain to the patient what you plan to do.

To reassure the patient and obtain the patient's assistance if possible.

Procedure 22-3. Cont'd

2. Wash hands.	Microorganisms will not be spread to the patient.
3. The nurse stands at the side of the bed to which the patient will move.	
4. The nurse assumes a broad stance, one foot in front of the other.	To provide balance.
5. The nurse's knees are flexed.	To bring the nurse to a working level by using the femoral muscles.
6. The patient places the arm nearest the nurse across the chest.	The arm will not stop the patient's movement or fall off the bed.
7. The nurse places an arm under the patient's far shoulder and neck.	To support the patient's head and shoulders.
8. The other arm is placed under the patient's waist.	To support the upper trunk.
9. The nurse rocks backward, shifting body weight to the rear leg, at the same time flexing knees. The nurse's hips come downward.	The nurse's weight moves the upper portion of the patient toward the side of the bed.
10. This action is repeated to move the patient's buttocks, legs, and feet.	One arm is placed under the waist, the other under the thighs to move buttocks.
11. The patient is assisted to a comfortable positon.	
12. If the nurse is not remaining at that side of the bed, a siderail is elevated.	To prevent the patient from falling off the bed.

Procedure 22-4.   Assisting a Patient to a Lateral Position

This particular movement is most easily accomplished if the patient is lying in a flat bed; however, it can also be accomplished if the head or the foot of the bed is raised. It is most easily carried out if the patient is in a straight-lying (supine) position (see section later in this chapter). Prior to turning the patient, it is frequently necessary to first move the patient to the opposite side of the bed. After the procedure, then, the patient will still be in the center of the bed.

When the nurse is assisting a patient to turn, care must be taken to control the roll so that the patient does not fall off the bed to the floor. The nurse can stop the patient's roll effectively by placing his or her elbows on the surface of the bed at the mattress's edge. In this position the nurse's forearms will brace the patient. In this movement the nurse's weight is used as the force that assists the patient to roll, and thus minimal muscular effort is required.

Action	**Explanation**
1. Explain to the patient what you plan to do.	To reassure the patient and gain cooperation if possible.
2. Wash hands.	To transmit no microorganisms.
3. The nurse stands facing the side of the bed to which the patient will turn.	
4. The nurse stands with a broad stance opposite the patient's abdomen.	The broad stance provides a stable base of support, and the abdominal area usually is the heaviest body area.

5. The patient places the arm nearest the nurse away from the body.

The patient will not roll on to the arm.

6. The patient places the far arm across the chest and the far leg over the near leg (Figure 22-5, A).

To aid in rolling.

Figure 22-5.

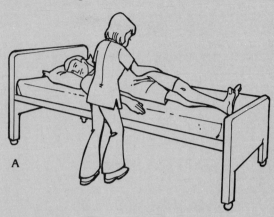

A

7. The nurse places one hand on the patient's far hip and the other hand on the far shoulder.

8. The nurse's weight is shifted from the front leg to the rear leg. The knees flex and the hips come down (see Figure 22-5, B).

The nurse's weight turns the patient to the side.

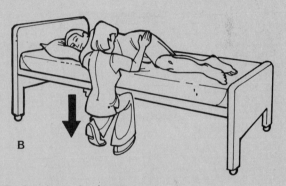

B

9. The nurse's elbows come to rest on the edge of the mattress.

To stop the patient's turn.

10. The patient is assisted to a comfortable position.

11. If the nurse is not remaining at that side of the bed, a side rail is elevated.

To prevent the patient from rolling off the bed.

Procedure 22-5.   Assisting a Patient in Bed to Raise His or Her Buttocks

This position is frequently used to assist the patient who remains in bed onto a bedpan. In this movement, the nurse's arm acts as a lever with the elbow on the bed surface as the fulcrum. The nurse's body weight is the force applied to the lever and hence to the patient.

Action

Explanation

1. Explain to the patient what you plan to do.

To reassure the patient and gain the patient's assistance if possible.

Procedure 22-5. Cont'd

2. Wash hands.

   To transmit no microorganisms to the patient.

3. The patient assumes a supine position, the head only elevated by a pillow. Adjust height according to the patient's needs.

4. The nurse stands at the patient's side opposite the buttocks. A bedpan is within easy reach if it is to be placed under the patient. Other needed supplies are also within reach.

5. The nurse assumes a broad stance with one foot in front of the other.

   To provide stability because the center of gravity falls between the feet.

6. The patient flexes the knees to bring the feet close to the buttocks.

   To use the femoral and gluteal muscles to raise the buttocks.

7. The patient places the arms at the sides, the elbows slightly bent, and the palms facing down against the bed (Figure 22-6, *A*).

   The arms will aid with the deltoid and latissimus dorsi muscles assisting in elevating the trunk. For patients who are on restricted bed rest, a trapeze may be helpful and require less effort.

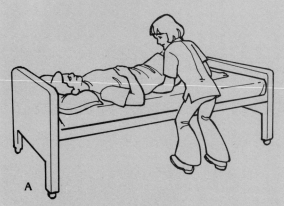

Figure 22-6.

A

8. The nurse's arm nearest the head of the bed is placed under the patient's sacrum palm upward.

9. The nurse's elbow rests on the mattress.

   It serves as the fulcrum and the arm as the lever.

10. The nurse's knees flex and buttocks lower (Figure 22-6, *B*).

    The patient's buttocks raise at the same time.

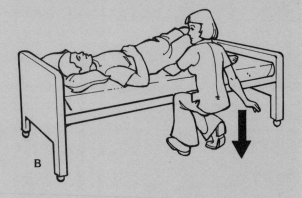

B

11. With the other hand the nurse puts the bedpan in place or massages the sacral area.

12. Assist the patient to a comfortable position.

Procedure 22-6.   Assisting a Patient to a Sitting Position in Bed

In these movements the nurse's weight is again used to counteract the patient's weight, and in one method the nurse's arm serves as a lever, the elbow as the fulcrum of the lever.

Action	**Explanation**
1. Explain to the patient what you plan to do.	To reassure the patient and to gain the patient's assistance if possible.
2. Wash hands.	To transmit no microorganisms to the patient.
3. Stand at the side of the patient's bed facing the head. Stand opposite to the patient's buttocks.	
4. Assume a broad stance with the foot nearest the bed behind the other foot.	To provide stability.
5. The patient assumes a supine position with arms at the side.	
6. If the patient is helpless, the nurse's arm farthest from the patient is placed over the near shoulder (Figure 22-7, *A*). The free arm rests on the bed surface. If the patient can assist, he or she flexes the knees, and the nurse's arm nearest the patient grasps the posterior aspect of the upper arm (Figure 22-7, *B*).	The free arm serves as a balance. The patient's arm assumes a similar position. The nurse's arm acts as a lever.

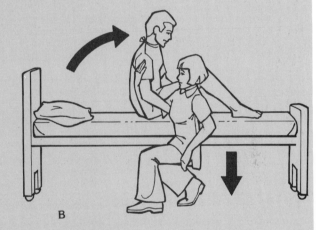

Figure 22-7.

B

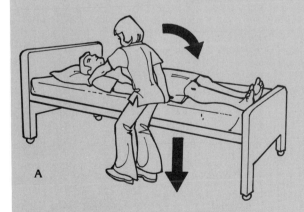

A

7. The nurse's weight shifts to the back leg, and the knees flex. The nurse's hips come downward.	The nurse's weight counteracts the patient's weight.
8. The patient's shoulders raise, and the patient assumes a sitting position.	

Procedure 22-7.   Assisting a Patient to a Sitting Position on the Edge of the Bed

In this movement the nurse's weight is again used to counterbalance the patient's weight. It is crucial in this movement that the nurse's balance is maintained while shifting weight from the front leg to the rear one.

Action	Explanation
1. Explain to the patient what you plan to do.	To reassure the patient.
2. Wash hands.	To transmit no microorganisms to the patient.
3. Assist the patient to a side-lying position facing the nurse.	See Procedure 22-4.
4. Raise the head of the bed to about 60°.	To assist raising the patient. Care must be taken that the patient does not fall.
5. The nurse stands at the side of the bed toward which the patient is facing.	
6. The nurse takes a broad stance opposite the patient's hips and faces the bottom far corner of the bed.	To provide for balance.
7. The nurse places the foot nearest to the bottom of the bed to the rear of the other foot.	To use the nurse's weight to move the patient.
8. The nurse places one arm under the shoulders of the patient and the other arm over the far thigh with the hand resting upon the posterior aspect of the thigh (Figure 22-8, *A*).	

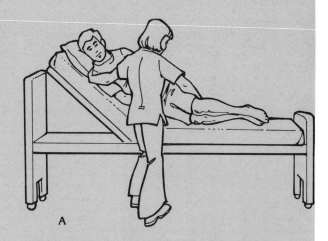

Figure 22-8.

A

9. The nurse assists the patient to place the feet and legs over the edge of the bed.

10. The nurse pivots so that the patient's legs swing downward and the nurse's weight shifts to the rear leg (Figure 22-8, *B*).

The nurse's weight counterbalances the patient's weight.

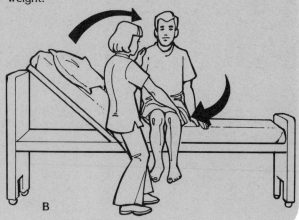

B

11. The patient assumes a sitting position.

Procedure 22-8.   **Assisting a Patient to Move Between a Bed and a Chair**

For this movement, the bed should be in the low position so that the patient can step easily to the floor. If the bed is not adjustable in this way, then a broad-based and stable footstool can be used. The patient needs to understand that he or she will step initially onto the stool and will next need to step down to the floor.

Action	Explanation
1. Explain to the patient what you plan to do.	To reassure the patient. To identify the patient.
2. Wash hands.	To transmit no microorganisms to the patient.
3. Obtain dressing gown, slippers, or shoes for the patient. Slippers or shoes should have a sole that is unlikely to slip.	
4. The patient assumes a sitting position on the side of the bed.	See Procedure 22-7.
5. Assist the patient to put on dressing gown and slippers.	
6. The chair in which the patient will sit is placed at the side of the bed with its back toward the foot of the bed. The front of the chair should be as close to the patient as possible.	
7. The nurse stands in front of the patient facing the patient. The leg of the nurse closest to the chair is in front of the other leg.	To provide smooth, balanced movement when turning.
8. The patient places the hands on the nurse's shoulders, and the nurse holds each side of the patient's waist.	To provide support for the patient.
9. When the patient steps to the floor or to a footstool, the nurse's front knee is braced against the patient's knee. Use a footstool if the bed is too high for the patient.	To prevent the patient's knees from buckling and the patient from falling.
10. After the patient feels steady, the nurse steps back with forward leg and guides the patient to the chair.	
11. The nurse's knees and hips flex as the patient lowers himself or herself to the chair.	To use the gluteal and femoral muscles and avoid back strain.
12. Assist the patient to a comfortable position.	

Two-Nurse Assist Between a Bed and a Chair

Another method of assisting a patient from a bed to a chair requires two nurses. In this method, the bed is left in the raised position.

The patient is assisted to a sitting position on the side of the bed and suitably attired for sitting out of bed. The chair for the patient is placed at the side of the bed with its back toward the foot of the bed and about 30–60 cm (1–2 ft) away from the bed.

Each nurse assumes a broad stance on opposite sides of the patient with knees flexed. Each nurse places an arm under the patient's nearest axilla, behind the back of the farthest axilla. The nurses can either hold the patient on his or her back just below the far axilla or grasp each other's forearms. The nurse's other arm is placed under the patient's thighs, where each nurse grasps the other's forearm.

The patient places his arms around each of the nurses' shoulders if possible. The nurses together extend their knees to lift the patient and then move the

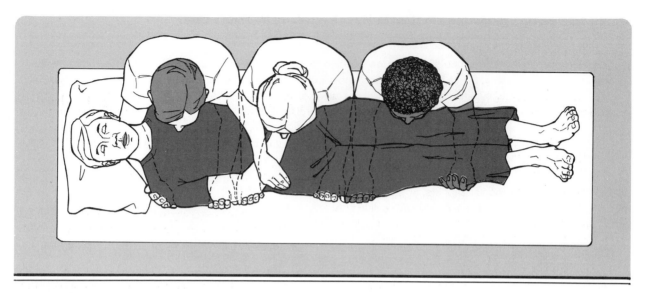

Figure 22-9.   The three-person carry. Note position of the lifters' arms.

patient to the chair with coordinated movements. The nurse nearest the chair side steps in front of the chair to the side opposite the bed while the other nurse moves forward to the side of the chair nearest the bed. The patient is now over the chair. Each nurse's knees flex as the patient is lowered into the chair.

Lifting a Patient Between a Bed and a Stretcher (Three-Man Carry)

Lifting and carrying the average adult from a bed to a stretcher or to another bed and at the same time maintaining a horizontal position generally requires three people. A child, on the other hand, may be more easily moved by just two persons and a baby by one person safely.

In the three-man lift for adult patients, the tallest person takes the upper part of the patient. This person probably has the longest reach and can thus best support the patient's head and shoulders. The second person will support the middle third of the patient, which is usually the heaviest portion. The first and third persons should place their arms next to the second person's arms in order to assist with this weight. The third person will support the patient's legs and feet. Where two people are moving a child, the first person supports the head, shoulders, and waist, and the second person supports the hips and legs.

The stretcher or bed to which the patient needs to move is best placed at right angles to the patient's bed with the head near to the foot of the bed. The wheels of both (stretcher and bed) should be locked

so that they will not slip out from under the patient.

For the three or two people to coordinate their movements, the first person at the head calls the numbers by which they move.

1. The three nurses face the side of the patient's bed. Each person assumes a broad stance with the foot closest to the direction of the movement forward, that is, if the stretcher to which the patient needs to move is to the nurse's right, the right foot of each nurse is placed in front of the left foot.

2. If the patient cannot move the arms, they need to be placed across the chest to avoid injury to them during the move.

3. At the count of "one," the nurses flex their knees and then slip their arms under the patient. The first nurse's arms are positioned under the patient's neck and shoulders and under the waist. The second nurse's arms are placed under the patient's waist and hips. The third nurse puts one arm under the patient's hips and the other arm under the lower leg (Figure 22–9).

4. At the count of "two," the nurses turn the patient slightly toward them with their elbows resting on the bed until the patient lies against them.

5. At the count of "three," each person rises, steps back with the forward foot, and walks in unison to the receiving bed or stretcher.

6. At the count of "four," the nurses flex their knees and rest their elbows on the second bed.

7. At the count of "five," the nurses extend their forearms, thus permitting the patient to gently and slowly roll to his or her back.

8. At the count of "six," the lifters withdraw their arms from beneath the patient.

DEVICES USED TO ASSIST PATIENTS TO MOVE

The Hydraulic Lifter

The hydraulic lifter is also known as a patient lifter or by the name of the particular model, such as a Hoyer lift. Each model has its own instructions regarding use, and the nurse should become aware of these in the individual setting. There are also rachet lifters available.

Some models have canvas straps, which fit under the patient in a lying position or under the buttocks and around the back of a patient in a sitting position. Two nurses are generally required when using a patient lift; one nurse guides the patient while the other operates the lift.

Lifters are used chiefly for patients who cannot help themselves, particularly those patients who are too heavy for others to lift (see Figure 22–10). Transfers are commonly made from a bed to a stretcher and from a wheelchair to a bathtub. For example, to operate a hydraulic lifter:

1. The wheelchair to which a patient is to be moved is placed nearby, allowing enough room for the lifter to be turned. The wheelchair brakes are then set.

2. The lifter is then wheeled to the bed in such a way that the wheel base is under the bed and at right angles to the bed. The height of the lifting bar is adjusted so that the canvas straps can fit under the patient.

3. The nurse then closes the hydraulic pressure valve to hold the lift bar in place.

4. The nurses then place the canvas straps under the patient, one under the buttocks and upper thighs and the other strap under the patient's back just below the level of the axillae (Figure 22–10).

5. The canvas straps are then fastened to the appropriate hooks on the lifting bar.

6. The nurse then releases the hydraulic pressure valve and pumps the lever. The lifter will then lift the patient. When the patient is clear of the bed, the nurse closes the hydraulic pressure valve.

7. One nurse then rolls the lifter to the wheelchair; the other nurse steadies the patient and guides him or her to a position over the wheelchair.

8. The hydraulic pressure valve is then released and the patient lowered into the wheelchair. The straps are then unhooked from the lifting bar and removed from beneath the patient.

The Drawsheet

A drawsheet can also be used to assist a patient to move in bed.

1. To assist a patient to move up in bed:

   a. Two nurses are required. Each nurse flexes the knees and grasps the drawsheet from opposite sides of the bed.

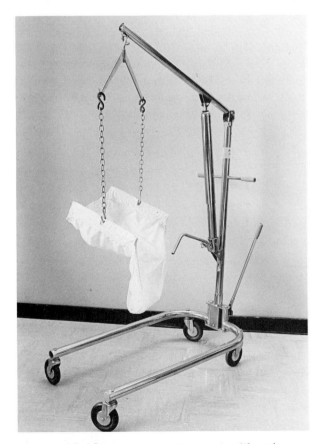

Figure 22-10.   A ratchet lifter used to lift and move patients.

b. The drawsheet should extend from the axillae to the inferior aspects of the buttocks.

c. The nurses then extend their knees and pivot, moving their weight from the foot nearest the foot of the bed to the other foot, moving the patient up toward the head of the bed.

2. To assist a patient to turn on his or her side:

a. The patient lies on his or her back, the arm nearest the nurse over the chest or slightly away from the patient's body.

b. The nurse loosens the drawsheet on the far side of the bed.

c. Standing at the side of the bed to which the patient will turn, the nurse grasps the far side of the drawsheet and pulls it over the patient in such a manner that the patient will roll over toward the nurse.

d. The nurse can use the elbows on the bed surface edge to stop the patient's turn and prevent falling if the patient is too near the edge of the bed.

HELPING PATIENTS ASSUME POSITIONS

In health a person generally assumes the position that is most comfortable. Although health is generally associated with good posture, some healthy people may require assistance to correct poor postural habits. For example, a teenage girl who has grown taller than her classmates may bend her shoulders forward to appear shorter. Even ill patients who are ambulatory will normally assume comfortable positions and may need assistance from nurses. For example, a patient with an abdominal incision may bend forward. A nurse's help is frequently required in the following situations:

1. When a patient needs to assume a specific position for therapeutic reasons. An example would be a patient who needs to assume a specific side-lying position to facilitate drainage from a wound or a patient with respiratory distress who needs to rest in an upright position.

2. When a patient is weak or paralyzed and unable to move independently.

3. When a patient is in discomfort and requires assistance to find a comfortable position.

In some situations, a physician orders a specific position for a patient. However, assisting the patient with this problem is usually a nursing function. Most patients will be most comfortable when they most closely approximate good body alignment. Many bed patients, however, will require additional supports such as pillows and sandbags. A firm mattress is essential to good alignment and a basic requirement for all positions that patients assume in a bed. The use of bed boards under the mattress is becoming increasingly frequent.

BED POSITIONS FOR PATIENTS

Bed Sitting Positions

Fowler's position (semisitting position) is frequently assumed by patients in bed for both comfort and therapeutic purposes. In this position, the head of the bed is raised to at least 45°. This position is convenient for patients when they are eating in bed, and it is a comfortable position from which to see visitors, to read, or to watch television. If it is not therapeutically contraindicated, it is a refreshing change for a person from any lying position.

In this position, the hips may or may not be flexed. Nurses will need to clarify criteria of Fowler's position in a particular agency because in some hospitals Fowler's position refers to elevation of the upper part of the body without hip flexion. The term *semi-Fowler's* in these agencies is then used to refer to the sitting position with hip flexion.

In Fowler's position, the main weight of the body is borne by the buttocks, that is, the inferior aspects of the pelvis, the ischium, which is the inferior aspect of the ilium bone. Other areas that bear less weight are the heels, the sacrum, and the scapulae.

There are two adaptations of the Fowler's position: the high Fowler's and semi-Fowler's positions. *High Fowler's* is a position in which the head of the bed is elevated to 90°, that is, at a right angle to the foundation of the bed. This position is the one most closely analogous to sitting in a chair, where the back

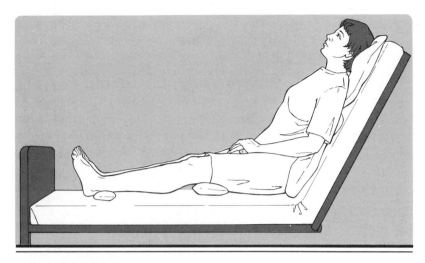

Figure 22-11.   The Fowler's position.

of the chair is in an upright angle. In this position, patients in bed can be supported by an overbed table placed in front of them. The patient then puts the arms on pillows that are placed on the table. This permits the patient to maintain body alignment and allows maximum chest expansion. This position is particularly helpful to a patient who has problems exhaling because the patient can press the lower part of the chest against the table.

Semi-Fowler's position usually refers to the elevation of the head of the bed to about 30°. This is a particularly comfortable position for patients who must remain in bed. It also provides for some chest elevation and is thus often indicated for patients who have cardiac and respiratory problems.

Patients who assume either of the Fowler's positions usually require some supportive pillows in order to support normal alignment (Table 22–2):

1. A pillow is first placed at the patient's lower back to support the lumbar spinal curve.

2. A second pillow is placed above this pillow; it should support the upper area of the back including the head. With good body alignment the patient's head should be upright, neither flexed nor hyperextended. If a patient is very thin, a third pillow may be needed to support the back and head.

3. A small pillow can be placed under the patient's thighs (Figure 22-11). This will provide slight flexion

Table 22-2.   Fowler's Position

Unsupported position	Corrective measure	Problem to be prevented
Bed sitting position with the upper part of the body elevated 30° to 90° commencing at the hips; head rests on the bed surface	Pillow at the lower back (lumbar region); second pillow to support the upper back, shoulders, and head	Posterior convexity of the lumbar curvature
Legs lie flat and straight on the lower bed surface	Small pillow under the patient's thighs to flex knees	Hyperextension of the knees
Legs externally rotated	Trochanter roll lateral to the femur	External rotation of the hips
Heels rest on the bed surface; feet in plantar flexion	Footboard to provide support for dorsal flexion	Plantar flexion
Arms fall at the sides	Pillows to support arms and hands if the patient does not have normal use of them	Shoulder muscle strain, possible dislocation of the shoulders, and edema of the hands and arms with flaccid paralysis; flexion contracture of the hand at the wrist

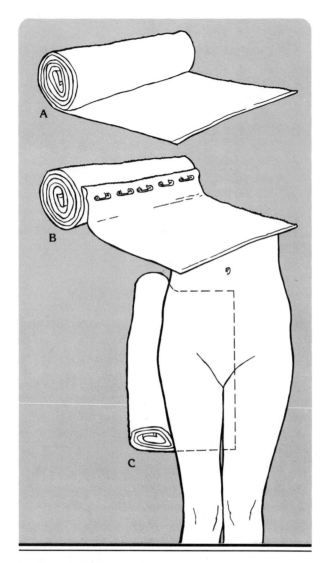

Figure 22-12.   Trochanter roll. **A,** Roll a towel to 12 inches from one end; **B,** secure roll with safety pins; and **C,** place roll against thigh with pins away from the patient.

of the knees. Supports should be used with great care under the popliteal spaces. The popliteal artery, which supplies blood to the lower leg and foot, can be occluded with continual pressure, thus inhibiting the circulation of blood and the delivery of oxygen and nutrients to the cells in those areas.

4.   A small pillow or a roll can also be used to support the ankles, thus raising the heels and reducing pressure on them from the bed. This measure is particularly important when a patient cannot move the legs or when the heels have become irritated from the prolonged pressure. A foot board will support the feet in the dorsal flexion position.

5.   A towel support, referred to as a *trochanter roll,* is placed firmly against the hips to prevent external rotation of the lower limb. A trochanter roll can be prepared by first folding a towel in half longitudinally. Then the towel is rolled tightly from one end to about one foot from the opposite end (Figure 22–12 *A*). Safety pins may be used to secure the roll (Figure 22–12, *B*). This trochanter support is then inverted with the roll lying inferior to the end of the towel. The straight part of the towel is placed under the patient's hip laterally at the area of the trochanter (Figure 22–12, *C*), and the roll is tightened securely until the thigh is well aligned.

6.   If a patient does not have movement or use of the arms, pillows at each side will support them effectively. If the arms are permitted to hang downward for a length of time, frequently the return flow of blood will be inhibited. Also, in paralyzed patients the continual pulling upon the shoulders by the weight of the arms can eventually result in dislocation of the joints and limited functioning.

Bed Lying Positions

Dorsal Recumbent Position (Supine Position)

In the dorsal recumbent position, a person lies on his or her back; the head and shoulders are usually slightly elevated with the support of a small pillow (Table 22–3). In the dorsal position, referred to as the *supine position,* the head and shoulders are not elevated. These positions are usually specifically ordered for patients by the physician, for example, after surgery upon the spinal vertebrae or after a spinal anesthetic.

In the dorsal recumbent position:

1.   The patient's head is erect or slightly flexed. It is not hyperextended with the support of a pillow. In the dorsal position (without a pillow for support), that is, the supine position, the head would be slightly hyperextended, particularly with persons who have thick chests. Although slight flexion of the cervical vertebrae helps the patient to see and eat while lying on his or her back, prolonged lying in this position can result in a permanent flexion of the cervical vertebrae and limited movement of the head.

2.   The lumbar curvature will usually be apparent. It will usually require the support of a small pillow over a firm mattress. A firm mattress will not give to the weight of the patient, thus providing good support.

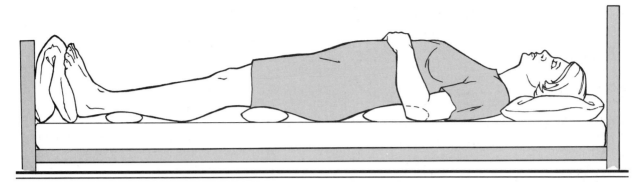

Figure 22-13.   The dorsal recumbent position.

Table 22-3.   Dorsal Recumbent Position

Unsupported position	Corrective measure	Problem to be prevented
Head flat on bed surface; may be slightly hyperextended in a thick-chested person	Pillow of suitable thickness under head and under shoulders if necessary for alignment	Hyperextension of the head and flexion of the head
Lumbar curvature of the spine apparent	Roll or small pillow under lumbar curvature	Flexion of the lumbar curvature
Legs externally rotated	Roll or sandbags placed laterally to the trochanter of the femurs	External rotation of legs
Legs extended	Small pillow under thigh to slightly flex legs	Hyperextension of knees
Feet assume plantar flexion position	Footboard or rolled pillow to support feet in dorsal flexion	Plantar flexion and footdrop

3. Normally, in this position the thighs of the patient will rotate externally. By placing a roll at the lateral aspects of the thighs opposite the femoral trochanters, the patient's legs will stay in alignment.

4. In good body alignment, the knees are normally slightly flexed. To attain this and thus support a comfortable position, small pads or pillows are placed under the thighs superior to the popliteal spaces (Figure 22–13). The avoidance of direct pressure upon these spaces has already been explained.

5. Without support, the feet in this position will normally assume a plantar flexion position. If this is maintained for a prolonged period, the gastrocnemius and soleus muscles of the lower legs become

involuntarily contracted, resulting in a condition known as *footdrop.* With this condition a person is unable to put the heel of the foot on the floor and thus is unable to walk appropriately.

Prone Position

In the prone position a person lies on his or her abdomen, legs extended and head turned to the side. This position is often used by children and adults as a comfortable sleeping position. In some instances, people flex one or both arms over their heads. This prone position is the only position other than the supine position in which the patient does not have the hips flexed. For this reason it is recommended as an alter-

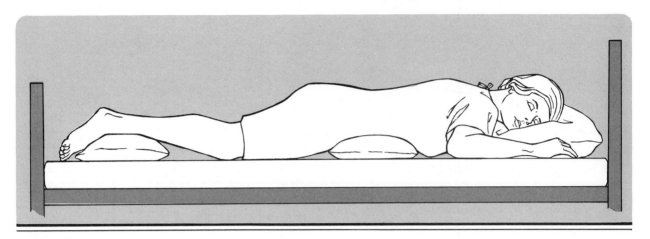

Figure 22-14.   The prone position.

Table 22-4.   Prone Position

Unsupported position	Corrective measure	Problem to be prevented
Head turned to the side and slightly flexed	Small pillow unless contraindicated because of promotion of mucous drainage from the mouth	Flexion or hyperextension of the head
Lying flat on abdomen accentuating lumbar curve	Small pillow or roll under abdomen just below the diaphragm	Hyperextension of the lumbar curvature; difficulty breathing; pressure on breasts of a woman
Toes on bed surface; foot in plantar flexion; legs extended	Pillow under lower legs to raise toes off the bed surface and flex leg slightly	Plantar flexion of feet

native position for patients on prolonged bed rest since it maintains normal alignment of the hips (Table 22–4).

In the prone position:

1. The patient's head is turned to the side and rests either on the flat surface of the bed or on a small pillow. A thick pillow will probably hyperextend the head.

2. Another small pillow under the patient just below the diaphragm will serve to support the lumbar curvature of the spine, ease breathing, and at the same time take some of the weight of the body off the breasts of a woman (Figure 22–14).

3. A pillow placed under the lower legs will serve two purposes. It will raise the toes off the surface of the bed, thereby eliminating the discomfort of weight borne by the toes, and at the same time reduce plantar flexion. The pillow will also slightly flex the legs at the knees.

Lateral Position (Side-lying Position)

The lateral position is a comfortable position for most people and a welcome change for the patient who spends a good deal of time in the dorsal recumbent position. The advantages of this position are that (a) pressure is taken off the back of the head, scapulae, sacrum, and heels, and (b) the legs and the feet without support are in a state of flexion rather than the state of extension of the supine position. The major disadvantage is the tendency for the upper shoulder and upper thigh to rotate inward unless adequately supported.

In the lateral position, the patient lies on his or her side, and most of the body weight is borne by the lateral aspect of the lower scapula and the lateral aspect of the lower ilium. Support is provided in the following ways (Table 22–5 and Figure 22–15):

1. A pillow under the head will support the head in good alignment and prevent flexion of the head

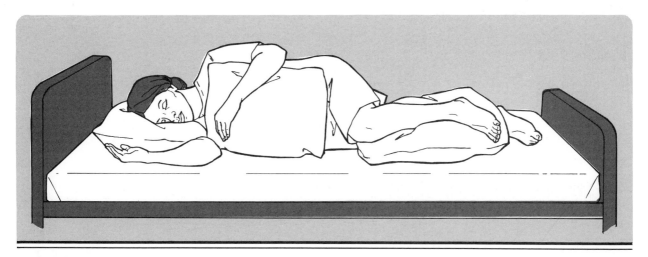

Figure 22-15.   The lateral (side-lying) position.

Table 22-5.   Lateral Position

Unsupported position	Corrective measure	Problem to be prevented
Body turned to the side, both arms in front on body, weight resting primarily on lateral aspects of the scapula and the ilium	Pillow under head to provide good alignment	Lateral flexion and fatigue of sternocleidomastoid muscles
Upper arm and shoulder rotate internally and adduct	Pillow under arm to place it in good alignment	Internal rotation and adduction of shoulder and subsequent limited function
Upper thigh and leg rotate internally and adduct	Pillow under leg and thigh to place them in good alignment	Internal rotation of thigh and adduction and subsequent limited function

laterally and fatigue of the sternocleidomastoid muscles.

2. In this side-lying position, both arms are in a slightly flexed position in front of the body. A pillow is generally needed to support the upper arm and shoulder, which tend to rotate internally. Supporting the shoulder and arm also permits the chest to expand more easily, thus facilitating breathing.

3. The upper leg will also require a pillow in order to prevent internal rotation and adduction of the hip.

4. A rolled pillow is placed at the patient's back.

Sim's Position (Semiprone Position)

Sim's position is similar to the lateral position in that the patient lies on his or her side. The main difference

between the two positions is that in Sim's the patient's weight is borne by the anterior aspects of the ilium (hip) and the humerus and clavicle (shoulder) rather than the lateral aspects of the ilium and by the scapula. Therefore, in Sim's position, the points of pressure of the body differ from those in the lateral, Fowler's, dorsal recumbent, and prone positions (see Figure 22–16).

Sim's position is frequently used for patients who are unconscious because it facilitates the drainage of mucus from the mouth. It is also a comfortable position for many people, including women who are in the last trimester of pregnancy.

In Sim's position, the patient's lower arm is behind him or her, and the upper arm is flexed at both the shoulder and the elbow. Both legs are also flexed in front of the patient. The upper one is more acutely flexed at the hip and the knee than the lower one.

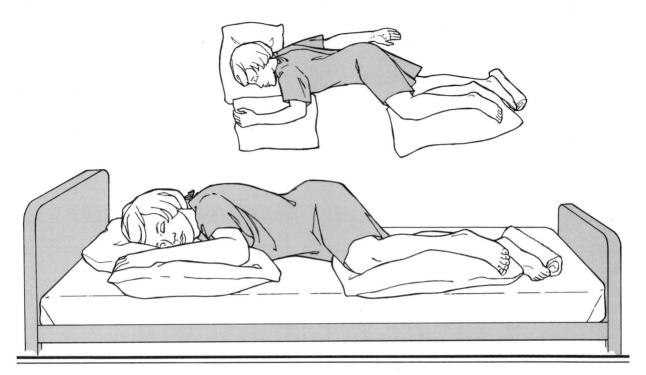

Figure 22-16.   Sim's position.

Table 22-6.   Sim's Position (Semiprone Position)

Unsupported position	Corrective measure	Problem to be prevented
Head rests upon the bed surface, weight borne by the lateral aspects of the cranial and aacial bones	Pillow supports the head, maintaining it in good alignment	Lateral flexion of the neck and head
The upper shoulder and arm are internally rotated	Pillow under the arm places it in alignment	Internal rotation of the shoulder and arm; pressure upon the chest restricting expansion during breathing
The upper leg and thigh are adducted and internally rotated	Pillow under the leg to support it in alignment	Internal rotation and adduction of the hip and leg
Plantar flexion of the feet	Sandbags to support the feet in dorsal flexion	Foot drop if position is maintained for a prolonged period

Support is provided in the following ways (Table 22-6):

1. A pillow placed under the patient's head will keep the head in good alignment, thus preventing lateral flexion of the head and neck. This is generally indicated unless mucus drainage from the mouth is to be facilitated by the laterally flexed position.

2. A pillow under the patient's upper arm will per- mit internal rotation of the shoulder and arm and permit chest expansion necessary for breathing.

3. A pillow under the upper leg will prevent ad- duction and internal rotation of the hip and leg.

4. The feet normally assume a plantar flexed posi- tion. If Sim's position is to be maintained for a prolonged period, supports to promote dorsal flexion of the feet are indicated. Sandbags are fre- quently used for this purpose.

GUIDELINES TO NURSING CARE

Each patient has specific needs related to personal health. These needs are identified by the patient and various members of the health team. Some of these are best met with the assistance of nursing personnel, for example, those related to movement and to body position. Although each patient has personal needs and a plan of care, there are certain guidelines that the nurse can use to assist in planning care related to body positions.

1. A pillow beneath the head, unless contraindicated, should be of sufficient thickness as to support the patient's head in an aligned position, neither flexing, hyperextending, or laterally flexing it.

2. The feet need to be supported with a footboard, sandbags, or rolls in a dorsal flexion position if the patient is to remain in bed for a prolonged period or if the patient is unable to move the feet freely.

3. The extremities should be in positions in which they can move freely whenever this is possible. For example, the top bedclothes need to be loose enough so that the patient can move the feet.

4. The elbows, hips, and knees should be slightly flexed.

5. The shoulders and the hips should be supported away from the body.

6. A patient should change position fairly frequently, at least every two hours.

7. Joints need exercise, either active or passive, regularly—generally, at least once each day. (See Chapter 23.)

8. Pressure areas of the body need special care with each change of position (See Chapter 20 "Decubitus Ulcers").

9. See Table 22–7 for some postural deviations.

Table 22-7.   Some Postural Deviations

Deviation	Description	Cause	Solution
1. Torticollis (twisted or wry neck)	Limitation of the range of motion of the neck with lateral inclination and rotation of the head away from the midline of the body	Congenital muscular contraction of the sternocleidomastoid muscle due to birth injury or vascular insufficiency	Daily stretching of involved muscle is effective in most situations; surgical release of one of the muscle attachments is occasionally needed
2. Scoliosis	Lateral curvature of the spine, which increases during active growth periods	May be secondary to other deformities such as a discrepancy in leg lengths or other defects of spinal supporting tissues (a functional scoliosis); most common cause of structural scoliosis is heredity, which produces an idiopathic structural scoliosis, a condition occurring five times more often in females than males, between the ages of 8 and 15	Treatment of underlying cause or bracing or casting from occiput to pelvis; surgical fusion of the spinal vertebrae may be necessary

Table 22-7. Cont'd

Deviation	Description	Cause	Solution
3. Kyphosis (roundback or humpback)	A fixed flexion deformity of the thoracic spine	Cause is unknown	Exercises to extend thoracic spine; sleeping without a pillow; occasionally bracing or spinal fusion may be required
4. Lordosis (swayback)	A fixed extension deformity of the lumbar spine	Most often occurs secondarily to other abnormalities such as kyphosis or muscular dystrophy	The underlying disease is treated
5. Hip dislocation	A bilateral or unilateral instability of the hip in infants with adduction contracture and limited abduction of the hip; after walking starts, the foot may be externally rotated, the thigh shortened due to proximal dislocation of the head of the femur; the knee joint is higher on the affected side, and the inguinal and gluteal creases may be asymmetrical	Congenital abnormality; breech deliveries	Treatment varies with age; infants are double diapered to abduct the hips, or abduction splints may be used; in young children a closed reduction and casting may be necessary; in older children, open reduction (surgery) may be required
6. Genu valgum (knock-knees)	The medial aspects of the knees touch each other in the standing position and the feet remain apart; normal between 3 and 4 years of age	Usually a developmental variant if not due to rickets or a congenital bone disorder	Corrected by growth; in some cases knee braces are used if knee ligaments become stretched
7. Genu varum (bowlegs)	The feet are held together but the knees remain apart; bowlegs are normal until the age of 2 to 2½ years	Same as for genu valgum	Corrected by growth; measurement of distance between the knees when inner ankles are held together gauges the process
8. Pronation (flatfoot)	The medial longitudinal arch of the foot is relaxed, and weight is borne on the medial side of the foot; in most cases what appears to be flatfootedness is the normal appearance of the infant or toddler's foot; fat pads create a fullness suggestive of a flatfoot	Familial occurrence	Young children are taught to stand on tiptoes 5 to 10 minutes daily; older children are taught to walk pigeon-toed 5 to 10 minutes daily with weight thrown on the lateral border of the foot; mechanical supports for the arch such as medial heel wedges or shoe inserts may be necessary
9. Talipes equinovarus (clubfoot)	The foot is malpositioned in plantar flexion (equinus) at the ankle with adduction and inversion of the heel and forefoot	Males are affected twice as often as females; cause is unknown; it is thought to be partly due to heredity and partly due to abnormal intrauterine position	Casts and splints such as Denis Browne splint; surgical correction may be needed in difficult situations

Deviation	Description	Cause	Solution
10. Toeing-in (pigeon-toe)	The entire foot or the forefoot only is rotated inward; some degree of toeing-in is common with all infants from their intrauterine position	Three Common Causes: 1. Metatarsus adductus (adduction of the forefoot with no deformity of the hind foot), a congenital disorder 2. Inward tibial torsion, which is always associated with a tibial bow; this can be aggravated by infants sleeping on their knees with feet turned inward or sitting on top of inturned feet 3. Inward femoral torsion	1. Passive stretching, reverse shoe, or casts and wedging started as early as possible 2. Growth corrects tibial torsion; train children to avoid harmful postures; wearing reverse shoes for a time may be helpful 3. No treatment required; correction does not occur with growth, but the development of an outward tibial torsion compensates for the defect

EVALUATION GUIDE FOR BODY POSITIONS

When nurses assist patients to maintain certain positions, some facts can assist in determining the adequacy of the position for the patient. The following guide should be considered for each patient:

1. The posture of the patient reflects good anatomical relationships between the various parts of the body. The body of the patient is as close to good body alignment in a standing or sitting position as possible.

2. The muscles are not becoming strained and tired.

3. The position of the hands is similar to that used to grasp a ball.

4. The position of the feet is dorsal flexion (that position assumed when standing).

5. The pressure points of the body (points on which body weight rests), for example, the sacrum, appear healthy; that is, they have the same color as the other parts of the skin, are intact and free of abrasions, are warm to touch, and convey a normal sense of feeling to the patient.

6. The joints can move through their normal ranges of motion.

7. The patient appears comfortable.

SUMMARY

For patients who are ill, moving even a little in bed can be a major challenge. Some patients are completely unable to move and rely upon nursing personnel to change position. A knowledge of body mechanics will assist nurses to help patients without injuring themselves or the patients.

Good posture is essential to normal physiologic functioning. There are characteristics of the well-aligned person both standing and sitting. The woman who is pregnant also needs to maintain correct body alignment. Beginning with the second trimester the postural changes of pregnancy start. Correct posture is important in preventing strain upon the spinal muscles and joints. Characteristically posture changes with age. It is important to know normal posture to assess abnormal alignment.

Specific guidelines can be applied to assist a patient to move. By employing the guidelines the nurse can assist patients in various ways in bed and out of bed. Two devices that are used to assist patients to move are the lift and the drawsheet. The use of these will often decrease the effort required by the patient and the nurse.

Patients assume a variety of positions in bed for both comfort and therapeutic reasons. Assisting a patient to assume a position and providing the required support are nursing functions. Once a patient has assumed a particular position, nurses need to provide care in terms of exercise, skin care, and change of position.

SUGGESTED ACTIVITIES

1. Observe the normal posture of individuals in each of the seven age groups: the newborn or infant, the toddler, the child, the adolescent, the adult, the pregnant woman, and the aged. Note similarities and differences.

2. In a hospital note the bed positions assumed by the patients. Analyze the positions in terms of body alignment. Draw up a plan to correct any poorly aligned position.

3. Using a student as a patient, assist the patient to move in bed as described in this chapter. Ask another student to observe your body mechanics while you are doing this.

SUGGESTED READINGS

Ford, Jack R., and Duckworth, Bridget. January, 1976. Moving a dependent patient safely, comfortably. Part I. Positioning. *Nursing 76* 6(1): 27–36.

These authors, a remedial gymnast and an occupational therapist, respectively, offer step-by-step procedures for positioning patients who are paralyzed and dependent upon others for movement. A photo story enhances the content. It is emphasized that no one method of moving patients works for everyone, since nurses vary in size, weight, and strength, and patients vary in their dependency needs.

Ford, Jack R., and Duckworth, Bridget. February, 1976. Moving a dependent patient safely, comfortably. Part 2. Transferring. *Nursing 76* 6(2): 58–65.

This second article emphasizes transfer techniques and presents a wide variety of methods for transferring a paralyzed patient from bed to wheelchair or from wheelchair to toilet and back. The nurse is advised to practice a variety of techniques to find which method works best in specific situations.

SELECTED REFERENCES

American Rehabilitation Foundation. 1962. *Rehabilitative nursing techniques. 1. Bed positioning and transfer procedures for the hemiplegic*. Minneapolis, Minn.

Bilger, Annetta J., and Greene, Ellen H., eds. 1973. *Winters' protective body mechanics*. New York: Springer Publishing Co.

Clausen, Joy Princeton, et al. 1973. *Maternity nursing today*. New York: McGraw-Hill Book Co.

Dickason, Elizabeth J., and Schult, Martha O., eds. 1975. *Maternal and infant care. A text for nurses*. New York: McGraw-Hill Book Co.

Drapeau, Janine. September, 1975. Getting back into good posture: how to erase your lumbar aches. *Nursing 75* 5(9): 63–65.

Helms, Donald B., and Turner, Jeffrey S. 1976. *Exploring child behavior*. Philadelphia: W. B. Saunders Co.

Mitchell, John J. 1973. *Human life: the first ten years*. Toronto: Holt, Rinehart and Winston of Canada, Ltd.

Nordmark, Madelyn T., and Rohweder, Anne W. 1975. *Scientific foundations of nursing*, 3rd ed. Philadelphia: J. B. Lippincott Co.

Nursing 74. October 1974. How to negotiate the ups and downs, ins and outs of body alignment. *Nursing 74* 4(10): 46–51.

Rantz, Marilyn J., and Courtial, Donald. 1977. *Lifting, moving and transferring patients: a manual*. St. Louis: The C. V. Mosby Co.

Smith, David W., and Bierman, Edwin L. 1973. *The biologic ages of man: from conception through old age*. Philadelphia: W. B. Saunders Co.

Stevens, Carolyn B. 1974. *Special needs of long-term patients*. Philadelphia: J. B. Lippincott Co.

CHAPTER 23

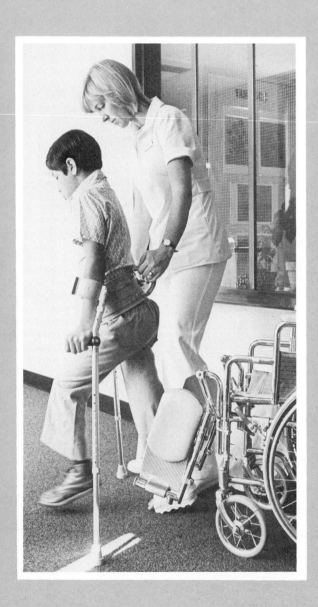

EXERCISE AND AMBULATION

PRENATAL AND POSTNATAL EXERCISES

   Prenatal Exercises

   Postnatal Exercises

EFFECTS OF EXERCISE

COMMON PROBLEMS OF JOINT AND MUSCLE MOVEMENTS

AMBULATION

   Exercises Preparatory to Ambulation

   Assisting a Patient to Walk

   Mechanical Aids for Walking

IMMOBILITY

   Kinds of Immobility

THE PROBLEMS OF IMMOBILITY

   Psychologic and Social Effects

   Physical Effects

THE CONCEPT OF REHABILITATION

OBJECTIVES

- Explain the various factors that affect mobility.
- Discuss how mobility develops from birth to 5 years.
- List the types of synovial joints.
- Describe the major range-of-motion exercises.
- Identify physical fitness.
- Assess the needs of individual people in relation to joint flexibility exercises, muscle tone exercises, and endurance exercises.
- Explain the kinds of exercises.
- Assist a patient to select and carry out appropriate exercises.
- Advise about isometric, prenatal, and postnatal exercises.
- Describe the effects of exercise.
- Assist a patient to prepare for ambulation.
- Assist individual patients to ambulate.
- Describe the types of immobility.
- Explain the problems of immobility.
- Describe the concept of rehabilitation.

Activity has been described as energetic action or being in a state of movement. Being mobile and able to move freely is essential and normal for most people. The loss of mobility even for a short time generally requires tremendous adjustments on the part of the person and family.

This chapter will discuss the need for mobility and activity by people of all ages and conversely the effects that rest in bed (immobility) and inactivity can have upon people. A description of the physically fit person will assist nursing students to identify problems that people may have when they exercise inadequately. The kinds of exercise are described together with guidelines for nurses when they are assisting patients to meet their exercise needs. The six different types of joints are described together with the types of movements which are normally possible. Specific exercises for special situations are also included.

Because many sick people spend more time in bed than they would normally, ambulation can become a major problem to them. Helping patients retain or regain their ambulatory skills can be an important area of nursing function. Not only does ambulation usually mean to patients that they are closer to resuming their normal activities, it also can mean that many problems connected with immobility are likely to be avoided.

Although most physical activity also serves as a stimulus to the mind, diversional activities are chiefly directed to this end. Not only do they help patients pass the time, they can also serve to meet needs for accomplishment and serve as vehicles for socializing for people who may otherwise have few common interests. These stimulation needs will be discussed subsequently in Chapter 34. In this chapter it will be seen that physical activity is a basic need of people and one with which the nurse is frequently called upon to assist patients.

MOBILITY

Being mobile, that is, being able to move about freely, is a basic need of people. To be able to carry out most of life's daily activities a person needs to be able to move. However, movement is not just moving one's self from place to place; a person's gestures, facial expressions, and mannerisms also depend upon the ability to move.

Mobility is altered chiefly by one or more of four reasons:

1. The age and developmental status of the person.
2. A disease process or injury.
3. Restriction by external factors such as a physician's prescription or a traction device.
4. Voluntary restriction of activity so that the person maintains psychologic equilibrium or conserves energy.

Age and Developmental Status

The mobility of a person varies according to age and individual development. The newborn baby has uncontrolled movement; many elderly persons have a typical stance (see "Developmental Variations in Body Movement").

Disease Process or Injury

To be able to move, a person needs to have a functioning musculoskeletal system and central nervous system. Disease processes such as multiple sclerosis or injuries such as those which affect the spinal cord will impede a person's mobility.

Restriction by External Factors

A person who has a disease or is injured is often restricted in activity on a physician's advice. Bed rest is not uncommon in illness. It usually has two purposes: (a) to conserve the body's energy so that a diseased or injured part of the body will heal and (b) to prevent further damage to a body part. A person who has had a myocardial infarction (an infarct in the heart muscle) usually requires bed rest for both these purposes. A person with a fractured hip may be confined to bed with the leg in traction until adequate healing has taken place. Even when people enter the hospital their activity is generally restricted by regulations of the institution.

Voluntary Restriction

Sometimes people voluntarily restrict their activity, without always knowing why or without feeling ill. The reason is generally that the person requires withdrawal from physical and psychologic stressors to maintain physical and psychologic equilibria. A student, after final examinations, may only want to go to bed and to sleep to regain energy and stability.

DEVELOPMENTAL VARIATIONS IN BODY MOVEMENT

The Neonate (Birth to 28 Days)

In neonates the function of the central nervous system is immature for some time after birth. Control of their motor activity thus lacks coordination. As a result their extremities move in a random fashion, and they cannot direct their movements toward any purpose. However, their muscles are firm, and when an extremity is extended passively, flexor muscles will offer assistance. Many of the newborn's activities present at birth are reflexive. These are:

1. coughing and sneezing
2. yawning
3. hiccupping
4. blinking
5. shivering
6. withdrawal from pain
7. crying when uncomfortable
8. sucking
9. rooting
10. swallowing, gagging, vomiting
11. grasp reflex
12. walking or stepping (dance) reflex
13. Moro reflex
14. tonic neck reflex

The last four are discussed in this chapter.

The Moro Reflex

The Moro reflex is also referred to as the *startle response* and is present from birth until about the fourth or fifth month. When the baby is lying quietly and then is suddenly jarred, the baby responds symmetrically by drawing the legs up and by throwing the arms forward. The response can be elicited by jerking a blanket beneath the baby, jarring the crib, or suddenly removing head support after holding the baby quietly. Lack of the Moro reflex or asymmetrical responses suggests some neurologic damage.

The Tonic Neck Reflex

The tonic neck reflex is alternatively called the *fencing position*. The infant lying on his or her back assumes a position similar to the stance of a fencer. The head is turned either to the left or the right, and the arm and leg on the side that the baby faces is extended. The opposite arm and leg are flexed. This reflex gradually disappears in several months as the nervous system develops. With increased motor control a symmetrical position is assumed.

The Stepping (Walking or Dancing) Reflex

The stepping reflex soon disappears after birth. In this reflex the newborn responds with dancing movements of the legs when the infant is held in the upright position and the feet touch a solid surface. Absence of the dance reflex suggests central nervous system or peripheral nerve damage.

The Grasp Reflex

The normal newborn has a well-developed grasp reflex. The fist automatically clenches around any object that touches the palm of the hand, such as the mother's index finger. Some newborns, not all, are able to be pulled into an upright position. This response is referred to as the *Darwinian reflex*. As motor control increases the infant soon learns to grasp and then release objects voluntarily.

The Infant (28 Days to 1 Year)

Movement of the Head

When placed in a prone position, newborn infants can turn the head readily from side to side and by 4 weeks of age can lift it off the surface.

At 3 months of age infants can lift their head and chest from the surface with arms extended in front, and at 4 months they can raise the head to the vertical position and turn it easily from side to side. By 7 months infants in the prone position can pivot when pursuing an object.

When in the supine position infants lie with the head turned to one side. In this supine position at 6 months they can lift the head up and spend much time showing interest in their legs.

Head control is lacking when infants are placed in a sitting position or an upright position until about 5 months of age. In the first 2 months the head falls backward when they are pulled from a supine to a sitting position, and it bobs around without control in the upright position. For this reason, when picking

Table 23-1.   Summary of Motor Skills From Birth to 5 Years of Age

	Motor Skill		Motor Skill
	First Month		**At Seven Months**
Prone:	Lies in flexed position; turns head from side to side	Prone:	Can pivot and roll over
Supine:	Generally flexed and somewhat stiff	Supine:	Lifts head; rolls over; squirms
Active reflexes:	Moro response; grasp reflex; dance reflex; tonic neck reflex	Sitting:	Sits briefly leaning forward on hands; spine is rounded from head to buttock
	At One Month	Standing:	May support most of weight and bounces
Prone:	Holds chin up; turns head; lies with legs more extended	Manual:	Reaches and grasps large objects with thumb to palm; transfers items from hand to hand; rakes at small objects
Supine:	Tonic neck posture is predominant; body is more relaxed and supple; head falls backward when pulled to sitting position		**At 10 Months**
		Sitting:	Sits up alone without support; spine is straight
	At Two Months	Standing:	Pulls to standing position
Prone:	Raises head farther; active infants may roll over	Moving:	Creeps or crawls
Supine:	Same as 1 month		**At 12 Months**
	At Three Months		Walks with one hand held or by holding onto furniture
Prone:	Arches back, lifts head and chest with arms extended forward; makes crawling movements with legs		**At 15 Months**
			Walks alone; crawls upstairs
Supine:	Tonic neck posture still predominant; reaches toward but misses objects; indicates a preference for prone or supine position		**At 18 Months**
			Runs awkwardly; sits on small chair; walks upstairs with one hand held, one foot at a time; explores all objects in reach
Sitting:	Head lag partially controlled on pull to sitting position; back is rounded		**At 24 Months**
Manual:	Clutching and scratching movements		Runs well; walks up and down stairs with one hand held; one step at a time; climbs on furniture; opens doors; can tower building blocks; can scribble in circular manner
Active reflexes:	Moro response is absent; makes some defensive withdrawal reactions		**At 30 Months**
			Jumps
	At Four to Six Months		**At 36 Months**
Prone:	Lifts head and chest; head is held in a near vertical axis; legs are extended; intentional rolling over by 4 months		Goes upstairs alternating feet; rides tricycle; stands on one foot
Supine:	Symmetrical posture predominates; hands held in midline; reaches and grasps objects; objects brought to mouth		**At 48 Months**
			Hops on one foot; throws ball; climbs well; manipulates scissors
Sitting:	Head is held erect, steady, and forward on pull to sitting position; enjoys sitting with spinal and head support		**At 60 Months**
Standing:	Pushes with feet when held upright		Skips
Manual:	Arm and hands progress to coordinated reaching and grasping; picks up objects at 4 months; intentionally releases them at 6 months		

up or holding a newborn, the nurse must support the head and back (which bows forward).

By 3 months of age some head control is evident when infants hold the head forward in the upright position. At 4 months they can hold the head fairly erect in the sitting position but tilt the head slightly forward in the upright position. By 5 months, the head is held steadily in the erect position.

Movements of the Hands

The grasp reflex continues for about two months until eye and hand coordination develop sufficiently for an active grasp to become possible. At 3 months of age, infants attempt to hold an offered object briefly and can purposefully get their hand to their mouth to satisy sucking needs. At 4 months infants can grasp objects of moderate size and move them to their mouth for exploration. Small objects are not properly visualized. By 6 months they can extend a hand toward a desired large object such as a rattle, grasp it, and transfer it from hand to hand. By 7 months they can visualize small objects, and although they may pursue these small objects by raking motions of the fingers, they are unable to pick them up.

After 6 months the hand movements primarily involve the radial side. At first the thumb is used in conjunction with the palm of the hand. Between 6 and 9 months the movements are more clearly refined into pincer motions of the thumb and forefinger. At 9 months the index finger is used to poke at objects. At 9 months an infant might release an object upon request if another person grasps the object. By one year most infants will independently release an object into an offered hand.

Sitting

By 4 to 5 months of age infants enjoy being in a sitting position but must be supported. Not until after 6 months are infants able to sit alone as they lean forward on their hands. By 8 to 9 months they can assume a sitting position from the supine position without help.

Standing, Creeping, and Walking

At 5 to 6 months infants will support their weight upon extended legs when pulled from a sitting to a standing position. After 6 months they will often flex their knees and return to the standing posture with help. By 8 months they are able to stand steadily for a short while as long as their hands are held. By 9 to 10 months most infants have mastered creeping or crawling and can walk a few steps if both hands are held.

The One- to Five-Year Old

During the second year children begin to reveal a high degree of locomotor control, progressing from an awkward upright stance to taking a few steps with assistance. Children develop the ability to walk alone by 15 months. The skill of running is acquired at about 18 months although the motion at first appears awkward and stiff. Between 18 and 24 months children are very active and run about, often into dangerous environments unless safeguarded. This is the age that has been so aptly called the "terrible twos," in which children actively and vigorously exploit all objects in their environment. Everything within reach is grasped and examined; waste baskets, drawers, and shelves will all be emptied. Motor control of the hand is also refined. For example, they will place small objects into small containers, balance building blocks one on top of the other, and scribble on paper, eventually producing some vertical, horizontal, and circular lines.

The ability to climb stairs begins at the age of 18 months when children can ascend one step at a time with one hand held. Going downstairs in the same manner soon follows. By 3 years of age children can alternate feet when ascending stairs and descend in the same manner by the age of 4. Standing on one foot is mastered by most children at the age of 3 and by the age of 5 most can hop on one foot and skip. See Table 23-1 for Summary of Motor Skills from Birth to 5 Years of Age.

MOVEMENT OF THE JOINTS

Range of Motion

The range of motion of a joint is the maximum movement that is possible for that joint. Not all people possess a similar range of motion. Each person's range of motion is determined by genetic inheri-

tances, developmental patterns, the presence or absence of disease, and the amount of physical activity in which the person normally engages.

The body has six types of synovial joints and certain specific movements that are normally possible for each type. A *synovial joint* is freely movable and characteristically has a cavity enclosed by a capsule. Within this capsule is a lining of synovial membrane, which secretes synovial fluid to lubricate the joint. Cartilage of a joint provides a smooth surface upon which a bone can glide during movement. Thick bands of collagenous fibers extending from one bone to another are called *ligaments*; these provide strength for the joint, and they are usually stretched tautly when the joint is in the position of greatest stability. The muscles surrounding the joint provide the most stability for the joints. Synovial joints of the body serve primarily to bear weight and to provide for movement.

Types of Synovial Joints

Ball and Socket

The ball-shaped head of one bone fits into the concave socket of another bone or bones. This type of joint provides for the greatest movement in all planes. Examples are the hip and shoulder joints.

Hinge

In the hinge joint the bone with a convex surface fits into a concave surface. The motion of this type of joint is limited to flexion and extension; examples are the elbow and knee joints.

Pivot

The motion of the pivot joint is limited to rotation only. The joint is made up of a process that rotates within a bony fossa around a longitudinal axis. Examples are the axis and atlas joints of the vertebral column.

Condyloid

In the condyloid joint an oval-shaped bony projection fits into an elliptical cavity. This kind of joint does not permit rotation; it only permits movement in two planes. An example of a condyloid joint is the wrist, which permits all movements but rotation.

Saddle

In the saddle joint each bony surface has a convex and concave surface so that the two bones fit together. This kind of joint does not permit rotation, but movement is possible in the two planes at right angles to each other. For example, the carpometacarpal joint of

the thumb and hand permits flexion and extension, abduction and adduction.

Gliding

The gliding joint is formed when the two bone surfaces are flat or when one is slightly convex and the other is slightly concave. The motion of the joint is a gliding one, such as the joint between the tibia and fibula and the intervertebral joints.

Synovial Joint Movements

Each type of synovial joint has specific movements of which it is capable. These movements are described in relation to the anatomical body position and the three body planes: sagittal, transverse, and coronal.

The following are movements of synovial joints:

1. *Flexion.* Decreasing the angle of the joint (between two bones), that is, the act of bending, as in bending the arm at the elbow joint.

2. *Extension.* Increasing the angle of the joint (between two bones), that is, the act of straightening, as in straightening the arm at the elbow joint.

3. *Hyperextension.* Further extension or stretching out at a joint, as in bending the head backward.

4. *Abduction.* Movement of the bone away from the midline of the body, as in raising the arm at the shoulder joint laterally.

5. *Adduction.* Movement of the bone toward the midline of the body, as in lowering the arm held laterally toward the side of the body.

6. *Rotation.* Movement of the bone around its central axis, for example, turning one's head as if to look over the shoulder. Internal rotation is turning away from the midline. An example of these kinds of rotation occurs at the hip joint. In the back-lying position a person's leg normally rotates externally at the hip.

7. *Circumduction.* The distal part of the bone moves in a circle while the proximal end remains fixed. An example would be describing a circle with the arm, moving the shoulder joint.

8. *Eversion.* Turning the sole of the foot outward by moving the ankle joint.

9. *Inversion.* Turning the sole of the foot inward by moving the ankle joint.

10 *Pronation.* Moving the bones of the forearm so that the palm of the hand is moved from anterior to

posterior in anatomic position or turning them face downward when held in front of the person.

11.   *Supination*. Moving the bones of the forearm so that the palm of the hand is moved from posterior to anterior in anatomic position or turning them face upward when held in front of the person.

12.   *Protraction*. Moving a part of the body forward in the same plane parallel to the ground, for example, pushing the lower jaw outward.

13.   *Retraction*. Moving a part of the body backward in the same plane parallel to the ground, for example, pulling the lower jaw inward.

Procedure 23-1.   Major Range of Motion Exercises

Action	Explanation

Neck

1.   Flex the neck by bringing the chin to rest on the chest (Figure 23-1, *A*).

2.   Extend neck by returning the head to an upright position (Figure 23-1, *B*).

3.   Hyperextend the neck by bending the head back as far as possible (Figure 23-1, *C*).

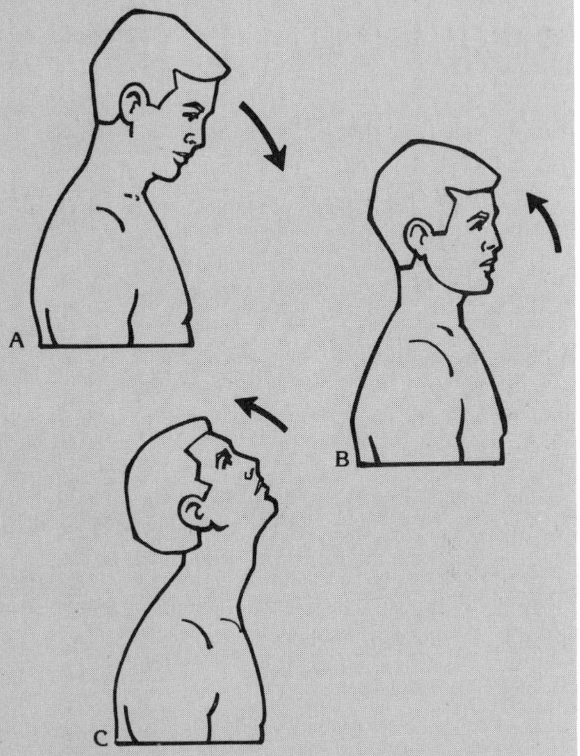

Figure 23-1.

4.   Laterally flex the neck by tilting the head as far as possible toward each shoulder (Figure 23-2).

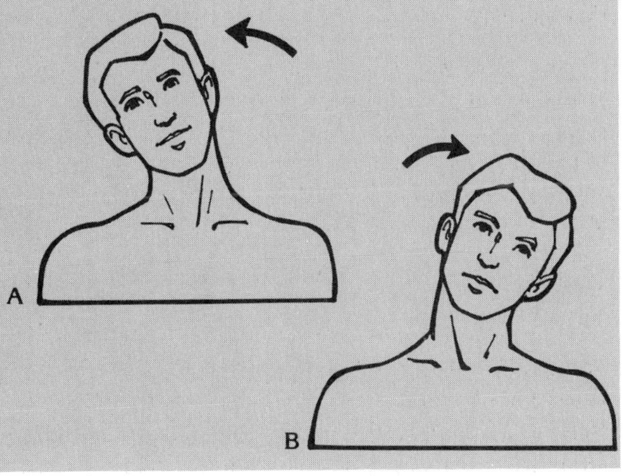

Figure 23-2.

Procedure 23-1. Cont'd

5. Rotate the neck by moving the head in a circular manner (Figure 23-3).

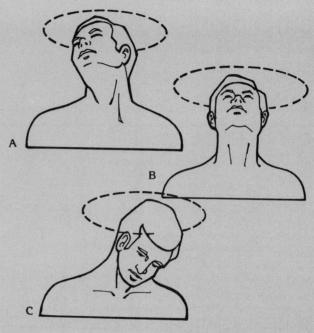

Figure 23-3.

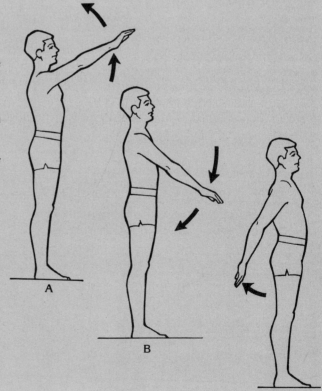

1. Extend the shoulder by raising the arm from the side position forward to a position above the head, palm facing downward (Figure 23-4,*A*).

2. Flex the shoulder by returning the arm to position at the side of the body (Figure 23-4,*B*).

3. Hyperextend the shoulder by moving the arm behind the body (Figure 23-4,*C*).

Figure 23-4.

Procedure 23-1. Cont'd

4. Abduct the shoulder by raising the arm to the side until it is above the head, palm facing downward (Figure 23-5,*A*).

5. Adduct the shoulder by lowering the arm sideways to the body (Figure 23-5,*B*).

Figure 23-5.

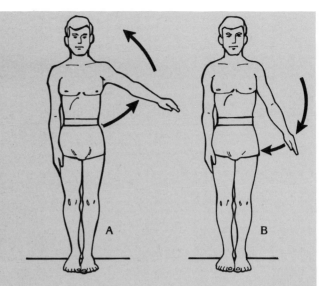

6. Circumduct the shoulder by moving the arm in a full circle (Figure 23-6).

Figure 23-6.

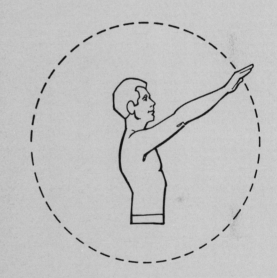

7. Outwardly rotate the shoulder by moving the arm until the thumb of the hand is laterally positioned (Figure 23-7,*A*).

8. Inwardly rotate the shoulder by moving the arm at the shoulder until the thumb of the hand is turned inwardly and to the back (Figure 23-7,*B*).

Figure 23-7.

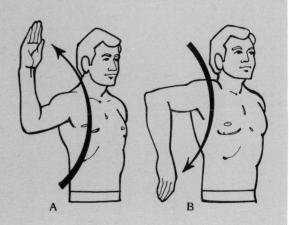

Procedure 23-1. Cont'd

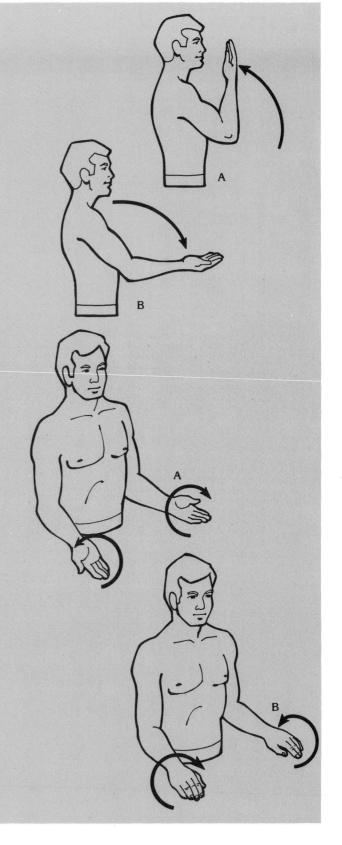

Elbow

1. Flex the elbow by bending the arm so that the hand is at the shoulder (Figure 23-8,*A*).

2. Extend the elbow by straightening the arm (Figure 23-8,*B*).

Figure 23-8.

3. Rotate the elbow for supination by turning the hand so that the palm is facing upward (Figure 23-9,*A*).

4. Rotate the elbow for pronation by turning the hand so that the palm is facing downward (Figure 23-9,*B*).

Figure 23-9.

Procedure 23-1. Cont'd

Wrist

1. Flex the wrist by bringing the fingers toward the inner aspect of the forearm (Figure 23-10,*A*).

2. Extend the wrist by straightening the hand to the same plane as the arm (Figure 23-10,*B*).

3. Hyperextend the wrist by bringing the fingers back as far as possible (Figure 23-10,*C*).

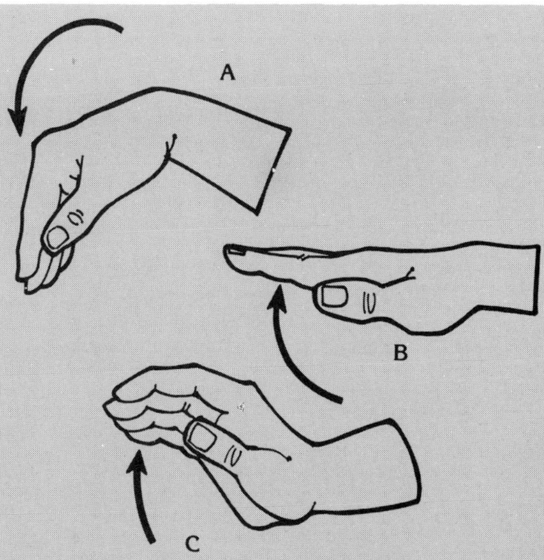

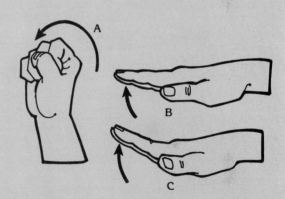

Figure 23-10.

Hand, Fingers, and Thumb

1. Flex the hand and fingers by making a fist (Figure 23-11,*A*).

2. Extend by straightening and hyperextend (Figure 23-11,*B*).

3. Hyperextend the hand (Figure 23-11,*C*).

Figure 23-11.

4. Abduct it by spreading the fingers and thumb (Figure 23-12,*A*).

5. Adduct it by bringing the fingers and thumb together (Figure 23-12,*B*).

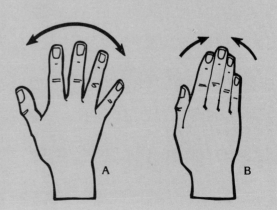

Figure 23-12.

Procedure 23-1. Cont'd

6. Oppose the thumb by touching each finger with the thumb (Figure 23-13).

7. Rotate the thumb by moving it in a circle (Figure 23-14).

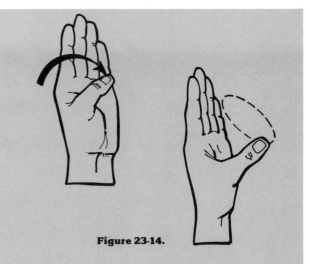

Figure 23-13.

Figure 23-14.

Hip

1. Flex the hip by moving the leg forward and up (Figure 23-15, A).

2. Extend the hip by moving the leg back down beside the other leg and beyond (hyperextension) (Figure 23-15, B, C).

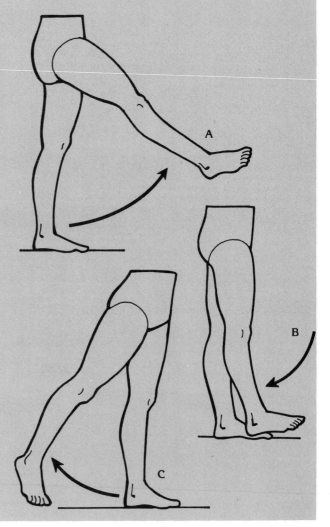

Figure 23-15.

Procedure 23-1. Cont'd

3. Abduct the hip by moving the leg out to the side (Figure 23-16, *A*).

4. Adduct the hip by moving the leg back to the other leg (Figure 23-16, *B*).

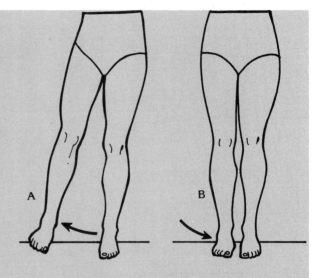

Figure 23-16.

5. Circumduct the hip by moving the leg in a circle (Figure 23-17).

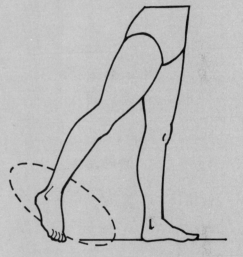

Figure 23-17.

6. Inwardly rotate the hip by turning the leg so that the toes are as far in as possible (Figure 23-18, *A*).

7. Outwardly rotate the hip by turning the leg so that the toes are turned laterally (Figure 23-18, *B*).

Figure 23-18.

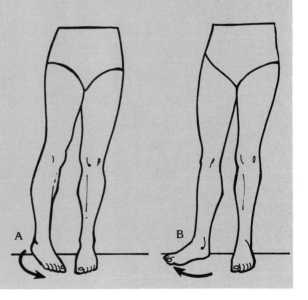

Procedure 23-1. Cont'd

Knee

1. Flex the knee by bending the leg, bringing the foot close to the posterior aspect of the thigh (Figure 23-19, A).

2. Extend the knee by straightening the leg (Figure 23-19,B).

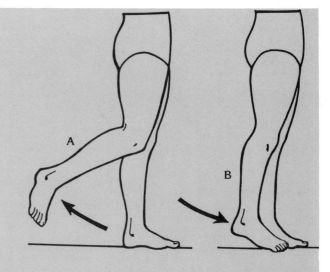

Figure 23-19.

Ankle

1. Move the ankle to plantar flexion so that the toes are pointing down (Figure 23-20, A).

2. Move the ankle to dorsal flexion so that the toes are pointing up (Figure 23-20, B).

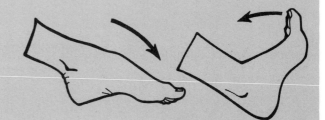

Figure 23-20.

Foot and Toes

1. Eversion of the foot turns the sole of the foot laterally (Figure 23-21, A).

2. Inversion of the foot turns the sole of the foot medially (Figure 23-21, B).

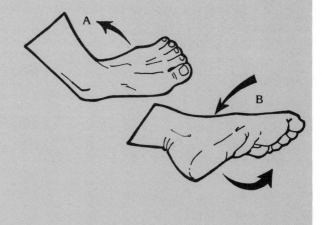

Figure 23-21.

3. Flex toes by bending them downward (Figure 23-22, A).

4. Extend the toes by straightening them (Figure 23-22, B).

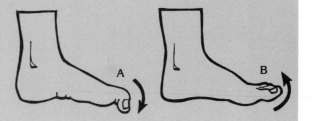

Figure 23-22.

Procedure 23-1. Cont'd

5. Abduct the toes by spreading them (Figure 23-23, *A*).

6. Adduct the toes by bringing them together (Figure 23-23, *B*).

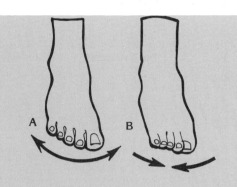

Figure 23-23.

Trunk

1. Flex the vertebral joints by bending the trunk at the waist to touch the toes (Figure 23-24, *A*).

2. Extend the vertebral joints by straightening the trunk (Figure 23-24, *B*).

3. Hyperextend the vertebral joints by bending the trunk backward (Figure 23-24, *C*).

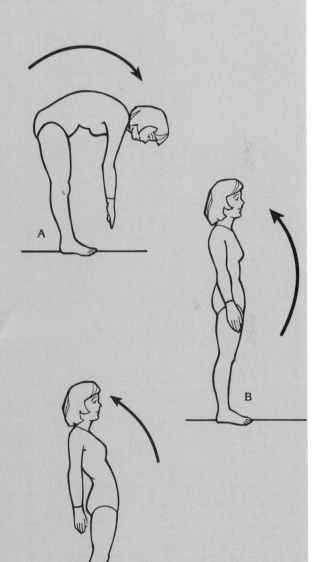

Figure 23-24.

Procedure 23-1. Cont'd

4. Laterally flex the vertebral joints by bending to each side (Figure 23-25, A,B).

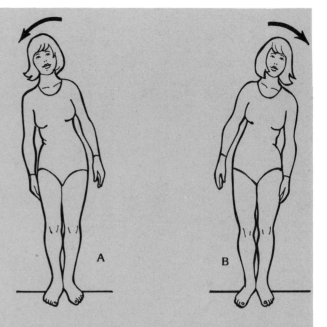

Figure 23-25.

5. Rotate the vertebral joints by moving the upper part of the body in a circle from the waist (Figure 23-26).

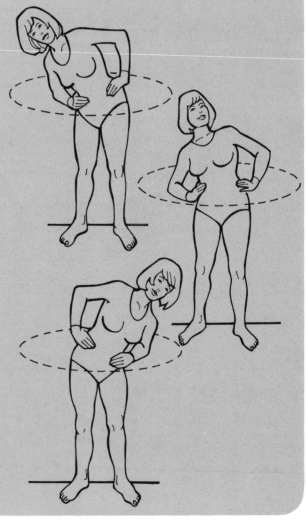

Figure 23-26.

PHYSICAL FITNESS

Regular exercise is necessary in order for a person to maintain good health. Physical fitness in daily life encompasses both caloric balance and functional fitness. The former is concerned with balancing the number of calories taken in daily with the number of calories expended. (See Table 23-2.)

Functional physical fitness has three aspects: joint flexibility, muscle tone, and endurance. A purposeful program can be designed to maintain each of these aspects of physical fitness. Examples of exercises to maintain these follow.

Joint Flexibility Exercises

1. Circumduction of the shoulder joints: Standing with a broad stance, full circles are made with both arms to the front, the rear, and across the body. (See Figure 23-27, A.)

2. Rotation of the hips: Standing again with feet apart, the hips are rotated through a full circle while feet stay on the ground and knees are slightly flexed. (See Figure 23-27, B.)

3. Twisting the trunk: With a semibroad stance and arms extended at the side, one slowly twists around each side, following the leading hand with the eyes. Feet remain fully on the floor, knees slightly flexed. Movement should be slow and smooth, not sudden. (See Figure 23-27, C.)

4. Rotating the head and neck: Rotate the head slowly through a full circle and repeat in the opposite direction. (See Figure 23-27, D.)

5. Flexing and hyperextending the shoulder and hip joints: Standing on one leg, one supports oneself with one hand and swings an arm and leg backward and forward in opposite directions. This is then repeated with the other arm and leg. (See Figure 23-27, E.)

6. Flexing the back: Sitting with legs spread apart, one places hands on the floor palms down between the thighs, then slowly bending forward, the hands are slid along the floor toward the feet. Movement is to be smooth without bouncing. Return to the sitting position. (See Figure 23-27, F.)

Table 23-2. Daily Balance of Calories

To Take in 100 Calories One of the following (approximate):		To Burn up 100 Calories* One of the following:	Female	Male
Apple	1¼	Clean windows	30 min	25 min
Banana	one	Bicycle 8 km/h (5 mph)	20 min	19 min
Ice cream	2/5 cup (100 ml)	Ping pong	30 min	24 min
Raw carrot stick	five	Run 15 km/h (9 mph)	9 min	6 min
Celery stick	twenty	Run (in place)	5 min	4 min
Whole milk	5/8 cup (155 ml)	140 counts per		
Skim milk	1 cup	minute		
Ground beef	2½ oz	Swim crawl	25 min	20 min
Hot dog	one third	20 meters/min		
French fried potato	8 pieces	Dance (moderate)	30 min	23 min
Baked potato	one	Walk (fast)	19 min	14 min
Cheddar cheese	one oz	Tennis (moderate)	16 min	13 min
Fried egg	1 small			
Bacon	2 slices			
Bread	1¼ slices			
Beer	8 oz (225 ml)			
Tea/coffee with milk and sugar 250 ml	2 cups 1 cup			

*To lose 2.2 lb (1 kg), approximately 3500 calories must be burned.

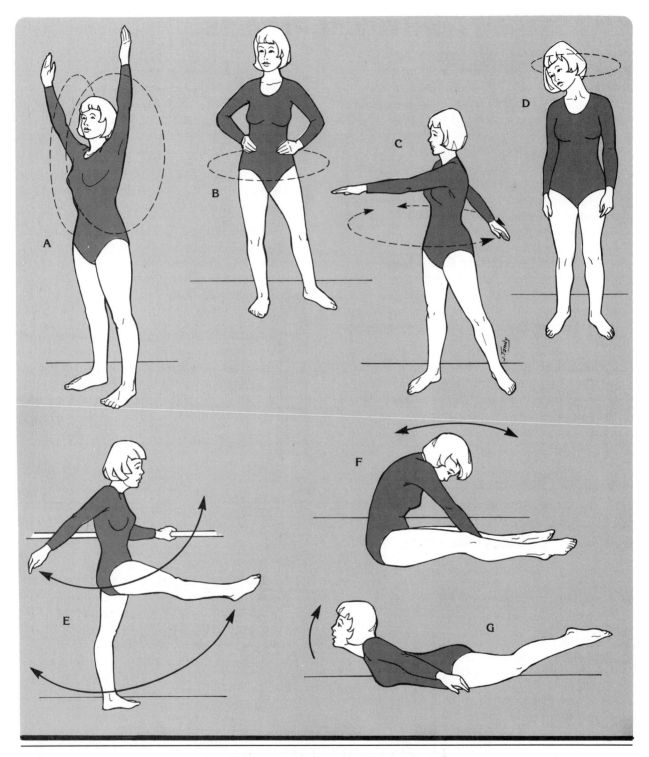

Figure 23-27.   Joint flexibility exercises. **A,** Circumduction of the shoulder; **B,** rotating the hip joints; **C,** twisting the trunk; **D,** rotating the head and neck; **E,** flexing and hyperextending the shoulder and hip joints; **F,** flexing the back; and **G,** hyperextending the shoulders, head, legs, and hips.

7. Hyperextending the shoulders, head, and legs at the hips: Lying on the stomach, one puts one's arms at the sides or stretches them outward. Tighten the back muscles so that the legs and upper body are lifted from the floor at the same time. (See Figure 23-27, G.)

Table 23-3.   Endurance Exercises*

Age (both sexes)	Target heart rate per minute
20–29	133
30–39	127
40–49	125
50–59	120
60–69	115

Frequency: 3 to 5 times per week

Intensity: Work up to and sustain target heart rate (for age during exercise)

Time: Attempt to keep moving for at least 15 minutes even if it is necessary to slow down

Type: Any endurance exercise—walking, cycling, jogging

To cool down, keep moving with light activities for at least 5 minutes after the endurance exercise

*From Collis, Martin. September, 1974. Prescription for fitness. *British Columbia Medical Journal* 16:262.

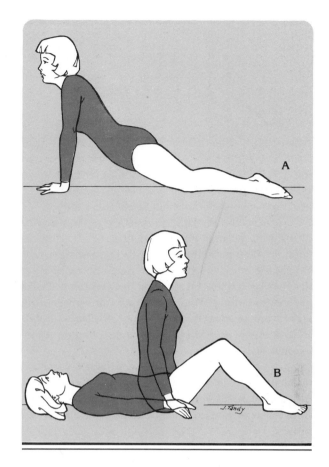

Figure 23-28.   Muscle tone exercises. **A**, Push-ups and, **B**, sit-ups.

Muscle Tone Exercises

1.   Push-ups: For push-ups one lies on one's stomach, placing the hands beneath the shoulders, palms down. Push up until the arms are straight, then lower the body to the floor. Beginners may keep the knees on the floor; advanced ones may pivot at the toes keeping the entire length of body straight (see Figure 23-28, *A*).

2.   Sit-ups: One sits on the floor with knees bent and feet supported (feet may be placed under the edge of a sofa). One then lies down and sits up; when individual ability improves, hands can be interlocked behind the head while lying and sitting. (See Figure 23-28, *B*.)

Endurance

There are a number of methods of assessing endurance, that is, the response of the body to exercises. One of the simplest is by taking the pulse rate. For suggested target heart rates, see Table 23-3.

As fitness level improves, a person can elect either one of two courses: to go on to higher heart rates or to continue longer at the same level.

KINDS OF EXERCISES

There are a number of kinds of exercises. The choice of which kind is appropriate to the individual patient depends upon the health and strength of the person and upon the purpose to be accomplished by the exercises.

Active or *isotonic* exercises are carried out by the patient, who supplies the energy to move the body parts. This type of exercise serves to both increase and maintain muscle tone, to maintain joint mobility, and to provide the additional effects discussed earlier.

Passive exercises are those in which the energy required to move the body part is provided by a nurse or by mechanical equipment. These exercises maintain joint mobility only. Because the muscles do not contract during passive exercises, muscular atrophy is not prevented.

Active-assistive exercises are carried out by the patient with some assistance from a nurse. The patient moves the body part as far as personally possible, and then the nurse moves it through the remainder of the normal range of movement. These exercises encourage normal muscle function.

In *isometric* or *static* muscle exercises no joint movement occurs, but the length of the muscle changes. The patient consciously increases the tension of the muscles without moving joints by holding the tension for several seconds, then relaxing. These exercises maintain muscle strength, thus preventing significant atrophy, but they do not affect joint mobility. Patients who have casts frequently require these exercises.

Resistive exercises consist of contraction of a muscle against an opposing force. The force may be manual or mechanical, for example, lifting a weight. Resistive exercises increase muscle size, strength, and power.

Providing Passive Exercises

In passive exercises the energy is *not* provided by the patient but by other people or mechanical equipment. Passive exercises are normally done to meet the patient's needs in regard to specific muscle problems; for a leg that rolls outward, emphasis is placed on rolling the leg inward. For passive exercises the patient assumes a position that will permit free movement of the joint to be moved. Often a supine position is advised if the patient can tolerate it.

There are three major factors in providing passive exercises: (a) the range of motion of the joint being exercised, (b) support for the joint against gravity and unwanted movement, and (c) the movement provided by the other hands to exert effort and control. Normally a joint is supported both above and below.

There are two ways in which a nurse can provide control and support of a joint: cradling and cupping. Where control is a problem, cradling will probably be used. It affords more support and frees the other hand to stabilize the joint proximal to the one being exercised. (See Figure 23-29.)

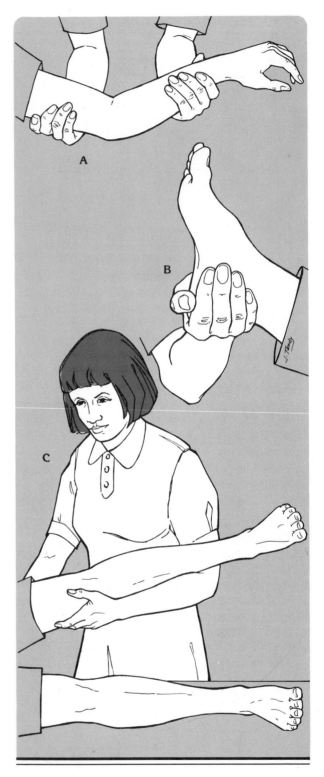

Figure 23-29. **A**, For passive exercises the joint is supported above and below. **B**, Cupping supports the joint and, **C**, cradling uses one hand to support, freeing the other to stabilize the joint proximal to the one being exercised.

The Value of Isometric Exercises

In isometric exercises an effort is made to use the whole muscle as a unit. It is specific in that all skeletal muscles can be exercised in a short time and without special equipment. With maximum effort all fibers in a muscle will shorten. With resistance the muscle will not measurably shorten because muscles use only sufficient fibers to carry out the given work.

Isometric exercises increase muscle strength, and they require very little time. They should be used in conjunction with other exercises. The technique is to maintain tension in a muscle for a given period of time. It is recommended to make maximal muscular effort for 6 seconds once a day. In the breaking-in period it can be done in two ways: a three-quarter effort for 6 seconds or a full effort for 2 to 4 seconds. This 6-second effort is carried out once a day to avoid fatigue. All muscles should be exercised for general conditioning, which takes less than 2 minutes (Russek et al. 1964:3).

PRENATAL AND POSTNATAL EXERCISES

Prenatal Exercises

During pregnancy the woman needs to learn Kegal exercises to strengthen her pubococcygeal muscle. This muscle is the master sphincter of the bladder, bowel function, and vaginal perception and response during intercourse. The exercise consists of 3 aspects: (a) contracting the anal sphincter, (b) contracting the introitus, and (c) contracting the meatal sphincter, then holding for a count of 10 before relaxing. This exercise is done 3 or 4 times per day.

Pelvic rocking can be done prenatally in order to relieve low backache. The woman assumes a hands-and-knees position, a standing position, or a supine position. The abdominal wall is tightened while

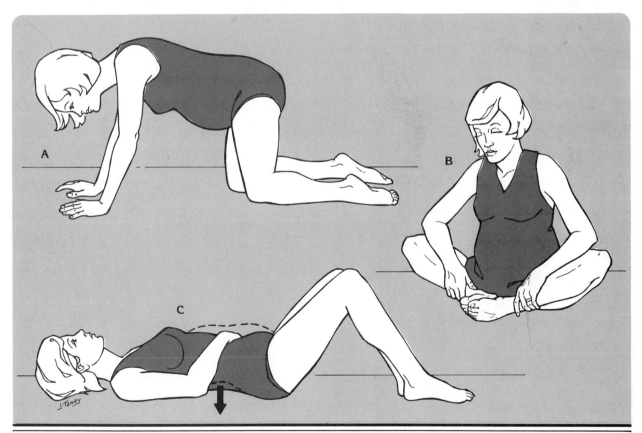

Figure 23-30.   **A,** Pelvic rocking can be carried out standing, sitting, lying down, or on the hands and knees as shown. **B,** Tailorsitting. **C,** Pelvic tilting.

tucking in the buttocks. This rocks the pelvis upward, flattening the lower back. The abdomen and buttocks are then slowly relaxed; this allows the hollow to return in the back. The exercise is repeated four to six times (see Figure 23-30,A).

Tailorsitting is done prenatally to stretch the thigh and pelvic floor muscles. The woman sits with her legs crossed in front and feet drawn toward her. The knees are comfortably extended toward the floor. This position needs to be assumed as often as possible (see Figure 23-30,B).

Postnatal Exercises

Postnatal exercises serve to trim the woman's figure and improve the tone of the muscles. If the delivery was uncomplicated, these can be started 2 or 3 days postpartum. It is usual to start with simple exercises and progress to more strenuous ones. The exercises should not be tiring. The following postpartum exercises are often practiced:

1. Abdominal tightening. Take a deep breath, let it out, then tighten the abdominal muscles, pulling in and up. Hold to a count of 3, then relax.

2. Chin lift. While tightening the abdominal muscles, lift the chin so that it is on the chest. Relax and let the head return to the pillow.

3. Leg raising (modified). Tighten the abdominal muscles, press the lower back into the bed, and raise the right leg and foot until it rests on left toes. Relax and lower. Repeat with left leg.

4. Pelvic tilting. Lying in the supine position with knees flexed, inhale, and while exhaling, flatten the back against the bed. While doing this, tighten the muscles of the abdomen and buttocks (see Figure 23-30,C).

5. Deep breathing. This exercise is designed to promote relaxation in order to prepare for exercises. Take a deep breath, then let it all out, relaxing all the muscles of the body.

Kegal exercises are also carried out in order to strengthen the pubococcygeal muscle postnatally. An exercise schedule postpartum permits for gradual increased exercise. The following schedule is used in some areas.

Delivery day

1. deep breathing
2. abdominal tightening

First day postpartum

1. repeat of above
2. chin lift

Second day postpartum

1. repeat of above
2. pelvic tilt

Third day postpartum

1. repeat of above
2. leg raising (modified)

EFFECTS OF EXERCISE

Exercise has a number of positive effects for people and can prevent a number of health problems. The latter benefit is of particular importance to patients who are ill and need to avoid further problems and complications.

Musculoskeletal System

Since use of an organ tends to maintain its normal state, exercise will maintain the tone and strength of muscles, including the heart muscle. The change in a muscle size is in proportion to its use; an unused muscle will atrophy, whereas an overused muscle will hypertrophy. Exercise will also maintain joint mobility. Joints that lose their normal range of motion may develop problems such as ankylosis and contractures.

Bone density is maintained through weight bearing and is therefore facilitated with exercise and activity.

Cardiovascular System

The blood circulation, especially the venous flow, is improved with exercise. This assists in the elimination of waste products from the muscles and in the delivery of oxygen and nutrients to the tissues. As muscles contract, superficial veins are milked or compressed, thus assisting the return flow of blood against gravity to the heart. This muscular action in the lower extremities is often likened to a pump and thus is referred to as the second pump of the body, the heart being the prime pump.

Metabolism

The metabolic rate is increased, thus providing good lung expansion in the body's effort to inhale the additional oxygen needed. It also stimulates the appetite.

Gastrointestinal System

Appetite is improved, and the gastrointestinal tract tone is increased.

Psychoneurologic Effects

Exercise assists in restoring a sense of relaxation and equilibrium.

Urinary System

Exercise promotes urinary function by improving the blood flow to and from the kidney; thus body wastes are excreted more effectively.

COMMON PROBLEMS OF JOINT AND MUSCLE MOVEMENTS

Common problems of body movement include the following:

1. *Ankylosis* refers to a stiffening of a joint. This is generally caused by scar tissue or bony growth and it can result in complete immobility of the joint and in some cases deformity.

2. *Contracture* is permanent shortening (contraction) of a muscle. The flexor muscles are stronger than the extensors. This is usually seen in situations where a patient's muscles are contracted for a prolonged period of time. An example is a patient who stays in bed for a year with knees flexed most of the time. Eventually the flexor muscles contract permanently, and the knee joints are permanently flexed. Contractures of the knees, hips, elbows, wrist, and ankles will be seen by nurses. In these cases it is the flexor muscles that are permanently contracted, and the extensor muscles are extended.

3. *Tonus* refers to the slight continual contraction of muscles. This is a normal state of muscles; healthy muscles have good muscle tone. *Hypertonicity* refers to excessive muscle tone and *hypotonicity* to decreased muscle tone. A muscle that possesses no tone is referred to as an atonic muscle, which is in a state of *atony.*

4. *Atrophy* refers to wasting away or a decrease in size, and it can refer to a cell, tissue, or other organ of the body as well as to a muscle. *Hypertrophy* is an increase in size of an organ or tissue, such as a muscle. It is due to an increase in the size of the cells. People who are confined to bed tend to develop atrophy of their muscles as a result of disuse. An athlete, on the other hand, often develops hypertrophied muscles from continual use, for example, the hypertrophied femoral muscles of the distance runner or the hypertrophy of the biceps muscles of the boxer.

AMBULATION

Ambulation is the act of walking. Most people who are ill require only a brief period of bed rest, and then they are walking about and able to gradually increase their activity. The more physically fit a person is before becoming ill, the quicker the person is likely to return to health. This is particularly true for the elderly person who has fewer reserves to call upon at a time of illness.

Even though a patient may have stayed in bed only a day or two, the person may feel weak and be unsteady. Just remaining in bed for a few days because of a cold can weaken muscles sufficiently that a person feels shaky when first getting up. A patient who, in addition to staying in bed, has had surgery or even a fever, is likely to feel more pronounced weakness. The elderly person, in addition, is likely to experience some joint stiffness as a result of immobility. The possible problems of bed rest and immobility will subsequently be discussed. There is no question that problems are less likely to occur in most instances when a patient becomes ambulatory as soon as possible.

Because of a person's age, general physical condition, or the length of time spent on bed rest, the person may need to prepare for becoming ambulatory by carrying out some conditioning exercises to improve muscle tone and strength and to improve the flexibility of the joints.

When a person walks, the joints of the hips and the lower extremities are used the most, and the muscles of the hips, thighs, and legs are required to provide the movement of these joints. The chief muscles that move the femur of the leg are the two iliopsoas, the three gluteal, and the adductor muscles. The biceps femoris and quadriceps femoris are largely responsible for moving the leg; the quadriceps femoris also assists in flexing the thigh. Since these muscles together with others in the abdomen, buttocks, and the lower extremities maintain the balance of a person in the upright postural position, they are the muscles that lose their tone most rapidly when a patient remains in bed.

Exercises Preparatory to Ambulation

Hip Flexion and Extension

Lying on the bed the patient extends the leg in front of him, then flexes the knee and brings it to the chest, pointing the toes upward in a dorsal flexion position. When the knee is as close to the chest as possible, the knee is extended (straightened), then the leg is returned to the fully extended position. This exercise is then repeated with the other leg.

Hip Rotation

1. With both the knee and ankle extended, roll the leg inward and then outward from the hip.
2. With both legs extended at the knee and the ankle, turn both legs inward until the toes touch and then outward until the heels touch.

Abduction and Adduction of the Hips

With the leg extended at the knee and with the toes in dorsal flexion, move one leg over to the side of the bed, then over to the other side of the bed over the other leg. Repeat for the other leg.

Knee Extensions

With the leg extended the patient pushes the back of the knee against the bed surface and raises the heels off the bed as far as possible. Repeat for the other leg.

Ankle Flexion, Inversion, and Eversion

1. Rotate the foot in a circular motion clockwise and counterclockwise.

2. Starting with the foot in plantar flexion, circle to the side, then circle bringing foot into dorsal flexion, then circle to the other side.

Toe Flexion and Extension

Flex and extend toes upward and downward.

Strengthening Muscles of the Abdomen, Buttocks, and Thighs for Walking

1. Set muscles of the abdomen, then relax them.
2. Breathe deeply to tighten abdominal muscles.
3. Tighten buttocks and then elevate hips while lying in the supine position.

These exercises should not be done to tire the patient. As a rough guide, a patient may be able to carry out these exercises three times each, twice or three times a day.

In addition to learning specific exercises in preparation for ambulation, some of the activities that are carried out by patients while they are in bed can be used for this therapeutic purpose. One example is the bath patients give themselves.

Assisting a Patient to Walk

Normally when people walk they move their arms and legs alternately; that is, the right arm swings forward as the left leg moves forward, and conversely the left arm moves with the right leg. Techniques that will support a patient and facilitate this normal body movement are usually best. This is particularly true for patients who have sufficient muscle and bone development and strength in both legs to stand and move themselves.

Assisting a Patient to Walk (One Nurse)

After the patient is assisted from bed and has balance, the nurse goes behind the patient, supporting the patient at the waist with both hands. The nurse may wrap a towel folded lengthwise around the patient's waist or use a walking belt, which also fits around the patient's waist. The advantage of this position is that the patient is assisted to maintain a center of gravity in the middle of the base of support (between the feet); that is, the patient is not encouraged to lean to one side or the other.

The patient should take only a few steps at first to assess steadiness and ability to balance. If the patient feels confident about continuing, the nurse follows behind, supporting the patient at the waist.

If the patient feels faint or thinks he or she may fall, the nurse assumes a broad stance, one foot in front of the other, and brings the patient back so that the patient is supported by the nurse's body. The patient can then be gently lowered to the floor without harm if additional assistance is not available.

If the patient feels unsteady and has a weakness in one leg, such as after a stroke, the nurse may find it advantageous to assume a position at the affected side. In this position the nurse places the near arm under the patient's arm and grasps the inferior aspect of the patient's upper arm. The nurse can then grasp the patient's lower arm or hand with the other hand. In this position the nurse can assist the patient in a fall by sliding the near arm up to the patient's axilla and then, after taking a broad stance, supporting the patient's body against the nurse's body with much of the weight against the nurse's hip. Again the patient can be gently lowered to the floor if additional assistance is not available.

Another position that a nurse can assume to assist a patient to walk is particularly effective when the patient has a distinct body weakness. In this position the nurse goes to the patient's unaffected side and places the near arm around the partient's waist. The patient places the near arm over the nurse's far shoulder, and the nurse grasps this with the free hand. The patient and nurse then step forward together. As the patient advances the weak far leg forward, the nurse's opposite leg is advanced to provide as wide a base of support as possible.

Assisting a Patient to Walk (Two Nurses)

Each nurse stands at a side of the patient and grasps the inferior aspect of the patient's upper arm with the nearest hand and the lower arm or hand with the other hand. The two nurses and the patient then walk in unison. Again the nurses can slide their hands up to the patient's axillae to give additional support if it is required. This technique provides more support than can be given by one nurse.

A second two-nurse support for a walking patient provides more support than the previously mentioned position. Again the nurses stand at each side of the patient. They slip their near arms under the patient's arm to the back and grasp each other's arms. The patient's arms are placed over the nurses' far shoulders, and they grasp the patient's hands with their free hands. For this technique to be effective, both nurses and the patient need to be about the same height.

Mechanical Aids for Walking

Cane

If a patient requires the use of a cane that provides only minimal support, the patient should hold it with the hand that is on the stronger side of the body. For example, it should be held with the left hand if the patient has a right-leg weakness. The position of the tip of the cane in a standing position is about 14 cm (6 inches) to the side of the foot. The patient moves the cane forward about 28 cm (1 ft), then moves the weak leg forward to the cane, and finally, moves the strong leg forward. This pattern of moving provides at least two points of support on the floor at any one time. As the patient becomes stronger, the patient may feel comfortable moving the cane and weak foot forward together, and then the strong foot, thus having only one point of support (the strong leg) during one part of the movement.

Tripod Cane

This supportive device has three legs to support the handle, which the patient holds on the weak side. It offers more support than a cane. However, it is not as readily moved because of the three legs.

Walker

A walker is a mechanical device with four legs for support. It is usually made of a light-weight metal such as aluminum so it can be easily lifted and moved.

The patient holds the upper bar of the walker at each side, lifts the walker forward, then steps into it. Because walkers are designed in such a way that the bars are in front of and around the sides of the patient, they provide a feeling of security as well as providing assistance with balance. Their disadvantage is that normal body alignment and walking motion are not encouraged, since the patient must bend forward to move the walker.

Braces

Sometimes patients are provided with braces for their weak legs. These are generally made of a light-weight metal with leather straps, which attach the brace to the leg. Some braces will support the ankle and lower leg; others can extend to the upper leg thus offering support to the knee. Patients who have braces usually learn to take these on and off themselves.

Crutches

Sometimes it is necessary for a patient to use crutches for a period of time. Although there are several types of crutches, two of the most commonly used types are the underarm and the forearm support crutches. Nurses may often need to assist patients in measuring for the underarm crutches. This can be done with the patient either in bed or standing.

Measuring for Crutches.   In bed, measure from the anterior fold of the patient's axilla to the heel of the foot. To this distance add 5 cm (2 inches).

While standing, measure again from the anterior fold of the axilla, but this time to a point 14 cm (6 inches) lateral to the heel. When being measured this way, it is best if the patient wears the shoes that will be regularly used (see Figure 23–31).

Appropriate Length of Crutches.   The top of the crutch is 5 cm (2 inches) below the axilla. Weight

should not be borne by the axillae. Prolonged pressure on the axillae can create damage to the underlying nerves, producing what is called a *crutch paralysis.* The axilla is protected poorly by a layer of fat, which does not support against pressure.

The hand grips need to be placed in a position so' that the patient's elbows are slightly flexed when holding them.

Pointers on Crutches.   When a patient initially obtains crutches, the axillary bar should not be padded because it encourages leaning on it while walking, thus increasing the danger of pressure upon the brachial nerve plexus. However, some patients who have learned to crutch walk may like a small pad on the crutch that does not touch the axilla when they move but that provides a little softer support when they lean on the crutches for short periods of time while standing. Patients who use long (underarm) crutches need to understand why pressure on the axillae needs to be avoided. Because the person's hands carry most or all of the patient's weight, the hand bars may be padded. It is important that padding be applied so that it does not rotate or slip.

Before using crutches, the patient who has been in bed may well need to carry out some exercises to strengthen the shoulder and upper arm muscles. In particular, the triceps, trapezius, and latissimus muscles are used in crutch walking. Simple exercises that a patient can carry out in bed to strengthen these muscles are push-ups from a sitting position. The patient places both arms at the sides, palms flat on the bed surface, and raises the buttocks. This exercise is excellent for developing the tricep muscles. Raising oneself off the bed with the use of a trapeze attached to a Balkan frame can also develop arm and shoulder muscles. The legs also need strengthening for standing and walking. For balance and posture the abdominal and back muscles need to have good tone.

Crutch Stance (Tripod Position).

Before crutch walking is attempted, posture and balance are of utmost importance. The proper standing position with crutches is called the *tripod (triangle) position* (see Figure 23–32). The crutches are placed about 14 cm (6 inches) in front of the feet and out laterally about 14 cm (6 inches), thus producing a wide base of support. The feet are slightly apart. To provide stability, a greater height requires a broader base. Thus a tall person requires a wider base than a short person. Hips and knees are extended, the back is straight, and the head is held straight and high. There should be no hunch to the shoulders and thus

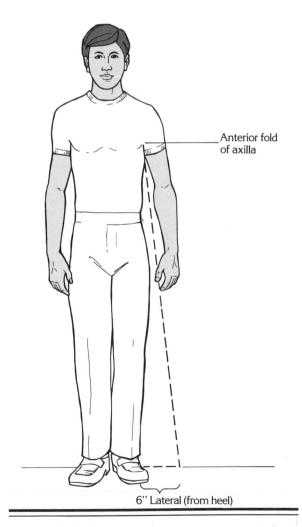

Anterior fold of axilla

6'' Lateral (from heel)

Figure 23-31.   Measuring for crutches in a standing position.

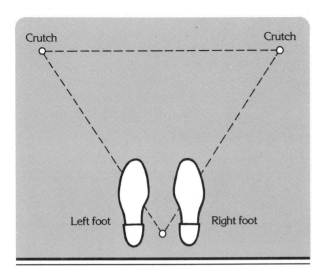

Figure 23-32.   The crutch stance. Tripod position.

no weight borne by the axillae. The palms are positioned lateral to the feet, and the elbows are extended sufficiently to allow weight bearing on the hands.

Sometimes patients are discouraged when crutch walking commences because the limitations with crutches become apparent. Weakness that was not apparent in bed can become prominent when standing or walking. Patients realize that balance can no longer be taken for granted with the weight of a heavy cast or a paralyzed limb. Frequently, progress may be slower than anticipated, and thus encouragement and the setting of realistic goals are especially important.

Crutch Gaits

There are four standard crutch gaits, which all begin with the tripod position. Physiotherapists usually teach crutch walking, and they will teach the gait or gaits particularly suitable for the·patient. However, in situations where there is no physiotherapist, for example in a small hospital in a rural setting, nurses will teach crutch walking.

Four-Point Alternate Crutch Gait.   This gait is used by patients who can bear partial weight on both their feet, for example, arthritic or cerebral palsy patients. It is a particularly safe gait in that there are three points of support on the floor at any one time. The gait has the following foot sequence: right crutch, left foot, left crutch, right foot (see Figure 23–33). This gait provides for a normal walking pattern and makes some use of the muscles of the lower extremities.

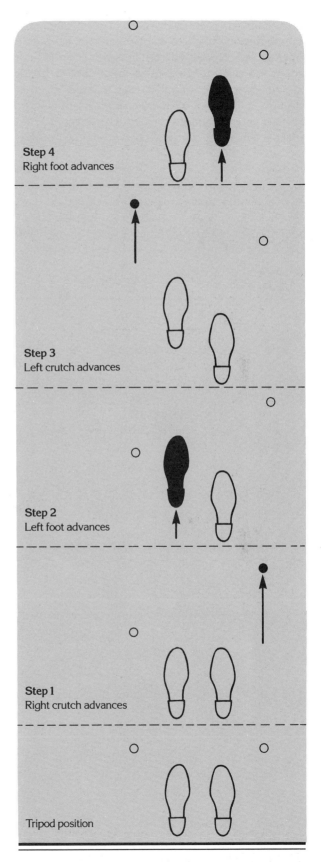

Figure 23-33.   Four-point crutch gait.

Three-Point Alternate Crutch Gait.   For this gait the patient must be able to bear the total body weight on one foot; the affected foot or leg is either partially or totally non–weight bearing (see Figure 23–34). In this gait the two crutches are moved forward together with the injured leg while the weight is being borne by the patient's hands on the crutches. The unaffected leg is then advanced forward.

Two-Point Crutch Gait.   The patient can bear partial weight on both feet for this gait and with practice can frequently move relatively quickly. The right crutch and the left foot move forward simultaneously as in normal walking (see Figure 23–35). Then the left crutch and the right foot advance forward.

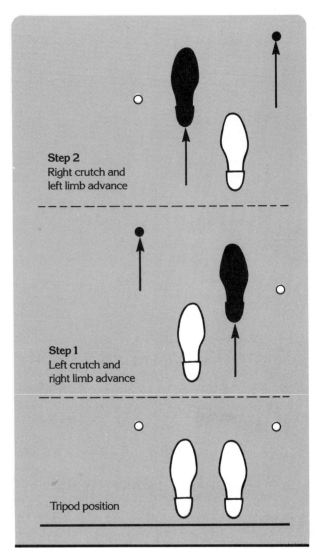

Figure 23-35.   Two-point crutch gait.

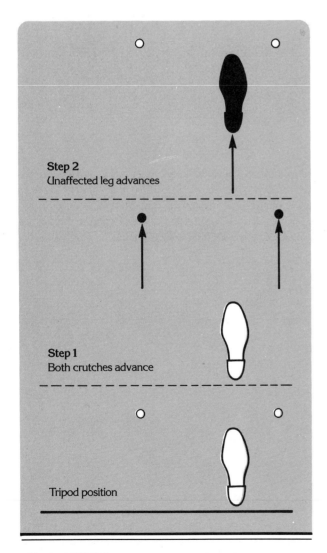

Figure 23-34.   Three-point crutch gait.

Swing Gaits.   There are two main swing gaits: the swing-to-crutch and the swing-through gaits. These gaits do not use the quadriceps and other lower extremity muscles a great deal because they do not simulate the normal walking motion. They are indicated when a patient is paralyzed or cannot move the lower extremities although the patient may be able to bear weight. Prolonged use of these gaits results in atrophy of the unused muscles. The advantage of these gaits is that they allow rapid movement.

In the *swing-to-crutch gait,* both crutches are placed forward, and then the patient swings forward to the crutches. This is then repeated in order for the patient to move forward (see Figure 23-36,A). This

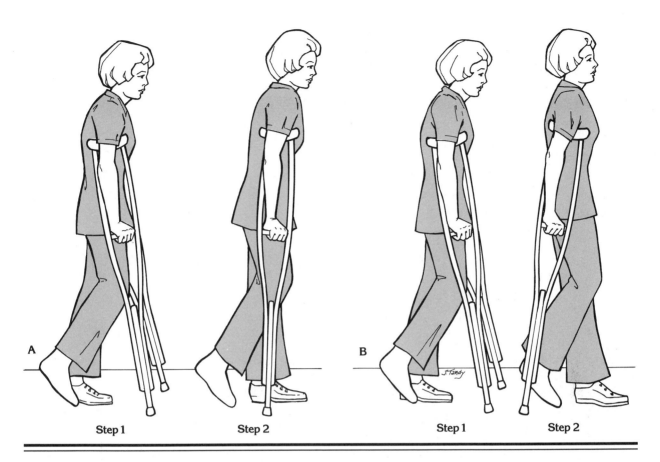

Figure 23-36.   Swing gaits. **A**, Swing-to-crutch gait. **B**, Swing-through gait.

is similar in motion to the three-point gait except that equal weight can be borne by both feet.

For the *swing-through gait*, the crutches are placed ahead of the patient, and the patient then swings through to the crutches and beyond to a position in front of them. Weight is shifted from the palms of the hands to the feet. This process is then repeated (see Figure 23-36,*B*).

IMMOBILITY

The concept of immobility is relative rather than absolute by definition. It does not necessarily mean complete lack of movement; it refers to a decrease in activity from that normally carried out. It has been described as "the prescribed or unavoidable restriction of movement in any area of the patient's life" (Carnevali et al. 1970: 1502).

Kinds of Immobility

The areas of immobility have been described as physical, intellectual, emotional, and social (Carnevali et al. 1503–1506).

Physical Immobility

Immobility in which the patient is physically restricted is frequently seen. Either the patient or factors in the environment may cause this immobility. It may be a limitation in physical movement or a limitation of some physiologic processes, such as breathing.

Intellectual Immobility

Immobility can be due to a lack of knowledge of how to function. As a result the person is constrained from acting. Some people who have brain damage due to a disease process or injury may be unable to act or to learn how to act appropriately in a given setting. Mentally retarded people who have a limited capacity to learn may be immobilized for that reason.

Emotional Immobility

People who are highly stressed, perhaps because of impending surgery or the loss of a loved one, may become immobilized emotionally and sometimes even physically. This can happen as a result of a sudden change that has not permitted the person time to adjust and to cope with the situation. Nurses will frequently see this in the hospital where a patient learns, for example, of a terminal malignancy.

Social Immobility

This type of immobility refers to changes in social interaction, which so often occurs as a result of illness. Patients who are admitted to the hospital may experience decreased interaction when separated from their family, or, in the case of elderly persons who live alone, the normal interaction is also decreased.

THE PROBLEMS OF IMMOBILITY

Healthy people are generally active people; however, when people are ill, they frequently face some degree of immobility. This restriction is frequently a physical one and can be prescribed by a physician or even by the person when faced with a problem such as a fever or a headache. Other reasons for immobilization can be psychologic and intellectual. For example, a very frightened person can be immobilized, or a boy who decides to stay at his desk and study rather than go to play football is restricting his mobility for intellectual reasons.

A person who is immobilized for a prolonged period is faced with a number of stressors and problems. These stressors can be classified as psychologic, social, and physical, each of which has a number of effects.

Psychologic and Social Effects

1. Motivation to learn is decreased; learning ability and retention of material are decreased.

2. Motivation to solve problems is decreased, including a loss in the ability to receive content to discriminate. For example, a patient may hear only a few of the nurse's statements and may be unable to differentiate between that which is important and that which is unimportant.

3. Drives such as hunger are generally diminished, and emotions are expressed in a variety of ways, including apathy, withdrawal, and aggression.

4. The person's body concept changes as does concept of self as a whole person and worthwhile being.

5. Immobility can also produce exaggerated emotional reactions that are often inappropriate to a situation and not normal for that particular person. For example, a patient may express sudden anger over an error in his dinner, a reaction the person normally would not have.

Because of immobility people receive a reduced quality and quantity in sensory stimuli. The male patient in a hospital bed for months may see only the nurses, patients, and a few visitors. He no longer meets with the people at work and friends on Saturdays. His life is much narrower and the variety of stimuli are less. As a result, his perception of time intervals may deteriorate. For example, he may think of the period of time he waited for his lunch as a long time (hours), when in effect it was only 15 minutes. The ability to estimate time intervals is largely related to the person's attitudes. For example, "time flies" often when people are busy and happy.

Another psychologic change for this immobilized person is related to role activities. As a father who normally attends his son's baseball games he now is unable to do so; he, as husband, is unable to earn a salary, and, as employee, is unable to contribute on the job. All of these can be stressors and as a result bring out feelings of fear, anxiety, and worthlessness. For further information see Chapter 34, "Stimulation Needs and Problems."

Physical Effects

Physical problems from immobilization can result even in those body systems which were healthy before the inactive period. Just as exercise can be good for all parts of the body of a healthy person, immobility can affect every organ and system of the body. The physical problems of immobility can be categorized as musculoskeletal, urinary, metabolic, gastrointestinal, respiratory, and cardiovascular (Olson 1967: 780–797).

Musculoskeletal Problems

Deterioration of muscles and bone function due to inactivity can result in a number of problems:

1. Demineralization of the bones (*osteoporosis*).
2. Contractures of the muscles and muscle atrophy.
3. Stiffness and pain in the joints.
4. Skin breakdown.

Demineralization of bones, that is, a depletion chiefly of calcium, which gives bones their strength and solidity, results from immobility. In the healthy person bone is continually being built and at the same time being broken down at similar rates. With inactivity the building process is interfered with, but the breakdown process continues. This is because the osteoblasts, which form the bony matrix, require the stress and strain of weight-bearing activity to function.

Continual demineralization causes bones to become spongy, and they may gradually deform or compress and fracture easily. Regardless of the amount of calcium in the diet of a person, this process of demineralization will take place with immobility. The unneeded calcium will only be excreted or deposited in the muscles, in the joints, and in the kidney pelvis. Deposition of calcium in the joints contributes to the stiffness and pain in these areas.

Contractures involve the muscles and the soft tissues areound the joints. All these tissues become atrophied with disuse, and the muscles eventually lose most of their strength and normal function. Contractures occur when the muscle fibers are unable to shorten and lengthen. These contractures can also occur with muscle imbalance, that is, when one muscle is much stronger than its opposite muscle. In a contracture the fibers of the muscle involved shorten and atrophy, thus limiting the range of motion of the affected joint. This process can eventually involve the tendons, ligaments, and capsule of the joint and become irreversible except by surgical intervention.

Skin breakdown and the subsequent occurrence of decubitus ulcers also may occur as a result of inactivity. Muscle activity is required for normal venous and arterial blood circulation. With the impeded circulation that can result from immobilization, nour-ishment to specific areas is impeded, thus resulting in the formation of decubitus ulcers (see Chapter 20 for further information).

Urinary Problems

The urinary system functions best when a person is in an upright position. Backlying positions and immobility predispose to such problems as (a) calculi (stones), (b) bladder distention, (c) involuntary micturition, and (d) infection.

In the backlying position the patient's kidney pelvis does not completely empty. Normal emptying is dependent upon the force of gravity in the upright position and the peristaltic action of the ureters. Stasis of urine occurs in the kidney pelvis even after just a few days in the supine position.

This stagnation of urine in which there are increased levels of minerals (see "Musculoskeletal Problems") can result in the formation of calculi, which are often composed of calcium salts. Urinary infections can also occur as a result of the elevated pH of urine due to increased alkalinity from calcium excretion. Normally urine is slightly acid (pH of 4.5 to 7.5).

A further problem that may occur is the lack of micturition control. This reflex action is not initiated due to the patient's inability to relax the perineal muscles and the external sphincter in the supine position. Therefore the bladder may become distended with urine, and urinary incontinence can result (see Chapter 27, "Urinary Incontinence").

Metabolic Problems

Problems arising from changes in the body's metabolism as a result of inactivity include (a) tissue atrophy and protein catabolism (breakdown), (b) a reduced metabolic rate, and (c) fluid and electrolyte imbalances.

The metabolic rate of a patient who is inactive or immobilized is reduced because of the reduced energy demands of the body cells. Thus *anabolism* (metabolic buildup) is reduced, but the rate of *catabolism* is increased. The process of protein breakdown can lead to a protein deficiency in the body and the subsequent formation of decubitus ulcers.

Other problems can result from the sweating of the patient in bed and the subsequent loss of essential electrolytes such as sodium, potassium chloride, and calcium (see Chapter 30).

The effects of stress upon the immobilized patient can also be reflected in fluid and electrolyte imbalances and in observable behavior.

Gastrointestinal Problems

Bed rest and immobility affect all three chief functions of the gastrointestinal tract (ingestion, digestion, and elimination), resulting in (a) anorexia, (b) diarrhea, and (c) constipation.

Patients who are immobilized are in a state of negative nitrogen balance due to the accelerated catabolic process. As a result they are frequently anorexic (lack an appetite). When the anorexic patient fails to eat, a condition of malnutrition can result, which may well affect any healing required for a disease process. The prolonged stress of immobility also results in the stimulation of the parasympathetic nervous system, which produces symptoms such as anorexia, dyspepsia, and diarrhea or constipation. These states can also have an effect upon the patient's appetite and subsequent intake of food and its digestion.

Elimination from the bowel is also affected. The immobilized patient may lose the defecation reflex and/or fecal expulsive power due to interference with the skeletal muscle activity and the visceral reflex patterns used in defecation. The patient then is likely to become constipated because of these weakened muscles and because of ignoring the defecation reflex. Certainly a supine position for defecation interferes with this reflex and with the muscles normally used in the defecation process.

Constipation is frequently accompanied by the symptoms of headache, anorexia, abdominal distention, malaise, and vertigo. All these symptoms can interfere with the person's ability to ingest and digest food.

Respiratory Problems

The immobilized person is also vulnerable to potential respiratory problems. These are basically of three different types:

1. Decreased respiratory movement.
2. The accumulation of secretions in the respiratory tract.
3. An imbalance in the oxygen–carbon dioxide ratio.

The chest of the person with limited mobility may be restricted in its movement by the loss of muscle coordination, perhaps through muscle disuse, and by certain pharmacologic agents such as sedatives and anesthetics.

Chest expansion can be further limited by the sitting or lying position of the patient; the Sim's position without shoulder or upper arm support can compress the lateral part of one side of the chest. It can also be limited by abdominal distention due to indigestion or for other reasons, which puts upward pressure on the diaphragm, or by the use of tight chest or abdominal binders.

Secretions may also accumulate in the respiratory tract and further interfere with respiration. Normally secretions are moved by coughing or by changing position or posture. In patients who find it uncomfortable to cough and who do not change their position, these secretions may well accumulate and inhibit the diffusion of oxygen and carbon dioxide in the alveoli. Lack of fluid intake can result in these secretions becoming thickened and even more difficult to cough up.

The oxygen–carbon dioxide imbalance is the third type of problem. Where there is decreased respiratory movement there may be a decreased intake of oxygen and a decreased output of carbon dioxide. Although increased carbon dioxide in the blood and decreased oxygen initially stimulate respirations, eventually they depress respiration (see Chapter 28).

Cardiovascular Problems

Immobility has three major effects upon the cardiovascular system. They are (a) orthostatic hypotension, (b) increased work load upon the heart, and (c) thrombus formation.

When a person has been in a lying position for a prolonged period, the autonomic nervous system is unable to equalize the blood supply to the body when the person gets up. This results in a condition known as *orthostatic hypotension* (low blood pressure in the standing position). Two underlying factors for this condition are the generalized loss of muscle tone and the decreased ability of the blood vessels to react to nervous stimuli. Normally, active muscle action of the body exerts pressure upon the veins and assists in the return of the venous blood to the heart. When there is poor muscle tone, this blood tends to pool in the dependent areas of the body, that is, areas lower than the heart such as the feet and legs in a standing position.

When a person lies in a supine position, the heart needs to work harder than when one is in the erect position. Becuase of the altered distribution of blood in the supine position, the heart rate is increased, and the stroke volume (the amount of blood ejected from the heart with each ventricular contraction) is increased.

Another factor that affects the heart and that nurses need very much to be aware of is the Valsalva maneuver. When patients in bed use their arms and upper trunk muscles, either to move up in bed or to sit on a bedpan, they tend to hold their breath. This builds up pressure, thus interfering with the blood entering the large thoracic veins. When they then release their breath, the blood suddenly flows to the heart. This sudden surge can result in serious cardiac problems for the patient who already may have a cardiac pathologic condition.

Thrombus formation is the third problem faced by immobilized patients. A *thrombus* is a solid mass of blood constituents, which forms in the heart or vessels. This tendency may be due to the pooling of the blood in the veins from inactivity mentioned earlier, the possible increased viscosity of the blood, perhaps due to dehydration, or to external pressure upon the veins, which can be exerted by the knee gatch of a bed.

THE CONCEPT OF REHABILITATION

The concept of rehabilitation has gained considerable acceptance during the past 20 years. Before that time it was generally associated with vocational help and social guidance for people who had physical injuries, not infrequently as a result of employment accidents. Today, the concept is applied to all health and illness (physical and mental) and to injury. It also involves every age group and every segment of society. A contemporary definition of *rehabilitation* is "the restoration through personal health services of handicapped individuals to the fullest physical, mental and social and economic usefulness of which they are capable, including ordinary treatments and treatments in special rehabilitation centres" (Krusen 1964:1). Rehabilitation, then, is a process of assisting the restoration of people to their previous level of health, that is, to their previous capabilities or to that level which is possible for them. Patients must actively participate in the process if it is to be effective.

The rehabilitation process involves the patient and a team of health personnel who have various specialized skills. A physician usually heads the team and is usually a specialist in rehabilitation medicine; this physician is referred to as a *physiatrist*. Also on the team there may be a nurse, a social worker, an occupational therapist, a physical therapist, and sometimes a psychiatrist and a speech therapist. These people together with the patient and often the family plan a program to assist the patient to make maximum use of capabilities.

Rehabilitation programs usually take place in independent centers in the community or in special units in hospitals. However, rehabilitation really starts the moment a patient enters the health-care system. Thus nurses are highly involved in the rehabilitation process whether they are employed on pediatric, psychiatric, or surgical units of hospitals, for example, or in the community. A rehabilitation process usually has three broad objectives to help a patient:

1. To return those abilities which have been affected to the highest level possible.
2. To prevent further disability.
3. To protect the patient's present abilities.
4. To assist the patient to use abilities.

Rehabilitation is frequently a long process, and the need for rehabilitation programs and facilities is steadily increasing. The growing incidence of chronic disease and disability and the increasingly large groups of elderly persons in North American society mean an increased need for rehabilitation.

SUMMARY

Mobility and exercise are essential to the health of humans. Mobility allows for movement from place to place and the ability to carry out most of life's daily activities. Even gestures and facial expressions rely upon the ability to move body parts. Alterations in mobility generally occur because of four reasons: the age and developmental status of the person, a disease process, prescribed restrictions by a physician or medical therapy, and voluntary restrictions imposed by the person to conserve energy.

Developmental variations in body movement are notable. The neonate lacks control and coordination of motor activity and moves in response to reflexes. Some of these include the Moro reflex, the tonic neck reflex, the walking or stepping (dance) reflex, and the grasp reflex. Infants need to learn head control, hand movements, and how to sit, stand, creep, and walk. During the second year of life increased locomotor control occurs. By the age of two years a child is able to run, walk up and down stairs with assistance, and enjoy climbing onto furniture. The progression of motor skills is outlined in Table 23–1.

Mobility is dependent upon adequate movement of the body joints. Six types of joints are present in the body, and each has a normal range of movement depending upon its type. These six joints are classified as ball and socket, hinge, pivot, condyloid, saddle, and gliding. Thirteen joint movements are described in relation to the anatomical body positon. Examples are flexion, extension, rotation, abduction, and adduction. The normal major range of motion exercises of each body joint are described and illustrated in the text.

Physical fitness requires regular exercise in balance with daily caloric intake. Three aspects of functional physical fitness include joint flexibility exercises, muscle tone exercises, and endurance exercises. Suggested target heart rates for endurance exercises are outlined.

There are various kinds of exercise, which may be used in accordance with an individual person's health and strength. These are (a) active (isotonic), (b) passive, (c) active-assistive, (d) isometric, and (e) resistive exercises. The purposes and indications for use for each of these vary. The nurse's role in providing passive exercises and the value of isometric and prenatal and postnatal exercises are emphasized.

Exercise has many positive effects. Muscle tone of the skeletal muscles and internal organs is maintained, blood circulation is facilitated, metabolism and appetite are increased, body wastes are excreted effectively, and a sense of mental equilibrium results. Common problems of joint and muscle movements include ankylosis, contracture, hypertonicity, hypotonicity, and atrophy.

Ambulation requires movement of the joints and muscles of the hip and lower extremities. Muscles of the abdomen and buttocks also assist these muscles in maintaining balance. When patients are bedridden, these muscles weaken, and exercises preparatory to ambulation are necessary. Significant exercises include those which flex and extend the hip, extend the knee, and strengthen the muscles of the abdomen, buttocks, and thighs.

When assisting patients to walk, the nurse needs to employ the use of body mechanics. Various positions and methods may be used to offer security and balance to the patient. Various mechanical aids can offer the patient independence of movement without the nurse's assistance. These include canes, walkers, limb braces, and crutches. The use of crutches offers the most versatility in that four different gaits can be achieved for varying degrees of mobility.

Limitations in mobility vary in degree but are generally described as immobility even though there is not complete lack of mobility. Broadly speaking, immobility includes physical, intellectual, emotional, and social aspects. Many problems ensue with prolonged immobility. Included are decreased ability to learn, decreased motivation to solve problems, exaggerated emotional reactions, osteoporosis, muscle atrophy, urinary calculi, constipation, accumulation of respiratory secretions, and orthostatic hypotension.

SUGGESTED ACTIVITIES

1. Observe a 2-year-old and a 5-year-old. Compare their motor development.

2. Assess your physical fitness in the areas of joint flexibility, muscle tone, and endurance.

3. Observe a physiotherapist with a patient. Identify the kind and purpose of the exercises being carried out.

4. Identify patients who require passive exercises. Carry out the appropriate exercises for one patient.

5. Visit a setting where people require assistance with their ambulation. Identify specific problems the patients encounter and the measures taken to assist the patients.

SUGGESTED READINGS

Brower, Phyllis, and Hicks, Dorothy. July, 1972. Maintaining muscle function in patients on bedrest. *American Journal of Nursing* 72:1250–1253.

The effects of bed rest on skeletal muscle are described. The article describes the usefulness of isometric exercises in instances when joint mobility is contraindicated. Isotonic exercise is also described together with a planned exercise program for a patient.

Gordon, Margory. January, 1976. Assessing activity tolerance. *American Journal of Nursing* 76:72–75.

The author discusses how to determine an individual person's appropriate exercise level. Assessment includes heart rate; heart rhythm; pulse strength; blood pressure; respiratory rate, depth, and rhythm; skin temperature and moistness; posture and equilibrium; activity rate; and emotional state.

Kamenetz, H. L. August, 1972. Exercises for the elderly. *American Journal of Nursing* 72:1401.

The article describes lying down, sitting up, and standing exercises recommended for the elderly.

SELECTED REFERENCES

Carnevali, D., and Brueckner, S. July, 1970. Immobilization—reassessment of a concept. *American Journal of Nursing* 70:1502–1507.

Diebel, A. W. July, 1975. Geriatrics. *Journal of Psychiatric Nursing and Mental Health Services* 13(7):20–23.

Drapeau, Janine, et al. September, 1975. Getting back into good posture: how to erase your lumbar aches. *Nursing 75* 5(9):63–65.

Huston, J. C. Sept. 1975. Overcoming the learning disabilities of stroke. *Nursing 75* 5(9):66, 68.

Jones, Phyllis E. November–December, 1974. Nursing needs of ambulatory patients with chronic disease. *Canadian Journal of Public Health.* 65:422–426.

Maternity Center Association. 1973. *Preparation for childbearing.* New York.

Olson, Edith V. April 1967. The hazards of immobility. *American Journal of Nursing* 67:780–797.

Krusen, Frank H. 1964. *Concepts in rehabilitation of the handicapped.* Philadelphia: W. B. Saunders Co.

Ranalls, J. December 1972. Crutches and walkers. *Nursing '72* 2:21–24.

Russek, A. S., et al. 1964. *Isometric exercises for physical fitness.* Rehabilitation monograph XXV. New York: Institute of Rehabilitation Medicine, New York University Medical Center.

Toohey, P., et al. 1968. *Range of motion exercise: key to joint mobility.* Rehabilitation Publication Number 703. Minneapolis: American Rehabilitation Foundation.

CHAPTER 24

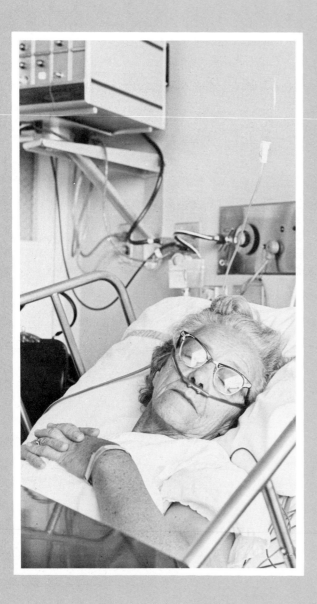

REST, SLEEP, AND RELIEF FROM PAIN

OBJECTIVES

- Discuss the meaning of rest.

- Describe the conditions that must be met to promote rest.

- Name and discuss the kinds of sleep and describe the stages of sleep.

- List and describe the way in which six factors affect sleep.

- Identify signs (behavior) that result from sleeplessness or sleep deprivation.

- Discuss nursing interventions that promote sleep.

- Describe common sleep problems and nursing interventions required.

- Describe how pain occurs and the physiologic signs.

- Discuss the gate control theory.

- Describe four types of pain in relation to source.

- Discuss three components of the pain experience.

- Identify factors that need to be considered in assessing pain.

- Relate specific nursing interventions that relieve pain to the five aspects of the pain experience.

Rest, sleep, and comfort are all essential for health. Everyone needs a certain amount of rest and sleep to function at an optimal level. During sleep the body repairs itself for the next day. People who are ill frequently require more rest and sleep than normal. Often, unusual amounts of energy are required just to maintain the activities of daily living, resulting in increased and frequent fatigue, and thus more rest and sleep are needed. In addition the ill person's normal sleep schedule is usually changed, which necessitates a need for nursing assistance to promote the sleep required.

Comfort can be thought of in both physical and emotional contents. *Physical comfort* includes freedom from pain and the person's harmony with the environment. For example, in a very hot environmental temperature, most people experience physical discomfort. *Emotional comfort* is freedom from mental distress such as anxiety or depression.

In this chapter comfort will be considered as it relates to pain and freedom from pain. Pain is frequently a problem for patients, and as such it challenges the nurse to provide individual measures that help patients obtain relief.

REST

Rest is often advised for people when they are ill. It is not always easily provided in that rest is not merely inactivity. *Rest* implies: freedom from anxiety; calmness; or relaxation without emotional stress (Ford 1965:11). Therefore rest does not always imply inactivity; in fact, changing one's activity can be restful to some people. For example, a student who is studying for examinations may find it restful to have a walk in the fresh air. The meaning of rest and the requirements for rest vary among individuals. Providing a restful environment for patients is an important function of nurses. In order to assess the patient's need for rest and to evaluate how effectively this need is met, nurses need to consider the following conditions that promote rest.

Conditions that Must Be Met to Promote Rest

Six characteristics of rest have been outlined that are applicable to most people. These provide a summary for the meaning of rest (Narrow 1967:1645) and a guide for the nurse in assessing and promoting rest for patients.

One can rest when one:

1. Feels that things are under control.
2. Feels accepted.
3. Feels that one can understand what is going on.
4. Is free from irritation and discomfort.
5. Has a satisfying amount of purposeful activity.
6. Knows that one will receive help when it is needed.

The patient needs to feel that both the situation in the hospital or other health care agency and the patient's personal life are under control. This has many implications for the nurse. By providing competent care, the nurse allows the patient to feel more relaxed and to have peace of mind. By listening to concerns about personal affairs and providing assistance in alleviating them, a nurse can often promote the patient's need to rest. For example, a patient who is hemorrhaging and is taken to an emergency ward may require assistance in making a phone call to inform family members before being able to relax. A busy lawyer who suffers a heart attack may be more worried about the papers that were to be delivered to a client than about pain and discomfort. Even when the person comes prepared for hospitalization, personal concerns and worries need to be considered. For example, the patient admitted for elective diagnostic surgery such as a cystoscopy may also be recovering successfully from a fractured hip. Routinely the patient has been walking prescribed distances each day, and is worried that progress will be disrupted if this routine is not maintained. Many patients have well-established routines that are important to them. These include countless activities, such as reading oneself to sleep, drinking hot water each morning to promote bowel evacuation, or following certain religious practices. Children often have security rituals for napping. For those patients who are hospitalized for long periods, the routine of sleeping in on a Saturday or Sunday morning or scheduled daily routines of quiet or privacy may be important. Most people need some time alone to themselves.

Feelings of being accepted are also essential for rest. Patients need to feel acceptable to themselves and to others. Grooming is often one important aspect of self-acceptance. Women may be concerned about the growth of body hair on their legs or the need for a shampoo or manicure; men may be concerned about the state of their beard or mustache. The nurse therefore needs to be sensitive to and attend to these aspects of care. Acceptance by the staff is also important to the patient. This can be conveyed in various ways such as by recognizing both the patient's limitations and progress or recognizing individual idiosyncrasies.

The need to understand what is happening is another essential condition for rest. The unknown always generates varying degrees of anxiety and interferes with rest. Explanations about diagnostic tests, surgery, agency policies or routines, and the patient's progress need to be offered frequently. Information that is given freely to patients prevents the tension associated with having to ask questions.

Freedom from irritation and discomfort includes both physical and emotional aspects. Generally the physical discomforts are readily recognized, such as pain, insufficient supports for body positions, dampness of a bed sheet, or a noisy environment. Emotional discomforts may include too many visitors or too few visitors, lack of privacy, being hurried, having to wait long periods, being alone, or concern about the life problems of self or others.

Purposeful activity often provides a sense of being worthwhile and can be relaxing. The grandmother who knits a scarf for her child, the person who helps make the bed, the adolescent who makes a wallet for her father, or the child who makes a toy puppet generally have a sense of contentment and peace of mind. The activity often promotes rest throughout the day and an undisturbed sleep at night.

The last condition for rest is the security of knowing that help is available when needed. Most people have experienced the sense of isolation and fear associated with being alone or helpless. Friends and family members often provide comfort when assistance is needed to make decisions or when help to perform daily tasks is required. During illness, patients feel reassured when the nurse anticipates and identifies these needs. Knowing that the call bell will be answered or that help will be given to walk, for example, may seem trivial, but can be exceedingly important to the patient. Nurses will encounter many situations in which patients require support and understanding to make major decisions. These may include questions such as "Shall I place the baby for adoption?" or "Shall I move to a nursing home?" Such situations need to be faced, and nurses can often be instrumental in offering additional information about referral agencies or by allowing the patient to express feelings.

SLEEP

Sleep is a basic physiologic need of people. It is identified by minimal physical activity, variable levels of consciousness, changes in the body's physiologic processes, and decreased responsiveness to external stimuli.

Individuals differ in their sleep habits, and on an average adults need between five and eight hours of sleep each 24 hours, usually at night. The sleep pattern can be affected by age, fatigue, illness, anxiety, medications, and alcohol. These will be discussed later in the chapter.

The purpose of sleep appears to be both integrative and restorative. The release of hormones, the biochemical changes, and the cellular nourishment all assist the body to become ready for another day's activities. During sleep, repair and reorganization occur within the neuronal system together with the formation of new connections. Consequently the day's learning is filed with other pathways for future use. Hence the importance of sleep for the learner. A third function of sleep is to mediate stress, anxiety, and tension and to assist the person to regain energy for concentration, coping, and interest in daily activities.

The Circadian Rhythm

Biorhythmology, the study of the biologic rhythms of the body, is receiving increasing attention from biologists. Rhythmic biologic clocks (biorhythms) exist in plants, animals, and man. In man these are controlled from within the body and are synchronized with environmental factors such as light and darkness, gravity, or electromagnetic stimuli. The rhythms in human beings are demonstrated biologically and behaviorally. Examples of biologic rhythms in humans are the repetitive rhythmic contractions of the heart muscle, the waking and sleeping cycles, and body temperature changes. Each biorhythmic cycle has peaks and troughs. When applied to individuals, these cyles vary somewhat. For example, the waking and sleeping cycle normally averages eight hours sleep at night for adults. However, some people, referred to as "night owls," seem to be more alert during the late evening hours and retire late. Others, referred to as "early birds," prefer to retire early and perform well in the early hours of the morning.

Biorhythms are classified according to the time involved for the cycle. The most common cycle is the *circadian rhythm*, which involves one day. The term circadian is from the Latin origin, *circa dies*, meaning "about a day." A second rhythm is the *infradian rhythm*, which cycles monthly. An example is the menstrual cycle. A third rhythm is the *ultradian rhythm*, which cycles during minutes or hours. An example is the REM (rapid eye movement) cycle of sleep. All biorhythms can be altered by changes in the environment. For example, the circadian rhythm of the nurse who changes to night shift is altered, or the menstrual cycle of a woman becomes dyssynchronized with anxiety or illness.

The circadian rhythm starts about the third month of life, and it may be inherited from the mother's cycle. While a person sleeps, a number of cycles of sleep are experienced, each one of which lasts about 90 minutes. Thus when one sleeps, one goes through about five cycles in a normal seven to eight hours of sleep. Each sleep cycle can be further subdivided into identifiable stages, although the person may not go through every stage in each cycle.

The use of the *electroencephalogram* (EEG) has provided a better picture of what occurs during sleep. Electrodes are placed on various parts of the person's scalp. They transmit the electrical energy produced by the cortex of the brain onto graph paper, producing what is known as brain waves. Each pen of the electroencephalogram corresponding to an electrode moves up when the electrical change is negative and down when it is positive.

Kinds of Sleep

There are two different types of sleep: slow-wave sleep and paradoxical sleep (REM sleep). *Slow-wave sleep* is also called deep restful sleep. In this type of sleep brain waves are slow, and it accounts for most sleep during the night. *Paradoxical sleep* is also called REM sleep, referring to the rapid eye movements that occur during this sleep. Paradoxical sleep is imposed on slow-wave sleep, and a person will have several bouts of it during a period of sleep. Each period of paradoxical sleep lasts 5–20 minutes. The first period generally occurs 80–100 minutes after the person falls asleep. The more tired the person, the shorter the first period of paradoxical sleep. There are a number of characteristics of this type of sleep that are of impor-

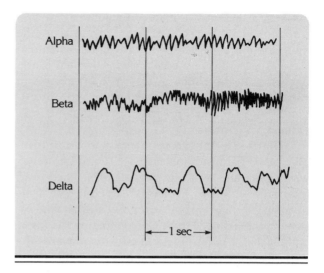

Figure 24-1.   Brain waves recorded on an electroencephalograph.

tance to nurses:

1. The person is difficult to arouse.
2. Muscle tone throughout the body is depressed.
3. Heart and respiratory rate usually become irregular.
4. Irregular muscle movements occur, especially in the eyes (REM) (Guyton 1976:739).

Before one goes to sleep, one feels drowsy and relaxed. The electroencephalograph will reveal a regular rhythm of alpha waves (Figure 24–1), which occur in almost all normal persons who are awake but in a quiet resting state.

Stages of Sleep

Stage I

Alpha waves continue to be present in Stage I, although they are more uneven and smaller than when the person is awake and resting. One feels that one is drifting off to sleep. One has fleeting thoughts and can be readily awakened. If awakened, one may not realize that one has been asleep.

Stage II

Stage II is a light sleep in which the brain waves slow down and assume a delta pattern (Figure 24–1), interspersed with alpha waves called sleep spindles. The person is more relaxed but can still be awakened readily.

Stage III

In Stage III, deep, slow delta waves occur with continued sleep spindles appearing on the EEG. The person becomes more relaxed, and body physiologic processes slow down: the heart rate decreases, the pulse decreases, and the respirations decrease. The person is more difficult to awaken during this stage.

Stage IV

Stage IV is the deep sleep stage during which delta waves dominate the EEG readout. The person is very relaxed and rarely moves. The person is difficult to awaken during this stage and if awakened will respond slowly. It is during this stage that dreams, which are often related to the previous day's events, usually take place. It is also at this time that most *somnambulism* (sleepwalking) and *enuresis* (bedwetting) take place.

After one falls asleep, one generally passes from Stage I through Stages II and III to Stage IV in about 20–30 minutes. The process is then reversed, and one ascends through Stages III and II to Stage I again, taking about 60–90 minutes. At this time (Stage I), REM sleep usually occurs. One's eyes move and often parts of the body twitch although the body muscles are relaxed. During this time vivid dreams often occur that are colorful and busy.

During this period, also, reflexes are diminished but the brain is active. After this Stage I REM activity, which takes about 10 to 15 minutes, one moves through Stages II and III to Stage IV again. The total cycle takes about 60–90 minutes. As the night progresses and one becomes less tired, less time is spent in Stages III and IV, and the time in Stage I REM sleep increases.

Factors that Affect Sleep

A number of factors affect sleep. Some of these are age, fatigue, illness, anxiety, medications, and alcohol.

Age

Age affects not only the pattern of sleep but the need for sleep. The nurse is referred to Table 24–1 for the variable needs of people for sleep and to "Developmental Variations of Rest and Sleep."

The infant spends about 50% of the time in REM sleep, whereas the adult spends about 23%. Elderly people have less Stages III and IV sleep and less REM than infants and adults. Thus elderly people have more frequent awakenings during the night. It is also during the Stage I REM that an elderly person will wander.

Fatigue

Fatigue also affects the sleep pattern in that the more tired the person is the shorter the first period of paradoxical (REM) sleep. As the person rests, the REM periods become longer.

Illness

People who are ill frequently require more sleep than normal, and the normal rhythm of sleeping and being awake is also disturbed. When people have been deprived of REM sleep, they subsequently spend more sleeping time in this stage than normal.

Anxiety

Anxiety and other emotional disturbances can also affect a person's ability to obtain sleep. When one is emotionally upset, one is often preoccupied with problems that do not allow relaxation prior to sleep.

Medications

Medications, especially hypnotics and sedatives, affect the sleep pattern. Hypnotics and barbiturates decrease the REM sleep even though they may increase the total sleep experience. The amphetamines also abnormally decrease REM sleep. Long-term use

Table 24-1. Estimated Average Sleeping Hours per Day by Age

Age	Average hours
Newborn	16–20
1 year	14–16
3 years	10–14
5 to 11 years	9–13
Adolescence	12–14 (some is rest)
Young adult	7–9
Middle-aged adult	7–9
Elderly adult	6–8 (less sleep, more rest)

can produce abnormal, speedy behavior, which can be attributed to long-term REM deprivation.

When a patient is withdrawing from any of these drugs, the patient has a very high amount of REM sleep and as a result may experience upsetting nightmares. Nurses need to be aware of this possible phenomenon and provide the patient with the support and help needed during this period.

Alcohol

Alcohol also affects sleep in that it also depresses the normal REM stage of sleep. While making up for this lost REM sleep after withdrawal from the alcohol, these people will also experience terrible nightmares.. Tolerance to alcohol can result in *insomnia* (inability to sleep) and subsequent irritability.

DEVELOPMENTAL VARIATIONS OF REST AND SLEEP

The amount of sleep that individual people require decreases not only with age but also as the growth rate decreases.

The Newborn and Infant

The newborn, regardless of gestational age or type of delivery, is awake, alert, and active during the transition from intrauterine to extrauterine life. This activity only lasts for about one half hour, however, and a sleep period follows for four to eight hours, depending upon the stresses of birth. After this initial phase, the waking periods become stabilized to every three or four hours. For the first few weeks these are dictated largely by hunger. As time progresses a need to socialize appears. On the average, newborns sleep for 17 hours per day, and by the end of the first month the periods of wakefulness gradually increase. For example, some may stay awake during the day from one feeding to another and sleep a longer interval at night. Sounds in the environment seem to have minimal, if any, effect on the newborn while asleep. This can be observed in nurseries where one newborn cries loudly in one crib and another newborn sleeps soundly in an adjacent crib.

Newborns can usually be aroused easily from sleep, and they just as easily return to sleep provided they are comfortable. Frequent movements of the body and facial grimaces are normal during their sleep periods and indicate REM sleep. When newborns do not sleep well and cry or fuss for long periods, it is usually because of hunger, a wet diaper, or temperature extremes. If comfort measures offer no relief, illness may be the cause.

By two months of age a preference for sleeping position is often noted but may actually have occurred from birth onward. By three months of age, routines before sleeping are established such as crying, sucking on fingers or toys, or attempts to find a suitable position. By four months most infants sleep through the night and have a scheduled pattern of nap periods that vary with individuals during the day. They generally awaken early in the morning, however. During waking periods the infant at this time begins to be content with short intervals alone. At the end of the first year, an infant usually has one or two naps per day and sleeps about 14 hours per day. The infant also begins to show fear about being deserted by the mother and being left alone.

The measures to promote sleep and rest for infants also include some safety and security measures. They are as follows:

1. Provide a firm mattress covered with thick plastic material that cannot be pulled over the face and cause suffocation. A flat surface provides the best alignment for bone development.

2. Avoid the use of pillows. They, too, can be a source of accidental suffocation.

3. Position the infant appropriately according to age. Newborns should not be placed on their abdomens unless they are observed very closely. They are unable to turn their heads from side to side and may suffocate if their noses press down firmly against the mattress. A safe position is the side-lying position but it needs to be alternated from one side to the other every two to three hours (Figure 24–2). This prevents flattening of the bones of the skull. The back-lying position is also avoided for newborns and young infants, since vomiting and subsequent aspiration of vomited fluids may occur. When able to turn the head from side to side, the infant may be positioned on the back, abdomen, or side. It is recommended that various positions be used.

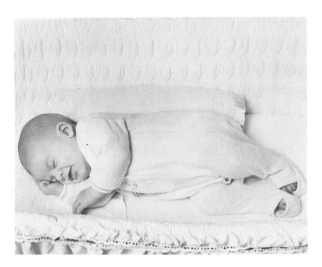

Figure 24-2.   The side-lying position is a safe sleeping position for an infant.

4. Ensure that the room temperature is adequate, approximately 21–23.5° C (70–75° F) in the daytime and 15.5–18.5° C (60–65° F) at night. Avoid drafts and tuck surplus blankets under the mattress to avoid danger of suffocation.

5. Soft lighting directed away from the eyes is preferred to darkness or bright light. Infants tend to like facing the light, so when changing their position it may be necessary to alternate their head from the top of the crib to its foot.

6. Ensure that the infant is dry and comfortable. Provide dry diapers and warm soft clothing.

7. Provide quieting activities before putting the infant down to sleep. Cuddle and/or rock the infant and talk in soothing tones. Give the infant a soft toy to hold and to take to bed, and establish consistent routines.

The Toddler

During the toddler period (one to three years), sleep requirements decrease to 10 to 14 hours per day. The need for an afternoon nap continues for most children, but the necessity for midmorning naps gradually decreases. However, the problems associated with going to sleep often increase with the toddler. Frequently parents seek guidance during this period to develop ways to handle sleeping problems. During toddlerhood dreams and nightmares are common.

At bedtime toddlers frequently resist sleep, feel tense, may be irritable, may cry and just not want to leave the company of adults or older siblings. Naptime and bedtime battles of autonomy and acquiescence normally occur. The mother may put the toddler to bed, but the child inevitably will climb out. These events are associated with the toddler's developmental needs of growing independence, self-control, curiosity, and endless vigor for exploration. On the other hand, toddlers like to set rituals and will insist upon them. For example, bedtime clothing is put on, the child is told that bedtime is in half an hour, a story is told, goodnight hugs are given, the child is taken to the bathroom, is provided with a security toy and given a drink of juice, the shades drawn, and the lights dimmed. Firm adherence to these schedules is essential. Consistency is of more importance than the ritual itself.

Toddlers often develop their own ways of going to sleep. They may talk to themselves for awhile, roll their heads, rock in bed, or play with a toy. These habits are important in relieving tension and are normal. Some of these behaviors will also occur during the daytime naps, and prenap rituals should be consistent. Often mothers at this time require an afternoon nap that can be scheduled with the toddler's.

Measures to promote sleep for toddlers include:

1. Provide consistency of bedtime or naptime rituals.

2. Adhere firmly to sleeping schedules.

3. Encourage quieting activities before sleep.

4. Support tension-reducing activities such as head-rolling or talking and providing one toy. Too many toys create too much stimulation.

5. Avoid using the bed as a disciplinary measure at any time.

The Preschooler

The preschooler from three to six years is similar to the toddler in that the preschooler is not aware of when rest or sleep are needed. Preschoolers are more interested in what is happening around them and also may resist sleep. The difference is that the preschooler requires more privacy, not only for sleep but also for the restful activities of fantasy, sexual explorations, enjoyment of possessions, or for intervals to deal with disappointments and hurts. At this time a private room or portion of a room is recommended for the preschooler.

Three-year-olds frequently have nightmares associated with real or imagined fears. Sometimes it is difficult for them to differentiate between what is real and what is not. It is not unusual for children at these times to wander into their parents' bedroom and to want to sleep with them. For those children who have difficulty sleeping at night, naps during the day can decrease their restlessness. Sleeping near older siblings or near the parents' room can also be comforting.

Four-to-five-year-olds reach a stage at which they resist daytime sleep. Although sleep may not be possible in the daytime, often a rest period is necessary. Parents should encourage some rest periods at this age level. The room can be darkened and restful or quiet activities promoted. Child day-care centers or kindergartens commonly schedule rest periods with mats on the floor for children of this age. By the age of five, children usually sleep restfully throughout the night, but they may require occasional naps in the daytime if activities are overly stimulating. Nightmares may persist but are to be expected.

Measures to promote sleep and rest for preschoolers are similar to those for the toddler. Increasing independence of the presleep ritual activities

occurs, and expression of fears increases and needs to be encouraged. When the parent listens to these fears and parental presence and availability is assured, the child is generally reassured.

The School-Age Child

A peaceful night's sleep for school-age children can not be guaranteed. Although the sleep requirements are less (9 to 13 hours), the schoolchild often has nightmares. These are often associated with fears of death, a concept about which the child now has a better grasp. Questions, discussions, and confidences with parents are common with this age group.

Growing children will increasingly begin to vocalize the time they wish to go to bed. Parental judgment is still required, however. Parents need to set limitations on the child's activities and schedule specific bedtimes to ensure sufficient rest. More flexibility for schedules will gradually occur with older children.

COMMON SLEEP PROBLEMS

The nurse will no doubt encounter a number of the following common sleep problems in nursing practice.

Insomnia

This is one of the most common problems in North American society. Most nurses can remember instances of their own *insomnia,* which is the inability to obtain sufficient sleep. It is not the total lack of sleep, and in fact, people having insomnia often obtain more sleep than they are aware of.

There are basically two types of insomnia: the inability to fall asleep and the inability to stay asleep. It can result from physical discomfort but more often is a result of mental overstimulation due to anxiety. People have even been known to become anxious because they think they might not be able to sleep. Insomnia also develops in people who become habituated to drugs or who drink large quantities of alcohol.

Treatment for insomnia frequently requires a physician's intervention and often the development of new behavior patterns on the part of the patient to

induce sleep. For example, one woman who had been unable to sleep without a sedative learned to take her dog for a long walk before retiring, thus relaxing and becoming somewhat physically fatigued.

Nocturnal Enuresis

Enuresis is involuntary urination; *nocturnal enuresis* is involuntary urination at night and is often called *bed-wetting.* It can occur in preadolescent children and its cause is unknown, although in preschool children it may be due to too severe training, too early training, or overtraining (Marlow 1977:619). In children over three or four years, environmental factors such as a dark hall may contribute to the child's reluctance to go to the bathroom. In the schoolchild enuresis may be caused by inadequate bladder capacity or jealousy over a new brother or sister. In most of these situations parents are advised to rule out physical abnormalities first and to provide a positive environment for the child in which the child feels loved. Restricting fluids before bedtime may assist with the obvious problem but not with the cause of the problem.

Somnambulism

Somnambulism is commonly known as *sleepwalking*, and it is not uncommonly seen in children. The condition is normally outgrown without incident. The walking generally takes place in sleep Stage IV when the person is unaware of walking.

The main concern in somnambulism is to protect the person from injury. Usually the sleepwalker can be awakened and quietly led back to bed.

ASSESSMENT OF THE NEED FOR SLEEP

When nurses assess the need of a patient for sleep, they need to consider the person's age, normal sleep habits and patterns, as well as any extenuating circumstances that affect sleep, such as an exhausting illness or anxiety.

The person who needs sleep will show some of the following signs:

1. Expression of a feeling of fatigue.
2. Exhibition of withdrawal, depression, and apathy.
3. Periods of irritability and aggressiveness.
4. Marked periods of inattention.
5. Confusion and hallucinations with total sleep deprivation.

Sleep Deprivation

Sleep deprivation or sleeplessness is accompanied by certain biochemical changes in the body. The person's behavior and personality also change. Initially sleep deprivation causes periods of inattention, irritability, apathy, and aggressiveness. With prolonged sleep deprivation the person may become confused and disoriented.

Patients who have been deprived of REM sleep periods become irritable, fatigued, and increasingly sensitive to pain, and may have a feeling of pressure around the head and momentary illusions (Long 1969:1898).

Sleeplessness also lowers the seizure threshold. Consequently, people who have epilepsy and are ill are advised not to go for prolonged periods without sleep. Sleep deprivation can also occur when sleep is repeatedly interrupted, for example when a patient is in an intensive care unit of a hospital and receiving constant medical or nursing care.

NURSING INTERVENTIONS TO PROMOTE SLEEP

There are a number of nursing measures that a nurse can choose to assist the individual patient to meet the need for sleep. The measures selected should meet the needs of the individual patient. Some of the measures are:

1. Provide a relaxing environment prior to the sleep time. This may include measures such as diversional activity, the relief of pain, and the provision of a fresh, clean environment. The latter can involve the removal of obnoxious odors and provision of a clean, comfortable bed.

2. Assist the patient to maintain usual before-sleep routines. People often establish routines that assist them to sleep. Some people like a tub bath before a night's sleep, others like to read or perhaps have a small snack. It is usually helpful for the sick person to maintain these activities when ill even if in a hospital unless the measures are contraindicated for health reasons. In talking to a patient who has difficulty getting to sleep, the nurse may discover the reason, for example, the patient could not brush his teeth—a lifelong habit!

3. Eliminate extraneous noises if possible. Banging bedpans, moving noisy equipment in the hallway, or loud laughter can all hinder sleep.

4. Provide an environment in which the patient feels safe and assured that care will be provided if the patient becomes more seriously ill while asleep.

5. Provide sufficient covers so that the patient will not become cold while sleeping. Elderly people often

require more covers at night than others because their body temperatures often drop lower than those of other people.

6. Children may require special comforting such as reading a favorite bedtime story or providing a night light to allay fear. A strange environment can be even more frightening to a child who does not understand what is happening.

7. Provide a hypnotic or sedative if this is ordered by the physician and if it is needed by the patient. If the patient also requires an analgesic, provide this in advance of the sedative so that the patient will feel comfortable when becoming sleepy.

8. Assist a patient to his or her normal position for sleeping if this is possible.

PAIN

Pain is a highly unpleasant sensation. It is also personal in that only the person who has pain really experiences it; it cannot be shared with others. Pain can also occupy all of one's thinking, direct one's activities, and change one's life. Pain is an important sign that there is something physiologically wrong. As such it can serve a useful purpose in that it may be the reason a person seeks help for a health problem of which the person would otherwise be unaware. Pain is usually accompanied by other bodily sensations such as pressure, heat, or perhaps cold. Pain then has been defined as "a basically unpleasant sensation referred to the body which represents the suffering induced by the psychic perception of real, threatened or phantasied injury" (Engel 1970:45).

Because pain is a highly personal sensation nurses are really dependent upon the patient's description to obtain pertinent data about it. Only a patient can say exactly where the pain is felt or the kind of pain experienced. Pain can be thought of as either acute or chronic. *Acute pain* is generally of short duration, such as that which occurs with a finger cut or a broken bone. *Chronic pain* lasts much longer, even years. Acute pain may develop into chronic pain. Chronic pain may gradually develop in such a manner that the person finds it difficult to remember when it first started.

Intractable pain is pain that is resistant to cure or relief. An example is with arthritis, for which narcotic analgesics are contraindicated because of the long-term duration of the disease and the danger of addiction. In some cases of intractable pain, behavior modification techniques have been used. In these programs behavior that is not pain oriented is rewarded, and pain-oriented behavior is ignored. The aim of this technique is to change one's behavior to that which will assist one to live more comfortably and effectively.

Pain Perception

The first step in the perception of pain by a person is the stimulation of receptors, which are located in almost every tissue of the body. They are most prevalent in the skin and body surface tissue such as mucous membrane. There are a number of kinds of receptors that are sensitive to pain, including temperature receptors, which pick up extremes in temperature. Sensory receptors are also sensitive to painful stimuli.

There is a difference in the sensitivity of various areas of the body. For example, the skin, the arterial walls, and the periosteum are abundantly supplied with receptors; the brain and the alveoli of the lungs, on the other hand, have none.

Once the receptors are aroused by a painful stimulus, the impulse travels along the sensory nerves to the spinal cord. At the same time a reflex action often occurs, withdrawing the body part from the source of the pain. Once at the spinal cord, the impulses cross to the opposite side of the spinal cord and ascend by the lateral spinothalamic tracts to the thalamus of the brain. At this stage the autonomic nervous system is activated. Superficial pain usually stimulates the sympathetic system, whereas deep (internal) pain stimulates the parasympathetic system (see Table 24–2). From the thalamus the impulses travel to the sensory area of the cerebral cortex. At this time the person becomes aware of the pain and takes action to avoid or eliminate the cause.

Sometimes pain is perceived to be in an area of the body other than its actual location. This is called *referred pain*. For example, cardiac pain may be perceived radiating to the left shoulder and down the left arm, or the pain from an inflamed appendix may be perceived as occurring throughout the abdomen. With referred pain the nerve fibers that carry the pain

Table 24-2. Physiologic Responses to Pain

Superficial pain (primarily sympathetic reaction)	Deep pain (primarily parasympathetic reaction)
1. Hyperalgesia	1. Nausea, in cases such as gallstones, angina
2. Tickling, itching	2. Pallor
3. Brisk movement	3. Sweating
4. Tachycardia	4. Fall in blood pressure
5. Increased respiratory rate	5. Bradycardia
6. Increased blood pressure	6. Decreased respiratory rate
7. Increased alertness	Increased alertness

impulse join with other nerve fibers in the spinal cord. When the pain is sufficiently intense, the impulses spread over to other areas that normally perceive impulses from the skin. Hence the person perceives the pain as originating in the skin rather than at its real source.

Phantom pain is pain that is perceived to be from a part of the body that no longer is present, such as an amputated foot. This type of pain is not well understood; however, if the gate control theory is applied, it has been suggested that the pain impulse originates higher up in the spinal pathway and that the gate control mechanism has failed.

The *gate control theory* proposes that pain impulses can be altered in the spinal cord, brainstem, and cerebral cortex of the brain. Certain cells along the transmission route can block the impulses, resulting in an altered pain perception or no perception at all (Siegele 1974:499). Closely packed cells extending the length of the spinal cord provide the blocking action for the impulses, in effect closing the gate. If the activity of these fibers is not sufficient to block the pain impulses, then the person perceives pain.

There are other control systems concerned with pain in the thalamus and cerebral cortex of the brain. Activation of a central control center can also initiate a descending blocking action to incoming pain impulses. This central control system affects the attention the person gives to the pain. Anxiety related to the experience, anticipation, suggestion, and memory of past experiences can affect one's perception of pain. They also affect the meaning that the person attaches to the pain. For example, a man who had a

heart attack three years previously may perceive any epigastric pain as cardiac pain.

Types of Pain

Pain is always ascribed to a body location, and it can be categorized as follows:

Superficial Somatic Tissues

Superficial somatic tissue areas, such as the skin, subcutaneous tissue, fibrous tissue, ligaments, and tendon sheaths are all well supplied with pain receptors and fibers. Therefore pain impulses arising from these structures will be well localized.

Deep Somatic Tissues and Viscera

Deep somatic tissues and viscera are less well supplied with pain fibers, and they do not have a direct connection with the sensory-discriminative system (Engel 1970:52). Thus when a person perceives pain of this type it is generally diffuse and less well localized. However, the closer an organ is to the body surface, the easier it is to localize. The pain from deep structures is often referred to a superficial body part rather than being perceived from the precise area affected. The term *radiating* is also used to describe such pain. For example, pain from the heart is felt to the left of the sternum and radiates down the left arm; pain from the gallbladder is felt in the right upper quadrant of the abdomen and radiates to the scapula. Many specific patterns of radiation commonly occur and are useful for diagnostic purposes. Sometimes past experiences or concurrent painful experiences can affect the place where the person locates the pain. For instance, the person who has a gastric ulcer may perceive concurrent anginal pain in the same area as the ulcer pain.

Neurogenic Pain

Neurogenic pain results when the peripheral or central nervous system has been damaged so that any sensation is perceived as pain (Engel 1970:60). The pain may result from abnormal processing of the afferent impulses or from paroxysmal activity that originates within the nervous system.

Psychogenic Pain.

Psychogenic pain, that is, pain originating in the mind, can have a number of sources: fantasies, wishes, needs, or impulses involving ideas of injury or punishment. The psychologic mechanism involved is conversion. See Chapter 8, "Mental Defense Mechanisms."

Components of the Pain Experience

The pain experience can be thought of as having three components:

1. Initiation of the pain impulse.
2. Perception of the pain.
3. Response to the pain.

Initiation of the Pain Impulse

According to the gate control theory, a stimulus may or may not result in the perception of pain. There are, however, a number of stimuli that can be perceived as pain. Some of these are chemical irritants such as hydrochloric acid in contact with a gastric ulcer; ischemia resulting in the accumulation of waste products in the tissues; mechanical trauma that contracts or distends body tissues or puts pressure on body tissues such as is caused by an excessively tight arm cast; and extremes of heat and cold.

Perception of Pain

The *pain perception threshold* refers to the amount of stimulation required for pain to be perceived. Pain thresholds are generally fairly uniform in people, although they can be dramatically altered by a state of consciousness. A patient who is anesthetized will not feel pain; a patient who is unconscious may or may not react to suborbital pressure, that is, pain on the lower aspect of the eye. The latter test is one way of testing the level of consciousness.

Perception involves understanding something new and then making it part of one's previous experience or knowledge. The process of the perception of pain involves interpretation of the sensory input in terms of previous experience. This is influenced by the person's previous and current psychologic experiences. For example, a person who is tired may attach a different meaning to a throbbing leg than he does when he is rested. It also explains why two people can react very differently to the same stimulus.

Children often perceive pain with fear because they do not understand what is happening to them. One study on what pain means to 10- and 11-year-old children found replies such as "it hurts" and that

their fear of bodily damage was exaggerated (Schultz 1971:672). Children of this age view pain in terms of what they cannot do, that is, in terms of hindrance to their needs and wants, such as "I can't play football."

Pain is sometimes perceived as being more severe when there is inadequate environmental stimulation. The person who is alone in a room at night or the person who is immobilized are two examples. The person alone is more likely to think about her pain and is not distracted by the conversation of others. The immobilized person is unable to physically move, and this creates a feeling of helplessness, which can contribute to the perception of pain.

Response to the Pain

People vary widely in their reactions to pain. The physiologic responses to pain were shown in Table 24-2. Behavioral responses to pain vary also. Different cultures have very different learned responses to pain. Some groups such as the North American Indian and the Chinese show stoical behavior in response to pain. Other groups such as the Italian and the Jewish people tend to be more expressive in their reactions (Blaylock 1968:270).

It is important that nurses recognize that there are a wide variety of learned responses that are considered appropriate by different cultural groups. The more stoical response is largely accepted in North American society, however, because many ethnic groups exist in North America, various responses to pain are observed by the nurse. Nurses need to avoid judging responses as good or bad in relation to their own beliefs. It is also important to realize that a stoical person probably will not state when he or she does have pain, thus making nonverbal clues an important part of nursing assessment.

Pain will usually create anxiety in a person. This largely occurs because of the person's realization that something is wrong and because of a subsequent change in normal activites. It is also not unusual for people to attach a value judgment to pain. Nurses may hear a patient say "What have I done to deserve this?" When a person believes that the pain is undeserved, the person may react with increased anxiety, stress, and even anger.

Sometimes people believe the pain is deserved. These people may feel guilty and see the pain as justified punishment. Others may use the pain as a means of obtaining attention. They will find the pain experience to be rewarding, thus reducing their anxiety.

ASSESSMENT OF PAIN

Because pain is such a personal experience nurses must rely to a large degree upon the patient's ability to verbally communicate about pain. In addition there are often nonverbal actions that can convey information about the pain. Pain is assessed according to its location, intensity, time and duration; qualitative characteristics; the nonverbal behavior of the patient; and the patient's previous experiences and precipitating factors.

Location

Superficial pain can usually be accurately located by a patient; however, pain arising from the viscera is perceived to be more general. Nurses need to ascertain where the patient experiences pain. The various abdominal sections, which the nurse can use when describing the location of abdominal pain, are shown in Chapter 14. In addition, the nurse needs to use vocabulary such as "proximal, distal, medial, lateral" when describing the location of pain in the body (see Chapter 23, "Synovial Joint Movements"). The term *diffuse* usually refers to pain that is perceived over a large area.

When assessing the location of pain experienced by a child, it is important to understand the child's vocabulary. For example, "tummy" might refer to the abdomen or part of the chest. It is wise for a nurse to ask a child to point out where the pain is rather than to rely on words, which may be highly individualistic. Often parents can assist nurses with the meaning of a child's words. For a smaller child and a baby, observation of when the child cries in response to movement can often assist in establishing the location of a pain.

Intensity

The intensity or severity of pain is also important. Although this is a subjective value, it is also true that certain tissues are more sensitive than others. There are several factors that affect the perception of intensity. One is the distraction or concentration of the person upon another event, another is the state of consciousness of the person, and a third is the person's expectations.

Pain may be described as slight, mild, medium, severe, or excruciating. What is perhaps of greatest importance is any change in the intensity of the pain.

This may indicate a change in the patient's pathologic condition and needs to be reported. For example, acute abdominal pain that abruptly decreases in intensity may indicate a ruptured appendix.

Reports of pain by a patient must be considered in relation to the patient's ability and need to report. The elderly, confused patient may distort the intensity of the pain, while a child may minimize pain to avoid admission to the hospital or unpleasant tests.

Other factors relating to the perception of pain such as central nervous system pathologic conditions, anxiety, and previous experiences have already been discussed in this chapter.

Time and Duration

The time and duration of the pain include the time of onset, how long it lasts, whether it recurs and, if so, the interval without pain, and when the pain last occurred. Often there are important factors that relate to the occurrence of the pain, such as cardiac pain that occurs upon physical exertion. Sometimes pain occurs after a meal or before a meal. If may last a few seconds or extend for hours or even weeks.

The interval between pains can also be very important. In obstetrical nursing the intervals between labor contractions are important in assessing the patient's progress in her labor. As the birth of the baby becomes more imminent, the labor pains become more severe and closer together.

Quality

Pain can also be described according to certain disruptive characteristics. Often the terms patients use are those familiar to them. A headache may be described as "hammer-like" or an abdominal pain as "piercing like a knife."

In some instances patients have difficulty describing pain because they have never experienced any sensation like it. This is particularly true of children and of adults who have pain originating within the nervous system. Following is a list of some of the terms used to describe pain.

Aching	Crushing
Burning	Cutting
Constant	Diffuse
Cramping	Dull

Excruciating	Pounding
Gnawing	Prickly
Hammering	Radiating
Heavy	Searing
Intermittent (spasmodic)	Sharp
Irritating	Shifting
Jabbing	Squeezing
Knifelike	Stabbing
Knotting	Tearing
Lancing	Throbbing
Piercing	Tingling
Pinching	Vicelike

When recording the description of the pain given by the patient, it is best to use the exact words used by the patient. In this way the description is more accurate than if the nurse interprets using the nurse's words.

Nonverbal Behavior

This is of particular importance in assessing pain experienced by patients who are unable to communicate verbally. The very young, the aphasic, and confused or disoriented persons will often communicate their experiences of pain only nonverbally. The nurse can obtain data by several types of nonverbal behavior.

Facial expression is often the first indication of pain and may be the only one. There are a variety of aspects that may be observed: clenched teeth, tightly shut eyes, open sombre eyes, biting of the lower lip, or a number of facial grimaces.

Body movement can also indicate the presence of pain. Immobilization of the body or a part of the body is frequently seen. The patient who is experiencing chest pain often holds the left arm across the chest. A person who had abdominal pain will assume a position of greatest comfort, often with the knees and hips flexed, and will move reluctantly. Even babies will flex their hips and legs when experiencing abdominal pain, although they do not tend to remain in that position (McCaffery 1972:21).

Purposeless body movements can also indicate the presence of pain. The person may toss and turn in bed or fling the arms about. Involuntary reflex movements also can indicate the presence of pain such as may happen when a needle is inserted through the skin. An adult may be able to control this reflex; however, a child may be unable or unwilling to control this response.

Rhythmic body movements or rubbing can also indicate pain nonverbally. The baby who is teething will like to chew on an object; an adult or child may assume a fetal position and rock back and forth when experiencing abdominal pain. During labor the woman may rhythmically massage her abdomen with her hands.

Another clue to the presence of pain is the speed of the speech and the pitch of the voice. Accelerated speed and elevated pitch reflect anxiety, while intense pain can be reflected in a slow speech and monotonous tone. For additional information on nonverbal behavior see Chapter 18.

Previous Experience

The way in which a patient reacts to pain depends to a large degree upon previous experiences. A woman in labor who had a painful, difficult time giving birth previously will probably anticipate and experience considerable pain during the next labor, reacting in a similar way as previously. Sometimes measures that were previously found to be effective in the relief of pain will again be effective for that reason. For example, one patient may be pleased to receive a nasogastric tube, which previously relieved his abdominal pain, rather than an analgesic. For another, an antispasmodic medication, which relieved abdominal pain previously, again may be helpful in relieving pain due to a burn on the leg.

Precipitating Factors

Precipitating factors are also important when reporting about pain. Sometimes particular activities precede pain; for example, physical exertion may be followed by chest pain, or eating may be followed by abdominal pain. These observations are helpful not only in preventing the occurrence of the pain by changing the patient's activities but also in determining the cause of the pain.

There are also environmental factors that can increase pain in people who are well or ill (McCaffery 1972:40). Extreme cold and extremes in humidity can affect some types of pain. For example, sudden exercise on a hot day can cause muscle spasm. In addition, the presence of physical and emotional stressors can precipitate pain. Emotional tension frequently precipitates a migraine headache. Intense fear or physical exertion can precipitate anginal pain.

NURSING INTERVENTIONS TO RELIEVE PAIN

Nursing intervention to relieve pain can take many forms depending upon the individual patient and the pathologic condition. One approach to nursing intervention is to determine at which point in the pain experience the intervention is most likely to be effective for that person. The five aspects of the pain experience to which nursing intervention can be directed are (a) the pain stimulus, (b) the reaction of the pain receptors, (c) the transmission of the pain impulse along the nerve fibers, (d) the pain perception, and (e) the interpretation and response to the pain.

Removing the Pain Stimulus

The removal of the pain stimulus is a highly effective and often long-lasting method of relieving pain. Removing a wet, irritating dressing, smoothing a wrinkled bed, and loosening a bandage that restricts circulation are all examples of removing the pain stimulus. Sometimes medications are also used in this manner; for example, antispasmodic drugs can relieve muscle spasm. The application of heat to a body area can increase circulation and thus relieve localized ischemia (see Chapter 17 for an explanation of the physiologic mechanism).

In some instances the stimulus can be removed by a change in activity. The patient who experiences cardiac pain may prevent this by restricting physical activity. The person with a gastric ulcer may often prevent pain by taking milk regularly. Pain upon voiding after a prostatectomy can often be eliminated by ingesting larger quantities of fluid.

Reducing the Reaction of the Pain Receptors

Sometimes the pain receptors can be protected from the pain stimulus. An ointment applied to the irritated labia can prevent further irritation by urine. Local anesthetics can prevent the transmission of pain at the receptors of the skin. Another example is padding a bony prominence before applying a bandage in order to prevent irritation and pain from the bandage.

Blocking the Transmission of the Pain Impulse

It is also possible to block the passage of the impulse along the nerve pathway. This can be done by injecting a local anesthetic into the nerve. Most nurses are familiar with the administration of a local anesthetic for dental work. The drug is injected to nerve pathways of the painful tooth, thus blocking the transmission of the pain impulse to the brain.

Pain pathways can also be interrupted surgically; the surgical procedure is called a *chordotomy*. The anterolateral nerve tracts in the spinal cord are severed. This is done sometimes in situations in which there is intractable pain.

Electrical stimulation is also carried out in some instances of intractable pain. There are several methods: in *transcutaneous electrical stimulation* electrodes are placed on the surface of the skin. In the *percutaneous method* needles are inserted near a major peripheral nerve. In both methods an electrical charge blocks the pain impulse. There are also two implantable devices: the *peripheral nerve implant* and the *dorsal column stimulator*. For the former the electrode is attached to a major sensory nerve, and in the latter instance the electrode is attached to the dorsal column of the spinal cord. In both types a transmitter is worn externally, sending the desired impulse to block the transmission of the pain impulse (Gaumer 1974:504–505). The blocking of the pain impulse is generally considered to be a physician's responsibility except in some instances in which the nurse is functioning in an expanded role.

Altering the Pain Perception

The perception of pain can be changed primarily in three ways: distraction, analgesics, and hypnosis. Pain is perceived in the thalamus of the brain, but by raising the threshold of perception the pain is not perceived. *Distraction* that draws the person's attention away from the pain can serve to reduce pain perception and in some instances can eliminate pain perception entirely from awareness. For example, a patient who is recovering from surgery may be entirely unaware of any pain while watching a football game on television only to have it return when the game is over. In this instance the pain is not perceived because the impulses from the thalamus are blocked by the cerebral cortical activity related to the football game. Distraction is most effective in instances of relatively mild pain, and it is only in instances of extreme concentration that acute pain is not perceived. An example of the latter is the adolescent who only after finishing a basketball game discovers she has a fractured bone in her foot. When a person is anxious, lonely, or bored, pain will tend to be perceived as greater. In addition if there are disturbing stimuli in the environment such as loud noises, bright lights, unpleasant odors, or an argumentative visitor, it can increase pain perception. The nurse therefore needs to reduce disturbing stimuli.

Analgesics also block pain perception. When an analgesic is given prior to the occurrence of severe pain, perception is more effectively decreased than when it is given after the pain has increased in severity. This is the reason analgesics are given at regular intervals, such as every four hours (q4h) after surgery.

Hypnosis has been used as a treatment of pain of a psychogenic nature and for anesthesia. The susceptible person accepts positive suggestions, which tend to alter perceptions. The success of hypnosis depends to a large degree upon the person's "openness" to suggestion, emotional readiness, and faith in the effectiveness of the hypnosis (American Journal of Nursing 1974:515).

Acupuncture has been practiced for centuries in China and is receiving increasing attention in North America. In acupuncture long slender needles are inserted into the body at various sites, which are not necessarily near the body parts that are anesthetized. The needles can be heated, attached to a mild electric current, or twirled continuously with the hand. Acu-

puncture is thought to provide an analgesic effect. It is currently being used selectively in North America for the treatment of chronic pain.

Altering the Interpretation and Response to Pain

Pain is interpreted in the cerebral cortex, to which the impulse travels from the thalamus of the brain. Narcotic analgesics also play an important role in changing the interpretation and response of a person to pain. Narcotics given to people experiencing pain tend to act at this level rather than changing pain perception. Hypnotics such as phenobarbital tend to change pain interpretation and decrease reaction when given in small doses. For example, the patient may still perceive the pain, but no longer regards it as important or disturbing.

Interaction between the nurse and the patient can also change the interpretation of the pain. Patients who obtain satisfaction from pain because of the extra attention they are given can be helped by receiving assistance to meet these needs in other ways. For additional information on the helping relationship, see Chapter 18.

Evaluation of Pain-Relief Measures

It is important for the nurse to assess the effect of nursing intervention upon the pain experienced by the patient. The nursing student is referred to the sections in this chapter, "Components of the Pain Experience" and "Assessment of Pain," to establish the presence or absence of pain. As a result of the nurse's assessment, other nursing measures may need to be employed.

SUMMARY

Providing for rest, sleep, and comfort needs is a frequent function of nurses. Often rest is prescribed as a therapy by the physician, but it is not always easily accomplished. Before a person can rest, at least six conditions need to be met. These include feelings that the illness situation and personal concerns such as business or family affairs are under control, feelings of being acceptable to self and to others, feelings of knowing what is happening, freedom from physi-

cal and emotional discomfort, purposeful activity, and knowing that help is available when needed.

Sleep is necessary to restore and reorganize the neuronal system, to mediate stress and anxiety, and to help the body prepare for daily activities required. Sleep patterns and requirements vary in accordance with the individual, with age, and with circadian biorhythms. Sleep cycles have been measured by electroencephalograms. Two different types of sleep occur: slow wave and paradoxical (REM), the latter being superimposed upon the other. Four stages of sleep occur with associated alpha and delta brain wave changes, changes in vital signs, and different levels of arousability. These four stages occur in cycles of about 90 minutes throughout sleep.

Several factors affect sleep. Age determines the amount of sleep required, and the proportion of REM sleep decreases with age. Fatigue shortens the first period of REM sleep. Illness often increases the time needed for sleep and alters the person's normal sleep patterns. Emotional problems result in insomnia. Hypnotics and sedatives increase the total sleep experience but decrease REM sleep. Overuse of sedatives can lead to REM deprivation.

The need for sleep is evident when a person expresses a feeling of fatigue or exhibits periods of depression, apathy, irritability, aggressiveness, and inattention. With increasing sleep deprivation, confusion and hallucinations can occur.

Nursing interventions to promote sleep need to be adapted to the individual patient. Some measures include provision of a relaxing environment prior to sleep, maintenance of individual before-bedtime routines, elimination of noise, attending to safety and security needs, provision of adequate warmth, and administration of hypnotics or sedatives as prescribed. Three common sleep problems are insomnia, enuresis, and somnambulism. Additional nursing measures are needed to assist with these.

Pain is probably the most common symptom of disease that nurses encounter. Regardless of whether the pain is acute, chronic, or intractable, it is a highly personal sensation, which only the patient can describe. The physiologic processes involved in pain perception include the pain receptors that vary in number among tissues, the sensory nerve pathways to the spinal cord, the ascending lateral spinothalamic tracts, the thalamus, and specific sensory areas of the cerebral cortex. Also involved are the sympathetic nervous system for superficial pain and the parasympathetic nervous system for deep (internal) pain.

Pain is sometimes perceived to be in an area other than its source. Examples are referred pain and phantom pain. The perception of pain is also sometimes blocked or altered. The gate control theory and theories of other control systems in the thalamus and cerebral cortex provide some explanations for these alterations. In addition, individual perceptions of pain vary.

Types of pain are categorized in accordance with body locations. Included are superficial somatic pain, deep somatic (visceral) pain, neurogenic pain, and psychogenic pain.

Three components of the pain experience are (a) initiation of the pain impulse, (b) perception of the pain, and (c) response to the pain. Various stimuli can initiate the pain impulse such as chemical irritants, ischemia, mechanical trauma, and extremes of heat or cold. The pain perception threshold is generally fairly uniform in people but can be altered by states of consciousness. However, the perception (interpretation) of pain often involves the person's current and past experiences and the meaning attached to the pain experience. Thus the perception of the pain is variable among individuals even when the stimulus is identical. Behavioral responses to pain vary considerably. These responses are learned from parental socialization and from cultural expectations. Acceptance of these differences by nurses is essential.

The assessment of pain relies heavily upon explicit data from the patient. Data collected need to include the location of the pain, its intensity, the time of its onset and duration, its quality or description, and associated nonverbal behavior. Previous experiences with the pain and any precipitating factors also need to be described.

Nursing interventions to relieve pain are directed toward relieving or alleviating the five aspects of the pain experience. These are (a) removing the pain stimulus, (b) reducing the reaction of the pain receptors, (c) blocking the transmission of the pain impulse, (d) altering the pain perception, and (e) altering the interpretation and response to pain.

SUGGESTED ACTIVITIES

1. Interview one person in each of the following age groups: five to six years, adolescence, young adult, elderly adult. Collect the following information and take this back to a student group in order to compare data and assess differences by age group.

   a. How much sleep does the person need?

   b. When does the person go to bed?

   c. What rituals, if any, assist the person to sleep?

   d. Does the person ever have difficulty sleeping? If so, what helps the person get to sleep?

2. Talk to a patient who has had pain recently. By what means was the pain relieved? What nursing activities helped relieve the pain and what did not? How did the patient describe the pain?

3. Carry out a complete assessment of a patient having pain using the assessment guide in this chapter.

SUGGESTED READINGS

Binzley, Veronica. January, 1977. State: overlooked factor in newborn nursing. *American Journal of Nursing* 77:102–103.

In caring for the newborn, nurses need to be aware of the normal sleep-wake cycles. Stages in the sleep-wake cycle are provided together with corresponding behavior.

Blaylock, Jerry. 1968. The psychological and cultural influences on the reaction to pain: a review of literature. *Nursing Forum* 7(3):262–274.

The author describes the findings of studies about pain. Included are the psychologic components, the influence of culture, and some implications for nursing. A reference list for additional readings about pain follows the article.

Fass, Grace. December, 1971. Sleep, drugs, and dreams. *American Journal of Nursing* 71:2316–2320.

The stages of sleep are described and then the effects of deprivation in the stages and how these stages are affected by some medications. Note the reasons some patients are unable to sleep and what the author suggests.

Schultz, Nancy V. October, 1971. How children perceive pain. *Nursing Outlook* 19:670–673.

The article describes a survey of fifth graders' concepts of pain. Drawn from this data are some implications for nursing care.

SELECTED REFERENCES

Rest and Sleep

Diekelmann, Nancy L. August, 1976. The young adult; the choice is health or illness. *American Journal of Nursing* 76:1274–1277.

Ford, Amasa B. 1965. The meaning of rest. *Cardiovascular Nursing* 1:11–14.

Guyton, Arthur C. 1976. *Textbook of medical physiology*, 5th ed. Philadelphia: W. B. Saunders Co.

Long, Barbara. September, 1969. Sleep. *American Journal of Nursing* 69:1896–1899.

Marlow, Dorothy R. 1977. *Textbook of pediatric nursing*, 5th ed. Philadelphia: W. B. Saunders Co.

Narrow, Barbara W. August, 1967. Rest is . . . *American Journal of Nursing* 67:1646–1649.

O'Dell, Margaret L. 1975. Human biorhythmology; implications for nursing practice. *Nursing Forum* 14(1):43–47.

Pain

American Journal of Nursing. March, 1974. Hypnotic suggestion. *American Journal of Nursing* 74:515.

Engel, George L. 1970. Pain. In MacBryde, Cyril M., and Blacklow, Robert S., eds. *Signs and symptoms: applied physiologic physiology and clinical interpretation.* 5th ed. Philadelphia: J. B. Lippincott Co.

Gaumer, William R. March, 1974. Electrical stimulation in chronic pain. *American Journal of Nursing* 74:504–505.

McCaffery, Margo. 1972. *Nursing management of the patient with pain.* Philadelphia: J. B. Lippincott Co.

Schultz, Nancy V. October, 1971. How children perceive pain. *Nursing Outlook* 19:670–673.

Siegele, Dorothy S. March, 1974. The gate control theory. *American Journal of Nursing* 74:498–502.

Stewart, Elizabeth. June, 1976. To lessen pain: relaxation and rhythmic breathing. *American Journal of Nursing* 76:958–959.

CHAPTER 25

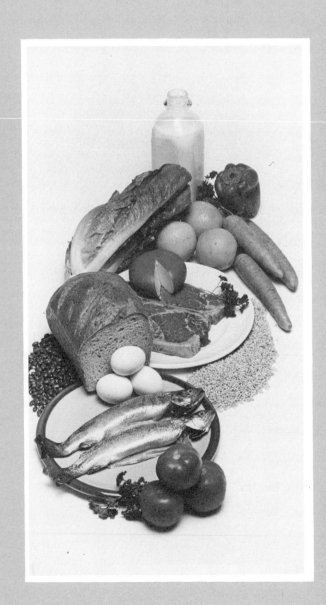

NUTRITION

FACTORS AFFECTING EATING HABITS

ASSESSING NUTRITIONAL STATUS

COMMON PROBLEMS RELATED TO NOURISHMENT

Factors Underlying Malnutrition and Undernutrition

Food Fads

NURSING INTERVENTION

Assisting Patients to Obtain Nourishment

Motivating Patients to Eat

Counseling about Nutrition

Instructing Patients with Special Dietary Problems

OBJECTIVES

- Describe the essential nutrients required by people and their food sources.
- Discuss factors that alter individual caloric requirements.
- Describe a balanced diet as recommended by the United States Department of Agriculture and the Canadian Department of Health and Welfare.
- Discuss variables in dietary needs according to age.
- Describe nutritional needs during pregnancy and lactation.
- Discuss factors that affect a person's eating habits.
- List criteria that may be used to assess a person's nutritional status.
- Describe common nutritional problems and factors contributing to them.
- Discuss the nurse's responsibilities in relation to food fads.
- Discuss four broad areas of nursing intervention related to the need for nutrition.

Food and water are two basic necessities for human survival. People can go without water for a few days and without food for a little longer, but they must obtain nourishment once their own stores of fat and protein are used up. The need for fluids is discussed in Chapter 29. This chapter will deal specifically with the need of people for nourishment.

In most societies food has other meanings in addition to providing nourishment. Food is closely related to the traditions and superstitions of most cultures. In this country turkey is associated with Thanksgiving and Christmas, and to spill salt is considered by some to mean bad luck. The taking of food has certain ritualistic practices associated with it, and these to some degree are culturally determined. In North America people sit at tables to eat a meal, and there is a general order in which different foods are eaten. For example, the dessert part of a meal is taken after the meat course. The variations in eating are numerous, and nurses need to establish what a patient is accustomed to eating and any other related practices when planning nursing care with the patient.

ESSENTIAL NUTRIENTS REQUIRED BY PEOPLE

The body requires essential nutrients for the growth and maintenance of all body tissues and the normal function of all body processes. A *nutrient* is an organic or inorganic substance found in food that is digested and absorbed in the gastrointestinal tract and then used in the body's metabolic processes. The essential nutrients are carbohydrates, proteins, fats, vitamins, and minerals. An adequate diet consists of a balance of these nutrients.

Carbohydrates

Carbohydrates are composed of carbon, hydrogen, and oxygen and are found in the sugars and starches of a diet. Carbohydrates are primarily used as a source of energy for the body. Excess carbohydrate is either converted into glycogen in the liver and stored there or converted into body fat (adipose tissue).

Foods high in carbohydrates are relatively low-cost foods readily accessible to most people. They include fruit, vegetables, cereal grain products (such as bread and oatmeal), and sugar. Carbohydrates are the chief source of calories, and hence a low-calorie diet generally has restricted carbohydrates. A *calorie* is a unit of heat. A *small calorie* is the amount of heat required to raise the temperature of 1 gm of water 1°C. A *large calorie (kilocalorie)* is the amount of heat required to raise the temperature of 1 kg of water 1°C and is the unit used by nutritionists.

Proteins

Proteins are necessary for growth and the repair of the body tissues. Excess protein is broken down into nitrogen and carbohydrate. The nitrogen is excreted, and the carbohydrate is stored as the dietary carbohydrate. The protein that is needed by the body is broken down into amino acids and then reformed into human protein. The major sources of protein are meat, fish, eggs, milk and milk products, poultry, cereals, and legumes (beans and peas). Protein foods are relatively expensive to purchase; however, even at times of tissue injury, excessive amounts of protein are rarely required. Increased amounts above normal intake are indicated in instances such as during pregnancy, lactation, and with burns and infections (Boykin 1975;146).

Fats

Fats are also necessary for the energy needs of the body. They are a quick source of energy, and they serve as a vehicle for the transportation of fat-soluble vitamins. The most common dietary sources of fat are butter, margarine, and cooking oils. Excessive intake of the *saturated* fats is considered to be a factor in the occurrence of coronary artery disease. Nutritionists recommend that fat provide from 25% to 30% of the total dietary calories and that *polyunsaturated* fats be used where this is feasible (Boykin 1975:109).

Vitamins

Vitamins increasingly have been recognized as essential nutrients, particularly during the past decade. Vitamins are organic compounds that help regulate the body processes. There are two types of vitamins, water soluble and fat soluble. The water-soluble vitamins are the B and C vitamins. These are not stored in the body, hence there must be a daily supply in the diet. The fat-soluble vitamins include A, D, E, and K. These can be stored in the body, although the storage of vitamins E and K has limitations. A daily supply of these vitamins, therefore, is not absolutely necessary. A balanced diet of carbohydrate, fats, and protein will contain the necessary vitamins.

Vitamin A is necessary for normal growth and healthy skin, hair, eyes, and mucous membranes. Major food sources include liver, kidney, dark green leafy vegetables, deep yellow vegetables, and whole milk. Vitamin B can be broken down into thiamine (B_1), riboflavin (B_2), niacin (B_3), pyridoxine (B_6), and cyanocobalamin (B_{12}). The vitamin B complex is necessary for healthy skin and mucous membranes, metabolism of various body tissues such as nervous tissue (B_{12}), and formation of red blood cells (B_{12}). Good dietary sources of the B vitamins include meat, liver, whole grains, and yeast. Vitamin C (ascorbic acid) is involved in the metabolism of amino acids and in enhancing iron absorption. It is necessary for healthy gums, which tend to bleed readily with ascorbic acid deficiency. Good food sources of vitamin C include citrus fruits, tomatoes, and raw cabbage. Vitamin D (calciferol) promotes normal skeletal development and normal tooth development. Sources include direct sunlight and fish liver oils as well as vitamin D-fortified milk. Vitamin E (antisterility factor) serves to aid in hematopoiesis. Major food sources include oils from vegetables, wheat germ, and legumes. Vitamin K (antihemorrhagic factor) also aids in blood clotting. Signs of deficiency include hemorrhages in the skin and mucous membranes. Food sources include green leafy vegetables, especially cabbage and spinach. In addition to these vitamins, there are others such as folic acid, pantothenic acid, and vitamin H (biotin). Dietary sources of vitamin H include liver, milk, and mushrooms.

Minerals

Minerals are found in organic compounds, as inorganic compounds and as free ions. They leave an ash upon oxidation, which can be acid or alkaline. Calcium and phosphorus are two minerals that make up 80% of all the mineral elements in the body (Boykin 1975:162). There are two categories of minerals: those which are found in the body in larger amounts and those trace elements (micronutrients) which are present in minute amounts. The former group includes calcium, phosphorus, potassium, chlorine, sodium, sulfur, and magnesium. The latter group includes iron, copper, iodine, and manganese. Minerals are involved in many body processes, including the regulation of the acid-base balance of the body. For further information the student is referred to Chapter 30. One common mineral deficiency that occurs frequently in women is iron deficiency.

Food sources of minerals include green leafy vegetables, milk and milk products, eggs, and organ meats. Liver is an excellent source of iron. Whole-grain cereals and brown rice are also good sources. Iodized salt is a major source of iodine.

Another part of food that is also essential for health is fiber (cellulose). It is nondigestible but forms the bulk for the stool. Fiber or roughage is found chiefly in fresh fruits and vegetables and in whole-grain cereals and their products.

Calories

Most foods supply energy to the body. The measurement of the energy is the calorie, which has been defined earlier in the chapter. Calories are required to maintain the basal metabolic rate of the body and to provide energy for activities such as running and walking. The *basal metabolic rate* (BMR) is the rate at which food is metabolized in order to maintain body functions such as breathing at rest.

The caloric requirements of individuals vary according to age and growth, sex, climate, state of health, sleep, food, and activity (Boykin 1975: 201–205).

Age

During periods of growth the body uses more energy. During the first 2 years of life, adolescence, and pregnancy, the rapid growth demands more calories than normal. For example, an active adolescent boy may need 3600 calories, whereas a 70-year-old woman may require only 1200 calories (Anderson et al. 1972:92). See Table 25-1 for caloric intake variables by age.

Sex

Men usually have a higher basal metabolic rate (BMR) than women. This is largely explained by the greater proportion of muscle in the body. Pregnant women also have a higher BMR than normal.

Climate

The climate also affects heat production in that people who live in cold climates average a higher (about

Table 25-1. Calorie Intake by Age*

Age	Weight kg	lb	Energy (calories)
Newborn to 6 months	6	14	kg × 117
6 months to 1 year	9	20	kg × 108
1 to 3 years	13	28	1300
4 to 6 years	20	44	1800
7 to 10 years	30	66	2400
Males			
11 to 14 years	44	97	2800
15 to 18 years	61	134	3000
19 to 22 years	67	147	3000
23 to 50 years	70	154	2700
51 years and over	70	154	2400
Females			
11 to 14 years	44	97	2400
15 to 18 years	54	119	2100
19 to 22 years	58	128	2100
23 to 50 years	58	128	2000
51 years and over	58	128	1800
Pregnancy			+300
Lactation			+500

*Adapted from Food and Nutrition Board, National Research Council, Academy of Sciences. 1974. *Recommended dietary allowances.* Washington, D.C.

Table 25-2. Recommended Daily Food*

United States	Canada
Milk Group Children, three or more glasses; smaller glasses for some children under 8 years; teenagers, four or more glasses; adults, two or more glasses; cheese, ice cream, and other milk-made foods can supply part of the milk	**Milk** Children (up to about 11 years), 2½ cups (20 fl oz); adolescents, 4 cups (32 fl oz); adults, 1½ cups (12 fl oz); expectant and nursing mothers, 4 cups (32 fl oz)
Meat group Two or more servings of meats, fish, poultry, eggs, or cheese with dry beans, peas, nuts as alternatives	**Meat and fish** One serving of meat, fish, or poultry; eat liver occasionally; eggs, cheese, dried beans, or peas may be used in place of meat; in addition, eggs and cheese at least three times a week
Vegetables and fruits Four or more servings; include dark green or yellow vegetables citrus fruit or tomatoes	**Vegetables** One serving of potatoes; two servings of other vegetables, preferably yellow or green and often raw **Fruit** Two servings of fruit or juice, including a satisfactory source of vitamin C (ascorbic acid) such as oranges, tomatoes, and vitaminized apple juice
Breads and cereals Four or more servings, enriched or whole grain; added milk improves nutritional values	**Breads and cereals** Bread (with butter or fortified margarine); one serving of whole-grain cereal Vitamin D, 400 International Units, for all growing persons and expectant and nursing mothers

*Courtesy National Dairy Council. *A guide to good eating.* Washington, D.C., and Canada, Department of Health and Welfare. *Canada's food guide,* Ottawa.

20%) metabolic rate than people in hot climates. This is thought to be because of the increased secretion of thyroxine in cold climates.

State of Health

Some illnesses, such as those accompanied by a fever or an infection, increase the BMR. In instances of malnutrition, however, the BMR is lowered.

Sleep

The need for energy is decreased during sleep, when the muscles are relaxed and physiologic processes are slowed. The BMR drops about 10% to 15% during sleep (Boykin 1975:204).

Food

The body's metabolism is stimulated by all foods but to varying degrees. Proteins increase heat production about 30%, carbohydrates and fats about 5%.

Activity

Muscular activity has the greatest effect upon a person's BMR. The greater the activity the greater the stimulation. Mental activity provides very little stimulation, using about 4 calories per hour.

A Balanced Diet in Health

In both the United States and Canada there are recommended daily requirements of foods. In the United States the Department of Agriculture has issued *A Guide to Good Eating*. In Canada the Department of Health and Welfare publishes *Canada's Food Guide*. There is only slight variation between these guides. See Table 25-2.

When referring to nutritional requirements, one is usually referring to the *minimal* requirements for health. There are many variations related to individual need. Activity, size, rate of growth, and so on must be taken into consideration when advising on requirements for a particular person at a specific time.

VARIABLES IN DIETARY NEEDS ACCORDING TO AGE

The Infant

Breast Feeding

When an infant is breast fed, nutritional requirements are normally met with the exception of fluoride, iron, and vitamin D. These are then provided as supplement feedings. Drops or crushed tablets may be placed directly on the baby's tongue or dissolved with water or milk. Later they may be mixed with food or juice. See Table 25-3 for a schedule.

Breast feeding usually begins within 24 hours after the infant's birth. To start the baby, express a little milk on the baby's lips. Stroke the cheek nearest the nipple to encourage the child to turn the mouth toward the breast. Some infants will obtain sufficient

Table 25-3. Typical Feeding Schedules for Normal Babies during the First Year*

Hour	Food	1 month	3 months	6 months	10 to 12 months
6 AM	Formula	3 or 4 oz	5 or 6 oz	7 or 8 oz	*6 AM* Orange juice, 3 oz
8 AM	Orange juice Vitamin D	1 oz 400 IU	3 oz 400 IU	3 oz 400 IU	Zwieback, ½ piece *Breakfast, 7:30 AM*
10 AM	Formula Cereal	3 or 4 oz	5 or 6 oz ¼ to 2 tbsp	7 or 8 oz 2 to 4 tbsp	Cereal, 2 to 5 tbsp Milk, 8 oz
2 PM	Formula Egg yolk Vegetable	-3 or.4 oz	5 or 6 oz	7 or 8 oz 1 yolk 2 or 3 tbsp	Chopped fruit, 1 or 2 tbsp Vitamin D, 400 IU *Dinner, 11:30 AM to 12 noon*
6 PM	Formula Cereal Fruit	3 or 4 oz	5 or 6 oz	7 or 8 oz 2 to 4 tbsp ¼ to 2 tbsp	Meat, ½ or 1 oz, or egg, 1 whole Potato, 2 to 4 tbsp
10 PM	Formula	3 or 4 oz	5 or 6 oz	Discontinued	Chopped vegetable, 2 to 4 tbsp Milk, 8 oz
2 AM	Formula	3 or 4 oz	Discontinued		*Supper, 5:30 PM* Cereal or potato, 2 to 5 tbsp Milk, 8 oz Chopped fruit, 1 or 2 tbsp Toast or zwieback

*From Robinson, Corinne H., and Lawler, Marilyn R. 1977. *Normal & therapeutic nutrition,* 15th ed., New York: Macmillan Publishing Co., Inc., p. 309.

nourishment by feeding on one breast, while others will need to feed from the other breast as well. For the next feeding, then, the breast that was emptied first with the previous feeding needs to be left until the other breast has been emptied.

Infants normally establish their own schedules for feeding. A very young infant may require 10 to 12 feedings per 24 hours; however, before long the infant establishes intervals usually of 3 to 4 hours between feedings. If a child is hungry and cries within 3 hours, the child may well be receiving insufficient nourishment or may have swallowed too much air during the previous feeding. By the age of 2 months most infants will sleep through the night without a feeding, and by the fourth or fifth month they will no longer require a 2200-hr. feeding.

It is important for the mother to sit comfortably and be relaxed when breast feeding. Anxiety and tension can be communicated to the baby.

Weaning usually starts between the fifth and ninth months. This is usually done by substituting a cup feeding for a breast feeding and increasing the cup feedings as the baby becomes accustomed to them. If breast feeding must be terminated earlier, then a bottle feeding is substituted.

Bottle Feeding

The most commonly used substitute for breast milk is cow's milk. The chief differences are as follows:

1. Cow's milk contains about three times as much protein.
2. Cow's milk contains a higher proportion of short-chain fatty acids, which are more irritating than the long-chain fatty acids found in human milk.
3. Human milk contains about twice as much lactose as cow's milk.
4. Both types of milk contain about 70 kilocalories per 100 ml (Robinson and Lawler 1977:304).

Bottle-fed babies are chiefly provided with commercially prepared formulas. In some instances the formulas require dilution with an equal volume of water. Some of these come in disposable bottles; others are measured into a bottle. Formulas can be prepared in the home; however, it is important when preparing these to maintain sanitary conditions, thus not contaminating the formula or the bottles (see Chapter 16 for definition of contamination). Formulas usually contain milk (often evaporated milk), sugar, and water.

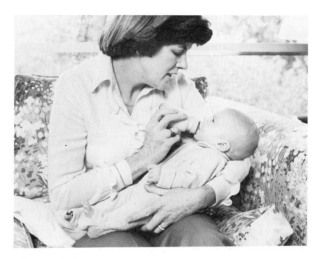

Figure 25-1.   An infant is supported comfortably during feeding.

When bottle feeding a baby, the feeding is warmed to body temperature. The baby is held in much the same way as for breast feeding with the nipple touching the lips (Figure 25-1). The nipple should be kept full of formula in order to minimize the intake of air.

Periodically with both types of feeding the baby will need to burp in order to release air that may have been swallowed. Two common positions for burping are over the shoulder or in sitting position with chin supported by a hand. Often, patting the back or rubbing it gently facilitates burping.

There is considerable variance of opinion about the addition of supplementary nourishment for the infant. Some physicians advise early introduction, while others wait until the third or fourth month.

Vitamins

Vitamins A and D are usually already added to premodified formulas. If they are prescribed as a supplement, the type that is dissolved in water is preferred in case it is aspirated. These vitamins can be added to a formula or given separately in water. At about the age of 3 weeks, orange juice may be introduced for its ascorbic acid.

Cereals

Cereals are semisolid foods. There are specially formulated cereals for babies that are enriched with iron.

Egg yolk

At about the third to fifth month, hard-cooked egg yolk can be added to the diet. It is mashed and often mixed with formula, cereal, or vegetable. It is advisable to start with a small amount, about ¼ tsp, in case the child is allergic to the egg yolk.

Fruits

Strained orange and grapefruit juice and ripe banana are the raw fruits given during the first year. Cooked or canned pears, applesauce, peaches, and other fruits can be started about the third to fourth month. These are strained when first given, but by the end of the first year they will only need to be chopped.

Vegetables

Strained vegetables such as carrots, spinach, squash, and peas are suitable at about the fourth month. Like fruits, strained vegetables are replaced by chopped vegetables at about 1 year.

Meats

Canned, strained baby meats are generally given about the fifth month. Later the infant can tolerate ground lamb, beef, pork, chicken, and liver. Another source of protein that is inexpensive is a variety of bean seen most commonly in the southwestern United States. It needs to be cooked and strained before serving.

The Toddler and the Preschooler

During the second year of life the child gains 3 to 4 kg (6.6–8.8 lbs), and thereafter will gain 2–3 kg (4.4–6.6 lbs) each year until the preadolescent period (Robinson and Lawler 1977:315). The nutritional requirements during the childhood period are much greater than those of an adult in proportion to body size. This is largely due to the body's growth and the physical activity of the child. The recommended energy requirements are given in Table 25-1.

The amount and type of food should be adjusted to the child's age and appetite. A sample menu, which can be adjusted, is shown in Table 25-4.

During these early years, it is important that children develop good food habits. They should be seated comfortably. The appetite will vary from time to time, so it is better to serve less than more of what they will eat. Too large helpings can discourage chil-

Table 25-4.   Sample Menu, Adjustable for Child's Age and Appetite*

Breakfast	Dinner	Supper
Orange juice	Beef patty	Cream of
Oatmeal porridge	Baked Potato	tomato soup
with milk	Green beans	Soft cooked egg
Milk	Carrots	Bread and
Toast and margarine	Milk pudding	margarine
	Milk	Canned peaches
		Milk

Midmorning	Midafternoon
Apple juice	Small glass of milk
	Cookie

*From Canada, Department of Health and Welfare. 1971. *Up the years from one to six.* Ottawa, p. 41.

dren from eating. Children need to be provided with forks and spoons that they can handle; the fork needs blunt tines to prevent harm (see Figure 25-2).

When children are served a new food, this should be at the beginning of the meal and in association with foods that are well-liked. When children refuse to eat a food, it is best removed without discussion. Children can learn quickly to attract attention through not eating.

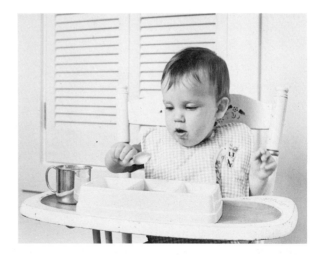

Figure 25-2.   A toddler has her own chair and utensils to use for meals.

The School-age Child

Many of the suggestions appropriate to the preschool child also apply to the school-age child. At this time the children encounter peers with eating habits different from those they have encountered at home. Children often try foods eaten by their friends to broaden their experience.

There are a number of nutrition programs in schools. The school lunch program has expanded since its inception in the United States in the 1930s, and the school breakfast program serves about one million children in the United States each day. Many of these meals are served free or at a reduced price.

The Teenager

In the teen years, growth accelerates and the need for calories increases (see Table 25-1). Some teenagers develop unusual food practices or follow food fads. Obesity in particular in teenage girls is not unusual.

Teenage boys and girls have high energy requirements, and thus meat, milk, and green leafy and deep yellow vegetables are important. Nutritional snacks are also important. The adolescent boy will require about one quart of milk or its equivalent each day. Girls will need additional iron because of the loss of body iron in the menses.

Pregnancy and Lactation

Daily food guides for the adult were mentioned earlier in this section. Of special consideration, however, is the pregnant and lactating woman. See Table 25-5 for recommended dietary allowances. In addition to the basic diet for an adult, the diet for a pregnant woman includes the following:

1. Increased protein is needed because of the growth of the fetus and accessory tissues of the woman.
2. Calcium and phosphorus are doubled to meet the needs of the fetus and the pregnant woman.
3. The magnesium requirement increases by 150 mg day.
4. Iron is needed to build sufficient hemoglobin and provide iron for the fetus.
5. Iodine is required for the pregnant woman, 25 mg over the normal requirement.

Table 25-5.   Recommended Dietary Allowances Before and During Pregnancy and Lactation*

Nutrient	11–14 years	15–18 years	19–22 years	23+ years	Pregnancy	Lactation
Energy (kcal)	2400	2100	2100	2000	+300	+500
Protein (gm)	44	48	46	46	+30	+20
Vitamin A (RE)	800	800	800	800	1000	1200
(IU)	4000	4000	4000	4000	5000	6000
Vitamin D (IU)	400	400	400	400	400	400
Vitamin E (IU)	12	12	12	12	15	15
Ascorbic acid (mg)	45	45	45	45	60	80
Folacin (μg)	400	400	400	400	800	600
Niacin (mg)	16	14	14	13	+2	+4
Riboflavin (mg)	1.3	1.4	1.4	1.2	+0.3	+0.5
Thiamin (mg)	1.2	1.1	1.1	1.0	+0.3	+0.3
Vitamin B_6 (mg)	1.6	2.0	2.0	2.0	2.5	2.5
Vitamin B_{12} (μg)	3.0	3.0	3.0	3.0	4.0	4.0
Calcium (mg)	1200	1200	800	800	1200–1600†	1200–1600†
Phosphorus (mg)	1200	1200	800	800	1200–1600†	1200–1600†
Iodine (μg)	115	115	100	100	125	150
Iron (mg)	18	18	18	18	18+	18
Magnesium (mg)	300	300	300	300	450	450
Zinc (mg)	15	15	15	15	20	25

*From Robinson, Corrine H., and Lawler, Marilyn R. 1977. *Normal and therapeutic nutrition,* 15th ed. New York: Macmillan Publishing Co., Inc., p. 291.
†The higher levels are indicated for the teenage girl.

Table 25-6. Sample Menus for Pregnancy*

For Pregnant Women of Normal Weight	For Pregnant Adolescent Girls of Normal Weight
Breakfast	**Breakfast**
Orange juice, 4 oz	Orange juice, 4 oz
Scrambled egg	Cornflakes or grits
Toast, 1 slice	Scrambled egg
Butter or margarine	Toast, 1 slice
Coffee	Milk, ½ pint
Midmorning	**Midmorning**
Milk, ½ pint	Milk, ½ pint
Lunch	**Lunch**
Meat, cheese, or peanut butter sandwich	Hamburger on a bun
Carrot sticks	Cole slaw
Oatmeal cookies	Oatmeal cookies
Milk, ½ pint	Milk, ½ pint
Midafternoon	**Midafternoon**
Milk, ½ pint	Frankfurter on a bun
	Milkshake or fruit juice, ½ pint
Dinner	**Dinner**
Roasted or broiled beef, pork, liver, fish	Roasted or broiled beef, pork, liver, fish
Broccoli or greens	Broccoli or greens
Baked potato	Baked or French-fried potatoes
Butter or margarine	Butter or margarine
Green salad with French dressing	Green salad with French dressing
Fresh or canned fruit	Fruit
Coffee, tea, or milk	Milk, ½ pint
Bedtime	**Bedtime**
Milk or cocoa, ½ pint	Fruit juice or cocoa, ½ pint

*From Mitchell, Helen S., et al, 1976. *Nutrition in Health and Disease,* 16th ed. New York: J.B. Lippincott Co., p. 241.

6. The zinc requirement is 5 mg above the normal daily requirement to meet the needs of newly forming maternal and fetal tissue.

7. Increased amounts of vitamins A, E, B complex, and C are advised. The pregnant woman may require additional folic acid to protect the fetus and maternal tissue. Folic acid is considered to be essential for DNA synthesis; with vitamin B_{12}, it regulates the formation of normal red blood cells (Robinson and Lawler 1977:188).

For a suitable diet for the pregnant woman and the pregnant adolescent, see Table 25-6.

The Elderly Adult

The elderly adult requires fewer calories than the younger adult. An adult requires 2% less energy per decade after maturity. Thus the elderly adult requires fewer calories than when younger, and yet fixed food habits often make the needed diet changes difficult.

Protein

Protein requirements change very little with age, and yet the elderly tend to eat less protein than previously. Often this is due to the cost of meats as well as the lack of available facilities for cooking meats and similar products. Denture problems and lack of appetite also contribute to this situation.

Carbohydrate

Because carbohydrates are a major source of calories it is apparent that carbohydrate needs are reduced for the elderly, yet many older people love sweet foods, maintain this high caloric intake as they become less active and thus tend to become obese.

Fat

The fat requirement for the elderly remains similar to that of the younger adult, or it is reduced because of the calorie content mentioned previously.

Minerals

The need for calcium intake appears to be similar to that of younger adults. Inadequate calcium intake is thought to be responsible for increased osteoporosis and subsequent fractures. The needs for other minerals appear to be similar to those of other adults.

Vitamins

Elderly people appear to require similar vitamin quantities as those of younger adults.

Cellulose and Water

Cellulose and water are important constituents of the elderly person's diet. Both fiber (cellulose) and water are necessary to maintain normal elimination, especially to prevent constipation. The elderly person tends to be inactive and to choose smooth, soft foods, both of which contribute to constipation.

Meals for the Elderly

The following guidelines can assist in the provision of appropriate meals for the elderly, thus encouraging them to eat:

1. Serve food attractively, providing color contrast.
2. Cook food well so that it can be easily chewed if the person has denture problems.
3. Serve essential foods first and provide sweet foods (carbohydrates) in moderation after.
4. Note foods that cause indigestion and do not serve them.
5. The heaviest meal can be served at noon if the person has difficulty sleeping at night after a heavy meal.
6. Avoid stimulants such as tea or coffee in the evening if the person has difficulty sleeping.

FACTORS AFFECTING EATING HABITS

There are a number of factors that affect a person's eating habits. Some of these are culture, religion, socioeconomic status, personal preference, emotions, and hunger and appetite.

Culture

The culture of a person can greatly affect eating habits. The examples are myriad and to a large degree are seen in the many ethnic groups in the United States. Rice is a staple food of many people of the world, including the Chinese. Curry is familiar to the Indian, whereas fish is important to the people from Scandinavia. North American foods include hot dogs and hamburgers as well as steak. The Spanish-American may be accustomed to tamales while the Italian-American often eats spaghetti, meatballs, and lasagna. The German ethnic people are accustomed to veal in its many forms, including veal scallopine and sauerbraten, whereas the Ukrainian ethnic people will eat cabbage rolls and borscht. For many people living in North America these kinds of foods are the staples in their daily diets.

Religion

A person's religion can also affect diet. The Orthodox Jew will not eat any part of a pig, and certain foods can be eaten only when they are specially prepared; the term *kosher* is used to describe such food.

For Roman Catholics, meat may not be eaten some days during Lent; people belonging to some Protestant faiths are forbidden tea and coffee or alcoholic beverages. People following the Islamic faith will celebrate some religious holidays by practicing periods of fasting followed by feasting. See Chapter 32 for additional information.

Socioeconomic Status

What a person eats and how much the person eats as well as how often are frequently affected by social and economic status. Poor people and the elderly may not be able to afford beef and vegetables. Through limitations of money they may be able to eat only tinned fish and bread. Social groups also affect food habits. Appetizers such as pâté and snails are the foods of some, while others will be accustomed to hamburgers and beans.

Personal Preference

What an individual person likes and dislikes is a significant factor affecting eating habits. People often grow up with preferences that arise from childhood. Father dislikes curry, thus does his son; mother loves oysters, and so does her daughter. People also develop likes and dislikes based upon associations with a typical food. A child who loves to visit his grandparents loves pickled crabapples, which they always serve. Another child who dislikes a very strict aunt grows up to dislike the special chicken casserole that she often prepares. Individual likes and dislikes can also be related to familiarity, particularly for children. Unfamiliar foods may be disliked before they are even tried. Sometimes people have indigestion from certain foods; onions and cabbage are common offenders resulting in the expression of dislike.

Emotions

Sometimes people associate certain foods with specific emotional reactions, which often originate in childhood. Desired food that was withheld as a punishment may be associated with feelings of guilt. Food used as a reward may elicit pleasant feelings. If a meal time is accompanied by expressed anger by a parent, a child may associate specific foods with this anger and reject them.

Hunger, Appetite, and Satiety

Hunger is largely an unpleasant sensation due to the deprivation of food. *Appetite* is a pleasant sensation in which a person desires food and anticipates it. An appetite can be general, or it may focus on specific foods. A mythical appetite often described is the pregnant woman's desire for pickles.

Satiety is the feeling of fullness that results from satisfying one's desire for food. Hunger, appetite, and satiety are controlled by the central nervous system, including the hypothalamus, and by hormones and gastric secretions. When these mechanisms are faulty, the person may never experience satiety and thus overeat, resulting in obesity. The lack of an appetite is known as *anorexia*. Prolonged anorexia can prevent a person from eating needed food, resulting in body *emaciation* (excessive thinness).

ASSESSING NUTRITIONAL STATUS

A person's nutritional status can generally be determined by assessing the following areas:

1. Weight in relation to height, age, sex, and build.
2. Daily food intake.
3. The condition of the eyes, skin, mouth, hair, and glands.
4. Level of energy in relation to normal activity; the presence of fatigue and lethargy.

Weight

The assessment of weight is discussed in Chapter 14. Normal weight ranges by age, sex, and frame are given in Tables 14-3 and 14-4. An inadequately nourished person may be underweight, or may be overweight, even obese.

Daily Food Intake

A record of a person's food intake over a 3-day period will provide information about the adequacy of nourishment. If eating habits vary on a weekend, it is sometimes advocated to include an assessment of a weekend day's meals (Malasanos et al.1977:60). An analysis of the food intake will provide information as to the nutrients taken by the person.

Eyes, Skin, Mouth, Hair, and Glands

Dryness of the cornea and conjunctiva, and corneal opacity are often associated with vitamin A deficiency. Infiltration by the blood vessels into the cornea can be associated with vitamin B_2 deficiency. The mouth may show cracks, fissures, or redness on the lips reflecting riboflavin deficiency. The hair can lack luster and become depigmented as a result of protein deficiency, and enlargement of the thyroid gland can indicate iodine lack.

Energy Level

An adequately nourished person will have sufficient energy for usual daily activities, taking age into consideration. A poorly nourished person may be underweight or even overweight, but energy quickly dissipates, making it difficult to carry out normal activities.

Fatigue and lethargy can indicate inadequate nourishment. The person may not show specific signs of deficiency diseases but may complain of lethargy and fatigue. These people are considered to be marginally undernourished. *Malnutrition* can be considered to be any disorder connected with nutrition. It usually manifests itself in specific disorders of nutrition such as *scurvy,* a vitamin C deficiency.

COMMON PROBLEMS RELATED TO NOURISHMENT

There are three broad areas of problems related specifically to nutrition. These are *malnutrition,* which results when there is a deficiency, excess, or imbalance of essential nutrients; *undernutrition,* which is an inadequate caloric intake and a deficiency of one or more essential nutrients; and *overnutrition,* which is the oversupply of calories and an excess of one or more nutrients (Robinson and Lawler 1977:5).

Malnutrition can be evidenced by specific deficiencies as was explained previously in this chapter. Some of these disorders are shown in Table 25-7. Undernutrition is chiefly evidenced by a lowered energy level and is not likely to be demonstrated by specific nutrient deficiencies. Overnutrition is largely evidenced by overweight and obesity. In North America, where high-carbohydrate foods are relatively inexpensive and inactivity is at epidemic levels, obesity is a common health problem. Generally persons are considered to be obese if their weight is more than 20% over the normal weight for their age and build.

Obesity is a complex problem related to a person's need to eat, difficulty experiencing satiety, reduced physical activity, and socioeconomic class. It is thought that the greater prevalence of obesity among people of lower classes is somewhat related to social values and group fashions.

Factors Underlying Malnutrition and Undernutrition

There are a number of factors that underlie malnutrition and undernutrition.

Economics

The cost of nutritious foods is one of the major reasons for poorly nourished people. The relatively high cost of protein foods such as meat has already been mentioned. For this reason primarily, malnutrition is a widespread problem among the lower class.

Education

Lack of knowledge about nourishment and nutritious foods also contributes to malnutrition. People with minimal or no education are frequently unaware of nutritional needs and the foods that best supply nourishment.

Social and Class Values

A person will often eat the food that is eaten by others of the same social class. Ethnic groups in the United States and Canada often maintain the eating customs of their original countries even after immigration. Sometimes these customs grew out of the unavailability of some foods, and people continue these diets even though more nourishing foods are now available to them. Another social influence is evident among teenagers. They often consider it more important to socialize with peers and to eat chips and drink beer than to eat a more nourishing meal. Their fads in regard to eating can, over a period of time, lead to nourishment problems.

Physiologic Factors

Once food is taken into the body, it is necessary that it be digested and absorbed so that it can be used. There are many physiologic factors that can impair this process. The lack of teeth, poorly fitting teeth, or a sore mouth may make the mastication of food difficult. To *masticate* is to chew, one of the first steps in the digestive process.

Difficulty swallowing due to a painfully inflamed throat or a stricture of the esophagus can discourage a person from obtaining adequate nourishment.

Impairment of the digestive process in the stomach and gastrointestinal tract may have a variety of causes. Pathologic processes such as tumors or ulcers are not uncommon. Impairment in the flow of the

Table 25-7.   Deficiencies and Disorders*

Deficiency	Disorders	Deficiency	Disorders
Vitamin A	Poor growth, poor tooth and bone development, poor adaptation to light and night blindness	Vitamin C (ascorbic acid)	Soreness of mouth, gums, cutaneous bleeding, anorexia, restlessness, irritability, scurvy
Vitamin B₁ (thiamine)	Polyneuritis, anorexia, constipation, nervousness, gastrointestinal disturbances, beriberi	Vitamin D	Rickets in children, stunted growth, osteomalacia
		Vitamin E	Anemia
Vitamin B₂ (riboflavin)	Cheilosis, inflamed tongue, blurred vision, itching eyes	Vitamin K	Slow blood clotting time, hemorrhages in the newborn
Niacin (nicotinic acid)	Pellagra	Carbohydrates	Underweight, overweight, hypoglycemia, diabetes mellitus
Vitamin B₆	Anemia, mucous membrane lesions, weakness, convulsions in infants		
Vitamin B₁₂	Neurologic degeneration, poor growth, pernicious anemia	Fat	Decrease in amount of adipose tissue around vital organs, low heat and energy thresholds, constipation
Folic acid	Diarrhea, glossitis, anemia	Protein	Kwashiorkor, marasmus, greater likelihood of developing infections during pregnancy and following surgery, slow wound healing
Pantothenic acid	Anorexia, indigestion, nausea		

*For deficiencies related to minerals see Chapter 30.

digestive juices can also affect digestion. Gallstones, resulting in blockage of the flow of bile, are a common cause of impaired digestion of fat in the diet. Once the food enters the stomach, it is normally moved along the gastrointestinal tract, where the nutrients and water are absorbed and the waste products are collected in the sigmoid colon for subsequent excretion. When the movement of the tract is either slowed or accelerated, digestion and absorption can be affected. Decreased motility results in excessive absorption of water and subsequent formation of hard fecal material, resulting in constipation. Excessive motility can be evidenced by diarrhea and the loss of abnormally large amounts of water and other nutrients. See Chapter 26, "Diarrhea," for further discussion.

People who take certain medications also may have their digestion impaired. Iron in some forms taken orally is a common cause of indigestion, *nausea* (the urge to vomit), and even vomiting. Anorexia and nausea can affect a person's eating and consequently nourishment.

Psychologic Factors

Anorexia and weight loss, which have already been discussed, can also be indicative of depression (Solomon and Patch 1974:58). *Anorexia nervosa* is a disease that is most frequently seen in adolescent women. With this condition the patient refuses to eat, often loses a great deal of weight, and in some instances starves herself to death.

Food Fads

Food fads of one sort or another are continually being practiced in North American society. A *fad* is an interest or a practice of many people that is followed with considerable zeal for a period of time. Some fads are related to improving a person's nutritional status, such as the practice of eating only natural foods or ingesting excessive amounts of vitamin E or C. Others are directed toward health problems. Some of the most common are those practices designed to help obese people lose weight. An example that has received considerable publicity is the liquid protein diet, which appears to have accounted for several deaths.

A nurse does have responsibilities in regard to food fads. Some of these are as follows:

1. If a person is thinking about following some advertised practice, it is the nurse's responsibility to suggest that this be discussed with the physician.

2. Fads that are contrary to recognized nutritional practices need to be investigated further, perhaps with a nutritionist.

3. Fads that promise results that are not within normal expectations need to be considered in light of advice from a person such as a physician or nutritionist.

4. People who believe in fads based upon false statements require correct information. For example, the belief that pesticides poison food requires corrective information such as that government controls now make sure that the amount of any pesticides remaining in the food is at a minimal level that is safe for consumers.

NURSING INTERVENTION

Nursing intervention in regard to nutrition can be considered in four broad areas. These are (a) assisting patients to obtain nourishment either through feeding or assisting with eating, (b) motivating patients to eat, (c) assisting patients to obtain needed nourishment through counseling about nutrition, and (d) assisting patients with special problems through counseling about therapeutic diets.

Assisting Patients to Obtain Nourishment

Very young children will require assistance in a hospital just as they do at home. Such patients probably will require more assistance than normal, as will people of all ages. When people are ill, they usually have little energy and often need more time than usual to eat. Very weak children and adults may need to be specially supported in their usual eating positions. Sometimes small children are best held on the nurse's knee, or they can be assisted to maintain position in the high chair or crib with pillows. People usually like to assume the normal sitting position while eating. If they are unable to sit in a chair even with the support of pillows, raising the head of the bed is often possible, thus assuming the eating position as closely as possible (see Figure 25-3). It is difficult for most people to eat while lying in the supine position. If they cannot assume a sitting position, the next best

position is a lateral one. In this position the patient is less likely to choke, and swallowing is facilitated.

Feeding persons means assisting them with a basic activity that, except for the infant, they usually had been able to do themselves. For young children who have learned to feed themselves, being helped by a nurse may be necessary, but the nurse needs to be sensitive to any negative feelings because children are generally proud of this new accomplishment. Sometimes a simple explanation by a nurse together with praise about what children have learned to do are helpful. Older children and adults can find feeding embarrassing and resent being fed, since it represents to them a degree of dependency to which they are unaccustomed. Whenever possible, patients should be helped with eating rather than have feeding completely taken over by the nurse.

There are special utensils that can assist a patient to eat. Straws used for liquids are helpful to many people who have difficulty drinking from a cup or glass. They often permit the patient to obtain liquids with less effort and with less spillage, which can be embarrassing to many patients. Other special utensils are weighted cups and glasses, which are easier to handle, and forks and spoons that have wide handles, allowing them to be gripped more easily than the usual utensils. Special drinking cups are also available to assist people. One model has a spout; another is especially designed to permit drinking with less tipping of the cup than is normally required.

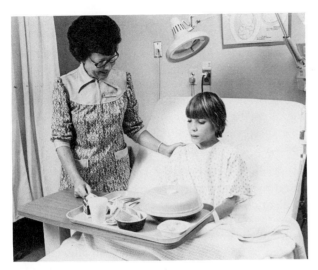

Figure 25-3.   A patient confined to bed in a hospital is supported in Fowler's position for a meal.

A nurse who is assisting a patient with a meal should ask the patient which food the patient wants first; if the patient is blind, the food should be described. For blind patients who can feed themselves, orienting them to where the food is on the tray is helpful.

Patients who are hospitalized are frequently served their meals on trays. Food is frequently prepared and dished out in central locations and then delivered to a nursing unit to be served. In some settings patients are given a menu from which to choose their meals for the next day. When a tray is delivered to a patient, the nurse needs to check it for the following:

1. The name on the tray card corresponds with that of the patient to whom it is given.

2. The patient has received the food requested if menu service is provided.

3. Hot foods are hot and cold foods are cold.

4. Liquids have not been spilled and the tray is attractively and conveniently arranged.

For patients who are unable to eat, such as the unconscious patient, there are alternative feeding methods.

Nasogastric Feeding

A feeding administered through a nasogastric tube is referred to as a *gastric gavage*. The tube is usually made of flexible plastic and is long and narrow. The tube is initially lubricated with water and then inserted through an unobstructed nostril and passed through the nose and nasopharynx into the esophagus, terminating in the stomach. Inserting a nasogastric tube requires a physician's order, and it does require considerable skill in order to ensure that it does not terminate in the patient's lungs. A nasogastric feeding must never be administered until the nurse confirms that the tube is in the stomach. See Table 25-8 for ways of determining when the tube is in the stomach or in the lungs. See Chapter 37 for insertion of a Levin tube.

Nasogastric fluids may be prepared commercially, or they may be prepared by the dietary department in accordance with the physician's orders. The preparations are liquid and contain a variety of nutrients, depending upon the physician's order. The amount of the feeding and the frequency of administration are also ordered by the physician. The feeding itself should be at room temperature in order to avoid irritation of the stomach mucosa due to very hot or cold fluids. It is important that the feeding not be administered with undue pressure, which could cause the formation of flatus and reflex vomiting. For this reason the tube is usually attached to a container placed about one foot above the patient's head, allowing the liquid to slowly enter the stomach by the force of gravity. If the nurse inserts the gavage fluid by syringe, care must be taken to inject it slowly with minimal pressure.

Another method by which gavage feedings are administered is through a surgically made opening on the abdomen (a *gastrostomy*) that leads directly to

Table 25-8.   Methods of Differentiating the Placement of a Nasogastric Tube

Stomach	Lungs
1. Place distal end of tube in glass of water. A few bubbles may show initially as gas in the stomach is released or no bubbles will occur.	Bubbles will show as patient breathes.
2. Listen to the distal end. No noise will be apparent.	A crackling sound will be heard.
3. Attach distal end of tube to a syringe and withdraw. Some gastric fluid will be withdrawn.	No fluid will be withdrawn.
4. During insertion of the tube the patient will experience no distress upon breathing.	The patient may experience dyspnea.
5. Listen over the stomach with a stethoscope after injecting 10 ml of air into the tube. Air can be heard entering the stomach.	

the stomach. A tube is inserted into this opening, and the fluid is inserted in much the same way as it is through a nasogastric tube.

Hyperalimentation

Another more recently developed method of administering nutrients to a patient is hyperalimentation. The student is referred to Chapter 30 for a discussion of parenteral hyperalimentation.

Motivating Patients to Eat

The lack of appetite (anorexia) is a frequent occurrence accompanying illness. There are a number of reasons for anorexia, some of which are:

1. An accompanying physical illness.
2. The presence of food with which the person is unfamiliar or finds unpalatable.
3. Environmental factors such as unpleasant odors or an elevated room temperature.
4. Psychologic reasons such as anxiety or depression.
5. Physical discomfort such as pain.

A lowered food intake that lasts for only a few days is not often a problem for an adult; however, a prolonged decreased food intake is reflected by loss of weight, decreased strength and stamina, and subsequent nutritional problems. A decreased food intake is often accompanied by a decreased fluid intake, thus resulting in fluid and electrolyte problems. See Chapter 30 for specific information in regard to problems.

Increasing a person's appetite generally involves determining the reason for the lack of appetite and then dealing with the problem. Some specific nursing interventions that may improve a person's appetite are:

1. Dealing with the patient's symptoms accompanying a physical illness prior to meal time by giving an analgesic for pain or an antipyretic for a fever or by allowing rest for fatigue.

2. Providing food that the person likes and with which the patient is familiar, such as rice for a Chinese patient. Often the relatives of patients are pleased to bring food from home even if they require some guidance as to requirements for a special diet. It is also important to present the food in sufficiently small quantities so as not to discourage the anorexic patient.

3. Arranging the environment so that it is conducive to eating. It needs to be fresh and free of unpleasant odors. Unpleasant or uncomfortable treatments should not be carried out immediately before or after a meal. A tidy, clean environment that is free of unpleasant sights is also important. A soiled dressing, a used bedpan, an uncovered irrigation set, or even used dishes may not be conducive to a good appetite.

4. Reducing psychologic stress. A lack of understanding as to therapy, the anticipation of an operation, and fear of the unknown can be causes of anorexia. Often discussion with the patient about feelings, the provision of information, and assistance offered by the nurse to the person to alleviate concerns are helpful measures.

Counseling about Nutrition

People frequently need counseling at times in their lives on nutrition. Nurses need to know the special nutritional needs of different age groups and the food sources of nourishment, especially inexpensive sources.

Nurses may also be asked about common problems experienced by people such as feeding problems of babies and children and nutritional needs during pregnancy and lactation.

Instructing Patients with Special Dietary Problems

Assisting patients with therapeutic diets is a nursing function often shared with the nutritionist and the dietitian. In some communities there are also specially trained community workers who can help with nutritional problems.

There are a number of kinds of therapeutic diets that are frequently prescribed by physicians. Some of these are the low-calorie diet for obesity, the high-calorie diet for underweight, the low-sodium diet for cardiovascular problems, the regulated diet for diabetics, and special diets for people with allergies.

Once a diet has been prescribed, patients often need assistance adapting the diet to their own cultural, religious, ethnic, and economic patterns. Helping the patient adapt the diet to food habits is of great importance. Most diets are written using Anglo-American foods with which the Chinese-American or Italian-American may be unfamiliar. Nutritionists and dietitians can often assist nurses to adapt a diet to one better suited to a person's lifestyle.

Another important aspect is adapting a diet to a person's economic status. Often less costly foods can substitute for recommended foods, such as fish for beef or powdered milk instead of fresh milk.

Motivation is highly important for the success of a diet. If any person, a child or an adult, does not want to follow a diet or accept the need to follow it, the therapeutic value is lost. Understanding is also important. A patient may understand that sugar in coffee is not allowed on a low-calorie diet, but may not

understand that bread also contains sugar and is also restricted. A teenager may understand that a diet applies to what is eaten at mealtime, but may not understand that it also applies to between-meal snacks. An example is the elderly hospitalized patient who understands that she is not to have salt added to foods during cooking but borrows her neighbor's salt during meal hour. This patient does not really understand the importance or the reason for salt restriction.

SUMMARY

Food is essential to survival but is also related to various traditions, customs, superstitions, and pleasures of man. When planning measures to meet nutritional needs of patients, the nurse therefore needs to consider the variations in food practices and habits among individuals.

The essential nutrients required for health include carbohydrates, proteins, fats, vitamins, and minerals. Carbohydrates are the chief source of calories, are abundant in grain products, fruits, and vegetables, and are the major source of energy for the body. Proteins are essential for growth and repair of body tissues. Major sources are dairy products and meat. Fats, in addition to meeting energy needs, are essential as a vehicle of transport for fat-soluble vitamins. These vitamins, A, D, E, and K, have important functions, respectively, maintenance of healthy skin, hair, eyes, and mucous membranes; skeletal and tooth development; aid in hematopoiesis; and blood clotting. The water-soluble vitamins B and C require daily replenishment, since they are not stored in the body. The B vitamins include thiamine (B_1), riboflavin (B_2), niacin (B_3), pyridoxine (B_6), and cyanocobalamin (B_{12}) and are essential for metabolism and red blood cell development (B_{12}). Vitamin C is essential for the metabolism of amino acids and enhances iron absorption. The major minerals required include calcium, phosphorus, potassium, sodium, chlorine, sulfur, and magnesium. Micronutrient minerals include iron, iodine, copper, and magnesium. Cellulose is also an essential part of food for health maintenance.

Sufficient calories are required to maintain the body's basal metabolic rate and to provide energy for activity. These caloric requirements vary in accordance with age, growth rates, sex, climate, state of health, and activity.

Daily food requirements are recommended by the United States Department of Agriculture and the

Canadian Department of Health and Welfare. These guides refer to minimal requirements for health and need to be adjusted in accordance with individual requirements.

Infants who are breast fed require supplements of vitamin D and fluoride if the water supply is not fluoridated. Formulas usually include vitamin D, but bottle-fed infants also require fluoride. Iron-fortified cereals are introduced at about 3 months when the infant stores are depleted. Feeding schedules are generally established by each individual infant and vary from every 2 to 3 hours initially to every 4 hours with progressively decreasing night feedings. Recommendations for the introduction of foods vary among physicians. Orange juice containing vitamin C may be prescribed as early as 3 weeks, egg yolk from the third to fifth month, pureed fruits and vegetables at about 6 months, and meat about 10 months.

The toddler and preschooler require well-balanced diets to meet their growth needs. A recommended menu that can be adjusted to the child's needs includes all of the essential foods. Teenagers have increased energy and growth requirements necessitating additional foods such as meat, milk, and vegetables. Snacks are often necessary but need to be nutritious. Females may need additional iron when menses commence.

Pregnant and lactating women require several increases in specific nutrients to meet the growth demands of the fetus. These increases include protein, calcium and phosphorous, iron, magnesium, iodine, and vitamins A, B, C, and E.

The elderly person requires fewer calories than the adult but needs the same amounts of protein, minerals, and vitamins. The carbohydrate and fat intakes need to be reduced, but cellulose intake needs to be maintained or increased.

Many factors affect a person's eating habits. Included are culture, religion, socioeconomic status, personal preference, emotions, and hunger or appetite.

When assessing a person's nutritional status, the nurse needs to consider the person's weight; daily food intake; the condition of skin, hair, and eyes, which reflects the adequacy of specific vitamins; the level of energy; and the degree of fatigue or lethargy. Common problems related to nutrition are classified broadly as malnutrition, undernutrition, and overnutrition. The factors contributing to malnutrition and undernutrition include economics, education, social or class values, and physiologic or psychologic problems. Food fads may also contribute to malnutrition, although some fads may positively influence health.

Nursing interventions related to nutritional needs are categorized as those which (a) assist patients to obtain nourishment, (b) motivate patients to eat, (c) provide counseling about needed nourishment, and (d) assist patients who have special problems with instruction about therapeutic diets.

SUGGESTED ACTIVITIES

1. List your own dietary intake over a 3-day period. Analyze it for caloric and nutrient value. Compare your intake with the food intake recommended by the government.

2. Interview a child, a pregnant woman, and an elderly adult. Compare each of their dietary intakes against recommended intakes.

3. Identify any problems as a result of the interview in activity 2 and plan for corrective nursing intervention.

4. In a clinical setting observe a group of patients who are eating a meal. Identify factors that facilitated and factors that inhibited eating.

5. In a clinical setting select a patient who requires assistance with a meal. After assisting the patient, identify the problems you and the patient encountered.

SUGGESTED READINGS

Caghan, Susan B. October, 1975. The adolescent process and the problem of nutrition. *American Journal of Nursing* 75:1728–1731.

The development of the adolescent personality and the use of food as a defense is discussed. Also included are recommendations as to how to assist the adolescent to be well nourished.

Crim, Sarah R. September, 1969. Nutritional problems of the poor. *Nursing Outlook* 17(9):65–67.

Nutritional problems and poverty are interrelated. Malnutrition is due to many factors as well as poverty. Understanding the prevalence of poverty among particular groups and in particular areas of the country is an important consideration for nurses when planning and implementing care.

Kroog, Emily. April, 1975. Helping people stretch their grocery dollars. *American Journal of Nursing* 75:646–648.

This article explains how a family can buy nourishing food and stretch their dollars. Best buys such as those concerned with milk, meats, fruits, vegetables, and cereals are discussed.

Rubin, Reva. Spring, 1967. Food and feeding: a matrix of relationships. *Nursing Forum* 6(2):195–205.

The role of food in early learning and early socialization is described as well as a person's response to offered food and to giving food.

SELECTED REFERENCES

Anderson, Linnea, et al. 1972. *Nutrition in nursing.* Philadelphia: J. B. Lippincott Co.

Bass, Linda. February, 1977. More fiber—less constipation. *American Journal of Nursing* 77:254–255.

Boykin, Lorraine Stith. 1975. *Nutrition in nursing.* New York: Medical Examination Publishing Co., Inc.

Caly, Joan C. October, 1977. Helping people eat for health: assessing adult's nutrition. *American Journal of Nursing* 77:1605–1609.

Crow, Rosemary A. 1977. An ethnological study of the development of infant feeding. *Journal of Advanced Nursing* 2(2):99–109.

Dansky, Kathryn H. October, 1977. Assessing children's nutrition. *American Journal of Nursing* 77:1610–1611.

Fulmer, Teresa T. October, 1977. On vitamins, calories, and help for the elderly. *American Journal of Nursing* 77:1614–1615.

Grenby, Mike. April, 1977. Living to eat: nutrition for senior citizens. *The Canadian Nurse* 73(4):42–44.

Maclean, Gaynor D. 1977. An appraisal of the concepts of infant feeding and their application in practice. *Journal of Advanced Nursing* (2):111–126.

Malasanos, Lois, et al. 1977. *Health assessment.* St. Louis: The C. V. Mosby Co.

Manning, Mary Louise. April, 1965. The psychodynamics of dietetics. *Nursing Outlook* 13(4):55–59. Reprinted in Meyers, Mary E. 1967. *Nursing fundamentals.* Dubuque, Iowa: William C. Brown Co., Publishers, pp. 174–181.

Markesbery, Barbara Abram, and Wong, Wendy M. October, 1977. Helping people eat for health: points for maternity patients. *American Journal of Nursing* 77:1612–1614.

Robinson, Corinne H., and Lawler, Marilyn R. 1977. *Normal and therapeutic nutrition,* 15th ed. New York: Macmillan Publishing Co., Inc.

CHAPTER 26

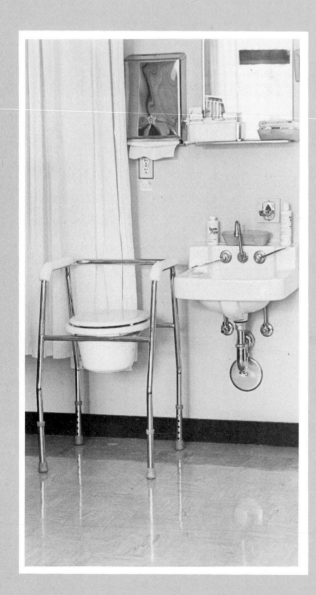

BOWEL ELIMINATION

OBJECTIVES

- Discuss the physiology of defecation.

- Explain the stages of bowel training.

- Describe the factors involved in normal defecation.

- Discuss the factors that promote defecation.

- Describe the factors that affect normal bowel elimination.

- Assess a patient's bowel elimination.

- Describe common problems in fecal elimination and relevant nursing intervention.

- Secure a stool specimen.

- Evaluate the effectiveness of nursing interaction.

The elimination of feces (stool) from the bowels is a subject that is always before people in North America. The advertising concerned with laxatives and descriptions such as feelings of tiredness due to irregularity are continually before us. Some elderly people also are preoccupied with their bowels. Often it is a matter of great concern to them when they are hospitalized. For people who believe they have had a bowel movement once a day for seventy-five years, missing one day can be seen as a serious problem, even though they may not have eaten anything for two days.

In this chapter the physiology of *defecation* (the discharge of feces from the bowels) is discussed. Measures to promote defecation are outlined. The factors that affect normal defecation are provided to assist the nurse in health teaching.

Nurses will frequently be consulted or be involved in assisting patients with elimination problems. These problems are often embarrassing to patients and can cause them considerable discomfort. An understanding, competent nurse can frequently provide patients with much needed assistance, thereby relieving discomfort.

THE PHYSIOLOGY OF DEFECATION

Essential to health is the elimination of the waste products of digestion from the body. These excreted waste products are referred to as *stool* or *feces.*

Large Intestine

The large intestine extends from the ileocecal (ileocolic) valve, which lies between the small and large intestines, to the anus. The colon (large intestine) in the adult is generally about 125 to 150 cm (50 to 60 inches). It has seven parts: the cecum; ascending, transverse, and descending colons; sigmoid colon; rectum; and anus or external orifice (see Figure 26-1).

The waste products leaving the stomach through

the ileocecal valve are referred to as *chyme.* Usually about 450 ml of chyme enter the adult cecum each 24 hours. Of this amount only about 100 ml remains for excretion by the time it reaches the rectum; the remainder is reabsorbed into the capillaries of the large intestine (Nordmark and Rohweder 1975:145).

The constituents of the colon normally represent a mixture of foods ingested over the previous four days, although most of the waste products will be excreted within forty-eight hours of *ingestion* (the act of taking in food).

The colon has two kinds of movement: a mixing movement and a movement that propels the chyme along its tract. The mixing movement helps the absorptive process take place. Water, sodium, and chlo-

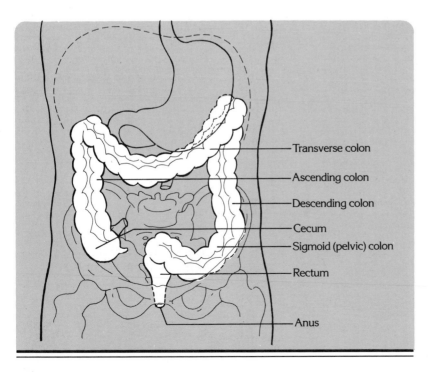

Figure 26-1.   Diagram of the large intestine.

- Transverse colon
- Ascending colon
- Descending colon
- Cecum
- Sigmoid (pelvic) colon
- Rectum
- Anus

ride ions are normally absorbed from the colon, whereas potassium and bicarbonate ions are normally excreted into the chyme. The propulsive movements are called *peristalsis*, and they normally occur only a few times a day. Mass peristaltic waves in the duodenum and colon are caused by the gastrocolic and duodenocolic reflexes, which are initiated after meals by the filling of the duodenum by food from the stomach.

The muscles of the colon are innervated by the autonomic nervous system. The parasympathetic nervous system stimulates movement, and the sympathetic system inhibits movement.

Peristaltic waves occur in the large intestine anywhere from one to four times during twenty-four hours. With these waves the mass of feces moves along the colon to the sigmoid colon and rectum, where it stays until defecation. Most feces remain in the sigmoid colon until just prior to defecation.

Rectum and Anal Canal

The rectum in the adult is usually 10–15 cm (4–6 inches) in length; the most distal portion, 2.5–5 cm (1 to 2 inches), is the anal canal.

Within the rectum itself there are three folds of tissue that extend across the rectum and folds that extend vertically. Each of the vertical folds contains a vein and an artery. It is believed that these folds assist to retain feces within the rectum. When the veins become distended, as can occur with repeated pressure, a condition known as *hemorrhoids* occurs.

The anal canal is bound by an internal and an external sphincter muscle. The internal sphincter is under involuntary control, and the external sphincter normally is voluntarily controlled. The external sphincter's action is augmented by the levator ani muscle of the pelvic floor. The internal sphincter muscle is innervated by the autonomic nervous system; the external sphincter is innervated by skeletal motor nerves.

Defecation

Defecation or the expulsion of feces normally takes place in people from several times per day to only two or three times per week. There is a wide range of the frequency of defecation between normal, healthy individuals.

The act of defecation can be described in a number of steps.

1. Movement of feces into the rectum from the sigmoid colon. The sensory nerves in the rectum are stimulated as a result of the presence of the feces, and impulses travel by the nerves to the spinal cord and hence to the sacral nerves. Other impulses travel to the brain by the spinothalamic tract. They arouse the person's perception of the need to defecate.

2. The internal sphincter muscle relaxes and at the same time more feces move from the sigmoid colon to the rectum.

3. The person, aware of the need to defecate, finds a toilet or bedpan and voluntarily relaxes the external sphincter. Additional pressure is exerted to expel the feces by contraction of the abdominal muscles and the diaphragm, which increases the abdominal pressure. Contraction of the levator ani muscles in the pelvic floor lifts the anal canal over the feces in the canal. The feces are expelled.

Normal defecation can be facilitated by (a) thigh flexion, which places pressure on the abdomen, and (b) a sitting position, which increases the downward pressure upon the rectum.

If the defecation reflex is ignored or if defecation is consciously inhibited by contraction of the external sphincter muscle, the reflex generally disappears for a few hours before occurring again. Most people after the age of about four years have sufficient neuromuscular development and control that they are able to do this; however, irregular bowel habits can lead to constipation.

BOWEL TRAINING

Bowel training can usually begin after children learn to walk at about the age of one and one half to two years. It is at this time that they can ask to go to the toilet during the day when they feel the need. It is also at this age that their nervous and muscular systems are sufficiently well developed so that they will have some degree of control.

When children are in the process of toilet training, it is important that they are able to be as independent as possible in this function. In this regard the following measures are helpful:

1. They need to wear pants that they can remove easily themselves.

2. An easily accessible training toilet needs to be available. This may be a portable toilet or a special seat on the toilet with steps up to it so that the toddler can reach it.

When children are admitted to the hospital, it is important that the nurse learn from the parents at what stage the children are in their toilet training. In particular it is important to know what words they use to indicate their needs and their usual routine for defecation. It is important that children continue the habits that are being established at home. On the other hand, if the child is not trained, initiation of training in the hospital setting is normally avoided for two reasons: a sick and anxious child will not readily tolerate the stress of learning new habits, and the child's mother or a significant person is not present in the hospital. Pleasing the significant person is the motivating factor behind learning toilet training for children.

Stages of Bowel Training

1. Awareness of the discomfort created by an incontinent bowel movement.
2. Identification that the elimination function is the reason for the discomfort.
3. Awareness of the body sensation that indicates the need for defecation.
4. Desire to avoid the discomfort caused by involuntary defecation. This discomfort can be physical and sociologic. The latter is demonstrated by the disapproval expressed by others and the social isolation sometimes given to an incontinent child. *Incontinence* in this context is the inability to restrain defecation.

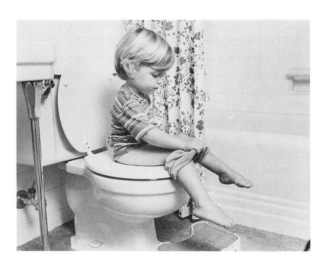

Figure 26-2.   A toddler being toilet-trained has his own potty.

The methods used to accomplish toilet training vary; usually they must incorporate five aspects:

1. The involvement of a significant person in the child's life whom the child wishes to please.
2. Sufficient time and a consistent pattern.
3. A method of communication between the child and the significant person.
4. Praise and reinforcement of successful behavior.
5. Lack of punishment or disapproval when the child is unsuccessful so that the situation does not become too stressful.

If any of these is absent, the child may encounter difficulty in becoming trained. Daytime bowel control is normally attained by the age of 30 months (Figure 26-2).

NORMAL DEFECATION

Defecation has two aspects, the pattern of defecation of an individual person and characteristics of the feces.

Pattern

The pattern of defecation is highly individualistic just as is the frequency of defecation. It has already been mentioned that some people normally defecate once a day; others only defecate three or four times a week. For some, defecating after breakfast is normal, whereas for others an evening defecation pattern has been developed. Often the pattern followed by a person will largely depend upon early training and convenience in one's daily living. Most people develop the habit of defecating after breakfast, when the gastrocolic and duodenocolic reflexes cause mass movements in the large intestine.

Feces

Normal feces contain about 75% water if the person has an adequate fluid intake. The other 25% is made up of solid materials. The student is referred to Table 26-1.

Color

Normal feces are brown. The color is due to two main factors: the bilirubin derivatives stercobilin and urobilin, and the action of the normal bacteria within the intestine. *Bilirubin* is a red pigment in the bile.

Feces may have other colors, usually due to the presence of abnormal constituents. For example, black, tarry feces may indicate the presence of old blood, clay-colored *(acholic)* feces usually indicate the absence of bile, and green or orange stools may indicate the presence of an intestinal infection. Food may also affect the color of feces; red beets can color stool red or sometimes green.

Consistency

Normally feces are formed but soft. Their shape is usually that of the rectum. Therefore any abnormalities in the shape of the stool other than those which the person considers normal need to be noted. A stringlike stool may be indicative of a pathologic condition of the rectum.

Watery stools contain more than the normal 75% water. The stool has moved more quickly than normal through the intestine, hence less water and fewer ions were reabsorbed into the body.

Table 26-1.   Content of Normal Feces (Solid Materials)*

Constituent	Percent
Dead bacteria	30
Fat	10 to 20
Inorganic matter	10 to 20
Protein	2 to 3
Undigested roughage and dried constituents of digestive juices (for example, bile pigment and sloughed epithelical cells)	30

*From Guyton, Arthur C. *Textbook of medical physiology*, 5th ed. © 1976 by The W. B. Saunders Co., Philadelphia, Pennsylvania, p. 892.

Hard stool contains less water than normal and in some instances may be difficult and painful to excrete. Some people, in particular, babies and young children, may pass stools in which there is undigested food.

Odor

The odor of feces results from the action of bacteria in the intestine, and it normally varies somewhat from person to person. It is important for the nurse to note any changes in odor that the patient notices. A putrid (rotten, distasteful) odor may well indicate a digestive disorder.

MEASURES THAT PROMOTE DEFECATION

There are a number of measures that can be employed to assist defecation in addition to those which are highly individualistic, such as the need to drink hot lemonade before being able to defecate. In this instance the individual is probably stimulating the gastrocolic reflex. The following measures should assist in promoting regular defecation:

1. Balanced diet that contains adequate bulk (fiber content).
2. Adequate fluid intake.
3. Regular meals.
4. Regular time for defecation and adequate time to defecate.
5. Regular exercise.
6. Privacy for defecation.
7. Taking a rectal suppository, enema, or laxative when necessary.

FACTORS THAT AFFECT NORMAL BOWEL ELIMINATION

Age

The age of a person can affect not only the character of fecal elimination but also the control. The very young are unable to control their elimination until the neuromuscular system is developed. This occurs between the ages of two and three years. There are also changes in the elderly person's body that can also affect bowel evacuation. Two of these are *atony* (lack of normal muscle tone) of the smooth muscle of the colon, which can result in a slower peristalsis and hence hardened (drier) feces, and decreased tone of the abdominal muscles, which also decreases the pressure that can be exerted during bowel evacuation. Some elderly people also have a problem of decreased control over the anal sphincter muscles, which can result in an urgency to defecate.

Diet

The food a person eats is a major factor affecting bowel elimination. Sufficient bulk (cellulose, fiber) in the diet is necessary to provide fecal volume. Some foods are also difficult or impossible for some people to digest. This results in digestive upsets and, in some instances, the passage of watery stools.

Fluid

The volume of fluid taken by a person also affects bowel elimination. When fluid intake is inadequate or output (urine or vomitus, for example) is excessive for some reason, the body reabsorbs the needed fluid from the chyme as it passes along the colon. As a result the chyme becomes drier than normal, resulting in hard feces.

Exercise

A program of exercises for people of all ages serves to maintain muscle tone. The abdominal and pelvic muscles and the diaphragm are important for defecation. Activity also stimulates peristalsis, thus facilitating the movement of chyme along the colon. Conversely, immobility depresses colonic mobility.

Stress

Excessive stress can also affect bowel elimination. Some people, when they are anxious, afraid, or angry, experience increased peristaltic activity and subsequent diarrhea, whereas others experience constipation. The latter is most likely to occur when the person is depressed.

Regular Time for Elimination

Establishing a regular time for bowel elimination and taking sufficient time to provide for elimination are important. By establishing a regular time and by utilizing the defecation reflex that is stimulated at that time, regular and complete defecation is facilitated.

Regular Mealtimes

Eating at regular times also affects defecation, just as irregular eating times can impair regular defecation. The body with regular meal times becomes accustomed to a regularly timed, physiologic response to the food intake and a regular pattern for peristaltic activity in the colon.

Medications

Some drugs have side effects that can interfere with normal elimination. Some will cause diarrhea; others will cause constipation, such as large doses of some tranquilizers and repeated administration of morphine and codeine.

There are also medications that directly affect elimination. *Laxatives* are medications used to stimulate bowel activity, hence to assist fecal elimination. There are also laxatives that soften stool, thereby facilitating defecation. There are also medications that slow colon function and can be used to treat diarrhea, such as Kaolin, Donnatal, and diphenoxylate (Lomotil).

ASSESSMENT OF FECAL ELIMINATION

The following data need to be gathered and recorded when making an assessment of a person's fecal elimination.

1. The character (color, odor, consistency) of the stool and the presence of abnormal constituents such as mucus.

2. The frequency of defecation and the amount of feces.

3. Whether the person perceives the character and frequency (and amount) as different from usual.

4. The presence of flatus and any distention of the abdomen. *Flatus* is gas or air in the stomach or intestines.

5. The person's medical diagnosis.

COMMON PROBLEMS OF FECAL ELIMINATION

The most frequent problems related to bowel elimination are constipation, fecal impaction, diarrhea, anal incontinence, and flatulence leading to intestinal distention.

Constipation

Constipation refers to the passage of small, dry, hard stools or the passage of no stool for a period of time. It occurs when the movement of feces through the large intestine is slow, thus allowing time for additional reabsorption of fluid from the large intestine. Associated with constipation is the difficult evacuation of stools and increased effort or straining of the voluntary muscles of defecation. It is important that constipation is determined in relation to the person's regular elimination pattern. Some people normally defecate only a few times a week and therefore are not necessarily constipated when they miss a day or two. On the other hand, some people defecate more than once a day, and to them a movement only once a day can indicate constipation. A careful assessment of the person's habits is necessary before a diagnosis of constipation is made.

Causes of Constipation

There are many causes for constipation:

1. *Irregular bowel habits.* One of the most frequent causes of constipation is irregular bowel habits. When the normal defecation reflexes are inhibited or ignored, there is a tendency for these conditioned reflexes to become progressively weakened. With habitual neglect, the urge to defecate is ultimately lost. Children may tend to ignore these reflexes in preference to play; adults ignore them because of the pressures of time related to work or catching a bus. Hospitalized patients who are on bed rest may suppress the urge because of embarrassment about using a bedpan or because defecation is too uncomfortable. The change of routine and diet can also contribute to constipation. The prevention of constipation is largely due to the establishment of regular bowel habits throughout life.

2. *Overuse of laxatives.* Frequently laxatives are resorted to for bowel irregularity. Persistent use of these has the same effect as ignoring the urge to defecate; natural defecation reflexes are inhibited. The habitual user of laxatives eventually requires larger or stronger doses of laxative, since they have a progressively weakening effect on the nervous system.

3. *Emotional tension.* Strong emotion is thought to cause constipation by inhibiting intestinal peristalsis through the action of adrenalin and the sympathetic nervous system. Tension can also cause a spastic bowel (spastic or hypertonic constipation or an irritable colon). Associated with this type of constipation are crampy abdominal pains, increased mucus formation, and alternating periods of constipation with diarrhea.

4. *Dietary alterations.* Bland diets and low-roughage diets are lacking in bulk and therefore create insufficient residue of waste products to stimulate the reflex for defecation. Low-residue foods such as rice, eggs, or lean meats move more slowly through the intestinal tract. Increasing the fluid intake with these foods will increase their rate of movement.

5. *Medications.* Many drugs have side effects that cause constipation. Some of these, such as morphine or codeine as well as adrenergic and anticholinergic drugs, slow the motility of the colon through their action on the central nervous system, thus causing constipation. Others act more locally on the bowel mucosa to cause constipation, such as oral iron, which has an astringent effect. Iron also has an irritating effect and can cause diarrhea in some people.

6. *Insufficient exercise.* The effects of lack of exercise were discussed in Chapter 23. For patients on prolonged bed rest, generalized muscle weakness extends to the abdominal, diaphragmatic, and levator ani muscles, which are used in defecation. Indirectly associated with lack of exercise is the lack of appetite and possible subsequent lack of roughage food, which is necessary to stimulate defecation reflexes.

uscle weakness and poor sphincter
n elderly people contributes to con-

esses. Several disease conditions of
the bowel can produce constipation. Among these are
bowel obstruction originating from painful defecation due to hemorrhoids, which provokes the person
to avoid a movement; paralysis, which inhibits the
patient's ability to bear down; or pelvic inflammatory
conditions, which create paralysis or atony of the
bowel.

Nursing Intervention for Constipation

Nursing intervention to relieve constipation is determined by first assessing the specific factors
contributing to the constipation for that person. If
there are no pathologic causes such as a bowel
obstruction, the nurse and patient can together establish a plan of action. Some suggestions are as follows:

1. Increase the daily fluid intake, or take a hot drink
when arising.

2. Include bulk in the diet such as prunes, raw fruit,
and bran products.

3. Increase the person's physical activity by planning ambulation periods if possible.

4. Provide a regular time for fecal evacuation such
as after breakfast each day or in accordance with the
person's usual time.

5. Provide for privacy and comfort. For bedridden
patients, offer a warm bedpan and assist them to assume a high Fowler's position with knees flexed. Cur-
tain off the area, and allow them privacy and time to
relax.

6. Promote measures to relieve tension, and try to
prevent factors that make the patient suppress the
urge to defecate.

Other specific measures may need to be employed for constipation such as the administration of
cathartics and enemas.

Cathartics. *Cathartics* are drugs that induce defecation. They vary in their degree of action and method
of action. Cathartics can have a laxative effect or a
purgative effect; a laxative effect is mild in comparison to the purgative effect, which produces frequent
movements of the bowel, soft liquid stools, and sometimes abdominal cramps. Different cathartics have
different effects, but even the same cathartic may

have either a purgative or laxative effect depending
upon the dosage taken. A large dose of a cathartic may
have a purgative effect while a small dose of the same
cathartic may have a laxative effect, producing a normal bowel movement.

There are several ways in which cathartics act to
induce defecation:

1. *Bulk-forming cathartics.* These act by increasing
the fluid, gas, or solid bulk of the intestinal content.
The increased bulk stimulates peristalsis, and thus
defecation occurs. Adequate fluids need to be taken
with this type of cathartic. An example is Metamucil.

2. *Emollient cathartics* such as liquid petrolatum.
These act to soften and delay the drying of the fecal
mass. Prolonged use of liquid petrolatum is contraindicated, since it inhibits the absorption of some fat-
soluble vitamins.

3. *Chemical irritants.* Some cathartics have an irritating effect on the bowel mucosa, which causes rapid
propulsion of the contents from the small intestine.
Considerable fluid is passed with the stool because of
the rapid movement of the feces, which does not allow the normal diffusion of fluid from the bowel.
Castor oil is an example of a chemically irritating cathartic. It causes complete evacuation of the bowel so
that no movements may occur for a day or two after
its administration. Another example is cascara, although its irritant effect occurs primarily in the large
intestine.

4. *Moistening or wetting agents.* These act by lowering the surface tension of the fecal matter, thus allowing water to penetrate and become well mixed with
the feces. A soft-formed stool is the result. An example is Colace.

5. *Saline cathartics.* These cathartics are soluble
salts, which are not absorbed or only slightly absorbed in the intestine. The fluid bulk is increased,
since water absorption is decreased with the salt solution in the large intestine. Examples of these are
magnesium hydroxide (milk of magnesia) and magnesium sulfate (Epsom salts).

The administration of cathartics is prescribed
with caution and in many instances is ordered by the
physician. There are a number of reasons for prescribing cathartics other than for constipation, such as
prior to radiologic examinations or surgical procedures when the bowel contents must be evacuated.

The nurse's unique function with constipated
patients is to help them understand how laxatives can
be effectively used but not abused. Some patients

come to rely on laxatives and need help to learn how to change this habit. Others may require periodic or regular use of laxatives, such as elderly persons who have difficulty increasing the bulk in their diet because of being edentulous or not having the physical health to carry out appropriate exercise.

The nurse also needs to be aware of any other pathologic condition the patient may have when administering laxatives. The classic example is the person who has an inflamed appendix. Ingestion of a laxative by this person can bring about rupture of the appendix as a result of increasing the peristaltic action of the bowel. Some other contraindications are ulcerative conditions of the intestine, obstructions, or severe debilitation from electrolyte imbalances.

Suppositories.   Some laxatives are given in the form of suppositories. These act in various ways: by softening the feces, by releasing gases such as carbon dioxide to distend the rectum, or by stimulating the nerve endings in the rectal mucosa. Suppositories need to be inserted beyond the internal anal sphincter. A finger cot or disposable glove is worn by the nurse, and the suppository is well lubricated prior to insertion to prevent friction and tissue damage. The suppository is inserted gently about three to four inches or the length of the nurse's index finger for an adult and less for a child and baby, while the patient is instructed to breathe through the mouth. Mouth breathing usually relaxes the anal sphincter. The suppository needs to be placed along the wall of the rectum rather than through the feces to be effective. After insertion the glove or finger cot is removed by turning it inside out and is discarded. Nondisposable gloves are rinsed in soap and water. Immediately after insertion the nurse can help dispel any urge the patient has to expel the suppository by pressing the patient's buttocks together for a few seconds. See Chapter 36, "Rectal Insertion," for further information.

Generally, suppositories are effective within half an hour. The best results can be obtained by inserting the suppository half an hour before the patient's usual defecation time or when the peristaltic action is greatest, such as after breakfast.

Fecal Impaction

Fecal impaction can be defined as a mass or collection of hardened, puttylike feces in the folds of the rectum due to prolonged retention and accumulation of fecal material. In severe conditions the feces accumulate and extend well up into the sigmoid colon and beyond. Fecal impaction is recognized by the passage of liquid fecal seepage (diarrhea) and no normal stools. The liquid portion of the feces seeps out around the impacted mass. Impaction can also be assessed by digital examination of the rectum during which the hardened mass can often be palpated.

Along with fecal seepage and constipation, the patient often has a frequent desire to defecate to no avail as well as some rectal pain. A generalized feeling of illness results, and the patient becomes anorexic, the abdomen becomes distended, and nausea and vomiting may occur.

The causes of fecal impaction are usually poor habits concerned with defecation and constipation. Certain drugs previously described in connection with constipation can also contribute to impactions. The barium used in radiologic examinations of the upper and lower gastrointestinal tracts can be a causative factor. Therefore, after these x-ray examinations, measures are taken to ensure removal of the barium. In the elderly a combination of factors contribute to impactions such as poor fluid intake, insufficient bulk intake, lack of activity, and weakened muscle tone for bearing down at defecation. In some people, impactions tend to occur regardless of the measures taken to prevent them.

Nursing Intervention for Impactions

Ideally, the occurrence of fecal impaction can be prevented. However, therapeutic measures are sometimes necessary to disimpact a patient. Often an oil retention enema is given followed by a cleansing enema two to four hours later and daily follow-up with additional cleansing enemas, suppositories, or laxatives.

The technique for giving an oil retention enema is similar to that for a cleansing enema (see "Enemas"). Because small amounts of oil are administered, the oil is usually placed in a small pitcher and then administered directly through the rectal tube with an Asepto syringe or through a small funnel that is attached by a connecting tube to the rectal catheter.

Digital removal of the fecal impaction is sometimes necessary. This involves digitally breaking up the fecal mass and then removing portions of it. This is distressing and uncomfortable to patients, and they may desire the presence of another nurse or family member for support. Care must be taken to avoid injuring the bowel mucosa and thus prevent bleeding. For this reason, agency policies vary in regard to who may digitally break up impactions. Usually follow-up measures to encourage normal defecation, such as enemas or suppositories, are implemented for a few days after disimpaction.

Procedure 26-1.   Digital Removal of a Fecal Impaction

Action	Explanation
Assemble Equipment	
1. Pair of plastic or rubber gloves.	For the nurse to wear.
2. Bedpan and cover.	To receive the feces.
3. Disposable bed pads.	To protect the bed.
4. Toilet tissue.	
5. Lubricant and tissue.	
To Remove an Impaction	
1. Explain to the patient what you plan to do. Adjust the explanation to the patient's needs.	To reassure the patient through knowledge of what will happen. To identify the patient.
2. Provide the patient with privacy.	To prevent unnecessary embarrassment.
3. Wash hands.	To transmit no microorganisms to the patient.
4. Assist the patient to a side-lying position with knees flexed and back toward the nurse or to a Sim's position.	Some patients may prefer to sit on a toilet, but disimpacting can be exhausting; therefore a side-lying bed position is advised for most patients.
5. Place the bed pad under the buttocks.	
6. Place the bedpan nearby.	To receive the stool.
7. Put on gloves.	
8. Lubricate the index finger to be inserted.	To prevent irritation of the rectal mucosa.
9. Gently insert the index finger into the rectum, following the wall of the rectum. The angle should be directed toward the umbilicus.	
10. Gently massage around the stool.	To loosen and dislodge it.
11. Work finger into the hardened mass.	To break it up.
12. Work the stool downward to the end of the rectum, and remove in small pieces.	To avoid injury to the mucosa of the rectum.
13. Continue to remove as much fecal material as possible. Watch patient for signs of fatigue such as skin color changes, changes in pulse, or diaphoresis.	
14. Assist the patient to wash the anal area and buttocks if needed.	These will probably have become soiled.
15. Assist patient onto a bedpan for a short time.	A commode or toilet can be used if the patient is strong enough. Digital stimulation of the rectum can induce the urge to defecate.
16. Assist the patient to a comfortable position.	
17. Wash hands.	

18. Record the characteristics of the fecal material, the results of the evacuation.

19. It is sometimes indicated to follow up a fecal evacuation with an enema or suppository.

Diarrhea

Diarrhea refers to the passage of liquid feces and an increased frequency of defecation. It is the opposite of constipation and results from rapid movement of fecal contents through the large intenstine. This reduces the time available for the large intestine to reabsorb water and electrolytes. Some people pass stools with increased frequency but diarrhea is not present unless the stool is relatively unformed and excessively liquid. The person with diarrhea finds it difficult or impossible to control the urge to defecate for very long, a source of concern and embarrassment with fears of accidental defecation. Often spasmodic, piercing, abdominal cramps are associated with diarrhea. Sometimes the passage of excessive mucus and blood, and nausea and vomiting also occur. With persistent bouts of diarrhea, irritation of the anal region extending to the perineum and buttocks generally results. Fatigue, weakness, malaise, and emaciation are the end results of prolonged diarrhea.

When the cause of diarrhea is irritants in the intestinal tract, it is thought to be a protective flushing mechanism. On the other hand, it can create serious fluid and electrolyte losses in the body. These can develop within frighteningly short periods of time, particularly in infants and small children. See Chapter 30 for further information concerning fluid and electrolyte losses in the body.

Causes of Diarrhea

As with constipation there can be numerous reasons for the development of diarrhea.

1. *Intestinal infection (enteritis).* Infectious diarrhea can be caused either by bacteria or viruses. Generally, the distal end of the ileum and the large intestine are involved in the infectious process. When the bowel becomes exceedingly irritated, both the rate of secretion of ileal juices and the motility are increased substantially. The increased fluid flushes the infectious agent toward the anus and is assisted by the strong propulsive movements of the colon.

2. *Nervous tension.* Probably everyone has experienced periods of diarrhea associated with increased emotional tension such as prior to final examinations. This type of emotional or psychogenic diarrhea results from excessive stimulation of the parasympathetic nervous system, which increases both the motility and secretions of the distal colon. Previously mentioned with constipation was the occurrence of alternating bouts of constipation with the diarrhea in prolonged anxiety states.

3. *Dietary indiscretions.* Individual people vary in their tolerance of some foods and fluids. Temporary diarrhea may occur after the ingestion of rich pastries, coffee, alcoholic beverages, or strong seasonings. Some people may have allergies to certain foods and respond with diarrhea to the allergen.

4. *Abuse of cathartics.* Excessive irritation of the colon from overuse of cathartics leads to diarrhea. The person who has irregular bowel habits and becomes constipated may be inclined to overuse laxatives periodically.

5. *Medications.* Some medications are irritating to the gastrointestinal tract and can cause diarrhea as a side effect. A few examples of these are the antibiotic tetracycline, the iron preparation ferrous sulfate, and the antihypertensive drug reserpine.

6. *Other disease conditions.* Malabsorption syndromes such as congenital celiac disease or ulcerative colitis interfere with the bowel's ability to reabsorb water, thus creating diarrhea. Other diseases such as electrolyte imbalances and neuromuscular disorders can also cause diarrhea.

Nursing Intervention for Diarrhea

Nursing measures for diarrhea vary according to the contributing factors and the severity. With excessive fluid and electrolyte loss a major responsibility is to replace the fluid and electrolytes. In some instances intravenous therapy is prescribed. Oral intake of fluids and food needs to be encouraged when possible. Because ingestion of foods and fluids stimulates the gastrocolic and duodenocolic reflexes, thus inducing more stool, the patient may be reluctant to eat or drink. The provision of small, frequent feedings of bland foods can be helpful, since they are more easily absorbed. Potassium losses may be great with diarrhea, and therefore food or fluids containing potassium should be encouraged (see Chapter 30, "Hypokalemia"). Excessively hot or cold fluids should be avoided because they stimulate peristalsis.

Because the patient with diarrhea has difficulty controlling the urge to defecate, a bedpan or commode must be placed in a convenient accessible place. Liquid feces are often malodorous and therefore can be embarrassing to patients. If possible, these patients need rooms that can be well ventilated, and prompt emptying of their bedpans. Skin excoriation around the anal region can be prevented by using soft tissues and by proper cleansing and drying of the area after defecation. Protective creams such as petroleum jelly and zinc oxide or nonirritating powders are also used.

In some instances the patient may accidentally soil the bed or clothing. The nurse needs to provide linen changes and convey understanding and support for the distress or embarrassment that the patient might feel. Encouraging adequate rest and reducing physical activity are also helpful in lessening bowel activity.

If the cause of the diarrhea is sustained anxiety, the nurse may assist by helping the patient to talk about those life situations which are stressful and to consider ways in which these stresses can be reduced. Referral for psychiatric counseling may be indicated.

The nurse will also be involved in medical therapies employed to treat the cause of the diarrhea. Antidiarrhetics may be ordered by the physician. Some of these act by mechanically coating the irritated bowel and act as protectives (demulcents). Others absorb gas or toxic substances from the bowel (adsorbents) or shrink swollen and inflamed tissues (astringents). Antiseptics such as the sulfonamides that are poorly absorbed from the intestine and other antibiotics may be taken. In certain situations, sedatives and antispasmodics may also be taken.

Anal Incontinence

Anal incontinence refers to loss of voluntary ability to control the fecal and gaseous discharges through the anal sphincter. The incontinence may occur at specific times such as after meals, or it may occur irregularly.

The causes of anal incontinence are generally those which impair proper functioning of the anal sphincter or its nerve supply such as neuromuscular disease, spinal cord trauma, and tumors of the external anal sphincter muscle.

Anal incontinence is an emotionally distressing problem that can ultimately lead to social isolation. Involved persons withdraw into the confines of their home or, if in the hospital, the confines of their room to minimize the embarrassment associated with soiling. The desire to dress in street clothes may be replaced by dressing in easily washable night garments. Skin irritation and excoriation around the anal region can become a serious problem, which warrants preventive measures. These were discussed previously for diarrhea.

Bowel Retraining

Many patients with anal incontinence can be helped to regain bowel control with a planned program of bowel training. This plan is usually initiated by the physician, who determines the possibility of success in accordance with the underlying causes. The measures used will vary with the individual person concerned but can include the following:

1. Determining with the patient the time of day for evacuation such as after breakfast. After breakfast the gastrocolic reflex is stimulated, and this enhances defecation.

2. Arranging to have the patient on the commode or toilet at the specified time, since defecation is facilitated by gravity and by the more efficient muscular contraction in this position.

3. Providing a drink of hot coffee or tea in the early morning to stimulate peristalsis.

4. Administering oral stool softeners daily or a laxative suppository 30 minutes prior to the prescribed defecation time. These serve to stimulate the rectal mucosa.

5. Teaching the patient while on the toilet to lean forward at the hips, to apply pressure on the abdomen with the hands, and to bear down as is normally done. These measures increase the pressure on the large colon and help achieve the best possible results. Straining should be discouraged, however, because hemorrhoids may occur.

6. Providing privacy and a time limit for defecation. Some patients find that reading a book or smoking a cigarette helps them to relax. A suggested time limit for defecation is twenty minutes.

7. Ensuring that the patient's diet has sufficient roughage and that permitted exercise is encouraged.

Bowel training requires patience by the patient. The nurse needs to offer praise for the patient's efforts and encouragement to consistently pursue the program.

Flatulence Leading to Intestinal Distention

Flatulence is the presence of excessive amounts of gases (flatus) in the intestines and leads to stretching and inflation of the intestines (intestinal distention). This is also referred to as *tympanites*. Large amounts of air and other gases can also accumulate in the stomach, resulting in gastric distention.

A certain amount of gas in the gastrointestinal system is normal. Sources of intestinal gas are swallowed air and gas that originates from the bacterial decomposition of food residue and diffusion from the bloodstream. Swallowed air accounts for approximately two-thirds of flatus normally, and bacterial decomposition and diffusion from the bloodstream account for the remaining third. Normally the gas is propelled by peristalsis along the tract and is absorbed. The swallowed air is usually *eructated* (belched).

Flatus may be expelled orally or anally, offering relief to the distention, or it may be retained. With increasing distention the abdomen becomes progressively swollen, and the patient may complain of crampy pain and shortness of breath. The latter occurs when the diaphragm is elevated as a result of intraabdominal pressure.

Common causes of flatulence and distention are constipation, medications that decrease intestinal motility such as codeine or barbituates, and anxiety states in which large amounts of air are swallowed. Most people have experienced some flatulence and distention related to certain gas-forming foods such as beans or cabbage. Postoperative distention after abdominal surgery is commonly seen in hospitals. This type of distention generally occurs about the third postoperative day and is caused by the effects of anesthesia, narcotics, dietary changes, and reduction in activity (see Chapter 37).

Nursing Intervention for Flatulence

Several nursing measures can be employed to relieve flatus and abdominal distention depending upon the cause. Minimizing the amount of swallowed air may be necessary. If the patient is anxious and hyperventilating, and swallowing large amounts of air, appropriate breathing patterns may need to be learned as well as planning ways to reduce the anxiety. Limiting the ingestion of carbonated beverages, the use of straws to drink, or the chewing of gum will also reduce the amount of air ingested. For some abdominal surgeries, nasogastric tubes are present postoperatively. These tubes in addition to removing fluid also enhance the passage of gas from the upper gastrointestinal tract. Movement in bed or ambulation will facilitate even more efficient removal of the flatus.

Insertion of a Rectal Tube.   The insertion of a rectal tube can provide temporary relief from flatulence. This is usually implemented when other measures fail. Standard size rectal tubes are used (no. 22 to 30 French for adults, 16 to 24 for children in accordance with age.) The rectal tube is lubricated prior to insertion to reduce resistance during passage of the tube through the anal sphincters. It can be inserted further than the distance recommended for enema insertion, since fluid will not be administered. For adults about six inches is recommended, for infants and small children, two to four inches, depending upon their age. Prior to this an absorbent pad should be placed under the patient's buttocks.

After insertion of the rectal tube the patient is instructed to lie quietly in bed in the lateral position so that the tube is not dislodged. If necessary the tube may be taped to one buttock. The open end of the tube is then placed in a folded or rolled absorbent pad or towel to catch any seepage of liquid fecal material. Some agencies advocate attachment of the open end of the rectal tube to some connecting tubing, which is attached to a collecting receptacle containing water. In this way, the passage of flatus can be determined by noting the presence of the gas bubbles in the water. The distal end of the connecting tubing must be placed below the level of the water in the collecting receptacle for bubbles to be noted.

Prolonged insertion time of rectal tubes can reduce the responsiveness of the anal sphincters and can also irritate the rectal mucosa. It is recommended that rectal tubes remain inserted for no longer than thirty minutes and are then again reinserted as needed every two to three hours.

After removing the rectal tube, the patient's response should be noted. If no flatus is expelled and the patient continues to be distended after several attempts, the physician needs to be notified.

ENEMAS

An *enema* (pl. enemas, enemata) is the introduction of a solution into the rectum and sigmoid colon. Its function is to remove feces and/or flatus. Enemas are commonly given for the following purposes:

1. To remove feces in instances of constipation and/or impaction.
2. To remove feces and cleanse the rectum and colon in preparation for an examination.
3. To remove feces prior to a surgical procedure or a delivery to prevent inadvertent defecation and subsequent contamination of a wound.

Enemas are less frequently given for other reasons, such as to reduce body temperature (ice water enema) and to reduce cerebral edema (magnesium sulfate enema).

Enemas can be classified according to their action:

1. *Cleansing enemas.* These primarily act by stimulating peristalsis through irritation of the colon and rectum and by distention by volume. A volume of 1000 to 1500 ml is instilled into the adult. Infants normally receive no more than 250 ml. Some agencies differentiate between high and low cleansing enemas. A *high enema* is given to cleanse as much of the large bowel as possible. Usually about 1000 ml of solution is administered. It is administered at a higher pressure, and the patient changes position in order for the fluid to follow the bowel during its administration. A *low enema* is used to cleanse only the lower bowel. About 500 ml of solution is administered at a lower pressure.

2. *Oil enemas.* The action of oil serves to lubricate the rectum and colon and to soften the feces, thus making defecation easier. About 150 to 200 ml of oil is instilled in an adult. For small children, 75 to 150 ml of oil is considered suitable.

3. *Carminative enemas.* These are primarily given to expel flatus, and they act primarily by releasing gas that distends the colon and rectum. Usually only 60 to 180 ml of fluid is instilled into the rectum and colon.

Enemas come commercially prepared for adults and children, or they can be made up in the home and hospital. Tap water is commonly used for adults but should not be used for infants because of the danger of electrolyte imbalance. The colon does absorb water, and repeated tap water enemas can result in cardiovascular overload and subsequent electrolyte imbalance. The symptoms of this overload include dizziness, pallor, sweating, and vomiting.

Soap suds and physiologic saline are also used for cleansing enemas. Too strong a solution or repeated use can result in irritation of the lining of the colon and damage to the mucous membrane.

If a commercially prepared product is used, the strength should not be greater than 5 ml of soap per 1000 ml of water. When a solution of soap is made up, it is more difficult to gauge the strength of the solution. Only white bland soap should be used. The common household detergents are considered to be too strong for the colon and rectum. Caution should be taken to use only bar soap that has not been used before to prevent the instillation of pathogenic microorganisms into the patient. Soap packets of Castile soap are available commercially. They are convenient and permit a more accurate measure of the strength of the enema.

Physiologic saline acts to distend the colon and rectum, thus stimulating peristalsis. One problem with repeated saline enemas is the absorption of fluid and electrolytes into the bloodstream. Most agencies have a policy regarding the strength of a saline enema. One guide is 8 ml of sodium chloride to 1000 ml of water.

Some commercially prepared disposable enemas come as hypertonic solutions. Their action is to both distend the colon and rectum and to irritate the mucous membrane, thus stimulating peristalsis. The amount of solution that is instilled is about 120 ml (4 oz). Because it is hypertonic it draws fluid into the bowel from the circulation, thus increasing the fluid volume in the colon and rectum. A hypertonic solution is usually left for 5 to 7 minutes before the patient defecates. This time allows the fluid volume within the colon to increase sufficiently to stimulate defecation.

Oil retention enemas are administered to patients to soften the feces and lubricate the lining of the colon and rectum as an aid to defecation. Salad oil or liquid petrolatum are commonly used at a temperature of 33° C (91° F). There are also commercially prepared retention enemas. Once the oil has been administered (adults usually receive about 180 ml of oil), it is retained for from 1 to 3 hours before it is expelled.

Carminative enemas are given primarily to expel flatus. There are number of kinds, and many agencies have a preferred type. Three commonly used types are the 1–2–3 enema, the milk and molasses enema, and the Mayo enema.

The 1–2–3 enema contains 30 gm of magnesium sulfate, 60 gm of glycerine, and 90 gm of warm water.

The milk and molasses enema contains equal amounts of milk and molasses. The amounts vary from 180 ml to 2400 ml, depending upon the type of enema (low or high).

The Mayo enema contains 240 cc of water, 60 cc of white sugar, and 30 cc of sodium bicarbonate. The last ingredient is added immediately before the enema is administered, while the solution is bubbling.

Nursing Guidelines for Administering Enemas

1. The appropriate size rectal tube needs to be used. For adults this is usually no. 22 to no. 32 French. Children use a smaller size (smaller number) catheter such as a no. 12 French for an infant and a no. 14 to 18 French for the toddler and school-age child.

2. Rectal tubes need to be smooth and flexible with one or two openings at the end through which the solution will flow. They are usually made of rubber or plastic. Any tube with a sharp or ragged edge should not be used because of the possibility of damaging the mucous membrane of the rectum. The rectal tube is lubricated with a water-soluble lubricant to facilitate insertion and decrease irritation of the rectal mucosa.

3. The temperature of the enema solution is normally 40.5° to 43° C (105° to 110° F) for adults and 37.7° C (100° F) for children.

4. The amount of solution to be administered will depend upon the kind of enema and the age and size of the person.

  Infant: 250 ml or less
  Toddler and preschooler: 500 ml or less
  School-age child: 500 to 1000 ml
  Adult: 750 to 1000 ml

5. When an enema is administered, the patient usually assumes the left lateral position (see Figure 26-3). In this position the sigmoid colon is below the rectum, thus facilitating the instillation of the fluid. For a high cleansing the patient changes position during the administration of the enema from left lateral to dorsal recumbent and then to right lateral. In this way the entire colon will be reached by the fluid.

6. The distance to which the tube is inserted depends upon the age and size of the patient. For an adult it is normally inserted 7.5–10 cm (3–4 inches). For children it is inserted 5–7.5 cm (2–3 inches), and for infants it is normally inserted only 2.5–3.75 cm (1–1.5 inches). If any obstruction is encountered upon insertion of the tube, it should be withdrawn and reported.

7. For most enemas the container for the solution should be no higher than 30 cm (12 inches) above the level of the bed. The higher the container the greater the force with which the solution flows into the patient. For a high cleansing enema the solution container is usually 30–45 cm (12–18 inches) above the bed level because the fluid is to be instilled further to cleanse the entire bowel.

8. Prepacked enemas will have their own instructions, which need to be followed unless there are other instructions from the physician or the agency.

9. The time it takes to administer an enema largely depends upon the amount of fluid to be instilled. Large volumes such as 1500 ml may take ten to fifteen minutes to instill, and small volumes will require less time.

10. The length of time that the enema solution is retained will depend upon the purpose of the enema and the ability of the patient to contract the external sphincter to retain the solution. Oil retention enemas are usually retained two to three hours. Other enemas are normally retained five to ten minutes. To assist a baby to retain the solution the nurse can press the baby's buttocks together, thus providing pressure over the anal area.

11. While the enema solution is being held by the patient, a feeling of fullness and some abdominal discomfort may be experienced.

12. When it is time for the patient to defecate, the nurse may assist him or her to a commode or bathroom, depending upon the patient's preference and physical condition.

Procedure 26-2.   Administering an Enema

Action	Explanation
Assemble Equipment	
1. Disposable enema unit	
or	
2. Tray.	
3. Container.	For solution.
4. Solution as required.	
5. Bath thermometer.	To measure temperature of solution.
6. Bedpan, commode, or toilet.	
7. Tubing with clamp.	
8. Rectal tube.	
9. Bed pad.	To protect bed.
10. Lubricant.	To facilitate insertion of rectal tube.
To Administer Enema	
1. Explain to the patient what you plan to do. Adjust the explanation to the patient's needs.	To reassure the patient by knowledge of what will happen. To identify the patient.
2. Provide for privacy.	Patient will be embarrassed because of exposure to buttocks.
3. Wash hands.	To transmit no microorganisms to the patient.
4. Assist the patient to a left lateral position and drape with blanket (see Figure 26-3). The dorsal recumbent position is frequently used by children, and some commercial products recommend the lower chest position.	The descending colon is on the left side, and therefore the fluid will flow downward.

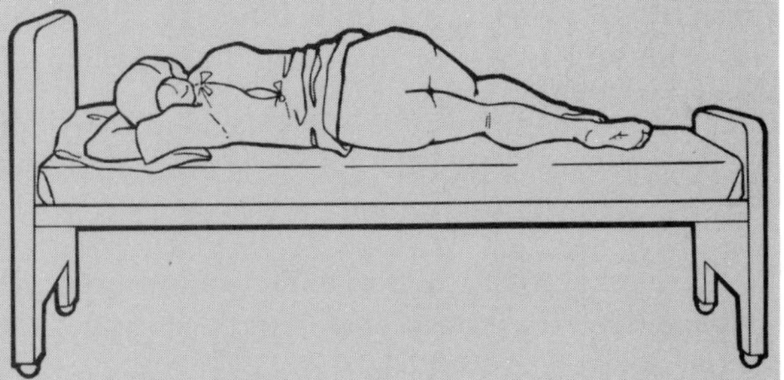

Figure 26-3.   The left lateral position is assumed for the administration of an enema to an adult.

5. Lubricate the tube.	For an adult, 3 inches; 2 inches for a child; 1 inch for an infant or small child. To ease insertion of tube.

6. Insert the tube smoothly and slowly into the rectum. The direction of the insertion should be toward the umbilicus. Distance for insertion: adult, 7.5–10 cm (3–4 inches); child, 5–7.5 cm (2–3 inches); infant, 2.5–3.75 cm (1–1.5 inches).

To follow the direction of the rectum. The tube should be inserted just beyond the internal sphincter.

7. Instill the solution by raising the solution container to 30 cm (12 inches) above bed level or by compressing the pliable commercial container by hand.

At this height the pressure exerted on the walls of the rectum will not damage the mucous membranes.

8. Administer fluid slowly.

Slow administration decreases the likelihood of intestinal spasm and subsequent premature ejection.

9. Remove tube when all the solution has been administered or when the patient feels distended and has a strong desire to defecate.

This usually indicates sufficient fluid has been administered to cleanse the lower bowel.

10. Advise the patient to hold the solution for 5 to 10 minutes depending upon the type of enema.

This permits additional softening of the feces.

11. Collect and remove equipment.

12. Assist the patient to a sitting position on the commode, bedpan, or toilet.

The sitting position permits use of perineal and abdominal muscles for defecation.

13. If a stool specimen is required or if the stool is to be observed, caution the patient not to flush the toilet.

14. Wash hands.

15. Record the enema, the amount, color, and consistency of returns, and any complaints of discomfort by the patient.

SPECIAL ENEMA ADMINISTRATION PROBLEMS

Administering an Enema to an Incontinent Patient

Occasionally a nurse may need to administer an enema to a patient who is unable to contract the external sphincter muscle and hold the solution. Some elderly people do have this problem. In this instance the patient will need to be seated on a bedpan during the administration of the enema. The head of the bed can be raised to about 30° for the patient's comfort, and pillows will be needed to provide additional support for the patient's lumbar region and head.

The nurse needs to use a glove for the hand that holds the rectal tube in place because the solution and feces will be expelled over the hand into the bedpan while the solution is being administered.

This technique is also used when administering an enema to a baby or small child. The infant-size bedpan is usually padded to prevent injury to the skin of the child.

Siphoning an Enema

In some instances a patient may be unable to expel the solution after the administration of an enema. The solution will need to be siphoned off. In siphoning, the nurse uses the force of gravity to draw the fluid out of the rectum.

The equipment required includes a bedpan, a funnel and rectal tube, lubricant, and a container of water at 40° C (105° F). For this the patient assumes a right side-lying position so that the sigmoid colon is uppermost, thus facilitating the drainage of the solution from the rectum and the colon. The patient lies on the bed with hips toward the side of the bed. A bedpan is placed on a chair at the side of the bed near the patient's hips. The rectal tube is lubricated and attached to the funnel. The tube and half of the funnel are filled with solution, then the tube is pinched and gently inserted into the rectum as was done to administer the enema. Holding the funnel about 10 cm (4 inches) above the anus, release the pinched rectal tube and quickly lower the funnel over the bedpan. This action should draw the fluid from the colon and rectum, permitting it to flow through the rectal tube and funnel into the bedpan. The nurse then notes the amount of fluid siphoned off as well as the color, odor, and presence of any feces or abnormal constituents such as blood or mucus.

SECURING A STOOL SPECIMEN

Stool specimens are frequently required so that they can be analyzed for abnormal constituents. Agencies usually provide special containers in which to place a fecal sample. It is important that the nurse know why the specimen is being secured and that the correct container is used. There are several containers that contain preservatives specific to the tests to be performed. There may well be special directions on the container, which need to be followed in obtaining the specimen.

Often a patient can obtain the specimen if given adequate information. The feces to be collected should not have been mixed with urine or water, thus the patient will need to use a bedpan or a commode for defecation.

A wooden or plastic tongue depressor is used to collect the specimen, and about 2.5 cm (1 inch) is placed into the container. If the stool is liquid, between 15 ml and 30 ml needs to be collected. The container is then closed securely, and the appropriate requisitions are completed. The fact that the specimen has been taken also needs to be entered on the patient's chart.

In some instances it is necessary for the laboratory to receive the stool specimen while it is warm. When this is necessary, the specimen needs to be taken immediately to the laboratory. A stool specimen should not be left at room temperature for any length of time because of the bacteriologic changes that take place. Specimen containers usually have directions for storage and should be followed if the specimen cannot be delivered immediately for examination. In some instances refrigeration is indicated.

To secure a stool specimen from a baby or young child who is not toilet trained, a specimen is taken from newly passed feces. Usually a sterile applicator is used when the stool is being cultured for microorganisms.

SUMMARY

Elimination of the waste products of digestion from the body is essential to health. Although patterns of bowel elimination vary, regularity is important to most people. When any irregularity occurs, the person may become preoccupied about reestablishing regularity and may resort to the use of laxatives. Nurses are frequently involved in assisting patients with bowel problems brought about by illness or age or any number of factors such as dietary changes or diagnostic tests.

Adequate elimination of the body's waste products from digestion involves proper functioning of the small and large bowel. As chyme moves through the small bowel, many nutrients are absorbed, and the waste products proceed through the ileocecal valve to the large bowel. More absorption of substances occurs in the large bowel (water and electrolytes) until a firm stool is formed and retained in the rectum. The act of defecation is facilitated by the gastrocolic reflex and by a sitting position. It is consciously controlled and learned by about the age of 2 years. Effective bowel training involves a significant person to please and offer praise, sufficient time, and a consistent pattern.

Normal defecation has two aspects, the pattern or frequency of defecation and normal color, odor, and consistency of the stool. Important measures that influence defecation include a balanced diet, adequate fluid intake, regularity of meals, regular exercise, privacy, and a regular time for defecation. Individual practices that stimulate the gastrocolic reflex such as a hot drink in the morning are also helpful, particularly for the aged.

Common problems of fecal elimination include constipation, fecal impaction, diarrhea, anal incontinence, and flatulence leading to intestinal distention. The causes for each of these and the specific nursing intervention required are outlined. Some of the interventions include the administration of cathartics, antidiarrhetics and suppositories, digital removal of impactions, bowel retraining programs, insertion of rectal tubes, and enemas.

Enemas are given for a variety of reasons and are classified according to their action: cleansing, oil, and carminative. Soapsuds and normal saline are commonly used solutions for cleansing enemas in amounts that distend the bowel (500 to 1000 ml) and stimulate peristalsis. Oil enemas of 100 to 200 ml serve to lubricate the rectum and to soften feces and thus need to be retained for a few hours. Carminative enemas are used primarily to expel flatus. Commonly used types are the 1–2–3, the milk and molasses, and the Mayo enema. Guidelines for the nurse when administering an enema and the technique involved are outlined in point form. Siphoning an enema is occasionally necessary for those who are unable to expel the solution.

SUGGESTED ACTIVITIES

1. Interview a young mother and a grandmother about bowel training methods used for their children. Compare the methods.

2. In a clinical setting note the methods used to maintain regular bowel function for elderly patients. Discuss and compare your findings with a group of classmates.

3. For a patient who has a specific elimination problem, outline a nursing care plan that reflects the health instruction required.

SUGGESTED READINGS

Corman, Marvin L., et al. February, 1975. Cathartics. *American Journal of Nursing* 75:273–279.

The authors discuss the use of different cathartics and recommendations as to improving bowel function. Over-the-counter laxatives are listed together with sites of action.

Habeeb, Marjorie C., et al. April, 1976. Bowel program for institutionalized adults. *American Journal of Nursing* 76:606–608.

This article describes a program for retaining stool for patients who have fecal incontinence. The care includes low residue diet, medications, rectal examinations, and enemas when needed.

Stahlgren, Leroy H., et al. June, 1977. Intestinal obstruction. *American Journal of Nursing* 77:999–1002.

An overview of the reasons for obstruction and the clinical assessment are included as well as the treatment. There are two photographs of abdominal and intestinal radiographs.

SELECTED REFERENCES

Keusch, Gerald. June, 1973. Bacterial diarrheas. *American Journal of Nursing* 73:1028–1032.

Lewin, D. March 25, 1976. Care of the constipated patient. *Nursing Times* 72:444–446.

Nordmark, Madelyn T., and Rohweder, Anne W. 1975. *Scientific foundations of nursing.* 3rd ed. Philadelphia: J. B. Lippincott Co.

Sheridan, J. L. March, 1975. Nursing care of the stroke patient. *Nursing Clinics of North America* 10:147–155.

CHAPTER 27

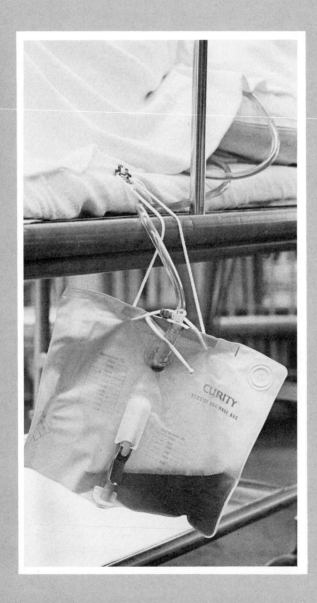

URINARY ELIMINATION

OBJECTIVES

- Discuss the physiology of urination.
- Describe normal patterns of voiding.
- Explain the physiology of micturition.
- Explain the factors influencing urinary elimination.
- Explain the importance of adequate urinary elimination in health.
- Assess the urine elimination of individual patients.
- Identify common urinary problems.
- List the common causes of urinary problems.
- Apply the guidelines of urinary care in planning and implementing nursing.
- Plan nursing care to patients with common urinary problems.
- Demonstrate beginning skill in various nursing techniques related to the urinary system.

In North American society, elimination, both bladder and bowel, is generally considered to be inappropriate as a social topic. Although bowel habits are discussed in various advertising media in relation to the sale of laxatives, urinary elimination is seldom discussed.

Elimination from the urinary tract is generally taken for granted by most people. It is only when there is a problem that one usually becomes aware of one's urinary habits and any adjunctive symptoms.

The urinary habits of a person are dependent upon both social culture and personal habit. In North America most people are accustomed to privacy while they urinate as well as clean surroundings, which may also be even decorative. The lack of privacy that is normal in many European and Far Eastern countries is surprising and frequently disturbing to North Americans traveling there.

Personal habits regarding urination are affected by the social propriety of leaving to urinate, the availability of a private clean facility, and initial bladder training. Urinary elimination is essential to health, and voiding can only be postponed for just so long before the urge normally becomes too great to control.

THE PHYSIOLOGY OF THE URINARY TRACT

For an adult the desire to void is normally experienced when the bladder contains between 250 and 450 ml of urine. Normal output of urine for an adult is about 1500 ml per day. The age of a person, however, also affects urinary output (see Table 27-1).

Urinary Tract

The urinary tract is only one route whereby body wastes are eliminated from the body. Urination permits the elimination of the following products:

1. Nitrogenous wastes—urea, uric acid, ammonia, and creatinine, for example.
2. Electrolytes—sodium, potassium, ammonium chloride, bicarbonate, phosphate, sulphate, and some minerals.

3. Pigments.
4. Hormones.
5. Toxins—produced by bacteria within the body.
6. Abnormal products—glucose, blood, and albumin, for example.
7. Water (96%).

The learner is referred to the constituents of feces, Table 26-1, and Chapter 29, "Normal Fluid Output."

The urine is formed in the kidneys, which are situated in the retroperitoneal space within the body. The kidneys filter out those products from the blood for which the body has no use. It is estimated that in the average adult 1200 ml of blood passes through the kidneys every minute. This figure represents about 21% of the cardiac output (5600 ml per minute). From this blood the functional unit of the kidney, the nephron (Figure 27-1), forms glomerular filtrate (about 180 liters per day). About 99% of this filtrate is reabsorbed into the blood stream. The remainder forms the urine to be excreted from the body (Guyton 1976:440–443).

Once the urine is formed in the kidneys it enters the ureters and then passes on to the bladder (Figure 27-2). The ureters are from 25 to 30 cm (10 to 12 inches) long in the adult and about 1.25 cm (½ inch) in diameter. The upper end of each ureter is funnel shaped as it enters the kidney, forming what is referred to as the *renal pelvis*. The lower ends of the ureters enter the bladder at the posterior corners of the floor of the bladder. At this junction between the ureter and the bladder there is a fold of mucous membrane,

Table 27-1.   Average Daily Excretion of Urine

Age	Amount
First and second day of life	15 to 60 ml
Third to tenth day	100 to 300 ml
Tenth day to 2 months	250 to 450 ml
2 months to 1 year	400 to 500 ml
1 to 3 years	500 to 600 ml
3 to 5 years	600 to 700 ml
5 to 8 years	700 to 1000 ml
8 to 14 years	800 to 1400 ml
Adult	1500 ml

which acts as a valve to prevent the back flow of urine up the ureters to the kidneys.

The bladder serves as a reservoir for urine and as the organ of excretion. It is made up of three layers of muscle, which collectively are called the *detrusor muscle.* From the bladder there is a third opening in the anterior inferior corner, the urethra. The amount of urine that is normally stored in the bladder is to some degree an individual matter and one that varies with age.

The urethra has two sphincter muscles, which control the retention and excretion of the urine. The internal sphincter is located at the base of the bladder and is under involuntary control. The urinary bladder and the internal sphincter are innervated by the autonomic nervous system. The sympathetic branch carries nervous impulses, which basically have two functions: (a) constriction of the internal sphincter muscle and (b) relaxation of the detrusor muscle. Thus the urine is held within the bladder as a result of this innervation.

The parasympathetic nervous system also inner-ⁿates the internal sphincter muscle and the detrusor

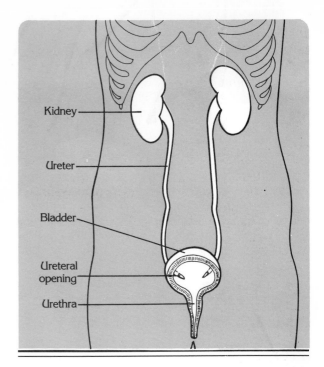

Figure 27-2.   A diagram of the anatomical struc-tures of the urinary tract.

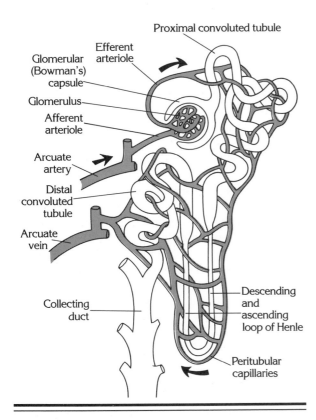

Figure 27-1.   A diagram of the nephron unit of the kidney.

muscle. In this case its actions are the opposite to those of the sympathetic branch. It has the following actions: (a) relaxation of the internal sphincter muscle and (b) contraction of the detrusor muscle. As a result, urine is released from the bladder.

There is also an external sphincter muscle. In the male this muscle is situated distal to the prostate por-tion of the urethra. In the female it is situated about midpoint in the urethra. This sphincter muscle is un-der voluntary control, thus enabling the person to consciously retain or eliminate urine.

The urethra extends from the bladder to the urin-ary meatus and is the passageway for the urine. In the adult male it is about 20 cm (8 inches) in length. It is divided into three parts: the prostatic urethra, which starts at the bladder and extends through the prostate gland; the membranous urethra, which extends from the prostatic section to the third section; and the cav-ernous urethra, which extends from the triangular ligament to the urethral orifice (Figure 27-3).

In the adult female the urethra is about 3.7 cm (1.5 inches) in length (Figure 27-4). Because of its shortness it is particularly prone to bacterial invasion. The urethras of both the male and female are lined with mucous membrane.

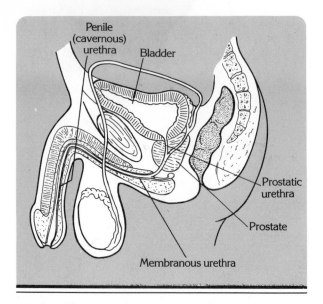

Figure 27-3.   The male urogenital system.

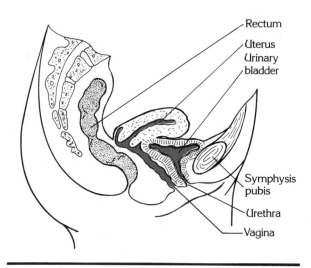

Figure 27-4.   The female urogenital system.

Urinary Control

Babies are born without urinary control; however, they soon learn during the second year that it is essential to gain bladder as well as bowel control to obtain parental approval.

Toddlers must be sufficiently mature physiologically before they can learn this control. Usually it is started when they are able to hold their urine for 2 hours and occurs generally after bowel control has begun. Usually children will communicate when they are ready to begin bladder training, perhaps by pointing or gesturing before urinating.

Most children are able to control their urination during the daytime by the time they are two years old. Nighttime control might not be learned until three or four years of age.

Urinary control in adults is sometimes lost because of disease processes. This usually is an embarrassment to the adult, and yet it is something about which little can be done. Tumors of the brain, strokes, and urinary infections are just a few of the reasons that can result in loss of urinary control.

Normal Patterns of Urination

The patterns of urination are highly individualistic, affected by some of the factors mentioned earlier.

Most people take for granted their normal pattern for urination, but they are quick to recognize any abnormalities; people who normally sleep through the night without the need to urinate are quickly aware when they must arise twice for that purpose. The pattern and frequency of micturition (voiding) is dependent upon many of the factors discussed later in this chapter.

Physiology of Urination

Micturition, voiding, and *urination* all mean the process of emptying the urinary bladder. Urine collects in the bladder until the pressure stimulates stretch sensory nerves within the bladder wall and the person becomes aware of the need to void. This occurs when the adult bladder contains between 250 and 450 ml of urine. For the child a considerably smaller volume, 50 to 200 ml, stimulates these nerves.

The impulse then travels from the stretch receptors to the spinal cord, specifically to the voiding reflex center located at the level of the second to fourth sacral vertebrae. Some impulses continue up the spinal cord to the voiding control center in the cerebral cortex. If the time is appropriate to void, the brain then sends impulses through the spinal cord to the motor neurons in the sacral area, causing stimulation of the parasympathetic nerves and subsequent relaxation of the internal sphincter muscle and contraction of the detrusor muscle. Conscious relaxation of the external sphincter muscle also takes place through the motor nerves, and thus voiding occurs. If voiding is not appropriate, the stimuli travel through the sympathetic branch, causing relaxation of the detrusor muscle and constriction of the internal sphincter muscle. In this case also the external sphincter is constricted voluntarily.

DEVELOPMENT OF BLADDER CONTROL (TOILET TRAINING)

Bladder control develops when children learn to use voluntary muscle groups that manipulate intra-abdominal pressure and when they learn to inhibit or enhance stimuli of the autonomic involuntary smooth muscles. The age at which control is achieved varies but usually occurs between the ages of 2 and 4½ years. Boys are slower than girls in gaining control.

The skill of bladder control can be considered to be learned in four steps:

1. Children first become aware that they have already urinated and will point to their diapers.

2. They then learn to hold their urine for a brief period beyond the urge to void and will warn their parents of the urge to void.

3. Children then acquire daytime control, which usually becomes well established by 2 years of age.

4. Children learn last to acquire nighttime control by 3 to 4 years of age. At this point all involved muscle groups are coordinated, and they can urinate at almost any degree of bladder filling.

Training for bladder control needs to be a gradual process, started when children are physically mature and have a desire to learn. Children are physiologically ready when they are able to retain their urine for a two-hour period. As with bowel training (see Chapter 26), toddlers learn to control their urination in response to their mother's approval. Trusting relationships developed between the child and the mother thus facilitate the motivation to succeed. Older siblings can also be an influencing factor. A young child may see older children using the toilet and want to mimic their behavior or may even be laughed at about puddles on the floor. As young children become more active they also find wet clothing increasingly uncomfortable.

Praise should be offered when the child first shows awareness of having urinated. However, a period of time must pass before the child will indicate the need to void prior to urinating. As with bowel training, specific words will be used to communicate what is expected, such as "pee" or "wee-wee." When the child has been dry for a few hours, he or she needs to be put on the toilet. This generally occurs at about 18 months of age. Those who say their children are trained before this age have probably trained themselves to catch the child's movements at regular times. The child can be assisted in keeping dry during the day by observing the usual times of urination and by taking the child to the toilet at these times. Such times might include before or after meals, before or after the nap, before or after going outside, and before bedtime. It is not necessary for the child to remain on the toilet for longer than a few minutes. The bladder will empty relatively quickly, since it is just starting to fill up to near capacity. Training pants during the day and suitable clothing also assist the child. Changing the pants even when they are slightly wet helps the child to become accustomed to being dry, and being out of diapers can make him or her feel more grown up. A sense of independence is achieved by the use of pull-down trousers that the child can manage alone. Steps for the child to reach the adult toilet and an attachable child's seat may be helpful. Little boys first learn to urinate sitting down and learn to stand up to urinate by watching other males urinate. Thus the age at which boys stand to urinate varies with their contact with males. Little girls may also want to urinate in the standing position but soon realize the problems this creates.

A casual, patient, matter-of-fact attitude is required on the part of parents for bladder training. It is learned more slowly than bowel training, and it has periods of success alternating with periods of failure or accidents. Growing children are active and busy, and although they may have learned the signals of a full bladder, these signs may go unnoticed during play until an accident occurs. They will inevitably run to their mother and tell her about it, an indication of learning some responsibility about urinating. Wetting may occur also when children are excited.

Each time children urinate in the training chair, praise and cuddling should be given. When the child fails to do so, it is best to withhold disapproval or disappointment, or the child may develop feelings of fear or inferiority.

Nighttime bladder control takes even more time than daytime control. It is recommended that it not be hurried. Some advise that fluids be restricted in the late afternoon and evening; however, the child may then cry of thirst during the night. Getting the child up during the night is not advised unless the child wakens on his or her own. The child who is wakened may be unable to sleep for a long period after being awakened and may become antagonized. Increasing maturity generally takes care of nighttime control. Even when the child has acquired good control, there normally may be continual lapses in control when the child is overly fatigued or is suffering emotionally.

FACTORS INFLUENCING URINARY ELIMINATION

The following factors affect a person's urinary elimination:

1. Amount of *fluid intake.*

2. *Diet.* Coffee, for example, increases the amount of urine formed.

3. *Response to the initial urge to void.* Some people ignore the initial urge and void only later when the urge is stronger.

4. *Stress.* During times of stress the person may perceive the need for increased frequency of urination due to the feeling that the bladder is full or to the increase in the amount of urine produced.

5. *Activity.* Increased activity generally results in increased frequency of voiding. The activity increases the person's metabolism, thus resulting in increased urine production.

6. *Pathologic conditions.* A wide variety of conditions can increase or decrease urination. A fever and excessive perspiration may decrease urine production because of the excessive loss of fluid by the skin. Inflammatory conditions and irritation of the urinary organs can promote retention of urine in the bladder.

7. *Medications.* Certain medications can cause a change in urine production, both in amount and character. Some medications such as diuretics increase urine output, whereas others such as some analgesics can cause urinary retention. Other medications cause urine to change in color.

ASSESSMENT OF URINARY ELIMINATION

To make an assessment of a patient's urinary functions it is necessary to collect data in regard to urinary habits, urine, and any particular problems. The following data are collected:

A. Urinary habits
1. Frequency
2. Volume
B. Urine
1. Color
2. Odor
3. Specific gravity
4. pH
5. Protein
6. Abnormal constituents
C. Particular problems

Urinary Habits

Frequency

It is not unusual for a person to void five or more times a day depending upon individual habits and the opportunity. Most people void about 70% of their daily urine during the waking hours and do not need to void during the night. People usually void when they first awake in the morning, before they go to bed, and around meal times. The urine voided upon wakening is the most concentrated urine excreted during the 24 hours.

Volume

The volume of urine excreted varies because of a number of factors, which have already been discussed. The student is also referred to Table 27-1. For an adult a volume of under 500 ml or over 3000 ml in a 24-hour period is unusual and needs to be reported.

Urine

Color

Normal urine is straw colored or amber colored. The latter is most likely early in the morning when it is most concentrated. The color of urine can be altered by certain drugs such as phenazopyridine (Pyridium), which turns urine a dark orange color. Any abnormal color needs to be reported. Red, brown, or orange urine may be indicative of disease processes; red or brown may indicate the presence of blood in the urine.

Odor

Normal urine has a characteristic faint aromatic odor. A strong odor may be indicative of some problem such as an infection or in some cases the ingestion of certain medications.

Specific Gravity

The specific gravity is a particularly important characteristic, since it can indicate kidney dysfunction when it is abnormal. The normal range for specific gravity is 1.010 to 1.025 (French 1975:26).

To measure specific gravity, a hydrometer is placed in a tube of urine. The instrument is made of glass and has in it a mercury bulb and a specific-gravity scale at the top. By displacing the amount of urine, the concentration as related to water can be measured. The more concentrated the urine the more of the instrument is displaced upward. The nurse then reads the scale at the level of the urine.

Table 27-2.   Characteristics of Normal Urine

Color	Straw, amber, or transparent
Odor	Faint aromatic
pH	4.5 to 7.5
Specific gravity	1.010 to 1.025
Amount (adult)	1200 to 1500 ml per day

pH

Normal urine is slightly acid with a pH of 4.5 (greater acidity) to 7.5 (lesser acidity). This can be tested by dipping in the urine a reagent paper such as a Nitrazine stick. The paper stick will change color reflecting the pH. See Table 27-2 for normal values.

Urine that is left at room temperature for several hours will gradually become alkaline because of bacterial action. Vegetarians normally excrete a slightly alkaline urine.

Protein

The presence of protein in the urine can also be tested with a reagent strip. Normally large protein molecules such as albumin are not filtered through into the urine; however, a small amount of smaller protein molecules normally does filter through. Large amounts of protein can indicate bleeding or an inflammatory process.

Normal and Abnormal Constituents

For normal constituents of urine see Table 27-3. Abnormal constituents are also tested for if it is

Table 27-3.   Normal Constituents of Urine

Constituent	Percentage
Water	90% to 95%
Nitrogenous wastes	3.7%
Inorganic wastes	
Electrolytes (sodium, potassium, ammonium, etc.)	1.3%
Toxins	
Pigments	
Hormones	

indicated. Some of these, glucose and acetone, are frequently tested for by the nurse. Again, reagent sticks are frequently used indicating by color the presence of the glucose or acetone. These tests are frequently done for patients who have diabetes mellitus.

The presence of other abnormal constituents of urine is tested by the use of a microscope. Some of these are white blood cells, red blood cells, casts, and fat bodies.

A number of words are used to describe the presence of abnormal constituents in the urine. Some of these are as follows:

1. *hematuria:* blood in the urine
2. *pyuria:* pus in the urine
3. *albuminuria:* albumin in the urine
4. *proteinuria:* protein in the urine
5. *glycosuria* (glucosuria): glucose in the urine

Common Urinary Problems

The nurse is likely to encounter some of the following common problems of the urinary tract.

Urinary Retention

Retention is the holding of urine in the bladder because of the inability to excrete it. This can occur postoperatively and in situations in which the urethra is occluded such as by an enlarged prostate gland. The patient will normally tell the nurse he or she has not voided and measured output will also indicate this. The retention can be further affirmed by the appearance of a distended bladder just above the symphysis pubis and by percussion. By percussing the area of the bladder region the presence of fluid in the bladder will be indicated by a duller sound than normal. See "Percussion Technique" in Chapter 12.

Occasionally a patient will have urinary retention with overflow. In this situation the bladder is holding urine, and only overflow urine is excreted. The pressure of the urine becomes too great for sphincter control. The patient then voids small amounts of urine frequently or dribbles urine; however, the bladder remains distended.

Urinary Incontinence

Urinary incontinence is the inability of the sphincter muscles to control the flow of urine from the bladder. It is the opposite of retention. This condition is seen in elderly patients for whom this is part of the aging process. It is also seen in patients who have enlarged prostate glands, spinal cord injuries, or bladder infections, for example.

Stress incontinence is the inability to control urine flow at a time when the intraabdominal pressure increases, for example, when coughing, sneezing, or even laughing. It is generally caused by the inability of the external sphincter muscle to close, and it is seen in children who have not learned to control the external sphincter and in adults who have a disease process interfering with the sphincter action.

Frequency

This is generally considered to be voiding at frequent intervals, that is, more often than usual. Normally there is some increase in the frequency with which a person voids with an increase in fluids. Frequency, however, without an increase in fluid intake may be the result of a urinary infection, stress, or pressure upon the bladder, for example, because of pregnancy.

With frequency the amount of urine voided may not be above that normally voided. The amounts voided each time are small, such as 50 to 100 ml.

Nocturia (nycturia) refers to increased frequency at night that is not a result of an increased fluid intake. Like frequency, it is usually expressed in terms of the number of times the person gets out of bed to void, for example, "nocturia × 4."

Urgency

This is the feeling that the person *must* void. There may or may not be a great deal of urine in the bladder, but the person feels a need to void immediately. Often the person hurries to the toilet with the fear of being incontinent if he or she does not urinate. Urgency accompanies psychologic stress and urinary tract infections. It is also not uncommon in young children who have poor external sphincter control.

Dysuria

This refers to either painful or difficult voiding. It can accompany a stricture of the urethra, urinary infections, and injury to the bladder and/or urethra. Often patients will say that they have to push to void or that the process of voiding is painful.

Burning

Burning is not an uncommon complaint of patients with urinary tract infections. The patient may state that the burning accompanies voiding or that it follows voiding. In the former instance it is often due to an irritated urethra; in the latter it may be the result of a bladder infection when the irritated rugae of the bladder rub together. The burning may be described as severe like a hot poker or more subdued like a sunburn.

Anuria and Oliguria

The situation in which the kidneys are producing no urine is *anuria. Complete kidney shutdown* is a phrase with the same meaning. *Oliguria* is the production of abnormally small amounts of urine by the kidneys, for example, 30 ml per 8 hours.

Both anuria and oliguria can occur as a result of kidney disease, burns, and shock. These symptoms can be fatal if some other means, for example, an artificial kidney, is not used to remove the body wastes.

Polyuria

Polyuria refers to the production of abnormally large amounts of urine by the kidneys such as 2500 ml per day without an increased fluid intake. This can happen as a result of hormone imbalances. Another word, *diuresis*, also refers to the excessive production of urine.

Common Causes of Urinary Problems

There are a number of situations that can cause urinary problems. These can be grouped as (a) ob-struction, (b) abnormal tissue growth, (c) calculi, (d) infection, and (e) systemic problems.

An *obstruction* can occur almost anywhere in the urinary tract, the kidneys, ureters, bladder, or urethra. The cause of the obstruction can be abnormal cell growth (tumor), swelling as a result of an inflammatory process or local trauma, and calculi (stones), which are discussed later.

Abnormal tissue growth can occur without producing an obstruction. A tumor of the bladder may, for example, occupy part of the bladder space and yet not impede the flow of urine.

Calculi are stones that form in the urine and may be passed when voiding or lie in a space in the urinary system such as the kidney, pelvis, or bladder. Occasionally a calculus may be lodged in a ureter, for example, causing an obstruction.

An *infection* of the urinary tract may be secondary to one of the other common problems or singular in its occurrence. The urinary tract is lined with mucous membrane, which extends from the meatus of the urethra to the kidneys. This membrane provides an excellent medium for the growth of some pathogens and for the spreading of infection. Women are particularly prone to urinary infections because of their short urethras.

Systemic problems of the body such as heart disease and central nervous system problems can also present urinary problems. In particular, they can interfere with the formation of urine and/or the excretion of urine.

GUIDELINES FOR URINARY CARE

The kidneys eliminate most of the waste products of protein metabolism. These include urea, uric acid, and creatinine, which are organic compounds, and ammonium salts, which are inorganic compounds. They also eliminate excessive amounts of ketone bodies and electrolytes. The former are the result of the oxidation of fatty acids.

Normally the blood urea nitrogen (BUN) level is below 20 mg per 100 ml., and this is regulated by the kidneys. The BUN is one means of assessing kidney function.

The kidneys produce urine continuously, usually at the rate of from 60 to 120 ml per hour in the adult. Newborn babies need to start micturition from 24 to 36 hours after birth.

Critical signs of renal failure in the adult are a urine output of 300 ml or less in 24 hours, the pres-ence of uremic frost (urea crystals) on the skin, elevated BUN, aromatic odor to the skin, and symptoms of fluid and electrolyte imbalances (see Chapter 30).

An adult urinary bladder normally holds about 250 to 450 ml of urine when the micturition reflex is stimulated. However, some adult bladders can distend to hold 3000 to 4000 ml of urine.

Mucous membrane lines the urinary tract, thus facilitating the spread of an infection. Microorganisms are normally not present in the urinary tract beyond the lower urethra. Thus any procedures administered to the urinary tract are conducted with sterile or surgical asepsis.

After the age of 2 or 3 years the neuromuscular systems are usually sufficiently well developed that urinary control can be maintained.

NURSING INTERVENTION RELATED TO URINATION

In some instances nursing measures are required to facilitate the normal functioning of the urinary system and in some cases to also deal with a particular problem such as cystitis (inflammation of the urinary bladder).

General Measures

Appropriate Fluid Intake

Patients who have urinary problems often have their amount of daily fluid intake prescribed by the physician. The fluid may be provided for oral intake and/or it may include intravenous fluids.

For patients who have urinary infections, fluids are often forced. The adult patient usually needs to have an intake of between 3000 and 4000 ml over a 24-hour period. The exact amount is frequently ordered by the physician, or there is a related agency policy. Occasionally fluids may be restricted, for example, when the kidneys are being rested or when a patient has a large amount of edema.

Measurement of Fluid Intake and Output

If the male patient is able to go to the bathroom, he will need to understand to void into a urinal rather than the toilet and then to save the urine in order that it can be measured. For the female patient a bedpan is used instead of the toilet to collect the urine.

Many patients can also measure and record their own fluid intakes. For those who are unable to do so, it is important that the nurse record the intake volume in milliliters accurately. See Chapter 29, "Measuring Fluid Intake and Output."

Assistance to Maintain Normal Voiding Patterns

Some patients will need assistance in order to maintain their usual voiding habits. They can be assisted in a number of ways:

1. Assist the patient to his or her normal position for voiding. Male patients may find it easier to void when standing rather than when sitting or lying down; standing at the side of the bed with a urinal may be helpful. A female patient may find it easier to void using a commode at the side of the bed, providing this is feasible, rather than a bedpan in bed.

2. Provide privacy for the patient. Even children may be accustomed to privacy and may be unable to void in the presence of another person.

3. If a bedpan or urinal is used, make sure that it is warm. A cold bedpan may prompt contraction of the perineal muscles of the female patient.

4. Foster muscle relaxation by providing necessary physical support for the patient and freedom from pain.

5. Local application of heat to the perineum of the female or with a hot-water bottle to the lower abdomen of both men and women can foster muscular relaxation.

6. Pouring warm water over the genitals can also encourage voiding. If the urine volume is to be measured, the amount of water to be poured must first be measured.

7. Provide any assistance required when the patient first feels the need to void. By waiting, the desire to void may pass, and difficulty starting to void may result.

8. Turn on running water within hearing distance of the patient or provide water in which the patient's fingers can be dangled.

9. Set aside sufficient time.

10. Be reassuring to the patient and avoid producing anxiety. With emotional support the patient is more likely to be relaxed and able to void.

Hygienic Measures

Ensure that hygienic measures are taken to maintain the cleanliness of the genital area. Good hygiene is essential for two main reasons: to promote the patient's comfort and to prevent infection. A patient with a urinary tract problem may have a discharge or urine that has an unpleasant odor and that may be irritating to surrounding mucous membranes and skin. Normally the genital area is cleansed several times a day or more often if it is indicated. (See "Perineal and Genital Care" in Chapter 20.)

Cleanliness of the genital area can also help to prevent microorganisms from entering the urinary meatus, which subsequently can cause a urinary infection. Because of the continuous mucous membrane lining an infection of the urethra can extend into the kidney pelvis.

Bedpans and Urinals

Bedpans and urinals are receptacles used for urine and feces from patients who cannot go to the bathroom or for whom the urine volume needs to be measured. Bedpans are used for both urine and feces from female patients and feces from male patients. Urinals are used for urine from male patients.

Bedpans are made of metal and of nylon resins. Frequently stainless steel bedpans are used today. Metal bedpans have the problem of feeling cold and therefore should be warmed under running warm water before being given to a patient. There are two basic types of bedpans, one that is about 2 inches deep all around and a second type called a *slipper pan.* The latter slips more easily under a patient because it is no deeper than ½ inch at the upper end (the end that fits under the patient's sacrum).

If a patient is to use a bedpan in bed, it is easiest if the head of the bed is slightly elevated, thus providing a more normal position in which to urinate. From this position it is also easier for the patient to lift him or herself on the pan. If for any reason this exertion is contraindicated, then the nurse can assist by placing the patient's hand under the patient's sacrum and using that arm as a lever (see Procedure 22-5 in Chapter 22). Some patients can help to lift themselves up by the use of a trapeze attached to a bar above the bed.

When providing a patient with a bedpan, it is not necessary to expose the patient. Usually it is perfectly satisfactory just to turn back a corner of the top bedclothes and then slip the bedpan under the bedclothes and the patient. The bedpan is placed in such a manner that the curved smooth edge fits under the patient and the sharper edge is toward the foot of the bed.

After the bedpan is in place, the toilet paper is left near the patient and the signal cord is placed in reach. The patient is then left in privacy. When the patient signals that he or she is through with the bedpan, the nurse then removes it. For patients who cannot wipe themselves, the nurse will need to do this. Usually in removing the bedpan the patient raises and the nurse slips it out. If the patient is unable to move, it is often easiest if the patient rolls to a lateral position away from the nurse while the nurse holds the bedpan. The patient is then in a suitable position

for wiping and cleansing if this is required. The toilet paper roll is then put away, and the patient is provided with a moistened cloth to wipe the hands.

For the male patient the urinal is more easily used than a bedpan. Often a sitting position facilitates its use, or the patient may sit or stand at the side of the bed if this is possible.

For female patients who are in body casts and completely unable to move, some agencies have female urinals. These fit against the female perineum, permitting the patient to urinate without moving.

If a patient is able to use a bathroom, the nurse must make sure that the patient is safe. Often patients feel well enough while in bed to walk to the bathroom, but after getting up they do not feel as strong as they believed they were. If the patient is weak or at all unsteady, the patient should be walked by the nurse to the bathroom and assisted to the toilet. Often the nurse will remain just outside the bathroom and reenter when the patient indicates readiness to return to bed.

The frequency with which a bedpan or urinal needs to be offered depends upon the individual patient and the situation. Nurses cannot offer a bedpan too often, but not offering one often enough can result in problems for the patient such as discomfort or bedwetting. These are uncomfortable and embarrassing to patients so that extraordinary efforts to get to the bathroom may be taken, which may be contraindicated because of the patient's condition. Most nurses can recall at least one incident of the weak little old lady "who climbed over the bedside rails to go to the bathroom and then climbed back"!

Assisting the Hospitalized Child to Urinate

Children who are hospitalized and separated from their mother may regress in their ability to control their bladder and may wet occasionally. On admission to the hospital the nurse needs to record the child's stage of development and determine the methods of training that were or are being used. For example, the nurse needs to find out what equipment is being used, what words the child uses in relation to urinating, and the times the child habitually urinates sitting on the toilet seat each day. As much as possible the methods of urinating that the child is accustomed to should be continued in the hospital. It will be necessary for some children to use the bedpan or urinal

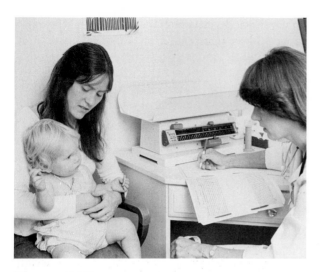

Figure 27-5. The nurse obtains pertinent information from a mother upon admission of her infant to the hospital.

for a period of time. This equipment is best shown to the child in the mother's presence, and hopefully with her approval the child will cooperate in their use (see Figure 27-5).

For children who are toilet trained the nurse should be prepared for accidents. Children who do wet accidentally in the hospital will generally be upset and will need understanding help and acceptance from the nurse. It is important that nurses examine their own feelings about children who wet or soil their bed or clothing. Feelings of repugnancy need to be controlled.

For children who are not toilet trained it is advised that toilet training not be started while in the hospital unless they are to have an extended or prolonged stay. Young children when hospitalized feel abandoned by their mothers and feel enough emotional strain without adding the stress of toilet training. In situations of prolonged hospitalization, toilet training is planned and carried out by the mother and preferably by a nurse who is liked by the child.

A few children in the hospital will use soiling as a means of gaining attention or as a means to get even with the parents for abandoning them. In these instances the nurse needs to avoid censure, accept this behavior matter of factly, and determine the reason for this behavior. Together the nurse and child need to work out a way in which the child's love and attention needs are more appropriately met.

Urinary Incontinence

Urinary incontinence is one of the more common problems encountered by patients who are in hospital. Disease processes such as strokes, enlarged prostates, and even just old age can help produce this problem. Often the patient is embarrassed about dribbling or about having an accident, and many normal activities are restricted for this reason even at home.

A number of measures can be employed to help reduce the problem of incontinence:

1. Regular voiding schedule. The patient is helped to maintain a regular voiding schedule, for example, every 2 hours, whether feeling the urge or not. Often when it is found that voiding can be controlled this way, the patient may be able to slightly lengthen the intervals between voiding and at the same time remain continent.

2. Regulation of fluid intake. This is often of particular importance before retiring so that the patient does not need to void as often during the night. Fluids may also be encouraged about half an hour before the voiding time, and at other times they are carefully regulated.

3. Increasing physical activity. This will improve muscle tone and blood circulation, thus helping the patient to control voiding.

4. Toilets and bedpans within reach. If the incontinent patient can get to a bedpan or toilet quickly, this will gradually help the patient gain control and at the same time develop confidence in the ability to control voiding.

5. Perineal exercises. These increase the tone of muscles concerned with micturition, in particular, the perineal and abdominal muscles. Periodic tightening of the perineal muscles and intentionally stopping and then starting the urine stream can also assist in gaining voiding control.

Urinary Retention

Just the opposite of urinary incontinence is urinary retention. Measures that assist the patient to maintain a normal voiding pattern have already been discussed in the section "Assistance to Maintain Normal Voiding Patterns" and are equally applicable when dealing with urinary retention.

Retention can be identified by several signs. With a distended abdomen, particularly in the lower aspect, percussion of the area will reveal kettle-drum-like sounds. Another sign is the disproportionately small amount of output in proportion to intake and, in some patients, frequent voiding of small volumes of urine.

Bedwetting

When wetting occurs in a child over the age of 4, it generally occurs at night and is referred to as *nocturnal enuresis*. It may happen once or several times during the night. Some children may wet in the daytime during periods of excitement or when absorbed with play, particularly on a cold, damp day. Still others may have not yet learned to be dry. In school-age children, wetting rarely occurs during the school hours but sometimes does occur during play hours at recess, during the lunch hour, or after school. Because of absorption in play the need to urinate is not realized until it is too late to reach a toilet. It is estimated that 15% to 20% of school-age children are bedwetters, with a definite male predominance (de Castro et al. 1972:91).

Children who are bedwetters need understanding help. Generally, it is corrected relatively easily with the appropriate steps.

The most common cause of persistent bedwetting is too early and too vigorous training before the child was physiologically ready. As a result, enuresis in the child may express an unconscious desire to regress and to receive the attention and care he or she had as a young child. It may also be an expression of a feeling of resentment toward the parent.

Many other explanations for nocturnal enuresis have been proposed, and no doubt there are several causes or contributing factors in each individual situation. Some of these are as follows:

1. The bladder capacity is smaller than normal.

2. The child is a sound sleeper, and signals from the bladder indicating the need to urinate go unnoticed until it is too late for the child to get out of bed and to the bathroom.

3. The bladder may be irritable and thus unable to hold large quantities of urine.

4. An unpleasant emotional climate in the home can result in a revenge type of enuresis for lack of love. Examples are sibling rivalry and quarrelsome parents.

5. Parents who have the idea that the child will outgrow the habit without help may not train the child.

6. There may be infections of the urinary tract or physical or neurologic defects of the urinary system.

7. Foods that are too rich in salts and minerals or spicy foods such as pickles or relishes are irritating to the urinary system.

8. The child may fear walking down a dark corridor to the bathroom at night.

The complexity of enuresis is obvious; therefore a comprehensive history with physical and psychologic assessment is warranted in determining the cause. The child's feelings about bedwetting need to be explored carefully. Some may think they have a weak bladder and feel totally disinterested. Others may be interested in their problem but feel utterly hopeless about it and react by fearing to go to sleep. Professional counseling may be necessary, and a referral by the physician is indicated.

A urinalysis is usually performed initially, and subsequent tests such as a culture and sensitivity are often carried out. Other urologic examinations are done when abnormalities are found to rule out infection or structural problems. In the majority of situations the cause is psychologic; thus the goal of therapy is to help the child and family find a comfortable way to cope with the situation.

Some practical methods include providing a waterproof pad on the bed to prevent soiling of the mattress and prevent worry and conflict for both parents and child. Restrict fluids at bedtime and arrange a time for the child to be awakened to get up to urinate. These methods frequently achieve the best results when the child is involved in the plans and encouraged to assume some responsibility for them. It is recommended that no punishment be imposed. Praise for success is the most effective reward. If something is upsetting the child emotionally, this needs to be considered, such as a change to a new neighborhood or too great expectations from the parents about manners or neatness. It is important to convey to the child the idea that the child can be helped.

Other therapies include a conditioning program to increase the child's bladder capacity. This is accomplished by increasing the child's fluid intake during the daytime and then encouraging the child to suppress the desire to void as long as possible. Sometimes medications such as tranquilizers or belladonna derivatives are prescribed, although their effectiveness is questionable. In many situations, continued family counseling is warranted.

URINARY CATHETERIZATION

Urinary catheterization is the introduction of a tube (a catheter) through the urethra into the urinary bladder. This is usually performed only when absolutely necessary, since certain hazards are involved. Because the urinary structures are normally sterile except at the end of the urethra, the danger of introducing microorganisms into the bladder exists. For those patients who have lowered resistance due to certain disease processes, this potential hazard is greatest. Once an infection is introduced into the bladder it can ascend up the ureters and eventually involve the kidneys. Even after the catheter is inserted and left in place for a time, the potential hazard of infection remains, since pathogens can be introduced through the catheter lumen. Thus strict sterile technique is used for catheterizations.

Another possible hazard is that of trauma, particularly in the male patient, whose urethra is long with a more tortuous path. Damage to the urethra can occur if a catheter is forced during insertion through strictures or at the incorrect angle. It is important therefore to insert catheters along the normal contour of the urethra. For females, the urethra lies posteriorly, then has a slightly anterior direction toward the bladder (Figure 27-6); for males the urethra is straightened by elevating the penis perpendicular to the body.

Types of Catheters

Catheters are commonly made of rubber or plastic. Some agencies provide other types of catheters made of woven silk or metal. Catheters are often referred to as straight catheters or retention (Foley) catheters. The *straight catheter* is a single lumen tube with a small eye or opening about ½ inch from the insertion tip. The *retention catheter* contains a second smaller tube throughout its length on the inside. This second inner tube connects to an inflatable balloon near the insertion tip, which, when expanded after insertion, holds the tube in place within the bladder. The opposite end of the retention catheter is bifurcated, that is, it has two openings, one to drain the urine, the other to inflate the balloon.

The size of catheters is the diameter of the lumen, which is graded according to a French scale of numbers; the larger the number, the larger the lumen. For children small sizes are used such as no. 8 or 10. For adults sizes no. 14, 16, and 18 are commonly used. Only even numbers are available.

Purposes of Urinary Catheterization

1. To obtain a sterile urine specimen for diagnostic reasons.
2. To measure the amount of residual urine when the bladder is incompletely emptied. This is the amount of urine remaining in the bladder after voiding.
3. To empty the bladder prior to surgery involving adjacent organs such as the rectum or vagina, thereby preventing inadvertent injury to the bladder.
4. To prevent bladder distention postoperatively or provide gradual decompression of an overdistended bladder when all other measures to facilitate voiding have failed.

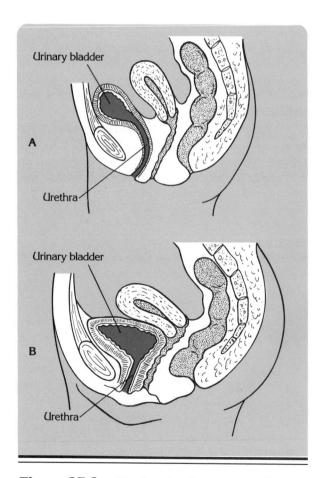

Figure 27-6. The female urinary system. Note the angle of the urethra in a child, **A**, and an adult, **B**.

5. To manage incontinency when all other measures to prevent skin breakdown have failed for a particular patient.

6. To provide for intermittent or continuous bladder drainage and irrigation.

7. To prevent urine from contacting an incision after perineal surgery.

A straight or single-lumen catheter is used for the first two purposes, whereas a retention catheter is usually used for the other purposes.

Procedure 27-1   Female Urinary Catheterization

Action	Explanation
Assemble Equipment	
All items must be sterile.	Equipment varies from agency to agency. Prepared trays may contain many or all of these items.
Wash hands before handling sterile equipment to maintain sterility.	
1. Pair of gloves.	
2. Towel drapes.	To place under the patient's buttocks and over her thighs.
3. Fenestrated drape (optional).	To place over the pubic area.
4. Antiseptic recommended by agency policy, for example, aqueous Zephiran 1:750.	To cleanse the labia and urinary meatus.
5. Cotton swabs in container.	To cleanse the labia.
6. Tissue or Kelly forceps.	To swab and cleanse.
7. Lubricant.	To lubricate the insertion tip of the catheter.
8. Catheter size 14 or 16 for an adult.	
9. Solution or K-basin.	To collect the urine.
10. Paper bag or other receptacle (not sterile).	To dispose of cotton balls used for cleansing.
11. Other items are required in accordance with the purpose, for example, a specimen container with label if a specimen is needed.	
To Catheterize the Female Urinary Bladder	
1. Explain to the patient the reason for the procedure and what it entails.	Some patients fear pain and may need to be told there should be no pain, only a slight sensation of pressure. To identify the patient.
2. Ensure privacy for the patient by screening the area well.	Exposure of the genitals is embarrassing and a culturally private matter. Relieving the patient's tension also facilitates easier insertion of the catheter, since the sphincters are more likely to be relaxed.
3. Assist the patient to a supine position with her knees flexed and her thighs separated. Pillows may be needed to support the knees and underneath the buttocks.	This elevates the pelvis and can make visualization of the urinary meatus easier.

Procedure 27-1. Cont'd.

4. Drape the patient by using a bath blanket to cover the chest and the abdomen. The patient's legs and feet can be covered by the bed sheet or by the use of another bath blanket.

The patient's gown needs to be pulled up over her hips.

This bath blanket can be placed diagonally on the patient with a corner around each foot.

5. Provide for adequate lighting.

An additional light such as a flashlight or gooseneck lamp may be necessary at the foot of the bed, focused on the genital area.

6. Wash the genital-perineal area well with soap and water, rinse, and dry well. Disposable gloves may be used.

Cleanliness reduces the possibility of introducing infection with the catheter. Appropriate rinsing prevents the possibility of the soap inhibiting the action of antiseptics used later.

7. Masks are put on in accordance with agency policy.

Some agencies also advocate the use of a clean gown and a surgical cap if the nurse's hair is long.

8. The hands are washed thoroughly using surgical aseptic technique.

This is done after the patient is draped if a sink is available in the patient's room and before sterile items are handled.

9. Open the sterile tray and put on the sterile gloves. The tray can be placed between the patient's thighs.

See "Donning Sterile Gloves" in Chapter 17.

10. Drape the patient with the sterile drapes, being careful to protect the sterility of the gloves.

The underpad is placed with the edges cuffed over the nurse's gloves. Thigh drapes are placed from the side farthest from the nurse to the side nearest. If an underpad is not available, the two thigh drapes can be placed so that they overlap between each thigh.

11. Pour the antiseptic solution over the cotton balls.

12. Open the lubricant and lubricate the insertion tip of the catheter liberally. Place it aside on the sterile tray ready for insertion.

Water-soluble lubricant facilitates the insertion of the catheter by reducing the friction. This step is important before cleansing is done, since the nurse will subsequently have only one sterile hand available.

13. Cleanse the labia minora on each side and finally the urinary meatus. Cleansing is done by separating the labia with two cotton balls under the thumb and forefinger of one hand while cleansing with the forceps held in the other hand. Use each swab only once, moving from the pubic area to the anus, and then discard it.

Note: It is important to expose the urinary meatus adequately. This is best done by retracting the tissue of the labia minora in an upward (anterior) direction toward the symphysis pubis (see Figure 27-7). Once the meatus is cleansed the labia must not be allowed to move over it.

Note that the hand that touches the patient is now contaminated, and it remains in position exposing the urinary meatus. Using forceps retains the sterility of the nurse's glove.

This cleanses from the area of least contamination to the area of greatest contamination.

This prevents the risk of added contamination.

14. Pick up the catheter with the sterile gloved hand, holding it approximately 2 to 3 inches from the insertion tip. The opposite end of the catheter is placed in the urine receptacle.

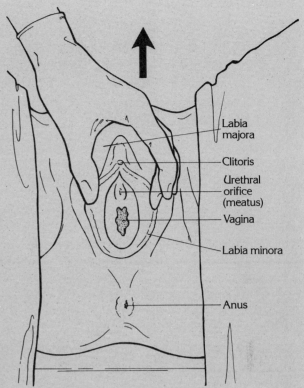

Figure 27-7. Exposing the urinary meatus of the female.

Labia majora

Clitoris

Urethral orifice (meatus)

Vagina

Labia minora

Anus

15. Gently insert the catheter into the urinary meatus about 2 inches or until urine flows. Direct the catheter in the direction of the urethra. If resistance is met during insertion, the catheter should not be forced. By asking the patient to take deep breaths, slight pressure may be relieved. If not, the procedure should be discontinued and reported.

Caution is needed to prevent the catheter tip from becoming contaminated. If it is contaminated, it needs to be discarded.

This may relax the external sphincter.

16. While the urine flows, the nurse's hand can be transferred from the labia to the catheter to hold it in place.

17. Collect a urine specimen if required after the urine has flowed for a few seconds. It is necessary to pinch the catheter before transferring the drainage end of the catheter into the sterile specimen bottle. Usually 30 ml of urine is sufficient for a specimen.

18. Empty the bladder and remove the catheter slowly.

For patients who have urinary retention it is recommended that no more than 750 ml be removed at one time. Removing larger amounts of urine too quickly can induce engorgement of the pelvic blood vessels and shock. Usually the physician will prescribe the amount and times at which urine is to be withdrawn.

19. Dry the patient's perineum with a towel or drape.

Procedure 27-1.   Cont'd.

20. Remove the equipment. Assist the patient to a comfortable position and leave the room in order.

21. Record the reason for catheterization and any other pertinent observations, such as the color and the amount of the urine.

Procedure 27-2.   Male Urinary Catheterization

The procedure for male urinary catheterization is similar to that for females with a few differences, which will be outlined. Usually a male catheterization is carried out by physicians, male nurses, or orderlies, but on occasion a female nurse may be required to do this. Competency, matter-of-factness, and understanding on the part of the nurse can help alleviate much of the patient's embarrassment.

Action	Explanation
Assemble Equipment	
Wash hands. Follow steps 1 to 11 as for female catheterization. A size 16 or 18 catheter usually is used.	
To Catheterize the Male Urinary Bladder	
1. Follow steps 1 and 2 for female catheterization.	
2. Assist the patient to a supine position. Flex the knees slightly and abduct legs. The patient may retain a pillow for his head.	
3. Follow steps 4 to 9 for female catheterization.	
4. Place a sterile water-resistant drape under the penis and a second drape above the penis.	To provide a sterile field.
5. To cleanse the meatus, the penis is grasped behind the glans and the urinary meatus spread between the thumb and forefinger. For uncircumcised males the foreskin is retracted. Cleanse the tissue surrounding the meatus in a circular fashion and then the meatus last. Discard each swab after only one wipe.	To avoid stimulating an erection, firm pressure rather than light pressure is used to grasp the penis.
6. Pick up the catheter (previously lubricated), holding it about 4 inches from the insertion tip.	
7. To insert the catheter, the penis is first lifted perpendicular to the body (90° angle), and slight traction is exerted (Figure 27-8). The catheter is then	This straightens the downward curvature of the prepubic (cavernous) urethra.

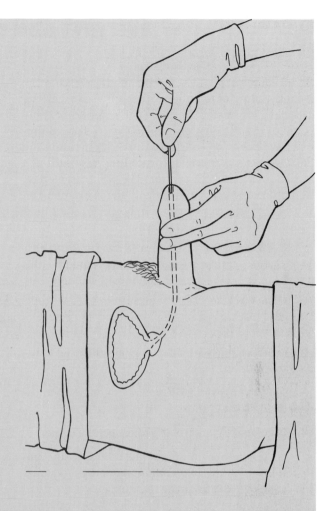

Figure 27-8. Elevation of the penis to a 90° angle for the insertion of a urinary catheter.

steadily inserted about 20 cm (8 inches) or until urine begins to flow. For a slight resistance at the sphincter, the catheter can be twisted to bypass it or held until a sphincter relaxes. The patient can also be asked to take deep breaths or to try to void. Discontinue the procedure and report it to physician if difficult resistances are met.

8. While the urine flows the penis can be lowered, and the nurse's hand is transferred to the catheter to hold it in place.

9. Follow steps 17 to 18 as for female catheterization.

10. Dry the patient's penis.

11. Follow steps 19 and 20 as for female catheterization.

Slight resistances are normally encountered at the external and internal urethral sphincters. Trauma can occur to the urethra if forceful pressure is exerted against major resistances.

RETENTION CATHETERS

Insertion

An indwelling or retention catheter is used when the catheter is to remain in place for a period of time. Some of the reasons for inserting indwelling catheters have been previously discussed. Commonly the Foley catheter is used. The procedure for inserting a retention catheter differs from the basic catheterization procedure only after the catheter is inserted.

Prior to the catheterization, however, additional equipment is needed as follows:

1. Retention catheter size 16 or 18 for an adult with a 5 ml balloon unless a larger size is ordered by the physician or has been used previously. Balloon sizes vary from 5 to 30 ml and are indicated in writing on each catheter along with the French size, for example, Foley no. 14, 5 ml.

2. 10 ml syringe with adapter or needle used to inflate the balloon.

3. Sterile water or sterile normal saline used to inflate the balloon.

4. Drainage bag and tubing to collect the urine.

5. Adhesive tape to attach the tubing to the patient's thigh and for open drainage setups to attach the catheter to the drainage set.

Some disposable retention catheter sets include all of the necessary equipment; others do not include the bag and tubing. Agency equipment thus needs to be checked when preparing for this procedure.

Testing the Balloon

It is important prior to the insertion of a retention catheter to test the balloon. This is done using sterile technique by prefilling the syringe with the prescribed amount of sterile water or normal saline, injecting it into the lumen of the catheter, which fills the balloon, and then leaving it in for a few seconds. If a leak is present, another catheter is selected, and it is tested also. When the nurse is assured that there is not a leak, the fluid is withdrawn, the catheter is detached from the syringe, and then the syringe is set aside on the sterile tray ready for use after the catheter is inserted. Whether an adapter or a needle is attached to the syringe to inflate the balloon depends upon the design of the catheter. Some have a self-sealing inlet so that a needle is used; others need an adapter and then must be clamped or clipped in some manner.

Inflating the Balloon

After the catheter is inserted and the bladder has been emptied of urine (not exceeding 750 ml), the balloon is then inflated in the bladder. Because the balloon is located behind the opening at the insertion tip, it is important first to insert the catheter an additional 2.5 cm (1 inch) after first obtaining urine. This ensures that the balloon is inflated in the bladder and not in the urethra (Figure 27-9). If the patient complains of discomfort or pain during the balloon inflation, the nurse should withdraw the fluid, insert the catheter a little further, and then again inflate the balloon. After the balloon is safely inflated in the patient's bladder, the nurse applies slight tension on the catheter to ensure that it is anchored well in the bladder.

Establishing the Drainage System

Urinary drainage systems are referred to as *open drainage systems* or *closed drainage systems*. The *open drainage system* is one in which the system can be disconnected or opened between the catheter and tubing and between the tubing and the drainage bag. This system is becoming obsolete because of the danger of using poor technique in opening the system and of introducing a urinary tract infection. As a result, the *closed drainage system* is now the preferred system. It is a continuous sterile system including disposable catheter, tubing, and drainage bag that cannot be separated at any point. Some of these are equipped with special air filters in the drainage bag that allow the air to escape but prevent the entrance of microorganisms.

Urinary drainage systems for indwelling catheters operate on the principle of gravity and are often referred to as *straight drainages*. Commonly, disposable clear plastic equipment is utilized, but rubber tubing and a glass drainage bottle with a rubber stopper that allows air to escape can suffice. The drainage receptacle must always be kept below the level of the patient's bladder so that urine can flow with gravity and urine is prevented from flowing back to the bladder. When the patient is in bed, the receptacle is usually attached to the lower side of the bed (Figure 27-10); when the patient is ambulating, it is carried by the patient below hip level or pinned to the dressing gown. When the patient is in a chair, it is often attached to the chair.

The drainage tubing must be of sufficient length to allow the patient freedom to move about in bed

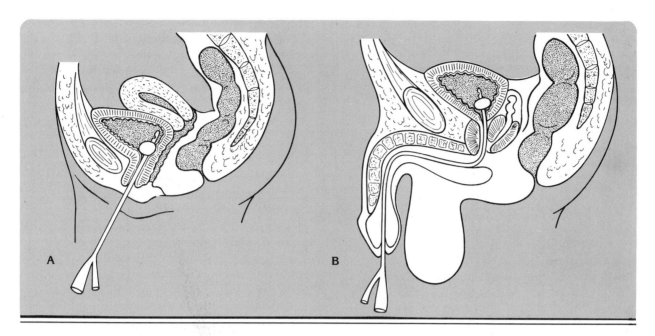

Figure 27-9.   Retention catheters in place. **A,** Female and, **B,** male.

and elsewhere. Because it is longer than the distance between the catheter and the bag, it needs to be coiled and pinned or taped in some manner to prevent kinks that would obstruct the flow of urine or loops that may fall below the drainage receptacle. In the latter case, urine then is required to flow against gravity and may pool in the tubing. The tubing can be attached to the bedding in a number of ways:

1. By pinching a piece of sheet on either side of the tubing and then pinning the sides over the tubing, still keeping it patent.

2. By taping the tubing to the sheet in a crisscross manner with adhesive tape looped under and over the tubing. This is the preferred method when safety pins cannot be used because of the danger of puncturing an alternating pressure mattress.

3. By looping an elastic band around the tubing and then pinning the elastic band to the bedclothes. This method allows even more freedom of movement, since any tension created on the catheter or tubing is absorbed by the elastic band, which stretches readily.

4. By using a special tubing clamp or clip provided with some disposable drainage sets.

5. By looping a piece of adhesive tape around the tubing and then pinning the tape to the bedclothes.

Figure 27-10.   A diagram of a closed urinary drainage system.

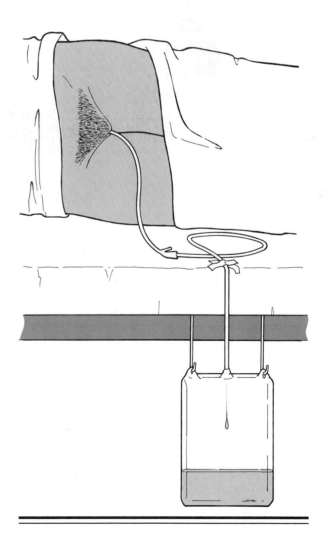

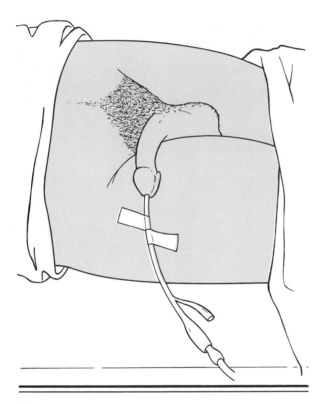

Figure 27-11.   Retention catheter taped to the thigh of a male patient.

It is important that the retention catheter is not pulled, subsequently creating pressure and trauma on the bladder and urethra. Commonly the catheter is taped with a nonallergenic tape to the patient's thigh. Some agencies advocate taping the catheter to the lower abdomen or upper thigh of a male patient with the penis directed toward his head (Figure 27-11). This is thought to prevent irritation and excoriation at the normal angle of the penis and scrotum.

The patient's position in bed can inhibit urinary drainage. When the patient is on his or her back, it is important that the tubing lies over the thigh and that it is not compressed by the patient's weight. When the patient is on the side facing the system, the tubing can rest on the bed in front of the patient and can thus be unobstructed. However, when the patient's back is to the drainage receptacle, the tubing is best placed directly back between the patient's thighs rather than over the thigh. In the latter instance the amount and pressure of urine in the bladder must increase sufficiently to force urine up into the tubing over the thigh for drainage to occur.

Other urinary drainage receptacles are available for ambulatory patients. These attach to the patient's

thigh. They are available in plastic or rubber and are so designed that the catheter fits directly into the top of the receptacle. The bag is equipped with straps that fasten around the thigh. With this type of system the patient can be fully clothed, and the system is concealed from view.

Care of the Patient

Nursing care of the patient with an indwelling catheter and continuous drainage is largely directed toward preventing infection of the urinary tract and encouraging urinary flow through the drainage system. It includes encouraging large amounts of fluid intake, accurate recording of the fluid intake and output, providing perineal-genital care, changing the retention catheter and tubing, maintaining the patency of the drainage system, preventing contamination of the drainage system, and teaching these measures to the patient. The first two measures have been discussed previously.

Perineal-Genital Care

Perineal-genital care is recommended at least twice daily for the patient with an indwelling catheter. It is considered to be one of the most significant measures to reduce the incidence of infection. Any secretions or encrustations that accumulate provide an excellent medium for pathogens, which can ascend up the tract. Most agencies recommend their own specific methods. Some advocate routine perineal-genital care be given with warm soap and water. For the male patient the foreskin is retracted if necessary to cleanse well under it. Any encrustations on the catheter are also removed. Then an antiseptic solution or aerosol is applied around the urinary meatus and around the catheter adjacent to the meatus. After this an antibiotic ointment such as a neomycin-hydrocortisone preparation is sometimes also applied with cotton balls or applicators around both the meatus and adjacent catheter. Disposable gloves are used for this nursing care.

Changing the Catheter and Tubing

Agency policies advise the frequency of catheter and tubing changes. Some agencies advocate that both be changed weekly; others advocate more frequent changes for the tubing and drainage bag, such as every 24 to 48 hours. Recommendations for changes are made on the basis of reducing the incidence of infection and on preventing the development of unpleasant odors. Some authorities recommend catheter changes as infrequently as possible.

When changing the tubing, strict sterile technique is essential to prevent contamination of the distal lumen of the catheter. A new drainage bag and tubing are acquired along with a sterile towel or sterile gauzes and a clamp. Steps involved are as follows:

1. Wash hands.
2. Open the sterile towel or sterile gauze.
3. Open the new drainage and tubing package.
4. Remove the protective cap from the drainage tube, and place the open end of the tubing on the sterile towel or gauze.
5. Clamp the catheter above the connector and disconnect the catheter from the old tubing, being careful to not contaminate the end of the catheter.
6. Connect the catheter to the new tubing.
7. Unclamp the catheter, and establish drainage by securing the tubing and drainage receptacle appropriately to the bed.
8. Waterproof tape may be applied around the connection site of the catheter and the tubing to ensure a continued closed drainage system.

Maintaining Patency of the Drainage System

Ensuring continual patency of the system has been discussed to some extent in the section on establishing the drainage system. The observations needed to be made by the nurse are summarized as follows:

1. Check that there are no obstructions in the drainage, for example, that there are no kinks in the tubing, the patient is not lying on the tubing, and the tubing is not clogged with mucus or blood (if the patient is bleeding or passing pus).

2. Check that there is no tension on the catheter or tubing, that the catheter is taped to the patient's thigh or abdomen, and that the tubing is fastened appropriately to the bedclothes.

3. Check that the gravity drainage is facilitated, for example, that there are no loops in the tubing before entry to the drainage receptacle.

4. Check that the drainage system is well sealed or is closed, for example, that no leaks are detectable at the connection sites in open systems.

Preventing Contamination of the Drainage System

Some agencies recommend the instillation of a 37% formaldehyde solution to the drainage bag. Although this solution has an unpleasant odor, it is germicidal against all forms of microorganisms and viruses and is not affected by organic matter. Agency policies vary, however, and need to be followed.

When emptying the drainage bag, the nurse must maintain aseptic technique. The bag is emptied usually at the end of each shift of duty, and the tube at the bottom of the bag is used to drain the bag. The amount of drainage is noted in accordance with the calibrations on the bag, or a graduated pitcher is brought to the bedside in order to accurately assess the output. It is important for the nurse to not contaminate the end of the tubing and to replace it appropriately when the bag is emptied.

Patient Learning

Teaching the patient some principles about the gravity drainage system and the importance of maintaining a closed system are advised. The patient needs to understand that the drainage tubing and drainage bag need to be kept lower than the bladder at all times. The patient also needs to know how to prevent tension on the catheter tubing, to prevent loops or kinks in the drainage tubing, and to avoid lying on the tubing. Understanding how to manipulate the system when ambulating can provide the patient with a sense of independence.

Obtaining a Sterile Specimen from a Foley Catheter

To obtain a sterile specimen from a Foley catheter connected to a closed drainage system, a nurse requires a sterile 21 to 25 gauge needle, a 3 cc syringe, and a cotton swab with a disinfectant. The needle can be inserted in catheters with self-sealing rubber (not Silastic, plastic, or silicone catheters). The seal area (distal area) is wiped off, and then with the needle at an angle it is inserted into the catheter lumen (Figure 27-12). Care is taken not to puncture the lumen leading to the balloon. If the urine is not available, lift the tubing slightly to return a little urine to the area. Care needs to be taken not to return the urine to the bladder. Another way to secure urine is to kink the tubing about 3 inches from the catheter and hold it with a rubber band until urine is visible.

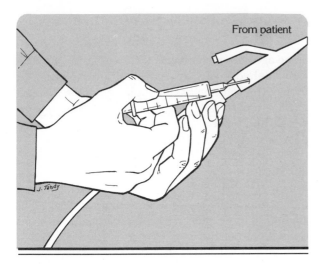

From patient

Figure 27-12.   Collecting a specimen of urine from a Foley catheter.

Some urine bags have a special sampling port in the tubing. The tubing is entered in the same manner to obtain the urine. After the urine has been drawn up into the syringe, it is transferred to a sterile container. Sterile technique is maintained at this time also. The container is closed, labeled, and sent to the laboratory.

Catheter Removal

To remove an indwelling catheter the nurse requires a receptacle for the catheter and a syringe with which to remove the sterile water from the balloon. The nurse first checks the label on the catheter to ascertain how much fluid is in the balloon (5 to 20 ml). All the fluid is then withdrawn. The catheter is then gently withdrawn from the urethra. If the catheter does not come out readily, it should not be forced; however, the physician needs to be notified.

A patient who has had a retention catheter in for weeks or months may well experience some frequency after its removal while the bladder regains its muscle tone. Encouraging the patient to force fluids will assist in this and at the same time flush out any microorganisms that may be present. Occasionally the urethra may have been irritated by the catheter, and as a result the patient may experience some burning when voiding. This usually passes in a few days and is helped by maintaining a dilute urine with a high fluid intake. Patients are sometimes reluctant to take fluids because of the burning upon urination, and thus an explanation by the nurse is important.

After removal of a retention catheter, the patient's intake and output are usually measured until any problems are over. It is also important to assess how often the patient is voiding, how much, and any unusual symptoms such as pain.

APPLICATION OF A CONDOM

The condom or condom catheter is a device that can be applied externally to the male penis as a means of catching urine and directing it to a drainage bag. It can sometimes be used to replace the indwelling catheter, which presents the risk of trauma to the urethra and microorganisms entering the bladder. The condom is usually made of soft pliable plastic or rubberized material, which fits snugly high up over the penis. When the patient is ambulating, the condom is often connected to a bag that is in turn attached to the patient's thigh, and when the patient is in bed the condom is connected to a straight drainage bag as for an indwelling catheter.

Condom appliances are available in commercially prepared packages, or they may be assembled by attaching a condom to a piece of rubber tubing 3 to 4 inches in length and about ½ inch in diameter. The two are attached by means of adhesive tape, elastic bands, or thin rubber rings that are cut from the piece of rubber tubing. Following is a method for assembling a condom appliance using rubber rings (Figure 27-13.

Making a Condom Appliance

1. Put a rubber ring around the rubber tubing midway along its length (Figure 27-13,*A*).
2. With the rolled edge of the condom on the inside, put the condom over one end of the tubing and over the rubber ring (Figure 27-13,*B*).
3. Place another rubber ring over the end of the condom, attaching it firmly to the rubber tube (Figure 27-13,*C*).
4. Then pull the condom back over the second ring. The condom will now have the rolled edge on the outside (Figure 27-13,*D*).

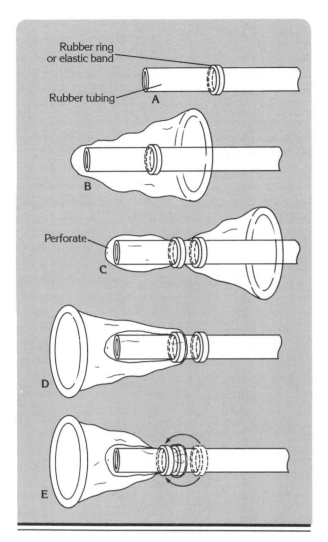

6. Make a small pinhole through the condom covering the lumen of the tube to allow for drainage.

Applying the Condom

Generally, condoms are applied by male nurses and orderlies, although in some instances, female nurses may be required to do so.

Before applying the condom the genital area is thoroughly washed and dried. Methods of attaching the condom vary. Some agencies apply a thin layer of tincture of benzoin, allowing it to dry well, followed by surgical cement around the foreskin of the penis. The condom is then rolled up over the entire penis, making sure that the tip of the tubing is about 1 or 2 inches below the tip of the penis. This prevents irritation of the glans penis. In addition to the above, some agencies independently attach the condom by applying a strip of elastic adhesive around the condom and penis. This adhesive needs to be applied snugly but not too tightly to cause construction of the blood supply. The nurse is advised to check with the agency about other methods that may be used.

Nursing Intervention for a Condom Appliance

Skin excoriation is a possible problem with the use of a condom appliance. Generally, the condom can be applied for about forty-eight hours before it is changed. At this time the skin is cleansed with soap and water, dried well, and inspected for signs of skin irritation. This is best done at the time the patient is bathed. The condom is removed before a bath and a new one applied after the bath.

Maintenance of free urinary drainage is important. Because the condom is pliable it sometimes becomes twisted at the tip of the penis, causing an obstruction to urinary flow. The nurse needs to check the patient's condom at periodic intervals throughout the day. Leakages sometimes occur also and require a change of the condom.

Figure 27-13.   Assembling a condom appliance. **A,** Place rubber ring at the midpoint around the tubing; **B,** pull condom over one end of the tubing and over rubber ring—rolled edge of condom needs to be on the inside; **C,** place another rubber ring over the end of the condom, attaching it firmly to the tubing; **D, E,** first rubber ring is then drawn over second rubber ring.

5. To further secure the condom to the tubing, draw the first rubber ring over the second rubber ring (Figure 27-13,*E*).

URINARY BLADDER IRRIGATION

A bladder irrigation is carried out on a physician's order, usually with the purpose of washing out the bladder and/or applying an antiseptic solution to the bladder lining. It is done using sterile technique.

In some instances a continuous bladder irrigation is set up using a three-way Foley catheter. With this type of Foley catheter, one lumen permits the drainage of urine, a second leads to the bag, which, when inflated, retains the catheter in place in the bladder, and the third lumen permits the passage of irrigating fluid into the bladder. The first lumen of the catheter is connected to a drainage tube, which leads to a closed drainage bag. In this way the system is entirely closed to the air, thus helping to prevent the entry of microorganisms into the bladder.

In the usual bladder irrigation a two-way Foley is usually in place, or the patient is catheterized with a straight catheter for the purpose of the irrigation. For a bladder irrigation the frequency of the irrigation and type of solution to be used will be ordered by the physician. It is not unusual to prepare about 1000 ml of irrigating solution at room temperature and to administer from 180 to 240 ml at one time.

The equipment used for an irrigation is sterile. It will include a container for the irrigation solution, a container for a solution to cleanse the end of the catheter, a receptacle for the solution returning from the bladder, a syringe such as a bulb syringe to administer the fluid, a sterile towel, and a protective towel for the bed. In some instances masks are indicated, and gloves are usually used. Some agencies also suggest that the nurse put on a clean gown.

The nurse first washes and sets up the equipment before taking it to the patient. The patient is draped appropriately, the protective towel is placed on the bed beside the patient's hips, and then the nurse opens the sterile set. Sterile gloves are then put on, the sterile towel is laid near the catheter, and the sterile receptacle is placed upon it. If the catheter is connected to tubing, sterile gauze is used to separate the two, and they are cleansed with an antiseptic solution such as aqueous Zephiran 1:1000 solution and placed on the sterile towel.

The irrigating solution is then drawn into the syringe and injected through the catheter into the bladder. The amount to be injected at one time is generally prescribed by the physician. After injecting the prescribed amount of the fluid, it is permitted to drain into the receptacle. If it does not flow back, it can be drawn out gently with the syringe. This procedure is repeated until the return flow is clear or until all the irrigating solution has been used. The catheter is then reconnected to the tubing or withdrawn.

In recording the bladder irrigation it is important to include the time of the treatment, the type and strength of solution used, and the character of the return flow.

The student is referred to the description of a catheterization if this is required prior to the bladder irrigation.

MEASURING RESIDUAL URINE

Residual urine has been previously defined in this chapter. The physician usually prescribes the measurement of residual urine, although it may be routinely done at the nurse's discretion in specific situations and in accordance with hospital policy. Normally, residual urine in adults is nil or only a few milliliters. Large amounts of residual urine can occur in situations of bladder outlet obstruction, for example, in prostatic hypertrophy or in loss of bladder muscular tone. The latter can result from disorders affecting the nervous control of the bladder or after surgery or indwelling catheterization of the bladder. Incomplete emptying of the bladder is generally suspected when small amounts of urine are voided frequently, for example, 100 ml during one voiding in the adult. The consequence of residual urine is ultimately a urinary infection.

To determine the amount of residual urine the bladder is first emptied by natural voiding, and then the patient is catheterized. Both the amount of urine voided and the amount of residual urine are noted and recorded. If the amount of residual urine exceeds 50 ml, the physician may order that an indwelling catheter be inserted for a period of time.

Residual urine is also frequently measured for patients with suprapubic catheters. This type of catheter is inserted through the abdominal wall above the pubic area into the bladder. To acquire the residual urine the suprapubic catheter is first closed with a clamp for 2 to 4 hours. The patient then voids by the normal route, emptying the bladder as completely as possible. After this the residual urine is obtained by releasing the suprapubic catheter and allowing any remaining urine to drain. Both the amount of urine voided and the amount of residual urine are measured. It is important to carry out sterile techniques when handling the suprapubic catheter.

COLLECTING URINE SPECIMENS

Kinds of Specimens

A number of kinds of urine specimens are requested by physicians for analysis. Four of these are (a) the early morning specimen, (b) the sterile specimen, (c) the sterile voiding, midstream, or clean-catch specimen, and (d) the 24-hour urine specimen.

Early Morning Specimen

An early morning specimen is one taken when the patient first arises in the morning. It is usually the most concentrated urine of the day and the one generally used for routine urinalysis. The specimen is put in a clean container, and thus it is not suitable for bacteriologic study.

Sterile Specimen

A sterile specimen is one required for bacteriologic study. To obtain this sample urine, the patient is catheterized unless a catheter is already in place, and the end of the catheter is placed in a sterile container. (See "Urinary Catheterization" in this chapter.)

Sterile Voided (Midstream or Clean-catch) Specimen

A sterile voided specimen is also referred to as a *midstream* or *clean-catch* specimen. The purpose is to obtain a specimen that is free of any microorganisms that may be at the urinary meatus.

For both male and female patients, thoroughly cleanse the area around the urinary meatus with soap and water. For the female patient it is important to wipe from the urinary meatus toward the rectum, that is, from the area of least contamination to the area of greatest contamination. The patient then starts to void; the first part of the urine is discarded, and the sample is taken from the midstream or the middle portion of the voiding. The sample is voided into a sterile bottle or test tube, which is immediately covered with a sterile top. The last portion of the urine stream is also discarded.

Once a urine specimen has been obtained, it should be immediately delivered to the laboratory for testing. Permitting the urine to stand for a time fosters the growth of any bacteria in the urine and the breakdown of the urea component, changing the urine to a more alkaline pH.

Twenty-four-hour Specimen

A 24-hour urine specimen is needed for some types of diagnostic study, for example, assessment of the corticosteroid levels excreted in certain kinds of adrenal or pituitary disease or assessment of the fluid and electrolyte excretion in infants. Adult patients need to know that all their urine is to be collected during a specified 24-hour period such as 0700 hours one day to 0700 hours the following day. A reminder that the urine is to be kept separate from the stool can be helpful. Usually the first specimen is taken and discarded, and then all urine is kept after this initial voiding. Because the reasons for 24-hour urine collections vary, it is important for the nurse to understand the specific test involved. Sometimes the urine is collected in one large receptacle; at other times, individual receptacles are provided for each voiding and labeled according to sequence and time. Refrigeration of the urine is generally warranted to prevent decomposition of the urine, and in some situations additional preservatives are added to the containers. For some tests a 24-hour urine specimen is first taken for control purposes. The patient is then given a medication at specified times, and a second 24-hour specimen is collected a day or so later. This latter urine is compared to the control sample.

Collecting Urine Specimens from Infants and Children

As with adults a urine specimen is routinely collected on admission to the hospital. For children who have not yet acquired bladder control, special plastic disposable collection bags are available in various designs. These bags generally have nonallergenic adhesive tape around the opening, which is attached securely around the genitals, and some are also equipped with a drainage tab that can be removed to drain the bag after the specimen is collected.

Prior to applying the bag the genital-perineal area is cleansed, rinsed, and dried. Cotton swabs are used for this. For girls the area is wiped from the clitoris to the anus using one cotton swab for each stroke. For boys the penis is wiped in a circular motion from the tip to the scrotum. The foreskin is retracted as necessary.

Two nurses may be necessary for this procedure, one to comfort and restrain the child, the other to apply the collecting device. The infant is positioned on the back; the hips are externally rotated and abducted and the knees flexed. The collecting device is then taped to the perineum. For girls it may be necessary to stretch the perineum around the vagina. The device is generally applied starting at the perineum between the rectum and vagina and working upward. For boys the bag is fitted over the penis and scrotum, and the flaps pressed firmly all around the perineum. It is important that the adhesive is applied without puckers to prevent leakage. A diaper may be applied over the bag to prevent the child from tampering with it. To assist urine drainage by gravity, the head of the crib can be elevated.

After the infant has voided, the bag is removed carefully to prevent skin injury. Depending upon the design of the collection device, the specimen is either transferred through the drainage tab to another collection container, or the adhesive surfaces are closed and the specimen is sent intact in the plastic bag to the laboratory. The child's perineum is inspected and cleansed prior to rediapering.

Routine urine specimens can readily be obtained from preschool or school-age children. As with adults, the genitalia are cleansed first. Then the female child is placed on a training chair and voids into a container or bedpan placed beneath. The male child uses the urinal. It is more difficult to collect a midstream or clean-catch specimen, however. The child needs careful explanations and encouragement to first void a small amount into an unsterile container and then the rest into a sterile container.

When continuous collections of urine are required from small children during certain illnesses, procedures vary in accordance with the equipment available. For example, some agencies have specially designed cribs for infants up to two years of age that allow the urine to flow through a mesh hammock into a collecting bottle below. The advantage of this system is that the infant does not need to be restrained. In other agencies, plastic devices similar to the one described for routine urine specimen collection are used. These devices are then attached to a collecting bottle beneath the crib. In this situation the nurse needs to check frequently that leakage of urine and skin excoriation are prevented.

Catheterization of Infants and Children

Catheterization is rarely performed on young children because of the possibility of introducing an infection. When catheterization is necessary, the presence of a second nurse is recommended to restrain and support the very young child or to console the cooperative older child. The procedure is identical to that described for the adult except that a small catheter is used, for example, no. 8 or 10 French. One other difference relates to the position of the bladder. The bladder of the young infant is located more anteriorly and higher than in the adult. See Figure 27-6 and note the C-shaped curve of the urethra. During the first 3 years of life the bladder descends relatively rapidly and then proceeds gradually until the adult position is assumed in late adolescence. Thus when catheterizing a female infant, the catheter should be directed downward on insertion even more than it is for the adult female.

SUMMARY

Urinary elimination is a need taken for granted by most people until a health problem occurs. The volume of urine eliminated each day varies according to age and has certain characteristics that need to be recognized by the nurse. Urinary control is a learned response, which occurs after bowel control is established. Daytime control is generally achieved by the age of two years, but nighttime control may not be achieved until the age of four years. The four steps involved in learning bladder control and ways that facilitate this learning process are outlined.

The normal process of micturition includes sufficient accumulation of urine in the bladder to stimulate the sensory stretch nerves in the bladder wall. In the adult, micturition generally occurs after 250 to 450 ml of urine have collected in the bladder, but in children the amounts are smaller (50 to 200 ml). Impulses from these stretch receptors then travel to the spinal cord to the voiding reflex center and to the voiding control center in the cerebral cortex, where conscious control of micturition is regulated.

Many factors influence a person's urinary elimination. Increased amounts of urine may be excreted when large amounts of fluid are ingested during stress, when activity is increased, or when diuretics are prescribed. Pathologic conditions may increase or decrease the amount of urine eliminated. When assessing a person's urinary function the nurse needs to systematically consider (a) the person's urinary habits such as frequency of urination and volumes, (b) the characteristics of the urine such as color and odor, and (c) the particular problems that the patient is experiencing, such as retention, incontinence, frequency, or dysuria. The common causes of urinary problems are categorized broadly as obstruction, abnormal tissue growth, infection, and other systemic problems such as cardiac disease that impair urinary function.

Nursing interventions related to urination are generally directed toward facilitating the normal functioning of the urinary system or toward assisting the patient with particular problems. These nursing interventions are outlined as those which (a) assist the patient to maintain an appropriate fluid intake, (b) assist the patient to maintain normal voiding patterns, (c) monitor the patient's daily fluid intake and output, and (d) ensure that cleanliness of the genital area is maintained. Frequently the use of bedpans and urinals is required for bedridden patients. Factors to consider in the use of these are outlined. Measures to assist the hospitalized child are also included.

Nursing interventions for patients with common urinary problems require specific measures relative to the problem. These specific measures are outlined for patients who have urinary incontinence, urinary retention, and childhood nocturnal enuresis. Urinary catheterization is frequently required for patients with urinary problems. The purposes of this technique and the technique itself are described. Sterile technique is essential to prevent ascending urinary infections. The differences between the male and the female catheterization technique are outlined.

The use of urinary retention catheters requires additional considerations by the nurse. Prior to insertion the nurse needs to test the balloon. After insertion the balloon must be safely inflated and a drainage system attached and maintained. Care of patients with indwelling catheters is directed toward preventing infection of the urinary tract and encouraging urinary flow through the drainage system. Measures include accurate recording of fluid intake and output, providing perineal-genital care, changing the catheter and tubing in accordance with agency policies, maintaining the patency of the drainage system, and preventing contamination of the system. Frequently the patient can be taught to assist with these measures. After removal of a retention catheter, the nurse needs to monitor the patient's

ability to void and to measure intake and output until it is established that these are satisfactory.

In lieu of a retention catheter, the condom appliance is frequently used. One way of assembling these appliances is described. Important points to consider to apply condoms and to maintain them are outlined. Frequent observations by the nurse are necessary to prevent the occurrence of skin excoriation, leakage, and obstruction to the patency of the system. Other techniques related to urinary elimination include bladder irrigation, measuring residual urine, and the collection of urine specimens. These techniques are described and outlined.

SUGGESTED ACTIVITIES

1. In a clinical setting, select a patient with a urinary problem. Compare the patient's urinary output in relation to fluid intake. Assess the characteristics of the urine as contrasted to normal, and take into account whether the patient's customary urinary habits have been altered.

2. In a hospital setting, note the policies and practices in regard to patients who have indwelling catheters. Justify the reasons for these.

3. In a laboratory setting, assemble a condom appliance.

4. Interview a mother who has a three- or four-year-old child. Determine how the child was or is being bladder trained.

5. Research why urine specimens are collected in a specific agency. Relate the method of collection to the reason for the specimen.

SUGGESTED READINGS

DeGroot, Jane, and Kunin, Calvin M. March, 1975. Indwelling catheters. *American Journal of Nursing* 75:448–449.

The article provides practical solutions to a number of urinary tract infections. Closed drainage systems, changing catheters, and perineal cleansing are included.

DeGroot, Jane. August, 1976. Catheter-induced urinary tract infections: how can we prevent them? *Nursing 76* 6:34–37.

When not to catheterize is discussed as well as when it is justified. Closed drainage helps to prevent infections if properly maintained. The limits of preventing infections conclude the article.

Khan, Abdul J., and Pryles, Charles V. August, 1973. Urinary tract infection in children. *American Journal of Nursing* 73:1340–1343.

> *The authors discuss the causes of urinary tract infections in children. Preventive measures are included as well as a list of antibacterial drugs and their side effects.*

SELECTED REFERENCES

Beaumont, E. January, 1974. Urinary drainage systems. *Nursing '74* 4:52–60.

de Castro, Fernando J., et al. 1972. *The pediatric nurse practitioner.* St. Louis: The C. V. Mosby Co.

French, Ruth M. 1975. *Guide to diagnostic procedures.* 4th ed. New York: McGraw-Hill Book Co.

Garner, J. February, 1974. Urinary catheter care: doing it better. *Nursing '74* 4:54–56.

Guyton, Arthur C. 1976. *Textbook of medical physiology.* 5th ed. Philadelphia: W. B. Saunders Co.

Tudor, L. L. November, 1970. Bladder and bowel retraining. *American Journal of Nursing* 70:2391–2394.

CHAPTER 28

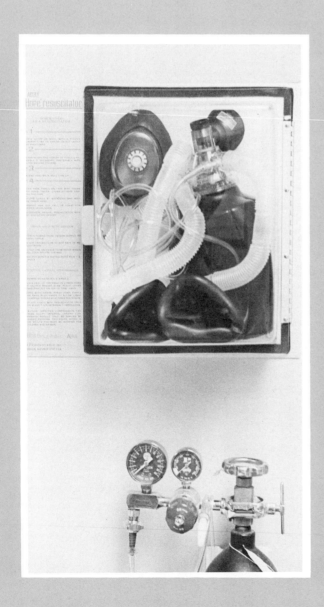

OXYGEN

Nebulization

Artificial Oropharyngeal Airways

Oral and Nasal Suctioning

Oxygen Therapy

Methods of Oxygen Administration

Intermittent Positive Pressure Breathing
Therapy

RESUSCITATION

Artificial Respiration

Cardiopulmonary Resuscitation

OBJECTIVES

- Name three physiologic phases of respiration.

- Discuss the basic mechanics of ventilation, including the pulmonary volumes, capacities, and pressures.

- Describe four requirements essential for adequate ventilation.

- Discuss four factors that influence the rate of diffusion of gases through the respiratory membrane, giving examples of each.

- Explain how oxygen and carbon dioxide are transported to and from the tissues.

- Define terms used to describe respiratory and circulatory status.

- Discuss general nursing interventions that maintain normal respirations.

- Describe postural drainage and its supportive techniques of percussion and vibration.

- Describe various types of humidifiers and their purposes.

- Identify the main parts of a nebulizer.

- List the safety precautions necessitated when oxygen therapy is administered.

- Describe how to administer and maintain oxygen therapy by a nasal cannula, a nasal catheter, an oxygen mask, and an oxygen tent.

- Identify the indications for IPPB therapy and ways to assist patients with this therapy.

- Describe two artificial respiration techniques and cardiopulmonary resuscitation.

PHYSIOLOGY OF RESPIRATION

Respiration is the transport of oxygen from the atmosphere to the body cells and the transport of carbon dioxide from the cells back to the atmosphere. The process can be subdivided into three parts:

1. Pulmonary ventilation, or the inflow and outflow of air between the atmosphere and the alveoli.
2. Diffusion of gases (oxygen and carbon dioxide) between the alveoli and pulmonary capillaries.
3. Transportation of oxygen and carbon dioxide between the alveoli and tissue cells.

Pulmonary Ventilation

Ventilation of the lungs includes the basic mechanics or act of breathing (inspiration and expiration). The degree of chest expansion during ventilation is minimal with normal breathing but can reach maximal capacities during strenuous activity. These normal pulmonary volumes and capacities are described and considered in this section. The relationship of the pulmonary pressures to inspiration and expiration are also included. Many factors are essential for adequate ventilation. These include adequate atmospheric oxygen, clear air passages, adequate pulmonary compliance, and regulation of respiration.

The Mechanisms of Breathing

The act of breathing is likened to a bellows mechanism. It includes *inspiration,* the inflow of air from the atmosphere to the lungs, and *expiration,* the outflow of air from the lungs to the atmosphere. Inspiration lasts normally one to 1.5 seconds, and expiration lasts two to three seconds, including a short resting phase. Normal breathing (eupnea) is silent and effortless. It is accomplished largely by movement of the diaphragm. The diaphragm contracts or flattens on inspiration, thus lengthening and pulling the lower chest cavity downward. On expiration the diaphragm simply relaxes or moves upward. This upward movement of the diaphragm can be enhanced significantly by actively contracting the abdominal muscles. These muscles push the abdominal organs up against the bottom of the diaphragm. (See Figure 28-1.)

Maximal breathing during strenuous exercises of illness requires greater chest expansion and effort.

This is accomplished by intercostal and other muscles that elevate or depress the rib cage. During inspiration the rib cage is pulled upward by the anterior neck muscles and contraction of the external intercostals. During expiration the rib cage is pulled downward by the anterior abdominal muscles. Active use of these muscles and noticeable effort in breathing are seen in patients with obstructive respiratory disease. See "Assessment of Respiratory Status: Chest Shape and Symmetry" in Chapter 14. The changes in thoracic diameters during ventilation are associated with changes in pulmonary volumes and pulmonary pressures.

Pulmonary Volumes.   The volume to which the lungs expand during ventilation varies, depending upon whether the breathing is normal or whether maximal inspiration and expiration occur. In the young male adult, the volume of air inspired and expired during normal breathing is about 500 ml. This value is about 20% to 25% less in the female but may be even less in small persons or greater in large or athletic persons. Subsequent values will also relate to the adult male, and in all cases the female values should be considered as 20% to 25% less. This normal volume of air inspired and expired is referred to as the *tidal volume*. Three other volumes are classified,

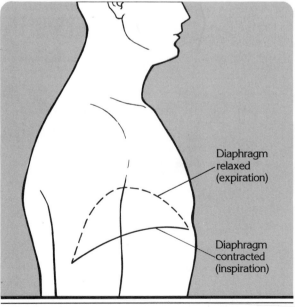

Figure 28-1.   Movement of the diaphragm during inspiration and expiration.

which, when added together with the tidal volume, produce the maximum volume to which the lungs can be expanded. These are as follows:

1. *The inspiratory reserve volume:* approximates 3000 ml and refers to the additional volume of air that can be inspired beyond the normal tidal volume.

2. *The expiratory reserve volume:* approximates 1100 ml and is the amount of air that can be forcefully expired after the normal tidal volume.

3. *The residual volume:* averages about 1200 ml and refers to the amount of air remaining in the lungs after exhalation of both the tidal and the expiratory reserve volumes. Residual air is important because it allows exchange of gases between the alveoli and the pulmonary capillaries between breaths (continuously). Thus the concentrations of oxygen and carbon dioxide do not rise or fall drastically.

All of these volumes added together average about 5800 ml and are referred to as the *total lung capacity* (the maximum volume to which the lungs can be expanded). This requires the greatest possible inspiratory effort.

Pulmonary Capacities.   The pulmonary volumes are often considered in combinations of two or more of the pulmonary volumes. These are referred to as the *pulmonary capacities* and include the total lung capacity already mentioned.

1. *The inspiratory capacity,* which comprises the tidal volume and the inspiratory reserve volume (3500 ml).

2. *The vital capacity,* which comprises the tidal volume plus the inspiratory reserve volume plus the expiratory reserve volume (4600 ml) or, in other words, all pulmonary volumes except the residual volume. The vital capacity of individual persons varies in accordance with (a) the anatomical build of a person, (b) the person's position, (c) the strength of the respiratory muscles, and (d) the distensibility of the lungs and thorax. A tall, thin person has a higher capacity than an obese person. Athletes may develop vital capacities up to 7000 ml. The standing position also increases the vital capacity, whereas lying down reduces it. In the lying position the abdominal organs tend to push against the diaphragm and the volume of pulmonary blood is increased, both of which reduce pulmonary space and air. Weakness or paralysis of respiratory muscles such as occurs in quadriplegics can decrease the vital capacity to a point that is just adequate to sustain life or lower (500 to 100 ml). Interferences with lung distensibility such as pulmonary edema or lung cancer can also seriously reduce the vital capacity.

3. *The functional residual capacity,* which comprises the expiratory reserve volume and the residual volume, is the total amount of air left in the lungs after normal expiration (2300 ml).

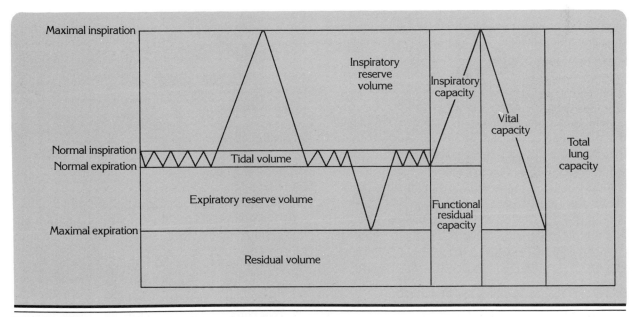

Figure 28-2.   Pulmonary volumes and capacities.

Measurement of the pulmonary volumes and capacities is frequently done by *spirometry* in clinical medicine. The patient breathes a mixture of air and oxygen through a mouthpiece from a drum that is suspended over a chamber of water. On breathing in and out, the gas drum rises and falls in the water, and a recording is made on another drum (spirogram). All lung volumes and capacities can be measured by spirometry except for the residual volume and thus the functional residual capacity and total vital capacity, which include the residual volume. (See Figure 28-2.)

Pulmonary Pressures.   The act of breathing also involves pressure changes within the lungs *(intrapulmonic)* and outside or around the lungs *(intrapleural)*. These pressure changes are related to the changes in the lung volumes in accordance with Boyle's Law of Physics. This law states that the volume of a gas varies inversely with its pressure, provided that the temperature of the gas remains constant. In other words, as the volume increases the pressure decreases, and vice versa.

Applying Boyle's Law to ventilation, on inspiration the volume of the lungs increases, and thus the intrapulmonic pressure decreases. This allows for atmospheric air to enter, since its pressure is greater. Conversely, on expiration the volume of the lungs decreases, and the intrapulmonic pressure increases. This allows the air to escape to the atmosphere, which now has a lower pressure than that contained in the lungs. At sea level the atmospheric pressure is about 760 mm Hg. Only very small pressure changes are required to move air in and out of the lungs. On inspiration the intrapulmonic pressure change is less than 1 mm Hg in relation to the atmosphere, whereas on expiration it rises to +1 mm Hg above the atmosphere (Guyton 1976: 517).

The intrapleural pressure is always negative unless the chest cavity is damaged or opened. This negative pressure is essential in providing a suction effect that holds the visceral pleura and the parietal pleura together as the chest cage expands and contracts. The recoil tendency of the lungs is a major factor responsible for this negative pressure. The fluid in the intrapleural space, however, provides even more negative pressure. It causes adherence of the pleura in much the same manner as water holds two glass slides together.

Essential Requirements for Ventilation.

Ventilation of the lungs is dependent upon (a) adequate atmospheric oxygen, (b) clear air passages, (c) adequate pulmonary compliance and recoil, and (d) regulation of respiration.

Adequate Atmospheric Oxygen.   The presence of oxygen in the atmosphere in adequate concentration is basic to adequate respirations. In high altitudes the concentration of oxygen is less than at sea level and in some instances requires the use of an oxygen tank.

Clear Air Passages.   During inspiration, air passes through the nose, pharynx, larynx, trachea, bronchi, and bronchioles to the alveoli and then back on expiration. The nose performs three important functions. It warms the air, moistens the air, and filters the air. These functions can be appreciated when a person is required to breathe directly through a tube into the trachea (tracheostomy). The drying effect and loss of filtration can lead to infections of the lung. Large particles in the air are filtered by the hairs at the entrance of the nares, and smaller particles are filtered by nasal turbulence. Each time air contacts the nasal turbinates or the septum it must change direction, and in the process small particles are precipitated.

Air passages are also cleared by the mucous membrane lining, which contains *cilia* (hairlike projections of the respiratory mucous membrane). Mucus entraps organisms or other small foreign material while the cilia move the material from the trachea, for example, toward the pharynx. Material can be moved as much as 1 cm per minute along the trachea (Guyton 1976:527). The cough reflex and the sneeze reflex are also essential cleansing mechanisms. The cough reflex is triggered by irritants that send nerve impulses through the vagus nerve to the medulla. Any foreign matter in the larynx, trachea, or bronchi initiates the cough reflex. A particularly sensitive area is the *carina*, the ridge or junction where the main bronchi meet at the trachea. The sneeze reflex is to the nasal passages as the cough is to lower respiratory passages. This reflex is initiated when irritating impulses pass by way of the fifth cranial nerve to the medulla.

Adequate Pulmonary Compliance and Recoil.   *Compliance* is expansibility or stretchability. It generally includes expansibility of both the lungs and the thorax but is sometimes referred to as compliance of the lungs alone. Expansibility of the lungs alone when placed outside of the thorax is almost double that of the lungs and the thorax together. Compliance can be measured by noting the amount of volume increase in the lungs that is produced by units of increased intraalveolar pressure. Expansibility is obviously essential for adequate inspiration.

Inadequate compliance can be caused by any condition that destroys lung tissue, such as edema or tumors, or any condition that inhibits thoracic expansion, such as paralysis or kyphosis.

In contrast to lung compliance is *lung recoil.* The lungs have a continual tendency to collapse away from the chest wall. Two factors are responsible for this recoil tendency: (a) elastic fibers present in lung tissue and (b) surface tension of the fluid lining the alveoli. The latter accounts for two thirds of the recoil phenomenon. Counterbalancing this surface tension in the alveoli is a lipoprotein mixture called *surfactant.* When surfactant is absent, lung expansion is exceedingly difficult, and the lungs collapse. Normally the secretion of surfactant by the alveoli is stimulated several times each hour by yawning, sighing, or deep breaths. Surfactant stimulation has important applications clinically for patients on automatic ventilation. The alveoli must be stretched several times every hour by a specific sigh mechanism on the respirator.

Regulation of Respiration.   Several factors regulate the respiratory process. The primary regulator is the *respiratory center* located in the medulla oblongata. This area maintains the normal smooth rhythm of respiration by mechanisms not fully understood. It is thought that two alternating circuits operate: one for inspiration and one for expiration. Each inhibits the other; thus when one is active, the other is inactive in an oscillating fashion.

Other specialized receptors throughout the body transmit impulses to the respiratory center to bring about changes in respiration. Included are stretch receptors, chemoreceptors, and proprioceptors. The *stretch receptors,* located principally in the bronchioles, are activated when the lungs become inflated. Impulses are transmitted through the vagus nerves to the brainstem and thence to the respiratory center. Inspiration is then inhibited, and overdistention of the lungs is prevented. This mechanism is commonly referred to as the *Herring-Brewer inflation reflex.* During expiration the *Herring-Brewer deflation reflex* operates. The stretch receptors are decreasingly stimulated until no impulses occur. This then allows inspiration to be triggered again. It is thought that compression receptors may also be present in the walls of the alveoli that control the amount of lung deflation. Expiration is inhibited in the same way that the stretch receptors inhibit inspiration.

Chemoreceptors (chemical receptors) that affect respiration are present in the respiratory center, along the arch of the aorta, and in carotid bodies at the bifurcation of the common carotid arteries. These receptors respond to changes in the chemical composition of the blood and tissue fluids, specifically to the changes in oxygen, carbon dioxide, or hydrogen ion concentrations. Changes in carbon dioxide and hydrogen ion concentrations stimulate receptors di-

rectly in the respiratory center. When the levels of carbon dioxide and hydrogen ions increase, the respiratory center is greatly stimulated. Changes in arterial oxygen concentrations exert their effects on the aortic and carotid bodies. A low level of oxygen stimulates the chemoreceptors, which then in turn stimulate the respiratory center to increase ventilation. The aortic and carotid bodies can also be stimulated to increase ventilation when the arterial blood pressure falls below 80 mm Hg even when the oxygen concentration is normal. Thus hypotension itself initiates reflexes that increase respiration. Vasoconstriction is also brought about to increase the blood pressure. Of these three factors that stimulate chemoreceptors (carbon dioxide, hydrogen ions, and oxygen), carbon dioxide has the most potent effect on stimulating respiration.

Proprioceptors present in the muscles and tendons of movable joints are stimulated by passive body movements and vigorous exercise. These receptors transmit impulses to the respiratory center and stimulate increased or intense respiration. This explains why an increase in ventilation occurs at the beginning of an exercise period. It was formerly believed that hypoxia of the muscles during and after exercise initiated increased respiration (Guyton 1976:567).

Diffusion of Gases

After the alveoli are ventilated with air, the second phase of the respiratory process is the diffusion of oxygen from the alveoli into the pulmonary blood vessels. In the opposite direction, carbon dioxide diffuses from the pulmonary blood vessels into the alveoli. Because the alveolar walls are very thin and are surrounded by a closely intertwined network of blood capillaries, these membranes are together often referred to as the *respiratory membrane. Diffusion* is the movement of gases or other particles from an area of greater pressure or concentration to an area of lower pressure or concentration.

Four factors influence the rate of diffusion of gases through the respiratory membrane. These are (a) the thickness of the membrane, (b) the surface area of the membrane, (c) the diffusion coefficient of the gas, and (d) the pressure difference on each side of the membrane (Guyton 1976:539).

The thickness of the respiratory membrane increases in some pulmonary diseases such as pulmonary edema. Any increase in the size of this membrane can seriously decrease gaseous diffusion. The surface area of the membrane can also be altered. Conditions such as emphysema, in which several alveoli coalesce, or lobectomy, the surgical removal of a portion of the lung, impede gaseous exchange. Under resting conditions the loss of some surface area is not a serious deficit. However, when more than 25% is lost or when increased demands are necessary as during exercise, even less than 25% can be a serious detriment. The *diffusion coefficient* of oxygen and carbon dioxide is also a significant factor. This coefficient is dependent upon the molecular weight and solubility of the gases in the membrane. Carbon dioxide diffuses about 20 times more rapidly than oxygen. Thus in some situations an oxygen lack is seen without a carbon dioxide build-up. For instance, carbon monoxide diffuses 200 times more rapidly than oxygen, which accounts for the rapidity of fatality by carbon monoxide poisoning.

The pressure differences in the gases on each side of the respiratory membrane obviously affect diffusion. When the pressure of oxygen is greater in the alveoli than in the blood, oxygen diffuses into the blood. The reverse happens with carbon dioxide. Normally the oxygen pressure gradient is about 40 mm Hg between the alveoli and the blood entering the pulmonary capillaries. The partial pressure of oxygen (P_{O_2}) in the alveoli is about 100 mm Hg, whereas the P_{O_2} in the entering venous blood of the pulmonary arteries is about 60 mm Hg. These pressures equalize very rapidly, however, so that the arterial P_{O_2} also becomes about 100 mm Hg. Carbon dioxide, on the other hand, has a partial pressure in the venous blood entering the pulmonary capillaries of about 45 mm Hg, whereas that in the alveoli is about 40 mm Hg. These partial pressures are used frequently as diagnostic measures to assess deficiencies or excesses of oxygen and carbon dioxide levels in persons with pulmonary disease.

Transportation of Oxygen and Carbon Dioxide

The third part of the respiratory process involves the transport of the respiratory gases. Oxygen needs to be transported from the lungs to the tissues, and carbon dioxide must be transported from the tissues back to the lungs.

Oxygen Transport

Normally most of the oxygen (97%) combines loosely with the hemoglobin in the red blood cells and is carried to the tissues as *oxyhemoglobin* (the compound of oxygen and hemoglobin). The remaining oxygen is dissolved and transported in the water of plasma and cells. The maximum amount of oxygen that the blood will absorb to become fully saturated is about

20 ml per 100 ml of blood. This is expressed as 20 vol%. As the hemoglobin releases oxygen to the tissues, it is referred to as *reduced hemoglobin*. Under normal conditions only about 25% or 5 ml of oxygen per 100 ml of blood is diffused to the tissues (utilization coefficient). However, this rate of release can be increased to 75% during periods of stress or increased exercise, since more oxygen is utilized by the cells. In situations of extreme oxygen lack by the tissues caused by a sluggish blood flow or a very high metabolic rate, all (100%) of the oxygen can be removed.

Carbon Dioxide Transport

On the return trip to the lungs the hemoglobin that released its oxygen does not travel empty handed. It is regarded as a fickle escort that also combines with carbon dioxide as *carbaminohemoglobin*. However, only a moderate amount (30%) of carbon dioxide is transported this way. The largest amount of CO_2 (about 65%) is carried in the form of bicarbonate (HCO_3^-) inside the red blood cells. Smaller amounts (5%) are transported in solution in the plasma and as *carbonic acid* (the compound formed when CO_2 combines with water). Under normal resting conditions about 4 ml of CO_2 in each 100 ml of blood is transported from the tissues to the lungs. Carbon dioxide is an important factor in the acid-base balance of the body. This function is discussed in Chapter 30.

Factors Influencing Oxygen Transport

Several factors affect the rate of oxygen transport from the lungs to the tissues. The major factors are: (a) cardiac output, (b) number of erythrocytes, (c) exercise, and (d) blood hematocrit.

The normal cardiac output is approximately 5 liters per minute, and under resting conditions 250 ml of oxygen is transported per minute. Any pathologic condition that decreases cardiac output diminishes this amount of oxygen delivered to the tissues. Disease such as myocardial infarction (heart attack) weakens the pumping motion of the heart and thus diminishes the transport of oxygen. Hemorrhage or dehydration can significantly reduce the blood volume and subsequently the cardiac output. The backlog of blood in the venous system for any reason prevents adequate return flow of blood to the heart. These all reduce cardiac output and thus diminish oxygen transport. Generally the heart compensates for inadequate output by increasing its pumping rate. Normally, compensatory cardiac output can increase the oxygen transport fivefold, but when disease conditions exist, this is not possible.

The second factor influencing oxygen transport

is the number of erythrocytes. The normal number of circulating erythrocytes in men is about 5 million per cubic mm, and in women it is about 4½ million per cubic mm. Reductions in these normal values can be brought about by anemia of any cause.

Exercise also has a direct influence upon oxygen transport. In well-trained athletes the oxygen transport can be increased up to 20 times the normal. This increase is due in part to an increased cardiac output and to increased utilization of oxygen by the cells (utilization coefficient).

The *blood hematocrit* refers to the percentage proportion of red cell mass to plasma. It is also referred to as the packed cell volume per 100 ml. Normally this proportion is about 40% to 50% in men and 35% to 45% in women. Excessive increases in the blood hematocrit increase the blood viscosity, reduce the cardiac output, and therefore reduce oxygen transport. Excessive reductions in the blood hematocrit, such as occur in anemia, also reduce the oxygen transport. It is interesting to note that persons who develop elevated hematocrits when acclimatizing to high altitudes do not have oxygen transport problems. This is thought to be due to an associated increase in the numbers and sizes of peripheral blood vessels, thus preventing a fall in cardiac output.

ASSESSMENT OF RESPIRATORY AND CIRCULATORY STATUS

Assessment methods of the vital signs of respiration and pulse are discussed in Chapter 13. Included also is assessment of the chest cage, lungs, and heart in Chapter 14. This section will emphasize common respiratory and circulatory problems and the terms used to describe these problems rather than the normal variations that occur with age.

Terms Used in Assessing Respiratory Status

The assessment of a person's respiratory status can be considered in the following categories: (a) breathing patterns, (b) breath sounds, (c) chest movements, and (d) secretions and coughing.

Breathing Patterns

Breathing patterns relate to rate, volume, rhythm, or degree of ease of respiration.

1. Rates
   Eupnea—normal respiration that is quiet, rhythmical, and effortless. Variations in rates according to age are discussed in Chapter 13.
   Tachypnea—rapid respiration marked by quick, shallow breaths.
   Bradypnea—abnormally slow breathing.
   Apnea—cessation of breathing.

2. Volumes
   Hyperventilation—an increase in the amount of air in the lungs characterized by prolonged and deep breaths; associated with anxiety.
   Hypoventilation—a reduction in the amount of air in the lungs characterized by shallow respirations.

3. Rhythm
   Cheyne-Stokes breathing—rhythmic waxing and waning of respirations from very deep breathing to very shallow breathing and temporary apnea; often associated with cardiac failure, increased intracranial pressure, or brain damage.

4. Ease or effort
   Dyspnea—a feeling of difficult and labored breathing in which the patient has a persistent unsatisfied need for air and feels distressed.
   Orthopnea—ability to breathe only in the upright position of sitting or standing.

Breath Sounds

Breath sounds include those which are obvious to the ear and those which require amplification by a stethoscope.

1. Sounds audible to the ear
   Stridor—a shrill, harsh sound heard during inspiration with laryngeal obstruction.
   Stertor—snoring or sonorous respiration, usually due to a partial obstruction of the upper airway.
   Wheeze—whistling respiratory sound on expiration that usually indicates some narrowing of the bronchial tree.

Bubbling—gurgling sounds as air globules pass through moist secretions in the respiratory tract.

2. Sounds audible by stethoscope
Râles—rattling or bubbling sounds generally heard on inspiration as air moves through accumulated moist secretions.
Rhonchi—coarse, dry, wheezy, or whistling sound more audible during expiration as the air moves through tenacious mucus or a narrowed bronchi.
Creps (crepitation)—a dry crackling sound like crumpled cellophane produced by air in the subcutaneous tissue or by air moving through fluid in the alveoli.
Pleural rub—coarse, leathery, or grating sound produced by the rubbing together of the pleura; also called *friction rub*.
Areas of decreased intensity or absence—sounds below normal or absent indicate inadequate ventilation or expansion; thus such areas also need to be noted.

Chest Movements

1. Retractions
Intercostal—indrawing between the ribs.
Substernal—indrawing beneath the breast bone.
Suprasternal—indrawing above the breast bone.
Supraclavicular—indrawing above the clavicles.
Tracheal tug—indrawing and downward pull of the trachea during inspiration.
2. *Flail chest* is the ballooning out of the chest wall through injured rib spaces. It results in *paradoxical breathing* where the chest wall balloons out during expiration but is depressed or sucked inward on inspiration.

Secretions and Coughing

1. Secretions
Hemoptysis—the presence of blood in the sputum. Determine amount, kind, color, and odor, for example, thick, frothy, pink, rusty, green, yellow.
2. Cough
Productive—secretions are expectorated when coughing.
Nonproductive—a dry harsh cough without secretions.

Terms Used in Assessing Circulatory Status

Anoxia—systematic absence or reduction of oxygen below physiologic levels in body tissues. This state is frequently accompanied by signs such as increased pulse rate, rapid or deep respirations, cyanosis, restlessness, anxiety, dizziness (vertigo), or faintness (syncope).

Hypoxemia—deficient oxygenation of the blood measured by laboratory means.

Hypoxia—diminished availability of oxygen for body tissues due to internal or external causes.

Tachycardia—excessively rapid heart rate, over 100 beats per minute in the adult.

Bradycardia—abnormal slowness of the heart rate, below 60 beats per minute in the adult.

Pulse deficit—the difference between the apical and radial pulse.

Cyanosis—bluish color of mucous membrane, nail beds, or skin due to excessive deoxygenation of hemoglobin.

GENERAL NURSING INTERVENTIONS TO MAINTAIN NORMAL RESPIRATIONS

Positioning

Normally, adequate ventilation is maintained by frequent changes of position, ambulation, and exercise. When persons become ill, however, some respiratory functions may be inhibited for a variety of reasons. A common reason is immobility, which may be induced by surgery or medical therapy. Lying too long in one position compresses the thorax and limits chest expansion and thus the movement of air throughout the lungs. Sitting in a slumped position also inhibits chest expansion, since the abdominal contents are pushed up against the diaphragm. Another frequent cause of limited chest expansion is abdominal pain or chest pain. The patient in these instances will voluntarily limit chest movements to relieve the pain. By making the respirations shallow, both diaphragmatic excursion and lung distensibility are inhibited. The result of inadequate chest expansion is stasis and pooling of respiratory secretions, which ultimately harbor microorganisms and become infected. This situation is often compounded for the hospitalized patient who receives narcotics for pain. Narcotics further depress the rate and depth of respiration.

Interventions by the nurse to maintain the normal respirations of patients need to include (a) appropriate positioning to enable maximal chest expansion, (b) encouraging or providing frequent changes in position for bed patients, (c) encouraging ambulation, and (d) measures to promote comfort such as the relief of pain. The semi-Fowler's or high Fowler's position encourages maximum chest expansion for bed patients, particularly those who are dyspneic. For patients unable to assume this position, frequent turning from side to side needs to be encouraged so that alternate sides of the chest are permitted maximum expansion.

Deep Breathing and Coughing

In addition to positioning patients, the nurse can facilitate respiratory functioning by encouraging deep breathing exercises and coughing to remove secretions. Deep breathing can be demonstrated to patients by the nurse. The nurse places the hands palm down on the border of the rib cage and inhales slowly and evenly until the greatest chest expansion is achieved. The breath is then held for a few seconds followed by slow exhalation of the air by blowing out through the mouth. Exhalation proceeds until maximal chest contraction is achieved. To assist the patient to deep breathe, the nurse then instructs the patient to do the same or the nurse's hands may be placed on the patient's chest border. The number of breaths and the frequency throughout the day for deep breathing vary in accordance with the patient's condition. Patients such as those who are on bedrest or who have had abdominal or chest surgery need to be encouraged by the nurse to perform deep breathing at least three or four times daily. Each session should include a minimum of five deep breaths. For patients who are prone to pulmonary problems, deep breathing exercises may be implemented every hour. Special breathing exercises are required for patients with chronic respiratory disease. Included are pursed-lip breathing and abdominal breathing exercises. Details

about these are included in the references at the end of the chapter.

Voluntary coughing in conjunction with deep breathing facilitates the movement and expectoration of secretions in the respiratory tract. Frequently the deep breathing exercises automatically initiate the cough reflex. Voluntary coughing, however, is encouraged for patients who are susceptible to accumulating respiratory secretions. An example is the postoperative patient. Medications given to these patients preoperatively and anesthesia itself depress the action of the cilia and the respiratory center. As a result, secretions accumulate, may become tenacious and thick, and eventually create obstruction to some airways. These patients require encouragement and assistance from the nurse to cough, particularly those with chest or abdominal incisions.

Effective coughing is best achieved in the sitting position. After a deep inhalation the patient is instructed to cough forcefully using the abdominal and other accessory respiratory muscles. If the patient has an incision, the nurse can provide support to it by placing the palms of the hands on either side of the incision during coughing. For patients with abdominal incisions the patient can be instructed to splint the abdomen with a firmly rolled pillow held against it.

Adequate Hydration

Adequate hydration maintains the moisture of the respiratory mucous membranes. Normally secretions of the respiratory tract are thin and therefore moved by ciliary action readily. However, when states of body dehydration occur or when the environment has a low humidity, the respiratory secretions can become thick and tenacious. The mucous membranes then become irritated and prone to infection. Nursing measures to increase and monitor fluid intake are discussed in Chapter 29. If the air lacks humidity, humidifiers may be necessary (see "Humidifiers" in this chapter).

Promoting Health Practices and a Healthy Environment

The effects of cigarette smoking and air pollution on health are well known. Chronic bronchitis associated with both can progress to disabling breathlessness and prolonged respiratory and cardiovascular ailments. The specific effects of smoking include (a) an increased incidence of lung cancer, (b) a prevalence of bronchitis and emphysema with recurrent episodes of respiratory infection, (c) development of premature coronary heart disease, (d) birth of babies with a lower than average birth weight, and (e) higher rates of cancer of the larynx, pharynx, oral cavity, esophagus, pancreas, and urinary bladder (World Health Organization 1975:8). In this respect, the nurse can be instrumental in providing health instruction to individual patients and the public.

Many communities now offer supportive programs to assist people to stop smoking. When young people stop smoking, pulmonary functions may return to normal. In persons with moderately severe obstructive lung impairments the return of normal function may never occur. However, dyspnea and cough can improve significantly.

SPECIFIC NURSING INTERVENTIONS TO ASSIST RESPIRATORY IMPAIRMENT

Postural Drainage

Postural drainage is the drainage by gravity of secretions from various lung segments by the use of specific positions. It is implemented (a) to assist the removal of secretions that have accumulated in patients such as those with chronic lung disease or (b) to prevent the accumulation of secretions for those patients who are unconscious or are receiving mechanical ventilation. Retained secretions facilitate bacterial growth and subsequent infection. They also can obstruct the smaller airways. Secretions in the major airways such as the trachea and the right and left main bronchi are usually coughed out or can be effectively removed by suctioning (see "Oral and Nasal Suctioning" in this chapter). However, the peripheral lung segments require postural assistance to drain their secretions into these main airways.

The lung segments involved and the airways (segmental bronchi) draining them determine the positions selected for postural drainage. Assessment of the areas involved is determined by auscultation, percussion, or radiologic means. Abnormal breath sounds such as râles can be heard on auscultation; hyperresonance or flatness can be determined by percussion. The appropriate position for drainage is then selected. Posturing involves placing the patient in a position that will allow drainage of the segmental bronchi by gravity (see Figure 28-3). These positions are generally subdivided into three major categories:

1. Positions that drain the upper lung segments or upper lobes.

2. Positions that drain the middle lung segments. Note that only the right lung has a middle lobe.

3. Positions that drain the basilar lung segments or lower lobes.

Drainage of the Upper Lung Segments

Sitting in the upright position in a chair provides drainage of the uppermost lung segments. To drain the anterior upper segments the patient needs to bend his or her body backward at about a 30° angle. Pillow supports can be provided for the lumbar region. This position can also be accomplished in bed by use of the semi-Fowler's position. To drain the posterior upper segments the patient needs to bend forward about 30° at the hips. A table with or without pillows is needed to support the arms at the elbows for this position. To drain the lateral upper segments the patient needs to bend sideways about 45° first to one side and then to the other. Leaning on an arm rest supports this position.

Drainage of the Middle Lung Segments

To drain the right middle segments the patient is positioned flat in bed on the left side with a pillow support for the patient's head. The right shoulder and body are swung forward. To drain the left middle lung segments the opposite position is assumed.

Drainage of the Basilar Lung Segments

Drainage of the lower lobes can be accomplished by positioning the patient's bed in the Trendelenberg position or by elevating the patient's hips with the use of several pillows. The hips must be positioned higher than the shoulders. To drain both the right and left anterior basilar segments, the patient lies on his or her back in the Trendelenberg position. If the hips are elevated with pillows, the patient flexes the knees and places the feet flat on the mattress. The shoulders should also rest flatly against the mattress. To drain the posterior basilar segments, the patient lies on the stomach in the Trendelenberg position or

672

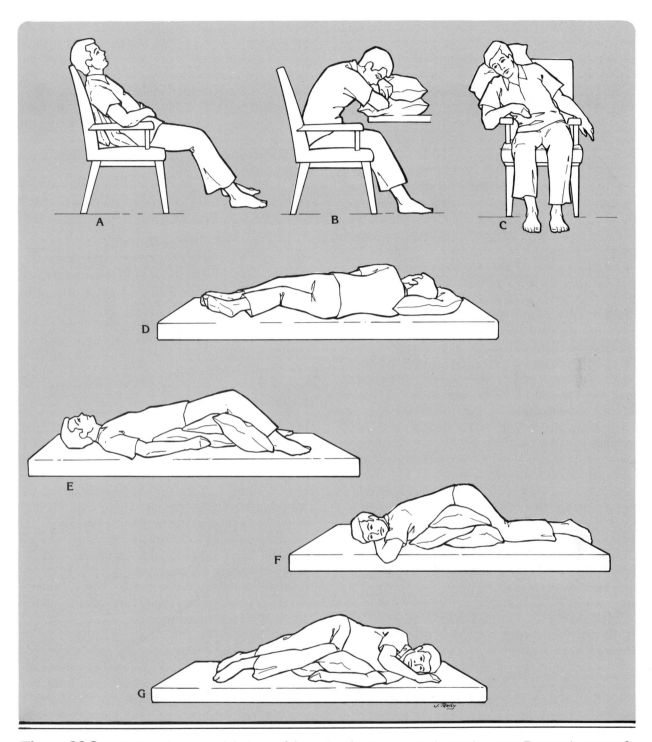

Figure 28-3.   Positions for postural drainage of the various lung segments. **A,** anterior upper; **B,** posterior upper; **C,** lateral upper; **D,** left middle lateral; **E,** anterior basal; **F,** posterior basal; **G,** lateral basal.

may have the hips elevated by three or four pillows to produce a jackknife position from the knees to the shoulders. To drain the lateral basilar segments the side-lying position is used as described in drainage of the middle lung segments. In this case, however, the hips are positioned higher than the shoulders.

Supportive Techniques to Postural Drainage

Prior to postural drainage, bronchodilator medications or nebulization therapy may be prescribed to encourage drainage and expulsion of secretions. The patient is also instructed to use diaphragmatic breathing throughout the drainage session. This was discussed previously. During postural drainage, the nurse or physiotherapist can also facilitate the loosening or dislodgment of secretions that are dry or tenacious by the use of percussion (cupping) techniques and vibration techniques.

Percussion is the technique of forcefully striking the chest wall over the involved area with cupped hands. In the cupped position the fingers and thumb are held together and then slightly flexed to form a cup of the palms as one would to scoop up water. With the hands in this position, the wrists are then loosely and rapidly flexed and extended to slap the thoracic cage. It is important to keep the hands cupped to maintain an air-cushioned impact and to avoid hurting the patient. Areas to avoid in percussion are over the spinal column, the breasts, and the kidneys. Percussion is usually done for 1 or 2 minutes and is usually confined to the most congested areas.

Vibration can be likened to a series of vigorous quiverings. This technique is used after percussion over the same areas but only while the patient exhales. The nurse places one hand flat on the chest wall and the other hand on top of the first. Using mainly the heel of the hand, the nurse tenses all hand and arm muscles and then presses and vibrates downward on the chest wall. The pressure is relaxed when the patient inhales. Vibration is generally done four or five times.

Periodically the patient is encouraged to cough up any secretions during postural drainage, percussion, and vibration. Tissues and a paper bag must be provided for disposal of secretions. After postural drainage, the nurse should provide the patient with a mouthwash for cleansing and comfort purposes. The effectiveness of the therapy is recorded, noting the color, character, and amount of sputum expectorated and the reaction of the patient to therapy. Many patients may require instruction to maintain these techniques at home.

Scheduling Postural Drainage

Frequently postural drainage treatments are planned for two or three times daily, depending upon the amount of secretions a patient has. The best times include before breakfast, before lunch, late afternoon, or before bedtime. These times avoid the meal hours and the hours shortly after meals. Fatigue and vomiting can be induced at these times if postural drainage is carried out.

The length of time of treatments must also be considered. Usually the entire treatment takes 30 minutes. This includes the prepostural drainage therapies of nebulization, deep breathing, and all

positions assumed during posturing. Some patients can tolerate long treatments less frequently. Others require shorter treatments more frequently. The nurse therefore needs to evaluate the patient's tolerance of these treatments. This can be done by observing the stability of the patient's vital signs, particularly the pulse and respiratory rates or any pallor, diaphoresis, or signs of dyspnea or fatigue.

Positions may also need to be compromised for some patients. For example, some may become dyspneic with the Trendelenberg positions and require only a moderate tilt or shorter time in this position.

Humidifiers

The provision of moisture for the respiratory mucous membranes is a common therapy for persons with respiratory problems. This is offered in a variety of ways and often is a necessary adjunct for other therapies such as oxygen inhalation and nebulization. Included are hot steam inhalators and the Croupette humidity tent.

Hot Steam Inhalators

Several types of steam inhalators are manufactured commercially. In the home, however, an ordinary electric kettle may be used. Steam when inhaled provides warmth and moisture to the mucous membrane. Both facilitate the expectoration of secretions. The warmth increases the blood supply and hydration of the respiratory membranes by *transudation*. It also relaxes the smooth muscles of the respiratory passages. The moisture liquefies secretions and decreases irritation. For optimal effectiveness steam inhalations must be inhaled deeply, slowly, and as directly as possible. Precautions are necessary, however, to avoid burns to the patient's face or elsewhere by accidental contact with the equipment. For continuous steam inhalations, such as for bedridden patients, the nozzle of the steam inhalator is directed so that the steam surrounds the patient's head but avoids the patient's face. Drafts need to be prevented or minimized, and linen needs to be changed when damp to avoid chills. Expectoration by the patient should be encouraged and tissues and a container provided for their disposal. For intermittent inhalations the patient may sit close to the inhalator and be instructed to breathe deeply.

Steam inhalation may be prescribed as a vehicle to administer medications. A common home remedy is tincture of benzoin. The steam may be directed over the medication, or the medication may be mixed with the water.

Croupette Humidity Tent

The Croupette humidity tent, a rectangular, clear plastic tent, is often used for infants and young children with respiratory problems. It provides high humidity levels and may also provide increased oxygen levels of 40% to 60%. The cooling and moisturizing effects are advantageous in reducing fevers accompanying respiratory infections and also in liquefying respiratory secretions. The temperature is maintained at below room temperature by 2° to 3° C (6° to 8° F). (See Figure 28-4.) The canopy of the tent (A) is supported by a metal frame, which is usually tied to the upper third of the bedsprings with gauze strips. One or two zippers (B) on each side of the tent are provided to allow for care of the infant or child with minimal disruption to the humidity or oxygen levels. At the end of the tent, which lies against the head of the bed, are the various mechanical parts, which provide for humidity and oxygenation. The largest container is the trough (C), which is filled with ice to the depth indicated by a line (about 10 inches). A drainage tube (D) connected to the trough is kept in an elevated notch or opening provided until drainage is desired, in which case it is detached and lowered into a receptacle below. A damper valve (E) is located on the large tube between the trough and the tent. This valve is opened periodically and then closed to minimize condensation or adjusted for continuous operation in accordance with doctor's orders. Another tube beneath the trough connects to the air or oxygen source (F). Before the infant is placed in the tent, it is flooded with air and oxygen if ordered. The flowmeter is then adjusted to deliver the required amount of oxygen. (See "Oxygen Therapy" for further information.) Alongside the air tube is a jar with a screw cap (G). This is filled with distilled water to a mark indicated by a black line. Its purpose is to moisturize the air or oxygen entering the Croupette, and it must be refilled at least every 8 hours to maintain this level. In addition, a nebulizer outlet (H) is provided to supply aerosol antibiotics or other aerosols as required. This outlet is attached to additional tubing and a secondary air or oxygen source. The front part of the canopy (I) is fan folded well into the bedclothes or into an additional overlying drawsheet to ensure closure of the tent. All sides of the canopy must be well tucked under the mattress.

The child in a Croupette needs physical protection and frequent observation. Warmth needs to be provided to protect the child from chilling and from the dampness of condensation. Additional gowns or a cotton blanket can be used. Some agencies provide gowns with hoods, or a small towel may be wrapped around the infant's head. The bed linen and clothing needs to be changed frequently. Padding in the form of a small pillow or rolled towel placed at the head of the Croupette can prevent bruising or bumping of the infant's head. This padding also absorbs the excess moisture by condensation. When administering nursing care, the humidity and oxygen therapy needs to be maintained. This can be accomplished by moving the canopy up around the infant's head and neck and securing it under a pillow when providing care. Emotional support to the child also needs to be provided, particularly for preschoolers who can be exceedingly anxious.

Maintenance of the equipment is essential. The water needs to be drained and the ice in the trough replenished as necessary. The distilled water in the screw-cap bottle must also be maintained. The air and oxygen flow must also be monitored frequently to maintain appropriate concentrations. All connections should be airtight.

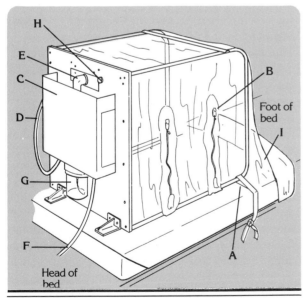

Figure 28-4.   A Croupette humidity tent. **A,** Metal frame supports canopy of tent and is attached to bed frame by gauze strips; **B,** zippers allow for provision of care; **C,** trough filled with ice; **D,** drainage tube for trough; **E,** damper valve; **F,** tube connected to air or oxygen source; **G,** distilled water to moisture the air or oxygen; **H,** nebulizer outlet; and **I,** canopy folded under bed linen.

Nebulization

A *nebulizer* is an atomizer or sprayer. These come in various designs and materials but in essence have four main parts. (See Figure 28-5.)

1. A cylindrical chamber (A), which holds the prescribed amount of aerosol.

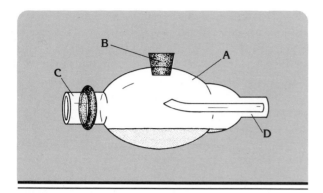

Figure 28-5.   The basic parts of the nebulizer include **A,** cylindrical chamber for aerosol; **B,** opening into chamber to insert aerosol is closed by cork or cap when filled; **C,** wide, open end that attaches to a patient's mouth piece or another air source, such as oxygen tank; and **D,** small, open end that is attached to pressure source, such as hand pump.

2. An opening at the top *(B)* of the chamber to insert the aerosol. A small syringe with or without a needle needs to be used to inject the aerosol into the chamber of some nebulizers.

3. A wide opened end *(C)* that may be affixed to a Croupette humidity tent or to a mouthpiece through which the patient inhales.

4. A smaller open end *(D)* containing a tube that is attached to a pressure source such as oxygen or a hand pressure pump.

Nebulization therapy is also referred to as *inhalation* or *aerosol therapy.* Frequently medications such as bronchodilators or mucolytic agents are administered by nebulization. These are inhaled directly through various commercially prepared aerosol containers or may be administered in conjunction with oxygen or compressed air or respirators (see "Intermittent Positive Pressure Breathing"). The latter method is useful when aerosol treatments need to be administered for 10- or 15-minute periods. Also smaller particles and fine mists of the aerosol can be delivered when IPPB equipment is used to administer drugs. When the patient takes deep, slow breaths, the drug is dispersed into the lower respiratory passages. Hand atomizers, on the other hand, deliver larger droplets and are more effective for the upper respiratory passages.

Artificial Oropharyngeal Airways

The oropharyngeal airway is the simplest type of artificial airway. It is a curved rubber or plastic device

that is used to bypass the obstruction of the tongue lying against the posterior pharynx in unconscious patients. This airway is available in a variety of sizes for children and adults. To determine the appropriate size for a person, the airway is placed externally along the side of the cheek. With the flange of the airway parallel to the front teeth, the airway should extend back to the angle of the jaw. Placement of too large an airway forces the epiglottis down onto the laryngeal opening, thus creating an obstruction.

Insertion of the airway is achieved by gently placing it over the tongue and first pointing it toward the cheek. Once it has passed over the back of the tongue, it is then gently turned so that it is pointing toward the patient's feet. When the flange of the airway is external to the teeth and the curved tip lies at the level of the epiglottis, the airway is correctly placed.

This type of airway is commonly used for patients recovering from anesthesia postoperatively. Once the patient regains consciousness, the mouth piece is dislodged naturally. Suctioning of the airway may be necessary to maintain its patency.

Oral and Nasal Suctioning

Suctioning of the oropharynx and passages is sometimes necessary for patients who have difficulty swallowing or expectorating secretions effectively. *Suctioning* is the aspiration of secretions by a rubber or polyethylene catheter connected to a suction machine or wall outlet. The purposes of this procedure are to maintain the patency of the airway through the mouth and/or nose to the trachea, to obtain secretions for diagnostic purposes, and to prevent the potential for infection that may result from accumulated secretions. Catheters used for suctioning vary in size from 14 to 18 French for adults and from 8 to 18 French for children. The tip of suction catheters has several openings along the sides. These openings distribute the negative pressure of the suction over a wide area, thus preventing excessive irritation to any one area of the respiratory mucous membrane. The suction apparatus includes a collection bottle, a tubing system, which is connected to the suction catheter, and a gauge that registers the degree of suction. These gauges are either portable or wall mounted. Indications to the nurse for suctioning of the upper respiratory airways include (a) inability to cough effectively, (b) inability to swallow, or (c) light bubbling or rattling breath sounds indicating the accumulation of secretions.

Procedure 28-1.   Suctioning Oropharyngeal and Nasal Passages

Action	Explanation
Assemble Equipment	
1. Portable suction machine or gauge to attach to wall suction.	
2. Y-connector (optional)	To facilitate opening and closing of the suction system.
3. Clean disposable suction catheter.	
4. Cup of tap water.	To moisten the catheter.
5. Clean disposable glove or gloves (optional).	
6. Paper bag.	To hold the contaminated catheters.
To Suction the Oral and/or Nasal Passages	
1. Wash hands thoroughly.	Microorganisms can be spread by direct contact.
2. Explain the procedure to the patient, including that the procedure is painless but may stimulate the cough, gag, or sneeze reflexes.	Knowing the procedure will relieve breathing often reassures the patient and elicits his or her cooperation.
3. Position a conscious patient who has a functional gag reflex in the semi-Fowler's position with the patient's head turned to one side for oral suctioning and head hyperextended for nasal suctioning. Position an unconscious patient in the lateral position facing the nurse.	These positions facilitate the insertion of the catheter. This position allows the patient's tongue to fall forward, thus preventing obstruction to the catheter on insertion. It also facilitates drainage of secretions from the pharynx and prevents the possibility of aspiration.

4. Set the pressure on the suction gauge and turn on the suction. For wall units the pressure is set at:
    a. 115 to 150 mm Hg for adults
    b. 95 to 115 mm Hg for children
    c. 50 to 95 mm Hg for infants
For portable units, use:
    a. 10 to 15 in. Hg for adults
    b. 5 to 10 in. Hg for children
    c. 2 to 5 in. Hg for infants (Hunsinger 1973:249)	

5. Moisten the catheter tip by dipping it in the cup of water.	A moistened catheter reduces friction and eases insertion.
6. Encourage the patient to cough if possible.	Coughing moves secretions into the pharynx.
7. Stop the suction pressure temporarily and gently insert the catheter into the mouth or nares. The suction pressure is stopped by (a) pinching the suction catheter between the thumb and forefinger, or (b) leaving the Y-connection, if used, open.	The suction pressure is stopped on insertion to minimize trauma or irritation to the mucous membrane.

Procedure 28-1.   Cont'd.

8. When the catheter is in place, start the suction and withdraw the catheter slowly with a gentle rotating motion. To start the suction release, pinch on the catheter or close the Y-connection with your thumb.

Rotating the catheter between the thumb and fore-finger prevents prolonged suction pressure on any one area of the respiratory mucosa and thus trauma.

9. Apply suction for 10-second periods or less.

Hypoxia can result with prolonged suctioning and the obstruction of the airway by the suction catheter.

10. When the catheter has been removed, rinse the catheter by flushing it with water.

Rinsing the catheter removes secretions from the tubing.

11. Steps 6 to 10 are then repeated until the airways are cleared.

12. Dispose of the catheter, the water, and container and glove if used.

13. Replace used equipment so that it is available for the next suctioning procedure.

Suction collection bottles and tubing are changed daily or more frequently as necessary.

14. Record the amount of secretion, its consistency, color, and odor, and observe the patient's breathing status.

For example, foamy white mucus, thick green-tinged mucus, or blood-flecked mucus.

Oxygen Therapy

Additional oxygen is indicated for numerous patients who have *hypoxemia* (poor blood oxygenation). The conditions that produce hypoxemia are many. Examples are lung congestion from any cause that reduces the diffusion of oxygen through the respiratory membrane, heart failure leading to inadequate transport of oxygen, loss of substantial lung tissue from tumors or surgery, narrowed or obstructed airways from infections, or other disease processes. In most situations, oxygen therapy is prescribed by the physician, who specifies the specific concentration, method, and liter flow per minute. The concentration is of more importance than the liter flow per minute.

In other situations the administration of oxygen is an emergency measure. In these situations the nurse initiates the therapy based upon observations indicating acute hypoxemia. These signs generally include, in order of occurrence:

1. Increased rapid pulse.
2. Rapid, shallow respirations and dyspnea.
3. Increased restlessness or lightheadedness.
4. Flaring of the nares.
5. Substernal or intercostal retractions.
6. Cyanosis.

Difficult breathing creates apprehension and panic. The nurse therefore needs to be competent in providing support and appropriate therapy.

Safety Precautions During Oxygen Therapy

Oxygen will not by itself burn or explode, but it does facilitate combustion. To exemplify, a bed sheet ordinarily burns slowly when ignited in the normal atmosphere; however, if saturated with free-flowing oxygen, it will burn rapidly and explosively when ignited by a spark. The greater the concentration of the oxygen, the more rapidly fires start and burn. Extinguishing such fires can be difficult. Because oxygen is colorless, odorless, and tasteless people are often unaware of the presence of oxygen and need reminding. Safety measures therefore must be taken by the staff, the patient, and visitors. These include the following:

1. Cautionary "No smoking: Oxygen in Use" signs are placed on the patient's door, at the foot or head of the bed, and on the oxygen equipment.

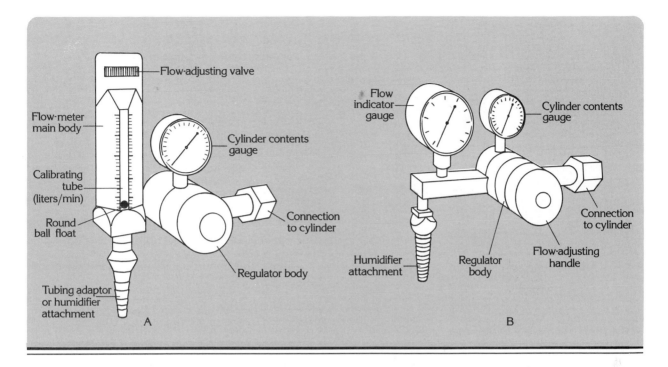

Figure 28-6. Two types of oxygen regulators. **A,** Thorpe tube and, **B,** Bourdon tube.

2. Matches and cigarette lighters are removed from the bedside.

3. Other patients in the room and visitors are requested to smoke in areas provided elsewhere in the hospital.

4. Electrical equipment, such as razors, hearing aids, radios, televisions, and heating pads are removed or put aside in case short-circuit sparks occur.

5. The use of materials that generate static electricity is avoided such as woolen blankets or synthetic fabrics. Cotton blankets are provided, and nurses are advised to wear cotton fabrics.

6. Volatile flammable materials such as oils, greases, alcohol, or ether should not be used on patients receiving oxygen. Lip ointments, if required, should have a water-soluble base such as K-Y Jelly or glycerine. Alcohol back rubs are avoided, and nail polish removers or the like should be removed from the immediate vicinity.

7. Electrical monitoring equipment, suction machines, and portable diagnostic machines should be appropriately grounded when used or not permitted in the vicinity. Oxygen therapy should be discontinued temporarily if portable radiographic equipment is required. Monitoring and suction equipment needs to be placed on the bedside opposite the oxygen source.

8. The location of fire extinguishers such as a carbon dioxide extinguisher and knowledge of their use is an essential precaution should fires occur.

Supply of Oxygen

Oxygen can be supplied from steel cylinders (oxygen tanks) that store 244 cubic feet of oxygen or smaller portable tanks that are commonly used for emergency or home use. The oxygen is stored under a pressure of 2200 psi (pounds per square inch). Many hospitals now provide piped-in oxygen that is supplied from wall outlets by each bed in the room. Piped-in oxygen is usually stored under low pressure, about 50 to 60 psi.

Using Oxygen Tanks.   Oxygen tanks are generally encased in metal carriers equipped with wheels for transport and a broad flat base to stand at the bedside to prevent danger of falling. A cap on the top protects the valves and outlets. Oxygen tanks should be placed beside the bedhead away from traffic areas and heaters. When using oxygen tanks a regulator and a humidifier must be attached. The regulator consists of two parts: a flowmeter and a cylinder contents gauge. The purpose of the regulator is to reduce the pressure in the oxygen cylinder to a safer level. The flowmeter regulates the gas flow in liters per minute. Two types of regulators are shown in Figure 28-6. To assemble the oxygen tank for use the following steps

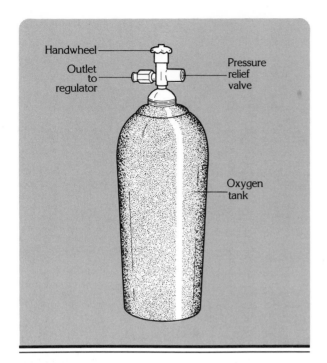

Figure 28-7. Diagram showing basic parts of an oxygen tank.

are required:

1. Remove the protector cap.

2. Remove any dust in the outlets by slightly opening the handwheel at the top of the tank slowly and then closing it quickly. This is referred to as "cracking the tank." People can be frightened if not forewarned of the loud forceful hissing sound that occurs when the tank is opened. To open the tank the handwheel is turned clockwise.

3. Connect the flow regulator gauge to the tank outlet shown in Figure 28-7, and tighten the inlet nut with a wrench, ensuring that the regulator is held firmly.

4. Stand at the side of the cylinder and open the cylinder valve very slowly until the needle on the cylinder gauge stops moving.

5. Regulate the flowmeter to the desired rate of flow in liters per minute. For the Thorpe tube this is done by turning the flow-adjusting valve. If the Bourdon tube is used, turn the flow adjusting handle slowly to the right.

6. Fill the humidifier bottle with distilled water to the mark indicated, and attach it below the flowmeter (see the next section).

7. Attach specific oxygen tubing and equipment prescribed for the patient, for example, a nasal catheter, a nasal cannula, or a face mask.

Using Piped-in Oxygen. To assemble the equipment for piped-in oxygen only a flowmeter and a humidifier are required. The following steps are followed:

1. Attach the flowmeter to the wall outlet, exerting firm pressure. The flowmeter should be in the *off* position.

2. Fill the humidifier bottle with distilled water (this can be done before reaching the bedside).

3. Attach the humidifier bottle to the base of the flowmeter.

4. Attach oxygen tubing and the oxygen device prescribed by the physician.

5. Regulate the flowmeter to the desired level.

Oxygen Humidifying Devices

Oxygen that is administered from a cylinder or from pipeline systems is dry. When dry gases are given to patients, dehydration of the respiratory mucous membranes occurs. Thus humidifying devices are an essential adjunct of oxygen therapy. All humidifiers employ the simple method of passing the gas through sterile water so that water vapor is picked up before being transmitted to the patient. The more bubbles created, the more water vapor produced.

Methods of Oxygen Administration

Oxygen can be administered by a variety of methods. Included are the nasal cannula, nasal catheters, oxygen masks, oxygen tents, including the Croupette, incubators, and respirators. Each method has different advantages and indications.

The Nasal Cannula

The nasal cannula is a relatively simple and comfortable method of supplying oxygen of low concentrations (22% to 30%) at liter flows of 1 to 5 liters per minute. The physician generally specifies the liter flow desired. The cannula does not interfere with the patient's ability to eat and does not bypass the natural respiratory functions of the nose. Freedom to move about in bed or from the bed to an adjacent chair is also possible.

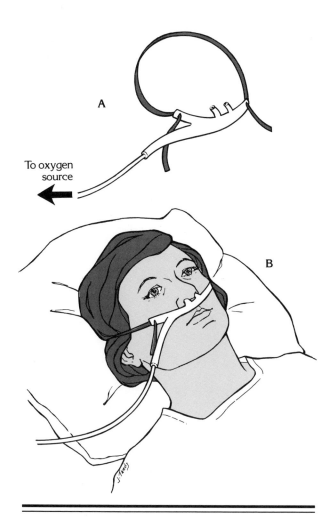

To oxygen source

Figure 28-8. A, A nasal cannula, and **B,** when it is in place.

The cannula consists of a rubber or plastic tube that extends from each cheekbone and has ¼- to ½-inch curved prongs that fit into the nostrils. It is held in place by an elasticized band that can be easily adjusted to fit around the patient's head. Although it is not usually necessary to secure the cannula in place with tape, small pieces may be put over the cannula on each side of the face for patients who are confused or particularly active. (See Figure 28-8.) One side of the tube connects to the oxygen tubing and oxygen supply.

Higher concentration and flow rates can be administered by the nasal cannula; however, with flow rates above 8 liters per minute there is a tendency for air swallowing and irritation of the nasal and pharyngeal mucosa to occur. Primary responsibilities of the nurse in caring for patients with a nasal cannula include the following:

1. Assembling the equipment, including the humidifier.

2. Orienting the patient to this therapy and instructing the patient to breathe through the nose. Mouth breathing dilutes the oxygen concentration received.

3. Instructing the patient about the safety precautions required for oxygen therapy.

4. Changing the cannula every eight hours or as dictated by agency policy to ensure proper functioning.

5. Inspecting the nares for encrustations or irritations and applying a water-soluble lubricant to the nares when necessary.

6. Inspecting the skin for signs of irritation if tape is used to hold the cannula in place.

7. Maintaining the liter flow and the level of the distilled water in the humidifier bottle.

8. Maintaining the patient in a position for optimal lung expansion and encouraging turning and deep breathing exercises every two to four hours.

9. Assessing the patient's vital signs and breathing patterns periodically to determine the patient's response to therapy.

The Nasal Catheter

The nasal catheter is also used to administer low to moderate oxygen concentrations but can deliver higher concentrations of oxygen than the nasal cannula. At flows of 1 to 5 liters per minute, concentrations of 30% to 35% can be achieved. This method of oxygen administration is used more frequently than the nasal cannula in some agencies. It is regarded as effective, allows the same mobility of the patient as the cannula, and is accepted without fear by most patients.

The nasal catheter is a rubber or plastic tube about 16 inches long with six or eight holes at the tip to disperse the oxygen. (See Figure 28-9.) It is inserted

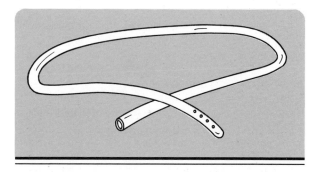

Figure 28-9. A nasal catheter, illustrating the holes through which the oxygen flows into the patient.

through the nares to the entrance of the oropharynx. Sterile disposable plastic catheters are preferred. Sizes vary from no. 8 to 14 French. Because the use of nasal catheters causes irritation and dehydration to nasal passages, lubrication of the tube is required prior to insertion, and humidification is essential during therapy. A doctor's order is required for this procedure indicating the flow rate desired. The specific method for inserting a nasal catheter is outlined in Procedure 28-2.

Procedure 28-2.   Initiating Oxygen Therapy by Nasal Catheter

Action	Explanation
Assemble Equipment	
Check doctor's order.	To determine flow rate desired.
1. Nasal catheter of appropriate size.	No. 8 or 10 French for children; 10 or 12 French for women; 12 or 14 French for men.
2. Oxygen connecting tubing.	
3. Flowmeter or regulator.	For piped-in oxygen; for oxygen cylinder.
4. Humidifier filled with sterile distilled water.	To moisten and vaporize the oxygen.
5. "No smoking" signs.	
6. Water-soluble lubricating jelly and a gauze square.	To facilitate catheter insertion.
7. Adhesive tape (nonallergenic preferred).	To secure catheter to the patient's face.
8. Flashlight and tongue depressor.	To help assess correct placement of the catheter.
9. Glass of water.	To test the oxygen flow.
Initiate Therapy	
1. Teach the patient about the therapy and the safety precautions required.	Answer questions and allay anxiety if present.
2. Put up the "No smoking" signs.	
3. Assemble the equipment.	
a. Attach the flowmeter to the wall outlet or the regulator to the oxygen tank after cracking the tank.	
b. Attach the humidifier to the flowmeter.	
c. Attach the oxygen connecting tubing to the humidifier and to the catheter.	
d. Test the oxygen flow by turning on the oxygen flowmeter to 3 liters per minute and inserting the tip of the catheter into the glass of water.	Bubbling in the water indicates that oxygen flow is satisfactory.
4. Measure the length to insert the catheter by placing the end of the catheter in a straight line between the tip of the patient's nose and the ear lobe. This distance can be marked with tape. (See Figure 28-10.)	

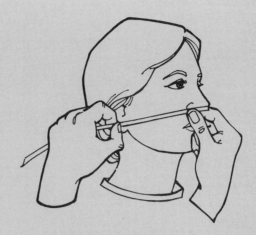

Figure 28-10.

5. Lubricate the tip of the catheter with water-soluble jelly. The lubricant can be squeezed into a square gauze and the catheter rotated over it.

Lubrication facilitates insertion and prevents injury to the nasal mucous membrane. Avoid the use of mineral oil or petroleum jelly, since, if aspirated, these can cause severe lung irritations or lipoid pneumonia.

6. Start the flow of oxygen at about 3 liters per minute prior to inserting the tube.

The flow of oxygen prevents the catheter from becoming plugged by secretions during insertion.

7. Introduce the nasal catheter slowly into the naris to the previously marked distance. The patient may prefer to hyperextend the head.

Never force the tube if an obstruction is encountered. Remove the catheter and insert it into the other naris.

8. Check that the position of the catheter is at the entrance to the oropharynx by (a) having the patient open the mouth widely, (b) depressing the tongue with the tongue blade, and (c) directing the flashlight into the throat. Be careful to avoid inducing the gag reflex. (See Figure 28-11.)

The tip of the catheter should rest at or beside the level of the uvula. If the patient gags or coughs, the catheter is positioned too deeply.

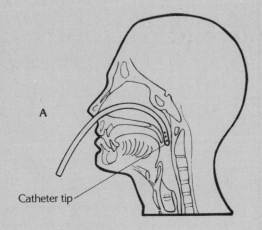

A

Catheter tip

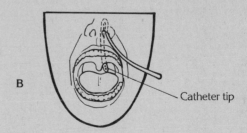

B

Catheter tip

Figure 28-11.

Procedure 28-2.   Cont'd.

9. Withdraw the catheter slightly until the tip is no longer seen.

10. Adjust the oxygen flow rate to the prescribed liters per minute.

11. Tape the nasal catheter to the patient's face (see Figure 28-12), (a) to the side of the nose and the cheek or (b) to the tip of the nose and the forehead.

This position prevents the patient from swallowing oxygen, which may result in gastric distention.

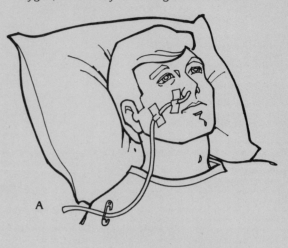

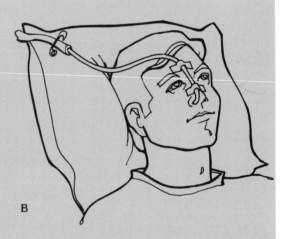

Figure 28-12.

12. Secure the connecting tubing to the bed or to the patient's gown with an elastic band and a safety pin.

13. Record the initiation of the procedure and the patient's response to therapy, including time, method, and liter flow rate.

Leave enough slack in the tubing to allow movement by the patient.

Nursing responsibilities when caring for patients with a nasal catheter are similar to those for the patient with a nasal cannula. The nasal catheter also needs changing every eight hours. The catheters should be inserted alternately in one naris and then the other. This prevents the development of encrustations and irritation of the respiratory mucosa.

The Oxygen Face Mask

A variety of face masks that cover the patient's nose and mouth are marketed for oxygen inhalation. Oxygen concentrations with masks generally range from about 25% to 60% at flow rates of 8 to 12 liters per minute. A few are designed to deliver 100% con-

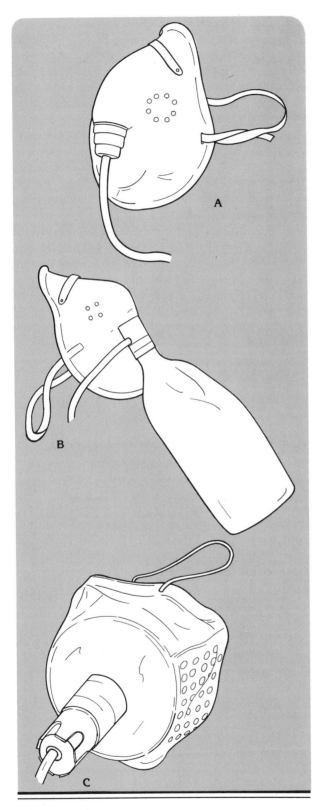

centrations. However, concentrations above 60% are rarely prescribed because of the danger of oxygen toxicity. Oxygen face masks are advantageous also for patients who are unable to breathe solely through their nose. Most masks are made of clear pliable plastic or rubber that can be molded to fit the face snugly. A metal clip is provided on some that can be bent over the bridge of the nose for a snug fit. They also have several holes in the sides (exhalation ports) to allow the escape of exhaled carbon dioxide. The masks are fastened to the patient's head with elasticized bands. See Figure 28-13 for various types of masks. Some masks have reservoir bags attached. These are also referred to as *partial rebreathing bags.* They provide for higher oxygen concentrations to the patient in that a portion of the patient's expired air is directed into the bag and rebreathed. Because this air is dead-space air, which does not take part in gaseous exchange, its oxygen concentration remains high. Thus when this air is added to the inflow from the oxygen source, an increased oxygen concentration is provided.

To initiate oxygen therapy by a face mask the nurse follows most of the same steps of preparation as for nasal cannula and nasal catheter except that an appropriate size of face mask must be obtained. Smaller sizes are available for children. To apply the face mask the following steps are recommended if the patient is conscious:

1. Familiarize the patient with the mask when possible. Allow the patient to hold the mask, guide it toward the face, and get used to the feel of it covering the nose and mouth. Instruct the patient to apply it from the nose downward during expiration.

2. Turn on the oxygen to the liter flow prescribed and allow the patient to adjust to the flow of the oxygen. When a reservoir bag is used, the bag should be first flushed with oxygen until it is partially inflated.

3. Gradually fit the mask to the contours of the face, and encourage the patient to breathe normally. The mask should be molded adequately to prevent oxygen escaping upward into the patient's eyes or around the cheeks or chin. If a reservoir bag is used, the oxygen flow must be adjusted to a level that prevents the bag from collapsing by a deep inspiration of the patient.

4. Secure the elasticized band around the patient's head, and adjust it for a comfortable but snug fit.

5. See that the patient is positioned comfortably in the semi-Fowler's or high Fowler's position.

Figure 28-13. Three types of oxygen masks. **A,** Oxygen mask, **B,** Oxygen mask with partial rebreathing bag. Note fewer holes at the sides than in **A, C,** Venturi mask used to control concentrations. Rebreathing is prevented by the high air flow that enters the mask.

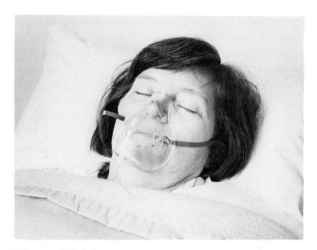

Figure 28-14.   An oxygen mask worn by a patient.

6. Stay until the patient is at ease. Some patients respond with panic, restlessness, and fear of suffocation. (See Figure 28-14 for an oxygen mask in place.)

7. Inform the patient of the frequency of your return visits in accordance with the patient's needs. This should be within minutes in the early part of therapy, such as every 10 to 15 minutes. Leave the call light within easy reach.

8. Assess the patient's pulse rate and breathing rates and patterns.

9. Record the initiation of therapy and the patient's response.

To maintain oxygen therapy by face mask, observe the same procedures as for the nasal catheter and cannula regarding (a) maintaining the flow rate, (b) maintaining the level of distilled water in the humidifier bottle, (c) positioning the patient appropriately, (d) encouraging adequate hydration, movement, and deep breathing exercises, (e) preserving safety precautions, and (f) observing the patient's progress. In addition, the face mask needs to be removed periodically (every two hours) to observe the status of the skin. Condensation occurs, and the patient's face needs to be sponged and dried. Mouth care to lubricate the oral mucous membranes is also essential, since mouth breathing has a drying effect.

The Oxygen Tent

The oxygen tent provides the patient with controlled oxygen concentrations and in addition an environment of controlled temperature and high humidity. It also provides the patient with a feeling of freedom to move about in bed. On the other hand, it also can incur feelings of isolation. Oxygen tents are currently used less frequently than other methods of oxygen administration, perhaps because high volumes of oxygen are required to maintain desired concentrations. A minimum of 10 liters per minute is required for an oxygen tent. Tents can supply concentrations up to 60%. However, loss of the desired concentration occurs each time the tent is opened to provide nursing care. Another disadvantage is that the equipment is nondisposable and requires cleansing and maintenance repairs. In some instances the oxygen tent may be used for its humidifying purposes only as is the Croupette for infants and children. This use, however, is rare.

Oxygen tents consist of a clear plastic canopy that is placed over the upper half of the bed and a motor unit driven by electricity. Two large round accordion-like hoses connect the motor with the canopy. The gauges on the motor unit include (a) a power switch that turns the machine on or off, (b) a temperature dial, and (c) a circulation dial that can be set between degrees of low and high.

To initiate oxygen therapy using a tent the following steps are required:

1. Place the tent to one side of the head of the bed with the control knobs away from it.

2. Plug the machine into the electrical outlet.

3. Attach the flowmeter to the wall outlet or the regulator to the oxygen tank, and then connect either to the oxygen outlet or the tent.

4. Set up the humidifier or nebulizer. Some units have a water tray at the back of the machine that requires filling; others use a separate nebulizer. Water pans are filled with 500 ml of distilled water.

5. Set up the canopy and place it loosely over the head of the bed.

6. Turn the power switch to the *on* position.

7. Set the temperature dial at about 21° to 22°C (70° to 72°F).

8. Set the circulation dial midway between high and low.

9. Flush the tent with oxygen (a) by setting the flowmeter at 15 liters per minute or (b) for tents that have flush button controls, by pressing the flush button for 1 minute.

10. Place the canopy over the patient, allowing as much space as possible inside. Tuck in all sides. The front may be fan folded with a drawsheet over the patient's thighs. Ensure that the side zippers are closed.

11. Regulate the flowmeter at a *minimum* of 10 liters per minute. This rate of flow is necessary to allow for adequate removal of carbon dioxide.

The same general nursing responsibilities apply for patients in oxygen tents, such as (a) turning the patient every two to four hours and positioning the patient to ensure adequate lung expansion, for example, in the high or semi-Fowler's position, (b) maintaining the oxygen flow rates and appropriate humidification and temperature, (c) preserving safety precautions, (d) encouraging adequate hydration and deep breathing exercises, and (e) observing the patient's progress by evaluating vital signs and color.

In addition, it is necessary to check the oxygen concentration in the tent at regular intervals (every four to seven hours). This is done with a special instrument called an *oxygen analyzer*. To acquire accurate readings the tent must be closed for 10 or 15 minutes prior to the analysis.

It is important also that nursing care measures for patients in oxygen tents are planned in such a way that the tent is opened as little as possible. Some agencies advise that the tent be flushed with oxygen for a minute or two after all nursing care measures. This compensates for the loss of oxygen concentration when the tent has been opened.

Some patients feel isolated and anxious in an oxygen tent. Planned regular visits by the nurse can be reassuring. A call bell within easy reach is also advised. Some agencies recommend the use of a manual call bell rather than the electrical bedside bell, which may become a fire hazard if short circuited. Many patients also complain of coldness. Providing additional cotton bed clothing or increasing the tent temperature usually suffices.

Intermittent Positive Pressure Breathing Therapy

Intermittent positive pressure breathing (IPPB) is a breathing pattern established by inflating the lungs with positive pressure (above atmospheric) during inspiration and by releasing the pressure so that expiration occurs passively. Positive pressure is also occasionally administered by some sophisticated machines during the expiratory phase, so that the abbreviations sometimes used to differentiate these methods are IPPB/I (inspiratory) and IPPB/E (expiratory). Generally, when the term *IPPB* is used, however, it refers to positive pressure therapy administered during inspiration, a safer and more common practice. As with most oxygen equipment, various types of

IPPB machines are marketed. Two commonly used ones are the Bird Respirator and the Bennett Respirator. Usually IPPB treatments are given by respiratory technicians or by nurses who have had special training programs. However, the general nurse needs to understand the reasons for its use and the principles of operation to assist patients as needed in the absence of special technicians. The nurse must also observe the patient's response and progress to such therapy. This discussion is limited to IPPB therapy that is patient activated and given on an intermittent basis rather than the controlled or time-cycled continuous therapy for patients who are unable to initiate inspiration. The latter therapy controls the patient's breathing artificially and entirely by machine. The learner is referred to more advanced readings for such material.

The Bird Respirator

There are several types of Bird Respirators; however, all are equipped with six basic controls (see Figure 28-15).

1. *Pressure control setting.* This control (A) sets the pressure that will be received at the height of inspiration before the patient enters the expiratory phase. It measures the pressure in centimeters of water pressure from 0 to 60 cm. Usually the pressure is started low at 15 or 20 cm water pressure. This control can be likened to placing one's finger over the end of a faucet to increase the pressure.

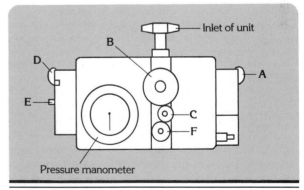

Figure 28-15. Bird respirator. **A,** Pressure control setting for the height of inspiration; **B,** flow rate control for rate of flow of air or oxygen; **C,** air mix plunger, when pulled out, delivers 40% oxygen and 60% air—when pushed in, 100% oxygen is delivered; **D,** sensitivity control which starts flow of air or oxygen in accordance with the inspiratory effort expended by the patient; **E.** manual control knob that can start ventilator; and **F,** expiratory time control that is turned to off position for patient-cycle ventilator.

2. *Flow rate control.* This control (B) adjusts the inspiratory time and switches the ventilator from *off* to *on*. Likened to a water tap, the more it is turned on the faster the flow of gas. Low numbers on this dial indicate slow rates, and higher numbers indicate faster rates. Since the aim of therapy is usually to achieve deep respirations and transfer of gases deep into the alveoli, the flow rate is generally set at about 10 or less. Fast flow rates tend to flood only the upper respiratory tract. Effective flow rates can be assessed by observing the patient's chest expansion during therapy.

3. *Air mix plunger.* This control (C) determines the proportion of oxygen and air delivered to the patient. When the plunger is pushed in, 100% oxygen is delivered. When it is pulled out, a mixture of 40% oxygen and 60% air is delivered. These proportions cannot be varied as on the more sophisticated respirators. Generally the oxygen/air mixture is used.

4. *Sensitivity control.* This control (D) adjusts the inspiratory effort required by the patient to trigger or trip the machine (start the flow of gas). Once the machine is triggered, the pressure automatically builds up to its peak pressure that was set by the pressure control knob. The smaller the number that is set on the sensitivity control the higher is the sensitivity. In other words, less effort is required by the patient to start the machine if a low number on the sensitivity control is used. Patients who are weak often require a high sensitivity control (low number) to start the machine, but patients who need to be encouraged to breathe deeply should use a low sensitivity control (high number) that offers more resistance and requires more effort. It is usually set at 15 when starting therapy.

5. *Manual control knob.* This pink knob or pin below the sensitivity control (E) can be manually pushed in to cycle the ventilator on. It is mostly used to check the respirator function before applying it to the patient.

6. *Expiratory time control.* This control (F) is turned to the *off* position for patient-cycled IPPB. It is used only for patients who are apneic or who require continuous assisted ventilation. When turned on, the expiration times cycle automatically.

Assembly and maintenance of respirators is usually done by oxygen therapists. The machine is connected to an oxygen supply and is equipped with an in-line humidifier, which must be filled with distilled water. The patient breathes through a mouthpiece or a mask attached to the end of the respirator tubing.

The Bennett Respirator

This respirator is different in appearance from the Bird Respirator, but its operation is similar. The PR-1 model, which is frequently used, has the same basic controls previously discussed (see Figure 28-16).

1. The pressure control knob (A), capable of delivering 0 to 45 cm of water pressure, is rotated clockwise and generally set at 15 to 20 cm water for adults or 10 to 12 cm water for children.

2. The control pressure gauge (B) records the pressure that is reached by turning dial A.

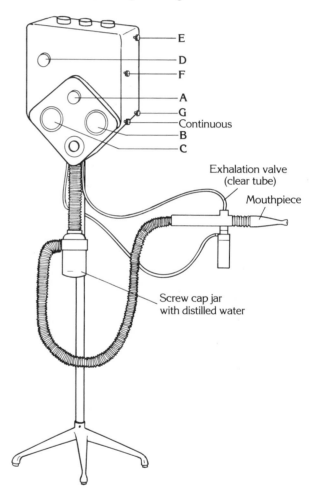

Figure 28-16. Bennet Respirator PR I. **A,** Pressure control knob; **B,** control pressure gauge that records pressure reached by setting the pressure control knob; **C,** system pressure gauge that should equal the pressure shown in B and the one required by the patient to start the machine; **D,** rate control for automatic cycled IPPB; **E,** sensitivity control; **F,** air dilution control that is pushed in for a mixture of oxygen and air; and **G,** nebulization control.

3. The system pressure gauge (C) records the pressure that is required by the patient and should equal that measured in B.

4. The rate control (D) controls the rate of automatic cycling and is turned to the *off* position for patient-cycled IPPB.

5. The sensitivity control (E) controls the amount of inspiratory effort required to start inspiration and is used only if the patient has difficulty triggering the machine. Indications of difficulty are determined when patients say they are sucking or drawing on the machine to no avail or when the system pressure gauge needle deflects to the negative side. In these instances the sensitivity control should be set higher so that less effort is required by the patient to trigger the machine.

6. The air dilution control (F) is usually pushed in to allow for an air-oxygen mixture. When it is pulled out, 100% oxygen is delivered.

7. The nebulization controls (G) provide power to the side steam nebulizer to deliver aerosol medications. One knob sets the nebulization for continuous therapy, the other for inspiratory nebulization. If the patient is receiving a medicated treatment, the inspiration knob is generally turned one revolution to ensure adequate nebulization on inspiration. The continuous nebulization valve is generally turned only a fourth of a revolution, since the delivery of medication on expiration is unnecessary.

Indications for IPPB

IPPB therapy is prescribed frequently for patients for 15- to 20-minute periods three or four times a day. The purposes of therapy include either one or a combination of the following:

1. To deliver aerosol medications such as antibiotics, bronchodilators, detergents, or mucolytics.

2. To periodically increase the depth of respiration and prevent accumulation of secretions that may result in infections or atelectasis (lung collapse).

3. To facilitate the clearing of bronchial secretions in patients who have difficulty coughing or inspiring deeply.

4. To orient patients preoperatively to the IPPB therapy that may be used postoperatively.

5. To provide moisture to the respiratory mucous membranes.

Assisting Patients with IPPB

For IPPB therapy the patient needs to be placed in the upright position, preferably in a chair or in the high Fowler's position. The upright position provides the most adequate ventilation of the lungs. The patient also needs to be taught to breathe through the mouth and not the nose. Nose clips are available but are not usually necessary with appropriate instruction. Have the patient practice with a mouthpiece prior to therapy. The mouthpiece must be completely sealed by the lips and made airtight for the IPPB system to operate efficiently.

Encouraging the patient to breathe normally is also helpful. Some patients have a tendency to force their respiration or to struggle with the apparatus. When advised against forcing breaths and to relax, to breathe slowly, and to allow time for expiration (this takes longer than inspiration), these patients normally adjust to the therapy readily. Remind patients that they control the respirator: each time patients breathe in, they start the machine; each time patients breathe out, they stop the machine. Extra effort is not required, nor is there need to be dictated by the machine. The machine will not start until the patient breathes in. It is often necessary in addition to encourage the patient to allow the maximum pressure to reach its peak before exhaling. The patient should try not to breathe out until the positive pressure respirator fills the lungs.

The nurse needs to observe the patient's lung expansion during therapy and the adequacy of the therapy. The degree of lung expansion can be visually observed; however, the gauges on the respirator can be more reliable measures. If the needle gauge on the respirator reaches the preset pressure levels as the patient inhales, then the adequacy of respiration can be considered satisfactory. However, if inadequate or no deflection of the needle gauges occurs, the nurse needs to assess the problem. Is the system airtight? Perhaps the patient has not sealed the lips around the mouthpiece adequately. Is the patient relaxed? Perhaps the patient is not breathing normally. Perhaps the patient is blowing back into the mouthpiece before the lungs are filled. Is the machine not triggering? Perhaps the patient does not have sufficient inspiratory effort to start the machine, in which case the sensitivity gauge needs to be adjusted. Perhaps the patient is sucking or using too much inspiratory effort, so that the needle deflection is too negative. By staying with the patient during IPPB therapy the nurse can provide constructive assistance and instruction.

RESUSCITATION

Resuscitation includes all measures that are applied to revive patients who have stopped breathing due to either respiratory or cardiac failure. *Artificial respiration* is used when the patient's breathing has stopped while the heart continues to beat. *External cardiac massage* is used when both the heartbeat and breathing have stopped. In such an instance both artificial respiration and external cardiac massage are applied at the same time. Thus it is often referred to as *cardiopulmonary resuscitation* (CPR). Other measures may include administration of oxygen and use of mechanical resuscitators such as the Ambu-resuscitator.

Artificial Respiration

The purpose of artificial respiration is to force air into and out of the lungs. This is achieved in three ways: (a) oral resuscitation, that is mouth-to-mouth or mouth-to-nose resuscitation, (b) intermittent manual compression of the chest and arm lifting by the revised Sylvester method, and (c) hand compressible breathing bags. The oral resuscitation method is the most effective method, since larger volumes of air can be moved in and out of the lungs than by either of the chest compression methods. It also has the advantage of being applied instantly wherever and in whatever position the victim is found. For children and for patients who have injured chests such as fractured ribs, oral resuscitation is particularly beneficial. On the other hand, the chest compression methods may be necessary when the victim has mouth or jaw injuries or when the rescuer finds it difficult to provide oral resuscitation for physical, emotional, or cultural reasons. Hand compressible breathing bags, such as the Ambu-resuscitator, are frequently supplied in hospitals or ambulances and are the preferred method if available.

Oral Resuscitation

Mouth-to-mouth breathing makes use of the large amount of air that a normal person can inspire and therefore can breathe into the victim's lungs. Although the oxygen content of expired air is slightly reduced, it is sufficient for revival.

Procedure 28-3.   Oral Resuscitation

Action	Explanation
1. Clear the patient's mouth and the back of the throat of any obstructive material.	This is done manually using the index finger. Remove fluids by turning the patient's head to the side or face down.
2. Place the patient in the supine position on a hard surface if possible.	A folded coat or pillow can be placed under the victim's shoulders.
3. Tilt the patient's head back as far as possible and lift the jaw upward (see Figure 28-17).	This position ensures an open airway. The tongue is prevented from falling back to obstruct the airway. The forehead is pressed backward with one hand while the neck is supported by the opposite hand. Spontaneous breathing may occur with the airway opened.
4. Pinch the patient's nostrils closed.	Use the index finger and the thumb of the hand on the patient's forehead.
5. Take a deep breath, place your widely opened mouth over the patient's mouth, and blow forcibly	Ensure an airtight seal over the patient's mouth. Observe the expansion of the patient's chest.

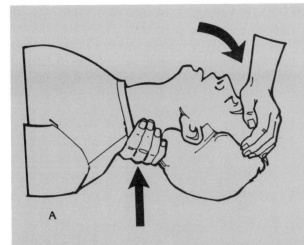

A

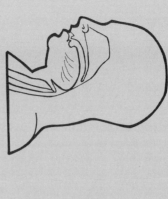

B

Figure 28-17.

enough to make the patient's chest rise; *or,* for mouth-to-nose resuscitation, cover the patient's mouth with two fingers and enclose the patient's nose tightly by making contact with the patient's cheeks around the nose. (See Figure 28-18.)

Figure 28-18.

6. After each inflation move your mouth away from the patient's mouth.

To allow for air to escape when the patient exhales and to allow for inhalation yourself.

7. Repeat inflation 12 to 20 times per minute about every three to five seconds, until the patient breathes spontaneously.

For children more gentle puffs of air are required about 20 to 30 times per minute, and the rescuer's mouth is placed over both the mouth and nose.

It is important to watch for chest expansion each time the lungs are inflated. If this fails to occur, ensure that the head is hyperextended and the jaw lifted upward, or check again for the presence of obstructive material, fluid, or vomitus.

The Revised Sylvester Method

The revised Sylvester method of resuscitation is recommended by the St. John Ambulance Association (1972:85). This method of resuscitation requires that the patient is flat on his or her back on a firm surface. The shoulders need to be elevated on a thick folded blanket or something similar. The head must tilt backward to raise the tongue off the back of the throat, thus opening the airway. Prior to resuscitation the mouth and throat should be cleared of foreign material. This revised Sylvester method includes two phases: the chest compression phase and the chest expansion phase.

Procedure 28-4.   The Revised Sylvester Method

Action	Explanation
Compression Phase	
1. Kneel at the patient's head facing the patient's chest.	
2. Grasp the patient's wrists and place them over the lower half of the sternum (breastbone).	
3. Rock forward and press firmly downward on the patient's chest for a few seconds. Exert just enough pressure to compress the patient's chest. (See Figure 28-19, A.)	This action forces the air out of the lungs. Counting "one and two and" during compression assures adequate timing.
Expansion Phase	
4. Next, lift and stretch the patient's arms upward, outward, and backward for a few seconds. (See Figure 28-19, B.)	This action pulls air into the lungs by expanding the chest wall. Counting "three and four and" during expansion assures adequate inhalation time.
5. On the count of "five" the patient's wrists are placed back across the sternum.	

Figure 28-19.

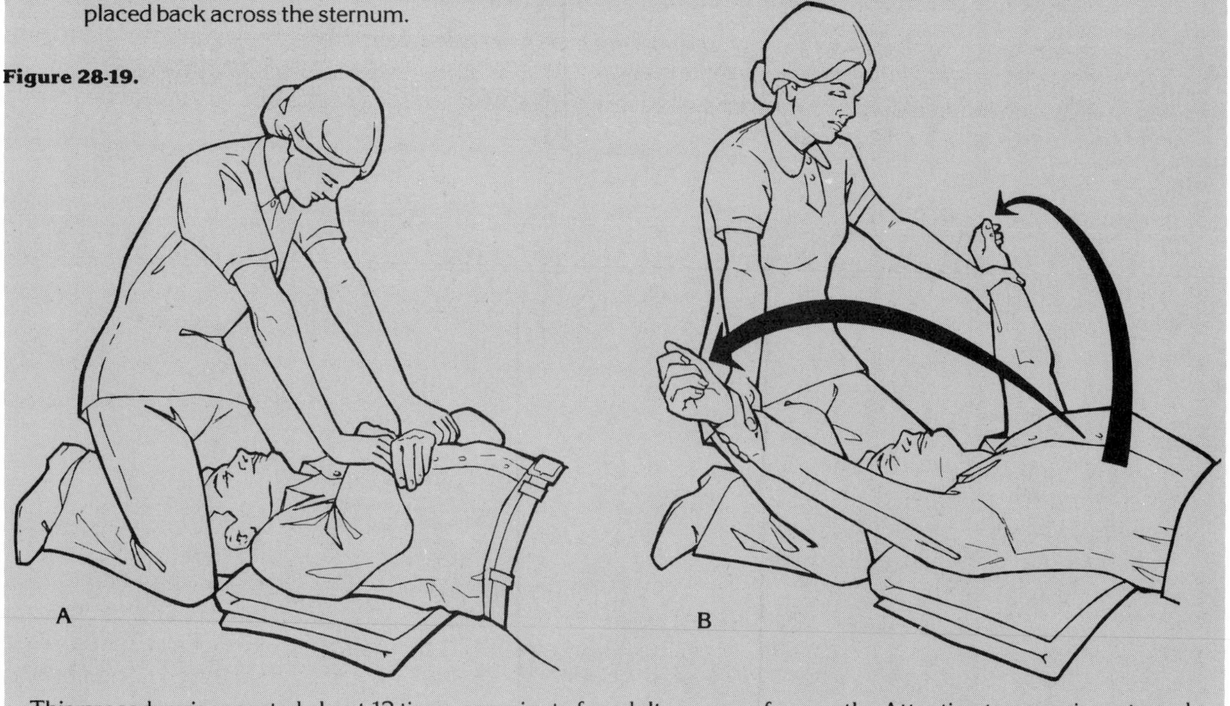

A

B

This procedure is repeated about 12 times per minute for adults or more frequently. Attention to a precise rate and rhythm is not essential.

Hand-Compressible Breathing Bags

Rubberized breathing bags that are attached to face masks are available in many agencies for respiratory resuscitation. A common one is the Ambu-bag. They are easily applied and used. The bags are compressed by the hand to deliver air into the mask and rapidly self-inflate through a valve system after compression. The exhaled air of the patient is released through an exhaust valve to prevent its entry back into the bag. One significant advantage to this method of resuscitation is that supplemental oxygen can be attached. Use of this method of resuscitation incorporates the same measures as other ventilation methods. The patient is positioned on the back, with the shoulders elevated, head hyperextended, and jaw upward. The resuscitator stands at the patient's head and nose. One hand is used to secure the mask at the top and bottom as well as hold the jaw forward (see Figure 28-20). The other hand is used to alternately squeeze and release the bag. The compression on the bag is released when sufficient elevation of the patient's chest is observed. Ventilation is repeated 12 to 15 times per minute. The same preliminary actions of clearing the mouth and throat are essential prior to this procedure or when insufficient lung expansion occurs.

Cardiopulmonary Resuscitation

Cardiac arrest refers to a sudden state of apnea and circulatory failure. It is a dramatic event that requires instant respiratory resuscitation and cardiac stimulation and massage. Within only four to six minutes after cardiac arrest, permanent brain and heart damage can result from the oxygen lack. Causes of cardiac arrest are many and include electrocution, myocardial infarction (heart attack), respiratory failure, extensive hemorrhage, and brain injuries. The three cardinal signs of cardiac arrest are (a) apnea, (b) absence of a carotid or femoral pulse, and (c) dilated pupils.

The person's skin will also appear pale or grayish and feel cool. Cyanosis is evident when respiratory function fails prior to heart failure. The three cardinal signs must be assessed prior to resuscitation.

The ABC's of cardiopulmonary resuscitation (CPR) are as follows:

A: clear the *airways*.

B: initiate artificial *breathing* (oral resuscitation).

C: initiate *cardiac* compression or artificial *circulation*.

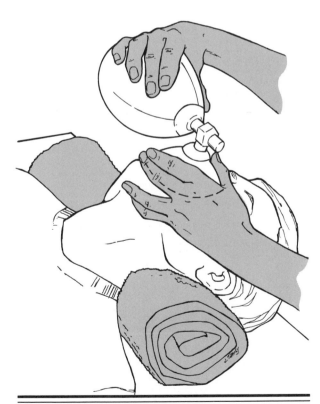

Figure 28-20. A diagram of the Ambu resuscitator in use. Note how one hand secures the mask and holds the jaw forward and how the other hand is used to compress and release the bag.

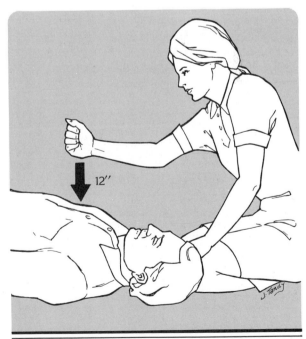

Figure 28-21. Providing a precordial thump to a patient's chest. Recommended for use only during witnessed cardiac arrest and only during the first minute of arrest.

These measures are provided in this sequence because spontaneous breathing may occur after any one action, such as after the airway is opened or after a few artificial respirations are provided. For the steps involved to clear the airway and to initiate breathing, see Procedure 28-3. If the arrest is witnessed, a *precordial thump* is recommended prior to initiating cardiac compression. It is administered by sharply hitting the middle of the sternum (breastbone) with the fist, the bottom fleshy part. In some instances the heart will resume beating and a carotid pulse will then be palpable after this blow is delivered. If the carotid pulse cannot be palpated after this thump, cardiac compression is started immediately. The precordial thump is not recommended for children or for arrests that are unwitnessed. Even in arrests that are witnessed the precordial thump is advised for use only during the first minute of the arrest. (See Figure 28-21.)

External Cardiac Compression

The purpose of external cardiac compression is to provide *artificial circulation.* It reproduces the normal intermittent heart contractions that pump blood throughout the body. *External cardiac compression* consists of manual intermittent rhythmical compression to the sternum using the heel of the hand. Thus the heart is squeezed between the sternum and the vertebrae lying posteriorly. The effectiveness of cardiac resuscitation depends equally upon simultaneous artificial respiration to oxygenate the bloodstream.

Procedure 28-5.   External Cardiac Compression

Action	Explanation
1. Position the patient on the back on a flat, firm surface.	A cardiac board is provided in some agencies to place under the back of a bed patient. If necessary, the floor may be used.
2. Kneel along one side of the patient's chest.	For bed patients it is often necessary to kneel on the patient's bed.
3. Place the heel of one hand in parallel fashion to the long axis of the sternum on the lower third of the sternum above the xiphoid process (the tip). Keep the fingers elevated from the chest wall.	Use of the heel of the hand exerts pressure only on the sternum. Pressure elsewhere can create rib fractures if excessive force is used. For children the heel of the hand is placed over the middle third of the sternum, and for infants the tips of the index and middle fingers only are used.
4. Place the heel of the other hand on top of the first hand. The fingers may be interlocked.	Your shoulders should be positioned over the patient's sternum and your elbows locked.
5. Press firmly downward on the sternum by rocking from the shoulders.	For adults the sternum should be depressed 1½ to 2 inches; for children, about 1 inch; and for infants, about ½ inch.
6. Release the pressure, taking care *not* to change the position of your hands *nor* to move them off the chest wall.	
7. Rhythmically continue cardiac compression at the rate of 60 per minute (for adults) until circulation is restored or until other assistance becomes available.	For young children and for infants the rate of compression is 80 to 100 per minute.

Note: Cardiac compression administered by one person must be interrupted periodically to inflate the lungs by mouth-to-mouth resuscitation. It is recommended that four lung inflations be given prior to cardiac compression, then two inflations are given after every 15 cardiac compressions. A rhythmical pattern needs to be maintained. To achieve a compression rate of 60 per minute, the single rescuer needs to compress at a rate of 80 compressions per minute. This accommodates for the times taken to inflate the lungs. Cardiac compression administered by two persons is easier. One person provides the cardiac compression at a rate of 60 per minute while the other provides artificial respiration. One ventilation is provided after every five cardiac compressions. These can be interposed without interruption of cardiac compression. See Figure 28-22.

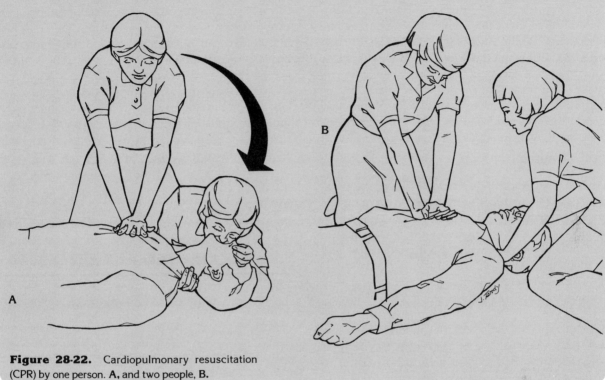

Figure 28-22. Cardiopulmonary resuscitation (CPR) by one person. **A,** and two people, **B.**

SUMMARY

Respiration is vital to the body's functioning and survival. Normally it occurs effortlessly without conscious awareness. However, when maximal demands for energy are required such as during strenuous exercise or when respiratory disease is present, a person becomes acutely aware of the mechanics of inspiration and expiration. The process of respiration can be subdivided into three phases: pulmonary ventilation, diffusion of oxygen and carbon dioxide, and transportation of these respiratory gases to and from the cells.

Ventilation includes the processes of inspiration and expiration, both of which are associated with changes in pulmonary volumes and pressures. The pulmonary volumes include the total volume, the inspiratory and expiratory reserve volumes, and the residual volume. All of these volumes added together are referred to as the *total lung capacity*. When two or more of the pulmonary volumes are considered in combination, they are referred to as *pulmonary capacities* (inspiratory, vital, and functional residual). These capacities are frequently assessed by spirometry to determine the degree of lung impairment in persons with respiratory disease. Changes in pulmonary pressures also occur during ventilation. These pressure changes are indirectly related to the volume changes and account for the movement of air into and out of the lungs. Four essential requirements for adequate ventilation are (a) adequate atmospheric oxygen, (b) patency of the air passages, (c) sufficient pulmonary compliance and recoil, and (d) satisfactory regulatory mechanisms.

Diffusion of the respiratory gases through the respiratory membrane is the second phase of respiration. Four major factors influence the rate of this diffusion. These are the thickness of the membrane, the surface area of the membrane, the diffusion coefficient of the gas, and the pressure difference on each side of the membrane. Disease conditions can affect any or all of these four factors and seriously impair this phase of respiration. Examples are pulmonary edema, carbon monoxide poisoning, and emphysema. In clinical situations the pressure gradients of oxygen and carbon dioxide are frequently measured to assess deficiencies or excesses.

The third phase of respiration includes the transport of oxygen to the cells and the transport of carbon dioxide from the cells. The rate of oxygen transport to the cells is influenced largely by the cardiac output, the number of circulating erythrocytes, exercise, and the blood hematocrit.

The assessment of the respiratory and circulatory status of patients is a frequent and essential function of the nurse. The methods used to assess the chest cage, lungs, heart, pulse, and respirations were discussed in Chapter 14. Emphasized in this chapter were the terms used to describe breathing patterns, breath sounds, chest movements, secretions and coughing, and circulatory status.

Four general nursing interventions implemented by the nurse to maintain normal respirations of patients are outlined. These are positioning patients to facilitate maximal lung expansion, encouraging frequent deep breathing exercises and coughing, providing adequate hydration to moisten the respiratory membranes, and promoting individual health practices and a healthy environment.

For persons who suffer respiratory impairment a variety of additional measures may be prescribed. Postural drainage along with percussion and vibration are implemented when secretions accumulate and are retained in various lung segments. Additional humidification may be provided by hot steam inhalators or the Croupette humidity tent for infants and young children. Nebulization therapy is an effective means of delivering required medications onto the respiratory membrane. Artificial oropharyngeal airways and oral and nasal suctioning may be necessitated to maintain airway patency in uncon-

scious patients or for those who have difficulty swallowing or expectorating secretions. Additional oxygen is frequently indicated for patients to relieve hypoxemia. A variety of methods are used to administer oxygen. These include the nasal cannula, the nasal catheter, the face mask, the oxygen tent, and positive pressure machines such as the Bird and Bennett Respirators. The safety precautions required during oxygen therapy are emphasized, since oxygen supports combustion. For each of the therapies just mentioned, the nurse's responsibilities in administering and maintaining the therapy and in caring for the patient are outlined.

Knowledge and skill in resuscitation techniques are mandatory for nurses. The resuscitation techniques include oral resuscitation, the revised Sylvester method, use of hand compressible breathing bags, and external cardiac compression. Nurses need to become skilled in performing cardiopulmonary resuscitation as a single rescuer and in partnership with another rescuer.

SUGGESTED ACTIVITIES

1. Assess and compare the respiratory and the pulse rates of an infant, toddler, school-age child, adult, and elderly person.

2. In a clinical setting determine what methods of administering oxygen are used most frequently, and determine why.

3. Observe a nurse or a physiotherapist helping a patient learn postural drainage, deep breathing, and effective coughing. Identify the points of emphasis.

4. In a laboratory, set up a Croupette and outline nursing intervention required.

5. Practice resuscitation techniques on a mannequin in a laboratory setting.

6. In a clinical setting identify patients receiving IPPB and determine the purpose and evaluate the effectiveness of this therapy.

SUGGESTED READINGS

Foley, Mary, et al. September, 1977. Pulmonary function screening tests in industry. *American Journal of Nursing* 77:1480–1484.

This article indicates that these tests are helpful in detecting early signs of pulmonary disease. However, individual variations need to be considered in calculating the test results. The tests are reviewed, and the steps are given for interpreting results.

Graas, Suzanne. October, 1974. Thermometer sites and oxygen. *American Journal of Nursing* 74(10):1862–1863.

This describes a small study that challenges the routine practice of taking rectal temperatures when a patient is receiving oxygen by nasal cannula.

Manzi, Catherine Ciaverelli. March, 1978. Cardiac emergency! How to use drugs and C.P.R. to save lives. *Nursing 78* 8:30–39.

In addition to the ABC's of life support, this article emphasizes the D step for life support, which is the definite treatment (diagnosis, drugs, and defibrillation). The rationale for giving drugs and the nurse's role in CPR are included.

Rau, Joseph, and Rau, Mary. April, 1977. To breathe or be breathed: understanding IPPB. *American Journal of Nursing* 77: 613–617.

This article outlines principles of IPPB, its treatment goals, some hazards of IPPB, and a procedure for administering this treatment. It also includes a comparison of the Bird and Bennett Respirators.

Waterson, Marian. Teaching your patients postural drainage. March, 1978. *Nursing 78* 8: 51–53.

This article includes a patient teaching aid showing six commonly prescribed positions. Patient reminders in a Do and Don't format are outlined.

SELECTED REFERENCES

Allcock, Muriel, and Wilson, Sandra. November, 1975. "Code 66!" from anxious "amateurs" to smooth-working code team. *Nursing 75* 5:17–20.

Canadian Heart Foundation. August, 1976. Cardiopulmonary resuscitation (CPR). Part I. Recommended standards for basic life support. Ottawa: The Foundation.

Chrisman, Marilyn. April, 1974. Dyspnea. *American Journal of Nursing* 74: 643–646.

Felton, Cynthia L. January, 1978. Hypoxemia and oral temperatures. *American Journal of Nursing* 78: 56–57.

Flatter, Patricia A. January, 1968. Hazards of oxygen therapy. *American Journal of Nursing* 68: 80–84.

Foss, Georgia. April, 1973. Postural drainage. *American Journal of Nursing* 73:666–669.

Garvey, Judith. April, 1975. Infant respiratory distress syndrome. *American Journal of Nursing* 75: 614–617.

Hunsinger, Doris L., et al. 1973. *Respiratory technology: a procedure manual.* Reston, Va.: Reston Publishing Co.

LeFort, Sandra. February, 1978. Cardiopulmonary resuscitation (CPR): step-by-step. *The Canadian Nurse* 74:38–47

Nussbaum, Gloria B., and Fisher, John G. January, 1978. A crash cart that works. *American Journal of Nursing* 78:45–48.

Razzell, Mary. September, 1975. "No thanks, I've quit smoking." *The Canadian Nurse* 71: 23–25.

Ryan, Mary Ann. August, 1974. Helping the family cope with cardiac arrest. *Nursing 74* 4:80–81.

World Health Organization. 1975. Smoking and its effects on health. Geneva. WHO Tech. Rep. No. 568.

CHAPTER 29

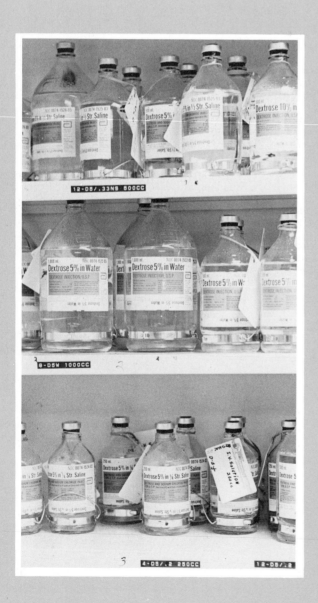

FLUID AND ELECTROLYTE NEEDS

ACID-BASE BALANCE

NORMAL FLUID INTAKE AND OUTPUT

Normal Fluid Intake

Developmental Variations in Daily Fluid Intake

Normal Fluid Output

ASSESSING THE WELL-HYDRATED PERSON

MEASURING FLUID INTAKE AND OUTPUT

Nursing Intervention for Patients on Measured Intake and Output

URINE ASSESSMENT

OBJECTIVES

- Explain total body fluid.
- Describe the distribution of body fluid.
- Describe the main electrolytes of body fluids.
- Explain the movement of body water and electrolytes between body compartments.
- Explain osmotic pressure and hydrostatic pressure.
- Discuss normal fluid intake and output and how it varies with age.
- Describe the well-hydrated person.
- Measure fluid intake and output.
- Plan and intervene for patients on measured fluid intake and output.
- Assess urine as to its color, specific gravity, pH, and presence of protein, glucose, and acetone.

Both fluids and electrolytes are necessary for a person to maintain good health. Not only are they necessary, but their relative amounts must be maintained in the body within a narrow range. The balance of fluids and electrolytes within the body is called *homeostasis*. (See Chapter 7, "Physiologic Homeostasis.")

A great deal has been learned about the roles of fluids and electrolytes in both health and disease. It is known that this delicate balance is maintained in health by the body's physiologic processes. In almost every illness, however, this balance is threatened. Even in normal daily living, excessive temperatures or excessive activity can disturb this balance if an adequate water or salt intake is not maintained. A nurse may observe that some therapeutic measures for patients, such as the use of diuretics, can also disturb the body's homeostasis unless replacement water and electrolytes are given.

This chapter will emphasize the normal aspects of the body's fluids and electrolytes. For nurses to appreciate the dangers of imbalances, they must first understand the normal amounts of fluid and electrolytes required to maintain health. The role of fluids in the body, their distribution, and variations in composition in the various compartments are included. Consideration is given to the maintenance of total body water volumes as it relates to body weight. One of the most common activities of the nurse is to measure patients' body weights in estimating fluid gains or losses. Two other common activities are the measuring and recording of a patient's fluid intake and output and determining the specific gravity of urine. Because of the frequency of the need to promote the intake of oral fluids in ill people, methods to promote oral intake are also included.

TOTAL BODY FLUID

The proportion of the human body comprised of fluid is surprisingly large, considering that the external appearance of man suggests a consistency of mostly solid tissue such as muscle and bone. Over half (60%) of the average healthy adult man's weight is comprised of fluid. In health, this volume of body fluid remains relatively constant. In fact, a person's weight varies less than ½ pound in 24 hours regardless of the amount of fluid ingested. In some diseases serious excesses or deficiencies of body fluid occur. For example, a patient with heart failure can retain fluid in the tissues and may suffer a fluid excess. Another patient with kidney disease may not be able to excrete the required amount of urine, and also suffer a fluid excess; yet another patient may not be able to drink because of a mouth injury and suffer a fluid loss.

The percentage of total body fluid varies according to the individual person's age, body fat, and sex. For variations by age, see Table 29-1. Humans begin life with the highest proportion of fluid, and as life progresses the proportion decreases. In the body, fat is essentially free of fluid. Therefore, the amount of body fat in an obese person alters the total amount of body fluid in relative proportion to body weight. In other words, the less body fat that is present, the greater is the proportionate amount of the total body fluid. For example, a thin man's body may contain 70% fluid, whereas an obese man's may contain only 55%. This variable of body fat also accounts for the difference in total body fluid between the sexes. After adolescence, women have proportionately more fat than men. Thus, they contain a smaller percentage of fluid in relation to their total body weight than do men.

DISTRIBUTION OF BODY FLUID

The body's fluid is divided into two major reservoirs, intracellular and extracellular. The *intracellular fluid*, also referred to as the *cellular fluid*, is that fluid found within the cells of the body. It comprises about two thirds to three quarters of the total body fluid. The *extracellular fluid* is that fluid found outside the cells; it is subdivided again into two compartments, the *in-*

travascular (plasma) and the *interstitial*. The *plasma* is that fluid found within the vascular system; the *interstitial fluid* is that fluid which surrounds the cells and includes lymph. These latter fluids comprise a third to a fourth of the body's total fluid.

Extracellular fluid is in constant motion throughout the body. Although it is the smaller of the two

Table 29-1.   Percentage of Body Weight Comprised of Fluid According to Age

Early human embryo	97% water
Newborn infant	77% water
Adult male	60% water
Adult female	55% water
Elderly	45% water (approx.)

Note: As age increases, total proportion of body water decreases.

Table 29-2.   Secretions of the Alimentary Tract in 24 hours

Saliva		1500 ml
Gastric juice		2500 ml
Bile		500 ml
Pancreatic juice		700 ml
Intestinal secretions		3000 ml
	Total:	8200 ml

compartments, it serves as the transport system of nutrients and waste products to and from the cells. The plasma carries oxygen from the lungs and glucose from the gastrointestinal tract, for example, to the capillaries of the vascular system. From there the oxygen and glucose move across the capillary membrane into the interstitial spaces and thence across the cellular membrane into the cells. The opposite route is taken for waste products, for example, carbon dioxide to the lungs and metabolic acid wastes eventually to the kidneys. One significant difference between plasma and interstitial fluids is that in the latter reservoir, fluid leaves by way of the lymph system in addition to the direct route back to the blood plasma through the blood capillaries. Lymph circulation does ultimately reach the vascular circulation, however, through the thoracic duct into the venous system.

The interstitial fluid comprises three quarters of the extracellular fluid. Normal body functioning requires that the volumes of each fluid compartment remain relatively constant. Regulating mechanisms are discussed later in this chapter.

Secretions and excretions are also a part of the body's total fluid volume and provide essential functions. They are part of the extracellular fluid. A *secretion* is the product of a gland, for example, the salivary glands. An *excretion* is the waste product produced by the cells of the body. Just as balances exist between cellular and extracellular compartments, so do special balances occur between the plasma and the body's secretions and excretions. Some specific secretions are cerebrospinal fluid, synovial fluid, pericardial fluid, and alimentary secretions. Alimentary secretions have been estimated to reach 8200 ml per day (see Table 29-2 for the daily amounts of body secretions for an adult).

Large volumes of fluid in the body also carry dissolved waste materials through the kidneys and through the gastrointestinal tract. However, in both instances, most of this fluid is reabsorbed into the vascular spaces and reused in the body. For example, of 8200 ml produced in the alimentary tract, only 200 ml are usually excreted in the feces, just enough to keep the feces lubricated. Of 180 liters of glomerular filtrate that filters through the kidneys per day, only 1500 ml is usually excreted from the body under normal conditions.

Nurses need to be aware of abnormal amounts of both secretions and excretions. Excessive losses can seriously deplete the extracellular fluid volume and subsequently the intracellular fluid volume. (See "Movement of Body Fluid and Electrolytes" later in this chapter.)

BODY ELECTROLYTES

Extracellular and intracellular fluid are similar in their content of electrolytes and other substances. These fluids contain oxygen from the lungs; dissolved nutrients from the gastrointestinal tract, which include glucose, fatty acids, and amino acids; the excretory products of metabolism, of which carbon dioxide is the most abundant; and salts.

Salts that dissociate in water, that is, break up into one or more electrically charged particles, are called *ions*. The salt sodium chloride breaks up into one ion of sodium (Na^+) and one ion of chloride (Cl^+). In clinical practice these charged particles are called *electrolytes*. Ions that carry a positive charge are called *cations*, and ions carrying a negative charge are called *anions*. Examples of cations are sodium (Na^+), potassium (K^+), calcium (Ca^{++}), and magnesium

(Mg^{++}). Anions include chloride (Cl$^-$), bicarbonate (HCO$_3^-$), phosphate (HPO$_4^{--}$), and sulfate (SO$_4^{--}$).

The Electrolyte Composition of Body Fluids

The electrolyte composition of fluids varies from one compartment to another. Principal ions of extracellular fluid are sodium and chloride; principle ions of cellular fluid are potassium and phosphate. (See Figure 29-1.) The composition of the two extracellular fluid reservoirs (intravascular and interstitial) is similar ionically. The main difference is the greater quantity of protein contained in the intravascular compartment (plasma) as compared to the interstitial fluid. This results because large particles of protein have difficulty passing through the vascular (capillary) membranes into the interstitial fluid. All other electrolytes move readily between these two extracellular compartments.

The higher quantity of protein in plasma plays a significant role in maintaining the intravascular fluid volume and blood pressure. When quantities of plasma protein are low in the body, the blood volume diminishes noticeably and results in a state of hypotension (low blood pressure). This is particularly noticeable in people with disease of the liver (the source of body plasma proteins), who are unable to produce sufficient quantities of plasma proteins.

Just as fluid volumes within compartments must be maintained, so too must the electrolyte composition of the various compartments. The balances are maintained in proportion to the quantities of fluid in the various compartments and the electrolyte composition. Although the specific numbers of cations and anions may differ in the various fluid compartments, the total number of cations equals the number of anions within each compartment in a state of homeostasis.

Measurement of Electrolytes

Electrolytes are measured in milliequivalents per liter of water (mEq/L) or milligrams per 100 milliliters (mg/ml). The term *milliequivalent* means one thou-

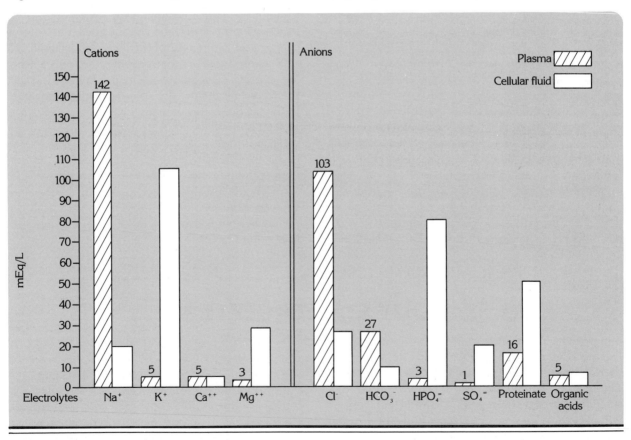

Figure 29-1.   The electrolyte composition of plasma and cellular fluids are measured in milliequivalents per liter. The composition of interstitial fluid (not shown) is similar to plasma except that it has a smaller amount of protein.

sandth of an equivalent. The latter part, *equivalent*, refers to the *chemical combining power* of a substance or the power of cations to unite with anions to form molecules. This chemical combining activity is determined in relation to the chemical combining activity of the hydrogen ion (H^+), the base measure. For example, sodium and chloride ions are equivalent, since they combine equally. One mEq of $Na^+ = 1$ mEq of Cl^-. However, these cations and anions are not equal in weight. One milligram (mg) of sodium (Na^+) does not equal one mg of chloride (Cl^-). If the two were to be compared in weight, it would take 3 mg of sodium to equal 2 mg of chloride.

Clinically, the milliequivalent system is commonly used. However, the nurse needs to be aware of the different systems of measurement when interpreting laboratory results. It is important to realize that laboratory examination usually indicates the findings of blood plasma, since the intracellular fluid is not easily accessible for examination. Examination of extracellular fluid (plasma), however, can frequently reflect the state of the intracellular fluid, even though it may not always be a precise indicator of it.

MOVEMENT OF BODY FLUID AND ELECTROLYTES

Movement of fluid and the transport of substances occur in three phases. First, blood plasma moves around the body within the circulatory system. Nutrients and fluids are picked up from the lungs and the gastrointestinal tract. Second, interstitial fluid and its components move between the blood capillaries and the cells. Third, fluid and substances then move from the interstitial fluid into the cells. In the reverse direction, fluid and its components move back from the cells to the interstitial spaces and thence to the intravascular compartment. This intravascular fluid then flows to the kidneys where the metabolic by-products of the cells are excreted.

Methods of Movement

The methods by which body fluids and electrolytes move are:

1. diffusion
2. osmosis
3. active transport

Diffusion

Diffusion is the continual intermingling of molecules in liquids, gases, or solids brought about by the random movement of the molecules. For example, two gases become mixed due to the incessant motion of their molecules. The process of diffusion occurs even when two substances are separated by a thin membrane. In the body, diffusion of water, electrolytes, and other substances occurs through the pores of capillary membranes and cell membranes.

The rate of diffusion of substances varies according to (a) the size of the molecules, (b) the concentra-tion of the solution, and (c) the temperature of the solution.

Larger molecules move less quickly than smaller ones, since they require more energy to move about. Molecules move more rapidly from a solution of higher concentration to a solution of lower concentration. Increases in temperature increase the rate of motion of molecules and therefore the rate of diffusion.

Osmosis

The term *osmosis* refers to the diffusion of water across cell membranes. The direction of flow is from the less concentrated solution to the more highly concentrated solution. In other words, water goes where the most salt is. The process of osmosis is important in maintaining proper balance in the volumes of extracellular fluid and intracellular fluid.

Active Transport

Movement of substances across cell membranes against a concentration gradient is referred to as *active transport*. This process differs from diffusion and osmosis in that metabolic energy is required to move substances against the concentration gradient. This process is of particular importance in maintaining the differences in sodium and potassium ion concentrations of extracellular fluid and intracellular fluid. Under normal conditions, sodium concentrations are higher in the extracellular fluid as contrasted to potassium, which is higher inside the cells. For more sodium to move into the cells, the mechanism of active transport, also called the *sodium pump*, is activated.

The Selective Permeability of Membranes

In the body, capillary and cellular membranes are described as being selectively permeable. This is because not all substances move with the same ease across the membranes. Compounds of very large molecular size such as proteins, lipids, and glycogen do not readily cross capillary and cellular membranes. On the other hand, organic compounds of molecular size such as urea, glucose, and amino acids move freely. Membranes that allow water molecules and particles (crystalloids) in true solution to move through but not particles in colloid dispersion are called *dialyzing membranes*. Most of the membranes that surround cells are dialyzing membranes.

Cellular (not capillary) membranes are particularly selective in regard to the electrolytes of sodium and potassium. Movement of potassium across cell membranes depends upon metabolic cellular activities. When glucose or insulin is administered, the movement of potassium into the cells is accelerated. Sodium enters the cells in greater quantities when cells lose potassium. Anything that alters the properties of the cell membranes brings about changes in the distribution of sodium and potassium. Some of these factors are excitation of nerve and muscle cells, changes in pH, and anoxia.

Fluid Pressures

A number of pressures are exerted within the body as part of the movement of fluid and electrolytes from one compartment to another. Two of these are osmotic pressure and hydrostatic pressure, which act to cause a flow of fluid through the capillary membranes.

Osmotic Pressure

Osmotic pressure is the drawing force for water exerted by solute particles. The solute particles may be *crystalloids* (salts that dissolve readily into true solutions) or *colloids* (substances like large protein molecules that do not readily dissolve into true solutions). Normally, the net movement of fluid across cell membranes is nil, that is, even, because of the even distribution of electrolytes on both sides of membranes. However, should the concentration of the solute on one side of a membrane become greater, the osmotic pressure and attraction for water will in-

crease. Water will therefore flow toward the solution of the greater concentration until the concentration gradient disappears.

The principle of osmosis can be applied clinically in the administration of intravenous solution. Usually, solutions are given that are *isotonic*, having the same concentration (osmolarity) as blood plasma. This prevents sudden shifts of fluids and electrolytes. In some cases, however, hypertonic or hypotonic solutions may be advisable. *Hypertonic* solutions are those which have a greater concentration of solutes than plasma; *hypotonic* solutions have a lesser concentration of solutes. An example of a hypertonic solution is 50% glucose. It may be given to reduce cerebral edema. The high concentration of glucose temporarily draws fluid from interstitial spaces in the brain into the blood compartment. Use of hypotonic solutions is rare.

The osmotic pressure of plasma is greater than the osmotic pressure of the interstitial compartment. The reasons for this are twofold: (a) the protein concentration (solute) in the plasma is greater than that in the interstitial fluid compartment; and (b) the protein molecule is large, resembles a colloid, and does not readily pass through the capillary membrane. This greater colloid osmotic pressure of plasma is an extremely important physiologic mechanism that maintains the intravascular fluid volume.

Hydrostatic Pressure

Counterbalancing the osmotic pressure of plasma, which attracts fluid, is the hydrostatic pressure of the blood flowing through the capillaries, which pushes fluid out of the vascular space. *Hydrostatic pressure* is the pressure exerted by a fluid within a closed system. Thus hydrostatic pressure of the blood is the force exerted by blood against the vascular walls such as the artery walls. It is also referred to as *filtration force*. The principle involved with hydrostatic pressure is that fluids move from the area of greater pressure to the area of lesser pressure. For this reason fluid moves out of blood vessels. The net movement of water from plasma to tissue spaces thus depends upon which force is greater: hydrostatic pressure, which forces fluid out of the blood vessels, or osmotic pressure, which draws fluid into the blood vessels. Normally, fluid moves out of capillaries at the arterial end where the intravascular hydrostatic pressure exceeds the colloid osmotic pressure. At the venous end of the capillaries, fluid is drawn from the interstitial compartment into the intravascular compartment, where the colloid osmotic pressure is the greater of the two.

Regulation of Fluids and Electrolytes

Health is usually maintained as long as the fluid volume and chemical composition of all the fluid compartments stays within narrow, safe limits. The kidney is largely responsible for maintaining these limits with help from the lungs and some body glands such as the adrenals, parathyroids, pituitary, and the hypothalamus of the brain. Generally, increases of fluid or food intake over and above body requirements are counterbalanced by an increase in output by the kidneys. A reduction in intake is counterbalanced by a reduction in urine output. The body signals the kidney to alter its fluid output by changes in the crystalloid osmotic pressure of the extracellular fluid. Osmotic pressure in the extracellular fluid is regulated by the concentration of sodium and proteins. Once changes in osmotic pressure occur in the extracellular fluid compartment, cells called *osmoreceptors* in the hypothalamus are alerted to release or withhold antidiuretic hormone (ADH), the so-called water hormone. When it is released, water is retained in the body; when it is withheld, water is excreted. A second hormone, aldosterone, which is secreted by the adrenal cortex, is the so-called salt hormone. Aldosterone responds by stimulating the kidneys to retain sodium in the body and excrete potassium.

ACID-BASE BALANCE

The body's cellular activity requires an alkaline medium. Body fluids are normally maintained at a pH of about 7.4. *pH* refers to the measure of hydrogen ion concentration indicating acidity or alkalinity. Alterations of pH within even a few tenths can be incompatible with cellular activity. However, opposing this alkalinity are cellular chemical processes that are constantly producing large amounts of acid as by-products of metabolism. Fortunately, precise control mechanisms operate to maintain this pH of body fluids within a very narrow range. The pH is controlled by buffer systems present in all body fluids and by respiratory and kidney regulatory systems.

Three major buffer systems of the body fluids are the bicarbonate buffer, the phosphate buffer, and the protein buffer. Discussion here will be limited to the bicarbonate buffer system, since the phosphate and protein buffer systems operate in almost the same manner.

The bicarbonate buffer system consists of sodium bicarbonate ($NaHCO_3$) or potassium bicarbonate ($KHCO_3$) and carbonic acid (H_2CO_3) in the same solution. Buffers do not neutralize. Acid-base buffers make strong acids and strong bases weaker; thus the pH of body fluids falls or rises only slightly. For example, if a strong acid such as hydrochloric acid (HCl) is introduced to a glass of water, the pH of the fluid would drop significantly to a pH of 1 or 2. However, if a bicarbonate buffer system is already present in the water, the HCl quickly combines with the buffer, producing a weaker acid (carbonic acid). Thus the pH drops only slightly. The above reaction is shown as follows:

$$HCl + NaHCO_3 \rightarrow H_2CO_3 + NaCl$$
(hydrochloric   (sodium   (carbonic   (sodium
acid)   bicarbonate)   acid)   chloride)

A strong acid is a compound that completely dissociates its hydrogen ions; for example, HCl yields H^+ and Cl^-. A weak acid is one that frees only some of its hydrogen ions; for example, H_2CO_3 yields H^+ and HCO_3^-. One hydrogen ion is free, the other is not.

In contrast, when a strong base such as sodium hydroxide is added to body fluids, it combines with carbonic acid to form a weaker base, sodium bicarbonate.

$$NaOH + H_2CO_3 \rightarrow NaHCO_3 + H_2O$$
(sodium   (carbonic   (sodium   (water)
hydroxide)   acid)   bicarbonate)

Although the bicarbonate buffer system is not the strongest buffer system in the body (the most powerful and plentiful one is the proteins of plasma and cells), it is important because the concentrations of both sodium bicarbonate and carbonic acid are regulated by the kidneys and by the respiratory system. The kidneys regulate the bicarbonate ions, and the respiratory system regulates the carbonic acid. How does the elimination of carbon dioxide by the lungs regulate acid-base balance? The carbon dioxide man exhales comes from carbonic acid as follows:

$$H_2CO_3 \rightarrow CO_2 \text{ and } H_2O$$

The more CO_2 that is exhaled, the more carbonic acid (H_2CO_3) is removed from the blood, thus elevating the blood pH to a more alkaline level. Hyperventilation is an example. Doubling the ventilation rate can raise the pH about 0.23 pH units; for example, a 7.4 pH can be raised to 7.63 (Guyton 1976:517). On the other hand, holding one's breath, or hypoventilating, retains CO_2, which is then available to form carbonic acid, leading to a reduced or more acid pH. Significant changes in the pH of body fluids therefore are made by altering respiratory activity.

The kidney's role in maintaining acid-base balance is more complex. To simplify, the kidneys excrete hydrogen ions and form bicarbonate ions in specific amounts as indicated by the pH of the blood. When the plasma pH drops (becomes more acidic), H^+ ions (acid) are excreted and bicarbonate ions (base) are formed and retained. Conversely, when the plasma pH rises (becomes more alkaline), H^+ ions are retained in the body and bicarbonate ions are excreted.

The normal pH range of extracellular fluid is 7.35 to 7.45. This precise balance is maintained as long as the ratio of one carbonic acid molecule to 20 bicarbonate ions is maintained in the extracellular fluid. The ratio is important rather than the specific amounts of each.

Imbalances in pH can result in either *acidosis* or *alkalosis*. To simplify, acidosis occurs with increases in blood carbonic acid or with decreases in blood bicarbonate. Alkalosis, on the other hand, occurs with increases in blood bicarbonate or decreases in blood carbonic acid. The patient will not become acidotic or alkalotic, however, unless the normal ratio of one carbonic acid molecule to 20 bicarbonate ions is altered. Compensatory (adaptive) mechanisms operate to maintain this balance. (See Chapter 30, "Acid-Base Imbalances.")

Two adjectives describe the general cause or origin of pH imbalances: metabolic and respiratory. *Metabolic acidosis* and *metabolic alkalosis* refer to imbalances brought about by changes in the bicarbonate levels as a result of metabolism. *Respiratory acidosis* and *respiratory alkalosis* refer to imbalances brought about by changes in carbonic acid levels as a result of respiratory alterations.

NORMAL FLUID INTAKE AND OUTPUT

In health, one's intake generally equates to one's output. This is regulated by the body in such a manner that a person is rarely aware that this balance is being maintained, nor does the person require assistance to maintain this balance. When debilitated or injured, however, a person often requires assistance to maintain this balance or in some situations specific measures to maintain an adequate intake and output.

Normal Fluid Intake

The average adult (moderate activity at moderate temperature) drinks about 1500 ml per day yet needs 2500 ml per day, an additional 1000 ml. This added volume is acquired from the ingestion of foods (referred to as *preformed water)* and from the oxidation of these foods during metabolic processes. Interestingly, the water content of food is relatively large, contributing about half of the amount of fluid that is ingested (750 ml per day). The water content of fresh vegetables is approximately 90%, of fresh fruits about 85%, and of lean meats around 60%.

Oxidative water, which is formed as a by-product of the body's oxidation of food, accounts for the remaining amount of water that is required. For each 100 calories of protein, fat, and carbohydrate, 14 ml of water is formed as the end product of metabolism. Thus a 2500-calorie diet would produce 350 ml of water ($\frac{2500}{100} \times 14 = 350$ ml). Oxidative water approximates, then, about half of the volume of water provided by food itself or about a quarter of the total amount of water a person drinks. These three amounts are easily recalled if a 4:2:1 ratio is applied.

Average daily fluid intake for an adult is as follows:

		Ratio
Water consumed as fluids	1500 ml	(4)
Water present in foods	750 ml	(2)
Water of oxidation	350 ml	(1)
Total:	2600 ml	

Developmental Variations in Daily Fluid Intake

Naturally, fluid intake requirements vary with age. Intake requirements have been determined for various ages in accordance with body surface area, metabolic requirements, and body weight.

Infants and growing children have much greater

fluid turnovers than adults, that is, greater water needs and greater water losses. This difference is due to the greater metabolic rate, which increases their fluid loss through the kidneys. (See "Normal Fluid Output.") Immature kidneys in infants are less efficient than adult kidneys, thereby increasing the loss of fluid through the kidneys. Infant losses in proportion to body weight are also greater from both the lungs and the skin, essentially because respirations are more rapid and the body surface area is proportionately greater. These more rapid turnovers of fluid plus the additional losses produced by disease can create critical fluid imbalances in children much more rapidly than in adults. See Table 29-3 for approximate fluid requirements at different ages according to body weight. A 70 kg adult requires 40 × 70 = 2800 ml of fluid per day, whereas a 1-year-old infant weighing 10 kg requires 100 × 10 = 1000 ml daily, that is, more than twice the amount per kilogram of body weight of the adult.

Fluid requirements are most accurately determined from metabolic rate, that is, the calories metabolized, or from the surface area of the body, which varies directly with the metabolic rate. Because neither of these is easily measured clinically, tables have been produced that relate body surface areas to body weight. See Figures 29-2 and 29-3.

Normal Fluid Output

Fluid losses counterbalance the adult's 2½-liter daily intake of water. The main channel of excretion is the kidneys, which are responsible for an output of 1500 to 1700 ml per day in the adult. This amount approximates the amount of fluid that an adult drinks per day. The oral intake and the output through the kidneys are frequently and easily measured in nursing practice.

Three other routes of fluid output are as follows:

1. Through the skin as insensible perspiration (independent of sweat gland activity).
2. Through the lungs as water vapor in expired air.
3. Through the intestine in the feces.

Refer to Table 29-4 for average daily output for an adult. The normal loss from skin and lungs accounts for about two thirds of the urinary loss, whereas loss in the feces is minimal. It is important to remember also that *daily intake = daily output*. For variations in total daily urine output in infants and children, see Table 27-1.

Obligatory loss refers to the essential fluid loss

Table 29-3.   Approximate Daily Fluid Requirements in Milliliters per Kilogram at Different Ages*

Age	Total Fluids (ml/kg)
Newborn	80 to 100
Infant to 1 year	100 to 150
1 to 2 years	100 to 125
2 to 4 years	90
4 to 6 years	100
7 to 10 years	75
11 to 18 years	50 to 75
Adult	40

*From Waechter, Eugenia H., and Blake, Florence G., 1976. *Nursing care of children*, 9th ed. (Philadelphia: J. B. Lippincott Co.), and Scipien, Gladys M., et al., 1975, *Comprehensive pediatric nursing* (New York: McGraw Hill Book Co.).

required to maintain body functioning. Water lost as vapor in expired air and as vapor from the skin (insensible perspiration) as well as a minimum volume of about 500 ml from the kidneys are required to excrete the solid metabolic wastes produced daily. These are the obligatory losses, totaling 1300 ml per day.

Since the vaporized losses are not readily measured, the measured obligatory kidney loss becomes of prime importance in critical illness. An hourly urine volume of less than 30 ml is serious, as is a daily volume of less than 500 ml. Patients with inadequate output require immediate attention. Such findings by the nurse must therefore be reported promptly. Although losses from the skin, lungs, and intestines in health account for approximately half of the daily loss, they can account for a much larger percentage of loss from a patient who has a fever or accelerated respiration.

These increases in respiratory rate, fever, *diaphoresis* (sweating), and diarrhea can magnify fluid loss from the normal routes immensely. Other routes of loss, such as from the stomach through emesis or suction, or from abnormal body openings such as fistulas or surgically implanted drainage tubes often also account for significant losses, all of which require equivalent intake replacements.

In health, output volumes shown above may vary noticeably from day to day and throughout one day. For example, sweat gland activity can increase when the environmental temperature or the humidity increases. Urinary volume automatically increases

Table 29-4.   Average Daily Fluid Output for an Adult

Urine	1500 ml
Lungs	400 ml
Skin	500 ml
Feces	200 ml
Total:	2600 ml

as amount of fluids ingested increases, as can occur on a hot summer day. On the other hand, if the fluid loss from the skin is large, the urinary volume may decrease to maintain the homeostatic fluid volumes in the body. Balance is maintained between the intake and output by the specific mechanisms already discussed.

ASSESSING THE WELL-HYDRATED PERSON

People who are well hydrated, that is, neither dehydrated nor overhydrated, exhibit certain signs. The nurse should be able to assess adequate hydration or problems in the hydration of patients. The following list describes some of the signs of adequate hydration. It is unlikely that any one person will have all the

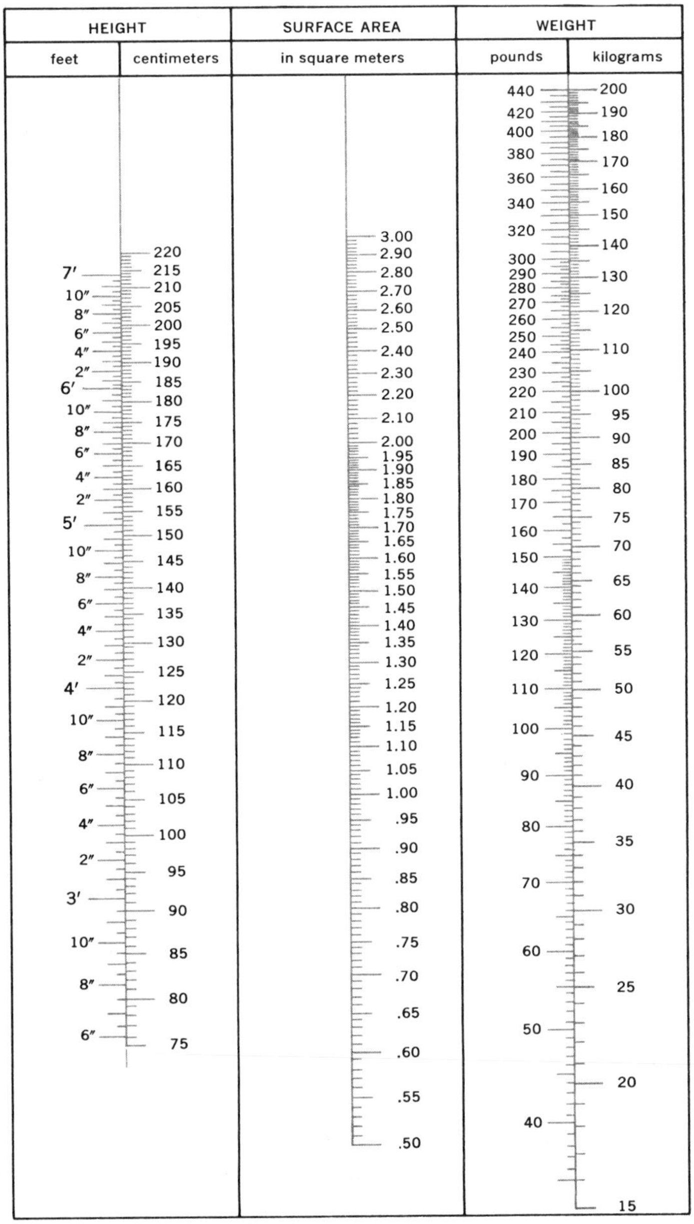

Figure 29-2.   To determine the surface area of older children and adults, a straight line is drawn between the point on the left vertical scale, which represents the patient's height, to the point on the right vertical scale, which represents the patient's weight. Point where this line intersects middle vertical scale indicates patient's surface area in square meters.

listed signs. Lack of any one of these signs may or may not indicate fluid problems. However, nurses should be familiar with the signs of normal hydration to be able to identify problems that patients can have.

The well-hydrated person shows the following signs:

1. Stable weight from day to day.
2. Moist mucous membranes.
3. An appropriate food intake.

4. Straw-colored urine (which has a specific gravity of 1.010 to 1.030).
5. Good tissue turgor.
6. Mental orientation.
7. No complaint of thirst.
8. Amount of excreted urine appropriate to intake.
9. No evidence of edema.
10. No evidence of dehydration, such as depressed periorbital spaces.

MEASURING FLUID INTAKE AND OUTPUT

It can be the nurse's function to assess the oral fluid needs of patients. For people who have a fever or an infection, the nurse should advise additional fluid intake of up to 3000 ml per day. If the physician orders the recording of intake (I) and output (O) for the patient, the physician may also prescribe the exact amount of fluid that the patient should have in a 24-hour period. In some situations the intake may be limited, for example, for a patient who has a pathologic condition of the kidney or heart. For dehydrated patients, fluids are frequently encouraged or forced.

To measure oral intake, household measures must be converted to milliliters or cubic centimeters. Most agencies provide conversion tables, since the size of the dishes used is variable. For example, 1 soup bowl = 180 ml, and 1 juice glass = 100 ml. Printed intake and output records are usually also available. Eight-hour records are generally kept at the patient's bedside and then converted to 24-hour records on the patient's chart. (See Figure 29-4.)

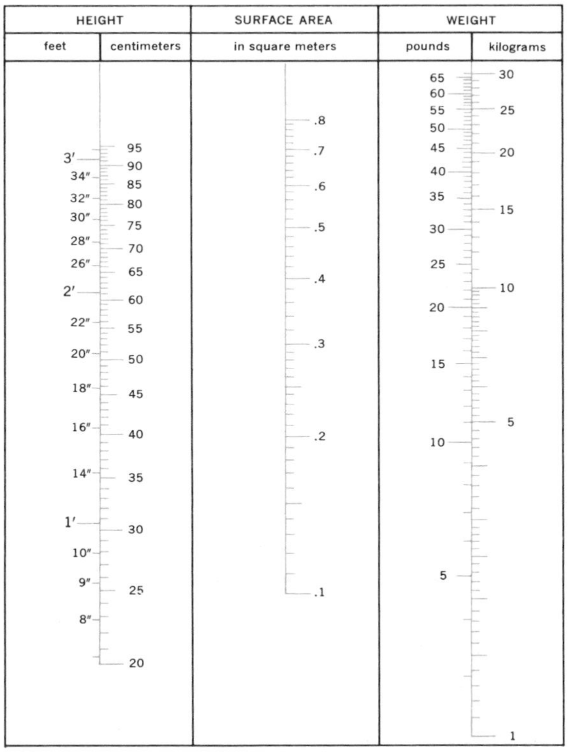

HEIGHT		SURFACE AREA	WEIGHT	
feet	centimeters	in square meters	pounds	kilograms

Figure 29-3.   The surface area of infants and young children is determined in the same manner as adults (see Figure 29-2).

LIONS GATE HOSPITAL

FLUID BALANCE SHEET

+ Slight
++ Moderate   Stool Disphoresis
+++ Profuse

	DATE:				DATE:			
	Nights	Days	Evening	24 Hour Total	Nights	Days	Evening	24 Hour Total
FLUID INTAKE								
Oral	90	180	150	420	170			
Blood								
Intravenous	500	1200	800	2500	300			
Gavage								
TOTAL INTAKE	590	1380	950	2920	470			
FLUID OUTPUT								
Urine: Voided	300	700	550	1550	480			
Catheter								
Ureteral								
Suprapubic				/				
Emesis:								
Levine								
T-Tube	90	150	100	340	80			
Wound Suction								
Stool								
Diaphoresis								
TOTAL OUTPUT	390	850	650	1890	560			

N.19 REV. 2/75
M-S-p

Figure 29-4. A sample of a 24-hour fluid intake and output record. (Courtesy Lion's Gate Hospital, Vancouver, B.C.)

Nursing Intervention for Patients on Measured Intake and Output

1. Place an intake and output record at the patient's bedside at beginning of each shift and a 24-hour record on the patient's chart.

2. Explain to the patient the reasons and importance of measuring and recording fluid intake and output. Emphasize that all fluids taken are to be measured. Include oral fluids, intravenous fluids, or any others that are pertinent to the patient's situation, such as a gastric feeding. Ambulatory patients need to save urine by voiding in a bedpan or urinal. Encourage patients to keep track of their own intake if they so desire.

3. With the patient, make a plan for providing the prescribed fluid intake; for example, if the goal is 2000 ml in 24 hours, allocate so much per shift:

Day shift	900 ml
Evening shift	900 ml
Night shift	200 ml

Consider the patient's fluid preferences and provide for these when possible.

4. Check and record the fluids taken at mealtimes and nourishment times. Often the patient will assist with this. When recording the intake of fluid, all obvious fluids must be measured as well as such foods as ice cream, gelatin, custard, soup, and infant cereals. Recording output when patients are incontinent of urine or feces presents problems for accuracy, but an assessment of amount should be recorded, for example, half a drawsheet saturated with urine × 2 (twice).

5. Record eight-hour and daily intake and output volumes on the appropriate records.

6. Note other excess losses such as vomiting, diarrhea, excessive perspiration, and losses from suctions, and measure and record these if possible.

URINE ASSESSMENT

The body's state of hydration can be determined by measuring the volume, appearance, color, and specific gravity of urine. For example, persons who have been on severely restricted fluid intake will have very little urine output, and the concentration of electrolytes and solids will be relatively high, thereby making the specific gravity high. The nurse needs to record the volume, appearance, and color of the urine. Report volumes that are less than 30 ml per hour or more than 500 ml per hour and concentrated or unusual appearances.

Specific Gravity

Specific gravity can be measured with a urinometer.

1. Check the calibration of the urinometer float by first placing it in distilled water.

2. Then fill the urinometer cylinder with urine that has been allowed to come to room temperature. Place the urinometer gently into the urine.

3. The float must not touch the sides of the cylinder; it must be in the center portion of the cylinder.

4. Specific gravity is determined by noting the reading of the float calibration scale, which is at the surface of the fluid.

5. Wash, rinse, and dry the urinometer thoroughly after each use.

6. Normal specific gravity ranges between 1.015 and 1.025 to 1.010 and 1.030.

pH

pH is the measure of hydrogen ion concentration in the urine. The complete pH range is from 1 to 14. pH is usually tested with nitrazine paper, which shows a variety of colors after being dipped in the urine. The colors range from yellow to green or blue depending upon the pH. There are commercial reagent strips available, which use a combination of dyes. By comparing the strip against a guide, a pH can be determined. Normal urine has a pH between 6 and 7.

Protein

Normal urine will have no protein present or a slight trace. The presence of the protein can be tested by adding a given amount of chemical to a given amount of urine and checking the subsequent cloudiness (coagulation), which is estimated on a scale: negative, tr (trace), $1+, 2+, 3+, 4+$. There are also reagent strips available; the presence of protein changes the color of the reagent.

Glucose

Normally there is no glucose present in the urine. The presence of glucose is reported as tr (trace), $1+$ to $4+$. There are reagent strips available, which, when dipped in the urine, will change color in the presence of glucose. Another method of testing is to add a stated amount of water to a stated amount of urine in a test tube and then add a Clinitest tablet. The solution will boil, and the color is read immediately when the boiling is completed. The color is compared with a color chart for a reading.

Acetone

Acetone is one of the ketone bodies, which are the products of fat and fatty acid metabolism. Normally there is none in the urine. Strip reagents are commonly used, which, when dipped in the urine, will turn purple in the presence of acetone.

SUMMARY

A balance of both fluid and electrolytes is necessary for health and life. The total body fluid of an adult comprises about 60% of his or her weight. The younger the person the higher this proportion. Body fluid is distributed in two major reservoirs: intracellular and extracellular. The extracellular can be subdivided into two compartments: intravascular (plasma) and interstitial. These comprise about a third to a quarter of the total body fluid.

The extracellular component is in constant motion and serves as the transport system for nutrients and wastes.

The body electrolytes (ions) are of two types: positively charged (cations) and negatively charged (anions). The principal ions of extracellular fluid are sodium and chloride, and the principal ions of intracellular fluid are potassium and phosphate. The amounts of electrolytes are measured in milliequivalents per liter of water (mEq/L).

Fluid moves between the body compartments by diffusion, osmosis, and active transport. The membranes of the cells and capillaries are selectively permeable; that is, not all substances can pass through them. The major fluid pressures of the body are the osmotic or drawing pressure and the hydrostatic or pushing pressure. The fluid of the body is largely regulated by the kidneys, influenced by aldosterone and antidiuretic hormones. The acid-base balance of the body is controlled by three buffer systems; bicarbonate, phosphate, and protein buffers. These buffers make strong bases weaker and strong acids weaker. Imbalances in acid-base can result in either acidosis or alkalosis.

Normal fluid intake for an adult is about 2500 ml per day, of which 1500 ml is liquid intake. Other sources of fluid are food and the oxidation of the food. The amount of fluid required varies according to age. A 1-year-old infant requires about 1000 to 1500 ml per day. These amounts are calculated according to body weight in kilograms and body surface area.

Normal fluid loss is through the urine, feces, skin, and breath. The average adult is required to lose approximately 1300 ml daily to maintain health.

Nurses are required to assess the fluid needs of patients. Basic to this is a knowledge of the signs of adequate hydration. Both oral intake and urine output are frequently measured as one way of assessing hydration. Urine can be noted for volume, color, odor, and clarity. It can be tested for specific gravity, pH, protein, glucose, and acetone.

SUGGESTED ACTIVITIES

1. Assess the daily fluid intake of a healthy adult, an infant, and a preschooler. Compare the results.

2. In a clinical setting, survey the intake and output records used. With a group of classmates from different clinical settings, note the similarities and differences in these records.

3. In a laboratory setting, determine the specific gravity of your own urine sample taken on arising.

SUGGESTED READINGS

Fenton, M. May, 1969. What to do about thirst. *American Journal of Nursing* 69:1014-1017.

Thirst may be created by the restriction of fluids. People may have a pattern of fluid intake that needs to be assessed, and then the allowed fluids need to be adjusted to this pattern. Other nursing assessment includes the condition of the oral mucosa, fluid output or loss, diet, motor ability, and mental state.

Sharer, J. E. June, 1975. Reviewing acid-base balance. *American Journal of Nursing* 75:980-983.

An overview of acid-base balance is presented, including acid-base control systems (buffers, respiratory mechanism, renal mechanism). Acid-base imbalances are explained with illustrations used to clarify the content.

SELECTED REFERENCES

Dickens, Margaret L. 1974. *Fluid and electrolyte balance: a programmed text.* 3rd ed. Philadelphia: F. A. Davis Co.

French, Ruth M. 1975. *Guide to diagnostic procedures.* 4th ed. New York: McGraw-Hill Book Co.

Grant, M. M., et al. August, 1975. Assessing a patient's hydration status. *American Journal of Nursing* 75:1306-1311.

Guyton, Arthur C. 1976. *Textbook of medical physiology.* 5th ed. Philadelphia: W. B. Saunders Co.

Metheny, Norma A. March, 1975. Water and electrolyte balance in the postoperative patient. *Nursing Clinics of North America* 10(1):49-57.

Reed, G. M. March, 1974. Confused about potassium? Here's a clear concise guide. *Nursing '74* 4:20-28.

Stroot, V. R., et al. 1974. *Fluids and electrolytes: a practical approach.* 2nd ed. Philadelphia: F. A. Davis Co.

CHAPTER 30

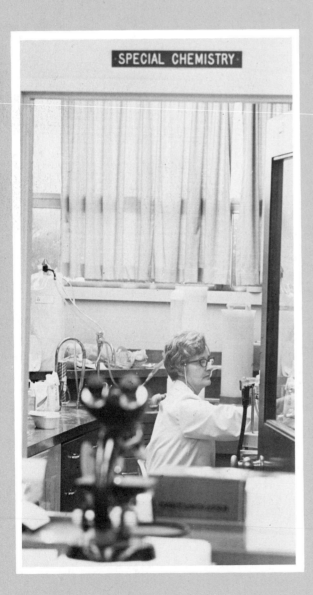

SPECIAL CHEMISTRY

OVERHYDRATION (EDEMA)

Kinds of Edema

Edema by Location

Formation of Edema

Effects of Generalized Edema

Assessment of the Overhydrated Person

UNDERHYDRATION (DEHYDRATION)

The Effects of Dehydration

Assessment of the Dehydrated Person

ELECTROLYTE IMBALANCES

Sodium Imbalances

Potassium Imbalances

Calcium Imbalances

ACID-BASE IMBALANCES

Assessing Acid-Base Imbalances

Acidosis

Alkalosis

FLUID AND ELECTROLYTE PROBLEMS

OBJECTIVES

- Describe various kinds of edema (overhydration) and dehydration (underhydration).

- List five factors involved in the formation of edema.

- Discuss the physiologic effects of generalized edema and dehydration.

- Outline common imbalances of electrolytes, reasons for them, and the therapies used to correct them.

- Assess patients for fluid and electrolyte imbalances.

- Describe the four acid-base imbalances.

- Interpret laboratory signs indicating acid-base imbalances.

- Describe the purposes of intravenous therapy and various types of solutions and equipment used.

- Discuss the nursing interventions required for patients receiving intravenous infusions.

- Explain four major complications of intravenous therapy.

- Describe the four major blood types of humans and the risks involved in transfusing blood products.

- Discuss the purposes and types of fluids administered for parenteral hyperalimentation and nursing interventions required.

Problems in a person's fluid and electrolyte balance frequently reflect other physiologic problems such as heart failure or kidney disease. To understand fluid and electrolyte imbalance and to make an accurate assessment of the patient's problems, data regarding a patient's fluids and electrolytes often need to be understood within the context of other pathologic conditions. By having a complete picture of the patient's health situation, nurses are better able to assess present and possible future fluid and electrolyte needs.

A patient who has considerable vomiting or diarrhea can reflect a triad of body disturbances in body water, body electrolytes, and the body's acid-base balance. Excessive vomiting over a period of time results in an excessive loss of hydrochloric acid (HCl) from the stomach and a resultant alkalosis. In some cases, excessive vomiting can also result in a loss of the alkaline duodenal secretions. Prolonged diarrhea, on the other hand, results in a body acidosis as a consequence of the loss of the bicarbonate ion (HCO_3^-) in the feces.

Another common situation that nurses will frequently encounter is a disturbed fluid balance as a result of excessive blood loss, such as after surgery or hemorrhage, and thus the depletion of extracellular fluid volume. Edema of the body has the opposite effect: the interstitial fluid spaces are overloaded with fluid.

This chapter will cover the common fluid and electrolyte imbalances and related concepts. The two kinds of fluid imbalance are overhydration (edema)

and underhydration (dehydration). Not all the individual electrolyte disturbances will be discussed. The signs and symptoms of sodium, potassium, and calcium imbalances will be presented for reference purposes. These are the cations most commonly considered in medical therapy. From a nurse's standpoint, most electrolyte disturbances are determined through laboratory examination of the blood plasma rather than through identifiable signs and symptoms. These laboratory values apply to extracellular fluid rather than to intracellular fluid, which is not readily available for study.

Because the magnitude of a fluid increase or deficit cannot be precisely determined by laboratory means, the following information can be helpful in assessing a patient's problems in hydration:

1. A reliable history from the patient or family.
2. A laboratory assessment of the blood plasma composition.
3. An estimate of fluid gains and losses.
4. The reasons for insufficient or excess fluid and/or food intake.
5. Specific losses from gastrointestinal tract, skin, or other routes.
6. Changes in urinary output.
7. Acute changes in body weight; previous body weight prior to present illness.
8. Time factor of the above.

OVERHYDRATION (EDEMA)

Edema refers to excess fluid in the interstitial compartment. It may be generalized throughout the body, called *anasarca,* or it may be localized to one part of the body. The source of edematous fluid is the blood plasma. Normally, the interstitial fluid compartment is relatively dry and compact, as well as elastic and expandable, not boggy. Normally, very little fluid is present except that which is needed to fill the crevices between the tissue substances. This relatively dry state is significant in facilitating diffusion of nutrient substances from the plasma to the intracellular fluid (ICF) and metabolic wastes in the reverse order, from the cells to the plasma. Any increase in the distance between the blood capillaries and the cells, such as happens in edema, invokes interference with the nutrition of the cells. See Figure 30-1.

Kinds of Edema

The two most prominent signs of water retention are a gain in a person's weight and swelling of the tissues. A person can accumulate up to 4.5 kg (10 pounds) of fluid before it becomes physically apparent. Edema of the tissues can be categorized as pitting, nonpitting, and/or dependent edema.

Pitting edema refers to edema that, after firm finger pressure on the skin, leaves a small depression called a *pit.* The pit is caused by movement of the edema fluid to adjacent tissue away from the applied pressure point. Within 10 to 30 seconds, the pit normally will disappear.

In *nonpitting edema* the fluid in edematous tissues cannot be moved by finger pressure to adjacent

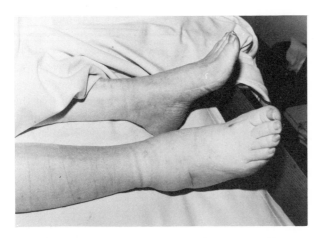

Figure 30-1. Note the excessive swelling of tissues of the extremity caused by edema. The movement of fluid, electrolytes, and nutrients to and from the tissues is impaired.

spaces. This occurs in infections and traumas that cause large quantities of fluid to collect and coagulate in the tissue spaces. The coagulation prevents displacement of fluid to other areas by pressure. *To coagulate* means to clot, as in the case of the blood.

Dependent edema refers to edema that collects in the lower parts or most dependent parts of the body. If a person is ambulatory, this type of edema may first be evident in the feet and ankles. On the other hand, if the person is continually in bed, the edema is more likely to occur in the sacral region.

Edema by Location

Other common descriptions of edema are made on the basis of the location of the edema in the body.

Cerebral edema refers to an excessive accumulation of fluid in the brain tissues. It has many causes such as a brain tumor, trauma, or infection. Increasing fluid pressure under the nonexpandable cranium (bony skull) is serious and can result in obstruction of the blood flow to the brain. Hypertonic glucose, mannitol, or sucrose solutions are often administered as an emergency measure to these patients. *Hypertonic solutions* (solutions with a greater tonicity than blood) increase the osmotic pressure of the blood and draw the fluid out of the intracranial interstitial and intracellular compartments. This therapy is not lasting because the plasma loses its osmotic properties within a few hours.

Pulmonary edema is fluid in the interstitial spaces of the lungs. It can rapidly rupture the alveoli of the lungs. Since pulmonary edema inevitably involves alveolar edema, a serious problem that can result is death by suffocation. Manifestations of pulmonary edema are frothy sputum, dyspnea, cough, and gurgling sounds on respiration. The most common cause of pulmonary edema is left-sided heart failure with resulting increase in the pressure of the pulmonary blood capillaries and the interstitial spaces of the lung tissue. Caution is therefore essential in administering intravenous fluids to prevent overload of the capillaries of the lungs of persons with cardiac problems. This is also true of infants who, because of the size of their lungs, cannot handle large amounts of fluid.

Ascites is the accumulation of fluid in the abdominal cavity. It occurs when the venous pressure is increased as in heart failure or when resistance to blood flow is increased by the liver.

Slight *ankle edema*, especially during the latter stages, is normally associated with *pregnancy*. One reason for this edema is the increased capillary pressure because of interference with the venous blood return from the legs. This interference is caused by partial obstruction of iliac veins by the unborn baby. Another cause is a tendency toward hypoproteinemia of the pregnant woman, particularly in a toxemic condition when the albumin concentration in the plasma falls, thus reducing the plasma osmotic pressure. A third reason can be electrolyte imbalances (Na^+ and Cl^- retention), which result from endocrine changes in a normal pregnancy.

Formation of Edema

Several factors may be involved in the formation of edema.

1. *Increased venous pressure.* The most common causative factor in edema formation is increased venous pressure, which results in increased pressure at the venous or reabsorptive end of the capillaries. This pressure is greater than the normal blood protein osmotic pressure and thus impairs the return of the interstitial fluid into the capillaries. Venous pressure can be increased in conditions such as cardiac failure, in which there is poor venous return to the heart, or when there are obstructions or interference in venous flow as may be produced by varicosities.

2. *Reduction of plasma proteins.* Deficiencies in the blood proteins (albumin, globulin, and fibrinogen) reduce the osmotic pressure of the plasma, thus re-

ducing the movement of the fluid from the tissue spaces into the plasma. This is seen in conditions such as kidney nephrosis, in which there is an excessive loss of albumin in the urine, and in severe malnutrition when the actual supply of protein to the body is insufficient for the formation of the blood proteins. Plasma protein refers to albumin, globulin, and fibrinogen. Serum protein refers to albumin and globulin.

3. *Increased capillary permeability.* In inflammatory reactions (see "The Inflammatory Adaptive Response," Chapter 8), the localized swelling of tissues is due to increased capillary permeability, which allows excessive amounts of fluid and other blood constituents into the tissue spaces. In conditions such as allergic reactions and in some infections, certain bacteria release substances such as leukocytoxin that increase capillary permeability.

4. *Obstructed lymphatic vessels.* The accessory route in which fluids can flow from the interstitial spaces into the bloodstream is the lymphatic system. The importance of the lymph channels in carrying away large proteins and other large substances from the tissue spaces that cannot be reabsorbed by the blood capillaries is obvious in obstructive conditions such as after the surgical removal of the lymph nodes. A common example is the radical mastectomy, after which a patient's arm can swell to twice its normal size until the formation of new lymph channels partially relieves the problem.

5. *Reduced kidney output.* Conditions that decrease glomerular filtration in the kidneys, such as nephritis, or conditions that decrease blood flow to the kidneys, as is seen in shock or renal arteriosclerosis, impair renal output. This results in the accumulation of fluid in the interstitial spaces. Increased concentration of fluid-regulatory hormones such as antidiuretic hormone (ADH) and aldosterone cause edema. The excessive amounts of aldosterone produced by adrenal hyperfunction cause increased reabsorption of sodium by the renal tubules. This in turn increases blood plasma concentration and osmotic pressure and favors fluid retention.

Effects of Generalized Edema

The blood volume drops when the fluid from the plasma moves into the interstitial spaces. Then the antidiuretic hormone (ADH) and aldosterone are released. This is a compensatory response in that the kidneys are stimulated to retain fluid and sodium. This response can add to an existing problem in that the retained fluid can also be lost to the interstitial spaces, thus augmenting the edema. Therefore generalized edema is considered a self-perpetuating condition.

Assessment of the Overhydrated Person

People who are overhydrated exhibit certain signs and symptoms. A nurse should be able to recognize early signs of overhydration or edema as well as those indicating a more progressive condition. People need not have all of the following signs and symptoms to be overhydrated, neither does the presence of just a few signs necessarily indicate overhydration. The nurse's assessment needs to be in correlation with the findings of the physician and other members of the health team to provide an accurate and meaningful nursing assessment.

1. Weight gain.
2. Generalized or localized swelling of the tissues (edema).
3. Puffy eyelids.
4. A decreased fluid output in comparison to intake.
5. Amber urine with elevated specific gravity if the kidneys are not excreting the excessive fluid.
6. Decreased hematocrit, hemoglobin, and red blood cell count of blood plasma.
7. Complaints of weakness and anorexia.
8. Mental confusion.
9. Slow or absent responses.
10. Apathetic appearance or complaints of apathy.

UNDERHYDRATION (DEHYDRATION)

Losses of 10% or more of the body water are incapacitating to the human body. Deficits of water alone may occur because of (a) inadequate intake of water or (b) excessive vaporization through losses from the lungs and skin in prolonged high fevers. If food intake is restricted, electrolytes are also depleted.

Many illnesses are characterized by excessive losses of gastrointestinal fluids (vomiting, diarrhea, fistulas, tube drainages, and bowel obstruction when fluids are not reabsorbed); urine and sweat losses also create deficits in electrolytes. For practical purposes, it is wise to assume that in dehydration of more than a slight degree due to excessive fluid loss the body also loses sodium, chloride, and potassium.

The Effects of Dehydration

The effects of dehydration depend upon the rate and volume of the fluid deficit. If patients are young or elderly or if their general condition is poor, the effects will be more acute. A baby with no water intake will lose a volume of fluid equal to his or her extracellular fluid volume in 5 days, whereas it will take an adult 10 days to lose the same proportion of fluid (MacBryde and Blacklow 1970:749). People who have less water in proportion to their body weight are also vulnerable to more rapid depletions.

With loss of body fluids, the primary result is a decreased loss of the interstitial fluid volume. As dehydration progresses and if it becomes severe, the plasma volume also decreases. Dehydration also involves the loss of excessive amounts of sodium and chloride (major ions of the extracellular fluid) in addition to water.

The great majority of people who are dehydrated have losses of water in relatively greater amounts than the loss of sodium (Na). Therefore when the body is deprived of H_2O, the extracellular fluid compartment, including interstitial fluid, is reduced, but water by the process of osmosis passes into plasma immediately from the intracellular compartments through interstitial fluid. This tends to preserve the circulating blood plasma volume. If the kidneys are functioning normally, they will attempt to retain water and salt by reducing the excretion of sodium chloride and water to minimal amounts. As dehydration progresses, the concentrations of the sodium ion (Na^+) and the chloride ion (Cl^-) in plasma rise with a developing blood concentration.

When the fluid compartments become greatly depleted, shock results, indicating that the deficits are so great that the regulatory mechanisms of the body can no longer maintain the plasma volume. This blood volume reduction (*hypovolemia*) is responsible for such manifestations as a rapid weak pulse, fall in blood pressure, and increased concentration of blood solutes. Since the kidneys rely upon sufficient arterial blood pressure to produce urine, hypovolemia results in decreased urine output. Oliguria progresses to anuria. As a consequence when metabolic wastes are allowed to accumulate, the patient quickly becomes disoriented and comatose; death ensues due to the effects of the acid waste products on the cells.

Wide variations occur in the electrolyte changes in dehydration. The nature of these changes is dependent upon many factors, some of which are as follows:

1. The volume and composition of the fluid lost. In vomiting due to pyloric obstruction, large amounts of chloride may be lost, whereas in severe diarrhea, large amounts of potassium can be lost.

2. The state of renal function. The function of the kidneys may be impaired as a result of dehydration or other underlying disease, thus altering the plasma electrolyte concentrations.

3. The underlying disease process and the amount of water and electrolyte intake. In diabetes mellitus large amounts of sodium, chloride, and water are lost with the diuresis associated with the disease. In addition, large amounts of water may be lost by vaporization from the lungs with hyperventilation. Large amounts of potassium are also lost from the intracellular compartment. These losses are magnified when the intake is also reduced.

4. The proportionate loss of electrolytes as compared to the water loss. Fluids and electrolytes are not necessarily lost in the same proportions. Any one of the following may take place:

    a. The loss of electrolytes is in excess proportionate to the loss of fluid.

    b. The loss of electrolytes is in the same proportion as the loss of fluids.

    c. The loss of electrolytes is proportionately less than the loss of fluid.

Assessment of the Dehydrated Person

People who are dehydrated manifest certain signs and symptoms. The nurse should be able to assess the initial signs and symptoms of dehydration as well as those indicating a more progressive condition. It is not necessary for a person to have all of these signs to be dehydrated; neither does the presence of one or two of these signs necessarily indicate dehydration:

1. Weight loss.
2. Dry skin, which may be flaky.
3. Sticky mucous membrane.
4. A decreased urine output.
5. Amber colored urine.

6. Increased hemoglobin, increased red blood cell concentration, and increased hematocrit and blood urea nitrogen (BUN).

7. Complaints of thirst.

8. A low fluid intake, or total fluid output disproportionately high to the intake.

9. Lethargy.

10. Loss of tissue turgor.

11. Sunken eyeballs; depressed fontanelles in children.

12. Low blood pressure (late sign).

13. Mental disorientation (late sign).

14. Coma (late sign).

ELECTROLYTE IMBALANCES

In health a person's body automatically maintains a state of homeostasis, that is, a balance in the electrolytes and the fluids within the three body compartments. In situations in which fluid is lost from the body, electrolytes are also lost. In disease conditions, major losses frequently occur from the body's secretions or excretions such as increased perspiration during fever or from intestinal secretions throughout suction therapy or diarrhea. See Table 30-1 for the normal electrolyte composition of body secretions as compared to plasma.

Usually electrolyte imbalances are determined through laboratory assessment of a patient's electrolyte levels in the blood plasma. Because the blood plasma has a composition and concentration of electrolytes similar to the interstitial fluid, plasma is used

Table 30-1.   Electrolyte Composition of Body Secretions and Excretions in mEq/L as Compared to Plasma

Electrolyte	Plasma	Gastric Secretions	Pancreatic Juice	Hepatic Duct Bile	Jejunal Secretions	Perspiration	Diarrhea in Children
Sodium (Na^+)	140+	70	140+	140+	140	80	15
Potassium (K^+)	5	5+	5	5	5	5	18
Chloride (Cl^-)	100+	140	35	100+	135	85	10
Bicarbonate (HCO_3^-)	25+	5	115+	40	30	—	No method of determining; thought to be as high as K^+

to measure the composition of extracellualr fluids. The one difference is that plasma contains plasma proteins called *colloids*, which interstitial tissue fluid does not contain. At this time, scientists are unable to measure the electrolyte concentrations of intracellular fluid precisely.

Imbalances can be described as excesses or deficits in electrolytes. Electrolyte imbalances of sodium, potassium, and calcium will be described. The bicarbonate imbalances are discussed with acid-base imbalances.

Sodium Imbalances

The sodium ion (Na^+), referred to in this section as sodium, plays a major role in the body's fluid balance and in therapy for fluid disturbances. Sodium is generally associated with water, in that where water is, there generally is sodium. The major source of sodium (salt) for most people is table salt (NaCl), which is used in cooking and is added to foods as a condiment.

Sodium is the major cation (Na^+) of the extracellular fluids, that is, blood plasma and interstitial fluid. The sodium ion moves rapidly between the plasma and the interstitial fluid. This movement is closely related to the movement of fluid between the two spaces. Under normal conditions the loss of sodium from the body is minimal; it is regulated chiefly by the kidneys. When the amount of sodium is decreased in the body, aldosterone is produced by the adrenal cortex as a result of stimulation by the pituitary gland. Aldosterone acts on the kidney tubules to cause increased reabsorption of sodium.

In illness, abnormally large amounts of sodium can be lost through the gastrointestinal tract and because of profuse sweating. The sodium content of pancreatic secretions and the gastric mucus is especially high. Conditions such as severe prolonged diarrhea or a draining pancreatic fistula can result in an abnormally high sodium loss, just as can gastric suction, which withdraws gastric fluids including gastric mucus.

Hypernatremia is an elevated level of sodium in the blood plasma. *Hyponatremia* refers to a lowered sodium level in the blood plasma. Either hypernatremia or hyponatremia can occur in dehydration. Hypernatremia suggests that the amount of water lost is in excess proportionate to the amount of sodium lost. Hyponatremia together with dehydration indicates that the amount of water lost is either proportionate to the loss of sodium or proportionately less than the amount of sodium.

Hyponatremia

Two situations that can precede a sodium deficit are as follows:

1. A loss of sodium in excess of the loss of water such as in prolonged excessive sweating or the prolonged use of strong diuretics.

2. The intake of water in excess of the intake of sodium as by drinking excessive quantities of water.

Nursing Assessment

1. Feelings of apprehension and impending doom.
2. Abdominal cramps and diarrhea.
3. Convulsions in extreme hyponatremia, which can precede death.

Laboratory Findings

1. The blood plasma level of sodium will be below 137 mEq/liter, as low as 20 mEq/liter.

2. The urine will have a specific gravity below 1.010.

Therapy.   Sodium chloride tablets are provided in situations where excessive losses are caused by increased sweating, such as for persons working in high environmental temperatures. In other situations, the underlying cause is treated, such as a draining fistula. Saline infusions may be necessary if oral ingestion of salt tablets is not possible.

Hypernatremia

Hypernatremia can occur in a person as a result of one of the following situations:

1. When sodium intake is greatly in excess of water intake, as in a person who mistakenly ingests a large number of sodium chloride tablets.

2. When a person's water loss is in excess of sodium loss as is caused by a draining intestinal wound from which an excess of fluid drains compared to the sodium loss through the wound. Nurses may also see hypernatremia about the fifth or sixth day after the onset of untreated diarrhea.

Nursing Assessment.   Nurses may observe some or all of the following signs in a hypernatremic patient:

1. Oliguria (decreased urine output).
2. Agitated behavior, which can lead to gross hyperactivity (mania) or convulsions.
3. Firm, rubbery tissue turgor.
4. Dry, sticky mucous membrane.
5. Fever.

Laboratory findings

1. The sodium level in the plasma will be above 140 mEq/liter.

2. The specific gravity of the urine will be above 1.030.

Therapy.   Treatment has two main objectives: first, to treat the reason for the excess sodium, that is, the diarrhea or the draining wound; and second, to administer fluids. If the sodium excess is not too severe, adminstration of oral fluids may be all that is necessary, but if the excess is extreme, an intravenous infusion such as water with 5% glucose is frequently given.

Depending upon the patient's condition, a diet that is low in sodium may be indicated. Often eliminating table salt in and on food is sufficient. This may include the provision of salt-free foods such as butter.

Potassium Imbalances

Potassium (K$^+$) is the principal cation of the intracellular fluids. Potassium is significant in maintaining the body's fluid and electrolyte balance, particularly the intracellular fluid. Just as with sodium, the intake and output of potassium is normally well balanced. The average adult's diet meets the daily need for potassium (about 2 to 4 gm).

Potassium affects the functions of most of the body systems such as the cardiovascular system, the gastrointestinal system, the neuromuscular system, and the respiratory system. Of particular relevance is the role of potassium in transmitting electrical impulses in muscles such as the heart, in lung tissues, and in intestinal tissues. Most of the body's potassium is found inside the cells. A proportionately small amount is found in the plasma and interstitial fluids.

Potassium is usually excreted by the kidneys. Unlike sodium, the kidneys do not regulate the excretion of potassium effectively. Therefore an acute potassium deficiency can develop rapidly. Of the body's secretions, the gastrointestinal secretions are high in potassium.

As is true of the other electrolytes, potassium is continually moving in and out of the cells. This movement from the interstitial fluid, which has less potassium, to the intracellular fluid, which has a greater concentration, is influenced by the adrenal steroids, testosterone, pH changes, glycogen formation, and hyponatremia. In situations where tissues are damaged, potassium can quickly be lost from the cells and from the body. It has been estimated that about a third of all hospital patients may show signs indicating a deficiency in potassium. People receiving diuretics are frequently deficient in potassium if the daily intake does not reach 30 to 45 mEq daily (Abott Laboratories Ltd. 1970:19). *Hyperkalemia* is an excess of potassium, and *hypokalemia* refers to a deficit of potassium in the body.

Hypokalemia

A potassium deficit is not an uncommon problem. Potassium can be lost rapidly as a result of diarrhea, vomiting, some kidney diseases, diuretic therapy, and increased stress.

Nursing Assessment

1. Muscle weakness, including skeletal, intestinal, and respiratory muscles.
2. Arrhythmias of the heart (variations in normal rhythm), which can be reflected in an irregular pulse.
3. Anorexia and abdominal distention.

Laboratory Findings

1. The potassium level of the blood plasma is repeatedly below 4 mEq/liter.

2. An electrocardiogram may show flattening of the T waves and depression of the S-T segment. (See the normal cardiogram shown in Figure 38-2.)

Therapy.   The therapy frequently prescribed is the administration of potassium by intravenous infusion or in some cases by mouth.

Hyperkalemia

An excess of potassium is usually a result of leakage of potassium out of the cells. It can also occur as a result of renal failure or excessive administration of potassium by intravenous infusion.

Nursing Assessment.   The following observations may indicate hyperkalemia:

1. Intestinal colic.
2. Oliguria, which may progress to anuria.
3. Diarrhea.
4. Heart muscle weakness, which may be reflected by an irregular pulse.

Laboratory Findings

1. The potassium of the blood plasma is repeatedly above 5.6 mEq/liter.
2. The electrocardiogram will show early high T waves and depressed S-T segments and later a disappearance of T waves and heart block.

Therapy.   The major objective in hyperkalemia therapy is to reduce the level of the serum potassium. This can usually be accomplished by employing all or some of the following measures:

1. Increase the output of potassium by the kidneys. It may only be necessary to provide increased fluid intake, and it may also be necessary to employ a method such as peritoneal dialysis.
2. Reduce the intake of potassium by eliminating the oral intake of all foods that contain potassium and any intravenous infusions that contain potassium.

Calcium Imbalances

More than 90% of the body calcium is contained in the bones. If the serum calcium level falls below normal (below 5 mEq/liter), then calcium is withdrawn from the bones to make up the deficit in the blood serum. *Hypocalcemia* refers to a calcium deficit, and *hypercalcemia* refers to an excess of calcium.

Hypocalcemia

Hypocalcemia occurs in a number of situations such as in the removal of the parathyroid glands and in the excessive loss of the intestinal secretions, which contain a great deal of calcium.

Nursing Assessment

1. Muscle cramps.
2. Tingling in the fingers.
3. *Tetany* (muscle spasms, sharp flexion of the wrists and ankles, cramps), which may lead to convulsions.

Laboratory Findings

1. The plasma calcium will be below 4.5 mEq/liter.
2. The electrocardiogram will show a prolonged Q-T interval.

Therapy.   The therapy includes the provision of calcium orally, intramuscularly, or intravenously. Seldom is calcium administered intravenously because of the reservoir of calcium in bone and the fact that intravenous infusion of calcium will not prevent the decalcification of bone.

Hypercalcemia.

The major reason for hypercalcemia is overactivity of the parathyroid glands. It may also be seen in malignant disease of the bone and in hyperthyroidism.

Nursing Assessment.   Hypercalcemia tends to effect nearly all the systems of the body.

1. Relaxed muscles.
2. Pain in the flank as a result of the production of kidney stones.
3. Deep pain in the thighs due to the honeycombing of the bones.
4. Pathologic fractures of bones.
5. In calcium crisis the heart arrests, and the patient experiences nausea, vomiting, and eventually stupor and coma.

Laboratory Findings

1. The serum calcium level will be above 10.5 mg%.
2. An electrocardiogram will reflect neuromuscular changes.

Therapy.   The therapy is designed to treat not only the reason for the excess calcium but also to reduce the intake of calcium. Persons who take large amounts of milk may experience some symptoms of hypercalemia, which readily disappear by reducing the milk intake. For patients who have hyperfunctioning parathyroid glands because of a tumor or enlarged gland, this is generally treated by surgical removal.

ACID-BASE IMBALANCES

Body fluids are maintained within a precise pH range of 7.35 to 7.45 (a slightly alkaline state, since neutrality is 7.0). The pH measurement reflects the hydrogen ion concentration of body fluids. Normally, the ratio of carbonic acid to bicarbonate is 1:20.

Normal metabolic processes are always pouring acids into the body fluids. A major acid resulting from metabolism is carbonic acid because carbon dioxide is one of the chief end products of metabolism.

$$CO_2 \quad + \quad H_2O \quad \longrightarrow \quad H_2CO_3$$
(carbon dioxide)   (water)   (carbonic acid)

Carbonic acid is sometimes considered a respiratory acid, since the lungs excrete it as carbon dioxide and water. Other acids produced as waste products of metabolism are sulfuric, phosphoric, and lactic acids, all of which enter the bloodstream and are normally excreted by the kidneys.

Imbalances in the pH of body fluid result in either acidosis or alkalosis. These are further subdivided into respiratory or metabolic imbalances. Thus the four acid-base disturbances are (a) respiratory acidosis, (b) metabolic acidosis, (c) respiratory alkalosis, and (d) metabolic alkalosis.

The respiratory imbalances are those brought about by changes in the blood carbonic acid, which is regulated by the lungs, whereas the metabolic imbalances are those brought about by changes in the blood bicarbonate, which is regulated by the kidneys.

Both respiratory and metabolic acidosis are more frequently encountered clinically than alkalotic conditions. Death can occur when the pH falls below 6.8 or rises above 7.8. (See Figure 30-2 for pH of body fluids.)

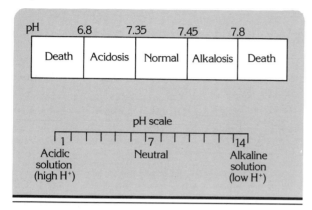

Figure 30-2.   The pH of body fluids in maintained at a slightly alkaline state between the precise range of 7.35 to 7.45.

Assessing Acid-Base Imbalances

The clinical signs indicating that patients have an acid-base imbalance are not as specific as the laboratory signs. Major clinical signs include changes in respirations and in mental alertness. The nurse needs to be alert to such signs as hypoventilation or hyperventilation and to signs of disorientation that progress to coma and stupor. These changes can occur rapidly or take several days.

The laboratory signs include the pH of plasma, the pH of urine, the P_{CO_2} level of plasma, the bicarbonate level of plasma, and the base excess. See Table 30-2 for normal values and explanations. Note that the P_{O_2} level of plasma is often taken in addition for patients with pulmonary problems. See Table 30-2 for laboratory indications of acid-base imbalances.

Acidosis

Acidosis, also referred to as *acidemia,* is a blood pH below 7.35.

Respiratory Acidosis (Carbonic Acid Excess)

Respiratory acidosis occurs when exhalation of carbonic dioxide is inhibited, creating a carbonic acid excess in the body. Its cause can broadly be considered to be hypoventilation. Two major conditions that cause hypoventialtion are central nervous system depression and obstructive lung disease. Morphine poisoning or anesthesia are examples of central nervous system depression, whereas disease processes such as asthma and emphysema are obstructive lung diseases. Hypoventilation for whatever reason retains carbon dioxide in the body and therefore carbonic acid. Thus a state of acidosis exists.

Table 30-2.   Laboratory Indications of Acid-Base Imbalance

Sign	Normal	Interpretation
Plasma pH	7.35–7.45	Less than 7.35 → acidosis More than 7.45 → alkalosis
Urine pH		Below 6 → acidosis Above 7 → alkalosis
PCO_2	About 40 mm Hg	Less than 40 → respiratory alkalosis More than 40 → respiratory acidosis
Bicarbonate (HCO_3^-)	22 to 29 mEq/liter (about 25 mEq/liter)	Less than 25 → metabolic acidosis More than 25 → metabolic alkalosis
Base excess	−2.5 to +2.5 mEq/liter	Positive results → alkaline excess Negative results → alkaline deficit These values do not always indicate a state of acidosis or alkalosis but show deficits or excesses of base.
PO_2	80 to 100 mm Hg	May be greater than 100 mm Hg if patient is on oxygen. May be less than 75 if there is a pulmonary problem.

Nursing Assessment

1. Hypoventilation that is seen by shallow respirations, poor exhalation, or respiratory embarrassment.

2. Loss of mental alertness and disorientation progressing to stupor, indicating central nervous system depression.

Laboratory Findings

1. Low plasma pH (below 7.35) or a normal pH if compensated (compensation is discussed subsequently).

2. Low urine pH (below 6).

3. High P_{CO_2} (above 40 mm Hg).

4. Normal or high plasma bicarbonate (HCO_3^-).
   a. Above 30 mEq/liter in adults.
   b. Above 25 mEq/liter in children.

5. Base excess is 0 or may be positive (for example, +6) with chronic conditions that are compensated.

Metabolic Acidosis (Base Bicarbonate Deficit)

Metabolic acidosis occurs when the levels of base bicarbonate are low in relation to the carbonic acid blood levels. The kidneys normally retain bicarbonate (HCO_3^-) or excrete hydrogen ions (H^+) in response to altered blood pH. Conditions causing metabolic acidosis are those which deluge the plasma with acid metabolites such as starvation, renal impairment, or diabetes mellitus. Prolonged diarrhea can waste bicarbonate.

Nursing Assessment

1. Kussmaul breathing (deep rapid breathing), which is a compensatory mechanism. This sign is absent in infants.

2. Weakness.

3. Disorientation.

4. Coma.

Laboratory Findings

1. Low plasma pH (below 7.35) or a normal pH if compensated.

2. Low urine pH (below 6).

3. Normal P_{CO_2} or low if compensated (the lungs attempt to blow off more acid).

4. Low plasma bicarbonate.
   a. Below 25 mEq/liter in adults.

   b. Below 20 mEq/liter in children.

5. Base excess shows negative results in a deficit (for example, –6).

6. Potassium excess is usually associated with metabolic acidosis.

Respiratory Alkalosis (Carbonic Acid Deficit)

Respiratory alkalosis occurs when exhalation of carbonic dioxide is excessive, resulting in a carbonic acid deficit. Its cause is, broadly, hyperventilation, which can be due to fever, anxiety, or pulmonary infections. Hyperventilation blows off abundant carbon dioxide, thereby resulting in lowered carbonic acid blood levels.

Alkalosis

Alkalosis, also referred to as *alkalemia*, is a blood pH above 7.45.

Nursing Assessment

1. Hyperventilation (deep and/or rapid breathing).

2. Unconsciousness.

Laboratory Findings

1. High plasma pH (above 7.45).

2. High urine pH (above 7).

3. Low plasma bicarbonate as a compensatory measure. Body compensation depends upon the kidneys and can be a slow process.
   a. Below 25 mEq/liter in adults.
   b. Below 20 mEq/liter in children.

4. Low P_{CO^2} (below 40 mm Hg).

5. Base excess: 0.

Metabolic Alkalosis (Bicarbonate Excess)

Metabolic alkalosis occurs when the level of base bicarbonate is high. Conditions causing metabolic alkalosis are those which flood the plasma with the bicarbonate anion such as excess intake of alkali (baking soda, sodium bicarbonate) and prolonged vomiting, in which the chloride anion is lost. This causes a compensating rise in the bicarbonate anion.

Nursing Assessment

1. Depressed respiration (compensatory).

2. Hypertonic muscles.

3. Tetany.

4. Mental dullness.

Laboratory Findings

1. High plasma pH (above 7.45).

2. High urine pH (above 7).

3. High plasma bicarbonate.
    a. Above 30 mEq/liter in adults.
    b. Above 25 mEq/liter in children.

4. Normal or high P_{CO_2} (above 40 mm Hg)—compensatory elevation.

5. Base excess—positive results indicating an excess (for example, +8).

6. Low K^+.

Compensation

In all acid-base imbalances, there is a corrective body response by both the kidneys and the lungs. Any given acid-base imbalance can be described as compensated until body reserves are used up. Then the condition is described as uncompensated.

In compensated acidosis or alkalosis, the kidneys and lungs are able to restore the altered ratio of one carbonic acid molecule to 20 bicarbonate molecules, thereby maintaining a normal pH. In respiratory acidosis, the plasma pH is maintained at normal even though there is an increase in the P_{CO_2} (carbonic acid) because the kidneys retain bicarbonate.

When the plasma pH is *not* maintained, the condition is described as *uncompensated*. Using the example of respiratory acidosis, there is an increase in the P_{CO_2} (carbonic acid), and the pH is lower than normal (more acid). In this case, the kidneys can no longer retain enough bicarbonate. (See Table 30-3 for an overview of fluid and electrolyte data.)

Clinical Situations

When interpreting laboratory results, the nurse can find a systematic method helpful. To determine whether the patient has acidosis or alkalosis it is necessary first to look at the plasma pH. If it is high or low, the interpretation is straightforward. However, if the pH of the plasma is normal, the patient may still have an acid-base imbalance, but it is probably compensated. The nurse needs then to note the P_{CO_2}. If the P_{CO_2} value is above or below normal, a respiratory

problem occurs (a respiratory acidosis or alkalosis). If the P_{CO_2} is normal, the nurse needs to look at the bicarbonate. An elevation of this value indicates a metabolic alkalosis, whereas a deficit indicates a metabolic acidosis. The nurse also needs to be aware that chronic disease conditions are usually compensated. Therefore the P_{CO_2} and bicarbonate values may be altered accordingly. Examples follow.

Problem 1. Respiratory acidosis

Acute

pH = 7.25	(low)
P_{CO_2} = 60 mm Hg	(high)
HCO_3^- = 25 mEq/liter	(normal)
Base excess (BE) = 0	(normal)
P_{O_2} = 60 mm Hg	(low)

Chronic (Compensated)

pH	7.36	(normal)
P_{CO_2}	70 mm Hg	(high)
HCO_3^-	32 mEq/liter	(high)
BE	+7	(excess)
P_{O_2}	80	(normal)

Problem 2. Metabolic acidosis

Acute

pH	=7.30	(low)
P_{CO_2}	= 40 mm Hg	(normal)
HCO_3^-	= 19 mEq/liter	(low)
BE	= −6	(deficit)
P_{O_2}	= 75	(low)

Chronic (Compensated)

pH	7.38	(normal)
P_{CO_2}	31 mm Hg	(low)
HCO_3^-	18 mEq/liter	(low)
BE	−6	(deficit)
P_{O_2}	80	(normal)

Problem 3. Respiratory alkalosis

Acute

pH	= 7.52	(high)
P_{CO_2}	= 31 mm Hg	(low)
HCO_3^-	= 25 mEq/liter	(normal)
BE	= 0	(normal)

Problem 4. Metabolic alkalosis

Acute

pH	= 7.50	(high)
P_{CO_2}	= 40 mm Hg	(normal)
HCO_3^-	= 31 mEq/liter	(high)
BE	= +8	(excess)

Table 30-3. Overview of Data Regarding Fluid and Electrolytes

Clinical Factor	Body Normal	Predisposing Conditions	Deficit Symptoms	Excess Symptoms	Food Source
Extracellular fluid	Infant: 29% of body weight Adult: 15% of body weight	*Deficit* Insufficient fluid intake, vomiting, diarrhea *Excess* Excessive administration or intake of fluid with NaCl	Weight loss, dry skin and mucous membrane, thirst, oliguria, low blood pressure, plasma pH above 7.45, urine pH above 7.0	Weight gain, edema, puffy eyelids, high blood pressure	Meats, fruits, vegetables, liquids
Base bicarbonate (HCO_3)	Plasma bicarbonates, 25 to 29 mEq/liter, urine pH 5.0 to 7.0, plasma pH 7.35 to 7.45	*Deficit* Uncontrolled diabetes mellitus, starvation, severe infectious diseases, renal insufficiency *Excess* Loss of Cl^- or K^+ through vomiting, gastric suction, hyperadrenalism, prolonged insertion of alkali	Metabolic acidosis, disorientation, weakness, shortness of breath, sweet fruity odor to breath, plasma pH below 7.35, HCO_3^- below 25 mEq/liter	Metabolic alkalosis, slow, shallow respirations, tetany, hypertonic muscles, plasma pH above 7.45, HCO_3^- above 30 mEq/liter	
Carbonic acid (H_2CO_3)		*Deficit* Oxygen lack, fever, encephalitis, hyperventilation *Excess* Pneumonia, emphysema, barbiturate poisoning	Respiratory alkalosis, deep rapid breathing, tetany, convulsions, plasma pH above 7.45, low P_{CO_2}	Respiratory acidosis, disorientation, respiratory embarrassment, cyanosis, weakness, plasma pH below 7.35, high P_{CO_2}	
Protein	14 to 18 gm/100 ml in plasma	*Deficit* Hemorrhage, burns,	Mental depression, fatigue, pallor, weight loss, loss of	No adverse effects	Dairy products, meat, fish, grains, poultry

Table 30-3.   **Cont'd.**

	(women), 12 to 16 gm/100 ml in plasma (men)	inadequate protein intake, draining wounds	muscle tone, edema		
Sodium (Na+)	135–145 mEq/L (plasma)	*Deficit* Excessive perspiration, gastrointestinal suction, diarrhea *Excess* Inadequate water intake.	Apprehension, abdominal cramps, rapid weak pulse, oliguria, plasma sodium below 135 mEq/liter	Dry, sticky mucous membrane, fever, thirst, firm rubbery tissue turgor, plasma sodium above 145 mEq/liter	Table salt (NaCl), cheese, butter and margarine, processed meat (ham, bacon, pork), canned vegetables, and vegetable juice
Potassium (K+)	3.5 to 5 mEq/liter (plasma)	*Deficit* Diarrhea, vomiting, some kidney disease, diuretic therapy, increased stress *Excess* Renal failure, burns, excessive administration	Muscle weakness, abnormal heart rhythm, anorexia, abdominal distention	Oliguria, intestinal colic, irritability, irregular pulse, diarrhea	Nuts, fruits, vegetables, poultry, fish
Calcium (Ca++)	5 mEq/liter (plasma)	*Deficit* Removal of parathyroid glands, excessive loss of intestinal fluids, massive infections *Excess* Overactive parathyroid gland, excessive ingestion of milk	Muscle cramps, tingling in the fingers, tetany, convulsions	Relaxed muscles, flank pain, kidney stones, deep bone pain	Dairy products, meat, fish, poultry, whole grain cereals

| Magnesium (Mg++) | 3 mEq/liter (plasma) | *Deficit* Diarrhea, vomiting, chronic alcoholism, gastric suction, renal disease *Excess* Chronic renal disease | Hallucinations, tremor, disorientation, hyperreflexia, rapid pulse, hypertension | Central nervous system depression, cardiac irregularities | Nuts, wheat bran, chocolate |

PARENTERAL FLUID THERAPY

Fluid therapy can be accomplished by the normal oral route, by nasogastric tube, or by the parenteral routes of intravenous infusion or subcutaneous infusion (*hypodermoclysis*). Oral fluid therapy was discussed in Chapter 29 and nasogastric feedings in Chapter 25. This chapter will include the intravenous route. Intravenous fluid therapy is a common practice in hospitals today. It is an efficient and effective method of supplying fluids directly into the extracellular fluid compartment, specifically the venous system. Hypodermoclysis is not as commonly used, but it is useful in the very young or elderly person whose veins are too small or difficult to enter.

Intravenous Therapy (IV Therapy)

Objectives

1. To supply fluids when patients are unable to take adequate fluids by mouth. Amounts of therapy must provide for average daily needs plus additional amounts for excessive losses. IV fluids are commonly available in 250, 500, or 1000 ml bottles.

2. To provide salts needed to maintain electrolyte balance. Common solutions used are isotonic normal saline (0.9% NaCl) or multiple electrolyte solutions discussed subsequently. Sometimes electrolytes are added to normal saline solutions such as 20 mEq KCl.

3. To provide glucose (dextrose), the main fuel for metabolism. Although many nutrient solutions are available, 5% glucose solutions, commonly referred to as D-5-W, are the most frequently used, or a solution containing glucose and saline (⅔—⅓) may be used. A ⅔—⅓ solution consists of 3.3% glucose and 0.3% sodium chloride solution. Each liter of 5% dextrose solutions provides about 200 calories. Sufficient carbohydrate (a minimum of 450 calories/day) is required to prevent catabolism of body fats for energy, a condition which can result in metabolic acidosis.

4. To provide some water-soluble vitamins such as vitamins B and C or other drugs intravenously. Berocca-C and Vi-Cert are two common vitamin pharmaceuticals. Several medications can be administered intravenously when rapid action is wanted or when the drugs are irritating to subcutaneous or intramuscular tissues. Administration of antibiotics intravenously is extremely common

Determining Dosages and Types of Fluid Administration

Volumes of fluid required are determined by considering the following:

1. Daily maintenance requirements.

2. Previous losses prior to therapy.

3. Concurrent losses that may occur throughout therapy such as may occur from a gastric suction, vomiting, or diarrhea.

For adults, the amount of fluid to be taken usually ranges from 2500 ml/day in moderate dehydration to 3000 ml/day in severe dehydration. For children, the amounts required vary in accordance with their size and metabolic requirements as well as their specific losses.

There are a wide variety of solutions available. In

most therapy situations the solutions of normal saline, glucose, or glucose in normal saline are used. Following is a regimen of solutions categorized in a framework of clinical application. Nutrient solutions, electrolyte solutions, alkalinizing solutions, acidifying solutions, and blood volume expanders are included.

Nutrient Solutions

The patient in bed has a daily caloric requirement of about 1600 calories. Intravenous solutions are now available supplying these calories in the form of carbohydrate, nitrogen (as amino acids), and vitamins that are essential to metabolism. Some commercial preparations also include ethyl alcohol to supply additional calories.

In recent years, lipids (fats) have been marketed with the advent of hyperalimentation (see "Parenteral Hyperalimentation"). The caloric content of nutrient solutions varies from approximately 200 to 1500 calories/liter. Nutrient solutions include the following:

A. Carbohydrate and water

    1. Dextrose (glucose)

    2. Levulose (fructose)

    3. Invert sugar (half dextrose and half levulose)

    4. Ethyl alcohol

B. Amino acid solutions, for example, Amigen, Aminosol, Travamine

C. Lipids, for example, Lipomul

Electrolyte Solutions

Electrolyte solutions are either saline solutions or multiple electrolyte solutions. Saline solutions are available in isotonic, hypotonic, and hypertonic concentrations. The isotonic concentration, called *normal saline*, is most frequently used. Many multiple electrolyte solutions are available, all with varying amounts of cations and anions. Some of these solutions are:

1. Ringer's solution containing Na^+, K^+, Cl^-, CA^{++}

2. Lactated Ringer's solution containing Na^+, K^+, Cl^-, Ca^{++}, HCO_3^-

3. Butler's solution containing Na^+, K^+, Mg^{++}, Cl^-, HCO_3^-

Normal saline solutions are used frequently as initial hydrating solutions. Multiple electrolyte solutions can be considered as balanced or maintenance solutions that approximate the ionic profile of plasma or as special solutions that restore or correct imbalances. Balanced solutions are the Ringer's solutions; Butler's solution is corrective.

Alkalinizing and Acidifying Solutions

Alkalinizing solutions produce alkaline substances and therefore are used to correct a state of acidosis in the body such as in a cardiac arrest or in diabetic coma. Examples of alkalinizing solutions are sodium lactate and sodium bicarbonate solutions. *Lactate* is a salt of lactic acid that is metabolized in the liver to form bicarbonate (HCO_3^-). Its effectiveness is dependent upon liver function.

Acidifying solutions provide acid substances and are used to correct states of alkalosis in the body. An acidifying solution is ammonium chloride. The ammonium is metabolized in the liver to increase urea and hydrogen ions. It is also dependent upon adequate liver function.

Blood Volume Expanders

Blood volume expanders are used to increase the volume of the vascular compartment when loss of blood or plasma has occurred. In severe hemorrhage when whole blood is not available, the administration of plasma maintains the blood volume. In severe burns, when large amounts of fluid shift from the intravascular compartment to the burn site, plasma is the preferred fluid to administer. Other blood volume expanders are human serum albumin and dextran, which comes in various concentrations. Both of these have significant osmotic properties that directly increase the fluid volume of blood.

Nursing Intervention for Intravenous Infusions

It is a nursing function to implement and maintain intravenous therapy. This involves several important measures such as:

1. Explanation and teaching for the patient.

2. Comfort and assistance with activities of daily living throughout the therapy.

3. Maintenance of the intravenous infusion, which involves:

a.   Frequent observation for possible complications.
b.   Changing bottles.
c.   Regulating flow rates.
d.   Changing tubing when necessary.

Explanation and Teaching for the Patient

Explanations can correct misconceptions, gain a person's cooperation, and offer emotional peace of mind. Explanations need to include terms the person understands, the purpose of the infusion, the equipment, the length of time involved, how the patient can help, activity permitted, and how the nurse will assist the patient to meet his or her needs. Explanations need to be adjusted to each patient's own requirements and concerns. Individual or developmental variables are important. Some elderly people may equate intravenous therapy with death and need to be informed of its purpose. Young children may equate it to punishment for not eating or drinking, and the very small child may just be aware of discomfort and fear.

Patient Comfort and Assistance with Activities of Daily Living

Depending upon the length of infusion time and placement of the needle, patients often require assistance with needs such as hygiene or ambulation. Often removing a hospital gown requires assistance from a nurse. Most gowns allow the passage of an intravenous bottle. To remove a soiled gown, remove it from the uninvolved arm first. Next, carefully remove the sleeve down over the infusion site and tubing until it is off the hand. Then remove the intravenous bottle from the stand and with your free hand lift the gown over and off the bottle. Rehang the bottle. To put on a new gown, reverse the order by putting the bottle and tubing through the sleeve of the new gown first. Restraints or splints should be removed periodically to check the state of the skin and circulatory status of the involved extremity. Patients with infusions will also require assistance to ambulate and to turn in bed. Ambulation is facilitated with portable intravenous stands. Turning bed patients may require movement of the intravenous bottle from one side of the bed to the other. When ambulating or turning patients, it is important to avoid placing tension on the tubing to safeguard the involved arm and to make sure that the flow rate is not altered with the movement.

Maintaining the Intravenous Infusion

Frequent observation is required to maintain the rate of flow of an intravenous infusion and to ensure that the patient is responding well to the therapy. It is helpful if the nurse develops a systematic routine in observing the status and progress of infusions. This should include observations of the flow rate, patency of the tubing, the infusion site, level of the fluid in the bottle, and the patient's comfort and reaction to the therapy.

Observation for Possible Complications of Intravenous Therapy   The major complications are infiltration, phlebitis, circulatory overload, and embolism. *Infiltration* is escape of fluid into subcutaneous tissue due to dislodgment of the needle. It is easily detected because the subcutaneous tissues swell, the skin becomes cold because intravenous fluid is at room temperature as contrasted to body temperature, and the patient may complain of pain at the site. Swelling can be checked by comparing the involved extremity with the other extremity. The earliest sign of infiltration can be a reduced rate of flow, and early recognition can prevent unnecessary discomfort to a patient. Some methods for identifying early infiltration are discussed later in this chapter (see "Factors Influencing Flow Rates").

Phlebitis is another potential complication of intravenous infusions caused by the mechanical trauma to the vein or the chemical irritation of some substances such as potassium chloride. Patients may complain of burning pain along the vein or a nurse may notice redness and increased skin temperature over the course of the vein. The venipuncture site needs to be changed and further use of the involved vein avoided.

Circulatory overload means that the intravascular fluid compartment contains more fluid than normal. It occurs when infusion rates are too rapid and results in cardiac failure and pulmonary edema. Signs of pulmonary edema are dyspnea, cough, frothy sputum, and gurgling sounds on respiration. Prevention is achieved by carefully monitoring flow rates so as not to exceed maximum volumes. Circulatory overload can occur if a nurse speeds up the flow rates for an infusion that is behind schedule.

Air embolism has been greatly overrated as a potential hazard of intravenous therapy. Sources vary as to the amount of air required to cause fatal embolism in the human, but amounts are far greater than the total volume of intravenous tubing (5 to 10 ml). Even so, its occurrence is often a matter of concern to patients, family members, and nurses. Embolism may also occur from thrombi formed at the end of the needle or intravenous catheter.

Changing bottles, regulating flow rates, and changing intravenous tubing   These measures are discussed subsequently in this chapter.

Intravenous Infusion Equipment

The design of intravenous infusion sets varies somewhat according to the commercial manufacturer. However, all are basically similar in the manner in which they function. The solutions and equipment are sterile and ready for use. A wide variety of solutions are marketed, each labeled with the specific contents.

Intravenous Solution Bottles

Solution bottles (see Figure 30-3) are vacuum sealed with nonpyrogenic solutions. The tops are fitted with solid rubber stoppers and sealed with metal caps. Covering the rubber stopper is a metal disc, which lies between the stopper and the metal cap. Once exposed, a marked circular area can be seen on the rubber stopper. It is through this area that the intravenous tubing is attached. It is important to note that some makes have two openings in the stopper, one to attach the tubing and the other to act as an air vent. The air vent is evident because a long tube extends from the stopper to the bottom of the bottle. This latter type of bottle also has a rubber seal directly over the stopper which must be removed prior to establishing the infusion to release the air vent.

Intravenous Tubing

Intravenous tubing is designed with an insertion spike at one end, a drip chamber, a clamp to regulate

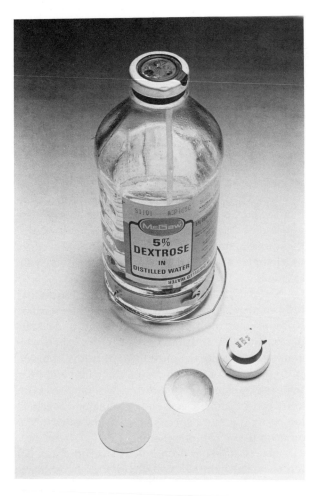

Figure 30-3.   Intravenous bottles with sterile solutions are vacuum sealed. The tops are fitted with solid rubber stoppers. Each one is covered with a metal disc, and a rubber disk, and sealed with a metal cap.

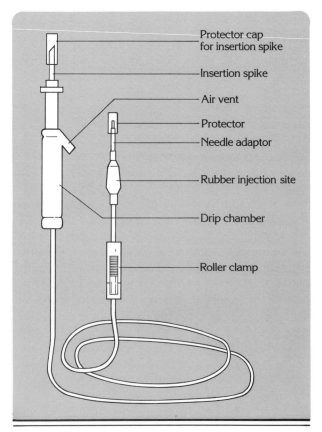

Figure 30-4.   Intravenous administration set consists of an insertion spike with an air vent, a drip chamber, plastic tubing with a control clamp, and a protective cap over the needle adaptor.

the flow and a connector at the end of the tubing, which is attached to the intravenous needle (see Figure 30-4). The sterility of each end of the tubing is maintained by protective plastic coverings. Insertion spikes may or may not have air vents; this depends upon whether the particular solution bottle is provided with one. The sizes of the openings into the drip chamber vary according to the manufacturer. The common sizes deliver 10, 15, or 20 drops per milliliter of solution. Each set has this information provided on the package.

In-line Devices

Special devices are sometimes attached below the insertion spike. These are commonly referred to as a *Volutrol* or a *Pediatrol (Buretrol)*. They are designed to deliver minute quantities of fluid (60 drops/ml). They are particularly useful for administering precise volumes of fluid to infants and children and to administer medications in the intravenous solution. (See Figure 30-5).

Intravenous Needles

Needles for an intravenous injection are usually packaged separately. Some are made of steel; others are made of plastic. The size of needle that is commonly used for intravenous infusions is no. 21 short bevel.

The age of the patient, and the type of infusion will determine the size of the needle. For blood transfusions larger needles are required because of the thickness of the blood; therefore larger veins are also used. For routine short-term intravenous infusions, smaller butterfly or wing-tipped needles may be used in smaller veins. For long-term therapy, intracatheters inserted into larger veins may be necessary. (See Figure 30-6).

Venipuncture Sites

The type of infusion, length of infusion time, and the age of the patient will determine the location of the site.

Adults

The most convenient veins for venipuncture in the adult are the basilic and median cubitus veins in the antecubital space. Since these veins are large and su-

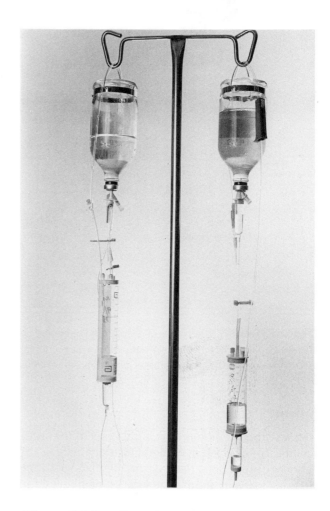

Figure 30-5.   Two in-line intravenous tubing devices.

perficial, they are frequently used by laboratory technicians to withdraw blood for examination. Unfortunately, use of these veins for prolonged infusions limits arm mobility for patients because splints are needed to stabilize the elbow joint. Thus for prolonged therapy other veins on the back of the hand and on the forearm are preferred. These sites are equipped with the natural splints of the ulna and radius and allow the patient more arm movement for activities such as eating. If a person is right handed, use of the left arm allows for more independence, and vice versa.

Ideally, sites for long-term therapy at the distal end of the arm should be used first. If these veins have been used for prolonged periods or if veins are thrombosed (bruised), other more proximal sites may be required. If arm veins are inaccessible, veins in the feet and legs may also be used. See Figure 30-7 for venipuncture sites of the arm, hand, and foot.

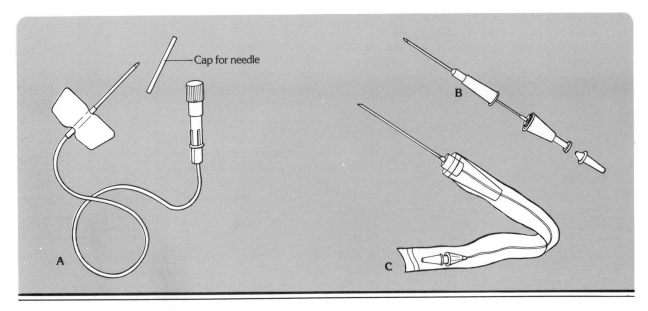

Figure 30-6. Three types of needles and catheters used to administer intravenous fluids. **A,** an intravenous butterfly needle. **B,** An angiocatheter is a needle within a plastic tubing. After insertion in the vein, the needle is removed and the plastic catheter remains. **C,** An intracatheter is a large bore needle with a plastic catheter that is threaded through it after venipuncture.

Infants

Because infants do not have large veins in the antecubital fossa, blood specimens for examination are usually taken from the external jugular vein and femoral veins. If an infusion is to be maintained for long periods, veins are selected in the temporal region of the scalp or sometimes in the back of the hand or the dorsum of the foot. See Figure 30-8 showing the use of the scalp vein for an infant.

Regulating Infusion Flow Rates

Maintaining a constant rate of flow for infusions is a nurse's responsibility. Too rapid infusion rates result in overloading the intravascular compartment, leading to serious cardiac and pulmonary complications. Too slow infusion rates result in inefficient fluid and electrolyte replacement. Methods used to regulate flow rates are based on hourly calculation in milliliters and on the number of drops (gtts) per minute according to the dripmeter. Since the design of intravenous equipment differs among commercial companies, there are variations in the size of openings of drip chambers and thus in the number of drops per milliliter. Fortunately, drops per milliliter are indicated on the container boxes of intravenous infusion sets. Common drop factors are 10, 15, 20, and 60 drops per milliliter.

Calculating the Number of Milliliters of Infusion per Hour

Hourly rates of infusion can be calculated by dividing the total infusion volume by the total time in hours for the infusion. For example, if 3000 ml are to be infused in 24 hours, the number of milliliters per hour of fluid to be infused is

$$\frac{3000 \text{ ml (total infusion volume)}}{24 \text{ hours (total time of infusion)}} = 125 \text{ ml/hour}$$

Hourly checks by nurses are needed to assure that the indicated milliliters per hour have infused. Some nurses add a strip of adhesive tape to the solution bottle marking the exact time and/or the amount to be infused. (See Figure 30-11.)

Calculating Drops per Minute

When an infusion is commenced, the drops per minute must be regulated to ensure that the prescribed amounts of solution will infuse. Calculating drops per minute is done by using the following formula:

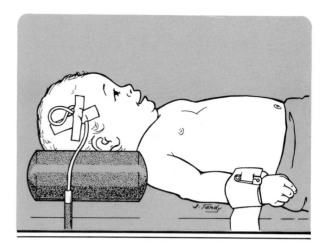

Figure 30-8. For infants, veins in the temporal region of the scalp are used to administer fluids for prolonged periods. Head and extremity restraints are needed to prevent dislodgement of the intravenous needle.

Drops per minute =

$$\frac{\text{Total infusion volume} \times \text{drops/ml (or drip factor)}}{\text{Total time of infusion in } \textit{minutes}}$$

If the requirements are 1000 ml in 8 hours (480 minutes) and the drip factor is 20 drops/ml, the drops per minute should be regulated as follows:

$$\frac{1000 \text{ ml (total infusion volume)} \times 20 \text{ drops/ml}}{480 \text{ minutes}} =$$

$$41 \text{ drops/minute}$$

Approximating this as 40 drops/minute, the nurse must then regulate the drops per minute by tightening or releasing the intravenous tubing clamp and counting the drops in much the same way as counting a pulse. New devices are now available such as battery-operated rate meters and infusion pumps with alarm systems to facilitate regulated flow.

Factors Influencing Flow Rates

No matter how often flow rates are regulated, several factors can change the rate of flow of IV infusions. If an infusion is not infusing as planned, several factors need to be considered. (Text continued on p. 739.)

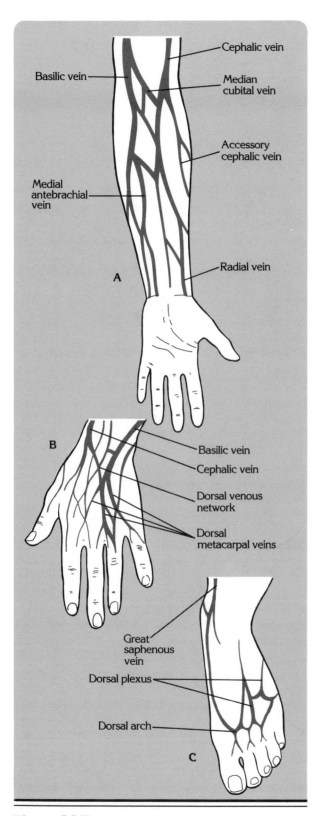

Figure 30-7. Commonly used venipuncture sites of the arm, **A;** hand, **B;** and foot, **C.**

Procedure 30-1.   Arm Venipuncture

Purposes

1. To start an infusion of fluid or blood.

2. To withdraw a blood sample.

3. To administer drugs.

Action	**Explanation**
Assemble Equipment	
1. Intravenous needle and syringe if other than wing-tipped needle is used.	
2. Alcohol swabs.	
3. Tourniquet.	
4. Receptacle.	For discarded fluid.
5. Adhesive tape.	
6. Parenteral solution ordered.	
7. Intravenous tubing and drip meter.	
8. Intravenous stand (pole).	
9. Check the intravenous solution and tubing. They should be clear and sterile.	Discolored or cloudy solutions may indicate contamination.
10. Select a needle size that is appropriate to the vein caliber and the solution. Lengths of needles used are 1 or 1½ inches.	More viscid solutions such as whole blood require large needles (no. 18 or 19); other solutions require no. 21 or 22.
Attach Intravenous Tubing to Bottle	
1. Explain to the patient what you plan to do. Adjust the explanation to the patient's needs.	To reassure the patient. To identify the patient.
2. Remove the metal cap from the intravenous bottle, being careful not to touch the bottle opening. Note that some preparations have a circular metal cap, which is easily removed. Others have a brown rubber insert that must also be removed. Two holes should then be exposed (one for the IV tubing spike, the other for the air outlet).	Sterile technique must be used to prevent contamination of the solution and the ends of the tubing. Variations in design of solution bottles occur with different commercial companies.
3. With the bottle upright, insert the dripmeter spike into the bottle opening.	
4. Hang the bottle on the intravenous stand 18 to 24 inches above the vein. Make sure the tubing is clamped first or fluid will be lost.	Sufficient height is needed for gravity to overcome venous pressure and facilitate flow of the solution into the vein.

5. Squeeze the drip chamber until it is two thirds full.

6. Flush the IV fluid through the tubing into the discard basin until all air is removed. Fluid will not flow until the clamp is released and the protective cap is removed at the end of the tubing.
   Once all the air is out of the tubing, reapply the protective cap, clamp the tubing, and hang it up on the IV stand until venipuncture is completed.

Large amounts of air act as emboli in the blood stream.

Sterile technique must be maintained in removing the protective cap and in reapplying it.

Select and Prepare the Venipuncture Site

1. First, prepare strips of adhesive tape to stabilize the IV needle once it is inserted.

2. Select a site starting at the distal end of the vein.

The remainder of the vein can be used for additional sites.

3. Shave the skin if necessary around the insertion site to remove hair where adhesive tape will be applied.

Dilate the Vein

1. Place the extremity in a dependent position (lower than the patient's heart).

Gravity impedes venous return and distends the veins.

2. Apply a tourniquet firmly 6 to 8 inches proximal to the venipuncture site.

The tourniquet must be tight enough to obstruct venous flow but not too tight to occlude arterial flow. If a radial pulse can be palpated, the arterial flow is not obstructed. Obstructing arterial flow inhibits venous filling.

3. Massage or stroke the vein distal to the site and in the direction of venous flow toward the heart.

This helps fill the vein.

4. Encourage the patient to rapidly clench and unclench the fist.

Contracting muscles compresses the distal veins, forcing blood along the veins and distending them to the point of the tourniquet.

5. Lightly tap the vein with your fingertips.

This distends the vein.

6. If steps 2 to 5 fail to distend the vein, remove the tourniquet and apply heat to the entire extremity for 10 to 15 minutes. Then repeat steps 2 to 5.

Heat dilates superficial blood vessels, causing them to fill.

Insert the Needle

1. Cleanse the skin with an antiseptic swab at the site of entry and pull the skin taut with the thumb below the vein site.

The latter stabilizes the vein and makes the skin taut for needle entry. It also makes initial tissue penetration less painful.

Procedure 30-1.   Cont'd

2. Holding the needle at a 30° angle with the bevel up, pierce the skin lateral to the vein. See Figure 30-9.

Figure 30-9.

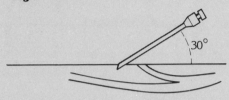

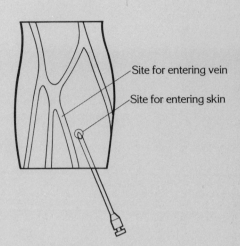

Site for entering vein

Site for entering skin

3. Once through the skin, lower the angle of the needle so it is parallel with the skin. Follow the course of the vein and pierce the side of the vein.

Lowering the angle limits the chances of puncturing both sides of a vein.

4. When back-flow of blood occurs into the needle tubing, insert the needle further up the vein (¾ to 1 inch) or to the hub of the butterfly needle.

Sudden lack of resistance can be felt as blood enters tubing or syringe.

5. Release the tourniquet and attach the infusion.

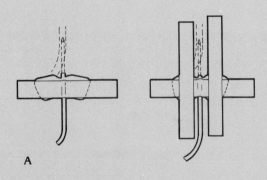

A

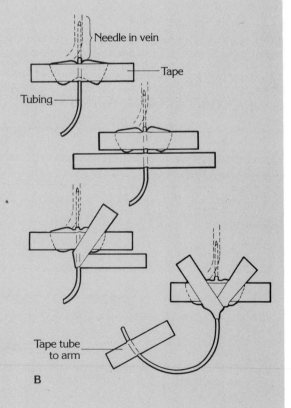

Needle in vein

Tape

Tubing

Tape tube to arm

B

Figure 30-10.   A, H-method and, B, Criss cross method.

6. Tape the needle securely by the H-method or criss cross method. See Figure 30-10. Support by a 2 × 2 gauze or cotton ball may be necessary under the needle to keep it in position in the vein.

7. Tape the tubing to prevent pull on the IV needle as shown in Figure 30-10.

8. Apply a padded armboard to splint the elbow or wrist joint if needed.

1. *Position of the forearm.* Sometimes having the patient change the position of the arm will facilitate flow, such as changing the position to slight pronation, supination, or extension. Elevating the forearm on a pillow also can help.

2. *Patency of the tubing.* Not infrequently, the tubing is obstructed by the patient lying on the tubing or by a kink. Readjusting the clamp on the tubing may be necessary.

3. *Height of the infusion bottle.* Elevating the height of the infusion bottle a few inches can hasten the flow by creating more pressure.

4. Possibility of *infiltration or fluid leakage.* Swelling, a feeling of coldness, and tenderness at the venipuncture site can indicate infiltration. If none are evident, the following measures can determine whether the needle is dislodged from the vein:

   a. Lower the infusion bottle below the level of the venipuncture site to see if blood returns. This will indicate that the intravenous needle is still in the vein, although it is not a foolproof method because the needle may be partially penetrating the vein wall.

   b. With a sterile syringe of saline, withdraw fluid from the rubber at the end of the tubing. If blood does not return, discontinue the intravenous.

   c. Try to stop the flow. Apply a tourniquet 4 to 6 inches above the insertion site and open the roller clamp wide. If the infusion continues to flow slowly, the needle is in subcutaneous tissue (it has infiltrated).

Changing Intravenous Bottles

It is the nurse's responsibility to change bottles when a small amount of solution is in the neck of the bottle before the drop chamber is empty. Sterile technique is essential. The procedure is as follows:

1. Prepare the new bottle prior to the old one running out. Remove the metal cap.

2. Some nurses clamp the intravenous tubing, although it is not always necessary if actions are conducted efficiently. However, it is better to clamp the tubing first when the air inlet is small, since fluid will be sucked up and the drip chamber becomes plugged with fluid. Then the drip count is impossible to regulate.

3. Remove the spike from the old bottle and quickly insert it into the new bottle.

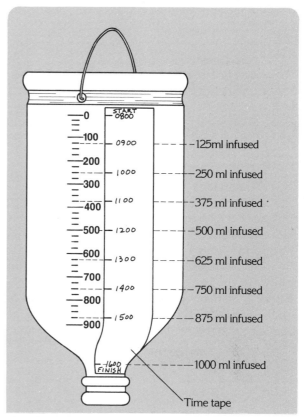

Figure 30-11. An adhesive marker placed on the solution bottle facilitates monitoring of the flow rate. Each hour, 125 ml of solution is to infuse up to 1000 ml. With a drip factor of 20, the solution is administered at 40 drops/min (125 ml/hr) for a total of eight hours.

4. Hang up the new bottle.

5. Release the tubing clamp if it was closed, and reestablish the infusion with the prescribed rate of flow.

6. Chart the amount and type of fluid that has infused and/or the amount and type of fluid added according to agency policy.

Changing the Intravenous Tubing

Agency policies should be checked about the recommended frequency of tubing changes. The change is most easily done when a new bottle is to be added. Specific times for tubing change should be recorded on the patient's record or Kardex. The procedure for attaching intravenous tubing to the bottle has already been discussed. The major difference in this instance is that the adhesive tapes securing the intravenous needle must be loosened to expose the needle hub. Then the old tubing can be removed and the new tubing (already prepared) attached. Reestablish the infusion and apply new tape to secure the needle and new tubing.

Discontinuing an Intravenous Infusion

Intravenous infusions are terminated when the prescribed volume of fluid has infused or when infiltration occurs (see Procedure 30-2.

Attaching Two or More Solutions

In some situations it is necessary to administer two or more different solutions to the patient such as whole blood and normal saline. Solutions can be attached in two ways. One method is to attach a small connecting tube from the air vent of one bottle and suspend the bottles in series. The second method is to use Y-tubing connections. The Y-tubing connection is advantageous in that it allows for simultaneous or inter-mittent infusion of the solutions. The former method using the connecting tube only provides for infusion in order of the series; that is, bottle A infuses first, followed by bottle B.

Blood Transfusions

A *blood transfusion* is the introduction of whole blood or components of the blood such as plasma, serum, erythrocytes, or platelets into the venous circulation.

The reasons for blood transfusions are as follows:

1. To restore blood volume after severe hemorrhage.
2. To restore the red blood cell level after severe and chronic anemias and to maintain blood hemoglobin levels.
3. To provide plasma factors such as antihemophilic factor (AHF) that are necessary to control bleeding.

Procedure 30-2   Discontinuing an Intravenous Infusion

Action	Explanation
1. Loosen the tape at the venipuncture site while holding the needle firmly. The tape does not need to be removed from the needle.	Moving the needle as little as possible prevents unnecessary trauma to the vein and discomfort to the patient.
2. Clamp the infusion tubing.	To stop the flow of fluid and prevent soiling the patient after the needle is removed.
3. Withdraw the needle by pulling on the needle hub in line with the vein. At the same time hold a dry sterile gauze or swab over the needle site.	To prevent vein trauma.
4. As soon as the needle is withdrawn, apply firm pressure to the site with a dry swab or gauze for 2 to 3 minutes.	Pressure helps to stop the bleeding and prevent hematoma formation.
5. Apply a small bandaid or sterile dressing over the needle site. (This dressing can be removed the following day.)	To stop further bleeding and prevent infection at the needle site.
6. Assist the patient to a comfortable position.	
7. Discard the administration set and dispose of the equipment appropriately.	
8. Wash hands.	
9. Record the amount of fluid infused.	Necessary for intake record.

Blood Matching

Human blood is classified into four main groups (A, B, AB, and O) on the basis of erythrocyte cell proteins that commonly cause antibody reactions. These proteins, type A and type B, are called *agglutinogens.* In other words, Group A blood contains type A agglutinogen. Group B blood contains type B agglutinogen, Group AB blood contains both A and B agglutinogens, but Group O contains neither agglutinogen.

In addition to the presence of agglutinogens in the erythrocytes, *antibodies (agglutinins)* are present in the blood plasma. The agglutinins are referred to as *alpha (anti-A) agglutinins,* which agglutinate type A cells, and *beta (anti-B) agglutinins,* which agglutinate type B cells. The antibodies each person has are different from the agglutinogen each has; otherwise the person's own cells would be attacked. Thus Group A blood does not contain agglutinin A but does contain agglutinin B. Group B blood does not contain agglutinin B but does contain agglutinin A. Group AB blood contains neither agglutinin, and Group O contains both anti-A and anti-B agglutinins. The most common blood types are type A and type O. More of the black population possess type B blood than does the white population, but almost 50% of both populations possess type O blood. See Table 30-4.

The Hemolytic Reaction

When similar agglutinins and agglutinogens come in contact with each other such as type A agglutinogen and anti-A agglutinin or type B agglutinogen and anti-B agglutinin, clumping (agglutination) and rupture (hemolysis) of the red cells occurs. This produces the fatal response called a *hemolytic reaction* (see Table 30-5.) When transfusions are given, it is essential that the blood used is of the same type as that of the recip-

ient. Otherwise the agglutinins present in the recipient's plasma will agglutinate the red cells being donated. Type A blood has anti-B agglutinins; therefore if type B blood is given to a person with type A blood, the anti-B agglutinins present will agglutinate the type B blood cells. Because type O blood has neither A nor B agglutinogens, it can be donated to recipients with any of the four types of blood; it is called the *universal donor.* Type AB blood, on the other hand, has neither anti-A or anti-B agglutinins in plasma and therefore is referred to as a *universal recipient,* being able to receive any of the four blood types.

In summary, similar agglutinins and agglutinogens react and produce agglutination and hemolysis of erythrocytes.

$$\begin{array}{ccc} \text{Type A} & + & \text{Type B} = \text{Hemolysis} \\ \text{(agglutinogen A)} & & \text{(anti-A agglutinin)} \end{array}$$

$$\begin{array}{ccc} \text{Type B} & + & \text{Type A} = \text{Hemolysis} \\ \text{(agglutinogen B)} & & \text{(anti-B agglutinin)} \end{array}$$

See Table 30-4 for possible donors.

Rhesus (Rh) Blood Groups

Other proteins are present in the blood that can lead to mismatching of blood. Of these, the Rh factor, which is present in about 85% of the population, can be a major cause of hemolytic reactions. Persons who possess the Rh factor are referred to as *Rh positive;* those who do not are referred to as *Rh negative.* Some other factors are the Hr, Kell, Lewis, M, N, and P factors. These latter factors rarely cause major reactions because their antigenic properties are poor. They have proved to be of more importance in forensic medicine than in transfusing blood. For example, it has been possible to determine fatherhood in situa-

Table 30-4.   Survey of Information on Blood Groups

Blood Type (Red Blood Cell Agglutinogens)	Agglutinins in Plasma	Possible Donors	Percentage of White Population	Percentage of Black Population
A	Anti-B (beta)	Types A and O	41	30
B	Anti-A (alpha)	Types B and O	9	20
AB	None	Types AB, A, B, and O	3	3
O (no agglutinogen)	Anti-A and anti-B	Type O	47	47

tions of disputed parentage by the presence of these factors. Usually half of the factors present in the child can be found in the mother's blood, the other half in the father's blood.

Rh Factor.   The Rh factor differs from the A and B agglutinogens in that it cannot cause a hemolytic reaction on first exposure of mismatched blood. This is because the Rh antibody is *not* present in those persons who are Rh negative. Although a person with type O blood does not have either A or B agglutinogen but does have anti-A and anti-B agglutinins, the Rh-negative person has no anti-Rh antibodies. This person, however, can develop Rh antibodies if exposed to the Rh factor. When Rh-positive blood is given to an Rh negative person the individual will produce Rh antibodies but will not manifest a reaction on first exposure. On second exposure, however, the agglutination process will occur.

Erythroblastosis fetalis is one of the major consequences of the Rh factor, which involves infants born by Rh negative mothers when the father is Rh positive. If the fetus inherits the Rh-positive factor from the father, some of this protein passes to the mother through the placental membrane. The mother then develops Rh antibodies, which in turn are passed back to the baby, in whom agglutination and destruction of the fetal red cells results. This process is fatal to many infants prior to birth. For those that do survive birth, exchange transfusions are necessary. The Rh-positive infant is transfused with Rh-negative blood, and the Rh-positive blood is removed. The Rh antibodies in the infant's body fluids cannot destroy this Rh-negative blood. Within approximately a month the Rh antibodies have been destroyed and the infant can then safely produce blood.

Risks of Blood Transfusion

Although technologic advances have made blood transfusions a relatively safe procedure, some risks are involved; therefore transfusions are given only when absolutely necessary. It has been estimated that 1 in 2000 persons receiving a blood transfusion dies.

Mislabeling Errors.   Faulty identification of containers can lead to a person receiving the wrong type of blood. Fatal hemolytic reactions can occur if, for example, a patient with type A blood receives types B or AB blood. See Table 30-5.

Transmission of Diseases.   Syphilis, malaria, and hepatitis can be transmitted by donors that are asymptomatic carriers. Although precautionary questions are asked when blood is donated, there is no foolproof method of detecting all carriers. The incidence of syphilis contracted through blood transfusions is rare now since the advent of serologic testing on all units of blood.

Hepatitis has *not* been known to follow the use of albumin, which, unlike all other blood products, is subjected to heating in the preparation process. This certifies albumin as free from all viral contaminants. Hepatitis remains a risk in the transfusion of all blood products, however, excepting albumin. Recipients of infected blood produce symptoms of the disease from 2 to 6 months after transfusion. The common signs are fever, jaundice, and lethargy.

Sensitivities.   In most blood transfusions the donor's red cells have some antigenic factor that the recipient does not have. For the most part these factors are poor antigens, but occasionally some can evoke intense antibody formation. This creates a risk for the recipient when subsequent transfusions are given. Sensitivities can also be produced to antigens of the donor's white cells, platelets, or some serum proteins.

Citrate Toxicity.   Citrate toxicity can occur when massive transfusions are required such as six units of blood in less than 24 hours. Each unit of whole blood contains approximately 50 ml of acid-citrate dextrose (ACD) solution. Its purpose is to serve as an anticoagulant and to provide the red cells with sugar for metabolism.

Iron Overload.   Each unit (500 ml) of blood contains 250 mg of iron. For patients who have chronic anemia and who must have frequent transfusions, hemosiderosis develops. *Hemosiderosis* is the deposition of iron in the skin, liver, spleen, and other organs, and it can interfere with normal physiologic function. See Table 30-6 for types of blood and blood products.

Parenteral Hyperalimentation

Hyperalimentation refers to parenteral nutrition; it is the administration of hypertonic solutions of carbohydrate, protein, and fats (lipids) by indwelling intravenous catheters into the superior vena cava through the jugular or subclavian veins. Some solutions may be given through superficial veins, and if

Table 30-5.   Survey of Information on Transfusion Reactions

Category and Description	Incidence and Cause	Signs and Symptoms	Medical Treatment	Nursing Actions
Hemolytic reaction Agglutination (clumping) of erythrocytes occurs first; blockage of capillaries and eventually disintegration of RBC's occurs; then hemoglobin is released into the circulation; this passes into the kidney tubulus, becomes concentrated, precipitates, and plugs the tubules; death ensues from renal shutdown (1 to 2 weeks)	Incidence is 1 in 5000; cause is mismatched blood of ABO incompatibility or Rh incompatibility on second and subsequent exposures	Chills, fever, headache, back pain, hemoglobinemia, hemoglobinuria (red urine), oliguria, jaundice, dyspnea, cyanosis, chest pain, vascular collapse, hypotension	1. Large quantities of fluid (for example, D-5-W) to promote diuresis and prevent hemoglobin from precipitating 2. Diuretics to increase flow of tubular fluids and prevent hemoglobin plugs (for example, mannitol) 3. Heparinization to combat intravascular coagulation 4. Alkaline substances to dilute hemoglobin, since acidic solutions hold less hemoglobin 5. Indwelling catheter to monitor urinary output 6. Oxygen and epinephrine for wheezing and dyspnea 7. Treatment of shock with matched blood and vasopressor drugs 8. Sedation for restlessness	1. Observe patient closely for first 10 minutes of transfusion, since these reactions occur rapidly 2. Discontinue blood immediately when reaction is assessed 3. Notify physician of patient's symptoms and vital signs 4. Notify laboratory to type and cross match blood and confirm diagnosis; the donor blood is sent back to the lab and a specimen of the recipient's blood is retested 5. Maintain intravenous infusion with D-5-W or saline 6. Monitor vital signs q15 minutes to assess shock and temperature 7. Record fluid intake and output to assess degree of kidney functioning 8. Save first voided specimen for laboratory analysis 9. Implement treatment as prescribed by the physician
Febrile reaction This is also referred to as bacterial reaction; the patient develops a fever and so-called red shock characterized by flushing of the skin due to massive peripheral dilatation	Incidence is rare with the advent of disposable plastic equipment and aseptic blood banking techniques Cause is: 1. Contaminated blood, particularly of the gram-negative bacteria, which can produce 50% fatality rates	Fever, shaking chills, warm, flushed skin, headache, backache, nausea, hematemesis, diarrhea, red shock, confusion or delirium	For acute reaction: 1. Vasopressor drug to maintain systolic pressure over 100 mm Hg 2. Corticosteroids to correct inflammation 3. Antibiotics in high dosages to combat pyrogens 4. Indwelling catheter to assess urinary	For acute reaction: 1. Observe patient closely for the first 30 minutes of transfusion 2. Stop the transfusion 3. Maintain intravenous infusion with saline or D-5-W 4. Monitor the patient's vital signs q30 minutes 5. Notify the physician 6. Notify the lab to

Table 30-5.   Cont'd.

			output	take a culture of
	2. Sensitivity to the donor's white cells or platelets, which is more common and less severe		5. Intravenous fluids in accordance with output 6. Antipyretics to abate fever For mild reaction: 1. Antipyretics for fever 2. Subsequent transfusions of leukocyte-poor blood	patient's and transfusion blood 7. Implement therapy as prescribed by physician 8. Alcohol sponges may be given for fever
Allergic reaction Reactions are usually mild; rarely does anaphylactic shock occur	Incidence is 1% to 2% (relatively common); cause is thought to be allergenic substances (drugs or foods) or antibodies in the donor's plasma	Urticaria (hives), occasional wheezing, arthralgia, generalized itching, nasal congestion, bronchospasm, severe dyspnea, circulatory collapse	For mild reactions: 1. Antihistamines 2. Antipyretics For severe reactions: 1. Epinephrine 2. Corticosteroids 3. Vasopressors	For mild reactions: 1. Slow the transfusion 2. Implement therapy as prescribed by physician For severe reactions: 1. Stop the transfusion 2. Notify physician immediately 3. Maintain intravenous infusion with saline or D-5-W 4. Monitor vital signs frequently

therapy is prolonged, external arteriovenous fistulas may be used. An arteriovenous fistula is created by a surgical procedure that *anastomoses* (joins) an artery in the arm to a vein in sideways fashion, thus making an opening between a large artery and a large vein. As the arterial blood flows directly into the large vein, it distends the vein and causes engorgement. The vein is therefore more easily punctured with larger needles such as 14 or 16 gauge.

The purposes of hyperalimentation are as follows:

1. To supply sufficient nutrients intravenously that will achieve *anabolism* (positive nitrogen balance) and tissue synthesis for patients who are unable to eat or absorb nutrients normally. Routine intravenous solutions normally do not deliver sufficient calories to promote wound healing or weight gain in adults or normal growth in children. For example, 1 liter of 5% dextrose provides 170 calories, which can be sufficient for short-lived maintenance therapy. Since the approximate minimum requirement for a normal resting adult is 500 calories, daily infusions of 2500 to 3000 ml can provide for this. However, caloric needs are increased with certain factors such as wound healing, fevers, and other disease conditions. If these are prolonged, daily needs can become greater than 3000 calories.

2. To permit rapid dilution of the hypertonic solution around the catheter tip, thus preventing phlebitis and thrombosis that occurs with concentrated solutions in superficial veins. The large volume of blood in the superior vena cava rapidly dilutes hypertonic solutions.

3. To free the extremities and permit more freedom for ambulation and activity. Use of the internal jugular vein only restricts the patient's neck mobility.

4. To allow for prolonged therapy, such as from two weeks to three months.

5. To protect the peripheral vascular epithelium from irritation during prolonged administration by administering intralipid solutions in conjunction with concentrated glucose solutions and amino acid mixtures.

Table 30-6.   Types of Blood and Blood Products and Indications for Use

Type	Indications
1. Whole blood Type A B AB O and/or Rh positive or negative	To treat blood volume deficiencies, for example, in acute hemorrhage; not indicated for correction of chronic anemia
2. Plasma	To expand blood volume; to restore circulation and renal blood flow when plasma volume is decreased but the red cell mass is adequate, as in acute dehydration or burns; it is being used more recently to replace deficient coagulation factors in bleeding disorders
3. Packed red cells have a high hematocrit, since approximately 80% of the plasma is removed	Used when blood volume is adequate but the red cell mass is inadequate, as in chronic anemia
4. Platelets	For patients with severe thrombocytopenia (reduced platelets); platelets plug small vascular leaks prior to clotting
5. Albumin	To expand the blood volume when blood volume is reduced in shock or burns; also to increase level of albumin in patients with hypoalbuminemia
6. Prothrombin complex (for example, Konyne, Proplex) contains Factors VII, IX, and XI and prothrombin	Used for bleeding associated with deficiencies of those factors
7. Factor VIII fractions	For hemophiliacs
8. Fibrinogen preparations	Used particularly for bleeding associated with congenital *hypofibrinogenemia* (a deficiency of fibrinogen in the blood); it is a necessary factor for blood coagulation

Types of Fluids

Carbohydrates.   Hypertonic solutions (10%, 20%, and 50%) of glucose can be given. The 10% solution is sometimes administered in superficial veins but is then given with an intralipid solution to reduce irritation to the veins. One liter of 10% solution provides approximately 400 calories.

Fats.   Fats provide about twice the number of calories per gram as carbohydrates or proteins (9 calories as contrasted to 4); thus they are excellent sources of energy. One liter of 10% intralipid solution provides 1100 calories, a large number of calories in a relatively small fluid volume. Intralipid solutions can be given in superficial veins. This prevents irritation and sclerosing of blood vessels when given in conjunction with concentrated glucose solutions and some protein solutions.

Proteins.   Several protein solutions are available. Some are categorized as *hydrolysates,* which are a relatively crude form of protein; others are categorized as *crystalline amino acids,* which are more refined and more expensive. Protein solutions are frequently prepared in combination with dextrose and alcohol, thus providing additional calories per liter. A 5% solution of protein hydrolysate provides 170 calories per liter.

Determining Dosages

The amount and type of solutions are in accordance with the patient's caloric requirements and proportions of carbohydrate, fat, and protein needed. The nurse regulates the flow in the same manner as for any intravenous solution such as by milliliters per hour and drops per minute. All bottles should be taped and calibrated for milliliters per hour.

Nursing Intervention during Hyperalimentation

1. The urine is checked regularly (q6h, every 6 hours) for glycosuria or acetone. If glycosuria does occur, the flow rate of the glucose solutions may be decreased, or insulin may be given on a sliding scale until the pancreas adjusts to accommodate the increased glucose supplied by the infusion.

2. An accurate record is kept of the patient's intake and output.

3. Daily weight is recorded to determine progress and weight gain.

Procedure 30-3.   Blood Transfusion

Action	**Explanation**

Assemble Equipment

1. Blood or blood product as required.

2. Hemo-administration set. See Figure 30-12.

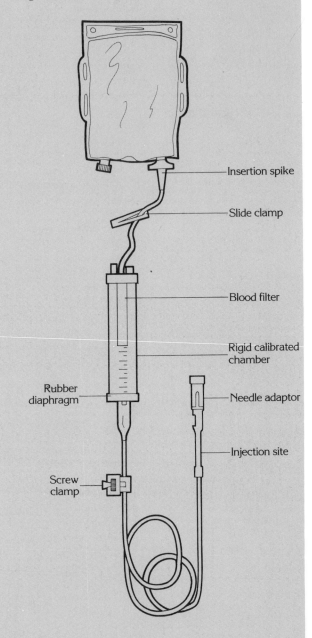

Insertion spike

Slide clamp

Blood filter

Rigid calibrated chamber

Rubber diaphragm

Needle adaptor

Injection site

Screw clamp

Figure 30-12.   A plastic blood container and blood administration set, which includes a filter.

3. Venipuncture equipment

See Procedure 30-1 to dilate a vein and for insertion of the needle.

To Start a Transfusion

1. Explain to the patient what you plan to do. Adjust the explanation to the patient's needs.

To reassure the patient. To identify the patient.

2. Wash hands.

746

3. Attach the hemoset to a plastic blood bag or glass bottle.

4. Partially fill the drip chamber and remove air from the tubing.

5. Adjust the rate of flow as prescribed by physician or at about 4 to 6 ml per minute for adults.

6. Record the time the infusion was commenced, the blood type and serial number, and by whom it was started.

7. After the transfusion:
   a. Detach the tubing from the blood bag and discard it.
   b. Fold the tabs over the outlet tube and secure them with an elastic band.
   c. Return the bag to the blood bank (a plastic bag may be used to transmit it).

8. Record the completion of transfusion, amount absorbed, time, and signature of nurse.

Directions are stated on the administration package.

Calibrated chambers that deliver precise volumes may be used. See Figure 30-12.

Start slowly.

4. A daily blood pressure is taken routinely.

5. Measurement of the serum electrolyte levels is initially done daily until they are regulated, and then they are measured on alternate days. Potassium is needed to transport glucose and amino acids across cell membranes. Commonly 40 mEq of potassium is added to each liter, but when the concentrations of protein and glucose are increased, the potassium must also be increased. It may be increased to 200 mEq liter. Sodium chloride is also administered as determined by serum analysis.

6. An ambulation and exercise program is planned, since inactivity encourages catabolism.

7. The patient is assessed for complications (see Table 30-7).
   a. Air embolism.
   b. Infection at the site.
   c. Circulatory overload.
   d. Glycosuria, osmotic diuresis, hyperglycemia.
   e. Brachial plexus injury.
   f. Pleural puncture.

8. The patient's psychologic needs are also important at this time.

9. Mouth care is provided to moisten the mucous membranes and the lips.

SUMMARY

Fluid and electrolyte problems are often an integral part of other physiologic problems. Tests of body fluids such as blood, vomitus, and urine can reflect these problems. It is chiefly through laboratory examination of the blood plasma that fluid and electrolyte imbalances are revealed.

Two types of fluid imbalance are overhydration (edema) and underhydration (dehydration). Edema is categorized as pitting or nonpitting and/or dependent. It can also be described according to its location, such as cerebral edema. A number of factors are involved in the formation of edema, including increased venous pressure, reduction of plasma proteins, increased capillary permeability, obstructed lymphatic vessels, reduced kidney output, and increased concentration of fluid regulatory hormones

Table 30-7. Potential Complications with Hyperalimentation

Complication	Cause	Signs and Symptoms	Prevention	Treatment
Infection A. At entry site B. At catheter tip from blood-borne bacteria C. Through solution infusion	Poor technique		Rigid asepsis when starting infusion, changing bottles and tubing, and preparing solutions	
Hypoglycemia	Infusion rate that is too slow	Ketonuria	Check urine for acetone q6h and maintain flow rates	Contact physician
Hyperglycemia	Infusion rate that is too rapid	Extreme dehydration, nausea, headache, lassitude	Check urine for sugar q6h and maintain flow rates	Give insulin as ordered or slow infusion rate
Osmotic diuresis	Hyperglycemia; the body eliminates excess glucose, taking fluid with it, and thus produces dehydration			
Air embolism	Air can be sucked into the intravenous system when the catheter is open and the patient takes in a deep breath (the pressure within the vena cava is decreased as thoracic pressure is reduced on inspiration)	Cyanosis, hypotension, rapid weak pulse, altered consciousness, restlessness	Have patient perform Valsalva maneuver during insertion of tubing and during tubing changes; check that all connections are secure; treat by clamping central venous line; have patient lie on left side to keep air in right ventricle and avoid pulmonary emboli	

such as aldosterone. Assessment of the overhydrated person by nurses includes determination of such factors as weight gain, puffy eyelids, and fluid output.

Underhydration, or dehydration, is also a problem encountered by nurses. The effects of dehydration depend largely on the rate and volume of the fluid deficit. Wide variations occur in the electrolyte changes with dehydration. These changes are due to a number of factors, including the volume and composition of the fluid lost, renal function, disease process, and the proportionate loss of electrolytes. Assessment of the dehydrated person includes such factors as weight loss, skin dryness, thirst, and loss of tissue turgor.

There are a number of electrolyte imbalances, the more common being sodium, potassium, and calcium imbalances. Acid-base imbalances occur when the pH of the body fluid is either higher or lower than the normal range of 7.35 to 7.45. There are two types of acid-base disturbances: respiratory and metabolic. With either type of disturbance, acidosis and alkalosis can occur. For any of these imbalances, there is a corrective body response by the kidneys or the lungs.

Parenteral fluid therapy includes the administration of fluids and electrolytes intravenously. A wide variety of solutions are available for administration. Nursing intervention for patients receiving intravenous infusions includes the following.

1. Explanation and teaching.

2. Comfort and assistance with activity as required.

3. Maintenance of the intravenous infusion, which includes observation for possible complications, changing bottles, regulating flow rates, changing tubing, and adding medications when needed.

   A number of venipuncture sites can be used. The choice usually depends upon the type of infusion, length of infusion time, and age of the patient. Blood transfusions are the introduction of whole blood or components of blood into a person. The blood to be transfused needs to be matched with the patient's blood.

Parenteral hyperalimentation is the administration of hypertonic solutions of carbohydrates, protein, and fats for nourishment. These are usually administered by intravenous catheter into the superior vena cava through the jugular and subclavian veins. Nursing intervention involves explanation and reassurance to the patient, maintenance of the infusion, record of intake and output, daily measurement of weight, daily blood pressure measurement, exercise, urine analysis, and assessment for complications as well as mouth care.

SUGGESTED ACTIVITIES

1. Select five patients in a hospital setting who have had laboratory tests for blood electrolytes. Compare the results with the normal values. If any of the readings are abnormal, assess patients for any symptoms.

2. In a laboratory setting, start an intravenous infusion as if for a patient, using sterile technique. Regulate the infusion so that 500 ml will be absorbed in eight hours. Label the bottle appropriately.

SUGGESTED READINGS

Kee, Joyce L., and Gregory, Anne P. June, 1974. The ABC's (and mEq's) of fluid balance in children. *Nursing 74* 4:28–36.

This article emphasizes the essential guidelines for assessing and monitoring correction of common imbalances in children. A checklist for nursing assessment of fluid imbalance is included.

Kurdi, William J. November, 1975. Refining your I.V. therapy techniques. *Nursing 75* 5:41–47.

Intravenous therapy procedures are outlined in a step-by-step format with accompanying photographs. Included are inserting the needle, taping needles and catheters, applying armboards, regulating flow rates, and changing bottles and tubing.

Scarlato, Michael. February, 1978. Blood transfusions today: what you should know and do. *Nursing 78* 8:68–70, 72.

This article outlines the nurse's responsibilities and nursing guidelines for transfusions. Checklists are provided to help the nurse minimize the risks of transfusing whole blood, packed red blood cells, platelets, and plasma fractions.

Snively, W. D., Jr., and Roberts, Kay T. 1973. The clinical picture as an aid to understanding body fluid disturbances. *Nursing Forum* 12(2):132–159.

A concise but comprehensive outline of 16 diagnostic classifications of body fluid disturbances. A resume of a few actual patients is included to emphasize the clinical picture approach for understanding the body fluid imbalance.

SELECTED REFERENCES

Abbott Laboratories, Ltd. 1970. *Fluids and electrolytes.* Montreal.

Beaumont, Estelle. July, 1977. The new I.V. infusion pumps. *Nursing 77* 7:31–35.

Borgen, Linda. February, 1978. Total parenteral nutrition in adults. *American Journal of Nursing* 78:224–228.

Brooks, Stewart M. 1968. *Basic facts of body water and ions.* 2nd ed. New York: Springer Publishing Co.

Brooks, Stewart M. 1970. *Integrated basic science.* 3rd ed. St. Louis: The C. V. Mosby Co.

Dickens, Margaret L. 1974. *Fluid and electrolyte balance: a programmed text.* 3rd ed. Philadelphia: F. A. Davis Company.

Grant, Marcia M., and Kubo, Winifred M. August, 1975. Assessing a patient's hydration status. *American Journal of Nursing* 75:1306–1311.

Guyton, Arthur C. 1976. *Textbook of medical physiology.* 5th ed. Philadelphia: W. B. Saunders Co.

Lee, Carla A., Stroot, Violet R., and Schaper, C. Ann. August, 1975. What to do when acid-base problems hang in the balance. *Nursing 75* 5:32–37.

MacBryde, Cyril Mitchell, and Blacklow, Robert Stanley, 1970. *Signs and symptoms: applied pathologic physiology and clinical interpretation.* 5th ed. Philadelphia: J. B. Lippincott Co.

Marlow, Dorothy R. 1973. *Textbook of pediatric nursing.* 4th ed. Philadelphia: W. B. Saunders Co.

Mitchell, Helen S., et al. 1976. *Nutrition in health and disease.* 16th ed. New York: J. B. Lippincott Co.

Mountcastle, Vernon, B., ed. 1974. *Medical physiology,* vol. 1. 12th ed. St. Louis: The C. V. Mosby Co.

Nordmark, Madelyn T., and Rohweder, Anne W. 1975. *Scientific foundations of nursing.* 3rd ed. Philadelphia: J. B. Lippincott Co.

Reed, Gretchen M. March, 1974. Confused about potassium? Here's a clear concise guide. *Nursing 74* 4:21.

Scipien, Gladys M., et al. 1975. Comprehensive pediatric nursing. New York: McGraw-Hill Book Co.

Sharer, Jo Ellen. June, 1975. Reviewing acid-base balance. *American Journal of Nursing* 75:980–983.

Snively, W. D., Jr. ed. 1962. *Body fluid disturbances.* New York: Grune & Stratton, Inc.

Tripp, Alice. July, 1976. Hyper and hypocalcemia. *American Journal of Nursing* 76:1142–1145.

Ungvarski, Peter J. December, 1976. Parenteral therapy. *American Journal of Nursing* 76:1974–1977.

Vaughan, Victor C., and McKay, R. James, eds. 1975. *Nelson textbook of pediatrics.* 10th ed. Philadelphia: W. B. Saunders Co.

Waechter, Eugenia H., and Blake, Florence G. 1976. *Nursing care of children.* 9th ed. Philadelphia: J. B. Lippincott Co.

UNIT VI

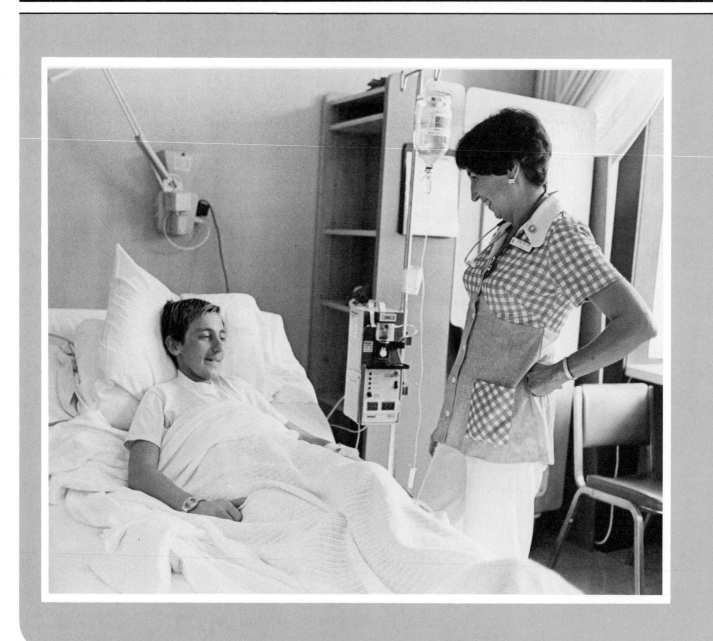

PSYCHOSOCIAL NEEDS

CHAPTER 31

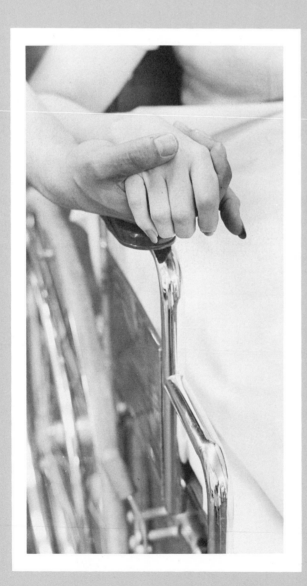

SEXUALITY

NURSING ASSESSMENT OF SEXUAL PROBLEMS

NURSING INTERVENTION FOR SEXUAL PROBLEMS

Assessment

Referral

Counselling

Education

CONTRACEPTION

OBJECTIVES

- Describe the structure and function of the male and female genitalia.

- Discuss the development of sexuality from the prenatal period to old age.

- Explain sexual stimulation and response patterns.

- Describe some sexual problems related to intercourse.

- Explain how some common illnesses affect sexuality.

- Assess patients for some sexual problems.

- Plan and provide nursing intervention for some sexual problems.

- Explain the different contraceptive methods.

Sexuality is essential to health. It facilitates the development of self, interpersonal relationships, intimacy, and love. In its broadest sense, human sexuality integrates the somatic, emotional, intellectual, social, and ethical aspects of sexual being and behavior. For example, in the physical sense, sexuality defines what constitutes male and female. It involves the physiologic events that occur when one becomes sexually aroused and experiences orgasm. In the social sense it includes the kind of relationships one participates in because of being male or female. In the ethical or moral sense, sexuality often involves decision-making about acceptable behaviors related to the sex act.

Human sexuality is frequently considered in terms of two components: the inherited and the learned. The inherited component refers to the structural and functional equipment with which one is born. The learned component is that which is learned by interaction with the social environment. However, every aspect of sexual behavior consists of both inherited and learned components. It is important therefore to consider the interaction of these two components in any given sexual activity.

Sexual dimorphism is the term used to describe the average differences between males and females in any given species. Males, for example, are generally taller, heavier, and physically stronger than females. However, these attributes are not always reliable indicators of maleness or femaleness. Some women are taller, heavier, or stronger than their male counterparts. The most reliable indicator is that males have a penis and females have a vagina and menstrual cycles and can become pregnant. Body hair distribution and length are another indication.

SEXUAL STRUCTURE AND FUNCTION

Male Genitalia

The male genitalia provide a system for transporting the male sperm to the vagina of the female. The organs involved in this system are two testes encased in the scrotum, a series of ducts (epididymis and vas deferens) that transport the sperm, several glands that secrete fluid (semen) to protect the sperm, and the penis to ejaculate the semen.

Testes

The testes, or male gonads, are oval-shaped organs about 3.75 cm (1½ inch) long and 2.5 cm (1 inch) wide. In each testes is a series of highly coiled tubules called *seminiferous tubules*, which manufacture the sperm. The outer layer of each testes consists of a smooth muscle capsule. Contractions of this muscle facilitate the transport of the sperm out of the testes into the transport ducts.

The two major functions of the testes are the production of the sperm and the production of sexual hormones. A *sperm* is a specialized type of cell consisting of a head, neckpiece, midpiece, and tail that contains *chromosomes* (genes). Chromosomes are responsible for a person's inherited characteristics. All cells of the body originally contain 23 pairs of chromosomes, referred to as the *diploid number*. These cells multiply by dividing in half and producing two new cells, each of which contain 23 pairs of chromosomes. This process of cell division is called *mitosis*. Sperm cells and egg cells, however, have only 23 single chromosomes, referred to as the *haploid number*. This occurs by a specialized type of cell division called *meiosis*. Thus when the sperm cell fertilizes the egg cell, the cell produced from their unification produces the required 23 pairs of chromosomes: 23 single ones from the female and 23 single ones from the male.

In the developing human, two of these chromosomes are the *sex chromosome pair*, which determine whether the person's gonads will develop as testes or ovaries. The female has two identical sex chromosomes, referred to as *XX*. The male has two different chromosomes designated as *XY*; thus one chromosome is the same as the female's (X) but the other is different (Y). Sperms therefore are of two types, since during meosis only one chromosome of the pair is present. An X-bearing sperm is called a *gynosperm*, and a Y-bearing sperm is called an *androsperm*. Thus if a gynosperm fertilizes the egg, a female results, but if an androsperm fertilizes the egg, the offspring will be male.

Androsperms are smaller in size, have longer tails, move or swim faster, and are more susceptible to changes in the environment such as vaginal pH than gynosperms. It is believed that for males to be conceived, intercourse must occur at the time of or as closely as possible to the time of the female's ovulation. Androsperms in this case move more quickly to the egg than gynosperms. Girls are thought to be conceived, however, a few days before the egg is ready to be fertilized. Gynosperms move more slowly and can withstand the relatively acid vaginal fluids secreted during this time and then unite with the egg once it is produced.

The second major function of the testes is the production of sexual hormones. The chief testicular hormone is *testosterone*, which stimulates the growth and development of the genital organs. It is also responsible for the secondary sexual male characteristics such as a deeper voice, larger musculature, and hair on the face and chest. Other hormonal secretions of the testes include estrogen and androgens other than testosterone. Estrogen seems to function in controlling spermatogenesis and is also produced by the adrenal galnds.

The control of male hormones is regulated by the hypothalamus. This organ secretes releasing factors that travel through the bloodstream to the pituitary gland. When stimulated by releasing factors, the pituitary gland secretes follicle stimulating hormone (FSH) and luteinizing hormone (LH). LH stimulates the secretion of testosterone, and FSH stimulates spermatogenesis. Both operate on the basis of a negative feedback system. (See Chapter 7.)

Scrotum

Because the testes are located outside of the body, protection from injury is provided by the *scrotum*, the sac suspended down and behind the penis. The scrotal sacs are located in the groin in humans and are outpouchings of the abdominal wall. The outer skin layer of the scrotum is wrinkled in appearance and relatively hairless. Beneath this layer of skin is a layer of smooth muscle and tough connective tissue called the *tunica dartos* and then another layer of striated muscle and connective tissue called the *cremaster*. Smooth muscles contract involuntarily, whereas striated muscles can be contracted voluntarily or involuntarily. Within these three layers of tissue the testes are protected. Usually the left testis hangs lower down in its scrotal sac than the right.

In the early stage of development of the male fetus the testes are located inside the abdominal cavity, but, before birth, male sexual hormones are porduced that facilitate the descent of the testes into the scrotal sacs. This descent occurs through the inguinal canal in the groin and is usually completed by the time of birth.

Failure of the testes to descend is called *cryptorchidism* and in the majority of males is bilateral. During the first year of life, spontaneous descent of the testes may occur, but by puberty, hormonal therapy with male hormones may be necessary to stimulate descent, or surgical intervention may be required. Although males with undescended testicles produce the normal amounts of male sex hormones, they are usually infertile because the abdominal body temperature is too high for sperm to be produced. Adequate sperm production requires lower temperatures.

Therefore, in addition to protecting the testes, the scrotum also plays a significant part in maintaining an appropriate temperature for the sperm. This cooler scrotal temperature is normally maintained by several factors:

1. The thin layer of scrotal skin, which has little or minimal underlying fat, thus offering little insulation.

2. The presence of many superficial small blood vessels in the scrotum, which facilitate heat loss as necessary.

3. The presence of abundant sweat glands, which enhance cooling by evaporation of sweat.

4. The presence of muscle receptors particularly in the tunica dartos muscle, which produce contraction when cooled and push the testes up toward the groin to be warmed.

Other factors that influence the temperature of the scrotum are garments which squeeze the scrotum up against the groin such as tight-fitting clothing or jockstraps. Continuous use of these can reduce sperm production by increasing the temperature. The cremaster muscle also can influence the scrotal temperature. Although this muscle is not largely involved in temperature regulation, it can alter the scrotal temperature. Strong contractions of the cremaster muscle brought about by sexual excitement, fear, anxiety, or stimulation of the cremasteric reflex by the stroking of the inner surface of the thighs increase the blood flow from the testes back into the body, thereby increasing scrotal temperature. These contractions, however, are not sustained for long periods.

Epididymis, Vas Deferens, and Ejaculatory Ducts

As mentioned previously, the testes contain coiled seminiferous tubules that manufacture the sperm. These tubules drain directly into a duct outside of the testis called the *epididymis*, a highly coiled duct. The epididymis then drains into the *vas deferens*, which is a long tube extending from the scrotum, curving around the urinary bladder, and emptying into *ejaculatory ducts*. The two ejaculatory ducts, one from

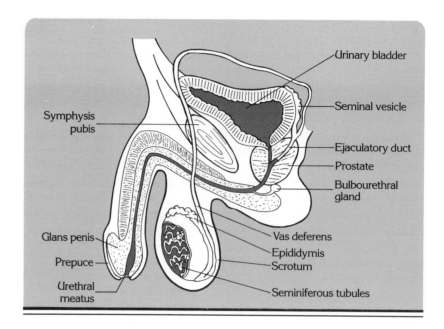

Figure 31-1. The male reproductive tract.

each testis, are short, and both connect with the urethra (See Figure 31-1).

Sperm are transported to the epididymis by mechanisms not fully understood. Transport may be facilitated by smooth muscle contractions of the capsule of the testes or by contractions of the seminiferous tubules. Cilia, which line the tubules, also move the sperm toward the epididymis.

The epididymis is thought to have a twofold function: (a) a chamber where ripening of the sperm occurs and (b) a chamber where abnormal sperm are selectively removed by the ameboid or phagocytic cells of the body. The vas deferens is known to serve as a holding tank for the mature sperm between ejaculations. Both the vas deferens and ejaculating ducts serve as vehicles by which the sperm and semen are propelled into the urethra and then out of the body during intercourse.

Seminal Vesicles, Prostate, and Cowper's Glands

These structures (see Figure 31-1) produce substances, collectively referred to as *seminal plasma,* which energize the sperm and enhance their transport but are not essential for mature sperm cells. Seminal plasma combined with sperm is referred to as *semen.* Normal characteristics of semen are as follows:

1. A creamy texture.
2. Gray or yellow in color.
3. Volume of 2 to 6 ml.

4. 120 million sperm per milliliter of seminal plasma.
5. Slightly alkaline pH (7.35 to 7.50)

Primary components of seminal plasma include the following:

1. Water to transport the sperm.
2. Mucus to lubricate the ducts.
3. Sugar (fructose) to energize the sperm.
4. Salts to maintain isotonicity of the seminal plasma with body fluids.
5. Base buffers to neutalize the acidity of the male urethra and subsequently the female vagina.
6. Coagulators to clot the semen in the vagina and prevent leakage of sperm out of the woman's vagina (Mann 1970:469–478).

Sperm that are ejaculated are concentrated in the first third of semen. Many sperm are also present from the secretions of these three glands at the opening of the male urethra prior to ejaculation. Thus persons who use withdrawal of the penis before ejaculation as a form of conception control need to know that pregnancy can occur without ejaculation from the male.

Penis

The penis consists of two parts: the shaft and glans. In uncircumscised males the skin of the shaft loosely encloses the glans and is referred to as the *foreskin* (prepuce). Between the foreskin and glans, *smegma*, a cheesy-like material, accumulates from a mixture of the oil secretions of the glans and dead tissue cells. This needs to be removed during hygienic practices.

Penile shapes and sizes vary considerably, not so much in circumference but in length. Males frequently experience a great deal of concern about the size of their penis, relating the size directly to their abilities as capable lovers. This concern about the relationship of size and ability, however, is unfounded. These fears can be equated to the emphasis placed on the size of the female breast, but size has little to do with functional abilities in either case. Fears about circumference also are unnecessary, since the female vagina accommodates to these differences. Females can contract the vaginal opening at will, thus narrowing it, or they can accommodate a wider penis, since the vagina has the capacity to stretch.

The function of the penis related to sexuality involves the transmission of semen to the female. This process includes (a) erection of the penis, (b) ejaculation of the semen, and (c) return of the penis to a flaccid state.

Erection is the lengthening, widening, and hardening of the penis as it becomes tumescent (congested) with blood. It is a spinal reflex that occurs when the erection center, located at the first to fourth sacral segments of the spinal cord, is stimulated. Erections commonly occur in response to sexual stimuli such as sexually stimulating thoughts or by the manipulation (touching) of the penis. However, occasionally erections occur without apparent sexual stimuli. These are referred to as *reflexogenic erections* and are often cause for embarrassment. For example, young teenagers whose nervous systems are immature often experience unexpected erections when taking a shower after playing sports. It is not uncommon for the nurse to encounter these types of erections in nursing practice. Nurses, for example, may encounter this while removing inguinal sutures on a young teenager. Morning erections are also common to both men and boys on awakening. The reason for these erections is not fully understood but may be attributed to the pressure of a full bladder, erotic dreams, friction against the sheets, or waking at the end of a paradoxical sleep phase.

Ejaculation is the propulsion of semen out of the penis and it is also a spinal reflex. However, the ejaculatory center is higher in the spinal cord than the erection center (from the third lumbar to the twelfth thoracic segment). The ejaculatory center is stimulated when an erect penis is intensely aroused by manipulation or intercourse. Ejaculation involves two stages: (a) the semen is transported to the urethra (emission stage), and (b) the semen is propelled out of the urethra (the expulsion stage). The expulsion of semen varies in force depending upon a number of factors, such as the degree of arousal, the time lapse between ejaculations, and age. Semen may ooze out over the glans penis or may be projected a certain distance.

After ejaculation the penis returns to a flaccid state. This process is referred to as *detumescence* and occurs whether or not ejaculation has occurred. The penile arteries constrict, thus reducing the blood flow to the penis, and the venous outflow allows the engorged blood vessels to empty.

Female Genitalia

The female genitalia include two ovaries, two fallopian tubes, the uterus, the vagina, the vulva, and the mammary glands. These structures provide a system for receiving the sperm, producing eggs, housing and nurturing the fertilized egg implant, delivering the mature fetus, and suckling the young.

Ovaries

The ovaries, or female gonads, are analogous to the testes in the male in that they produce eggs and secrete hormones, but they are located in the pelvic region of the abdominal cavity. (See Figure 31-2.) Adult ovaries are approximately 2.5 cm (1 inch) in length and have an oval shape. The inner portion of the ovary is called the *medulla*, and the outer portion is called the *cortex*. The cortex develops the eggs and secretes the hormones. The medulla consists of spirals, or coils, of blood vessels and connective tissue.

Like the testes, the ovaries have two primary functions (a) the production and expulsion of eggs (ova) and (b) the production of sexual hormones. In contrast to the male testis, which produces sperm throughout life, the female ovary contains all the primordial (primitive) ova at birth. These primordial ova originate on the outer surface (germinal layer) of the ovary but move from the outer layer of the cortex during fetal life into the main substance of the cortex. They then are surrounded by a single layer of cells referred to as *granulosa cells*. Once the ova are surrounded by these granulosa cells, they are referred to as *primordial follicles*. At birth about ¾ million primordial follicles are present in the two ovaries, but only about 450 of these follicles will develop sufficiently throughout the female reproductive life to expel their ova (Guyton 1976:1086). Primordial follicles undergo a process of degeneration throughout life

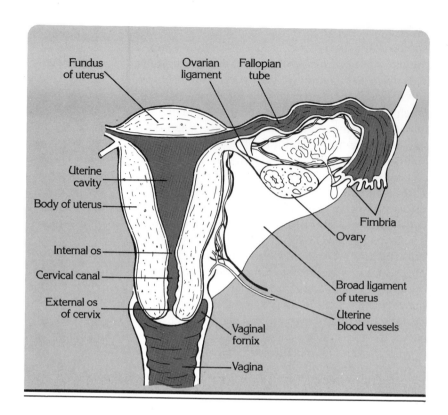

Figure 31-2. The female reproductive tract.

called *atresia.* By puberty only 400,000 follicles remain, and by menopause only a few remain (Guyton 1976:1086).

Two types of female sex hormones are produced by the ovaries: estrogen and progesterone. In addition, some male androgens are secreted. Estrogen has several effects such as regulating female fat distribution and breast development and neutralizing the vaginal pH during ovulation. Its primary control is exerted during the first half of the menstrual cycle. Progesterone, on the other hand, controls the second half of the menstrual cycle but also influences breast development. It is also responsible for inhibiting the uterine muscle contractions during pregnancy. The androgens are thought to increase sexual motivation.

The female sexual hormones are controlled by homeostatic negative feedback systems as are the male hormones, but they are cyclic in their production, (thus the female sexual cycle or the monthly menstrual cycle). These feedback systems also involve three different hierarchies of hormones: (a) releasing factors for FSH and LH from the hypothalamus, (b) the pituitary secretions of FSH and LH, and (c) the production of hormones (estrogen and progesterone) from the gonads (ovaries).

The duration of the female sexual cycle averages about 28 days, but can normally vary between 20 and 35 days. This cycle can be considered in terms of the following three stages:

1. The *preovulatory stage* extends for an average of 14 days (plus or minus three to five days), starting on the first day of menstrual flow and ending with *ovulation* (release of the ovum from the ovary). It is also referred to as the *proliferative* or *follicular stage.* On the first day of this stage the follicles begin to grow spontaneously without hormonal control. Then FSH from the pituitary gland, stimulated by the hypothalmic FSH-releasing factor, is produced, and only *one* of the follicles is stimulated to enlarge further. It is not known why only one follicle is stimulated. This enlarged follicle is called the *Graafian follicle* (maturing follicle). Estrogen secretion is then stimulated by this follicle under the influence of FSH. The effects of estrogen include the buildup of the endometrial lining of the uterus for anticipated conception and the final maturation of the Graafian follicle immediately before ovulation. Once estrogen reaches its peak level in the bloodstream, the production of FSH is decreased by negative feedback, but a sudden surge of LH is then released by the pituitary gland. This triggers ovulation.

2. The *postovulatory phase* of the female sexual cycle starts immediately after ovulation and averages about 13 days in the female whose cycle is 28 days. It ends when the woman begins her menstrual period. This

phase is also referred to as the *secretory* or *luteal* stage. The term *secretory* is used because the lining of the uterus secretes a substance (carbohydrate glycogen) to provide nourishment for a fertilized ovum (zygote). The term *luteal* is used because the Graafian follicle undergoes changes, forming a yellowish mass in the ovary known as the *corpus luteum*. This occurs under the influence of LH. If the ovum is impregnated, the corpus luteum grows and persists for several months. It secretes the hormone progesterone as well as estrogen. Progesterone is responsible for maintaining the uterine lining for the reception and development of the zygote. The estrogen enhances the action of progesterone. By negative feedback, progesterone inhibits the production of LH, and estrogen inhibits the production of FSH. These luteal hormones maintain the implanted zygote for about three months until the placenta is developed. It then secretes these hormones.

If fertilization does not occur, the corpus luteum gradually undergoes degeneration and becomes white and scarred in appearance. It is then referred to as the *corpus albicans*. Reductions in the production of progesterone and estrogen result, and menstrual flow is induced. The endometrium shrinks as the arteries collapse without hormonal stimulation. Deoxygenation of the endometrium results and the tissues die. Most of these dead tissues are reabsorbed, but bleeding occurs through the weak, collapsed capillaries due to hyperemia (blood vessels dilate under the influence of histamine and serotonin). Thus menstrual flow consists primarily of blood.

3. The *menses*, or menstrual flow extends for three to seven days. It overlaps with the beginning of the preovulatory phase. The first day of flow is considered to be the first day of the sexual cycle. The amount of menstrual discharge varies among persons and from cycle to cycle. The average discharge is about 90 ml (3 ounces) but can range from 30 to 180 ml (1 to 6 ounces). Women using the combination contraceptive pill tend to have less than the average discharge, whereas women with intrauterine devices (IUD) often have heavier flows.

Menarche, the first menstrual period, occurs between the ages of 9 and 17 years. For the first few years, ovulation and menses may be somewhat erratic. Eventually a stable rhythm is established until menopause occurs. Menstrual cramps are common, particularly during the first few days of menses because of contractions of the uterus and cervix. The cause of these is undetermined. Moods also change

before and during menses. A few days before menses, some women tend to feel tense, anxious, irritable, depressed, or hostile. As menses occurs most of these feelings are eased or disappear. However, until the estrogen levels are elevated during the preovulatory stage, depression is common. By the time of ovulation, when the estrogen levels are at their peak, women tend to feel happy and self-confident.

Thus mood swings during the female sexual cycle are influenced by the hormonal changes that occur throughout the cycle; conversely, a woman's emotional status can also directly influence her hormonal levels. For example, when a woman is experiencing a stressful situation such as illness or a work or family conflict, hormonal levels can be altered and subsequently change the menses. Menses may not occur throughout the cycle; conversely, a woman's degree of flow.

Fallopian Tubes

The two fallopian tubes (oviducts) are about 4 inches long and extend between the ovaries and uterus but are unattached to the ovaries. Their chief function is to provide an environment that is appropriate for the transport in opposite directions of the ova and sperm and that is appropriate for fertilization. Secretory cells in the mucosal lining of the tube are believed to provide nourishment to the ovum.

The mechanism by which the ova are transported from the ovaries into the fallopian tubes is not fully understood. Occasionally, because the two structures are unattached, an ovum is released into the abdominal cavity rather than into the fallopian tube. If this egg is fertilized and implanted in the abdominal cavity, the condition is referred to as an *ectopic pregnancy* (implantation of a zygote outside of the uterus). Ectopic pregnancies also occur occasionally in the fallopian tubes.

Fertilization of ova usually occurs in the upper third of a fallopian tube. The transport of the sperm is facilitated by muscle contractions of the tubes and by the sperm's active swimming movements. Transport of the zygote (fertilized ovum) is facilitated by the motion of cilia in the tube, which sweep toward the uterus, and also by tubal muscle contractions. Generally, the zygote is transported to the uterus in about three days. However, this rate of transport is influenced by the hormones progesterone and estrogen: progesterone retards the rate of transport, whereas estrogen accelerates it. Estrogen is therefore used to prevent implantation of the zygote. Large doses of estrogen administered postcoitus accelerate the transport of the zygote before it is ready for implantation. Estrogen also alters the endometrial lining, making it inappropriate to receive the zygote.

Uterus

The uterus, one of the most changeable organs of the body, lies between the rectum and urinary bladder. It is thick walled and hollow. The three layers of the wall are referred to as the *perimetrium*, the thin outer layer of serous membrane; the *myometrium*, the middle thick layer of smooth muscle; and the *endometrium*, the inner mucous membrane lining. The perimetrium of the uterus covers all the uterus except the *cervix* (the neck of the uterus). The myometrium contains many muscle fibers that run in different directions. Contractions of these fibers occur during childbirth, nursing, sexual tension, and orgasm. During pregnancy the uterus enlarges, and the muscle fibers increase in length; muscular contractions dilate the cervix and assist in expelling the fetus.

The endometrium is composed of two principal layers: the *functionalis*, the layer which is shed during menstruation, and the *basalis*, the layer closest to the myometrium. The basalis layer is maintained during menstruation and produces a new functionalis layer after menstruation. The endometrial lining is essential for the reception and maintenance of fertilized egg implants and for the development of the zygote. In the cervix the uterine lining differs in that special mucous-secreting glands are present. These glands produce mucus that plugs the opening into the uterus. During ovulation when estrogen levels are high the characteristics of this mucous plug change. The mucus becomes more copious and less thick, thus making it more penetrable by a sperm. Examination of the characteristics of the cervical mucous plug therefore may be used diagnostically to determine whether a woman is ovulating or infertile.

Vagina

The vagina has a threefold function. It serves as the lower part of the birth canal, the passageway for menstrual flow, and the receptacle for the penis during intercourse. The vagina, a muscular tubular organ lined with mucous membrane, is about 10 cm (4 inches) in length. The mucosa of the vagina is capable of a great deal of extension because it lies in a series of inwardly directed and transverse folds called *rugae*. The muscular layer of the vagina can also stretch considerably. This distensibility is important during the birth process and intercourse.

Large amounts of glycogen (a type of carbohydrate) are produced in the vagina. Glycogen is de-

composed by the normal bacterial inhabitants of the vagina (Döderlein's bacilli) into lactic acid. These acids create a low pH environment, which prevents many bacteria and yeasts from causing disease in the vagina. This acidity is also injurious to sperm cells, but the buffering action of semen ensures their survival.

Döderlein's bacilli can be destroyed by antibiotics. Thus it is not uncommon for women to get a vaginal infection when they are undergoing antibiotic treatment for some other infection.

Changes in the vaginal mucosa occur in response to estrogen during the menstrual cycle and in response to sexual tension and excitement. Normally the cells of the vaginal mucosa continually slough off and are replaced by new ones. During the menstrual cycle these cells, under the influence of estrogen, undergo *cornification* (hardening). Examination of these cells is done by observing them under a microscope. The cells are obtained by taking a vaginal swab of the secretions and transferring them to a glass slide. This is called a *vaginal smear*. Examination of vaginal smears taken when estrogen levels should be high at ovulation can be used to determine infertility problems.

During sexual excitement the numerous small blood vessels of the vagina become engorged with blood, and it develops a purplish hue. This congestion is also responsible for the lubrication of the vagina as sexual tension increases. Initially small droplets of fluid exude through the blood vessel walls (like sweating), and as sexual tension increases these droplets of fluid coalesce to form a shiny layer of lubricant over the mucosa.

At the *vaginal orifice* (the external opening of the vagina) there is a thin fold of vascularized mucous membrane called the *hymen*. It forms a border around the orifice, which partially closes it. Sometimes this membrane completely covers the orifice, and this is referred to as an *imperforate hymen*. This condition warrants medical intervention to permit the discharge of menstrual flow.

Vulva

The external female genitalia are collectively referred to as the *vulva*, or *pudendum*. The structures of the vulva include the mons pubis, two labia majora, two labia minora, the clitoris, and the vestibule.

The *mons pubis*, also referred to as the *mons veneris*, is a pillow of adipose tissue (fat) situated over the symphysis pubis and covered by coarse pubic hair. The mons pubis is a highly sensitive area that contains many touch receptors. Stimulation of the mons during intercourse or masturbation can lead to an orgasm.

The *labia majora* (meaning large lips) are the two longitudinal folds of skin extending downward and backward from the mons pubis. They serve to protect the labia minora and the openings of the vagina and urethra. The labia majora are covered by hair on their upper outer surfaces and contain an abundance of adipose tissue and sebaceous and sweat glands. Usually the labia majora form a deep cleft where they meet. However, during periods of sexual excitement these lips separate and flatten against the inner thighs to expose the minor lips and vaginal opening.

The *labia minora* lie inside the labia majora. They are devoid of hair and have relatively few sweat glands; however, they do contain numerous sebaceous glands. The labia minora extend upward to unite and form the prepuce (foreskin) of the clitoris and downward to protect the vaginal opening. Because the small lips undergo vivid color changes with mounting sexual tension, they are often called the "sex skin." The color changes are due to the increased influx of blood that occurs and vary in proportion to the level of arousal and depending on whether the woman is pregnant. In nonpregnant women the labia minora are normally pale pink and change to a bright red during sexual excitement. In pregnant women, the labia minora contain more blood vessels and thus are normally red in color. During sexual excitement the labia minora assume a deep wine color. These color changes are positive signs of approaching orgasm.

The *clitoris* is a small round mass of erectile tissue, blood vessels, and nerves located behind the junction of the labia minora (the prepuce). The exposed part of the clitoris is referred to as the *glans clitoris*. The clitoris is capable of enlargement upon tactile stimulation and is homologous to the male penis. Its principle function is as a receptor and transmitter of erotic stimuli during sexual excitement of the female. During sexual arousal the glans becomes tumescent and is elevated upward so that it is hidden behind the prepuce.

The *vestibule* is the cleft between the labia and contains the vaginal orifice, urethral orifice, hymen, and openings of several ducts. The vaginal orifice oc-cupies the major portion of the vestibule. Above the vaginal orifice and below the clitoris lies the urethral orifice. The ducts of glands that secrete mucus are located behind and on either side of the urethra (the lesser vestibular glands). These lesser vestibular glands are homologous to the male prostate. Larger glands (the greater vestibular glands) lie on either side of the vaginal orifice. Their ducts open into the space between the hymen and labia minora. These glands are homologous to the male Cowper's glands. They produce a mucoid secretion that acts as a lubricant during sexual intercourse.

The *mammary glands* (breasts) not only serve as vehicles of milk secretion but also as erotic organs. Internally each mammary gland consists of *lobes* (compartments) separated by adipose tissue, which is the primary factor determining the size of the breasts. Within each lobe are smaller compartments called *lobules*. These contain milk-secreting cells called *alveoli* that are clustered in grapelike arrangements. The milk from the alveoli is conveyed into a series of tubules and then into the mammary ducts, the *ampullae* (expanded sinuses where milk can be stored), and the *lactiferous ducts,* which terminate in the nipple. Each lactiferous duct conveys the milk from one of the lobes to the nipple. Surrounding the nipple is a circular pigmented area called the *areola*. It appears bumpy or rough because of the number of sebaceous glands present.

At birth the female mammary glands are underdeveloped. The breasts begin to develop with the onset of puberty under the influence of estrogen produced by the ovaries, progesterone, growth hormone from the pituitary, prolactin from the pituitary, and thyroxine from the thyroid gland.

The size and shape of the breasts are often of concern to the female as the size and shape of the penis are to the male. The size and shape, however, do not affect their functional abilities. Women often worry also about whether pregnancy and nursing will alter breast size. During pregnancy the breasts become heavier and some of the supporting ligaments may stretch, causing the breasts to hang slightly lower thereafter. However, nursing does not permanently alter breast size, shape, or "lift."

DEVELOPMENT OF SEXUALITY

The components or ingredients that contribute to the development of sexuality are numerous. From the beginning of life the human organism is designated as a sexual being. As has been previously discussed, sex is genetically determined at conception from the XX or XY chromosomal combination. Throughout life many biologic, psychosocial, and cultural components condition one's sexuality. From birth onward, gender affects the behavior expected within our culture and how we pattern our behavior throughout life.

Prenatal Period and Pregnancy

Biologic Components

When a fetus is 4 to 6 weeks old, its gonads are not recognizable as either ovaries or testes. Both genders (XX and XY) have internal genitalia consisting of two pairs of ducts. These are called the *müllerian* and *wolffian ducts*. The mullerian ducts are the genetic female pair, which eventually develop into the fallopian tubes, uterus, and upper one-third of the vagina. The wolffian ducts are the genetic male pair, which ultimately develop into the sperm ducts, seminal vesicles, and the epididymis. Externally the genitalia of both genders consist of a genital tubercle, genital folds, and genital swellings. The tubercles eventually develop into the clitoris or glans penis, the folds into the labia minora or shaft of the penis, and the swelling into the labia majora or the scrotum.

Sexual differentiation, or biologic sex, is fairly well determined by the 12th week of fetal life. The differentiation of these structures into male genitalia requires the presence of two substances: a testicular inductor substance (androgens) and a mullerian inhibitor substance. The androgens stimulate the development of the male structures internally and externally while the inhibitor substance suppresses the development of the mullerian ducts, causing them to degenerate. For a female to develop, these hormonal substances are absent. Thus the wolffian ducts degenerate, and the female genitalia develop.

Psychosocial Differences during Infancy

At birth, boys are generally larger, weigh more, and have greater musculatures than girls. Many other sex differences have been noted by authorities during infancy and childhood such as the following:

1. Boys show greater motor activity and can raise their heads earlier.
2. Girls are more physically passive and are more irritable during physical examination.
3. Girls show greater sensitivity to tactile stimuli and pain.
4. At 6 months of age girls have a longer attention span for visual stimuli such as a human face and show more responsiveness to social demands and parental wishes.
5. Boys have a longer attention span to a helix of light.
6. Boys prefer low-complexity stimuli
7. Girls prefer highly complex stimuli.
8. Girls demonstrate earlier language development.
9. Boys spend longer times away from their mothers and return less frequently.
10. Girls spend more time looking at and touching their mothers.
11. Boys are less frustrated with barriers in their path and will attempt to get around them.
12. Girls prefer toys with faces and toys requiring more motor coordination.
13. Boys spend more time playing with nontoys in a room.

What makes these differences between males and females is highly controversial. Exactly where heredity ends and learning from the social environment begins are difficult to determine.

Early and Late Childhood

Psychosocial Aspects

From the age of 2 years to the onset of puberty, several developmental changes occur related to sexuality. Although the genital organs are quiescent compared to the rapid physical growth in every other body system, the child's sexual self–identity is established, and sexual pleasure is discovered.

Sexual self–identity, or *gender identity,* is the feeling that one is male or female (or ambivalent). *Gender role* refers to all that a person says or does to indicate that one is male or female. The establishment of sex identity is critical between the ages of 18 months and 4 years. It begins with an awareness that one belongs to one sex or the other and is well established by 4 years of age. At 2 years of age a child can distinguish between a male and female. By 3 years of age, children can correctly answer the question "Are you a little boy or a little girl?" By age 5 or 6 years the child knows that gender is constant and that if the child is a girl, she cannot be changed into a boy.

Several factors influence the development of core gender. Some of these include communication, a sense of self, and imitation. Communication between parents and children provides children with many clues about their behavior and whether it is regarded as appropriate for the sex role. The term *sex-typed behavior* is used to refer to those behaviors that typically elicit different rewards for one sex or the other. Frequently, parents respond differently to girls than to boys beginning at birth. For example, parents may respond more to a baby girl's vocalizations than to a boy's. Nonverbal communication also may differ. Boys may be handled more roughly, whereas girls are fondled and caressed. Girls may be allowed to cry while boys are not. Even the choice of toys is significant. Many boys, for example, are discouraged from playing with dolls.

Learning appropriate sex-typed behaviors takes the child several years. Initially the child determines his or her gender. Frequent use of the labels *boy* and *he* or *girl* and *she* and rewards to the child for correct self-labelling from the parents assist the child in this process. After learning gender, the child then learns the gender role by the process of *imitation*, copying the behaviors and attitudes of adults. Freud referred to this process as *identification*.

The sense of self is another aspect of gender identity. The development of a sense of self is the ability to distinguish oneself from others. It begins during the first year of life from the child's interactions with the parents. The establishment of trust, the primary task of the infant according to Erikson (see Table 10-2), is basic to the development of a sense of self. Not until infants gain a sense of trust can they relax, be alone, and allow their mothers out of sight. This feeling of trust eventually merges with an awareness and sense of self and ultimately with the feeling that one is an acceptable person.

During early childhood, children develop a sense of pride and pleasure in their bodies, including the genital area. When exploring their bodies, children gain satisfaction in genital self-stimulation. They do not perceive this as masturbation but rather as a source of pleasure. However, parents may become alarmed, since they do perceive this activity as masturbation. The result is that parents then may respond in a negative manner, which conveys to children that the act is "bad." Subsequently children feel anxious, fearful, or guilty about such activity without knowing why. They may then associate pleasurable feelings with being bad.

Three- to 5-year-old children continue with this exploratory curiosity about their body parts. It is not uncommon for boys and girls to be found examining each other's anatomy and comparing the differences. Children need to be allowed to observe these differences at toilet or bathing time during the preschool years. This normal curiosity then subsides by the time the child starts school. In handling such situations, the mother or nurse needs to accept these behaviors. Often it is best to refrain from commenting about the behavior, to answer the child's questions (if there are any) in a matter-of-fact manner, and to direct the child to the next activity such as getting dressed and returning to a play activity. This conveys acceptance of the behavior to the child.

At about 3½ years of age, children become interested in the parental relationship such as their roles, sleeping arrangements, bathing arrangements, and similar matters. The father emerges as a special love object for the female child and the mother for the male child.

Between the ages of 4 and 5 years, children indulge in fantasies. This is the stage of initiative versus guilt, according to Erikson, and the phallic stage, including the castration complex, according to Freud. At this time children fear punishment for dreams or fantasies about their erotic genitals.

During the school-age years, children's curiosity about sexuality and the reproductive processes is high. This accompanies their tremendous broadening of interests and social contacts. Adults at this time receive many questions about sex such as, "Why do you have to go to the hospital to have a baby?" Another phenomenon of this age is social segregation of the sexes, which reaches its peak at about 12 years of age. This is often referred to as the *homosexual stage of development*, although there is no stage at which boys and girls do not show interest in each other. During this period, members of the same sex share genital explorations. The idea that sex is evil can be reinforced during these experiences if parents happen to discover them and react in a horrified manner.

Puberty and Adolescence

Biologic Changes

The physical changes in sexual anatomy and physiology brought about by puberty can be considered more profound than any other period of the life cycle. These changes were discussed in Chapter 12 and are summarized in the following lists.

For boys the changes include:

1. Enlargement of the penis and testes.
2. Appearance of straight pubic hair, which later becomes kinky.
3. Voice changes.
4. Ejaculation.
5. Growth of axillary hair and sweating.

6. Appearance of facial hair.

For girls the changes include:

1. Breast enlargement.
2. Appearance of straight pubic hair, which later becomes kinky.
3. Beginning of menarche.
4. Growth of axillary hair.

Psychosocial Components

Associated with these physical changes are vast psychologic changes. Included are the acceptance of altered body image, adjustment to different energy levels, the establishment of self-identity, and resolution of sexual conflicts.

Responses to altered body image among adolescents varies from feeling to anxiety about maturation to feelings of pleasure about assuming an adult body. Boys, for example, are often anxious about the size of their testicles and penis, equating this with virility and potency. Girls, on the other hand, are more concerned about their breast development and menses. Because the menstrual pattern for the first year is irregular, many girls become preoccupied about their menstrual timetables, particularly if they differ from their peers. Adolescents need to know that the size of the penis or breasts has no bearing on functional ability and that menses is normally irregular during the first year. Associated with these bodily changes in the adolescent is an awareness of sexual feelings. These feelings also have to be incorporated into an acceptable image of self.

Adjusting to different energy levels is another important aspect of development at this age. Increased physical activity and impulsive behavior are notable with adolescents. These behaviors are necessary at this time to cope with the tensions and anxieties associated with bodily changes. In contrast, rest and sleep are equally important to cope with the growth demands. Quiet activities such as reading or watching television offer respite from active physical endeavors.

The establishment of self-identity can become confusing and disconcerting. For example, with bodily changes and growth spurts, the sense of mastery of the body achieved earlier is often shaken. However, during this period the changes the adolescent undergoes eventually lead to a more stable existence. Adolescents acquire a new status. At 16 years of age they can obtain a driver's licenses; at 18 years of age they are allowed to vote. Heterosexual relationships are developed, and the peer group provides strong support. During this transition period, adolescents learn to become productive members of society and to assume the role of adulthood.

Sexual conflicts, however, remain a problem. Although adolescents are recognized by Western society as physically mature adults, they are denied the right to full adult privileges sexually. Thus this becomes a stressful period for adolescents. They experience intense sexual impulses that have to be controlled. During puberty, experimentation in erotic play (masturbation) and genital examination with members of the same sex continues, particularly among boys. This is simply a part of the developmental process. It is largely an attempt to learn about their own growth patterns and physical reactions as they compare themselves to other youths. Heterosexual activity varies widely among adolescents, moving from embracing, to kissing, to petting, and to intercourse. Guilt feelings are often associated with such experiences by adolescents. These feelings are frequently magnified by fears of pregnancy or venereal disease.

Adulthood and the Middle Years

A number of sexual behavior patterns occur during adulthood. These include heterosexual activities, masturbation, homosexuality, and abstention. Typically adulthood is considered to be devoted to parenting and the development of sexual intimacy with marriage partners. However, regardless of life-style arrangements, such as communal living or other alternatives to marriage, the sexual relationship is a crucial component of interpersonal relationships. The capacity to give and receive gratification heterosexually in a stable relationship prevails as a societal task. This not only encompasses the physiologic aspects of sexuality but also the concept of oneself as a sexual being with an associated sex role.

Biologic Changes

The process of aging begins in young adulthood and progressively continues. Physical changes occur that can threaten self-image and self-esteem, particularly in those adults who value their youthful image. Wrinkling of the skin, increased adipose tissue particularly at the waistline, graying hair, and baldness are changes that many find difficult to accept. Fears about loss of femininity or masculinity are magnified by the media, which advertise hair dyes, wrinkle creams, and products to reduce baldness.

During the middle years, menstruation wanes and ceases, and the breasts atrophy without the influence of estrogen. The vagina also atrophies. Vaginal lubrication is delayed, and the expansibility of the vaginal barrel decreases. Steroid therapy is often given to a woman during her middle-age years to compensate for these changes. For males, there is a delay in attaining erections, a decrease in the expulsive force of ejaculation, and a decrease in the volume of seminal fluid expelled.

Psychologic Aspects

In the early adult years, a number of factors must be considered related to sexuality. Pregnancy may alter the woman's self-image as a sexual being. Throughout pregnancy, sexual desire of both partners vacillates. The birth of a newborn often focuses the spouses' attention away from each other onto the infant. The presence of growing children also may decrease opportunities and privacy for sexual interaction. The physical and emotional strain placed on adults by their work or careers can often interfere with sexual desire. Because of the differences between the male and female sexual responses, many misunderstandings can arise. In light of these factors, the more each partner can learn about each other's unique responses and the more they can communicate their feelings, the greater the chance that compatible sexual relationships can be achieved by each.

During the middle-age years there is some decline in overall sexual interest and activity. However, sex continues to be important to middle-age adults, and many enjoy intercourse at least once a week. It is thought that the levels of sexual activity during youth and the older years are directly correlated. Another factor influencing sexual activity in the middle years is physical health. Disfiguring surgery or cardiac disease, for example, can alter sexual function. These are discussed later in this chapter.

The Elderly

Contrary to popular belief, the need for sexual expression and sexual intimacy remains into old age. The capacity for sexual performance often extends beyond the 80-year-old level. Some sexual adjustments, however, are often necessitated due to common disease conditions, including prostatic and cardiac conditions, senile vaginitis, and diabetes. At this time of life, aging persons find it necessary to nuture one another and to cope with bereavement and widowhood. Sexual activity and interest therefore may persist well into the eight and ninth decades, provided that health is maintained and that an interesting partner is available.

SEXUAL STIMULATION AND RESPONSE PATTERNS

Sexual Stimulation

Sexual stimulation may be of physical or psychologic origin. Erotic stimuli (those which cause sexual arousal) may be real or symbolic and are received by the sensory receptors of sight, hearing, smell, or touch.

Physical Stimulation

Physical stimulation refers to the activities of touch, pressure, or bodily contact. Nerve receptors then transfer these stimuli to the spinal cord and the brain. A variety of body contact activities are involved in physical stimulation. Included are stroking of the erogenous zones, kissing, breast stimulation, manual stimulation of the genitalia, oral-genital stimulation, anal stimulation, and pain. Purposeful physical contact or petting that increases sexual arousal prior to

intercourse is called *foreplay*, or *precoital stimulation*. Wide variations exist in the amount and methods of foreplay among persons in North America.

1. *Erogenous zones.* Certain areas of the body are richly supplied with nerve endings and, when stroked, stimulate sexual arousal. These areas are called *erogenous zones*. Obviously the genital organs of both sexes are highly erogenous. However, many other areas of the body such as the mouth, ears, breast, back, buttocks, anus, neck, abdomen, and thighs are also considered as erotic areas. For males the primary erogenous zones, other than the genitalia, are the thighs, lips, and ears; for females they are the breasts, thighs, and ears (Goldstein 1976:130). When stimulating erogenous zones, it is important to understand that rapid adaptation occurs with the touch and pain receptors of the skin. These nerve cells adapt rapidly to continuous stimulation by becoming decreasingly

responsive. Because touch and pressure receptors respond better to changes in stimulation, sexual arousal can be increased by moving the stimulation from place to place, such as from the clitoris to the nipples, rather than by maintaining continuous contact with one or two areas.

2. *Kissing.* To achieve erotic stimulation, kissing is unique to humans and varies in method from simple kissing to tongue kissing. It involves the senses of touch, taste, and smell. The use of simple or tongue kissing as an activity of foreplay varies among cultures. Some cultures tend to value oral contact with the genitalia during foreplay in preference to kissing.

3. *Breast stimulation.* Sexual arousal is also achieved by stimulation of the breasts either by manual manipulation or oral stimulation. Many women relate highly pleasurable sensations in response to mouthing and sucking of the nipples. The breast stimulation correlates with pleasurable contractions in the pelvic region. Stimulation of the breasts is associated with the release of the pituitary hormone oxytocin, which produces milk secretion and causes smooth muscle contractions of the uterus and related structures. Thus breast stimulation is often associated with feelings of sexual pleasure in women who are breast-feeding and can cause orgasm in some women. During foreplay, breast stimulation can maintain high sexual arousal levels and is significant to potential coital and sexual satisfaction.

4. *Manual stimulation of the genitalia.* This form of foreplay can by itself lead to orgasm. Manual stimulation may involve reciprocal stimulation between two partners or may involve *masturbation,* self-stimulation of the genitalia or other body parts that evokes erotic pleasure. The primary site of erotic stimulation for the majority of males is the penis rather than the scrotum. During manual stimulation the glans or the shaft of the penis can be stimulated by firm gripping and stroking techniques, or the *frenulum* (the fold on the lower surface of the glans penis that connects it with the prepuce) can be lightly touched or tugged. When sexual tension increases, the rapidity of manipulations is increased until the point of ejaculation occurs. After ejaculation the glans penis is often hypersensitive to touch or pressure.

Manual stimulation techniques of the female genitalia that create sexual arousal are more variable compared to those for the male. Direct stimulation of the glans clitoris is often considered to be the major erotic focus for females. However, this highly sensitive area rarely requires direct stimulation. Appropriate arousal levels are achieved by light touches or tugs on the prepuce and labia, which stimulate the clitoral shaft, and by pressure applied to the mons pubis or vulva.

Contrary to societal beliefs, masturbation is neither physically nor mentally harmful. The frequency of masturbation ranges from several times a day to several times per week, and the incidence is more than 80% of males and more than 50% of females. Most males tend to experience masturbation earlier in life (often before the age of 20 years) as compared to women, some of whom may not experience masturbation until the age of 40 years or greater. Sometimes genital substitutes are used during masturbation. Males may use vaginal substitutes that are made of lifelike inflatable plastic. These may be part of whole lifesize inflatable women. Women may use *dildoes* (artificial penises) or other accessories such as vibrators.

5. *Oral-genital stimulation.* Three types of oral-genital contact may be used in precoital stimulation: cunnilingus, fellatio, and soixante-neuf. *Cunnilingus* refers to oral stimulation of the female clitoris and labia by a partner. Kissing, sucking, and tonguing techniques are used. Lubrication is provided by saliva during the process. *Fellatio* is the act of stimulating the male genitalia by oral means. Licking, blowing, and sucking of the glans and shaft of the penis are involved. *Soixante-neuf,* the French term for "69," is simultaneous oral-genital stimulation between two persons. The use and desirability of oral-genital contact are an individual and perhaps a cultural matter. Many individuals have never performed oral-genital stimulation nor do they desire to. Oral-genital manipulation is considered by some to be a sex perversion, whereas others consider it highly desirable when performed voluntarily and in the privacy of their own homes.

6. *Anal stimulation.* When anal stimulation is provided orally, it is referred to as *anilingus.* Note that anilingus is different from anal intercourse. Anilingus is not a common method of precoital stimulation probably because of the association of the anus with the act of defecation. However, the anus is abundantly supplied with nerve receptors that are closely aligned to those of the genitalia. For sexual partners who are uninhibited and unrestricted by prior conditioning, the act of anilingus can provide sexual satisfaction. This area when kept clean has the same character as other healthy skin areas.

7. *Pain stimulation.* Scratching, pinching, or biting provided in certain degrees can increase sexual

arousal levels. For example, biting of the ear lobes or lips to the point of drawing blood is practiced by some people.

Psychologic Stimulation

Erotic stimulation through other sense organs such as those of smell, taste, hearing, sight, or fantasy is considered to be psychologic sexual stimulation. These stimuli affect a person primarily through psychologic associations related to previous experiences or to future hopes or desires. Psychologic stimuli include pleasing odors, visual attractions, and auditory media.

1. *Odors.* Body odors can be stimulating sexually or can in some situations be offensive. Perfumes when associated with a previous pleasurable sexual experience often produce a sexual response.

2. *Visual attractions.* Changes in light, certain colors, clothing, or the way a person moves can become erotic stimuli through the sense of vision. Variations occur among persons and between the sexes as to whether stimuli are erotic. Men tend to be aroused more by pictures of naked or clothed persons, whereas women tend to be aroused more by romantic themes such as persons embracing with affection or the decor and quality of the surroundings.

3. *Auditory media.* Sexual excitement is often enhanced by words or music. The sounds people find sexually pleasing or soothing vary considerably. For example, youths may respond to sensuous rock music, whereas adults may respond to soft singing or to a symphony. Erotic auditory stimuli often relate to previous positive sexual experiences.

Sexual Response Patterns

The physiologic response to sexual stimulation is basically the same for all individuals, male or female. However, the psychologic and sociologic aspects of the response to stimulation are highly variable. Variations occur between males and females, among members of the same sex, and even in the same person at different times.

Sexual Intercourse

Sexual intercourse can be physically stimulating and emotionally gratifying. Synonyms for the term sexual intercourse are *coitus* and *copulation. Coitus* is a term derived from the Latin word *coitio,* which means "a coming together." *Copulation,* also of Latin

origin, means "coupling or joining." Many slang terms are used by the public to convey the act of coitus.

Several positions may be used during sexual intercourse. Face-to-face, lying positions with either the male or female on top or side-by-side postures are commonly practiced. Variations of these face-to-face positions include a standing posture, which can allow more freedom of movement to each partner, and a sitting-kneeling position (the female sits on the edge of a bed or chair while the male kneels in front). In addition, several rear entry postures may be used. The number of coital positions used by any particular couple depends upon social influences, previous inhibitions, and their agility and imagination.

Because direct clitoral stimulation is important to the female during coitus, the side-lying positions and female-on-top positions are recommended (Masters and Johnson 1966:59). Although clitoral stimulation can also be provided by the male-on-top position with the male riding high over his partner, it is thought that during intromission in this position the penis is directed more toward the posterior vaginal wall and rectum rather than into the depths of the vaginal canal.

Physiology of Intercourse

Two primary physiologic changes occur during sexual intercourse: vasocongestion (congestion of the blood vessels) and myotonia (increased muscular tension). The physiologic changes during coitus are characterized as having four phases: (a) the excitement phase, (b) the plateau phase, (c) orgasm and (d) the resolution phase (Masters and Johnson 1966:4).

The *excitement phase* develops from any source of erotic stimuli and involves a gradual increase in the sexual arousal level. Signs of this stage in the male include the following:

1. Penile erection.
2. Tensing, thickening, and elevation of the scrotum.
3. An increase in size of the testes with elevation toward the perineum as the spermatic cord shortens. These signs are due largely to vasocongestion and parasympathetic nervous system effects.

In the female the signs of sexual excitement are as follows:

1. Enlargement of the clitoral glans.
2. Vaginal lubrication.
3. Expansion in width and length of the vaginal barrel.

4. Separation and flattening of the labia majora.

5. Reddening of the labia minora and vaginal wall.

6. Nipple erection, breast tumescence, and engorged areolae.

Other signs are common to both males and females during the excitement phase. These are increases in heart rate and blood pressure in proportion to the level of arousal, involuntary muscle tensing of the intercostal and abdominal muscles, and the appearance of the *sex flush*, a rashlike condition beginning on the abdomen and moving to the breasts, neck, face, and back. The sex flush is more common in females and increases with the level of arousal and high room temperatures.

The *plateau phase* is the period in which sexual tension becomes intensified to levels nearing orgasm, provided that adequate erotic stimulation is maintained. During this phase the influence of the sympathetic nervous system is evident in both sexes. Heart rates are accelerated to 100 to 175 beats per minute; breathing rates increase up to 40 breaths per minute, particularly in the late stages of the plateau phase; and the systolic and distolic blood pressures rise (20 to 80 mm Hg systolic and 10 to 40 mm Hg diastolic). Myotonia increases both voluntarily and involuntarily. Abdominal intercostal and facial muscles contract, and both males and females may voluntarily contract their rectal sphincters to enhance stimulation.

In the male, specific changes during the plateau phase include the following:

1. Increase in the penile circumference at the coronal ridge and inconsistent deepening in color.

2. 50% increase in testicular size and elevation closer to the perineum.

3. Appearance of a few drops of mucoid secretions from Cowper's glands.

4. Appearance of the sex flush late in the phase in some males.

In the female, further changes during the plateau phase include the following:

1. Retraction of the clitoris under the clitoral hood.

2. Appearance of the orgasmic platform, which is an increase in size of the outer one-third of the vagina and labia minora due to congestion. This platform prevents leakage of semen after ejaculation and also increases the friction on the penis.

3. Further increases in the depth and width of the vaginal barrel.

4. Increasing color change of the sex skin (labia minora) from bright red to a deep wine color.

5. Appearance of a few drops of mucoid secretions from Bartholin's glands, which correspond to the male Cowper's gland secretions.

6. Increasing engorgement of the labia majora.

7. Increasing engorgement of the breasts and nipples.

8. Spread of the sex flush over the entire body.

Orgasm is the involuntary climax of sexual tension in which a feeling of physiologic and psychologic release occurs. Although the total body is involved in orgasm, the pelvic area is perceived as the major focus. The orgasmic phase is of short duration compared to the previous phases, lasting only a few seconds. This stage involves rhythmic spasmodic contractions of the genitalia. The heart rate, breathing rate and blood pressure rise to peak levels during orgasm.

In the male, expulsive contractions of the penis occur, starting at less than one-second intervals. After the first three or four contractions, the frequency of contraction is reduced. The ejaculatory process can be divided into two stages. In the first stage, seminal fluid is expelled into the prostatic urethra. During the second stage, semen is then expelled from the prostatic urethra to the urethral meatus. The force of ejaculation diminishes after the first few initial expulsive contractions. Contraction of the secondary organs such as the vas deferens, epididymis, seminal vesicles, and prostate also occurs during orgasm. During ejaculation the internal bladder sphincter closes to prevent retrograde passage of semen into the bladder. Many males report feelings of pleasure about the amount of seminal fluid passing through the urethra.

In the female, approximately five to twelve contractions occur in the orgasmic platform during orgasm. The response is similar to the male in that contractions initially occur at frequencies of less than one second and then diminish in intervals and intensity. The muscles of the pelvic floor surrounding the lower one-third of the vagina and the uterine muscles also contract during orgasm. Greater variations exist in female orgasms. Common patterns of orgasm include (a) a minor orgasm in which the plateau phase fluctuates with only small surges toward orgasm, (b) a multiple orgasmic response and (c) a single orgasmic response comparable to the male. Changes in orgasmic response patterns occur in females after many coital experiences. The factors causing these changes are unknown. Females seem to start with a minor orgasmic pattern, progressing to a multiple and then a single orgasmic response, or they progress to a single and then multiple orgasmic response.

The *resolution phase* is the period involving a return to the nonsexually aroused state. Usually the length of this phase parallels the length of the excite-

ment phase. Many individuals perspire during this phase. Other responses vary from desire to sleep, feelings of relaxation, or emotional outbursts such as crying or laughing. Immediately after orgasm, males undergo a *physiologic refractory period* in which they cannot respond to continued sexual stimuli.

SEXUALITY PROBLEMS

Problems with Intercourse

It has been estimated that more than one half of married couples in North America have some sexual problems. Common concerns are that the woman lacks the ability to readily achieve orgasm or that the man lacks the ability to maintain an erection for coitus or cannot control his ejaculation for a sufficient length of time to satisfy his partner.

Impotence

The inability to achieve or maintain an erection sufficiently to perform intercourse is referred to as *impotence*. Numerous factors are involved in impotence. The major reasons underlying the condition are psychologic in origin. These factors include doubts about one's ability to perform or about one's masculinity. Fatigue and stress at work, in the family, and in interpersonal relationships are often factors. The treatment for impotence depends largely upon the cause. Implants in the penis have been used to treat biologically incurred impotence. Impotence of psychologic origin often requires a change in both partners' view of sexuality. Awareness of the cause of the condition and exercises designed to increase sensations are also used.

Premature Ejaculation

Premature ejaculation occurs when a man cannot control his ejaculation from 30 seconds to one minute after entering the female vagina. Another definition states that premature ejaculation occurs when the man cannot control his ejaculation long enough to satisfy his partner. The causes of this condition chiefly involve early conditioning in which rapid orgasm was desirable.

Treatment advocated by Masters and Johnson includes the development of increased sexual communication and responsiveness as well as decreasing performance demands. The couple together practice

sensate exercises (learning to enjoy the sensation of touch) and then work together to establish satisfying coitus.

Orgasmic Dysfunction

Orgasmic dysfunction is of two types: primary and situational. *Primary orgasmic dysfunction* refers to women who have never been able to achieve orgasm. *Situational dysfunction* refers to women who have experienced at least one orgasm but are at that time nonorgasmic. *Frigidity*, however, refers to a woman who has a low or nondetectable sex drive.

Orgasmic dysfunction can be caused by drugs, alcohol, aging, and anatomic abnormalities of the genitalia. However, most cases are psychologic in origin. Some of these can be poor sexual technique, hostility between partners, fear or guilt of a woman about enjoying the sexual act, or concern about performance. Therapy usually involves establishing new attitudes by both partners about sex. Pelvic muscle exercises (Kegal exercises) can also increase the capacity to achieve orgasm by increasing the strength of the pubococcygeal muscle (see Chapter 23, "Postnatal Exercises").

Vaginismus

Vaginismus is irregular and involuntary contraction of the muscles around the outer third of the vagina when coitus is attempted. Thus the vagina closes before penile penetration. The cause can be severe sexual inhibition, often associated with early learning such as in a family with strict religious beliefs. Other causes can be rape, incest, and painful intercourse.

Treatment often involves sensate focus exercises and psychologic changes. In some instances graduated vaginal dilators are also used.

Dyspareunia

Dyspareunia is pain experienced by a woman during intercourse. It can occur as a result of inadequate lubrication, scarring, vaginal infection, or hormonal imbalance. Treatment is aimed at the underlying cause such as supplying additional lubrication before intercourse.

Common Illnesses Affecting Sexuality

Medical Conditions

Heart disease and diabetes mellitus are two of the more frequently occurring long-term illnesses. For diabetic men impotency can be a problem. This can be treated with hormones such as testosterone.

Following a myocardial infarction some patients may fear sexual intercourse because of the increased heart and respiratory rates associated with sexual activity. Most patients can resume sexual activity four to six weeks after a myocardial infarction. The transient increases in heart and respiratory rates are generally within their capacities (Puksta 1977: 602). A prescribed program of progressive physical activity also improves the patient's tolerance for exercise and sexual activity. For postcoronary patients the on-bottom position during intercourse is considered less stressful than the on-top position. Thus couples may need to adjust to a position of less strain, although assuming a natural position is considered to be less stressful for some patients than a new position.

Spinal cord injuries can present special sexual problems to patients. Some individuals with paraplegia can be potent and fertile, depending on the type of injury. Some men are able to have erections with local stimulation; others can have erection from psychologic stimulation, and others are unable to have either reflexogenic or psychogenic erections. Sexual adjustments for patients who have spinal cord injuries are one of many complex adjustments faced by these patients and families. Special rehabilitative programs and counselling are frequently indicated.

Surgical Conditions

After certain surgical procedures such as a mastectomy, hysterectomy, or enterostomy, a person's concept of body image may be changed (see Chapter 35, "Accepting Loss and Dying"). The response of a loved one to any of these changes greatly affects the surgical patient's ability to reintegrate his or her self-image. Sexual relations can also be affected by the person's self-perceptions. The person who feels ugly and unloved may feel inadequate in a sexual relationship. This person may feel ashamed at having another see the body changes. Loss of one of the genitalia or reproductive organs can also be interpreted as making a person sexually inadequate, even if the organs related to sexuality are unaffected.

Accurate knowledge to clear up misconceptions is important. Sometimes the couple or marriage partners require assistance to express their feelings and to develop positive constructive attitudes toward each other and the sexual relationship.

The sexual significance of the female breast often requires special adjustments. Loss of a breast is often associated with anxiety about loss of femininity. The value a woman places upon a lost breast often reflects how much a woman relates her self-worth to her appearance.

Husbands may need assistance expressing any concern about the loss of the breast. Some men may feel revolted at the sight of the scar; others may fear harming their wives if they have sexual intercourse. If the relationship preoperatively is supportive, both partners find the adjustment less difficult postoperatively.

NURSING ASSESSMENT OF SEXUAL PROBLEMS

In assessing current or potential problems associated with sexuality, nurses should be aware of certain cues presented by patients and their families. Following are some of these:

1. Asks questions about normal sexual activity and what it is.

2. Refers to rigid upbringing in relation to sexual matters.

3. Reflects judgmental attitudes such as sex is dirty or evil or that it is a necessary but unpleasant part of marriage.

4. Expresses concern about sexual adequacy.

5. Perceives self as unattractive.

6. Reveals information about a previous rape, illegitimate pregnancy, incest, homosexual experiences, or abortion.

7. Refers to sexual partner in a negative manner.

8. Expresses feelings of lassitude, fatigue, and lack of interest in sexual matters after an illness.

NURSING INTERVENTION FOR SEXUAL PROBLEMS

The nursing intervention for sexual problems is primarily fourfold; assessment, referral, counselling, and education.

Assessment

That there might be a problem may be picked up by the nurse during interaction with a patient and/or the family. Some of the cues to possible sexual problems were listed in the previous section.

Referral

Sexual problems often require referral to the physician or counsellor. Conveying the patient's own words "I am disgusted by sex" is preferable to providing an interpretation of the words ("He states a dislike of sex").

Counselling

The nurse's counselling role with regard to sexual matters includes assisting in the expression of feelings, clarifying, assisting the patient relate feelings

with experience and knowledge, and the provision of information. The latter can often correct misinformation.

Patients and their families who are able to express their feelings in an accepting environment can often be helped to accept these feelings and to relate them to previous or current experiences. Once this relationship has been internalized, feelings and attitudes can often change to more positive constructive ones. Sometimes people have misinformation that they have believed for years such as eating garlic with meals will prevent conception. Nurses can often provide accurate information to replace outdated beliefs and at the same time reassure and support the patient in the acquisition of accurate information.

Education

Education about sexual matters is needed by children, adolescents, and frequently adults. Community agencies often have pamphlets for distribution to groups. Some schools conduct sex education programs geared to different age groups which are often provided by nurses. The nurse has a primary role to play in this education, both with groups and in one-to-one relationships.

CONTRACEPTION

Contraception is the voluntary prevention of conception or impregnation. To impregnate is to fertilize or to render pregnant. Contraceptive methods include the biologic or ovulation method, coitus interruptus, and hormonal, chemical, mechanical, and surgical procedures.

Biologic or Ovulation Method

The biologic method is often preferred by people whose religious beliefs conflict with artificial birth control methods and by those who do not believe in pharmacologic or mechanical devices, for example. Basic to this method is the identification of the days of the month when conception could take place and consequent abstinence from sexual activity during that time. Women must learn the following signs of ovulation, since that is when conception can take

place:

1. Secretion of mucus from the vagina. Initially the mucus is thick and yellow or sometimes cloudy. This secretion becomes clearer and thinner the nearer ovulation.
2. Breast tenderness.
3. Tenderness at either side of the lower abdomen.
4. Midcycle spotting of blood.
5. Rise in basal temperature. The temperature taken each morning upon arising will drop about 0.2°C or 0.3°F one or two days prior to ovulation and then rise 0.4° to 0.5°C (0.7° to 0.8°F) one to two days after ovulation. The fertile period around ovulation extends from one or two days before ovulation to two days after. These are the days of the mucous flow, or the "wet days."

The advantages of this method of contraception include economy, no pharmacologic or mechanic devices are used to interfere with body physiology, and it is readily learned by people. The disadvantages include abstinence from sexual activity for a period surrounding ovulation, and cooperation is required of both partners.

Coitus Interruptus

This method of contraception involves the withdrawal of the penis prior to ejaculation of the semen. This method requires considerable self-control. It has two primary disadvantages. Some semen may escape into the vagina prior to the climax, and it may decrease sexual gratification.

Hormonal Therapy

Single hormone therapy such as the administration of estrogen in daily doses for three weeks will suppress FSH and LH, thus preventing ovulation. One problem of single hormone therapy is nausea. As a result, combined hormone therapy is more popular. This therapy usually combines estrogen and progesterone. The "pill" is made up of synthetic preparations of these products. The high levels of these hormones block the release of FSH from the anterior pituitary and hence the ripening of the follicle and prevent ovulation.

The pill is taken once a day for 20 or 21 days starting on the fifth day of the menstrual cycle. The pill is provided in two forms: combined or sequential. In the combined form, estrogen and progesterone are combined in each pill. With the sequential form, estrogen only is contained in the first 15 pills and progesterone in the remaining seven pills.

The pill is usually supplied in a container in which the number of pills taken is easily seen (see Figure 31-3, D).

The pill is considered to be relatively safe. Annoying side effects are nausea, weight gain, and breast tenderness. If these persist, the patient should consult her physician. It is contraindicated for patients who are prone to heart attack, circulatory problems, severe migraines, liver pathology, and diabetes mellitus.

Chemical Methods

Chemical contraception includes the insertion of foam, jelly, creams, or suppositories into the vagina before intercourse. These products, which were in-

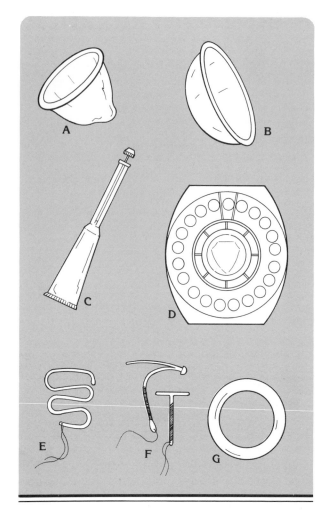

Figure 31.3   Some methods of contraception. **A,** Condom; **B,** diaphragm; **D,** the pill; **E,** Lippes loop (intrauterine device, or IUD); **F,** Cu7 and TCu(IUD); and **G,** vaginal ring.

troduced in the 1950s form a film over the surface o, the vagina that acts as a spermicide. A *spermicide* destroys sperm. These products are inserted using an applicator (see Figure 31-3, C). The applicator is filled and then inserted to the cervical os. It is then withdrawn about one-half inch, the plunger is depressed and the substance covers the os, preventing sperm from entering the uterus. These products must be inserted within one hour of intercourse to be effective and the application repeated if intercourse is repeated. Their chief disadvantages are the difficulty some women have inserting the substance up to the os and leakage from the vagina.

Mechanical Devices

There are three main kinds of mechanical contraceptive devices: intrauterine devices (IUD) or intrauterine contraceptive devices (IUCD), the vaginal diaphragm, and the condom. The IUD is a plastic ring, coil, loop, copper Tu, and Cu7 (see Figure 31-3, *F,G*), which is inserted into the uterus and prevents contraception. Lippes loop, which is made of plastic (see Figure 31-3, *E*) is popular.

These devices have the advantage of being economical, and, for those women who can retain them, no other action is required for contraceptive protection. Their chief disadvantage is that they cause cramping and excessive bleeding for some women and may be expelled spontaneously.

The vaginal diaphragm is a round rubber cup inserted into the vagina (see Figure 31-3, *B*). It must be properly fitted and used with a spermicide. It is left in place for six to eight hours after intercourse.

The condom, or sheath, is a plastic covering placed over the penis prior to intercourse (see Figure 31-3, *A*). It must be inspected for holes. The ejaculate is deposited in the condom rather than in the vagina. The cost of condoms may prevent some men from their consistent use.

Surgical Methods

Surgical contraceptive methods include tubal ligation for the woman and a vasectomy for the man. A *tubal ligation* is the tying of the fallopian tubes to interrupt tubal continuity. A small abdominal incision is made below the umbilicus, and with 20 to 30 minutes the procedure is complete. It is commonly done under local anesthetic.

A *vasectomy* is the ligation and cutting of the vas deferens on either side of the scrotum. The procedure is generally done under local anesthetic. A vasectomy does not affect potency.

SUMMARY

Sexuality is important in developing self-identity, interpersonal relationships, intimacy, and love. In its broad sense, sexuality involves physical, emotional, social, and ethical aspects of being and behaving. Every aspect of sexual behavior consists of learned and inherited components, which must be considered in any given sexual activity.

An understanding of the structure and function of the male and female genitalia is essential for nurses. The male genitalia include the testes and scrotum, a series of ducts (epididymis and vas deferens) that transport the sperm, glands that secrete seminal plasma, and the penis. The female genitalia include the ovaries, fallopian tubes, uterus, vagina, vulva, and mammary glands. All these organs have significant functions in reproduction and in sexual stimulation and intercourse.

The components that contribute to the development of sexuality are numerous. Both biologic and psychologic components are essential at all age levels. Biologic differences in the sexes are apparent at birth, but many behavioral differences are also notable throughout infancy and childhood.

The establishment of sexual self-identity and gender role are critical between the ages of 18 months to 4 years. The learning of sex-typed behaviors is dependent upon communication from parents and upon imitation of parental behavior. Learning appropriate sex-typed behaviors takes several years. During adolescence the establishment of self-identity can become disconcerting. Sexual conflicts are a major problem. Adults also often experience sexual problems. A major task of the adult is to develop an intimate relationship with a partner. During the middle and later years, physical changes in the genitalia occur. However, the desire and ability to maintain satisfying sexual relationships can be maintained.

An understanding of sexual stimuli and response patterns can enable individuals to experience satisfying sexual relationships. It can also assist nurses to understand the implications involved for patients who experience feelings of inadequacy, or medical problems such as spinal cord injuries or other illnesses such as myocardial infarctions. Common sexual problems of healthy adults are impotence, premature ejaculation, orgasmic dysfunction, vaginismus, and dyspareunia. Illnesses that commonly affect sexuality are myocardial infarction and diabetes mellitus. Many surgical procedures also affect sexual abilities and sexual self-image. Some of these are mastectomy, hysterectomy, and enterostomy.

Nursing intervention for sexual problems are categorized as fourfold: assessment, referral, counselling, and education. Several cues are outlined that may help the nurse determine potential sexual problems.

SUGGESTED ACTIVITIES

1. Observe a group of children at play. Identify those activities which are related to gender role and gender identity.

2. Interview the parents of a young child. Assess how they contribute to the development of the child's gender and gender role.

3. Discuss with an adolescent what he or she wants to know about sex. Where does the adolescent obtain information about sex.

4. Interview a physician in the community and determine what sexual problems he or she encounters in the medical practice.

SUGGESTED READINGS

Cowart, Marie and Newton, David W. June, 1976. Oral contraceptives: how best to explain their effects to patients. *Nursing 76* 6:44–48.

A description of the effects of oral contraceptives upon body physiology with information often requested by patients. Physical assessment prior to giving the pill is included as well as annoying and potentially serious side effects.

Schlesinger, Benjamin. October, 1977. From A to Z with adolescent sexuality. *The Canadian Nurse* 73:34–37.

Using a letter of the alphabet to start each paragraph, the issues related to adolescent sexuality are discussed. The need for education and research is included as well as basic issues about the male-female and parental roles.

Stephens, Gwen T. January, 1978. Creative contraries: a theory of sexuality. *American Journal of Nursing.* 78:70–75.

The author presents a theory of sexuality. Included is the motivational system, reward-need, and adaptive aspects of sexuality and sexual fantasies.

Timby, Barbara Kuhn. June, 1976. Ovulation method of birth control. *American Journal of Nursing.* 76:928–929.

The natural method of birth control is described. The physiologic changes in the female are described related to the menstrual cycle. Suggestions to women such as taking a morning temperature and maintaining a chart about vaginal mucous secretions as a means of determining safe days are given.

SELECTED REFERENCES

Andrews, Susan W. April, 1976. A college contraceptive Clinic. *American Journal of Nursing* 76:592–593.

Comarr, A. Estin, and Gunderson, Bernice B. February, 1975. Sexual function in traumatic paraplegia and quadriplegia. *American Journal of Nursing* 75:250–255.

Contemporary Nursing Series. 1973. *Human sexuality: nursing implications* New York: The American Journal of Nursing.

Costello, Marilyn K. August, 1975. Sex, intimacy and aging. *American Journal of Nursing* 75:1330–1332.

Easterbrook, Bonnie, and Rust, Beth. January, 1977. Abortion counselling. *The Canadian Nurse* 73:28–30.

Engel, June. January, 1978. Birth control update: what's new, what works and what's next in birth control devices *Chatelaine* 51:27–29, 78–80.

Evans, Ellis D., and McCandless, Boyd R. 1978. *Children and youth: psychosocial development,* 2nd ed. New York: Holt, Rinehart and Winston, Inc.

Goldstein, Bernard. 1976. *Human sexuality.* New York: McGraw-Hill Book Co.

Guyton, Arthur C. 1976. *Textbook of medical physiology,* 5th ed. Philadelphia: W. B. Saunders Co.

Hanlon, Kathryn. May, 1975. Maintaining sexuality after spinal cord injury. *Nursing 75* 5:58–59, 61–62.

Lief, Harold I., and Payne, Tyana. November, 1975. Sexuality—knowledge and attitudes. *American Journal of Nursing* 75:2026–2029.

Mann, T. 1970. The biochemical characteristics of spermatozoa and seminal plasma. In E. Rosenberg, et al., eds. *The human testis.* New York: Plenum Press, Inc.

Masters, W. H., and Johnson, V. E. 1966. *Human sexual response.* Boston: Little, Brown & Co.

Masters, W. H., and Johnson, V. E. 1970. *Human sexual inadequacy.* Boston: Little, Brown & Co.

Puksta, Nancy Sallese. April, 1977. All about sex . . . after a coronary. *American Journal of Nursing* 77:602–605.

Smith, Jim, and Bullough, Bonnie. December, 1975. Sexuality and the severely disabled person. *American Journal of Nursing* 75:2194–2197.

Stanford, Dennyse. April, 1977. All about sex . . . after middle age. *American Journal of Nursing* 77:608–611.

Sutterley, Doris Cook, and Donnelly, Gloria Ferraro. 1973. *Perspectives in human development.* Philadelphia: J. B. Lippincott Co.

Timby, Barbara Kuhn. June, 1976. Ovulation method of birth control. *American Journal of Nursing* 76:928–929.

Wood, Robin Young, and Rose, Karla. February, 1978. Penile implants for impotence. *American Journal of Nursing* 78:234–238.

Woods, Nancy Fugate. 1975. *Human sexuality in health and illness.* St. Louis: The C. V. Mosby Co.

CHAPTER 32

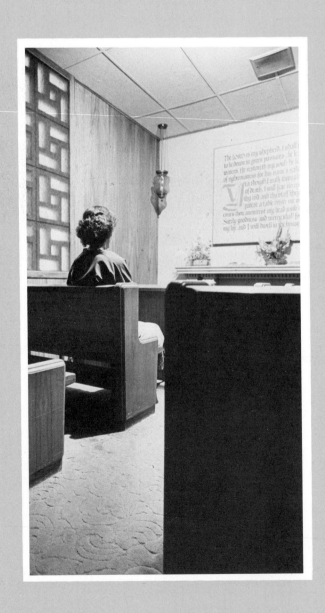

SPIRITUAL PREFERENCE

OBJECTIVES

- Discuss religious and moral development from birth through old age.
- Discuss spiritual needs in relation to illness.
- Describe the characteristics of people most likely to benefit from spiritual counsel.
- Describe the nurse's role in assisting patients to meet their spiritual needs.
- Describe how a hospital chaplain can assist patients.
- Explain the beliefs of religious groups related to health care.

Spiritual preference reflects a desire to understand one's relationship to the universe as well as the eventual direction and meaning of life. Most people have some type of spiritual belief. This belief usually provides guidance in issues involving mores and ethical values. It also serves as an integrating force in society and provides people with inner strengths that are closely associated with emotional and physical health.

At a time of illness many people who do not profess to have spiritual beliefs look to spirituality for assistance and consolation. The provision of spiritual guidance is in keeping with treating the whole person: assisting the patient emotionally, physically, and spiritually.

Religious and spiritual beliefs often assist people during times of stress. Some people look to religion to answer why they are ill, others look upon illness as a test of faith, and others look upon illness as punishment for sin. "What have I done to deserve this?" In these instances illness is looked upon as punishment by some outside force. In some instances, patients and families use prayer, promise, and even penance in an effort to treat the disease.

Sometimes religious beliefs can affect the course of an illness and how a person accepts the illness and therapy. Some religious groups such as the Church of Christ, Scientist (Christian Science) deny that illness really exists. People who strictly follow this religion will not accept a physician's consultation or accept medical treatment and rarely if ever enter a hospital. Other religious groups condemn modern medicine as false teaching. Some members of the Jehovah's Witnesses resist medical therapy and specifically blood transfusions. Other religious groups will accept medicine but avoid aspects of therapy such as drugs (the Seventh Day Adventists) or advocate dietary restrictions at specific times. Islam, also known as the Moslem Church, advocates fasting during the ninth month of the Mohammedan year (Ramadan).

RELIGIOUS DEVELOPMENT

Infants at birth do not have a sense of right or wrong. They do not have spiritual beliefs, nor do they have convictions that guide their activities. Toddlers may follow certain rituals such as saying their prayers at night, but they are only imitating to conform to the expectations of their parents. They may attend a nursery-type church school, but the emphasis will be on play and enhancing their positive self-image by accomplishing simple tasks and being told what they have accomplished.

The greatest influence on the preschooler is the parents. Their attitudes toward moral codes and religion convey to children what is considered to be good and bad. At this age children are imitators, and tend to copy what they see rather than what they are told. If what they see and what they are told are contradictory, problems arise.

Preschoolers often ask questions about morality and religion. Some of these may be, "Why is it (some action or word) wrong?" and "What is heaven?." Children at this age think that their parents are like God: omnipotent. Preschoolers can have two methods of spiritual education: indoctrination or choosing their own way. Children will follow a religion at this age, not because they understand it but because it is part of their daily life. Three-year-olds like prayers at night and before meals. Five-year-olds will often make up prayers themselves.

Children three to five years old believe that God or actual human beings are responsible for events such as the rain and the wind. Reasoning is that "The rain is God crying; the wind is God blowing air out of His mouth." It is at this age that children are old enough to go to church school and to participate in religious holidays. They ask many questions about the meaning of the holidays and need explanations about them. At this age children are more occupied with the ideas such as Santa Claus coming at Christmas rather than the reason behind a holiday. About this age children may begin to question myths such as the Easter Bunny associated with Easter. When they start questioning such things, they then are ready for a more sophisticated explanation about Easter.

Superego (conscience) development is also related to moral and religious development. Preschoolers identify with their parents and introject their standards and values. At this age children are exceedingly obedient and can be resentful if their parents do not live up to their own superego demands. The superego will continue to develop beyond these years. If the superego remains very strict, the child will grow up to be a self-righteous intolerant adult. If the superego does not develop, the adult subsequently will be unable to follow society's ethical and moral standards and will be unable to form mature relationships. Such a person is referred to as a *sociopath*.

During the school years children learn more about their religion. Six-year-olds expect that their prayers will be answered and that good is rewarded and bad is punished. It is at this age that children hold many thoughts and matters with reverence.

During the prepuberty stage children begin to be aware of disappointments. They realize that their prayers are not always answered. They now begin to reason rather than accept a faith blindly. At this age some children may drop religion entirely, others may continue to follow one because of their dependence upon their parents.

During the adolescent years youths compare the standards of their parents with those of others and determine which ones they want to incorporate into their own behavior. At this age parental standards may be kept. Adolescents also compare the scientific viewpoint with the religious viewpoint and try to bring the two together. By 16 years many adolescents decide whether to accept the family religion. They may experience their own religious awakenings such as being saved or converted. This awakening may be sudden or gradual. Adolescents with parents of dif-ferent faiths may choose one faith over the other or no faith. For some adolescents, a strong faith can serve as a strength during these turbulent years.

Young adults often take on a more mature attitude toward religion. They need to answer the questions of their own children, and they may find that the teachings of their own early childhood are more acceptable now. During the middle years adults may find that they have more time for religious activities such as church groups. Their children are older, and the striving for advancement in employment is replaced with acceptance that the alternatives now open are more limited.

Elderly persons who have developed religious beliefs will endeavor to broaden them and to understand the newer beliefs of younger people. They are comfortable with their own beliefs but appreciate those of others. Elderly persons who do not have mature religious beliefs may experience a feeling of deprivation as other activities such as employment are replaced with retirement. During these years they also face death, not only their own but also that of a spouse, which also makes them despondent. The development of a mature religious philosophy can often help in the acceptance of reality and assist elderly persons to participate in life and have feelings of self-worth. It can also assist them to face death and accept that as inevitable.

ASSESSING SPIRITUAL NEEDS

It is often the nurse who identifies a patient's spiritual needs and provides assistance in obtaining the desired help. Sometimes patients will ask directly for a visit from the hospital chaplain or their own clergyman. Others may want to discuss their concerns with the nurse and will ask about the nurse's beliefs as a way of looking for an understanding listener. Some people are embarrassed to ask for spiritual counsel, but they may question with statements such as, "I've been wondering what really will happen to me when I die" or hint at their concern by asking, "Do you go to a church?" The nurse may also obtain clues about a patient's concerns through observation. Does the patient read a prayer book or the Bible each day? Does he or she wear medals or have any religious medallions or symbols?

In a hospital the admission record will usually have information about the patient's religion, and it will also be recorded in the nursing history. The nurse also can ask if the patient follows a religious philosophy and if the patient would like a visit from the appropriate clergy. It is important to always ask the patient before obtaining assistance.

Some people profess to have no religious beliefs and may be angered if the nurse goes ahead and makes arrangements for a chaplain to visit. It is important that the nurse respect the patient's wishes and not make a judgment of right or wrong, good or bad.

As a guide for the nurse, a list of nine groups of people have been identified as those who may benefit from pastoral care (Westberg 1955:73). This list serves only as a guide for nurses and should not replace individual assessment. Nurses should not intrude on a patient's wishes and beliefs.

1. Patients who appear lonely and have few visitors.

2. Patients who express fear and anxiety.

3. Patients whose illness is related to the emotions or religious attitudes.

4. Patients who face surgery.

5. Patients who must change their lifestyle as a result of illness or injury.

6. Patients who are preoccupied about the relationship of their religion and health.

7. Patients who are unable to have their pastor visit or who would not normally receive pastoral care.

8. Patients whose illness has social implications.

9. Patients who are dying.

The nurse should not restrict the assessment of spiritual needs to the patient. At times of illness, families are often stressed and often want spiritual assistance. Facing death, the patient may have accepted this fate but the family may have not. Often relatives are grateful for spiritual support by a nurse or by a pastor. Assisting them can often indirectly assist the patient, who will see the family supported.

MEETING SPIRITUAL NEEDS

Meeting the spiritual needs of patients and their families is part of the function of nurses as well as that of members of the clergy such as priests, rabbis, and ministers. In many hospitals there are also special facilities for meeting spiritual needs such as quiet rooms and a chapel.

The Nurse's Role

Ministering to the spiritual needs of patients and their families involves assisting them to see meaning in their lives. Through the nurse-patient and nurse-family relationships a nurse can assist people to accept reality and discover practical solutions to problems.

If a nurse feels uncomfortable when asked to assist the patient spiritually this discomfort can be verbalized with an offer to obtain assistance for the patient. Again it is important to respect the patient's belief and maintain a supportive relationship. It is also equally important not to feel guilty because of feelings of discomfort.

A problem that nurses sometimes encounter is the patient who tries to convert the nurse and other health personnel. This can be dealt with by an honest reply telling the patient that you have other beliefs and feel uncomfortable with this request. At the same time you must acknowledge respect for the patient's beliefs to ensure that your relationship with the patient is unchanged.

Providing spiritual assistance involves the following:

- *Support:* being accepting of the person even though his or her beliefs may not agree with the nurse's.

- *Awareness:* being sensitive to what the patient is saying and not saying and to the patient's emotional tone.

- *Empathy:* understanding the patient and the patient's feelings.

- *Nonjudgmental understanding:* accepting and understanding the person without approving or disapproving.

Reaffirming a person's strengths, providing understanding listening, and helping the person develop emotionally are areas of spiritual intervention.

The Clergy

Many large hospitals have full-time chaplains who assist patients, family, and staff with their spiritual needs. The chaplains usually represent several faiths, including a rabbi of the Jewish faith, a priest of the Roman Catholic faith, and in some instances several Protestant ministers, who represent various denominations such as Episcopalian, Methodist, Baptist, and Presbyterian. Smaller hospitals that do not have chaplains will usually have clergy in the community who will provide this service. Many nursing units have an on-call list of clergy to be contacted when they are needed.

The chaplain functions in a variety of ways. Usually a newly admitted patient is visited and spiritual needs assessed. The chaplain then will do any of several things such as read spiritual literature aloud, conduct special sacraments, or simply visit, whatever is appropriate for the person. In some agencies regular religious services are held in the chapel for patients, families, and staff.

Some religious groups such as the Church of Latter-Day Saints and the Christian Scientists do not have ordained clergy. They usually do have people whose role it is to minister to the ill, and they must be recognized by nurses as having appropriate functions. In Christian Science the role of ministering to the sick is carried out by the practitioner (reader).

If the patient does not want a visit from representatives of any religious groups, it is important that the nurse respect this wish and communicate this tactfully to the visitors. In some instances members of religious groups will chant or wail at the patient's bedside. This can be disturbing to others and, if so, requires tactful intervention by the nurse.

Quiet Rooms and the Chapel

Most hospitals have quiet rooms or a chapel, which can be used by patients, families, and staff for meditation, counsel, and even worship services. Sometimes a patient will prefer to meet the chaplain in a quiet room where there is privacy. This is particularly true when a patient is sharing a room with others.

If a hospital holds religious services, these may be nondenominational, or there may be several services for different denominations. If a patient expresses a desire to attend one of these services, the nurse needs to help organize the patient's care so that the patient can attend.

RELIGIOUS BELIEFS RELATED TO HEALTH CARE

Four areas of particular significance relative to the spiritual needs of people are selected medical procedures, birth, death, and special religious observances.

Selected Medical Procedures

Abortion is prohibited by the Roman Catholic Church, the Greek Orthodox Church, and Jehovah's Witnesses. Other churches such as some Mennonite sects also oppose abortion. Some churches place the responsibility for an abortion upon the woman, thus possibly adding to her stress.

The loss of a body part such as an arm or leg also has religious significance for some people. To the Hindus it is a sign of wrongdoing in a previous life. The Orthodox Jewish tradition and some Roman Catholic dioceses require that the limb be buried. Some Orthodox Jews require any body tissue to be buried.

Birth

Infant baptism is practiced by the Eastern Orthodox, Greek Orthodox, Roman Catholics, and some Protestant groups such as Lutheran, Episcopalian, and Presbyterian. Other groups such as the Baptists, Jehovah's Witnesses, and Mennonites do not practice infant baptism.

For infants who are critically ill it is important in the Roman Catholic Church that they are baptized before death. In an emergency this can be done by a nurse, who sprinkles water on the infant's head and pronounces, "(Name of the child), I baptize you in the name of the Father, Son, and Holy Spirit." Once this sacrament has been performed the priest needs to be notified because it is performed only once.

For the Jewish, the rite of circumcision is performed on the eighth day after the birth of a male child. It can only be performed by a Mohel, who may be especially designated by the congregation, or a rabbi.

Death

Two important aspects of death are the last rites, which are required by some religions such as the Roman Catholic Church, and special care of the body such as in the Hindu faith. In the latter instance the priest will pour water into the mouth of the corpse and tie a thread around the wrist or neck to indicate blessing. This thread must not be removed. Before an Islamic patient dies he or she confesses sins and begs forgiveness. Only relatives and family can touch the body after death. They wash and prepare it and turn it toward Mecca. In the Jewish faith the body is washed by the Ritual Burial Society. Burial takes place as quickly as possible.

Some religious groups such as the Unitarian/Universalist group encourage their members to donate parts of their bodies to research and to banks such as the eye bank. Other religions such as Russian Orthodox Church discourage autopsy as well as donation of body parts.

Most religions discourage the prolongation of life in situations when the patient is terminally ill. Some leave the decision up to the family of the patient. The Islamic and Greek Orthodox churches encourage prolonging life.

Special Religious Observances

There are a wide variety of religious observances that are important. It is important for the nurse to learn those of importance to the patient and to assist in their observance. The Roman Catholic Church encourages anointing, which is mandatory before death. Some religions advocate confession, such as Episcopalian, Roman Catholic, and Greek Orthodox churches.

Some groups encourage fasting such as the Baha'i, Episcopalian, and Hindu churches.

Sunday is observed as the Sabbath by most religious groups, and there are no restrictions placed upon medical treatment on that day. Some Orthodox Jews may resist treatment on their Sabbath, which is sundown Friday to sundown Saturday.

Various Religious Groups

There are a large number of religious groups in the United States and Canada. The nurse cannot be expected to be familiar with all of them; however, it is important to be familiar with the major religious groups of the community. In most instances representatives of a religious group are pleased to give the nurse information that is required in the care of patients. Some of the larger religious groups are discussed briefly here.

American Indian

There are several hundred American Indian bands in the United States and Canada, each of which has its own culture. Most have medicine men or shamans, who perform various actions against illness and diseases. Protection from disease is looked for from superhuman powers.

Many Indians today follow the modern Christian religions; however, some still follow the traditional Indian beliefs. Some hold a combination of Christian and traditional beliefs.

Baha'i

People following the Baha'i faith use prayer at a time of illness and advocate fasting if the person's health permits. Their beliefs permit alcohol and drugs only on a physician's order. When a person becomes ill, it is written in the scriptures that the person seek competent medical assistance.

Baptist

At the time of illness some Baptists believe in cure by "laying on the hands." Although some Baptists believe in this faith healing as opposed to medical therapy, most Baptists seek competent medical help.

Some Baptists will not drink coffee or tea, and most Baptists will not take alcohol. The clergy ministers to patients and families at a time of illness.

Black Muslim (The Nation of Islam)

The Black Muslims have a special procedure for washing and shrouding the dead and special funeral rites. The practice of faith healing is not carried out except to raise morale.

Dietary considerations include prohibiting alcoholic beverages and pork. Traditionally Black Muslims eat food to which American blacks are accustomed such as corn bread and collard greens. Cleanliness of person is practiced.

Black Muslim is a separate religion from Islam although the beliefs are similar. Members emphasize black independence and are encouraged to obtain health care provided by the black community.

Church of Christ, Scientist (Christian Science)

Members of this religious group deny the existence of illness. Sickness and sin are errors of the human mind and can be changed by altering thoughts rather than by medicine. They do not, however, permit psychotherapy because the mind is altered by others. A Christian Scientist practitioner can be called to administer to the sick. Tobacco, alcohol, and coffee are also seen as drugs and are not used. Whether a person wishes to rely completely upon Christian Science is up to the individual. The church operates nursing homes in some areas of the country. Here there is complete reliance upon doctrine. Drugs and blood transfusions are not used, and biopsies and physical examinations are not carried out.

Church of Jesus Christ of Latter-Day Saints (Mormon)

Some adherents of this church believe in cure by "laying on the hands"; however, there is no prohibition to medical therapy. In fact, the church operates health facilities. Alcohol, tobacco, tea, and coffee are prohibited, and meat is eaten sparingly.

Some members of the church wear a special undergarment at all times, and patients in the hospital may request the Sacrament of the Lord's Supper by a Church priesthood holder.

Eastern Orthodox Churches

There are a number of denominations, most of which believe in infant baptism by immersion. The last rites are obligatory if death is impending. Dietary restrictions depend upon the particular sect. Their beliefs and practices are compatible with medical science.

Episcopalian (Anglican)

Some members of this church abstain from meat on Fridays, and some fast before receiving Holy Communion. Infant baptism is mandatory, but aborted fetuses are not baptized.

Greek Orthodox

Members of this church consider baptism to be important; it is usually done at least 40 days after birth. The last rites in this church are the administration of the Sacrament of Holy Communion. The church does advocate fasting periods; however, these can be foregone when a person's health is impaired. The usual fasting days are Wednesdays, Fridays, and during Lent.

Hindu

Hindus practice certain rites after death. Some injuries such as the loss of a limb are considered to be sins. The Hindus have many dietary restrictions about which the nurse needs to ask the patient or family. Most members of the Hindu church accept modern medical practices except artificial insemination because sterility reflects divine will to the church member.

Islamic (Muslim/Moslem)

Islam is a major religion of North Africa and the Near East. It emphasizes strict rituals and prayers.

All pork products are prohibited, and in some instances alcoholic beverages are disapproved. There is a fasting period, but people who are ill are exempt from it. The fasting period is the ninth month of the Mohammedan year (Ramadan).

If a fetus is aborted 130 days or more after conception, it is treated as a fully developed human being. Before that time it is looked upon as discarded tissue. The dying person must confess sins and beg forgiveness.

Jehovah's Witnesses

Adherents of the Jehovah's Witness church are opposed to blood transfusions, although some individuals do agree to them in a crisis. When parents refuse to have an infant transfused, a court order may be sought transferring custody to the courts or to an official of the hospital.

Members of the church eat meat that has been drained of blood. Some oppose modern medicine. The church opposes nationalistic ceremonies.

Judaism

There are several Jewish groups. The Orthodox group is the most strict; the Conservative and Reform groups are less strict. Jewish law demands that Jews seek competent medical care.

The Orthodox and Conservative Jews observe strict kosher dietary law, which prohibits pork, shellfish, and the eating of milk products and meat products in the same meal. Reform Jews usually do not observe kosher dietary regulations.

The ritual of circumcision is practiced by Orthodox and Conservative Jews on the eighth day after birth; the rabbi and male synagogue members are present. Therefore special arrangements generally need to be made for the ceremony including the physician's approval.

For Orthodox and Conservative Jews the Sabbath is observed from sundown Friday to sundown Saturday, and they may resist hospital admission or medical procedures during that period unless the procedures are necessary.

Lutheran

Baptism takes place 6 or 8 weeks after birth. A member who wishes may be anointed and blessed before death. They have no dietary restrictions.

Mennonite

Members of the Mennonite church are baptized in their middle teens. They advocate no special dietary restrictions, although some congregations require abstinence from alcohol.

Pentecostal (Assembly of God, Foursquare Church)

There is no doctrine against modern medical science, including blood transfusions. Abstinence from alcohol and tobacco and eating strangled animals is advocated. Some members will not eat pork.

Members may pray for divine healing, and in some congregations anointing with oil is practiced.

Orthodox Presbyterian

Orthodox Presbyterians have no dietary requirements or restrictions. The last rites are not a sacrament, but they read the scripture. Competent medical care is advocated.

Roman Catholic

Infant baptism is mandatory and urgent if the infant's health is critical. In death the Rite for the Anointing of the Sick is also mandatory. This is done for patients who are seriously ill in order to provide comfort. When in the hospital a patient is exempt from fasting or abstaining from meat on Ash Wednesday and Good Friday.

Holy Communion is administered by a priest. A patient may eat before the sacrament. Privacy is necessary during the Communion because the patient may wish to confess. If a patient is strictly not permitted food and fluids, Communion cannot be performed because it involves eating a bread wafer and drinking wine.

Seventh-Day Adventist (Church of God, Advent Christian Church)

This church is opposed to infant baptism but conducts baptism of adults by immersion. In dietary matters they prohibit alcohol, tobacco, narcotics, and stimulants, and some advocate ovolacto-vegetarian diets. Some sects practice divine healing, anointing with oil, and prayer. Saturday is considered to be the Sabbath by some. The members of this church believe in the second coming of Jesus Christ and believe it is their duty to warn others and to prepare for this.

Unitarian/Universalist

The members of this church emphasize reason and knowledge. They believe that each person is responsible for himself or herself and that values are individually established. There are no dietary restrictions or official sacraments.

SUMMARY

The spiritual needs of patients and their families often come into focus at a time of illness. It is during this time that a patient has time to think of spirituality when life is perhaps threatened. There are also patients who profess to have no religious beliefs. Just as nurses must respect the right of people to believe in certain religions, it is important also to respect the patient who has no religious beliefs.

Part of the nurse's function is to assist patients and families to meet their spiritual needs. The nurse may do this directly with the person through being supportive, empathetic, and having nonjudgmental understanding. All of this requires a particular awareness of the patient's needs. Scripture readings and prayers are also helpful to patients and can be carried out by the nurse. It is important that the nurse feels comfortable when doing this. If the nurse feels uncomfortable, it is appropriate, if the patient is agreeable, to ask another nurse or a clergyman.

There are many religions in the United States and Canada. It is important for the nurse to be aware of the various religious groups in the community and to have some knowledge of their beliefs and practices. Most patients or families when questioned will tell a nurse about any special religious practices they wish to observe such as a special diet. These practices related to religious belief largely center in three areas: birth, death, and some medical procedures such as abortion. There are many special religious observances associated with various religions. Nurses need to be aware of these and to assist the patient by arranging nursing care so that the practices can be carried out.

SUGGESTED ACTIVITIES

1. Each student in a group of ten or twelve chooses a specific religion to study. Visit the local church of the religion you have chosen, and obtain information regarding their beliefs and practices pertinent to health and illness. Share this with the group.

2. Visit a local hospital and find out what special arrangements are made in order to meet patients' spiritual needs, such as a chapel, services, and diet.

SUGGESTED READINGS

Piepgras, R. December, 1968. The other dimension: spiritual help. *American Journal of Nursing* 68:2610–2613.

This article suggests that little emphasis is placed upon spiritual needs of patients, yet for some patients this is the help that they need the most. Five manifestations of the need for spiritual help are outlined. Patient examples are included.

Morris, Karen L., and Foerster, John D. December, 1972. Team work: nurse and chaplain. *American Journal of Nursing* 72:2197–2199.

The authors describe a program in which nurses and clergymen worked together and the benefits to the patients and the personnel.

SELECTED REFERENCES

Berkowitz, Philip, and Berkowitz, Nancy S. November, 1967. The Jewish patient in hospital. *American Journal of Nursing* 67:2335–2337.

Dickinson, Sr. Corita. October, 1975. The search for spiritual meaning. *American Journal of Nursing* 75:1789–1793.

Murray, R., and Zentner, J. 1975. *Nursing assessment and health promotion through the life span.* Englewood Cliffs, N.J.: Prentice-Hall, Inc.

Naiman, H. L. November, 1970. Nursing in Jewish law. *American Journal of Nursing* 70:2378–2379.

Pederson, W. D. May, 1968. The broadening role of the hospital chaplain. *Hospitals* 42(9):58.

Pumphrey, John B. December, 1977. Recognizing your patient's spiritual needs. *Nursing 77* 7(12):64–69.

Westberg, G. E. 1955. *Nurse, pastor and patient.* Rock Island, Ill.: Augustana Press.

CHAPTER 33

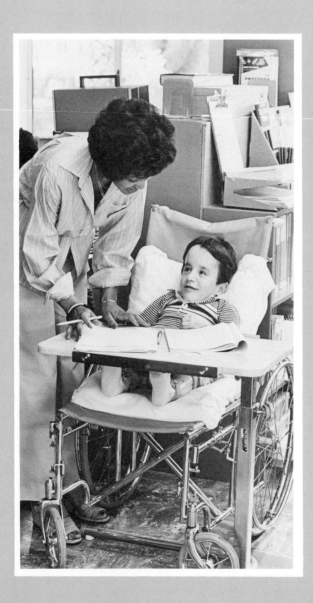

SELF-CONCEPT AND SELF-ESTEEM

NURSING INTERVENTION IN PROBLEMS OF SELF-CONCEPT AND SELF-ESTEEM

Guilt

Anxiety

Loss of Control over Events

Low Self-esteem

Role Conflict

Dependency Problems

OBJECTIVES

- Discuss the development of self-concept.
- Describe the factors that influence self-concept.
- Discuss the development of self-esteem.
- Explain the problems related to self-concept and self-esteem.
- Assess problems of self-concept and self-esteem.
- Plan and implement nursing action in regard to problems of self-concept and self-esteem.

Self-esteem and self-acceptance are used as synonymous terms in this chapter. *Self-esteem* is considered to be an aspect of the self-concept component related to the value or worth the person places on oneself. Self-esteem is experienced as a feeling; it is a part of every feeling experienced by a person, and it is experienced constantly.

Self-concept is a combination of the feelings and beliefs one holds in regard to oneself. Man has a need for psychic integrity, which is met by the person knowing who he or she is and feeling that this self is an adequate self (Roy et al. 1976:174). There are two basic components of the self-concept: the physical self and the personal self. Discussion of the physical self is covered in Chapter 35. The personal self can be further broken down into the moral-ethical self, self-consistency or integrity, and self-ideal/self-expectancy. The moral-ethical self sets the standards and evaluates the person's behavior. Freud referred to this aspect of the personality as the superego. *Self-integrity* is the consistent self-image that the person has a need to maintain, such as the thin person who becomes obese but continues to think of him or herself as thin. When any stressor threatens the integrity of the self-image, the person becomes anxious. Self-ideal/self-expectancy refers to what the person expects to be and to do. This image guides a person's behavior and assists one to set goals (Roy et al. 1976:175–176).

THE DEVELOPMENT OF SELF-CONCEPT

In psychosocial development there are three major tasks for the person: learning to live with tools, personal self-development, and learning to live with others (Roy et al. 1976:183). Living with tools includes acquiring skills appropriate for each stage of development. The tools can be the toys of a 2-year-old, the athletic skill of the adolescent, or the social skill of the executive in business. Personal self-development involves learning to live with oneself. It includes learning to live with impulses and drives and developing acceptable behaviors to deal with them. It also includes an awareness of one's own strengths, feelings, and resources. Learning to live with others includes relating to people in a variety of roles and learning to accept and respect others.

Throughout life there are developmental stages. Erikson proposed eight stages in life that describe stresses on the maturational process (see Table 10-2). The success with which one copes with these stressors largely determines the development of one's self-concept. Inability to cope with these stressors results in self-concept problems at the time and often later in life.

Trust versus Mistrust

During the first year of life the infant is entirely dependent upon others to meet needs. The infant requires nourishment, dryness, warmth, and safety that is positive and consistent. From these experiences of having needs met, the infant develops a sense of trust in the external environment. This trust is a feeling of confidence in the sameness, continuity, and predictability of the environment (Roy et al. 1976:185). From trust in the external environment the infant learns to trust him or herself. When the infant is uncomfortable and cries, someone will come and assist the child. The infant's cries can make something happen that will be satisfying.

For infants who do not develop trust in the environment and themselves, mistrust can affect the remainder of their lives. This mistrust can extend to others in future years. They will be unable to trust or rely on themselves. They will be unable to rely upon others or upon themselves to become what others trust they will become. The development of trust is basic to the development of the personality, in particular, to a person's self-concept.

Behavior Indicating Trust

1. Requesting assistance and expecting to receive it.
2. Saying you believe another person.
3. Sharing time, opinions, and experiences.

Behavior Indicating Mistrust

1. Restricting conversation to superficialities.
2. Refusing to provide a person with information.
3. Being unable to accept assistance.

Autonomy versus Shame and Doubt

An infant who has developed a sense of trust is then ready to develop autonomy or a sense of *I*. At this age the child will use words such as "no" or "I" a great deal. It is important that children have an area of living where they have control such as putting toys away. When a child says "no," this needs to be respected by others. The child requires some environmental limits so that self-confidence can be maintained. It is important that the children come to appreciate their impulses as good and not be shamed into appropriate behavior.

Behavior Indicating Autonomy

1. Accepting the rules of a group but also expressing disagreement when it is felt.
2. Expressing one's own opinion.
3. Accepting deferment of a wish fulfillment easily.

Behavior Indicating Shame and Doubt

1. Failing to express needs.
2. Not expressing one's own opinion when opposed.
3. Being overly concerned about being clean.

Initiative versus Guilt

With initiative the person can develop plans and ideas and put them into action. During the ages of 3 to 5 years most children undertake this developmental task. It is also an age of fantasy and imagination. The child questions what he or she can do and be. It is important that a child can explore the world and often through play live out various roles. Failure to achieve a sense of initiative can result in feelings of guilt. Some guilt feelings are normal, and they must be balanced with a sense of initiative. Also at this stage children start to develop a conscience. They attempt to sort out actions, which are labeled "good" or "bad." Discipline that uses shame creates feelings of guilt and decreases feelings of self-worth.

Behavior Indicating Initiative

1. Starting projects eagerly.
2. Expressing curiosity about many things.
3. Demonstrating original thought.

Behavior Indicating Guilt

1. Imitating others rather than developing independent ideas.
2. Apologizing and being very embarrassed over a small mistake.
3. Verbalizing fear about starting a new project.

Industry versus Inferiority

After the development of initiative the child has positive feelings in regard to "I." At this age the child is ready for school and the new experiences and routines associated with it. About the age of 5 years children begin to verbalize feelings about themselves and have an adult-like image with both positive and negative judgments. They are heavily influenced by the judgments of significant others.

During this maturational stress period the focus is upon learning to obtain recognition by producing things. The child learns to manipulate tools such as pencils and to concentrate upon a task. Completing the task is an objective that the child develops. At this time a child also learns to be active with others and to share.

Inadequacy can develop if children give up in the effort to handle tools and themselves in relation to given tasks. It is important that children receive guidance as to how to succeed and obtain recognition for their successes.

Behavior Indicating Industry

1. Completing a task once it has been started.
2. Working well with others.
3. Using time effectively.

Behavior Indicating Inferiority

1. Not completing tasks started.
2. Not assisting with the work of others.
3. Not organizing work.

Identity versus Role Confusion

During puberty and adolescence a person seeks answers to "Who and what am I?." The person will need to redefine trust, autonomy, initiative, and industry in terms of a new definition of self. Also included will be the sexual changes of adolescence and society's expectations of an adult. During adolescence the person is reassessing all his or her adaptive mechanisms. Because childhood responses are no longer appropriate, the adolescent must change relationships of the past, particularly that with parents. The new adult identity will assist the adolescent to cope with adult experiences and make adult decisions.

The person who is unable to form an adult identity will have role diffusion. Without a strong sense of self the person will feel confused and anxious and will find it difficult to respond to the demands of living in a realistic and stable way.

Behavior Indicating Identity

1. Establishing relationships with the same sex and then the opposite sex.
2. Asserting independence.
3. Planning realistically for future roles.

Behavior Indicating Role Confusion

1. Failing to assume responsibility for directing one's own behavior.
2. Accepting the values of others without question.
3. Failure to set goals in life.

Intimacy versus Isolation

Achieving intimacy involves achieving a close relationship with one special person. It includes committing oneself to another person. It also involves abandonment of self in close relationships. Failure to achieve intimacy can lead the person to a sense of isolation and self-absorption. When a person is self-absorbed, it is difficult to perceive feedback from others and subsequently to more fully develop a sense of self.

Behavior Indicating Intimacy

1. Establishing a close intense relationship with another person.
2. Accepting sexual behavior as desirable.
3. Commitment to that relationship even in times of stress and sacrifice.

Behavior Indicating Isolation

1. Remaining alone.
2. Avoiding the establishment of close personal relationships with the opposite sex.
3. Avoiding the sex role by mannerisms and dress.

Generativity versus Stagnation

Generativity is concern with establishing and guiding the next generation. It includes both productivity and creativity. Generativity is not restricted to producing children; it can also include producing something to be passed on to another generation such as writing, health, or ideas. When a person cannot pass along something, then stagnation results. The person becomes self-absorbed and chiefly concerned with self rather than others.

Behavior Indicating Generativity

1. Willingness to share with another person.
2. Guiding others.
3. Establishing a priority of needs recognizing both self and others.

Behavior Indicating Stagnation

1. Talking about oneself instead of listening to others.
2. Showing concern for oneself in spite of the needs of others.
3. Inability to accept interdependence.

Integrity versus Despair

This last stage in development is largely dependent upon the other previous stages. For the person who has some sense of trust, autonomy, initiative, industry, identity, intimacy, and generativity, feeling satisfied with one's life and decisions is the next developmental stressor. *Ego integrity* means feeling satisfied with one's lifestyle and accepting the inevitability of one's life cycle.

The person who does not acquire integrity feels despair and feels that the time left in life is too short to start another life.

Behavior Indicating Integrity

1. Using past experience to assist others.
2. Maintaining productivity in some areas.
3. Accepting limitations.

Behavior Indicating Despair

1. Crying and being apathetic.
2. Not accepting changes.
3. Demanding unnecessary assistance and attention.

FACTORS INFLUENCING SELF-CONCEPT

A number of factors influence the development of a self-concept in a person. Roy lists nine factors (Roy et al. 1976:189–190) in two groups. Contextual factors refer to environmental or milieu factors. Residual influencing factors are those held over from past experiences. These factors are discussed in this chapter.

Environmental Factors

1. Objects in the environment that can assist persons, such as the availability of a spoon for a child learning to feed him or herself.

2. Environmental feedback, which assists persons to learn who they are. These include feedback from significant people such as parents and all experiences in the environment such as the availability of team sports.

3. The present definition of the self-concept as a means of responding to stressors.

4. Learned coping mechanisms such as problem solving and ways of handling feelings.

5. The competence of self in areas which persons and other people value.

Past Experience Factors

1. Previous feedback from others, particularly people one considers significant.

2. Previous developmental and situational stressors and how the person coped with these.

3. The person's self-expectations and experiences with success and failure.

4. Particular experiences that create a sense of value and worth and those which do not generate this sense.

THE DEVELOPMENT OF SELF-ESTEEM

Self-esteem (self-acceptance, self-worth) is the value or worth one holds of oneself. *Esteem* is worth; people need to value who they are and what they are. The need for self-esteem was discussed briefly in Chapter 7, "Esteem Needs." Maslow's hierarchy of needs as adapted by Kalish presents esteem and self-esteem as fifth-level needs just below self-actualization. See Figure 7-3.

The way in which persons feel about themselves affects the way in which they deal with their environment. Persons with high self-esteem will deal more actively with their environment and feel secure. Persons of low self-esteem will see the environment as negative and threatening (Roy et al. 1976:233).

Self-esteem is closely related to self-concept. It is developed to a considerable degree as a result of feedback from others. In Chapter 35, feelings of loss as a result of changes in the physical self-concept will be discussed. Self-esteem is also closely related to the moral-ethical self, self-consistency and self-ideal, and expectancy. If a person's behavior is consistent with what one believes is moral and ethical, then the person sees him or herself as "good" and valued. On the

other hand, if one sees one's behavior as immoral or "bad," then the person's self-esteem is negatively affected. There is also a need to be consistent within a changing self-concept. When this consistency is threatened, anxiety results. *Self-expectancy* is the power that persons perceive they have to meet self-expectations. Those who are unable to meet self-expectations feel worthless, and their self-esteem is negatively affected.

One type of expectation that is important to self-esteem is learning to handle one's feelings of anger and aggression. People learn from others how to handle these feelings. A little girl who loses a favorite doll may react to her disappointment by angrily acting out behavior. Adults will try to assist the child to control her behavior by indicating that showing anger is bad. The child is reprimanded not only for the behavior but for the feeling. As this is reinforced repeatedly, the child learns that to feel and express feelings is "bad." Because situations repeatedly arise when one has these feelings, one feels guilty because one has learned that feelings are "bad." The adult then has the problem of dealing with loss by not showing feelings of anger and sadness. Consequently these feelings are turned inward, and the person feels less self-worth.

A second area in which children learn self-esteem is through the limitations placed on their behavior while growing up. Children who grow up within well-defined and enforced limits learn about reality because their behavior results in consequences. They learn to make decisions about their behavior and how to obtain positive and negative reinforcement. The child who does not have limits set does not have the opportunity to obtain positive reinforcement, hence does not have an opportunity to attain high self-esteem. As an adult, this person will probably have low self-esteem and have more difficulty setting limits on personal behavior and that of others.

Positive self-esteem is referred to as high self-esteem, the converse of which is low self-esteem or feelings of worthlessness.

ASSESSMENT OF PROBLEMS RELATED TO SELF-CONCEPT AND SELF-ESTEEM

Nurses need to be able to recognize problems basic to self-concept and self-esteem. These can be grouped into problems related to loss, guilt, anxiety, loss of control over events, low self-esteem, role conflict, and dependency. For assessment of loss as a problem, see Chapter 35.

Guilt

Guilt is the painful feeling associated with transgression of a person's moral-ethical beliefs. The development of the superego (Freud's term) takes place after the age of 3 years. Persons usually internalize the norms of the culture in which they live and control impulses contrary to these norms.

Some of the common manifestations of guilt are as follows:

Physical

- Stooped posture and slow movement.
- Decreased gastric functioning.
- Stammering.
- Blushing.
- Insomnia.

Personal self

- Statements of guilt such as "I am to blame."
- Apologizing.
- Depression.
- Self punishment such as encouraging reprimand by peers.
- Hypersensitivity.
- Crying.

Anxiety

Anxiety is a mental uneasiness due to an impending or anticipated threat. When a person's self-consistency is threatened, anxiety occurs. The manifestations of anxiety are highly individualistic and broad. Some of the common manifestations are as follows:

Physiologic

- Insomnia or somnolence. Somnolence is sleeping most of the day and evening as well as at night. The person cannot seem to get enough sleep.
- Polyuria.
- Diarrhea.
- Pallor, tachycardia, palpitations.
- Hyperventilation.
- Polyphagia (overeating), obesity.
- Nausea and vomiting.
- Cold, clammy skin.

Personal self

- Anger and denial. Denial is refusing to recognize reality, such as saying, "I do not want to talk about it."
- False cheerfulness, such as laughing while discussing a serious subject.
- Intellectualizing about a subject such as explaining the pathophysiology of leukemia rather than describing how one feels.
- Depression or the expression of sadness.
- Dependent behaviors such as demanding attention, crying, and behaving angrily.

Loss of Control over Events

The concept of being powerless involves the belief that one does not have control over events. Persons who believe they are powerless may manifest the following:

- Less alertness than normal to the environment.
- Lack of resistance to attempts to change the person.
- Less knowledge in regard to the area in which one feels powerless.
- Restlessness and sleeplessness.
- Depression and apathy.
- Anxiousness.

Low Self-Esteem

There are degrees of feeling low self-esteem, and individual people vary in their behavior. Some of the most common manifestations are as follows (Roy et al. 1976:236–7):

- Anorexia or overeating.
- Constipation or diarrhea.
- Difficulty sleeping or oversleeping.
- Withdrawal from activities and difficulty initiating new activities.
- Expression of feeling unloved, isolated, and unable to confront difficulties.
- Tendency to be a listener rather than a participant.
- Expression of self-depreciation or self-dislike.
- Sensitivity to criticism; self-conscious.
- Seeing self as a burden to others.
- Decreased motivation, interest, and concentration.

Role Conflict

Role conflict (intrarole conflict) occurs when a person experiences incompatible expectations from one or more persons in his or her environment in regard to expected behavior. Role conflict (interrole conflict) occurs when a person occupies two or more roles that require expected behaviors incompatible with each other (Roy et al. 1976:253). Roles change with growth and with the environment. The very young and the very old in North American society generally have less role function than people in the 30- to 65-year age group. During childhood there is a steady increase in the number of roles assumed by a person such as a sister, school member, club member, and team member. During the adult years there is usually the assumption of additional social responsibility. The primary role is that of a mature adult; however, there are secondary and tertiary roles assumed as a young adult. A *secondary role* is one that influences behavior in a variety of settings and is occupied according to the tasks that a person must accomplish to achieve autonomy at a particular time of life. A *tertiary role* is a temporary role of choice that a person assumes to accomplish some minor task associated with the current developmental stage (Roy et al. 1976:245–246).

For patients, role mastering is important. In it the patient demonstrates both expressive and instrumental behaviors appropriate to the patient's stage of illness. Instrumental behaviors include acknowledging that one is ill and seeking competent assistance. Expressive behaviors include expressing feelings about the illness and asking that special favors be performed because of the illness. For further information on the sick role see Chapter 3, "Stages of Illness" and "The Sick Role."

Nurses can observe a number of problems in relation to role. Problems with role distance occur when patients assume the patient role only at the last minute, when they have no choice. They also give up the patient role as soon as possible. These patients find that the patient role is incompatible with their self-concept, and they are uncomfortable in the role. Role conflict for patients occurs when they receive conflicting messages about behavior, such as being told by the nurse to move and exercise and being told by their families to rest.

Role failure occurs when there is an absence of instrumental and expressive behavior appropriate to the role. An example of this would be the patient who refuses to take the physician's advice on medications.

The following behaviors can be indicative of role problems:

Role distance

- Gets out of bed without assistance and against physician's advice.
- Tolerates pain without asking for help.
- Asks personal questions of nursing personnel.

Role conflict

- Is confused because of conflicting advice.
- Refuses to admit one is ill because of employment commitments.

Role failure

- Fails to take nursing and medical advice.
- Tells nurses how to carry out techniques.
- Advises other patients as to what to do.

Dependency Problems

Dependency problems include interdependence, dependence, and independence. *Interdependence* is a balance in relationships between dependence and independence. *Dependence* can be described as enjoying other people as satisfying and rewarding. *Independence* is manifested by self-reliance and self-assertiveness (Roy et al. 1976:291).

To be interdependent a person must be both independent and dependent. In North America interdependency is approved, and dependency is usually sanctioned during infancy, childhood, old age, and physical and mental illness. Traditionally the female role was considered to be a dependent role; however, the women's movement of the 1970s have done a great deal to change this.

Dependency and independency are manifested by the following:

Dependence

- Asks for physical assistance.
- Requests advice from another and follows the advice.
- Seeks attention by speaking loudly, overcommunicating, and asking irrelevant questions.
- Seeks affection by touching another with the hands or whispering.
- Seeks approval and praise by asking how a nurse likes a sweater or by providing gifts as a way of gaining recognition.

Independence

- Takes the initiative in beginning a task.
- Exhibits persistence and repeated effort in spite of obstacles trying to eat repeatedly in spite of position, fatigue, and difficulty reaching the food.
- Shows stubbornness by refusing to take medications until the physician tells the patient personally that these are necessary.
- Exhibits firmness by refusing to allow relatives to make a decision about changing one's place of living even though one is ill.

NURSING INTERVENTION IN PROBLEMS OF SELF-CONCEPT AND SELF-ESTEEM

Guilt

Behaviors that can be associated with guilt were described in the previous section. After the nurse has established that the behaviors of the patient are indeed manifestations of guilt, the patient may need assistance from the nurse to verbally express feelings. The patient may be able to explore the situations producing guilt with the nurse. This may be an uncomfortable experience for the patient, and emotional support and reassurance by the nurse are important. During the discussion the patient may see that some of his or her reasoning is irrational. The patient may be able to accept that personal expectations are unrea-

sonable. If unable to accept this, the patient may need psychiatric counselling to gain a more realistic idea of self-expectations and in some instances to change maladaptive behavior.

Anxiety

One way in which anxiety can be reduced or perhaps eliminated is by the establishment of goals that are attainable. Often patients need the assistance of a nurse to do this.

First, patients must recognize that they are anxious. This is best done in an atmosphere of warmth and trust. Sometimes patients who are anxious react negatively toward nurses as a manifestation of their personal frustration. It is important that a nurse understand this and react to the behavior in an unanxious manner.

After patients have agreed that they are anxious, it is important to discuss all the possible reasons for their anxiety. If patients can identify the cause of their anxiety, they will find it helpful to explore the cause, with the objective of learning better coping mechanisms. They may see that they have overestimated the threat or that they can reduce the source of the threat by specific action (for example, asking a teacher whether one is failing).

Loss of Control over Events

The feeling of loss of control over events is not an uncommon one for patients in a hospital setting. Nurses can assist patients with this problem in a number of ways. Including patients in the planning of their care allows them to feel that they can influence events. Encouraging patients to schedule their visiting hours, to choose their meals, and to assist in setting the goals for their care is helpful.

By personalizing nursing care, patients can feel important and that they do have control. Calling patients by name, being interested in them, and demonstrating concern about matters that patients are concerned with assist them to maintain a feeling of control over themselves and the events that affect them.

Low Self-Esteem

Patients who have low self-esteem need to explore those factors which they interpret as negative. They may need assistance seeing the positive aspects. Nurses can assist patients to explore their expectations, how these can be met, and how reasonable they are. Patients may also need assistance in understanding how past experiences are influencing the present. They may have developed a maladaptive pattern of behavior and need to learn how to change this. With the assistance of the nurse, patients can often learn to see life experiences in a more positive manner. Patients can be helped to feel hope; "Hope is opposed to despair" (Vaillot 1970:271). Patients can be assisted to identify their feelings at a particular moment and how they want to feel. The nurse can assist patients to

correctly perceive themselves and to choose activities that will help them to live up to their values.

Role Conflict

Nursing intervention with regard to role conflict is designed to assist patients cope with the role they have acquired, that is, the patient role. Often it is helpful if patients are related to in such a manner that is as compatible with the patient role as they perceive it. This may include patients' assisting with activities that they can master if this is important, thus making the patient role as nonthreatening as possible and supporting the common elements of any roles which are in conflict. Sometimes when patients manifest maladaptive behavior such as refusing to take medications, other stimuli can be introduced to change the situation. Patients may need to know that failure to take their medications can upset the healing process. The nurse can help patients to explore their fears, perhaps give them new information, and help them to understand the role of the nurse as a provider of care.

Dependency Problems

Elimination of problems of dependence–independence usually involves learning new ways of behaving. Patients can be encouraged to verbalize their feelings about a situation; identify the perceived and actual conflict; and be reeducated through teaching, translation, interpretation, and extrapolation of perceptual data (Roy et al. 1976:318–319). Basic nursing intervention in this situation is creative listening and responding as a means of establishing new behaviors.

Behavior modification is another method of changing behavior. *Behavior modification* is eliciting and rewarding externally desired behavioral responses to reduce, modify, or extinguish ineffective adaptive coping responses (Roy et al. 1976:320). One method is to provide the patient with a cue to a behavioral response. When a desired response is given, the patient is rewarded. For example, if a patient who does not want to eat is provided with a meal tray accompanied by a supportive statement from the nurse and then eats the meal the patient should be rewarded in a manner that the patient values. Such a reward might be a statement by the nurse that eating will help the patient to become stronger and to return home sooner.

SUMMARY

Self-esteem, an aspect of self-concept, is a feeling related to the value that persons place upon themselves. Self-concept is a combination of feelings (self-esteem) and beliefs that persons hold in regard to themselves. Both the physical and personal self comprise self-concept.

The development of a self-concept is an important aspect of psychosocial development. Erikson's eight stages of development describe the stresses of the maturational process. The success with which one copes with these stressors largely determines the development of one's self-concept. These eight stages are reviewed in this chapter together with a description of behavior that indicates successful or unsuccessful coping. The stages are as follows:

1. Trust versus mistrust
2. Autonomy versus shame and doubt
3. Initiative versus guilt
4. Industry versus inferiority
5. Identity versus role confusion
6. Intimacy versus isolation
7. Generativity versus stagnation
8. Integrity versus despair

A number of factors influence the development of the self-concept. These are divided into two groups: influencing factors and experience factors. The first group includes objects in the environment, feedback, the person's present definition of self-concept, learned coping mechanisms, and the competence of self in areas that the person and others value. Experience factors include previous feedback, previous stressors, the person's self-expectations, and experiences that create a sense of value.

The development of self-esteem is important in affecting how a person deals with the environment. An individual with high self-esteem will deal more actively with the environment and feel secure. A person of low self-esteem will see the environment as threatening. Self-esteem is largely developed as a result of feedback from others. Learning to handle one's feelings is important in the development of self-esteem. Children also learn from the limitations placed upon their behavior.

There are a number of behaviors related to problems in self-concept and self-esteem. These are guilt, anxiety, loss of control over events, low self-esteem, role conflict, and dependency problems.

Nursing intervention to assist patients with these problems often involves helping the patient to verbalize feelings, clarify data, identify the causes, and learn behavior to cope with the identified stressors.

SUGGESTED ACTIVITIES

1. Observe people in each age group described by Erikson. Identify behaviors that relate to developmental tasks.

2. Interview an elderly person in a long-term care agency. Assess how this person perceives and values him or herself.

3. Interview a mother of a newborn infant. Assess how she sees her role. Draw up a nursing care plan to assist her in adapting to her role.

SUGGESTED READINGS

Crary, William C., and Crary, Gerald D. March, 1973. Depression. *American Journal of Nursing* 73:472–475.

The physical, psychologic, and emotional changes that take place in depression are described. The descriptions can assist nurses to recognize depression in patients.

Rubin, Reva. Summer, 1967. Attainment of the maternal role. Part I. Processes. *Nursing Research* 16:237–245.

The article describes a study in which the processes of taking-in and the operating of the maternal role are described.

SELECTED REFERENCES

Anxiety—recognition and intervention. September, 1965. *American Journal of Nursing* 65:129–152.

Bee, H. 1975. *The developing child.* New York: Harper & Row, Publishers, Inc.

Erikson, Erik H. 1963. *Childhood and society.* 2nd ed. New York: W. W. Norton & Co., Inc.

Johnson, D. E. April, 1967. Powerlessness: a significant determinant in patient behavior? *Journal of Nursing Education* 6:39–44.

Lange, S. Shame. In Carlson, Carolyn E. 1970. *Behavioral concepts and nursing intervention.* Philadelphia: J. B. Lippincott Co.

Robinson, Lisa. 1968. *Psychological aspects of the care of hospitalized patients.* Philadelphia: F. A. Davis Co.

Robinson, Lisa. 1977. *Psychiatric nursing as a human experience.* 2nd ed. Philadelphia: W. B. Saunders Co.

Roy, Sr. C. et al. 1976. *Introduction to nursing: an adaptation model.* New Jersey: Prentice-Hall Inc.

Tiedt, Eileen. 1972. The adolescent in the hospital: an identity-resolution approach. *Nursing Forum* 11(2):121–140.

Ujhely, G. B. December, 1967. When adult patients cry. *Nursing Clinics of North America* 2:726.

Vaillot, Sr. Madeleine C. February, 1970. Living and dying. *American Journal of Nursing* 70:268, 270–273.

CHAPTER 34

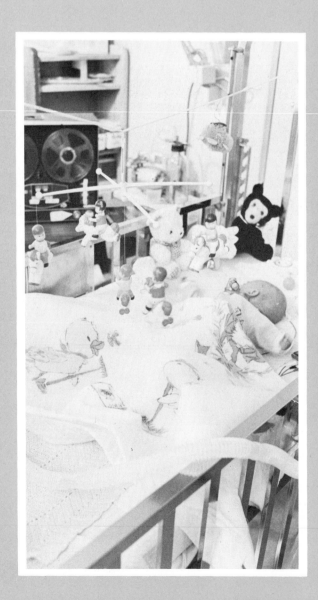

STIMULATION

ASSESSING SENSORY DISTURBANCES

Assessing Sensory Deprivation

Assessing Sensory Overload

Assessing Sensory Deficits

Changes in States of Awareness and Consciousness

NURSING INTERVENTION

During Growth and Development

During Illness

Evaluating Nursing Intervention

OBJECTIVES

- Discuss sensory stimulation as a basic need of people.
- Describe the role of stimulation in normal development.
- Explain normal sensory perception.
- Name and describe the types of sensation.
- Explain the kinds of sensory disturbances.
- Identify people who are prone to sensory disturbances.
- Assess symptoms indicative of sensory deprivation, sensory overload, sensory deficits, and changes in states of awareness.
- Plan and implement nursing intervention in regard to sensory deprivation, sensory overload, and sensory deficits.
- Evaluate the effectiveness of the nursing intervention.

The sensory-perception process is basic to learning about oneself and the world. Sensory stimulation is a basic need, which Kalish described in terms of second-level needs for novelty, manipulation, exploration, activity, and sex (see "Human Needs," Chapter 7).

It has long been recognized that, for children to develop normally, they require sensory stimulation. In recent years, sensory stimulation has received attention in relation to the needs of all people. The general public is becoming increasingly aware of stimuli such as noise levels and the visual surroundings of daily life. Problems in the perception of sensation can result in disturbances to a person's thinking and behavior. When one loses a function such as sight, one will develop other senses to a greater degree than normal in an effort to compensate for the loss. An-

other form of sensory deprivation is that encountered by the chronically ill and the elderly who are restricted in mobility and in their social interactions. Helping to meet these needs for sensory stimulation is part of the nurse's function.

The amount of sensory stimulus required for optimal functioning is a highly individual matter. An adult who lives alone may find that several visitors in a hospital provide more stimuli than tolerable; the mother of six children may find that the empty house provides sensory deprivation.

A person's state of awareness is important in one's ability to perceive the environment. States of awareness vary greatly in health and illness. The ability of an individual to respond to the environment is largely affected by the state of awareness.

STATES OF AWARENESS

Awareness is being able to perceive one's environment and one's own bodily reactions and to take this information and assimilate it into thought and action. The normal alert person can assimilate many kinds of information at one time such as by going to a restaurant with friends and appreciating the odors, tastes, conversation, and company at the same time. The normal person is able to perceive reality with considerable accuracy and to respond appropriately to it. One is able to separate necessary and extraneous stimuli and reach a logical conclusion by correlating in-

formation. Most people are able to do this with little or no awareness of the mental process involved. Occasionally normal persons do have abnormalities of thought; they become absent minded, lose their sense of direction, or even forget matters normally not forgotten. Often these episodes are due to intense concentration upon a subject to the extent that other stimuli are effectively blocked out, such as the student who is studying for a final examination and forgets to phone home as he had planned.

THE DEVELOPMENT OF SENSATION

Newborns have no perception of themselves and their environment. Initially through touch and later through hearing and vision they learn about their world. At the age of 2 months infants will play with objects and people. They will play with their toes, thereby differentiating themselves from their environment. By 3 months of age both eyes are coordinated and will follow objects. By 4 months they will recognize familiar objects. Their own body image will start to develop when they see themselves in a mirror.

The internal sensations they perceive also serve to differentiate themselves from others. They per-

ceive the sensation of hunger and eventually realize that food comes from an external source. Children use their senses to conceptualize and to discriminate. Through taste, sight, and touch children learn about oranges and how they differ from apples. Through imitation of sound they learn to speak.

The early responses of infants are chiefly reflexive. Later, sensations are perceived and interpreted, and sensations gain meaning. As children grow, they learn that certain sensations provide cues for behavior already learned, such as stopping and looking both ways before crossing a street. Adults have many learned responses to sensory cues. If one of these senses such as the sense of hearing is altered, it is likely to change the person's life considerably. A person uses his or her senses even without awareness, and they are integral to the ability to react to internal and external environments.

NORMAL SENSORY PERCEPTION

The process of sensory perception starts with an adequate stimulus, which triggers a specific sensory receptor and then travels by nerve pathways to the brain. Here the sensation is assembled and integrated. The mechanism in the brain that carries out these processes is thought to involve the thalamus, hypothalamus, and reticular activating system (RAS). The stimulus is then relayed to the cerebral cortex, where it is interpreted. It is at this stage that conscious awareness first takes place. It is also in the cerebral cortex that information is stored.

It is necessary to have constant and varied sensory stimuli for the process of sensory perception to take place. If the stimuli are insufficient or if there are too many of the same stimuli, the process of adaptation will take place, and the brain will no longer perceive the stimuli. Extreme concentration on any object or person will also produce the same effect. This is illustrated by some counterculture groups, who withdraw from the normal stimuli of society and follow a leader in all aspects of their lives.

The need for sensory stimulation has been referred to as *sensoristasis*. The human being appears to have a need for a certain level of sensory stimulation to function effectively.

Types of Sensation

Sensory stimuli are either external or internal in origin. External stimuli arise from outside of the person. They are *visual* (sight), *auditory* (hearing), *olfactory* (smell), *tactile* (touch), and *gustatory* (taste). The latter can be internal in origin as well. Internal stimuli are kinesthetic or visceral. *Kinesthetic* refers to the sense of awareness of the position and movement of body parts. *Visceral* refers to any large organ in the body's interior.

Sensations can be stimulated both internally and externally. This is important for nurses to realize in that a sound perceived by a patient may have an external stimulus, or it may be a result of a pathologic condition of the auditory nerve.

SENSORY DISTURBANCES

Kinds of Sensory Disturbances

There are a number of sensory disturbances. They can be developmental, thus affecting the infant or child, or they may occur for other reasons such as an illness or social isolation.

Sensory Deprivation (Restriction)

Sensory deprivation results when the sensory input is lower than the person requires to function. Persons who were experimentally isolated from stimulation changed the content of their thought; they became irritable but alternated these periods with times in which they were easily amused (Heron 1971:-355–356). Other symptoms reported in a study were

physical discomfort, space and time disorientation, sensory distortion, difficulty concentrating, and even hallucinations (Downs 1974:434–438).

Because of the increasing awareness about sensory deprivation, health agencies are providing visual stimulation in terms of colorful, attractive surroundings. Some agencies also provide background music or radios and television for the patients, thus also providing auditory stimulation.

There are three main reasons for sensory deprivation. It can result from lack of stimulation from the environment such as occurs when an elderly person is isolated in a room. It can also occur as a result of impairment of the senses such as deafness, and because of impairment of the brain centers that process sensory stimuli. The latter can be seen in an elderly patient who has had brain damage from a series of cerebrovascular accidents (strokes).

Sensory Overload

Sensory overload occurs when one receives more sensory stimulation in a given period than one can tolerate. A patient in a hospital may encounter sensory overload as a result of such stimuli as bright lights, noise, strange machinery, visits from health personnel, and visitors. A continuous barrage of these stimuli will result in the person showing many of the same behaviors associated with sensory deprivation. The person may appear fatigued or agitated or may experience psychologic disturbances such as hallucinations and confusion.

Sensory Deficit

A *sensory deficit* is an impairment in the functioning of the sensory or perceptual processes such as blindness or deafness. When only one sense is affected, other senses tend to develop to compensate for the loss. However, sudden loss of eyesight can result in total disorientation.

Some neurologic diseases result in changes in kinesthetic sense and tactile perceptions. With some inflammatory conditions the usual ability to inhibit background stimuli is weakened. As a result these persons can appear agitated and disturbed by bright lights, cold air, or normal voice levels.

Persons Prone to Sensory Disturbances

Nurses need to be aware of those patients who are particularly susceptible to sensory disturbances. By anticipating possible problems, nursing measures can often be implemented to prevent these problems from occurring. The following circumstances may predispose to sensory disturbances.

Persons Whose Activities Are Normally Carried Out in Isolation or in Nonstimulating Environments.

People who normally live alone and have little contact with other people may experience sensory overload upon entering a health agency as patients. This is particularly true of the elderly and of people who are employed independently with little social interaction such as writers. In their homes these persons require sensory stimulation.

Another group of people who are susceptible are those who live in institutions where the social and perceptual stimuli are unchanging.

Persons Who Are Therapeutically Isolated

In the hospital and home settings there are instances in which persons are isolated either for their own protection or for the protection of others. Patients for whom medical aseptic practices are instituted are usually socially isolated from others. When there is some contact, it is often only with health personnel, who will be gowned and masked.

Other patients are restricted when they are confined to a bed, particularly in a single room. They are unable to move about to find companionship and often must occupy themselves with minimal social interaction.

Persons Whose Environments Are Medically Intensive

Patients who are being treated in environments where staff are constantly present are often overloaded with stimuli. These patients, such as those in intensive care and coronary care units, are never left alone, and often there is machinery operating and a variety of medical personnel looking after them.

Persons Who Have Sensory Deficits

Patients who have various sensory perceptual deficits may encounter sensory deprivation or even sensory overload. Persons with visual problems may be unable to read, watch television, or even recognize nurses by sight. A strange environment can add to their confusion. These people probably have arranged structured environments, including furniture in specific places, and the new environment will require new learning, which can be taxing to ill persons. Because of impaired eyesight they will probably not move around readily or socialize with others in their new surroundings.

Deaf persons who have not learned to lip read are isolated from others because of their inability to communicate. Most people who have been deaf for some time are adept at lip reading. However, a person with whom the deaf person is communicating needs to face him or her while speaking.

Persons with Special Personality and Developmental Characteristics

There is a wide variety in the degree to which different people can tolerate some sensory deprivation.

People whose developmental levels are characterized by short attention spans, need for physical activity, and dependence upon others for amusement may have more difficulty than people who are more self-reliant and contemplative (Mitchell 1973:212). Persons who are stressed and anxious are also more prone to difficulty coping with sensory deprivation. The third factor that can affect a person's reaction to sensory deprivation is the use of drugs such as narcotics that decrease awareness of the environment.

ASSESSING SENSORY DISTURBANCES

To assess the sensory deprivation or overload of a person it is important to know the level of sensory input the person is accustomed to and tolerates best. This level is highly individual as was mentioned earlier in the chapter. The child who has five brothers and sisters may be accustomed to a different level of sensory input than the only child. Sensory deficit is related to the functioning of the various senses and the perception of these senses.

Assessing Sensory Deprivation

A person who is experiencing sensory deprivation may manifest boredom, inactivity, slowness of thought, daydreaming, increased sleeping, thought disorganization, anxiety, panic, or hallucinations (Cameron et al. 1972:33).

The person who is bored may be active or inactive. Activity will probably be with unimportant matters. The bored person may ask assistance from others for matters he or she could well take care of. An inactive person will probably appear apathetic and perhaps withdrawn. This person may also appear irritable and exhibit childish emotional responses (Heron 1971:358).

Slowness of thought is demonstrated by difficulty grasping ideas and slowness in communicating. One may demonstrate obvious difficulty in thinking about what one wants to say. Reaction time will be reduced, and physically the person will appear clumsy.

Persons who are *daydreaming* will appear absorbed in their own thoughts. They may even talk and laugh while daydreaming and may be difficult to arouse. These persons may even confuse a daydream with reality and imagine a conversation that really did not take place.

Increased sleeping is another manifestation of sensory deprivation. Lack of external stimulation may lead to difficulty staying awake and thus sleeping abnormally frequently or for long periods as a means of passing time.

Thought disorganization can be evidenced when one has difficulty remembering what one was saying. The person may start a sentence on one subject and end it with an unrelated subject. Thought disorganization may also be reflected in confusion about the time of day or the day of the week. The person may make inappropriate verbal responses such as laughing about a serious subject. The person may also experience sensory distortions such as seeing a physician when it is really a relative or smelling smoke that is really a steak cooking.

Anxiety and *panic* are similar. *Panic* is severe anxiety. See "Signs of Increased Stress," Chapter 8, for further information.

Hallucinations can also be a result of sensory deprivation. The person may hear voices that do not actually exist or see sights that are nonexistent. Illusions may also be present. An *illusion* is the false interpretation of some stimulus, such as a shadow that the patient believes is a man with a knife.

Assessing Sensory Overload

Sensory overload may be manifested by the same symptoms as sensory deprivation. In addition, the patient may appear agitated and restless. If by increasing the patient's social contacts the symptoms increase, this is an indication that he or she has sensory overload.

Assessing Sensory Deficits

Sensory deficits are generally assessed as part of the initial health assessment. In addition to that, nurses need to be observant and note behaviors that may reflect impairment of any of the senses. Particular observations of the various senses are outlined.

Auditory (sense of hearing)

1. Is the person able to locate the direction of sounds?

2. Can the person distinguish and differentiate voices?

3. Does the person have any unusual sensations such as humming, ringing, or buzzing?

4. Does the person speak more loudly than most people or shout?

Visual (sense of sight)

1. Is the person able to see objects or persons nearby and at a distance?

2. When reading, does the person hold the reading material closely or far away?

3. Does the person have any unusual distortions in vision?

4. Does the person have a full field of vision? Does the person only see objects directly in front of him or her?

5. Does the person experience any unusual sensations such as spots, colored areas, or halos around objects?

Gustatory (sense of taste)

1. Does the person experience unusual taste sensations such as bitterness or metallic tastes?

2. Is the person able to differentiate between sweet, sour, salt, and bitter tastes?

Olfactory (sense of smell)

1. Can the person distinguish between different odors of different foods?

2. Does the person experience unusual sensations for which there is no stimulus, such as smelling smoke when none is present?

Tactile (sense of touch)

1. Does the person discriminate between dull and sharp?

2. Does the person perceive heat, cold, and pain?

3. Does the person perceive unusual sensations such as so-called pins and needles?

Kinesthetic (awareness of position and movement)

1. Is the person aware of the position of his or her body parts?

Visceral (refers to large internal organs)

1. Does the person perceive any unusual sensations from the inner body such as pain or pressure?

Changes in States of Awareness and Consciousness

In illness a patient's awareness of the environment can also be affected. The elderly person whose environment is changed to a hospital suddenly can become confused by thinking he or she is at home. A mildly confused person is unable to perceive all significant stimuli in the environment. A woman may put away her shoes and forget where she put them, or a man might get dressed wearing two sweaters. The mildly confused person can wander away and become lost.

A severely confused (disoriented) person may not know family members or may think the nurse is a relative. Such a person may act in an untypical manner, such as the quiet old lady who became combative with nursing personnel in the hospital. This person is confused as to the time of the day, the day of the week, and the place.

The state of the consciousness of the person also affects awareness. (See Table 34-1 for stages of consciousness).

Table 34-1. Stages of Consciousness

Stage	Behavior
Full consciousness	Alert, aware of time, place, and person
Lethargy	Aware of stimuli, but senses are dulled and responses are slow
Somnolence	Barely awake, hardly aware of environmental stimuli; speech is muffled and slurred
Stupor	Occasionally aware of environmental stimuli; forceful stimuli needed to bring awareness
Semiconsciousness	Has occasional states of awareness; fluctuates in periods of awareness
Coma	Unconscious, variable response to stimuli such as pain; may be incontinent of feces and urine

NURSING INTERVENTION

The nursing intervention in regard to sensory disturbances has two aspects: the prevention of sensory disturbances and the management of existing sensory disturbances. Prevention involves education in regard to sensory needs and implementation of measures, particularly for people who are prone to sensory disturbances.

During Growth and Development

Children require sensory stimulation during their development. Mothering provides sensory stimulation in terms of tactile, auditory, and visual stimulation. It is important that nurses teach parents the importance of these stimuli. When infants and children are in a hospital, this need must continue to be met largely by nurses.

Sensory stimulation can be encouraged by the following:

1. Holding infants and talking and playing with them when they are not sleeping rather than leaving them in a crib alone.

2. Providing a number of bright objects of different designs to attract infants and toys for children that they can hold.

3. Changing the environment of infants by taking them for walks or arranging for them to be in a variety of areas such as the kitchen and the patio.

4. Providing music and auditory stimuli at suitable intervals.

5. Providing a variety of foods with different tastes, textures, and colors.

Constant sensory stimulation without adequate sleep and rest periods can result in sensory overload. A child needs to rest in a quiet room, free of odors and with reduced lighting.

During Illness

When an infant or child is admitted to a hospital or confined to bed at home, it is important that sensory development continue. Therefore the measures described in the previous section need also to be employed in a hospital setting.

For children and adults it is important to carefully assess individual needs. Included in this assessment is the person's need for structure and the degree of tolerance of monotony. A number of devices can offer assistance to the patient. Television and radio have some value. Toys of different textures, sizes, and colors assist children. Volunteers in some agencies will play with children. In some hospitals there are playrooms where a play therapist assists children to meet their play and stimulation needs. In hospitals for adults, particularly in long-term hospitals, there are often libraries and occupational and recreational facilities that provide stimulation for patients who otherwise might have no activities.

Nursing intervention in acute sensory deprivation indicates need for more interaction with nursing staff and health personnel as well as other stimuli such as television. For the patient who is hallucinating, intervention is twofold: recognizing the emotional aspect, such as saying, "I recognize that you are afraid," and explaining the experience in terms of the environmental stimuli, such as, "That shadow was made by the clothes hamper."

Touch is exceedingly important in sensory deprivation. Touch is the first sensation experienced by the infant, and it continues to be important throughout people's lives. Touch is a method by which people orient themselves to their environments. It also represents reassurance and caring on the part of the nurse. Some people touch others spontaneously with frequency, whereas other people seldom do this. The nurse needs to observe whether touching a hand or arm is offensive to the patient. Most frequently patients respond positively to this gesture of warmth.

Taste is another source of sensory stimulation. For patients who are unable to choose their own menu, nurses can help by choosing foods that offer a variety in color, texture, taste, and temperature. The sense of smell also offers stimulation. A light cologne, a bath powder, or an after-shave lotion can assist a patient in this regard.

For the patient whose senses are overloaded, less stimulation in the environment is required. This may be accomplished by restricting visitors on the length of time they stay. Reducing the number of lights in the room and reducing noise are also ways of reducing sensory stimuli. An additional method often employed in hospitals is establishing routines for each day, thus reducing novelty and surprise. Soft background music has also been known to reduce stimuli.

A nurse can also organize care so that the patient has long periods with low-level input. One way of doing this is to carry out several nursing measures together, thereby allowing a quiet period before the next activity.

Nursing intervention in regard to sensory deficits is primarily limited to reporting to the patient's physician observations about hearing or vision. Often the family may not have noticed that Grandfather no longer reads the newspaper, indicating that he needs new glasses. Other sensory deficits are likely to have implications in regard to medical diagnosis and therapy. These must also be communicated to the physician.

Evaluating Nursing Intervention

The effectiveness of nursing intervention can be evaluated in terms of the patient's symptoms. If the symptoms disappear or are diminished, then intervention is effective. If the symptoms continue to be present or are increased, then the intervention is ineffective and needs to be changed.

SUMMARY

Awareness of one's environment and bodily reactions is largely dependent upon one's state of awareness. Individuals develop the ability to perceive their environments and themselves. At 2 months of age, infants play with their toes. During the preschool years, children learn to take precautions against environmental dangers such as stopping at a street before crossing.

The need for sensory stimulation is sensoristasis. For sensory perception to take place, it is necessary to have constant and varied sensory stimuli. There are a number of kinds of stimuli: visual, auditory, olfactory, tactile, gustatory, kinesthetic, and visceral. The major types of sensory disturbances are sensory deprivation, sensory overload, and sensory deficit. Sensory deprivation occurs when the amount of sensory stimuli is less than a person requires. Sensory overload occurs when one receives more sensory stimulation than one can tolerate. Sensory deficit is an impairment in the functioning of the sensory or perceptual processes.

Nurses encounter a number of persons who are prone to sensory disturbances, such as the patient who is therapeutically isolated or the person with a sensory deficit. Assessing sensory disturbance is a function of nurses. Being aware of changes in behavior can assist the nurse. Behavior such as boredom, daydreaming, and increasing sleep may be indicative of sensory deprivation. Sensory overload can be manifested by some of the same symptoms. In addition, the patient may appear agitated and restless. Sensory deficit can be assessed in a systematic manner. Asking questions such as is the person able to locate the direction of sound can assist in assessing the auditory sense.

Nursing intervention involves the prevention of sensory disturbances and the management of existing sensory disturbances. During implementation, the nurse should also consider the individual's developmental status as well as individual needs.

SUGGESTED ACTIVITIES

1. In a laboratory setting, plan to provide a meal for a classmate who is blindfolded. Provide food on a tray. Interview the classmate as to how he or she felt. What other stimuli assumed importance?

2. Visit a health agency that cares for patients with long-term illness. Interview a patient and assess for symptoms of sensory disturbances. What types of activities are arranged to provide stimulation?

SUGGESTED READINGS

Bolin, Rose H. 1974. Sensory deprivation: an overview. *Nursing Forum* 13(3):240–258.

The author provides a theoretical framework by which concepts of sensory deprivation are discussed. Also included are an overview of clinical records of deprivation and the nursing implications.

Krieger, Dolores. May, 1975. Therapeutic touch: the imprimatur of nursing. *American Journal of Nursing* 75:784–787.

The article describes "laying on the hands." The importance of touch and a study in which nurses functioned as "healers" are described.

Perron, Denise M. June, 1974. Deprived of sound. *American Journal of Nursing* 74:1057–1059.

This article describes the problems of a deaf person who is admitted to a hospital. The importance of including these problems in the nursing care plan is pointed out.

SELECTED REFERENCES

Amacher, Nancy J. May, 1973. Touch is a way of caring and a way of communicating with an aphasic patient. *American Journal of Nursing* 73:852–854.

Burnside, Irene M. December, 1973. Touching is talking. *American Journal of Nursing* 73:2060–2063. Reproduced in *Contemporary Nursing Series, Nursing and the Aging Patient.* New York: The American Journal of Nursing Company.

Cameron, C. F. et al. November, 1972. When sensory deprivation occurs. *The Canadian Nurse* 68:32–34.

Chodil, J., et al. 1970. The concept of sensory deprivation. *Nursing Clinics of North America* 5(3):544–548.

Downs, Florence S. March, 1974. Bed rest and sensory disturbances. *American Journal of Nursing* 74:434–438.

Heron, W. January, 1957. The pathology of boredom. In *Readings from Scientific American. Physiological Psychology.* 1971. San Francisco: W. H. Freeman & Co.

McCorkle, Ruth. March–April, 1974. Effects of touch on seriously ill patients. *Nursing Research* 23:125–132.

Mitchell, Pamela H. 1973. *Concepts basic to nursing.* New York: McGraw-Hill Book Co.

Smith, M. J. March–April, 1975. Changes in judgment of duration with different patterns of auditory information for individuals confined to bed. *Nursing Research* 24:93–98.

Thomson, L. R. February, 1973. Sensory deprivation: a personal experience. *American Journal of Nursing* 73:266–268.

CHAPTER 35

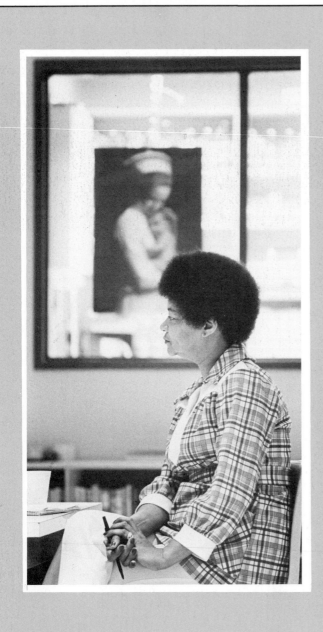

ACCEPTING LOSS AND DYING

OBJECTIVES

- Describe the types of loss.
- Explain the different reactions to loss.
- List and describe the stages of grieving and stages of dying.
- Discuss the kinds of grief.
- Assess needs of people related to loss.
- Identify the problems related to body image.
- Assess impending death.
- Discuss the special needs related to infants, children, and adolescents who are dying.
- Describe the components of nursing care for dying patients.

For all people, death is inevitable. It is a loss: the loss of life. All people have some concern about death, and this is often expressed in terms of concern over health. Another type of loss is that of body image. *Body image* (self-concept) is a view of one's body that includes physical appearance, kinesthetic feedback, sensory feedback, and emotion. The person who has *body image integrity* has an accurate perception of his or her body; the image changes as the body changes, and the person feels comfortable with the image.

Illness can threaten loss of both life and body image. The nurse's function in both of these areas is to identify the needs of the patient and the family and to provide support to them. Death is a lonely experience, which everyone ultimately faces alone. But even at death, as with any loss, people can grow both in perception of themselves and others and in acceptance of the reality of the situation.

TYPES OF LOSS

There are a number of types of loss. Three of these are as follows:

1. The loss of an aspect of oneself, a body part, a physiologic function, or a psychologic attribute.
2. The loss of objects external to oneself.
3. The loss of a loved or valued person.

The loss of an aspect of self changes a person's body image even though the loss may not be obvious to others. If a person has a scarred face as a result of a burn, this is generally obvious to all people who see it. Other losses may not be as obvious, such as the loss of part of one's stomach or the loss of the ability to feel emotion. The degree to which these losses will affect the person will largely depend upon the integrity of the body image (self-concept.) Sometimes changes in self-image affect a person in terms of social roles, such as employment or functions as a father or husband. Any change that is perceived by the person as a negative change in terms of the way he or she relates to the environment can be considered to be a loss of self.

Another aspect of loss of self is that which occurs as a result of growth and development. Failure of the person to develop a normal self-concept can occur for many reasons. The infant learns to distinguish self from the environment. To do this the infant requires tactile and auditory stimuli. Parents provide this sense of touch by holding, feeding, and bathing the infant. The auditory stimulation is provided through talking and other environmental sounds.

The toddler needs to learn about body parts through feeling them and requires an accepting attitude rather than a judgmental one. The child should not be told, "That is bad." Schoolchildren need contact and feedback from peers that they are normal. Failure of the toddler and schoolchild to receive this type of reassurance can result in the formation of a self-image that is negative or uncertain. Old age is another time when there are dramatic changes in physical and mental capabilities. Again the self-image is vulnerable, and support and reassurance are important.

Loss of objects external to oneself includes the loss of inanimate objects that have importance to the person, such as the loss of money for a businessman or the burning down of a family's house. The loss of objects that have symbolic meanings such as success or security can have a dramatic effect. Some people will become depressed and never recover, but others work through the loss and grow.

The loss of a loved one or a valued person through separation or death can also be disturbing. Even in illness some people are changed, such as through brain damage from a viral infection. Such a person may undergo personality changes that in effect result in a loss of that former person to friends and family.

Separation from an environment that provides security can also result in a sense of loss. The 6-year-old who up until the present has had the protection of home is likely to feel this loss when faced with first attending school and relating to more people. The university student who leaves home for the first time to study will also experience some sense of loss.

Loss through death is a permanent and complete loss. In primitive societies, death was considered to be a normal, natural event. Life was seldom prolonged. Grief was greatest for young men who died rather than for women, children, or elderly people.

In contemporary society, death usually does not occur in front of people unless there is an accident. It often happens in a hospital or in a home in front of immediate family members. Death in North American society is felt to be unacceptable. There is a tendency to prolong and preserve life. The culture reveres the young and youthful look. Although people expect to live to old age, this is not considered to be as attractive as youth.

Death is considered to be natural today only when it happens in old age. Any death that occurs before that is seen as unnatural. This is in contrast to the outlook of our ancestors, who expected some children to die of communicable disease and who themselves seldom expected to live to be old.

REACTIONS TO LOSS

There are a number of reactions to loss. *Grief* is emotional suffering often caused by bereavement. To *bereave* is to deprive, as in death. Grief is a psychologic process that permits a person to cope gradually after an overwhelming loss. The characteristics of grief are as follows:

1. There is a reaction of shock and disbelief.
2. The bereaved person has feelings of sadness and emptiness when the lost person is recalled.
3. The discomfort is often accompanied by weeping, tightness in the chest, choking, shortness of breath, and sighing.
4. The bereaved person has a preoccupation with the image of the deceased.
5. Feelings of guilt may be experienced early in the grief with thoughts such as "Maybe there is something I could have done."
6. The bereaved person tends to be irritable and angry (Burgess et al. 1976:421–422).

STAGES OF GRIEVING AND DYING

Engel has identified three stages of grieving:

1. Shock and disbelief.
2. Developing awareness.
3. Restitution and recovery (Engel 1964:94–96). See Table 35-1.

Kübler-Ross describes five stages of dying: denial, anger, bargaining, depression, and acceptance (Kübler-Ross 1969:34–121). These stages are similar to Engel's. They are separate emotional states, but they overlap. In the normal process the first stage is denial and the last is acceptance but the others vary considerably.

Reaction to any loss can be described in terms of these stages.

Denial

During this first stage of nonacceptance the person thinks, "This is not happening to me" or "There must be some mistake." At this time a person is not ready to deal with any related problems such as acquiring a prosthesis (an artificial body part) after the loss of a leg.

Some people act with artificial cheerfulness and prolong this stage. This is not always healthy in that the person is denying reality and not coping with it. In some instances where this continues and inhibits the person's progress, psychiatric counseling may be indicated.

Table 35-1.   Engel's Stages of Grieving*

Stage	Behavioral Responses
Shock and disbelief	Verbal and nonverbal denial
Developing awareness	Verbal acknowledgment of reality; Dreams and nightmares; Sense of guilt; Crying or loud lamenting; Anger
Restitution and recovery	Acceptance on the part of the dying person; Some physical discomfort such as shortness of breath, exhaustion, loss of appetite, or insomnia; Later in this stage: Return to prior level of functions; Establishment of new relationships; Enjoyment of pleasure without guilt; Remembrance of the loss realistically and comfortably

*From Engel, G.L., September, 1964. Grief and Grieving. *American Journal of Nursing* 64:93–98.

Anger

This second stage of anger is expressed in many ways. The patient may be angry at the hospital staff in regard to care or with friends for some reason. In reality the patient's anger is not directed specifically at these people but is general. The person is angry that "this has happened to me." It is during this period that a patient's family may also express anger in regard to matters that normally would not bother them. For both patient and family this is a normal reaction and indicates they are responding normally to the loss. It is important that this be recognized as normal and that the nurse be supportive and accepting.

Bargaining

This third stage is learned in childhood. Children learn at an early age that if they are good, they will be rewarded. They also learn bargaining such as, "If you eat your vegetables, you can have your dessert." Patients will often say "I will do anything to change this." Nurses need to listen attentively and convey supportive understanding at this time.

Depression

During the stage of depression the person grieves over what has happened and what cannot be. The man who loses an arm may be depressed about changing employment or his ability to play games with his children. A woman whose son has died will be depressed in regard to his death and the years of living he has lost. During this stage some people talk freely, but others withdraw and reject other people. Nurses can assist people by their presence and by listening when the person wants to talk. Sometimes sitting quietly not expecting conversation is helpful to the person. Consideration, touch, and other nonverbal communication are often helpful.

Acceptance

This is the last stage in the response to loss. Acceptance gradually develops as the person comes to terms with the changed body image or changed circumstances in life. At this time it is helpful for the person to talk about all his or her reactions and to make any plans that are indicated. For the dying person this may necessitate a will; for the woman who has lost a breast it can mean a fitting for her and discussion with her husband as to his feelings. Again support from the nurse is important, since this acceptance takes considerable time and should not be hurried.

KINDS OF GRIEF

Anticipatory Grief

Anticipatory grief is experienced in advance of the event. The wife who grieves before her husband dies is anticipating the loss. Because death often occurs over a long period, this grief is frequently seen. In terms of other losses, a beauty queen may grieve in advance of an operation that will leave a scar on her body.

Unresolved Chronic Grief

In chronic grief the person acts as if the event had never taken place. It is a denial of grieving. The person refuses to acknowledge the loss of a loved one and continues to act as if the deceased were alive. The painful effects of the loss are replaced by inappropriate good spirits and pleasure. Even though the death might be acknowledged intellectually, the person speaks and acts as if the loss did not affect him or her personally and he or she is unable to express sadness. For example, a man who carries on his life by taking a vacation as if nothing had happened after he had ac-

cidentally caused his brother's death when driving an automobile while drunk is probably denying the accident and any grief. The person who is experiencing chronic grief may need professional counseling if it continues for a prolonged period. From a nurse the person requires supportive listening and encouragement to verbalize feelings.

Absent or Inhibited Grief

In many situations absent or inhibited grief occurs, and this can be perfectly normal. The person may not have placed great value on the loss as others had anticipated. The elderly man may not grieve about his wife's death because he believes that she is finally free of pain. A woman who has lost the sight of one eye may have developed sufficiently strong coping mechanisms that she does not grieve the lost eye.

Sometimes grief is delayed until the person takes the time to realize the loss. After the death of a loved one, all the details of a funeral, visits from relatives, and legal matters may serve to delay the grieving process. Once all these matters have been attended to and people return to their normal activities, a widow realizes the implications of her loss.

Grief may also appear to be absent to others. The man who has lost a leg may feel that his family needs his support and that he cannot express his grief to them. In this situation he may find it easier to talk to an uninvolved person such as a clergyman or a nurse.

ASSESSING NEEDS RELATED TO LOSS

There are a number of factors to be assessed in regard to loss.

Developmental Status

The developmental status of the person is important in assessing needs. The adolescent needs peer approval, and thus any loss that interferes with this may present problems. The young adult who wants to have children may find that the loss of reproductive ability is a tragic loss. At each age there are developmental tasks that people may consider important. It is important to remember that one's developmental stage may not coincide with one's age; a 50-year-old man could be at an adolescent's developmental stage in terms of relations with the opposite sex. His appearance and ability to impress women is highly important to him, and any loss associated with this ability could present him with a problem.

Life-Style

Life-style includes such factors as employment, education, economic situation, and various social and cultural values. All of these to some degree will affect how a person accepts and deals with any loss. To a man who does physical labor for a living the loss of a leg may seriously affect his ability to support his family, whereas to a writer the same loss may be less traumatic.

Cultural and Social Values

The cultural and social values of the person also can affect how any loss is perceived. In a work-oriented culture such as that of many North Americans, the inability to work is viewed seriously. To the Italian woman the inability to have children may be a serious problem.

Coping Mechanisms

People develop coping mechanisms that they use at times of stress. These mechanisms are highly variable and of varying effectiveness. One person may cry and scream in the face of loss, whereas another will deal with the loss in a thoughtful manner. People who have developed effective mechanisms will use these in facing loss. Others whose coping mechanisms are minimal will require greater assistance in learning to deal with the problem.

Support Systems

A *support system* is those activities and people who can assist a person at a time of stress. At a time of death a person who belongs to a large, close family will see them as the support system. The person must be able to receive the support; this implies an emotional tie with the people providing support. The other extreme is the person who has no relatives and no close friends, which is not an uncommon situation for the elderly. This person may require more support from nurses because of a lack of other supportive people.

Part of a support system is certain activities such as religious rituals, reading books, or listening to music. To some people these activities provide a great deal of support at a time of loss.

INTERVENING IN PROBLEMS OF BODY IMAGE

Nurses can intervene in a number of ways to assist patients who have problems of loss related to body image. The following is a listing of some of these problems.

1. Supporting the strengths of patients and helping them look at these, such as supporting a man's ability to be an understanding father in spite of a physical handicap.

2. Assisting patients to look at themselves in totality rather than focusing upon limitations; this can be done by conveying interest in the patient rather than only the patient's activity, for example.

3. Providing perceptual feedback such as assisting a patient to touch a scar, then to describe the scar, and last to look at the scar. It is often very important to a patient to obtain this feedback in a positive way from family members. To do this effectively, family members can be assisted by some preparation from the nurse before they see the patient. Knowledge of the appearance of a scar before seeing it will assist family members to react positively rather than in shocked distaste.

4. Providing kinesthetic feedback to patients with a paralyzed limb by telling them "I am straightening your arm; now I am bending your arm."

5. Describing changes in functioning in realistic terms at a level appropriate to the patient. By encouraging discussion, misconceptions held by patients and their families are often revealed and can be corrected such as the misconception of the man who had a prostatectomy and believed he was now sterile.

6. Encouraging patients and their families to express their feelings and to understand them. Often understanding that these feelings are normal is reassuring to people.

IMPENDING DEATH

Awareness

People who are dying possess varying degrees of awareness. The amount of awareness of a patient and his or family is a factor in determining the nurse's role. Three types of awareness are closed awareness, mutual pretense, and open awareness (Strauss et al. 1970:300).

Closed Awareness

In closed awareness the patient and family are unaware of impending death. They may not completely understand why the patient is ill, but they believe he or she will recover. Physicians in these instances believe it is best not to communicate a diagnosis or prognosis. Nursing personnel are ethically bound to follow the physician's lead and not tell the patient or family. This results in a necessity of providing evasive or incorrect responses to questions. Ultimately the patient and family will know the truth and at that time may find the previous information given them to be out of context with reality.

Mutual Pretense

During mutual pretense the patient, family, and health personnel know that the prognosis is terminal. They do not talk about this and make an effort not to raise the subject. Sometimes the patient refrains from discussing death to protect the family from distress. The patient may also sense discomfort on the part of the nursing and health personnel and there-

fore not bring up the subject. Mutual pretense permits the patient a degree of privacy and dignity, but it does place a heavy burden on the dying person in terms of having no one to whom he can confide fears.

Open Awareness

In this setting, people around the patient know about impending death as does the patient. The patient and family feel comfortable about discussing the impending death even though it is difficult. This type of awareness often provides the patient with an opportunity to finalize affairs and even participate in planning funeral arrangements. Not all people can handle open awareness; a 45-year-old man struggled against dying to the end, which resulted in a difficult death for him and his family.

Assessment

Certain signs are indicative of impending death:

1. Reflexes gradually disappear.
2. Respirations become dyspneic and accelerated.
3. The facial expression appears pinched with some cyanosis.
4. The skin feels cold and clammy.
5. The pupils become dilated and fixed.
6. The pulse accelerates and becomes weaker.
7. The blood pressure falls.
8. The body temperature is elevated.

Special Needs of Infants, Children, and Adolescents Who Are Dying

Infants

A dying infant requires comforting and care just as do both the parents. The grief of parents about their infant's death goes beyond comprehension. Often parents internalize their feelings of helplessness and act out these feelings in their social life and marriage (Kavanaugh 1976:44).

Parents can become obsessed with many questions about genes, family heritage, and parental inadequacy. The nurse will hear questions such as, "Did I really want the baby?" or "Did he die because I smoked during pregnancy?" Both parents require encouragement in verbalizing these feelings and in finding their own answers. Often parents give vent to their anger at nurses and the care the infant is receiving. It is important to openly accept this anger and then assist the parents to see beyond this.

Children

Nursing the dying child should include the parents and siblings. Parents are generally exceedingly emotionally involved in the death of a child, more so than in the death of an elderly person who has lived a long life.

It is important to listen carefully to a child's questions and to answer them truthfully. To a question such as, "Will I be home for Christmas?" nurses can truthfully answer, "I really don't know, but I hope so." Children may ask questions about death, and often simple answers suffice such as, "It means not living anymore."

Parents of a dying child may have guilt feelings, and they may need to talk out their feelings to help each other and the child (Northrup 1974:1068). Parents often fear that as death nears the child will suffer more. Honest reassurance that the child will not suffer unduly is important.

Part of a young child's fear of death is aloneness, being away from Mother. Parents should be encouraged to spend as much time as possible with their terminally ill child. This calms the child's fears and helps the family work through the tragedy (Williams 1976:35).

Adolescents

Dying adolescents need to deal not only with the reality of dying but with developmental tasks of their age. Because hospitalization imposes many restrictions upon normal activity, it is important that adolescents receive supportive understanding for their behavior. Like children, adolescents require honest answers to their questions, support in their thinking, and encouragement in the process of accepting the reality of death.

Nursing Intervention for the Dying Patient

Emotional Intervention

The emotional needs of the dying patient are primarily those of reassurance. Some of these needs are as follows (Gray 1976:28–29):

1. Relief from loneliness, fear, and depression. The person requires someone who will spend time with him or her and listen, someone whom the patient feels cares.

2. Maintenance of security, self-confidence, and dignity. The patient should not be neglected or abandoned. Patients fear psychologic abandonment, which can occur such as when patients want to talk about dying and their families will not permit this. Sometimes with long terminal illnesses family members find it difficult to sustain the physical and emotional energy required to maintain contact with the dying person.

3. Maintenance of hope even in the last stages of dying. Hope makes the acceptance of death easier for patients and families. Even where death is highly probable, hope is important and not unrealistic. No one really knows what the future holds, and miraculous recoveries have been known.

4. The dying person may have spiritual needs, and these often arise during the night (Gray 1976:18). Frequently, nurses need to assist patients to meet these needs, particularly when clergy cannot be contacted.

Physiologic Problems

The physiologic needs are related to a slowing of body processes and homeostatic imbalances.

Slowing Blood Circulation. The extremities become cyanosed as the blood stagnates. Because of this poor circulation, analgesics may need to be administered by intravenous infusion rather than subcutaneously or intramuscularly.

Loss of Muscle Tone. The sphincters that control defecation and urination relax; thus absorbent padding is used and frequently changed. In some instances a retention catheter is inserted for the urine. The environment needs to be kept free of unpleasant odors, and deodorants can be used for this purpose as well as adequate ventilation.

Because of loss of muscle tone, the patient may be *dysphagic* (unable to swallow). Mucus tends to accumulate in the mouth and throat, necessitating the need for throat suctioning.

With reduced peristalsis, flatus tends to accumulate in the stomach and intestines. This can cause nausea and distend the patient's abdomen. Dying patients are usually anorexic but often request a few sips of water. Due to dehydration and an elevated fever the patient's mouth will become dry, requiring mouth care.

With the progressive loss of skeletal muscle tone, the patient will require increasing support to maintain a comfortable position. Loss of the power of motion and reflexes occurs first in the legs and then gradually in the arms. If the patient is conscious, Fowler's position is indicated to ease breathing, but if the patient is unconscious, a semiprone position will facilitate the drainage of mucus from the mouth and throat. It is important to avoid placing body parts in dependent positions because of the pooling of blood in them due to the slowing of the blood circulation.

Alteration of the Senses. As death approaches, the patient's vision becomes blurred; as a result the person will often prefer a lightened to a darkened room. The dying patient turns the head to the light. Although the sense of touch will be diminished, the patient will sense pressure. Secretions may gather in the eyes, requiring cleansing with absorbent cotton and normal saline. Hearing is thought to be the last sense to leave the body. A dying patient may hear what people are saying after he or she can no longer see or respond. When talking to a dying patient, care needs to be taken to speak clearly. Whispering should be avoided, since the patient tends to become disturbed when unable to hear.

Respiratory Distress. The symptom of respiratory distress is likely to bother a patient's family as well as the patient. The Fowler's or semiprone position in bed is indicated together with throat suctioning.

State of Consciousness. The state of consciousness will vary from full consciousness to drowsiness to stupor. It is a highly variable symptom. (See "States of Awareness," Chapter 34.)

SUMMARY

There are many kinds of loss. Two types faced by patients are loss of life (death) and change in body image (self-concept). Illness can threaten both of these. Loss of an aspect of self (change in self-concept) can occur as a result of scarring or loss of body parts, for example. Another aspect of loss is loss of loved or valued people. This type of loss is also encountered by nurses.

In growth and development, loss can occur when an individual does not develop a normal self-concept or when the person fails to develop normally physically.

Loss through death is a permanent and complete loss. The manner in which death is dealt with depends largely upon the particular society. In North America, death is feared; health and youth are revered.

Engel has identified three stages of grieving:

1. Shock and disbelief
2. Developing awareness
3. Restitution and recovery

Kübler-Ross describes five stages of dying; denial, anger, bargaining, depression, and acceptance. Reaction to any loss can also be described in terms of these stages.

There are many kinds of grief: anticipatory grief, chronic grief, and absent or inhibited grief. In assessing loss and grief, it is necessary to consider several factors such as developmental status, life-style, cultural and social values, coping mechanisms, and support systems. Nurses can intervene in a number of ways to assist patients who have experienced loss related to body image and in relation to death. The awareness of the individual may be closed, mutual pretense, or open.

Assessment of impending death can be made by nurses observing reflexes, respirations, facial expression, skin, pupils, blood pressure, pulse, and body temperature. An important aspect in the care of the dying is assisting with the special needs related to the death of an infant, child, and adolescent.

Nursing intervention for the dying patient involves emotional intervention and dealing with physiologic problems such as slowing blood circulation and loss of muscle tone. Support of the family as well as the patient is part of the nurse's function.

SUGGESTED ACTIVITIES

1. Interview a nurse who has assisted patients and their families during dying. What was identified as the patient's and family's needs? How did the nurse feel about providing this care?

2. Interview patients who have encountered some loss such as loss of mobility due to a fractured hip. How did the patient perceive this loss? What were the patient's greatest needs?

SUGGESTED READINGS

French, Jean, and Schwartz, Doris R. March, 1973. Terminal care at home in two cultures. *American Journal of Nursing* 73:502–505.

The terminal care of a Navajo Indian woman in Arizona is contrasted with that of an Italian man in Harlem. Cultural differences are noted, and values are pointed out.
Kavanaugh, Robert E. May, 1974. Helping patients who are facing death. *Nursing 74* 4:35–42.

This article describes the events and feelings surrounding a terminal illness. The actions of the physician, husband, and wife are revealed.

Loxley, Alice K. October, 1972. The emotional toll of crippling deformity. *American Journal of Nursing* 72:1839–1840.

A patient with deforming arthritis is described: her questions, fears, and verbalizations.

Rinear, Eileen E. March, 1975. Helping the survivors of expected death. *Nursing 75* 5:60–65.

The ways in which nurses can assist surviving family members are described. Practical guidelines such as summoning the family when death appears imminent are discussed.

Williams, Jane C. March, 1976. Understanding the feelings of the dying. *Nursing 76* 6:52–56.

The fears of the dying are described as well as how nurses can assist patients and their families.

SELECTED REFERENCES

Blaesing, Sandra, and Brockhaus, Joyce. December, 1972. The development of body image in the child. *Nursing Clinics of North America* 7(4):597–607.

Burgess, Ann W., and Lazare, Aaron. 1976. *Psychiatric nursing in the hospital and the community.* 2nd ed. Englewood Cliffs, N.J.: Prentice-Hall, Inc.

Corbeil, M. March, 1971. The nursing process for a patient with a body image disturbance. *Nursing Clinics of North America* 6:155–163.

Dempsey, Mary O. December, 1972. The development of body image in the adolescent. *Nursing Clinics of North America.* 7(4):609–615.

Encounters with grief. Series. March, 1978. *American Journal of Nursing* 78:414–425.

Engel, G. L. September, 1964. Grief and grieving. *American Journal of Nursing* 64:93–98. Reproduced in Meyers, M. E., ed. 1967. *Nursing fundamentals.* Dubuque, Iowa: William C. Brown Co., Publishers, pp. 88–100.

Gray, V. Ruth. 1976. Some physiological needs. In *Nursing skill book. Series: Dealing with death and dying.* Philadelphia: Intermed Communications, Inc., pp. 15–20.

Gyulay, J. E. March, 1976. Care of the dying child. *Nursing Clinics of North America* 11:95–107.

Hampe, Sandra O. March–April, 1975. Needs of the grieving spouse in a hospital setting. *Nursing Research* 24:113–119.

Kavanaugh, Robert E. 1976. Children's special needs. In *Nursing skill book. Series: Dealing with death and dying.* Philadelphia: Intermed Communications, Inc., pp. 33–46.

Kübler-Ross, E. 1969. *On death and dying.* New York: Macmillan Publishing Co., Inc.

Kübler-Ross, E. 1975. *Death: the final stage of growth.* Englewood Cliffs, N.J.: Prentice-Hall, Inc.

LaCasse, Christine M. March, 1975. A dying adolescent. *American Journal of Nursing* 75:433–434.

LeRoux, Rose S. 1977. Communicating with the dying patient. *Nursing Forum* 16(2):145–155.

Murray, R. L. December, 1972. Body image development in adulthood. *Nursing Clinics of North America* 7(4):617–630.

Northrup, Fran C. June, 1974. The dying child. *American Journal of Nursing* 74:1066–1068.

Strauss, A. L., et al. 1970. Awareness of dying. In Schoenberg, B., et al., eds. *Loss and grief.* New York: Columbia University Press.

Williams, Jane C. 1976. Allaying common fears. In *Nursing skill book. Series: Dealing with death and dying.* Philadelphia: Intermed Communications, Inc., pp. 27–32.

UNIT VII

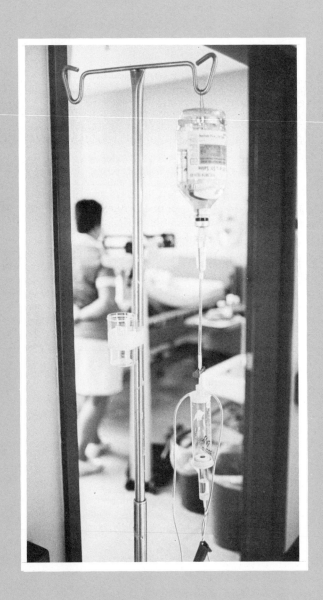

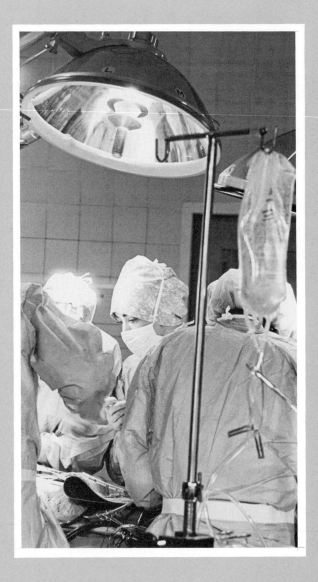

SPECIAL NURSING MEASURES

CHAPTER 36

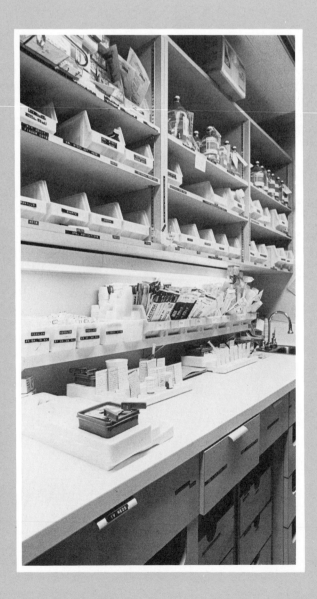

MEDICATIONS

OBJECTIVES

- Discuss drug standards using common terms.

- Explain the legal aspects of medications.

- Discuss the actions of medications and the variables that affect these actions.

- List and define the various kinds of effects of drugs.

- Compare the various routes of administration: oral, sublingual, intramuscular, subcutaneous, and intradermal.

- Describe the types of medication orders and the essential parts of an order.

- Explain the three systems of measurement: metric, apothecaries', and household.

- Calculate fractional dosages for infants and children.

- Discuss the guidelines for administering medications.

- Discuss the essential actions in administering any medication.

- Prepare and safely administer medications: oral, subcutaneous, intramuscular, intradermal, topical, instillation into eye, ear, nose, vagina, and insertion into rectum, vagina, and urethra.

- Mix different types of drugs, including insulin.

- Prepare powdered drugs.

- Explain medication errors.

- Discuss drug abuse.

Medicines have been known to man since the days of antiquity. Crude drugs such as opium, castor oil, and vinegar were used in ancient times.

Knowledge about these drugs was relatively limited then; what was known was gained chiefly by empirical observation. Over the centuries the number of drugs available has increased greatly, and knowledge about these drugs has become correspondingly more scientific. Today it is estimated that some 25,000 drugs and drug products are available in North America, and new ones are being added daily.

Drugs come from four main sources: (a) plants, such as digitalis and opium; (b) minerals, such as iron and sodium chloride; (c) animals, such as insulin and vaccines; and (d) chemical synthesis in the laboratory, such as the sulfonamides and dextropropoxyphene (Darvon, an analgesic compound). Early drugs were derived from the aforementioned three natural sources. During the past 40 years, however, more and more drugs have been produced synthetically.

DRUG STANDARDS

Drugs can vary in strength and activity. Drugs that come from plants, for example, may vary in strength according to the age of the plant, the particular variety, the place in which it is grown, and the method by which it is preserved. In order that drug dosage may be predictable in its effects it is important that the drugs be both pure and of a uniform strength. Drug standards have therefore been developed to ensure this quality.

In the United States, official drugs are those so designated by the Federal Food, Drug, and Cosmetic Act. These drugs are officially listed in the *United States Pharmacopeia (USP)* and described according to their source, physical and chemical properties, tests for purity and identity, method of storage, assay, category, and normal range of dosage. Two other publications, the *National Formulary* and the *Homeopathic Pharmacopoeia of the United States*, also list official

drugs. In Canada the *British Pharmacopoeia (BP)* is used for the same purpose, although some drugs used in Canada conform to the *USP* because they are obtained from the United States.

Under the auspices of the World Health Organization, the *Pharmacopoeia Internationalis (Ph. I.)* is published in Spanish, French, and English. It has served to improve drug standards among countries throughout the world.

The *National Formulary* in the United States and the *Canadian Formulary* are published in their respective countries. The *National Formulary* lists drugs based upon their therapeutic value and can include drugs that may still be used but that have been dropped by the *USP*. The *Canadian Formulary* lists drugs that are used extensively in Canada and that may not be listed in the *British Pharmacopoeia*.

Nursing students will find it valuable to know

about the official drug listings and the books regarding drugs that are available to them. Because of the thousands of drugs with which a nurse will be involved while assisting patients, either by administering the drugs themselves or by assessing their effectiveness and any untoward reactions, it is essential that a reliable reference be readily available. No longer is it possible for a nurse to recall all the essential information about all the drugs that are prescribed.

VOCABULARY

There are a number of special terms used in relation to medications.

1. *Drug* (medication): a chemical substance that is intended to have a therapeutic effect upon a patient.
2. *Pharmacology:* the science that studies the action of drugs upon living organisms.
3. *Pharmacy:* the art of preparing, compounding, and dispensing drugs. It can also refer to the place where drugs are prepared and dispensed.
4. *Pharmacist:* a person who is licensed to prepare and dispense drugs and to make up prescriptions.
5. *Prescription:* a written direction for the preparation and administration of a drug. In North America it is written by a physician.
6. *Pharmacopeia:* a book containing a list of products used in medicine with descriptions, chemical tests for determining identity and purity, and formulas for certain mixtures of the substances.
7. *Pharmacy assistant:* a member of the health team who in some areas of the United States and Canada administers the drugs to patients.
8. *Formulary:* a collection of formulas and prescriptions.

LEGAL ASPECTS OF MEDICATIONS

Under the law, nurses are responsible for their own actions regardless of whether there is a written order. If a physician writes an incorrect order, for example, Demerol 500 mg instead of Demerol 50 mg, a nurse who administers the written incorrect dosage is responsible for the action in making the error.

Another aspect of nursing practice that is governed by law is the use of narcotics and barbiturates. In both the United States and Canada, federal laws govern the use of these drugs. Narcotics are kept in a drawer or cupboard with a double lock in hospitals. Other medications, including barbiturates, are kept under one-lock safety, although in some places barbiturates are kept with the narcotics. Agencies have special forms for recording narcotics. The information that is required usually includes the name of the patient, date and time of administration, name of the drug, dosage, and signature of the person who prepared and gave the narcotic. The name of the physician who ordered the narcotic may also be included.

Included on the record should be any narcotics that were wasted in the process of preparation. In most agencies, narcotic and barbiturate counts are taken at the end of each shift. In the count the remaining narcotics of each kind are counted, and the total should tally with the number at the end of the last shift minus the number that were used. If the total actually left does not agree with the calculated remainder, this must be reported immediately.

The keys that lock the drug and narcotic cupboards are carried by a nurse who is on duty. They should never be left in the lock, even if a nurse leaves the cupboard for a minute.

Narcotics and barbiturates are closely controlled because of the problems of addiction in regard to these drugs. Heroin is the opiate that receives much publicity and that is illegally sold on the streets. It is more potent than either morphine or codeine. Heroin, however, is seldom used in health agencies because of the danger of a patient developing a dependence upon the drug. Related drugs such as morphine, meperidine (Demerol), dihydromorphinone (Dilaudid), and codeine are more frequently used in hospitals and prescribed by physicians generally.

NAMES, CLASSIFICATIONS AND TYPES OF MEDICATIONS

Names

One drug can have as many as four kinds of names: its generic name, official name, chemical name, and trademark or brand name. The generic name is given a drug before it becomes official. The official name is the name under which it is listed in one of the official publications. The chemical name is the name by which a chemist knows it; this name will precisely describe the constituents of the drug. The trademark or brand name is the name given the drug by its manufacturer. Because one drug may be manufactured by several companies, it can have several trade names; for example, the drug lithium carbonate (official name) is known by the trade names Carbolith, Lithane, Camcolit, Eskalith, Hypnorex, Lithonate, and Priadel.

Classifications

Drugs are classified in several ways: according to their overall effect upon the body, their composition, and their purposes. Most classifications according to action lack exactness because some drugs act on several systems of the body and may be used for different purposes for different people.

Types of Preparations

Medications come in different types of preparations. The preparations may determine the method of administration; an elixir, for example, is taken by mouth. When a medication is ordered for a patient, it is important that nurses use the correct preparation. The type of preparation is included in the order for the medication. (See Table 36-1.)

Table 36-1.   Pharmaceutical Preparations

Kind	Description	Example	Kind	Description	Example
Aqueous solution	One or more drugs dissolved in water.		Extract	Concentrated preparation of a drug from vegetables or animals; generally used to preserve a drug for use in a medication	Cascara dry extract
Syrup	An aqueous solution of sugar often used to disguise unpleasant-tasting drugs and soothe irritated membranes (demulcent effect)		Fluid extract	Alcoholic solution of a drug from a vegetable source; this is the most concentrated of all fluid preparations (100% concentration)	Casacara fluid extract
Aqueous suspension	One or more drugs finely divided in a liquid such as water	Penicillin G in water			
Spirit	A concentrated alcoholic solution of a volatile substance	Spirits of camphor	Elixir	Alcohol solution, sweetened and aromatic;	Phenobarbital elixir

Table 36-1. Pharmaceutical Preparations

Kind	Description	Example	Kind	Description	Example
	frequently mixed with another drug as a medicinal agent for children		Powder	chiefly replaced today by tablets and capsules A finely ground drug or drugs; some are used internally, some externally	
Tincture	Alcoholic or hydroalcoholic solution prepared from drugs derived from plants	Tincture of iodine	Ointment	Semisolid preparation of a drug or drugs in petrolatum	
Tablet	A powdered drug compressed into small, hard disks; some are readily broken along a scored line; some are enteric coated to prevent irritation to gastric mucosa or to prevent the effect of the gastric secretions upon the drug	Aspirin	Paste	Preparation like an ointment for external use; frequently thick and stiff; penetrates the skin less than ointments	Zinc oxide paste
			Lotion	Drug in liquid suspension intended for external use	Calamine lotion
			Plaster	Solid preparation used as a counterirritant or as an adhesive; used externally	Mustard plaster; adhesive tape
Capsule	A gelatinous container for powder, liquid, or oil drug form; it may be hard or soft and dissolves quickly in the stomach	Tetracycline hydrochloride	Poultice	Soft moist preparations that supply moist heat to the body; used externally	Linseed poultice
Lozenge (troche)	Flat, round, or oval preparation held in the mouth to dissolve and release the drug orally		Suppository	A drug or several drugs mixed with a firm base such as glycerinated gelatin and shaped for insertion into the body; the base dissolves slowly at body temperature, releasing the drug; kinds: rectal, vaginal, and urethral	Aminophylline suppository
Pill	Mixture of a drug or drugs with some cohesive material in oval, globular, or flattened shape;				

ACTIONS OF MEDICATIONS

Drugs act upon the body by either stimulating or inhibiting the function of certain tissues or organs. Tissues that are functioning abnormally can be stimulated or inhibited to function at normal levels, or if they are functioning normally, they may be stimulated or inhibited to function at abnormal levels. For example, atropine is frequently given to patients preoperatively to inhibit the normal production of saliva, and epinephrine (Adrenalin) may be given to stimulate the functioning of an inadequate heart muscle and conduction system.

The action of a drug can be described as a chemical interaction between the drug and the body cells. Most drugs are believed to interact with the cell membrane, the cell enzymes, or certain components of the cells. These interactions change the functioning of the cells, thus producing physiologic and biochemical changes in the body.

Physiologic Factors that Affect Drug Action

For a drug to act it must be present in the appropriate concentration at the site where the drug-cellular interaction is to take place. For example, for radioactive iodine to inhibit the functioning of the thyroid gland it must react with the gland and be there in a suitable concentration. Thus if it is ingested, it needs to be absorbed into the bloodstream and then travel to the thyroid gland. There are a number of factors that affect the action of a drug and hence its effects upon the body. Four of these are (a) absorption of the drug, (b) movement of the drug in the body, (c) the breakdown process, and (d) excretion of the breakdown products.

Absorption of Drugs

Absorption of a drug refers to the movement of the drug from the source of entry into the body to the bloodstream and lymphatic system. For example, in the case of orally ingested iron it is absorbed from the small intestine into the circulating systems.

The rate of absorption is affected by five main factors. First is the route of administration (see the next section). Second is the solubility of the drug; for example, orally administered drugs in a solution are generally more rapidly absorbed than are capsules and tablets. Third is the conditions at the site of administration; for example, good blood circulation to the site of an intramuscular injection will speed absorption compared to a site where the circulation is poor. The pH of the body fluid is the fourth consideration. For example, the pH in the stomach is about 1.0 to 1.4 (acid); thus drugs such as barbiturates, which are slightly acidic, are absorbed more quickly than codeine, which is slightly basic. On the other hand, in the small intestine the pH is higher, about 6 to 8 (alkaline), and there codeine will be absorbed more quickly than the barbiturates. The fifth main factor affecting absorption is the concentration of the drug or its dosage. A drug of high concentration or large dosage is more rapidly absorbed than one of weak concentration or smaller dosage. For example, digitalis 200 mg will be absorbed more quickly than digitalis 50 mg.

Movement of Drugs in the Body

After the absorption of the drug it is circulated throughout the body by the blood and lymphatic systems. The drug then moves out of the circulation through cell membranes in certain tissues. Some drugs are restricted to special tissues and body solutions, whereas others, for example, ethyl alcohol, can be found in all fluids of the body. Some drugs are also attracted to certain tissues of the body where they accumulate; for example, body fat and body muscle have affinity for certain drugs. These drugs are then released when the level of the particular drug drops in the blood plasma.

The movement of drugs to the appropriate tissue is highly dependent upon the circulation of the body fluids. Conditions that affect these fluid movements such as fluid and electrolyte imbalances and cardiac pathologic conditions can also affect the action of drugs in the body.

Breakdown Process

Once a drug has been circulated to the tissues where it interacts with the cells, it undergoes a breakdown into less active forms, which are more easily excreted. This breakdown process takes place chiefly in the liver, although some can occur in the blood plasma, the intestinal mucosa, and the kidneys. Most drugs are excreted in their less active forms. An exception is ether, which is excreted unchanged. For this reason a nurse can usually detect the distinctive odor of ether on a patient for some time after it has been administered. Because the liver is the major organ concerned with the breakdown of drugs, factors that affect liver physiology may also affect the drug metabolism (breakdown). For example, delayed drug metabolism as a result of hepatic diseases may result in a drug build-up in the body, whereas accelerated drug metabolism may appear as a drug tolerance.

Excretion of the Breakdown Products

After a drug is broken down, its products need to be excreted from the body. The major routes for excretion are the kidneys (urine), the intestines (feces), and the lungs (exhaled air). Once the drug metabolites are formed in the liver, they are excreted from the liver in the bile, which is emptied into the intestine. Some of the products are excreted from the intestine as feces; others are reabsorbed into the circulation and travel to the kidneys, where they are excreted in the urine. The lungs are chiefly responsible for excreting volatile substances such as anesthetics.

Variables that Influence Drug Action

There are a number of predictable variables that can affect the action of a drug upon a patient. Some of these main variables are (a) age and weight, (b) sex, (c) genetic factors, (d) psychologic factors, (e) illness and disease factors, (f) time of administration, and (g) the patient's environment.

Age and Weight

The very young and the elderly are often highly responsive to drugs. In the baby, the liver and kidney may be immature; in the elderly, diminished functioning can lead to an increased drug reaction. Body weight also directly affects drug action. The greater the body weight, the greater the dosage required.

Sex

Differences in drug reactions between men and women are chiefly due to two factors: the difference in size and the difference in the distribution of fat and water. Because women are usually smaller than men and weigh less, the same dosage of a drug is likely to have more effect upon a woman than upon a man. Women usually have more fatty pads than men, and men have more body fluid than women. Some drugs may be more soluble in fat, whereas others are more soluble in water. This will affect their action upon the patient.

Genetic Factors

Individual persons may react differently to drugs as a result of genetic factors. A patient may be abnormally sensitive to a drug or have a different drug metabolism due to genetic influences. Sometimes these reactions are mistaken for allergic reactions.

Psychologic Factors

The way a person feels about a drug and what one believes it can do are major factors in the effect of a drug. A traditional example of this is the reaction of some people to a placebo, which is an inactive substance such as normal saline given to a patient in order to satisfy his or her need for a drug. For some patients the placebo has the same effect as the drug itself.

Illness and Disease Factors

Illness and disease can affect the action of drugs upon a patient. For example, a person who has severe pain due to a kidney stone may tolerate large, repeated quantities of morphine before the pain is diminished. The same amount of morphine when the patient does not have this pain may well prove lethal. Another example is the use of aspirin. For a patient with a fever, aspirin can reduce the body temperature; for a patient without a fever, aspirin has no effect on the body temperature.

Time of Administration

The time of administration of oral medications is highly significant in relation to the time it takes a drug. A traditional example of this is the reaction of some people to a *placebo*, which is an inactive substance such as normal saline given to a patient in order to satisfy his or her need for a drug. For some taken after a meal. However, there are medications that are irritating to the gastrointestinal tract and need to be given after a meal, when they will be better tolerated. An example is iron (ferrous sulphate).

A patient's sleep-wake rhythm may also affect the action of a drug. The circadian variations in urine output and blood circulation, for example, may well affect a patient's response to a drug.

Environment

The patient's environment can also have an effect upon some drugs, particularly those which are used to treat the behavior and the mood of a patient. It is therefore important to consider the drug itself as well as the patient's personality and milieu when observing the effects of the medication. An example of a drug that needs to be considered in this context is Elavil Hydrochloride (amitriptyline hydrochloride).

The temperature of the environment may also affect drug activity. When the temperature is elevated, the peripheral blood vessels are dilated, thus intensifying the actions of drugs that are vasodilators. On the other hand, a cold environment and consequent vasoconstriction will inhibit the action of the same vasodilators.

Effects of Drugs

Drugs can be described as having several kinds of effects upon a person.

Therapeutic and Side Effects

The *therapeutic effect* is that effect which is desired, or the reason a drug is prescribed. *Side effects* are those effects which a drug has upon a person that are not intended. Digitalis increases the strength of myocardial contractions, but it can also cause nausea and vomiting (side effects). There are a number of kinds of side effects with which nurses need to be familiar in relation to drug therapy. Some of these are allergy, drug tolerance, cumulative effect, idiosyncratic effect, and synergistic effect.

Drug Allergy.   A *drug allergy* is the immunologic reaction of a person to a drug to which he or she has already been sensitized. When a patient is first exposed to a foreign body (antigen), the body may develop a reaction to this by producing antibodies. This is called an *immunologic reaction* (see Chapter 8). A patient can react to a drug as a foreign body and thus develop symptoms of an allergic reaction.

Allergic reactions can be either mild or severe. A mild reaction has a variety of symptoms from skin rashes to diarrhea (see Table 36-2). It can occur anytime from a few hours to 2 weeks after the administration of the drug.

A severe allergic reaction usually occurs immediately after the administration of the drug; it is called an *anaphylactic reaction*. This type of response can be fatal if the symptoms are not noticed immediately and assistance obtained. The earliest symptoms are irritability, extreme weakness, nausea, and vomiting, which then are followed quickly by acute shortness of breath, acute hypotension, and death (see Table 36-2).

Table 36-2.   Common Mild Allergic Responses

Sympton	Rationale
Skin rash	Either an intraepidermal vesicle rash or a rash typified by an urticarial wheal or macular eruption; rash is usually generalized over the body
Pruritus	Itching of the skin with or without a rash
Angioedemia	Edema due to increased permeability of the blood capillaries
Rhinitis	Excessive watery discharge from the nose
Lacrimal tearing	Excessive tearing from the eyes
Nausea, vomiting	Stimulation of these centers in the brain
Wheezing and dyspnea	Shortness of breath and wheezing upon inhalation and exhalation due to accumulated fluids and edema of the respiratory tissues
Diarrhea	Irritation of the mucosa of the large intestine

Drug Tolerance.   *Drug tolerance* exists in a person when there is decreased physiologic activity in response to the drug. For example, a person has developed a tolerance when furosemide (Lasix) 80 mg is required when previously Lasix 20 mg effected the same result.

Cumulative Effect.   A *cumulative effect* occurs when a person is unable to metabolize (break down) the previous dose of the drug. As a result the amount of the drug builds up in the patient's body unless the administered dosage is adjusted. High levels of the drug thus produce toxic effects, some of which can be prolonged.

Idiosyncratic Effect.   *Idiosyncratic effects* are unexpected and usually individualistic. Sometimes these reactions are an underresponse to the drug, an overresponse, a completely different effect from the normal one, or unpredictable and unexplainable symptoms.

Synergistic Effect.   In the synergistic effect, the combined effect of two or more drugs is different from the effects of each drug when taken alone. The combined effect may be less than what would be ex-pected or greater than the effect of each drug. Alcohol and barbiturates are potentially lethal; phenytoin (Dilantin) has an inhibitory effect upon digitalis.

ROUTES OF ADMINISTRATION OF MEDICATIONS

Pharmaceutical preparations are generally designed for one or two specific routes of administration. Normally physicians will order the route of administration when they order drugs for their patients. If a nurse is administering the drug, it is essential that the correct pharmaceutical preparation is used for the route ordered. For example, phenobarbital is taken orally; phenobarbital sodium may be taken parent-erally.

Oral Administration

The most common route used for the administration of drugs is by mouth (orally). It is the least expensive way and the most convenient for most patients. It is also a safe method of administration in that the skin is not broken as it is for an injection.

   The major disadvantages of oral administration of drugs are their unpleasant taste, the irritation of the gastric mucosa, the irregularity of absorption from the gastrointestinal tract, the time needed for absorption, and the harmful effect some drugs can have on a patient's teeth.

Sublingual Administration

A drug is given sublingually by placing it under the tongue and letting it slowly dissolve. Drugs such as nitroglycerine are commonly taken in this manner. (See Figure 36-1.)

Parenteral Administration

Parenteral administration refers to that type of administration accomplished by needle. Some of the more common routes for parenteral administration are as follows:

   Intramuscular: into a muscle

   Subcutaneous (hypodermic): into the subcutaneous tissue, just below the skin

   Intravenous: into a vein

   Intradermal: under the epidermis (into the dermis)

Some of the less commonly used routes for parenteral administration are *intraarterial* (into an artery), *intracardiac* (into the heart muscle), *intraosseous* (into the bone), and *intrathecal* or *intraspinal* (into the spinal canal). These latter parenteral injections are normally carried out by physicians. All parenteral therapy utilizes sterile equipment and sterile drug solutions. Parenteral therapy has the primary advantage of fast absorption of a measured amount of drug.

Insertions

Insertion means "putting in" a drug, for example, the insertion of suppositories into the rectum, the vagina, or the urethra. The suppository gradually dissolves at body temperature and releases the drug, which is then absorbed through the mucous membrane into the body circulation. Suppositories are not consid-ered to be as efficient vehicles for administration of drugs as are the parenteral and oral methods. Insert-ions do have great value for the administration of drugs to the local areas, for example, the administra-

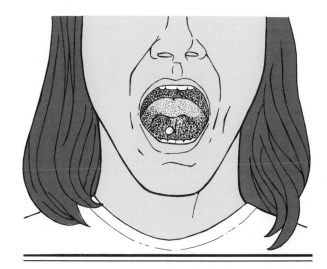

Figure 36.1.   The sublingual administration of a tab-let.

tion of suppositories rectally to promote the passage of feces.

Instillations

An *instillation* is putting a drug in liquid form into a body cavity, such as the urinary bladder, or into a body orifice, such as the ears, eyes, and the nose.

Topical Application

A *topical application* is an external application, for example, to the skin, the nails, or the hair. *Inunction* is the act of applying an ointment with friction. Many drugs are applied topically; astringents, emollients, and antiseptics are commonly used types applied either in liquid form or as ointments.

Inhalation

Inhalation is the administration of a drug into the respiratory tract. Nebulizers or positive pressure breathing apparatuses are generally used to administer the drug. The vehicles of air, oxygen, or steam are generally used to carry the drug into the lungs.

MEDICATION ORDERS

A physician is the person who usually determines the needs of patients for medications and orders them, although nurse practitioners in some settings now order some drugs. Usually the order is written, although telephone and verbal orders are acceptable in a number of agencies. Nursing students would be wise to know the agency policies regarding medication orders. In some hospitals, for example, only graduate nurses are permitted to accept telephone and verbal orders from physicians.

Types of Orders

There are two general types of orders: the standing order and the self-terminating order. A *standing order* is carried out until canceled by another order. Sometimes a physician writes a standing order and the conditions by which it is to be canceled; for example, "Give Reserpine 2.5 mg intravenously until blood pressure is 120/80."

Some hospitals and other health agencies have policies that govern standing orders. Many policies require review by the physician and reordering at intervals such as every 4 weeks, otherwise the order is automatically considered canceled. There are usually more standing orders in long-term care units than in acute care units of hospitals.

Some standing orders include the directions "prn," meaning "when necessary." In this instance it is usually the nurse's judgment as to when the specific medication is given; for example, "morphine 15 mg q4h prn" (morphine 15 mg every 4 hours as necessary).

Self-terminating orders are those which have the terminating time stated in the order itself. One type of self-terminating order is the stat order; it is to be carried out only once and immediately. Another type is one in which the number of doses or the number of days that the patient takes the drug are stated; for example, "digitoxin 0.1 mg daily for 5 days" or "pilocarpine gtts ♇ qh OD × 6" (pilocarpine two drops every hour in the right eye for six doses).

Policies regarding physicians' orders vary considerably from agency to agency. Generally, a physician orders which medicines are to be given to a patient by nurses and which medications a patient can keep at the bedside to self-administer after entering a hospital. Hospitals also have varying policies regarding orders. It is not unusual for a patient's orders to be automatically canceled after surgery or an examination involving an anesthetic after which new orders must be written. In this way the hospital is endeavoring to ensure that physicians are continually aware of their patients' conditions, particularly at more critical times such as after surgery. Most agencies also have lists of abbreviations that are officially accepted for use within the agency. Both nurses and physicians may need to refer to these lists if they have been working in a different agency. These abbreviations can be legally used on a patient's chart. The nursing student is referred to the Appendix, which gives commonly used abbreviations.

The Drug Order: Essential Parts

The drug order written by the physician has six essential parts: (a) the full name of the patient, (b) the date the order is written, (c) the name of the drug to be administered, (d) the dosage of the drug, (e) the method of administration, and (f) the signature of the physician. In addition, if the order is not a standing one, it should also contain the number of doses or the number of days the drug is to be administered.

The Full Name of the Patient

A patient's full name, that is, the first and last names and middle initials should always be used to avoid confusion between two patients who have the same last names. In some agencies as a further identification, the patient's admission number is also put on the order.

Some hospitals have a mechanism for imprinting the patient's name and hospital number on any forms as they are required, for example,

Lewis, Sharon R.
68793-39

This imprinter is usually available on the nursing unit; it is much like the credit card imprinters used in daily living.

The Date

The date an order is written is also included on the order. The date will include the day, the month, and the year. In some agencies, writing the time of the order is also practiced. By including the time, errors that may result from a change of nursing personnel between two shifts can sometimes be avoided.

In many agencies the 24-hour clock is used; this also clarifies time and can help avoid error. Time with the 24-hour clock starts at midnight, which is 0000 hours. Ten minutes after midnight is then 0010 hours, and 1 AM is 0100 hours; 12 noon is 1200 hours; 1 PM is 1200 hours plus 0100 hours or 1300 hours; 9 PM is then 1200 hours plus 0900 hours or 2100 hours, and so forth; 12 midnight is then 2400 hours.

Time has another importance in that it establishes the time when certain orders automatically terminate. For example, in some settings, narcotics can only be ordered for 48 hours after surgery. Therefore a drug that is ordered at 1600 hours February 1, 1979 is automatically canceled at 1600 hours February 3, 1979.

The Name of the Drug

The name of the drug that is ordered must be clearly written. In some settings only generic names are permitted; however, trade names are widely used in hos-

pitals and health agencies. Most settings where drug orders are written have drug reference sources available to nurses and physicians such as the *United States Pharmacopeia* or the *Compendium of Pharmaceuticals and Specialties (CPS)*. If nurses are unsure about a drug that is ordered, it is essential that they look it up in a suitable reference before preparing or administering the drug. Some hospitals provide their own formulary listing all drugs stocked in the hospital.

In some situations patients in a hospital may continue to take their own medications. So that the nurse knows what drug the patient is taking, it is necessary to confirm the name of the drug by checking the drug label or by checking with the physician or the pharmacy if the bottle is unlabeled.

The Dosage of the Drug

The dosage of the drug includes the amount, the times or frequency of administration, and in many instances the strength; for example, tetracycline *250 mg* (amount) *four times a day* (frequency); hydrochloric acid *10%* (strength) *5 ml* (amount) *three times a day with meals* (time and frequency).

Dosages are written in both apothecaries' or metric systems, but the metric system is being used increasingly frequently in some parts of the United States and in Canada.

The Method of Administration

Also included in the physician's order is the method of administration of the drug. Just as with the other parts of the order there are abbreviations that are frequently used when indicating the route of administration (see Appendix). It is not unusual for a drug to have several possible routes of administration; therefore it is important that this direction is included in the order. If the nurse considers that a patient's condition is such that the ordered route of administration is not suitable, the physician needs to be notified about this. Sometimes patients' conditions change so that a standing order needs to be changed before a drug can be administered. For example, an unconscious patient will be unable to swallow an oral medication.

The Signature of the Physician

The signature of the physician makes the drug order a legal request. An unsigned order has no validity, and the physician needs to be notified if this occurs, as it may on occasion, for example, if a physician is interrupted while writing an order.

In agencies where telephone orders are taken by nurses from physicians, the nurse usually indicates the name of the physician who phoned in the order. The nurse signs the order, and the physician cosigns or initials it when visiting the agency. Some hospitals have policies that telephone orders must be signed by the physician within a certain length of time, for example, 48 hours after they have been given.

The Five Rights

With reference to medications, five rights serve as guidelines for nurses: the right patient, the right medication, right time, right drug, and right route.

Problems with Orders

Although it is not common, a nurse may from time to time find there are problems with a physician's order. Generally, the problems are of three types:

1. The nurse is unable to read the directions.
2. The drug appears unsuitable for the patient, or the dosage is unsuitable.
3. The patient is unable to take or to tolerate the drug.

Nurses must be able to read all orders clearly and completely understand them. If a nurse cannot decipher or understand an order, it is necessary to ask for clarification from the physician before proceeding. In many situations nurses have learned to read the order while the physician is present so that they can ask questions immediately rather than try to find the physician an hour later.

Sometimes in the nurse's judgment a particular drug may seem unsuitable for a patient, or the dosage ordered is not within the usual range of dosages. Most physicians welcome questions in this regard. Often the nurse gains information from the physician about the drug therapy, thereby making the order more reasonable to the nurse. Sometimes an error has been made, and by questioning the physician the error is corrected before the patient is involved. In any case, questions from nurses in this context can serve to protect the patient and the physician from inadvertent error.

In some instances a patient is unable to take an ordered medication because of a change in his or her condition. This may occur in any setting, and it is the nurse's responsibility to notify the physician. This is also true when a patient cannot tolerate a certain drug and for some reason the physician does not know this.

If a nurse questions an order and is not satisfied with the answer and still believes the order is incor-

rect, the next step is to notify the nurse in charge of the hospital unit or agency. It is the nurse's responsibility to do this and the nurse's right to refuse to administer any drug that in the nurse's judgment is unsafe for the patient.

In some agencies there are lists of techniques and drugs that nurses and nursing students are not permitted to carry out or administer. It is the nurse's and nursing student's right and responsibility to decline to carry out techniques that are contrary to the agency's policy. The nurse in this situation should, however, convey this information to the nurse in charge. An example of a policy governing medications is one regarding heparin. Frequently this drug can be administered intravenously only by a physician.

Communicating a Medication Order

A drug order for a patient is usually written on the patient's chart or in a special book designed for that purpose. From there it is usually transcribed by a nurse to the Kardex and to a medication card (see Figure 36-2).

Medication cards in hospitals vary in form but include the patient's name, room and bed number, name of the drug, dose, times, and methods of administration. In some agencies the date that the order was prescribed and the date the order expires are also included, along with the signature of the person transcribing the order. The responsibility for transcribing medication orders is the nurse's; however, it may be delegated to a clerk.

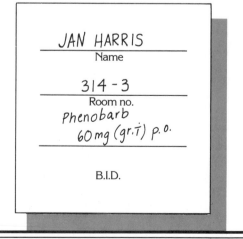

JAN HARRIS
Name

314 - 3
Room no.

Phenobarb
60 mg (gr. Ī) p. o.

B.I.D.

Figure 36-2.   A sample medication card with essential information.

SYSTEMS OF MEASUREMENT

Three systems of measurement are operant in North America: the metric system, the apothecaries' system, and the household system, which is similar to the apothecaries' system. It would be much simpler for everyone if one system were universally accepted; however, because all systems are in current use, it is necessary for nurses to become familiar with the three systems and to be able to convert from one to the other as it is necesssary.

The Metric System

The metric system, devised by the French in the latter part of the 18th century, is the system prescribed by law in most European countries. Its use is recently gaining momentum in North America. Canada is now in the process of converting to the metric system, and attempts are being made in the United States to legislate its use. The metric system is very logically organized into units of ten; it is a decimal system. Basic units can be multiplied or divided by ten in order to form secondary units. Multiples are made by moving the decimal point to the right, and subdivisions are made by moving the decimal point to the left.

Basic units of measurement are the meter, the liter, and the gram. Prefixes derived from Latin are used to designate subdivisions of the basic unit: deci (1/10 or 0.1), centi (1/100 or 0.01), and milli (1/1000 or 0.001). Multiples of the basic unit are designated by prefixes derived from Greek: deka (10), hecto (100),

and kilo (1000). For purposes of this chapter, only the measurements of volume (the liter) and of weight (the gram) will be considered. These are the measures used in medication administration (Figure 36-3). In medical and nursing practice the kilogram (kg) is the only multiple of the gram that is used, and the milligram (mg) is the only subdivision. Fractional parts of the liter are usually expressed in milliliters (ml), for example, 600 ml, and multiples of the liter are usually expressed, for example, as 2.5 liters or 2500 ml. See the Appendix for symbols and abbreviations of the metric system.

The Apothecaries' System

The Apothecaries' system was brought to the United States from England during the colonial period in the 18th century. It is an older system than the metric system. People are familiar with most units of measure in the apothecaries' system, since they have been used in everyday life. For example, milk is bought in pints or quarts, gasoline is purchased by the gallon, people weigh themselves in pounds, and distances are measured in feet or inches and miles.

The basic unit of weight in the apothecaries' system is the grain, likened to a grain of wheat, and the basic unit of volume is the minim, which derives from the quantity of water that would weigh a grain of wheat. The word *minim* means "the least." In ascending order the other units of weight are the scruple, the dram, the ounce, and the pound. Nowadays the scruple (℈) is seldom used, so it is generally omitted. The units of volume are, in ascending order, the fluid dram, the fluid ounce, the pint, the quart, and the gallon.

Quantities are often expressed in the apothecaries' system by lowercase Roman numerals, particularly when the basic units are abbreviated. The Roman numeral follows rather than precedes the unit of measure. For example, a fluid ounce is abbreviated as f ℥ . Two fluid ounces are written as f ℥ii , and 4 fluid ounces are written as f ℥iv . One-half fluid ounce is written as f ℥ss and 1½ fluid ounces f ℥iss. The relationships and equivalencies of the units of the apothecaries' system are shown in the Appendix.

The Household System

Household measures may need to be used in home situations when more accurate systems of measure

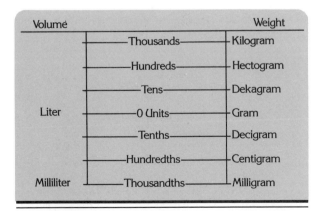

Volume		Weight
	Thousands	Kilogram
	Hundreds	Hectogram
	Tens	Dekagram
Liter	0 Units	Gram
	Tenths	Decigram
	Hundredths	Centigram
Milliliter	Thousandths	Milligram

Figure 36-3.   Basic measurements of volume and weight.

are not available. Included in household measures are drops, teaspoons, tablespoons, cups, and glasses. Although pints and quarts are often found in homes, they are defined as apothecaries' measures. For equivalents of units within the household system see the Appendix.

EXCHANGING UNITS OF WEIGHT AND MEASURE

Sometimes drugs are dispensed from the pharmacy in grams when the dosage ordered by the physician is ordered in milligrams, or they are dispensed in milligrams but they are ordered in grains. In another situation the nurse may be preparing a medicated irrigation only to find that the doctor has ordered the amount in an apothecaries' unit of measure (for example, a quart) and that the solution is dispensed only in metric or liter containers. In all situations it is the nurse's responsibility to exchange the units of measure or weight, and thus nurses must be aware of approximate equivalents within each system of measurement and between each system.

Exchanging Weights within the Metric System

It is a relatively simple matter to exchange units of weight within the metric system, since the system is based on units of ten. There are only two metric units of weight used in relation to drug dosages, the gram (gm) and the milligram (mg). Since 1000 mg is equal to 1 gm, exchanges between these two weights are done by dividing or multiplying by 1000. For example, to change milligrams to grams, the milligrams are divided by 1000. The simplest way to divide by 1000 is to move the decimal point three places to the left.

$$1000 \text{ mg} = 1 \text{ gm}$$
$$500 \text{ mg} = 0.5 \text{ gm}$$

Conversely, to convert grams to milligrams, the number of grams is multiplied by 1000, or the decimal point is moved three places to the right.

$$0.006 \text{ gm} = 6 \text{ mg}$$

Exchanging Weights and Measures between Metric, Apothecaries', and Household Systems

When preparing medications for patients, a nurse may find it necessary to convert weights or volumes from one system to another. As an example, the physician orders a drug using a unit of weight from the apothecaries' system, such as chloral hydrate grains vii $\overline{ss}$, and the pharmacy dispenses the drug in milligrams or grams (the metric system). For the nurse to prepare the correct dose for the patient, the equivalent measures from system to system must be known. The same example may be used to convert the metric or apothecaries' systems to household measures. Patients at home will often need a system of measure that is convenient for them such as teaspoon or a tablespoon. Again it is the nurse's responsibility to convert the metric or apothecaries' measure to a more realistic useful measure for a patient. All conversions are approximate, that is, not precisely accurate.

Exchanging Units of Volume

It is advisable for a nurse to learn some basic commonly used approximate equivalents for nursing practice such as those in Table 36-3.

By learning the equivalents in Table 36-3, many conversions can be readily made. For example, 15 minims = 15 drops; therefore 1 minim is approximately equivalent to 1 drop. Similarly, 1 quart approximates 1000 ml, and 1 gallon approximates 4000 ml; therefore 4 quarts is approximately 1 gallon.

Table 36-3. Equivalent Measures: Metric, Apothecaries', and Household

Metric		Apothecaries'		Household
1 ml	=	15 minims (mp or m)	=	15 drops (gtt)
15 ml	=	4 fluid drams (f℈)	=	1 tablespoon (tbsp)
30 ml	=	1 fluid ounce (f℥)	=	same
500 ml	=	1 pint (pt)	=	same
1000 ml	=	1 quart (qt)	=	same
4000 ml	=	1 gallon (gal)	=	same

Some practical applications of measures of volume are as follows:

1. The number of minims in a milliliter is frequently used to fractionize dosages.

2. Fluid drams and ounces are commonly used in prescribing liquid medications such as cough syrup, laxatives, antacids, and antibiotics for children. The fluid ounce is frequently converted to milliliters when measuring a patient's fluid intake or output.

3. Pints and quarts are the volumes commonly used to prepare solutions for enemas, irrigating solutions for douching, bladder irrigations, and for cleansing open wounds.

Exchanging Units of Weight

The most commonly used units of weight in nursing practice are the gram, milligram, and kilogram of the metric system and the grain and the pound in the apothecaries' system. Household units of weight are not applicable in this instance.

Table 36-4 shows metric and apothecaries' approximate equivalents. Learning these permits weight conversions readily.

Some common applications of converting or exchanging units of weight are the following:

1. Converting a person's body weight from kilograms to pounds and vice versa.

2. Converting grams and milligrams to grains and vice versa, for example, when preparing medications.

When converting units of weight from the metric system to the apothecaries' system, it is helpful for the nurse to first establish the fact that a milligram is smaller than a grain (1 mg = 1/60 grain or vice versa, 1 grain = 60 mg). When converting from a smaller unit (milligram) to a larger unit (grain), the outcome should be a smaller numerical value, thus the process of division (by 60) is involved (1 grain divided by 60 = 1/60 grain). Conversely, when converting from a

Table 36-4. Approximate Weight Equivalents: Metric and Apothecaries' Systems

Metric	Apothecaries'
1 mg	= 1/60 grain
60 mg	= 1 grain
1 gm	= 15 grains
4 gm	= 1 dram
30 gm	= 1 ounce
500 gm	= 1.1 pound (lb.)
1000 gm (1 kg)	= 2.2 lb.

larger unit to a smaller unit, the multiplication process (by 60) is required to acquire a larger numerical value. In other words:

Small units (mg) to large units = a smaller number

Large units (grains) to small units = a larger number

$$\frac{3000 \text{ mg}}{60} = 50 \text{ grains}$$

$$50 \text{ grains} \times 60 = 3000 \text{ mg}$$

The process of converting milligrams to grams was previously discussed, that is, moving the decimal point three spaces to the left.

$$3000 \text{ mg} = 3 \text{ gm}$$

When converting pounds to kilograms, the same rule applies. Since the pound is a smaller unit than the kilogram, conversions are divided or multiplied by 2.2.

$$\frac{110 \text{ lb}}{2.2} = 50 \text{ kg}$$

$$50 \text{ kg} \times 2.2 = 110 \text{ lb}$$

CALCULATING FRACTIONAL DOSAGES

The need to calculate fractional dosages from stock drugs arises chiefly when smaller dosages must be administered to infants and children. It may also be necessary in preparing preoperative medications, injectable analgesics, and intravenous medications for adult patients. Formulas have been devised to determine safe dosages for children. Three of these (Clark's rule, Fried's rule, and Young's rule) are based upon a child's age or weight in comparison to the average adult age or weight. Clark's rule, which is based on the child's weight, is thought to be more accurate than the age criterion, since the weight of children varies somewhat at the same age, and weight or size is directly pertinent to drug effectiveness.

Dosages for Children

According to Weight: Clark's Rule

Clark's rule calculates the dose for a child according to weight and therefore can be used for children of all ages. An average adult weight of 150 pounds (approximately 68 kg) is used. The amount for the child's dose is obtained by creating a fraction with the child's weight over the adult's weight (150 lb) and multiplying by the adult dose.

$$\text{Child's dose} = \frac{\text{Weight of child in pounds}}{150} \times \text{Adult dose}$$

If the adult dose of a drug is 1/6 grain, the amount a child weighing 30 pounds should receive is

$$\frac{30}{150} \times \frac{1}{6} = \frac{1}{30} \text{ grain}$$

Over 1 Year of Age: Young's Rule

The basic assumption underlying Young's formula is that a person under 12 or 12½ years of age is a child.

$$\frac{\text{Age of child (years)}}{\text{Age of child (years)} + 12} \times \text{Adult dose} = \text{Child's dose}$$

Using the same adult dose of the drug as illustrated above (1/6 grain), a child of 6 years of age should receive

$$\frac{6}{(6 + 12)} \times \frac{1}{6} = \frac{1}{18} \text{ grain}$$

Under 1 Year of Age: Fried's Rule

Fried's rule is similar to Young's rule except that the age of the child under 1 year must be considered in terms of months. Therefore the denominator or adult age is considered to be 150 months, the equivalent of 12½ years.

$$\frac{\text{Age of child (months)}}{150} \times \text{Adult dose} = \text{Infant's dose}$$

Again using the same adult dose of 1/6 grain, an infant of 6 months should receive

$$\frac{6}{150} \times \frac{1}{6} = \frac{1}{150} \text{ grain}$$

Fractional Dosages from Stock Drugs

The stock drug problem arises chiefly with the preparation of injectable drugs that are either available in tablet form and must be dissolved in water or that are already in solution and stored in ampules or vials.

Tablets

Determining a Smaller Dose of a Drug from a Tablet.
In recent years the availability of tablets for use in injections has decreased and has been replaced with individual-dose ampules or multidosed vials. However, it is still advisable for a nurse to learn how to fractionize dosages from tablets. Because it is impossible to divide a hypodermic tablet accurately, a whole tablet must be used and dissolved inside a syringe or sterile medicine glass. Sterile water or sterile normal saline from commercially prepared vials is used to dissolve the tablet, and then a fractional part of the entire solution is taken. This fractional part that is administered is determined by dividing the amount of the drug that is desired by the amount of drug on hand. Simply expressed in a formula this becomes

$$\frac{\text{D (amount desired)}}{\text{H (amount on hand)}} = \text{Fraction of tablet needed}$$

If morphine tablets are available in ¼ grain tablets but 1/6 grain is the dose ordered, the fraction of the tablet to be given would be

$$\frac{1/6 \text{ grain}}{1/4 \text{ grain}} = \text{Fraction of tablet}$$

Invert the divisor and multiply:

$$\frac{1}{6} \times \frac{4}{1} = \frac{2}{3} \text{ tablet} = \frac{1}{6} \text{ grain}$$

Dissolving and Preparing the Dose.   After the proportion of the tablet to be used is determined, it then becomes necessary to prepare the required amount in a syringe for injection. It was mentioned earlier that the entire tablet must be dissolved in sterile saline or sterile water, but using the last example, it has now been determined that only two thirds of the tablet and therefore two thirds of the total solution is required. To measure the volume of solution for dilution of the tablet it is necessary to consider two factors:

1. The amount of solution that is acceptable for administration.

2. The metric (milliliter) and apothecaries' (minim) calibrations on the syringe.

The recommended minimum amount of solution for injections is 8 minims or ½ ml, and the maximum amount is about 32 to 40 minims or 2 to 2½ ml. The maximum measures depend upon the site of injection and the size of the patient. A large muscular adult may safely absorb up to 5 ml intramuscularly.

Disposable syringes are usually available in a 3 ml size for medications.

Measurement of the solution can be done on the metric calibrations on one side of the syringe, which are divided into tenths, or on the minim calibrations on the other side, which are divided into sixteenths (16 minims = 1 ml). Thus to fractionize two thirds of a dose, the total amount of solution that may be used is 1 ml, and then two thirds of the solution (either 0.6 to 0.7 ml or 10 minims) is administered. In this case a third of the solution is discarded prior to administering the drug.

When preparing very small doses for children, it is frequently necessary to dilute the available tablets more. For example, to prepare 1/30 grain from 1/6 grain (the dose calculated previously by Clark's rule) it is first necessary to fractionize the amount of the tablet required.

$$\frac{\text{D (amount desired)}}{\text{H (amount on hand)}} = \frac{1/30}{1/6} \text{ grain} = \frac{1}{30} \times \frac{6}{1} = \frac{1}{5}$$

Because one fifth of a tablet or 1/5 ml (if the tablet is dissolved in 1 ml) is too small for administration, it is necessary to dissolve the tablet in a larger amount of solution such as 2½ ml. Then one fifth of 2½ ml is administered or ½ ml.

Prepared Vials or Ampules

Many medications are already in liquid form and ready for use, as for example, meperidine hydrochloride (Demerol). It is often distributed in large vials and prepared in dilutions of 50 mg per ml. Frequently it is a simple arithmetical matter to prepare multiples of 50 mg such as 75 or 100 mg, that is, 1½ and 2 ml, respectively. However, if, for example, 40 or 60 mg is required, it is necessary for a nurse to calculate the exact amount of solution required. In this case the same formula is used.

$$\frac{\text{D (amount desired)}}{\text{H (amount on hand)}} = \text{Amount (volume) wanted}$$

$$\frac{40 \text{ mg}}{50 \text{ mg}} = \frac{4}{5} \text{ ml}$$

Example problem: Prepare 4 mg of a drug from a vial containing 20 mg in a 5 ml solution.
Formula:

$$\frac{\text{Drug available}}{\text{Amount of solution}} = \frac{\text{Dose wanted}}{x \text{ ml}}$$

$$\frac{20 \text{ mg}}{5 \text{ ml}} = \frac{4 \text{ mg}}{x \text{ ml}}$$

Therefore: $\dfrac{20}{5} = \dfrac{4}{x}$

Cross multiply:
$$20\,x = 20$$
$$x = \frac{20}{20}$$
$$x = 1 \text{ ml}$$

GUIDELINES FOR ADMINISTERING MEDICATIONS

1. The method of administration that is prescribed usually determines the particular pharmaceutical preparation to be used.

2. The time between administering a drug and its effect upon the patient depends upon a variety of factors, including the route of administration.

3. People may have highly individualistic reactions to drugs.

4. Patients have a right to know the name and the action of the drug they are taking or receiving except in specific situations.

5. Patients are not legally required to take any drugs.

6. Understanding the effects of a drug requires a knowledge of physiology, pharmacology, and the patient.

7. Safety in medicinal therapy requires a knowledge of the symptoms of possible side effects.

8. The possibility of an error necessitates conscious thought in related nursing activities.

9. Patients will express their particular needs related to explanations about drug therapy in a variety of ways.

PREPARATION OF MEDICATIONS

Issuance of medications to a patient or for administration by another person to a patient is the responsibility of pharmacists. In some hospitals a senior nursing person may dispense drugs in the absence of a pharmacist, for example, on a holiday. Drugs are frequently dispensed now in an individualized dose for each patient called a *unit dose,* which refers to the amount of medication the patient receives at a prescribed hour. For example, on Monday at 1000 hours a unit dose may include three different medications for the patient. Previously medications were dispensed in packages or bottles according to the type of medication. In other words, the patient would have three envelopes of three different medications, and it was the nurse's responsibility to select the number of tablets required to be given. With the unit dose system the dosages are already prepared for the hour in one package.

It is believed that there is less likelihood of error with the unit dose method. However, although unit doses are being used in many settings, nurses still need to be able to prepare and calculate dosages when the need arises.

Drugs are prepared and administered by registered nurses, and in some settings licensed practical nurses also dispense oral medications. Pharmacy technologists also administer medications in some agencies.

In many settings there are now drug administration carts, which can be wheeled around a nursing unit and in which the patients' unit doses are kept. If trays are used to dispense drugs, the medication card and medication container are placed closely together. When a group of patients are receiving their medications at the same time, the cards and medications are best arranged on the tray in the order in which they will be dispensed.

Safety

If drugs are to be prepared in advance of giving them to the patient, for example, if liquids are to be poured from bottles or if tablets are to be dispensed from a stock supply, there are a number of guides to remember, which will help prevent drug errors.

1. The label of the drug should be read three times: once while reaching for the container; second, before pouring the medication or taking it out of its container (see Figure 36-4); and third, just before putting the container back in place. None of these three steps should be carried out automatically; a nurse must think and concentrate during this process.

2. The nurse should not be interrupted while preparing or giving any type of medication.

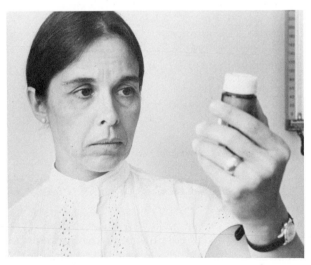

Figure 36-4.   A nurse holds a bottle of medicine at eye level while reading the label.

3. If a nurse must leave medications, they need to be locked safely in a cupboard to ensure that they will not be disturbed.

4. Before pouring or dispensing any medications, the nurse needs to check the physicians' orders to make sure that the medicine cards are up to date. Nursing notes also need to be checked to see whether medications should be withheld pending a physician's order; for example, the patient might have some symptoms that could indicate an allergic reaction to a drug. Some agencies have a system in which cards are checked daily, and the latter situation would be reported at shift change.

Time

The time at which medications are prepared and administered is ordered by the physician and governed by the agency. A physician orders a drug to be given to a patient, for example, four times per day. The hospital very often has a policy describing the exact time for dispensing, such as 1000, 1400, 1800, and 2200 hours or 0800, 1200, 1600, and 2000 hours. When a prn drug is ordered by the physician, nurses use their own judgment in administration and are not guided by specific hospital policies about times.

ADMINISTERING MEDICATIONS

In the dispensing of any drug, regardless of whether the route of administration is oral or parenteral, there are five steps to be followed:

1. Identification of the patient.
2. Administration of the drug.
3. Provision of adjunctive nursing care as indicated.
4. Recording.
5. Evaluation of the effectiveness of the drug.

Identification of the Patient

Identifying a patient sounds as if it is a simple matter and it usually is, but errors in the administration of drugs can and do occur because a patient gets a drug intended for another person. In hospitals most patients wear an identification such as a wrist band on which is printed their name and hospital identification number. Nurses are also advised to always ask the patient's name or state the name clearly and then listen to the patient's response before administering any medication.

Administration of the Drug

Equally important to identifying the patient is giving the correct drug. Again the medication card needs to be read carefully and checked with the name on the medication envelope or on the drawer or section of the drawer in which the patient's medications are kept if a medication cart is used. The medication is then administered in the amount and by the route ordered.

Adjunctive Nursing Intervention

Patients may have needs related to the dispensing of medications with which they require assistance. The needs may be physical ones, such as assisting them to positions for intramuscular injections, or they may involve explanations about the medications or guidance about other measures such as drinking fluids, which in some instances can enhance drug effectiveness and prevent complications. Some patients will convey fear about their medications. Careful listening by the nurse may provide answers to ways to assist patients. Patients may communicate information regarding their drugs, which needs to be communicated to physicians. Perhaps an analgesic is only effective for 10 or 15 minutes, another patient feels nauseated about 20 minutes after ingesting some drug, a third patient feels dizzy each afternoon at about the same time, and a fourth has pain in the right leg. This type of information needs to be noted. In some cases simple nursing measures such as the provision of milk with a medication can assist a patient with nausea; in other instances, it may be necessary for the physician to reassess the needs of the patient.

Recording

After the administration of the medications, this is recorded on the patient's chart on the appropriate record. Included in the recording should be the name of the drug, the dosage, the method of administration, specific relevant data such as the pulse rate of the patient, which is taken in most settings prior to the administration of digitalis, and any other pertinent information regarding the patient.

The recording should include the exact time of administration and in most agencies the signature of the nurse providing the medication. Often medications that are given regularly are recorded on a special flow record, whereas prn or stat medications are recorded separately on the nurse's notes.

Evaluation of the Effectiveness of the Drug

The effectiveness or lack of effectiveness of a medication can often be detected directly after its administration, as in the case of an intravenous administration, 10 to 20 minutes after an intramuscular or subcutaneous injection, and anywhere from immediately to several days after an orally administered drug. For example, the ingestion of aluminum hydroxide gel (Amphojel) often provides almost immediate relief for a patient who has epigastric pain; on the other hand, an antibiotic may need to be administered for 3 or 4 days before the patient or the nurse perceives any effect.

The kinds of behavior that reflect the action or lack of action of a drug are as variable as the purposes of the drugs themselves. For the anxious patient, a tranquilizer may show its effect by behavior that reflects a lowered stress level, for example, a slower pace of speaking or fewer random movements. The effect of a sedative can often be measured by how a patient slept; the effect of an antispasmodic can be determined by a patient's pain. In all nursing activities, nurses need to be aware of the medications that a patient is taking and communicate the effectiveness as assessed by the patient and the nurse on the patient's chart and in some cases to the senior nurse and physician directly.

DEVELOPMENTAL CONSIDERATIONS IN ADMINISTERING MEDICATIONS

A knowledge of growth and development is essential for the nurse when administering medications to children. The nurse needs to be aware of how to approach a child and to know what particular explanations and methods are required. Adolescents, pregnant women, and elderly patients also have special needs.

Infants and Children

Oral Medications

Oral medications for children are usually prepared in liquid sweetened forms such as syrups to make them more palatable. Some drugs are not palatable, and in this case the nurse can disguise the taste with honey, jam, juice, or any suitable sweetener. The parents can often provide suggestions about what method is best for their child. Use of a necessary food such as milk or orange juice should be avoided as a vehicle of disguise because the child may become conditioned to refusing that particular food in the future. Artificial sweeteners are available and may be necessary for diabetic children. It should not be assumed that sweeteners are required for all children; for some a disguise is not necessary, and they may be content with a sip of juice or a mint before and after a medicine. Nurses are encouraged to have an awareness of the taste of the medications they are giving, which allows them to answer questions honestly. For example, in response to "Will it taste bad?" the nurse may reply, "It tastes like strawberry to me" or ". . . like sour lemon." "Tell me what you think it tastes like." Most children will accept this challenge to experiment and to learn.

For toddlers who are in the independent "No" stage, the nurse's ability to gain the child's cooperation is of utmost importance. It is common for toddlers to push medications away or to seal their mouths in refusal. This can be due in part to dislike of medicines, to a need to control the situation, and to a desire to be able to take the medicine independently. Helping the child to take the medication is often facilitated by holding the child on your lap, acknowledging his or her distaste for the medicine, offering a simple explanation about why it is needed, and expressing faith in the child's ability to learn, that the child will soon be able to manage this situation independently. A spoon, a glass, or a straw can be used when giving oral medicines to toddlers. A few words of praise also go a long way. As soon as possible, the child should be encouraged to participate as much as possible, for example, by holding the glass or by choosing between a straw or a spoon. Forcing medications is a futile exercise; it communicates hostility and engenders distrust. If the child does not spit out the medication in response to force, the child will no doubt intentionally vomit the medication soon after. It is important, too, that nurses not convey any negative attitudes they may have about the medicine to the child. For example, if the nurse strongly dislikes the drug, this should not be expressed to the child verbally or nonverbally.

By the age of 4 to 6 years children are generally able to take pills, although some learn to swallow pills as young as the age of 2. When teaching children to swallow pills, instruct them to put the pill near the back of the tongue and then to wash it down with water, milk, or juice. Recognition and praise will elicit the cooperation of most young children, and seeing other children taking their medicines will help.

When older children refuse to take medications, it is wise for the nurse to encourage them to talk about their feelings about the medicines and to encourage any suggestions they may have about the situation. It is ill advised for a nurse to coax or bribe a child. It is better to convey a manner of expectancy and of helpful cooperation. For example, it is better to say, "I have your green pill for you, Johnny" rather than "Johnny, will you please take your green pill?" If given a few choices, for example, about whether to receive a pill or a liquid, most children will cooperate more readily. On rare occasions a child's cooperation may not be elicited, and in this case the situation needs to be analyzed individually. If all attempts fail, the physician needs to be consulted.

Injectable Medications

Any procedure in which a needle is used elicits reactions of fear in children due to the anticipation of pain or the unfamiliarity of the situation or both. The nurse needs to acknowledge that some pain will be experienced. Denying this fact will only enhance a sense of distrust. For very small infants, the painful stimuli may not be experienced with the same sensitivity, since they have delayed reactions to stimuli. They also have limited previous experiences to conjure up anticipatory fear or anxiety. By the age of approximately 6 months, infants have memory associated with past pain experiences and therefore will begin to anticipate pain and cry when they see a needle and syringe. By the age of 10 months or a year, the infant may make active attempts to wriggle away or to push the equipment aside. Thus when administering injections to young children, precautions need to be taken to hold or restrain them and protect them from injury. After the injection, it is important for the nurse (or the parent) to cuddle and speak softly to the infant and give the child a toy to dissuade any

thoughts that the nurse is associated only with painful situations.

The reasoning ability of toddlers and preschoolers is immature. Thus an injection is often equated with punishment for some "bad" behavior, real or imagined, particularly for hospitalized children. They may believe their parents abandoned them for some reason and that therefore they do not want them or that they want them punished. Although it is difficult for children of this age to understand exactly why the procedure is necessary even with simple explanations, children who are prepared can and usually do muster up coping mechanisms. For example, one child who was to receive an immunization injection found the situation easier to deal with when he was encouraged to tell the nurse, "You better be quick!" All injections should be given as rapidly as possible, and children must be adequately restrained. Even though a child says, "I'll hold still," another nurse needs to be present for safety purposes. For some 4-year-olds, two nurses may be required to restrain the child. For methods of holding and restraining children, see Chapter 21.

All children, adolescents included, should be encouraged to vent their feelings before and after the treatment. Young children may do this in play; adolescents may require support for open discussion.

The participation of parents can often be elicited, although many parents choose not to be involved in restraining their children. If they do participate, they can often console or divert their children by having them squeeze their hand or a toy during the injection. Involving children by giving them a choice as to which side they want the injection on or by allowing older children to swab the site is helpful in gaining their cooperation.

The Elderly

Older people can present special problems in relation to medications. Most of their problems are related to physiologic changes, to past experiences, and to established attitudes toward medications.

Physiologic changes in the elderly usually involve decrement of the function of some organs. Memory is frequently altered, hearing and vision are less acute, circulation is less active, excreting rates are decreased, liver function is impaired, and constipation is frequent. The latter four situations are responsible for poor absorption of some medications and the cumulative effects and toxicity. For example, with the impairment of the circulation, the action of medications that are given intramuscularly or sub-

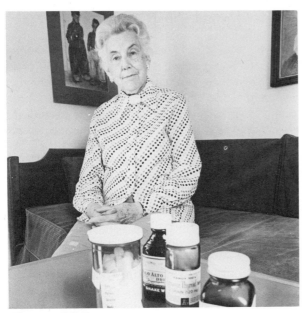

Figure 36-5. Elderly patients often receive many medications.

cutaneously can be delayed. Digitalis, which is frequently taken by elderly people, can accumulate to toxic levels and can cause a heart attack unless careful supervision is provided the patient.

It is not uncommon for elderly patients to take a dozen different medications daily. This number contributes to the incidence of increased errors in medications, regardless of whether the patient is taking medications independently at home or whether the medications are administered by nurses in an institution. The greater number of medications also compounds the problem of reciprocal drug interactions, because much is yet to be learned about the effects of drugs given in combinations. A general rule to follow is that elderly patients should take as few medications as possible (Figure 36-5).

The effects of certain drugs in the elderly are often increased but can also be decreased. Like the very young, the elderly person usually requires smaller dosages of drugs, especially of sedatives and other central nervous system depressants. Conversely, stimulants are required in higher doses. Reactions of the elderly to medications, particularly sedatives, are unpredictable and often bizarre in relation to the nature and dose of the drug. It is not uncommon to see irritability, confusion, disorientation, restlessness, and incontinence as a result of sedatives. Nurses therefore need to observe patients carefully for untoward reactions. Chloral hydrate and and paraldehyde have been found to be effective sedatives for these people. The use of alcohol (beer or brandy) as a bedtime relaxant and as an appetizer before meals is becoming more common. The moderate use of alcohol for people who are accustomed to it can contribute to their sense of well-being. Often elderly patients are advised to keep a supply of brandy in their homes.

Attitudes of elderly people toward medical care and medications vary from one person to another. It has been said that the elderly do not believe in the wisdom of the physician as readily as younger people. Certainly some are bewildered by the prescription of several medications because they grew up in an age when the number and availability of medications was limited. As a result some may passively accept their medications from nurses but not take them. Others may not believe in medications at all, thinking that they are not good for people, and may actively refuse them. This is one reason why the nurse is advised to stay with patients until they have taken the pills.

It is well for the nurse to remember, too, that the elderly are mature adults and capable of reasoning. Therefore explanations about the reason for the medicine and what effects they can expect should be offered, particularly for ambulatory geriatric patients. This can prevent the common occurrence of patients taking medications long after there is a need for them, or it can prevent patients from discontinuing the use of a drug when its continued use is essential to preserving their well-being. For example, patients should know that diuretics will cause them to urinate more frequently and will reduce ankle edema. Instructions about medications need to be given to all patients prior to discharge from a hospital. These instructions should include the times drugs are to be taken, the effects to expect, and when a physician should be consulted.

Because some patients are required to take several medications daily and because visual acuity and memory may be impaired it is important for the nurse, in consultation with the physician if necessary, to develop a simple but realistic plan for patients to follow at home. For example, most people, including the elderly, can have difficulties remembering to take drugs, but if they are planned to be taken with meal hours or at bedtime they are not as likely to forget. Some patients may take their medications and then an hour later not remember that they did take them. For these people the use of a special container or glass strictly for medications can be suggested. Then if the container or glass is empty, the person knows an hour later that he or she took the pills. Loss of visual acuity presents problems that can be overcome by writing out the plan in a large enough print that can be read. In some situations the help of a spouse or a son or daughter can be elicited advantageously.

ORAL MEDICATIONS

Oral medications are generally the least expensive and the most easily taken of all drugs. As long as a patient can swallow they are readily administered. Adjustments may need to be made if the patient is very young or very old or has difficulty swallowing solids. In these cases powders can often be mixed in a small amount of liquid for easier ingestion.

Most oral medications are absorbed in the small intestine, although small amounts can be absorbed through the oral and stomach mucosas. Sublingual medications, for example, are to a large degree absorbed into the capillaries under the tongue. Liquid medications are more readily absorbed in the stomach than are tablets or capsules. Some capsules are designed to dissolve in the stomach, whereas others dissolve in the presence of the intestinal juices. Some oral medicines are particularly irritating to mucous membranes. The unpleasant effects of such a drug can often be prevented by diluting the drug if it is a liquid or by advising the patient to take it after a meal when there is food in the stomach or with milk, unless the latter is contraindicated. For example, a drug such as tetracycline is less effective in the presence of milk.

The speed of absorption and degree of absorption of drugs from the gastrointestinal tract is to some degree unpredictable. It depends upon a number of factors, in particular the presence of food, which inhibits absorption. There are other disadvantages to the oral administration of some other medicines; for example, hydrochloric acid is irritating to oral and gastric mucosa and can damage a patient's teeth. This drug is normally well diluted with water and taken with a straw. Other drugs such as elixir of ferrous sulphate can stain a patient's teeth if these precautions are not taken in its administration. Some medications are inactivated to some degree by the gastrointestinal secretions, and therefore the length of time it takes for their absorption greatly affects the amount of effective drug absorbed.

Oral medications are contraindicated when a patient is vomiting, has a gastric or intestinal suction, or is unconscious and unable to swallow. Such patients in a hospital usually are on orders "nothing by mouth" (NPO, nothing per ora). For other patients who have difficulty swallowing, scored tablets can be broken, and other tablets can be crushed for easier swallowing. Enteric coated tablets and capsules should not be broken in this manner, however, because the coating is usually serving a purpose such as protecting the medicine from being inactivated by the gastric juices.

Procedure 36-1. Administration of an Oral Medication

Action	Explanation
Assemble Equipment	
1. Check the medication order for accuracy and recency. It should contain the following: a. The patient's name. b. The name of the drug dosage. c. Time for administration. d. Route of administration, for example, oral (p.o.), subcutaneous or hypodermic (H), intramuscular (IM), or intravenous (IV).	Records of medication orders include the physician's order, which is usually on the patient's chart, the Kardex record, and the medicine card. The medicine card needs to be checked against the physician's order. This is the safest check. In some settings a medication Kardex is used instead of medicine cards. This Kardex is usually kept in the medicine room or in the medication cart.
2. Clarify any discrepancies in the order with the senior nurse or the physician, whichever is appropriate in the agency.	
3. Arrange the medicine cards in a logical order for distribution.	To be efficient and avoid unnecessary work, nurses should distribute the drugs going from one room to another, not retracing steps.

Procedure 36-1.   Cont'd.

4. Wash hands.

This removes any microorganisms, thus assisting to keep medicine and equipment clean and helping prevent transfer of microorganisms from one patient to another.

5. After reading the medicine card, take the appropriate medicine from the shelf, drawer, or refrigerator.

The medicine may be in a refrigerator if it is to be kept cold. Medicines are dispensed in bottles, boxes, and envelopes.

6. Compare the label on the medicine container with the order on the medication card or order on the chart.

If these are not identical as to information, return to the patient's chart for a recheck. If there is still a discrepancy, check with the senior nurse.

7. Pour, select, or prepare the medication (see specific techniques). Capsules or tablets may be first poured into the cap, or, if not used, the cap is placed upside down. Liquid medication should be poured with the label next to the palm or up. Some special dispensers allow only one medicine to be poured at one time.

After preparation of the medication, again check the medicine card as to the patient's name, drug, dosage, route, and time of administration.

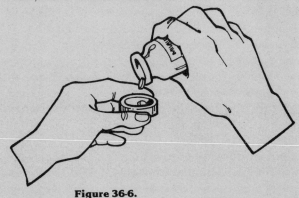

Figure 36-6.

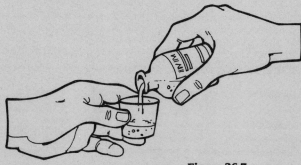

Figure 36-7.

8. Place the medicine or medication card on the tray or cart.

9. Return the bottle to its storage place.

Read the label again.

To Administer Oral Medication
1. Check the patient's identification band with the name on the medicine card. For unit dosages, check with the name or the package label.

Most patients will have an identification band on their wrist or have similar identification, which may also include a hospital number. An identification check may also be made in some instances by asking patients their names.

2. Explain the procedure to the patient as it is indicated. Adjust the explanation to the patient's needs.

3. Assist bed patients to a sitting position if possible. A lateral position is the next safest and easiest.

    A person lying on the back may aspirate the drug when swallowing.

4. Give water or fluid with oral medication, and give one medication at a time.

5. Stay with the patient until all medicines are swallowed.

    If patient has difficulty swallowing, suggest that the patient place the medicine on the back of the tongue before taking the water.

6. Wash hands.

7. Record the medication given, dosage, time, any complaints of the patient, and the signature of the nurse. If there are other patients who require medications, give these out before charting.

8. Replace supplies in the appropriate place.

    Wipe the tray, rinse medicine cups if they are to be washed, or dispose of disposable containers.

9. Return the medicine card to the slot of next time due.

Note: Some medications present special problems to patients.

1. For a medicine that has an unpleasant taste, provide orange juice, for example.

2. For a medicine that can stain teeth, advise the patient to drink water after the medicine.

3. For a medicine that can irritate the mucous membrane, dilute it with a liquid.

4. Some medications, such as aluminum hydroxide gel (Amphojel) and nitroglycerine, are normally left at the bedside; others should never be left there.

5. Do not return poured medicines to the stock supply. Either return them to the medicine cupboard with medicine care for a later administration, or dispose of them in their container in the medicine area.

SUBCUTANEOUS INJECTIONS

Subcutaneous administration is the injection of a drug into the subcutaneous (below the skin) tissue of the body. This method of administration has a number of advantages. The drug is almost completely absorbed from the tissues, provided that the blood circulation is normal. Thus the amount of drug that is absorbed is predictable. Subcutaneous injection does not depend upon a patient being conscious nor upon a patient who can swallow. The drug administered in this manner generally acts in 30 minutes. The chief disadvantage of this method, as is true of all methods of parenteral administrations, is that the skin is broken by the insertion of a needle. Breaking the skin barrier can potentiate an infection, particularly if aseptic technique is not employed.

Equipment

Syringes

There are several kinds of syringes that are used for subcutaneous injections. Three most commonly used types are the standard hypodermic syringe, the insulin syringe, and the tuberculin syringe. Most syringes used today are made of plastic, are individually packaged for sterility, and can be disposed of together with the needles once they have been used. Nondisposable glass syringes may be used in some areas. Once these are used, they need to be resterilized before further use.

Hypodermic syringes come in 2, 2.5, and 3 ml sizes. These syringes usually have two scales marked upon them, the minim and the milliliter. The milliliter scale is the one normally used; the minim scale is used for very small dosages, such as epinephrine minims ℥ "H."

Insulin syringes are similar to hypodermic syringes except that they have a scale especially designed for insulin. Insulin syringes have a 100-unit

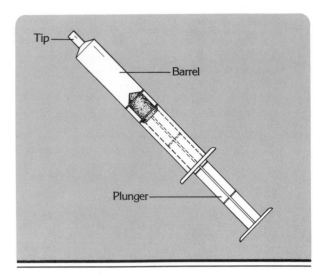

Figure 36-9.   The parts of a syringe.

calibrated scale intended for use with U100 insulin. This scale is replacing the U40 and U80 scales used for 40-unit and 80-unit insulin. These syringes are also available in both disposable and nondisposable types. (See Figure 36-8 for the three Types of Syringes.)

The tuberculin syringe was designed to administer tuberculin. It is a narrow syringe and is calibrated in tenths and hundredths of a milliliter (up to 1 ml) on one scale and in sixteenths of a minim (up to 1 minim) on the other scale. This type of syringe can also be useful in administering other drugs, particularly when small or precise measurement is indicated.

There are other sizes of syringes, for example, the 5, 10, 20, and 50 ml syringe. These are not generally used to administer drugs directly to patients but often are useful, for example, when adding sterile solutions to intravenous flasks or for irrigating wounds.

All syringes have three parts: the tip of the syringe, which connects with the needle, the barrel or outside part, on which the scales are printed, and the plunger or part that fits inside the barrel. (See Figure 36-9 for parts of a syringe.)

Needles

Needles can be made of stainless steel or other metals, and they also can be disposable. A needle has three discernible parts: the hub is the larger part of the needle, which fits onto the syringe, the cannula or stem is the long part, which connects to the hub, and the bevel of the needle is the slanted part at the end. The bevel may be short or long. The longer bevel pro-

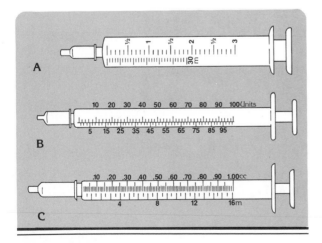

Figure 36-8.   Three kinds of syringes. **A,** Hypodermis; **B,** insulin; and **C,** tuberculin.

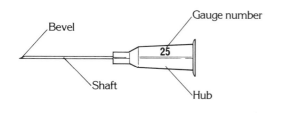

Figure 36-10.   The parts of a needle.

vides the sharpest needle, and it is used for subcutaneous and intramuscular injections. Short bevels are used for intravenous injections where a long bevel might become occluded if it rests against the side of a blood vessel. (See Figure 36-10 for the parts of a needle.)

Needles used for injection have three variables: the slant of the bevel, the length of the cannula, which varies from ⅜ to 5 inches, and the gauge or diameter of the cannula, which varies from no. 14 to 27. The larger the gauge number, the smaller the diameter of the cannula. For subcutaneous injections it is usual to use a needle no. 24 to 26 gauge, ⅜ to ⅝ inch long (1 to 1.5 cm). Obese patients may require a 1-inch

needle. For intramuscular injections a longer needle with a larger gauge is used, for example, gauge no. 20 to 22 and 1 to 1½ inches long. (See Figure 36-11 for relative sizes of needles.)

Syringes and needles can be obtained together or separately. Plastic disposable syringes and needles in their individual sterile plastic containers with a plastic needle protector are frequently used today.

Ampules and Vials

Ampules and vials are frequently used to package parenteral medications. An *ampule* is a glass container usually designed to hold a single dose of a drug. The ampule is made of clear glass, and it has a particular shape with a constricted neck. Some ampule necks have colored marks around them. Frequently the drug will be in the upper stem of the ampule above the neck as well as in the main portion of the ampule. Before opening, nurses need to flick the upper stem several times with their fingernails to bring all the medication down to the main portion of the ampule. Ampules that do not have a necklike constriction do not have this problem. (See Figure 36-12 for a vial, ampule, and ampule file.)

The neck is then scored with a small file if it has not been prescored on the colored line if one is present. If the neck of the ampule is scored on opposite sides, even thick ampules will open readily. The nurse then places a piece of sterile gauze on the far side of the ampule neck and breaks off the top by bending it outward. The sterile gauze serves to protect the nurse's fingers from the glass.

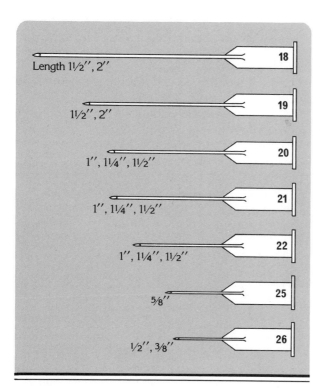

Figure 36-11.   The sizes of hypodermic needles commonly used.

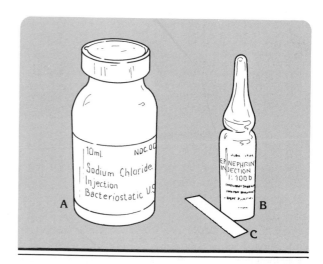

Figure 36-12.   A, vial; B, ampule; and C, ampule file.

Some ampules are prescored and do not require marking; however, a sterile gauze still needs to be used to prevent the nurse's fingers from being cut. To remove the medication from the bottom of the ampule, the hypodermic needle is inserted, and the amount of drug required for the dosage needs to be withdrawn. In a single-dose ampule this may necessitate holding the ampule slightly on its side to obtain the last milliliter of medication.

A *vial* is a small glass bottle with a sealed rubber cap. Vials come in different sizes from the single-dose vial to multidose, for example, 50 ml. Vials usually have a metal cap over the rubber one for protection of the rubber; it can be readily removed. The rubber cap is first cleansed with a disinfectant, often 70% alcohol on a swab, which is rubbed in a rotary motion. The needle is then inserted into the vial through the rubber cap. Air equal to the volume of fluid to be removed has already been drawn into the syringe. This air is then injected into the vial. The amount of drug is then withdrawn into the syringe by holding the vial upward at eye level.

Sites

The site of the subcutaneous tissue that is used for a hypodermic injection is usually the outer aspect of the upper arm and the anterior aspect of the thighs. These are convenient areas for injections, and they normally offer adequate area and have satisfactory circulation. Patients who administer their own injections, for example, those who have diabetes mellitus, will usually use the subcutaneous tissue of the anterior thighs and abdomen. Sites on the upper back below the scapulae are also used by nurses and physicians when administering subcutaneous injections. (See Figure 36-13 for sites commonly used for subcutaneous injections.)

It is often advisable to alternate sites if a patient is taking or receiving a number of injections. Often patients who administer their own injections will have a plan for alternative sites.

Administration

To administer a subcutaneous injection the skin site is cleansed; then the syringe is held so that the needle is at approximately a 90° or 45° angle with the skin. The bevel of the needle should be upward. A 90° angle is normally used with a ⅝ inch needle or longer for obese patients. A 45° angle is more commonly used with a needle ½ inch long or longer for the average patient. (See Figure 36-14 and Procedure 36-2.) The

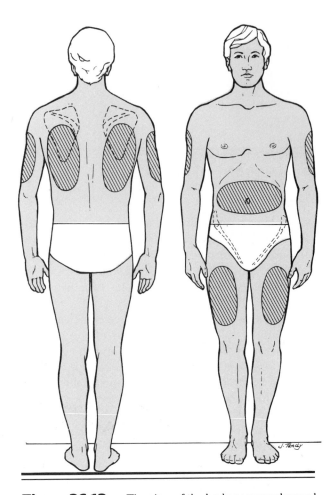

Figure 36-13.   The sites of the body commonly used for subcutaneous injections.

plunger is withdrawn, and if no blood appears, the medication is injected into the tissue. The needle is then withdrawn quickly, and the site is massaged with sterile antiseptic gauze.

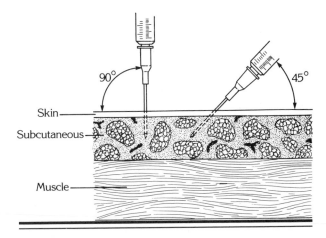

Figure 36-14.   For a subcutaneous injection the needle enters the skin at a 45° or 90° angle.

Procedure 36-2.   **Administration of a Subcutaneous Injection**

Action	**Explanation**

Assemble Equipment

1. Follow steps 1 to 5 of Procedure 36-1.

2. Select an appropriate needle and syringe. The needle size should be ⅜ to ⅝ inches (1 to 1.5 cm) long with a no. 24 to 26 gauge. The syringe size should be 2 or 3 ml unless an insulin or tuberculin syringe is indicated.

   The needle size is selected according to the depth of insertion and viscosity of the drug. A ½-inch needle will penetrate the subcutaneous tissues. The small bore allows nonviscous medications for subcutaneous use to pass easily.

3. Attach the needle to the syringe without removing it from its protective covering. (This step may not be necessary if the syringe and needle are packaged together as one unit.) Make sure the needle is on securely by grasping the needle hub and turning the syringe clockwise to tighten it.

4. Antiseptic swab.

   To cleanse the site.

5. Prepare the drug dose:
   From a vial:

   a. Cleanse the rubber stopper of the vial with an antiseptic swab (70% alcohol). Rub it in a rotary motion. Discard the swab.

   To decontaminate the stopper and lessen the chance of introducing microorganisms into the vial when the needle is inserted.

   b. Remove the needle cover by pulling it straight off the needle. Put it on the medicine tray or on the opened sterile syringe package.

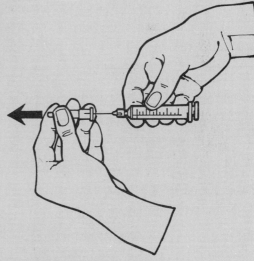

Figure 36-15.

   c. Put an amount of air into the syringe that is equal to the volume of the medicine to be withdrawn. This is done by grasping the syringe with one hand and pulling back on the plunger with the other hand. Hold the syringe inverted, erect, and at eye level.

851

Procedure 36-2.   Cont'd.

d. Inject the air through the rubber stopper into the vial. This is done by grasping and inverting the vial in one hand (between the thumb, index finger, and third finger) while holding the inverted syringe in the other hand. The barrel of the syringe is held between the thumb and index fingers. The fourth finger can be used to secure the plunger.

Air initially increased the pressure in the vial, thus facilitating withdrawal of the drug. After the drug is withdrawn, this air pressure returns to normal in the vial because the equivalent volume of medicine has been withdrawn.

Inversion of the vial and syringe allows the nurse to work at eye level and withdraw an accurate dose.

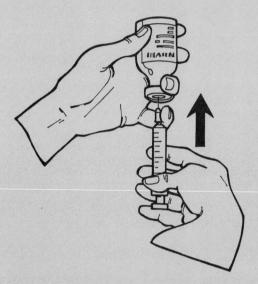

Figure 36-16.

e. Withdraw the prescribed amount of medication by keeping the bevel of the needle immersed in the solution.

Air will be drawn into the syringe if the bevel of the needle is not immersed in the solution.

f. Remove the needle from the vial while holding the barrel of the syringe securely.

Securing the barrel ensures that the dose is not changed.

g. Cover the needle immediately with its protective sterile cover. Place the needle straight into the center of the sheath without touching the outer rim. If a protective cover is not available, the needle may be protected between two sterile gauzes.

To prevent contamination of the needle during transport to the patient.

h. Place the syringe on the tray.

i. Dispose of the vial or return it to its storage place.

From an ampule:

a. First remove any medication that is lodged in the head of the ampule by flicking the head with your index fingernail or by grasping the top of the vial and shaking it down with a flick of the wrist.

b. Open the ampule by filing across the marked line and then breaking off the top. Protect your index finger with a piece of sterile gauze and break the top away from you.

To protect yourself from injury.

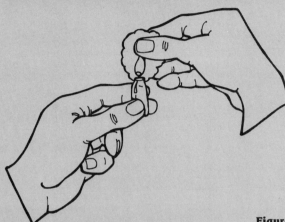

Figure 36-17.

c. Remove the needle cover as described.

d. Insert the needle into the ampule without touching the sides of the ampule. Insert the needle, if it is long enough, to the base of the ampule, without inverting the ampule. The ampule will need to be lifted if the needle does not reach the base. Once an ampule is opened, it is not airtight and therefore does not require air injection prior to withdrawal of the medication.

To maintain the sterility of the needle.

The medication will spill if the ampule is totally inverted.

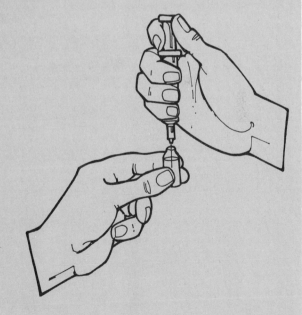

Figure 36-18.

e. Withdraw the medicine into the syringe.

f. Cover the needle as described.

g. Dispose of the ampule and any unused solution.

To Administer a Subcutaneous Injection

1. Explain to the patient what you plan to do. Adjust the explanation to the patient's needs.

To reassure the patient about what will happen. To identify the patient.

Procedure 36-2.   Cont'd.

2. Select the site.

Use a site that has not been used frequently. Check agency policy.

3. Provide privacy if the site necessitates exposure of the patient.

To avoid embarrassment.

4. Wash hands.

To avoid transferring microorganisms to the patient.

5. Cleanse the site with an antiseptic swab using a circular motion. Start at the center and widen the circle outward.

This step varies. Some think the antiseptic lessens the number of microorganisms; others think that cleansing destroys the normal antibacterial properties of the skin.

6. Remove the needle cover.

7. Expel any air bubbles from the syringe by inverting the syringe and gently pushing on the plunger until a drop of solution can be seen in the needle bevel. For some air bubbles it may be necessary to first flick the side of the syringe barrel. Some small bubbles that adhere to the plunger are of no consequence.

Expelling air ensures that the correct amount of solution is being administered.

8. Insert the needle by:
    a. Pinching or spreading the skin at the site with one hand.

Pinching the skin is thought to desensitize the area somewhat and thus lessen the sensation of needle insertion. Spreading the skin can make it more firm and facilitate needle insertion.

    b. Piercing the skin with the needle at a 45° angle with the bevel upward (for short needles such as for insulin injections a 90° angle may be used).
    c. Using a firm steady push on the needle.

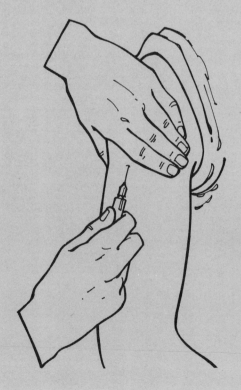

Figure 36-19.

9. Aspirate by pulling back on the plunger. If blood appears in the syringe, withdraw the needle slightly and aspirate again. If blood continues to appear, withdraw the needle and prepare a new injection. If blood does not reappear, it is safe to administer the medication.

To determine whether a blood vessel has been inadvertently entered.

10. Inject the medication by holding the syringe steadily and slowly pushing on the plunger.

Holding the syringe steady minimizes discomfort for the patient.

11. Remove the needle quickly, pulling with the line of insertion.

12. Massage the site with a sterile alcohol sponge.

This is thought to disperse the medication in the tissues and thus facilitate its absorption.

13. If bleeding occurs, apply pressure to the site until it stops, and apply an adhesive bandage if needed.

Bleeding rarely occurs with a subcutaneous injection.

14. Dispose of supplies according to agency procedure. Needle covers should be reapplied.

To protect yourself and others from injury and contamination.

15. Assist the patient to a comfortable position.

16. Wash hands.

17. Record the medication given, dosage, time, route, any complaints of the patient, and the signature of the nurse.

18. Replace supplies in an appropriate place.

Dispose of the needle and syringe according to agency policy.

INTRAMUSCULAR INJECTIONS

The intramuscular injection route is ordered frequently by physicians. It is generally indicated for medications that are irritating to subcutaneous tissue, for example, penicillin and paraldehyde. The speed of absorption is faster than by the subcutaneous route because of the greater blood supply to the body muscles. Muscles can also usually take a larger volume of fluid without discomfort than subcutaneous tissues, although the amount is highly variable between people, chiefly depending upon the size of the muscle and its condition.

Only healthy muscles should be used for injections. A normal healthy muscle has the following characteristics:

1. It is soft when relaxed and firm when tensed.

2. In the relaxed state there are no hardened masses palpable.

3. Firm palpation is not uncomfortable to the patient.

If a muscle is painful to touch or if there are any hardened areas in evidence, the use of that muscle for an injection is usually contraindicated. Areas with complications such as abscesses, necrotic and sloughing tissue including skin, and damaged nerves and bones are to be avoided. During the injection, damage to a nerve can cause the patient pain and perhaps permanent disability. Damage to bones by a needle can result in an inflammatory reaction such as periostitis (inflammation of the periosteum of the bone), but this is extremely rare even when a bone is stuck during an injection. These complications are the chief advantages of using intramuscular injections.

The exact amount of medication that any muscle can comfortably absorb will vary, but usually 5 ml is considered to be the maximum dose for a large muscle. Babies, the elderly, and emaciated patients are usually unable to tolerate this amount; usually 2 ml is the maximum volume for them. Nurses must use their own judgment as to the safe maximum volume, considering (a) the size of the muscle, (b) the health of the muscle, and (c) the adequacy of the blood supply.

Intramuscular Injection Sites

Selecting the appropriate site for an intramuscular injection is a critical factor in this type of administration. Not only should a large healthy muscle be used, but there are other considerations, such as the proximity of large nerves and blood vessels, the condition of the skin, its freedom from abrasions and infections, and the degree of irritation of the drug. When a person is receiving a number of injections, it is best to rotate the sites so that one muscle is not overused and overirritated. A number of sites are normally used. In babies and very young children the quadriceps muscles on the anterior and lateral aspects of the thighs are the sites of choice. The gluteal muscles of babies and children before they walk are not usually well developed for injections. The proximity of the large sciatic nerve and the danger of damaging it usually mitigates against the use of the gluteal muscles of the buttocks in all young children up to the age of about 3 years.

Dorsogluteal Site

The dorsogluteal site utilizes the gluteus maximus muscle for the injection. The exact site is the upper outer aspect of the upper outer quadrant of the buttock, about 2 to 3 inches below the crest of the ilium. To find the exact spot, the buttock can be divided into four quadrants with imaginary lines. The crest of the ilium can be palpated for the superior aspect, and the gluteal fold is the inferior aspect. The medial aspect is the medial fold, and the lateral is the side of the buttock. From these landmarks the upper outer quadrant is established. Then the upper outer aspect of this quadrant is established. (See Figure 36-20.)

A second method to establish this site is to draw an imaginary line from the posterior superior iliac spine to the greater trochanter of the femur. This line is lateral to and parallel to the sciatic nerve; therefore a site selected laterally and superiorly to this line will be away from the sciatic nerve and major blood vessels. (See Figure 36-20.) Again the landmarks should be palpated rather than estimated with the eye.

The dorsogluteal sites are generally used for adults rather than babies and children. The patient lies on the stomach, and when the toes are pointed medially, the muscles will generally be in a relaxed state for the injection.

Ventrogluteal Site

The ventrogluteal site uses the gluteus medius and gluteus minimus muscles for the injection. It is con-

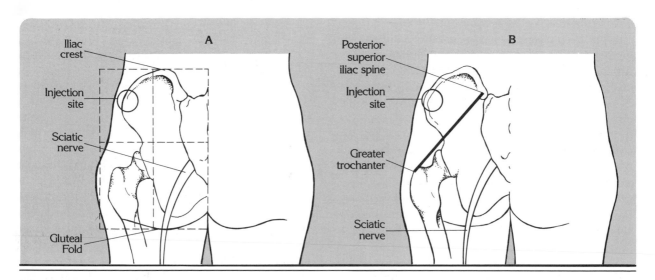

Figure 36-20.   Two methods to establish the dorsogluteal site for an intramuscular injection.

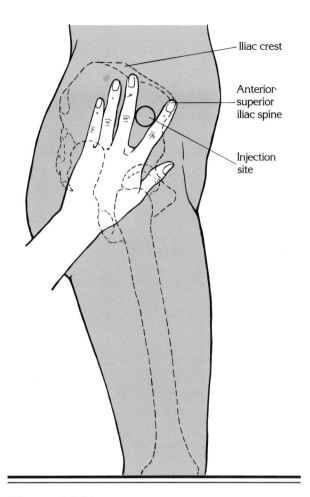

Figure 36-21. The ventrogluteal site for an intramuscular injection.

sidered to be a highly desirable site for babies, children, and adults. There are no large nerves or blood vessels in the area, and there is usually less fatty tissue than in the dorsogluteal site. Because it is more remote from the rectal area it tends to be less contaminated, which is a consideration for small babies.

To locate the exact site the nurse's hand rests on the patient's hip, the fingers pointing toward the patient's head. The opposite hand is used for the opposite buttock, for example, right hand for left hip and left hand for the right hip. With the index finger on the anterior superior iliac spine, the middle finger is stretched dorsally, palpating the crest of the ilium and then pressing just below it. The triangle formed between the index finder, the third finger, and the crest of the ilium is the injection site. (See Figure 36-21.)

The patient can lie on either the back or side for this injection. If the gluteal muscles feel tense, they can be relaxed by flexin~ the knees for the injection.

Quadriceps Site

The site of choice for babies and small children and sometimes for adults is the quadriceps. (See Figure 36-22.) It is a safe area in which there are no major nerves or blood vessels. It has the advantage for patients who administer their own medications in that it is easily reached. Its chief disadvantage is that an injection in that site causes discomfort for some people.

Rectus Femoris Site.   The muscle chiefly used is the rectus femoris muscle, which is located on the anterior aspect of the thigh.

Vastus Lateralis Site.   The vastus lateralis is usually a thick muscle and is situated on the anterior-lateral aspect of the thigh. The middle third of the muscle is suggested as the site. It can be established by dividing the area from the greater trochanter of the femur to just above the knee. Again there are no large nerves

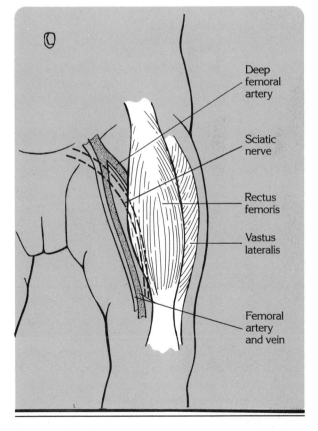

Figure 36-22. The vastus lateralis and rectus femoris muscles of the upper thigh used for intramuscular injections.

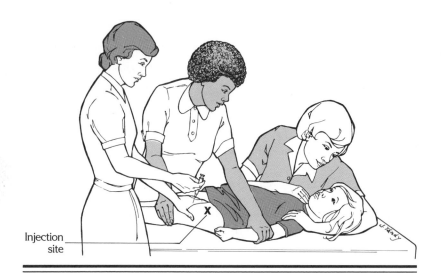

Figure 36-23.   The position of a child for an intramuscular injection.

Injection site

or blood vessels in the area. The patient lies on the back for an injection in this site.

Figure 36-23 shows the position of a child for an intramuscular injection.

Deltoid and Triceps Sites

The deltoid muscle is seldom used for intramuscular injections because it is normally smaller than the previously mentioned muscles. It can be found on the lateral aspect of the upper arm about 1 to 2 inches inferior to the acromion process. If it is to be used, only small volumes of medication should be injected, and care must be taken to avoid the radial nerve, which is in the area.

The posterior triceps muscle is located on the posterior aspect of the patient's upper arm. The site of choice is about midway between the acromion process and the olecranon process of the ulna (elbow).

Equipment

The equipment used for an intramuscular injection is similar to that required for subcutaneous administration. The major difference is the needle, which usually needs to be longer and of greater diameter to reach the muscle and so that it will not break. If a needle appears bent in any way, it should not be used, since the bent area is probably weakened and could break while it is in the patient's tissue. Usually a no. 20, 21, or 22 gauge needle is used, depending upon the thickness of the liquid medication. The lower gauge number is used for the thicker drug; however,

it causes more discomfort than a thinner needle. The length of the needle will depend upon the site of the injection and the amount of adipose tissue on the patient. For adults a 1½-inch needle is usually used, although 3-inch needles are manufactured. For babies and children a shorter needle, ¾ to 1 inch, is usually required.

Preparation

The injection is prepared much as for a subcutaneous injection. One difference is that a small bubble of air of 2 or 3 minims can be left in the syringe. This bubble will force the last drops of medication into the muscle before the needle is withdrawn. The advantage of this practice is that the dosage of drug received by the patient is exact and there is no spillage of a drug, which may be irritating, into the body tissue when the needle is withdrawn.

Administration

The patient is first assisted to a position that facilitates the relaxation of the muscle to be injected and that is comfortable. The area of the skin is cleansed, and then the syringe is held at a 90° angle and quickly and firmly inserted through the skin into the muscle. As in a subcutaneous injection it is then ascertained whether the needle is in a blood vessel; if it is not, the drug is then injected, the needle withdrawn quickly, and the area massaged with the antiseptic swab.

Procedure 36-3.   Administration of an Intramuscular Injection

Action	Explanation

Assemble Equipment

1. Follow steps 1 to 5 in Procedure 36-1.

2. Select an appropriate needle and syringe. The needle size should be 1 to 1 ½ inches (2.5 to 3.7 cm) long and a no. 21 or 22 gauge. Syringe size is commonly 2 or 3 ml, although 5 ml may be safely administered to adults in the iliac region.

The needle must be long enough to penetrate intramuscular tissue. For more viscous medicines, use larger gauges (smaller numbers).

3. See steps 3 and 4 under Procedure 36-2 for preparing the drug dose from a vial or from an ampule. Some agencies recommend that a small air bubble (1 or 2 minims) be left in the syringe, particularly for drugs that are irritating to subcutaneous tissue.

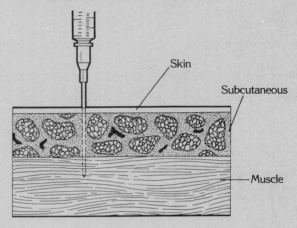

Figure 36-24.

4. Antiseptic swab.

To cleanse site.

To Administer an Intramuscular Injection

1. Explain to the patient what you plan to do. Adjust the explanation to the patient's needs.

To reassure the patient through knowledge of what will happen. To identify the patient.

2. Select the site.

Use site that has not been used frequently. Check agency policy.

3. Provide privacy if the site necessitates exposure of the patient.

4. Wash hands.

To avoid transferring microorganisms to the patient.

5. Cleanse the site with an antiseptic swab.

6. Remove the needle cover.

See step 3 under "Assemble Equipment."

7. Expel air bubbles unless one is to be left.

8. Insert the needle by:
   a. Stretching the skin at the site or displacing it to one side (Z-track technique). See "Z-track injection," which follows this procedure.
   b. Piercing the skin with the needle at a 90° angle.
   c. Using a quick dartlike thrust of the needle and syringe.

Stretching the skin makes it more firm and facilitates needle insertion. Moving the tissue to one side helps to enclose the medication in the muscle. As the needle is removed, subcutaneous tissue slides back over the needle opening of the muscle.
This angle must be used to penetrate the intramuscular tissues.

9. See steps 11 to 18 under Procedure 36-2 for aspirating, injecting the medication, removing the needle, and massaging the site.

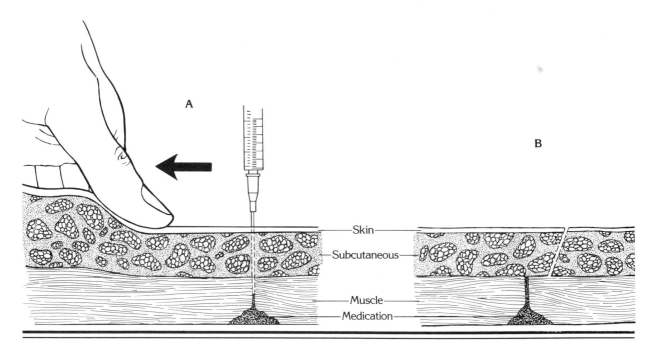

Figure 36-25. A Z-tract intramuscular injection. **A,** Skin pulled to one side for the injection; and **B,** the interrupted tract, which keeps the medication from seeping along the tract when the skin returns to its normal position.

Z-Track Injection

Pull the skin of the patient laterally, then insert the needle at a 90° angle as for a regular intramuscular injection. Withdraw the plunger; if no blood appears, inject the medicine. Wait 10 seconds. Remove the needle, then let the skin return to its normal position. Do not massage (see Figure 36-25).

INTRADERMAL INJECTION

An *intradermal (intracutaneous) injection* is the administration of a drug into the dermal layer of the skin just beneath the epidermis. Usually only a small amount of liquid volume is used, for example, 2 or 3 minims. This method of administration is frequently indicated when testing for allergies, for tuberculin testing, and for vaccinations.

Sites

Common sites for intradermal injections are the inner aspect of the lower arm, the upper aspect of the chest, and the back of the patient beneath the scapulae. See Figure 36-26.

Figure 36-26. Sites of the body commonly used for intradermal injections.

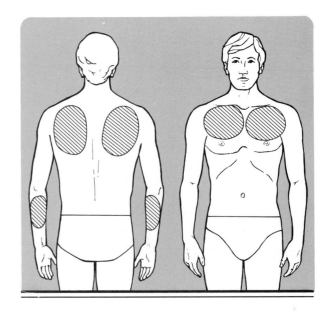

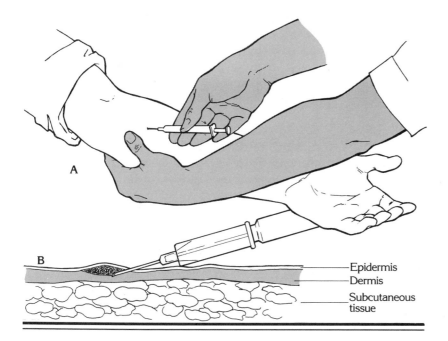

Figure 36-27. For an intradermal injection the needle enters the skin at a 15° angle, **A.** The medication forms a bleb under the epidermis, **B.**

Epidermis
Dermis
Subcutaneous tissue

Equipment

The equipment normally used is a small syringe as is used in a subcutaneous injection or a special syringe such as a tuberculin syringe (see "Subcutaneous Injections"). The needle used is a fine one, frequently a no. 26 gauge, ⅜ inch long.

Preparation

The preparation is similar to that described for a subcutaneous injection.

Administration

After the site is cleansed, the skin is held tautly, and the syringe is held at about a 15° angle to the skin with the bevel of the needle upward. The needle is thrust through the epidermis into the dermis, and then the fluid is injected. The drug will produce a small bleb just under the skin of the patient. (See Figure 36-27.) The needle is then withdrawn quickly, and the site is very lightly massaged with the disinfected swab. Intradermal injections are absorbed slowly through the blood capillaries in the area.

TOPICAL APPLICATIONS

Topical drugs come in a number of forms; emollients, lotions, powders, ointments, pastes, creams, and liniments are commonly used. The intention of a topical application is to have a local effect (upon the skin or mucous membrane at the site of the application). There are many reasons for the use of topical applications. The common actions are as follows:

1. To decrease itching (pruritus).
2. To lubricate and soften the skin.
3. To cause local vasoconstriction or vasodilatation.
4. To cause increased secretions or decreased secretions from the skin.
5. To provide a protective coating to the skin area.
6. To apply a drug such as an antibiotic or antiseptic for its effect upon bacteria that are present.

When topical drugs are applied to the skin or mucous membrane for the purpose of absorption, the process is called *inunction*. In applying such drugs the process of friction is involved, that is, they must be rubbed in. Drugs are not readily absorbed through the epidermis; however, they can be absorbed into the lining of the sebaceous glands and sweat pores. Absorption of the drugs is facilitated by washing the area well before the application, using a pharmaceutical preparation with a base such as alcohol, which mixes with fat, and using a drug that is fat soluble.

Emollients and Lotions

Both emollients and lotions are chiefly used to soothe irritated skin and mucous membranes. *Emollients* are oily substances, whereas *lotions* are liquids, which often carry an insoluble power, for example, calamine lotion. The lotion or emollient is poured onto sterile gauzes or cotton balls and then patted on the affected area. It is not rubbed on because rubbing serves to further irritate a rash or *pruritus* for which the lotion is being applied.

Powders

A powder is generally sprinkled on the area, usually after suitable cleansing, and then covered with a dressing so that it will stay on the site.

Ointments, Pastes, and Creams

Ointments and pastes are usually applied with a tongue blade or, for large areas, with gloves. Sterile technique is essential for any open wounds, and gloves should be worn in the presence of infected areas to protect the nurse and prevent transmission of the organisms.

The ointment or paste is taken out of the jar and placed on sterile gauze. Once the amount of ointment has been removed from the jar, the cap is replaced. The medicine is then spread on the area with firm, smooth strokes of the tongue blade. The affected area should be well covered but not overly covered. For opaque preparations no skin should be visible through the medicine. Some ointments need to be applied very thinly, such as cortisone.

Sterile dressings are often applied over the area so that the ointment or paste is not inadvertently wiped off, soiling the patient's clothes.

Creams are applied in the same manner as described above. In some situations nurses can use their hands rather than a tongue blade if there is no evidence of an open wound or an infection. In some instances creams are rubbed in with gentle firm strokes.

Liniments

Liniments are frequently applied to stimulate circulation to an area by vasodilatation of the capillaries. The liniment is poured onto the nurse's hands and then rubbed into the patient's skin with long, firm, smooth strokes. Gloves are normally not indicated for the application of a liniment.

The liniment should be at room temperature. A cold liniment will produce vasoconstriction of the area rather than dilation, and it is also uncomfortable for most patients.

INSERTIONS

An *insertion* is the placing of a medication into a body cavity such as the vagina, the rectum, or the urethra. Medications so administered are frequently prepared as suppositories; however, some tablets or ointments may also be used for insertion.

Vaginal Insertion

The patient voids before the procedure and then assumes a back-lying position with her knees flexed and hips rotated laterally. Vaginal medications can be administered by hand or with a special inserting device. Tablets and suppositories are usually inserted by hand, whereas ointments are usually inserted with a vaginal applicator. These applicators are either reusable or disposable. If the drug is to be inserted by hand, the nurse or patient should glove the hand to be used for the insertion, and the nurse should glove the other hand that exposes the orifice as well. The tablet or suppository is inserted about 3 ½ to 4 inches along the posterior fornix or posterior wall of the vagina in an adult. Note that the posterior wall of the vagina is about an inch longer than the anterior wall, since the cervix protrudes into the uppermost part of the anterior wall. To insert creams or jellies the applicator is normally inserted about 1½ to 2 inches, then the plunger is pushed forward, thus depositing the medication in the vagina. The applicator is gradually withdrawn as the cream is ejected. When the applicator is empty, it is withdrawn. (See Figure 36-28.) Usually

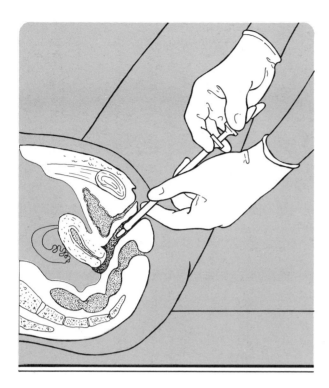

local effect, such as to reduce spasm. Sterile technique is used; however, the technique is not unlike that for the insertion of a rectal suppository. Refrigerating these suppositories prior to use facilitates their insertion. The urinary meatus and adjacent area are cleansed with a disinfectant. The nurse wears sterile gloves and gently inserts the suppository, which has been lubricated at the tip with a sterile water-soluble lubricant, into the urinary meatus. A sterile sponge is then placed against the urinary meatus to provide slight pressure until the spasms subside or until the suppository melts. This normally takes about 10 to 15 minutes.

Urethral suppositories can also be inserted using a sterile applicator. The end of the applicator is lubricated with a sterile water-soluble lubricant and then inserted about an inch into the urethra. The plunger is then pressed and the suppository ejected. The applicator is then withdrawn, and again pressure is placed on the urinary meatus with a sterile sponge for 10 to 15 minutes.

Figure 36-28.   A vaginal insertion using an applicator.

vaginal suppositories are kept in a refrigerator because they are more firm for insertion and they are designed to melt at body temperature.

Rectal Insertion

For a rectal insertion the patient best assumes a side-lying position with the upper leg acutely flexed. Usually suppositories rather than tablets are inserted into the rectum. They serve a variety of pruposes, such as softening feces, or they may be given for their systemic effect, such as aminophylline. The nurse gloves the hand to be used to insert the suppository and lubricates the suppository and the index finger with a water-soluble lubricant. The suppository is then removed from its wrapping and inserted smooth or rounded end first. The suppository is inserted past the anal sphincter (about 2½ to 3 inches) or the length of the index finger. The nurse's finger is then removed. (See Figure 36-29.)

Urethral Insertion

Urethral suppositories are longer and narrower than other suppositories. They are used primarily for their

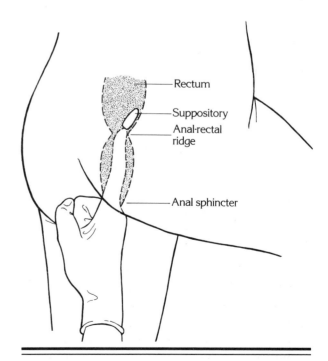

Rectum
Suppository
Anal-rectal ridge
Anal sphincter

Figure 36-29.   The insertion of a rectal suppository. Note correct placement of the suppository along the rectal wall beyond the anal-rectal ridge.

INSTILLATIONS

An *instillation* is defined precisely as the administration of a liquid drop by drop. In this section an instillation refers to the administration of liquids or ointments to the eyes, the ears, and the nose.

Eye Instillations

The cornea of the eye is a highly sensitive area, and yet drugs may need to act locally upon the cornea as well as the eyelids. These medications are administered in the form of liquid drops or ointments on the lower and in some cases the upper conjunctival sacs.

Instillation of Eye Drops

The patient best assumes a back-lying position with the head slightly hyperextended. The lids and lashes are wiped gently from the inner to the outer canthus. The eyes drain through the lacrimal apparatus situated in the inner aspect. The patient holds a piece of tissue in readiness to soak up the excess medication that leaves the eye.

The patient looks upward to the ceiling while the nurse places several fingers on the patient's cheek bone just below the affected eye. The number of drops of solution to be instilled are drawn into the eye dropper. The nurse draws the skin down by putting pressure on the cheek with a cotton ball. This exposes the lower conjunctival sac. The nurse then brings the dropper over the conjunctival sac using a side approach and instills the ordered number of drops in the center of the sac, holding the dropper 1 to

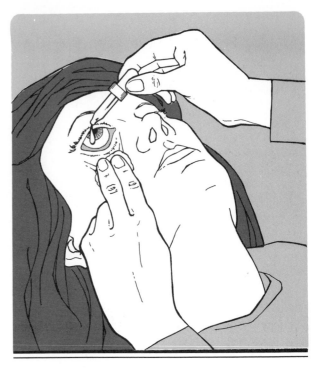

Figure 36-30.   Instillation of eye drops into the center of the lower conjunctival sac.

2 cm above the sac. (See Figure 36-30.) The drops are instilled into the central part or the outer part of the lower conjunctival sac. The dropper should touch neither the cornea nor the mucous membrane of the conjunctival sac. The skin is permitted to return to its normal position, and the patient closes the eye gently rather than squeezing it shut.

Procedure 36-4.   **Instillation of Liquid Drops in the Eye**

Action	Explanation
Assemble Equipment	
1. Sterile eye dropper.	To prevent contaminating the eye with foreign microorganisms.
2. Sterile cotton balls as needed.	
3. Saline solution as needed.	To cleanse the eyelids.

Procedure 36-4.   Cont'd.

4. Medication.

5. Treatment card or sheet.   To check the physician's prescribed medication.

6. Sterile eye dressings as needed.

7. Scotch tape as needed.   To secure eye dressing.

8. Tray or cart.   To carry equipment.

To Instill Eye Drops

1. Explain to the patient what you plan to do. Adjust   To reassure the patient through knowledge. To identify
    the explanation to the patient's needs.   the patient.

2. Assist the patient to a reclining or back-lying posi-   To facilitate instillation and ensure that the medication
    tion with the head slightly hyperextended.   will remain in the eye.

3. Wash hands.   To avoid transferring microorganisms to the patient.

4. Cleanse the lids and lashes of crusts by wiping   Lessens the chance of fluids spilling over to or con-
    from the inner to the outer canthus with a sterile   taminating the other eye and into the nasolacrimal
    gauze dampened with normal saline. This step is   duct.
    done only as required.

5. Prepare the number of drops of the ordered medi-
    cation into the eye dropper.

6. Instruct the patient to look upward to the ceiling   The patient is less likely to blink, and the cornea is
    and give him or her a piece of tissue to hold.   protected under the eyelid. The tissue can be used to
                                                              soak up excess medication.

7. Place fingers on patient's cheek bone just below   This minimizes the danger of touching the cornea and
    the eye or, if tissues are edematous, use cotton   prevents the patient from blinking or squinting.
    sponge.

8. The skin on the cheek is gently drawn down.   This exposes the lower conjunctival sac.

9. Using a side approach, instill the ordered drops   The patient is less likely to blink. The drops will not
    onto the outer third of the lower conjunctival sac.   harm the cornea as they might if dropped upon it. To
    Hold the dropper 1 to 2 cm above the sac.   prevent touching sac or the cornea of the eye. See
                                                              Figure 36-30.

10. Instruct the patient to close the eye gently.   This moves the medicine over the eye.

11. Wipe the lower lid from the inner cathus out.   To collect excess medication. The patient may also do
                                                              this with tissue.

12. Apply an eye pad as needed and secure it with   Cellophane tape is less irritating to the skin than adhe-
     Scotch tape.   sive tape and is removed more easily.

13. Assist the patient to a comfortable position.

14. Gather and dispose of equipment.

15. Wash hands.

16. Chart the name of the drug, number of drugs, eye   Include pertinent observations such as swelling, in-
     (right or left), time of instillation, and nurse's signa- flammation, discharge, or injection of eye.
     ture.

Instillation of Eye Ointment

For the insertion of an ointment into the eye, the patient assumes the same position and the nurse draws down the lower lid as described in Procedure 36-4. Holding the ointment in the other hand, the nurse approaches the eye from below, and the ointment (about 2 cm) is squeezed from the tube onto the conjunctival sac from the inner aspect to the lateral aspect. (See Figure 36-31, *B*.) The patient again closes the eye and moves it to spread the ointment unless this is contraindicated. The nurse discards a small amount of ointment on a clean cotton ball, wipes the top of the tube, and replaces the top.

Procedure 36-5. Instillation of Ointment in the Eye

Action	Explanation
Assemble Equipment	
1. Ointment.	As ordered by the physician.
2. Sterile cotton balls.	
3. Treatment card or sheet.	To check the physician's prescribed ointment.
4. Tray.	
To Instill Eye Ointment	
1. See steps 1 to 4 of Procedure 36-5.	
2. Discard the first bead of ointment from the container.	The top is considered potentially contaminated.
3. Draw the lower lid down.	

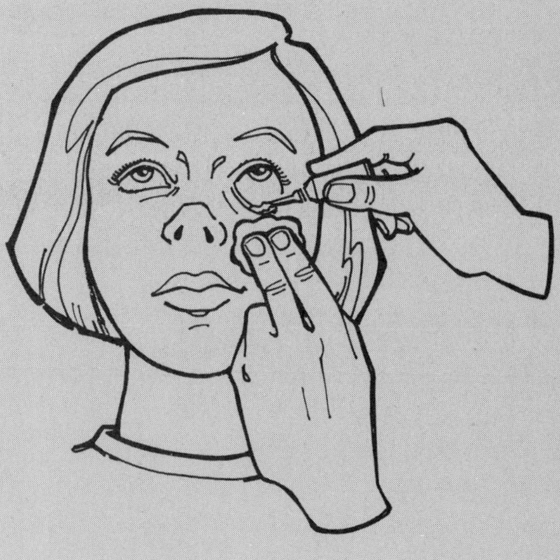

Figure 36-31.

4. Squeeze 2 cm of ointment from the tube into the lower conjunctival sac from the inner canthus out.	As for eye drops.
5. Discard a bead of ointment; replace the top.	To maintain the sterility of the remaining ointment.
6. The patient closes the eye gently and moves it if permitted.	Spreads medication.
7. Follow steps 7 to 11 of Procedure 36-4.	

Ear Instillation

Many ear instillations are done to insert a softening agent so that ear wax can be more easily removed later. The prescribed medication, the medicine dropper, and the medicine card are required.

The patient assumes a side-lying position. The external auditory meatus is wiped with a sterile cotton-tipped applicator. The ear is grasped in such a way as to straighten the ear canal. For adults the auricle is held up and back; for children it is held down and back. (See Figure 36-32.) The prescribed drops, which are normally at room temperature, are instilled. Then the tragus of the ear is pressed two or three times to assist the drops to move inward. The patient needs to remain in this position for about 5 minutes. A cotton ball in the external auditory meatus will catch the excess medication when the patient sits up.

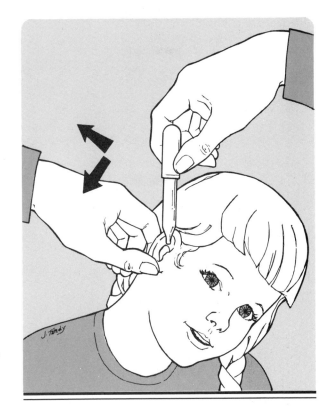

Figure 36-32.   Holding the ear for the instillation of drops into the external auditory canal of a child.

Procedure 36-6.   Instillation of Ear Drops

Action	Explanation
Assemble Equipment	
1. Bottle with dropper containing ordered medication.	
2. Medication card or treatment sheet.	To check the physician's order with the medication label. Check which ear.
3. Cotton-tipped applicators (sterile if needed).	To wipe the auditory meatus.
4. Tray or cart.	To carry equipment.
To Administer Ear Drops	
1. Explain to the patient what you plan to do. Adjust the explanation to the patient's needs.	To reassure the patient through knowledge of what will happen. To identify the patient.
2. Assist the patient to a backlying position with head turned to the side, affected ear turned upward.	So that the medication will enter the external ear canal.
3. Wash hands.	To transmit no microorganisms to the patient.

Procedure 36.6.   Cont'd.

4. Draw up into the dropper the amount of medicine to be instilled.

5. Straighten the ear canal.

For children, hold the lower ear lobe down and back. For adults, hold the upper auricle of the ear up and back.

6. Insert the tip of the ear dropper into the external ear canal.

Do not touch the canal, which may be sensitive or become irritated.

7. Instill the ordered number of drops. Drops should be at room temperature unless otherwise ordered.

To avoid discomfort for the patient.

8. Put the dropper on a tray with its top on a cotton ball.

To avoid contaminating the tray and transferring microorganisms.

9. Press gently but firmly on the tragus of the patient's ear two or three times.

To assist medication flow down the ear canal.

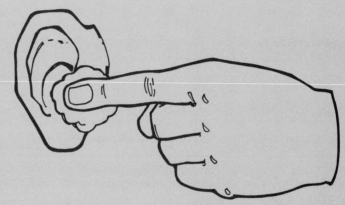

Figure 36-33.

10. Put a small cotton ball in the external ear. Remove it in 15 or 20 minutes.

To catch the excess medication that will flow out of the ear canal when the patient turns the head or sits up.

11. Assist the patient to a comfortable position.

12. Gather and dispose of equipment.

13. Wash hands.

14. Record the name of the drug, number of drops, ear (right or left), time of administration, and signature of the nurse.

Nose Instillation

Usually nose drops are instilled for their astringent effect (to shrink swollen mucous membranes) or to treat infections of the nasal cavity. The equipment required is the medication solution, which usually comes in a bottle with an attached dropper, disposable tissues, and a tray for the equipment. Sometimes an inhaler or atomizer is used instead of a dropper.

The patient assumes a dorsal recumbent position. A pillow under the shoulders will assist the patient to lower the head backward, thus facilitating the flow of the drops deep into the nasal cavity. The patient can also hang the head over the edge of the bed, where it needs to be supported by the nurse in order to avoid strain on the neck muscles. Once the head is lowered, it can remain in a straight line (Proetz position) or turn to one side (Parkinson position). The Proetz position is usually used for treating ethmoid and sphenoid sinuses. The Parkinson position is used to treat maxillary and frontal sinuses. (Figure 36-34 shows the two positions.)

Once the patient has assumed one of the above positions, the nurse administers the drops. The dropper is held just above the nostril, and the drops are directed toward the midline of the superior concha of the ethmoid. If the drops are directed toward the base of the nasal cavity, they will run down the throat instead of into the nasal cavity. The mucous membranes of the nostrils should not be touched to avoid injuring the tissue and contaminating the dropper. The patient needs to remain in this position for 5 to 10 minutes to permit the medication to be absorbed. Any additional medication in the dropper is discarded before being returned to the bottle. When an atomizer is used instead of drops, the patient assumes the same position and breathes through the nose with the mouth open.

After the absorption of the medication, the patient is assisted to a comfortable position. The instillation is recorded as for an ear instillation.

To administer nose drops to an infant, place a pillow under the infant's shoulders and allow the child's head to fall back over the edge of the pillow onto the nurse's arm. This arm can also be used to restrain the infant's arms. With the other hand administer the nose drops.

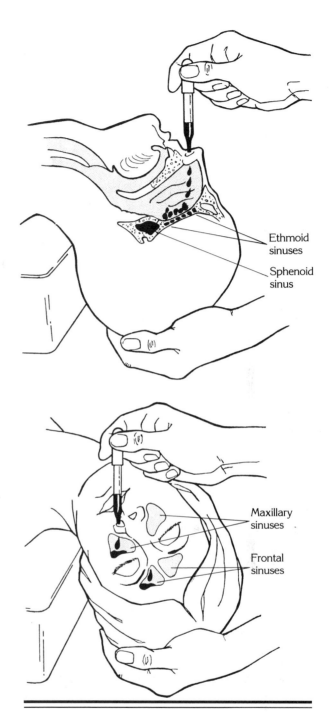

Figure 36-34. Positions assumed by a patient for the instillation of nose drops. **A,** Proetz position; and **B,** Parkinson position.

MIXING DRUGS

Frequently patients have more than one drug to be given by injection at the same time. To spare the patient from receiving two injections, two drugs (if compatible) are often mixed together in one syringe and given as one injection. The most common drugs given in this manner are two different types of insulin and injectable preoperative medications such as morphine or meperidine (Demerol) with atropine or scopolamine. Drugs are also mixed in intravenous solutions. Whenever a nurse is uncertain about drug compatibilities, a pharmacist should be consulted immediately.

Mixing Drugs from Two Vials

There are several types of insulin in vials, which have the same basic action in the body but vary according to their time of action. Some act within 2 hours and last for 8 to 10 hours, whereas others act within 6 hours and last for 24 to 36 hours. (See Table 36-5 for types of insulin and their actions.) Many hospitalized patients are given two types of insulin, short and long acting. These different types of insulin vary as to their content.

Chemically, insulin is a protein that, when hydrolyzed in the body, yields a number of amino acids. Some insulin preparations in addition have a modifying protein added such as globulin or protamine that slows the absorption. This fact is important when mixing two types of insulin preparations together for injection. Vials of insulins that do *not* have additional protein added should never be subjected to insulins from vials that do contain additional protein. For example, regular insulin (crystalline zinc insulin, CZ) should never be adulterated with other insulin such as protamine zinc, which has added protein.

To prepare two types of insulin in one syringe, the vial that has the protein added must first be prepared by injecting air into the vial, but it is drawn into the syringe last.

Example:	10 units of CZ (modified protamine zinc insulin) and 30 units of NPH insulin are to be administered to a patient at 0730 hours.
Step 1:	Inject 30 units of air into the NPH vial and withdraw the needle (there should be no insulin in the needle). The needle should not touch the insulin.
Step 2:	Inject 10 units of air into the CZ vial and immediately withdraw 10 units of CZ insulin.
Step 3:	Reinsert the needle into the NPH insulin vial and withdraw 30 units of NPH insulin (the air was previously injected into the vial).

Table 36-5.   Types of Insulin and Their Actions

Name and Classification	Onset of Action	Peak Action	Duration of Action	Time of Administration	Time When Hypoglycemic Reactions Can Occur
Rapid Acting					
Crystalline zinc (CZ)	Within 1 hour	2 to 4 hours	5 to 8 hours	Before meals and when needed	Between meals
Regular	Within 1 hour	2 to 4 hours	5 to 8 hours		Between meals
Semilente	Within 1 hour	6 to 10 hours	12 to 16 hours	Before breakfast	Around lunch
Intermediate acting					
Globin zinc*	Within 2 to 4 hours (faster as dose increases)	6 to 10 hours	18 to 24 hours (longer as dose increases)		Around dinner time or before bedtime
Lente	Within 2 to 4 hours	8 to 12 hours	28 to 32 hours		
Neutral protamine hasedorn (NPH) (isophane insulin)*	Within 2 to 4 hours	8 to 12 hours	28 to 30 hours		
Slow acting					
Protamine zinc (PZ or ZP1)*	4 to 6 hours	16 to 24 hours	24 to 36 hours or more		During night or early morning
Ultralente	8 hours	16 to 24 hours	36 hours or more		

* These insulins have a modifying protein added (protamine or globulin).

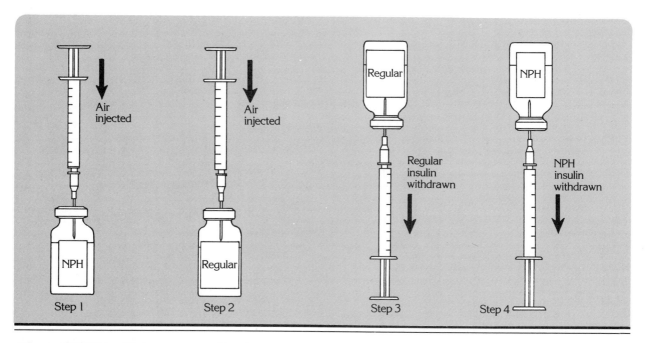

Figure 36-35. Mixing two types of insulin.

In this manner, NPH insulin is not added to the CZ insulin. This same procedure can be used when mixing other drugs from vials such as meperidine (Demerol) and dimenhydrinate (Gravol), provided compatibilities are first determined.

Mixing Drugs from One Vial and One Ampule

Because ampules do not require the addition of air prior to withdrawal of the drug, it is recommended that the medication from the vial be prepared first, and then the medication from the ampule can then be withdrawn.

PREPARING POWDERED DRUGS

Several drugs, such as penicillin, are dispensed in vials in a powdered form. A liquid (solvent or diluent) must be added to these powders to prepare them for injectable administration. The technique of adding a solvent to a powdered drug to prepare it for administration is referred to as *reconstitution.*

These powdered drugs usually have printed instructions enclosed with each packaged vial that describes the amount and kind of solvent to be added. A commonly used solvent is sterile water or normal sterile saline. Some preparations are supplied in individual-dose vials; others are multidose vials. When multidose vials are reconstituted, the nurse needs to label the vial as to the date it was prepared and the amount of drug contained in each milliliter. Once a vial is reconstituted, it is usually stored in a refrigerator.

Following are two examples of the preparation of powdered drugs:

1. *Single-dose vial:* Instructions for preparing a single-dose vial direct that 1.5 ml of sterile water be added to the sterile dry powder, thus providing a single dose of 2 ml. In this case the volume of the drug powder was 0.5 ml.

2. *Multidose vial:* A dose of 750 mg of a certain drug is ordered for a patient. On hand is a 10 gm multidose vial. The directions for preparation read, "Add 8.5 ml of sterile water, and each milliliter will contain 1.0 gm or 1000 mg." Thus after adding the solvent the nurse will give 750/1000 or ¾ ml (0.75 ml) of the medication.

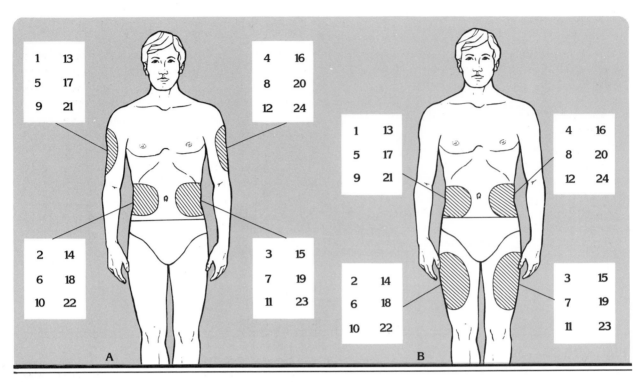

Figure 36-36.   A system of rotating injection sites on the body for the administration of insulin. **A,** Sites used by the nurse; and **B,** sites used by the patient.

PREPARING INSULIN

Insulin is prepared in units rather than milligrams or grains. It is available in units of 40, 80, and 100 per milliliter of solution. Insulin syringes have been previously described in this chapter. It is essential when preparing insulin that the appropriate calibrations on the syringe be used with the corresponding insulin preparation; for example, the 40-unit scale on the syringe is used only when administering 40-unit insulin and the 80-unit scale only for 80-unit insulin.

Because insulin is of watery consistency, the needle gauge used can be as small as possible (no. 26 gauge needle). The sites for administration are usually rotated (see Figure 36-36), and the injection is given at a 45° or 90° angle. The insulin is usually injected into the loose space between the fat and underlying muscle; therefore the skin is pinched up prior to administration. Insulin preparations are stored in the refrigerator in order to prevent deterioration. Cloudy preparations should never be used, and the solution should be well mixed prior to administration to ensure an accurate concentration and dose. Because shaking the vial can cause the medication to froth, a vial of insulin is usually rotated between the palms of the hands and inverted end to end to mix it thoroughly.

MEDICATION ERRORS

Medication errors do occasionally occur in health settings. Efforts are continually being made to decrease the incidence of errors by providing safer equipment and safer packaging of medicines. For example, the unit dose package system is a method of dispensing drugs designed to eliminate some errors of dosage.

When an error does occur, the nurse's first responsibility must be the patient. The error needs to be reported immediately and measures taken to correct the error if it is indicated. Errors are generally of two types:

1. A patient receives the incorrect drug or an incorrect dosage.
2. A patient does not receive an ordered medication.

In the event of an error it may be necessary to give a patient another drug to counteract the drug incorrectly taken, or it may be necessary to adjust subsequent dosages. In any case the physician needs to be notified of the error so that the steps necessary for the patient's health are taken.

Most agencies have policies regarding reporting errors, and incident or accident forms are filled out to report an error. These forms usually require complete information about the error and a description of any corrective measures that were taken for the patient. Over a period of time these reports may serve the purpose of pointing out problems in a particular situation with regard to medication preparation and administration. For example, several reports may indicate that the nurse was interrupted while preparing the medication. An assessment may indicate a need to change staffing patterns or change the location of a medicine cupboard.

DRUG ABUSE

Drug abuse is becoming an increasing problem in North America. It has two major facets, drug habituation and drug overuse.

Drug habituation or addiction is chiefly associated with narcotics and barbiturates. As such, it occurs in all areas of society and among all age groups. Drug addiction and the social problems connected with it are a part of twentieth century life, and nurses need to be aware of the problems and the conditions that facilitate addiction. Other drugs are also involved in habituation, such as tranquilizers and analgesics.

Some people become habituated to opiates as a result of a prolonged illness. Others become habituated because of unresolved emotional problems and the proximity of drugs as a compensating device. The latter is true of health professionals who are around drugs during their work and who tend to have highly stressful occupations.

Drug overuse occurs with over-the-counter drug preparations and with prescription drugs. Some people who are stressed or ill will tend to medicate themselves in the hope of saving time and money or perhaps in order not to bother the physician. Self-medication has the inherent danger of treating the symptoms but not always the cause. As a result real problems can go undetected for prolonged periods of time.

Drugs that are overused and are often self-prescribed are laxatives, antacids, vitamins, headache remedies, and cough and cold medications. For most people the use of these drugs is not harmful, but for some people it is. The persistent cough goes undiagnosed only until it is a far more serious and advanced problem. Persistent use of some of the over-the-counter or prescribed drugs can also result in damage to body parts that were initially healthy. For example, the prolonged use of some headache remedies containing phenacetin has been known to cause kidney damage and even death.

In regard to these problems, nurses have broad responsibilities:

1. To identify when a patient is becoming dependent upon a drug and to report this.
2. To observe for symptoms of habituation or addiction to drugs and to note withdrawal symptoms.
3. To assist patients with information pertinent to drug habituation and to assist them to develop healthy habits in regard to the use of drugs.

Symptoms of Drug Habituation

The physical and psychologic symptoms of drug habituation largely depend upon the particular drug taken. They are demonstrated when the drug is withheld and a withdrawal syndrome is exhibited. When taking opiates, the patient may demonstrate an elevated mood, relief of anxiety, and pinpoint pupils. Upon withdrawal, the patient will be restless, feel chilly, yawn, sneeze, and manifest increased nasal and lacrimal secretions, for example. Sometimes withdrawal symptoms are sufficiently severe to cause cardiovascular collapse.

SUMMARY

Drugs come from four main sources: plants, minerals, animals, and synthetics. Drugs derived from these sources must be pure and uniform in strength so that dosages derived are predictable. Official drugs are those designated by the Federal Food, Drug, and Cosmetic Act and are listed in pharmacopeias such as the USP and the BP. *National Formularies* are also published.

Legal aspects of medications include federal or national laws governing the control of drugs such as narcotics and an understanding on the part of the nurse to interpret safe dosages. Written records itemizing the drug, dosage, date and time of administration, recipient of the drug, and the signature of the nurse giving the drug are essential. For controlled drugs, additional policies are implemented such as double checks by two nurses prior to the administration of a drug and locked cupboards for narcotics and barbituates.

Drugs are classified according to their overall action in the body. Primary actions involve stimulation or inhibition of tissue or organ functions. Several factors influence these actions: drug concentrations, absorbability, circulation throughout the body, the breakdown process of the drug, and excretion of the breakdown products. Many other factors also influence drug action such as the age and weight of the individual, genetic factors, psychologic factors, specific illness, time of administration, and surrounding environment. The effects of drugs are characterized as therapeutic, side, and synergistic. Included in side effects are allergies, tolerances, cumulative, and idiosyncratic effects. Routes of administration of medications are sevenfold: oral, sublingual, parenteral (intramuscular, subcutaneous, intravenous, intradermal), insertions, instillations, topical, and inhalatory.

Two general types of medication orders exist: the standing order and the self-terminating order. Essential parts of the medication order are (a) the name of the patient, (b) the date and time of administration, (c) the name of the drug, (d) the dosage, (e) the method of administration, and (f) the signature of the physician. The dosage of drugs can be prescribed in terms of three systems: the apothecaries' system, the metric system, and the household system. It is important for the nurse to understand and to be able to relate and equate these three systems.

In nursing practice, the need to calculate fractional dosages is frequently necessary. Calculations are often necessary when preparing preoperative medications for adults or when measuring dosages for infants and children. When determining dosages for infants and children, Clarke's rule is commonly applied. Other rules are Fried's rule for infants (under 1 year of age) or Young's rule for children (over 1' year of age).

The administration of drugs involves five steps: (a) identify the patient, (b) administer the correct amount of drug by the appropriate route, (c) provide adjunctive nursing care, (d) record the measure, and (e) evaluate the effectiveness of the drug's action. Consideration also needs to be given to the age and individual needs of the patient. Recommended techniques for administering oral, subcutaneous, intramuscular, intradermal, and topical medications are outlined. Insertions and instillation procedures are also included. Supplementing knowledge about these techniques for the nurse is information about mixing drugs and the preparation of powdered drugs and insulin.

SUGGESTED ACTIVITIES

1. In a clinical setting, list the medications ordered for several patients that are self-terminating.

2. In a laboratory setting calculate fractional dosages for a child, using Clarke's rule for:

   a. a preoperative medication

   b. a narcotic analgesic

   c. an antibiotic

   d. another medication

3. In a clinical setting note some problems that patients of various age groups may have in taking or receiving medications by several different routes.

4. In a clinical setting, determine which medications are commonly provided in powdered forms for parenteral administration.

5. Interview some elderly patients who are taking daily medications. Assess their understanding of the medication in relation to effects.

SUGGESTED READINGS

Deberry, Pauline, et al. December, 1975. Teaching cardiac patients to manage medications. *American Journal of Nursing* 75:2191–2193.

A teaching program was planned and implemented for patients who would be taking medications upon leaving the hospital. Teaching techniques and learning difficulties are described. From this article students can obtain some ideas for assisting patients.

Kalant, Harold, and Kalant, Oriana J. 1972. *Drugs, society and personal choice.* Don Mills, Ontario: General Publishing Co., Ltd., Paperbacks, with the cooperation of the Research Division, Addiction Research Foundation of Ontario.

This small book is designed to assist all people, including nurses, to become better informed about drugs. The current problem is discussed together with special drugs, the reasons for nonmedical use of drugs, and the physical and psychologic consequences of drug use. Also included is a chapter on evaluating the effects of drug use.

Lambert, Martin L. March, 1975. Drug and diet interactions. *American Journal of Nursing* 75:402–406.

Included in this article are food malabsorption, drug malabsorption, and the interactions between drugs and food and fluids. A helpful list gives the nurse a guide at a glance as to how and when to administer certain drugs.

Willig, Sidnes, June, 1964. Drugs: dispensing—administering. *American Journal of Nursing* 64:126–131. Reprinted in Meyers, M. E., ed. 1967. *Nursing fundamentals.* Dubuque, Iowa: William C. Brown Co., Publishers.

The article discusses the position of the nurse when there is neither a physician nor a pharmacist during part of the 24-hour period. The position of the nurse in relation to the physician and laws governing labeling and repackaging are included. Drug lawsuit possibilities are also discussed together with insurance coverage.

SELECTED REFERENCES

Bergersen, Betty S. 1976. *Pharmacology in nursing.* 13th ed. St. Louis: the C. V. Mosby Co.

Brandt, Patricia A., et al. August, 1972. I.M. injections in children. *American Journal of Nursing* 72:1402–1406.

Budd, Ruth. February, 1971. We changed to unit-dose system. *Nursing Outlook* 19:116–117.

Burke, Elizabeth L. December, 1972. Insulin injection, the site and the technique. *American Journal of Nursing* 72:2194–2196.

Carr, Joseph J., et al. December, 1976. How to solve dosage problems in one easy lesson. *American Journal of Nursing* 76:1934–1937.

Drugs and alcohol. January, 1976. *American Journal of Nursing* 76:65. Reprinted from *The Medical Letter,* New Rochelle, N.Y. October 24, 1974.

Geolot, Denise H., et al. May, 1975. Administering parenteral drugs. *American Journal of Nursing* 75:788–793.

Hays, Doris. June, 1974. Do it yourself the Z-track way. *American Journal of Nursing* 74:1070–1071.

Keane, Claire B., and Fletcher, Sybil M. 1975. *Drugs and solutions: a programed introduction.* 3rd ed. Philadelphia: W. B. Saunders Co.

Lang, Susan H., et al. May, 1976. Reducing discomfort from injections. *American Journal of Nursing* 76:800–801.

Laugharne, Elizabeth. February, 1975. Insulin goes metric: a time for review. *The Canadian Nurse* 71:22–24.

Lawrence, Patricia A. September, 1973. U-100 insulin: let's make the transition trouble free. *American Journal of Nursing* 73:1539.

Schwartz, Doris. October 1975. Safe self-medication for elderly outpatients. *American Journal of Nursing* 75:1808–1810.

Stewart, Diane, Y., et al. August, 1976. Unit-dose medication: a nursing perspective. *American Journal of Nursing* 76:1308–1310.

CHAPTER 37

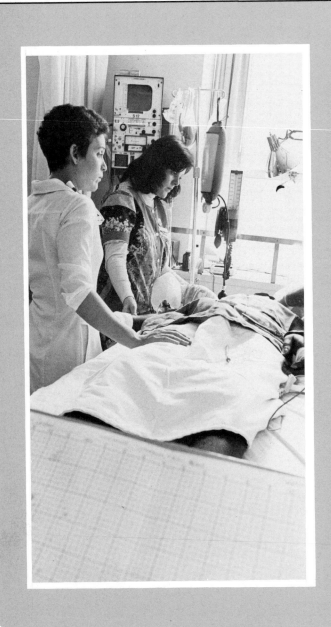

PREOPERATIVE AND POSTOPERATIVE CARE

REASONS FOR SURGERY

THE LEGAL ASPECTS OF SURGERY

ASSESSING A PATIENT PREOPERATIVELY

PREOPERATIVE NURSING INTERVENTION

SURGICAL SKIN PREPARATION

TYPES OF ANESTHESIA

SURGICAL PROCEDURES

ASSESSING A PATIENT POSTOPERATIVELY

POSTOPERATIVE NURSING INTERVENTION

OBJECTIVES

- Discuss the general reasons for surgery.
- Explain the legal aspects of surgery.
- Assess a patient preoperatively.
- Explain preoperative nursing intervention.
- Teach deep breathing and coughing.
- Teach leg exercises.
- Demonstrate beginning skill in surgical skin preparation.
- Describe surgical skin preparation areas.
- Explain inserting a Levin tube.
- Name common prefixes and suffixes.
- Assess a patient postoperatively.
- Explain postoperative nursing intervention.

Having an operation is a disrupting experience to both patients and their families. Today most operations take place in a hospital, a place which is often associated in people's minds with pain and death because many people go to a hospital to die. An operation implies to patients that their bodies will be maimed (damaged) and that they will endure pain. Surgery is seldom looked upon as a pleasant experience.

The nurse is an essential member of the health team caring for the surgical patient. The nurse prepares patients preoperatively, and often it is the nurse's responsibility to explain to the patient and family what will be happening. After surgery, the nurse's skills are required to assist the patient's return to health. Some patients have postoperative learning needs before leaving a hospital, such as learning to use crutches. It is the nurse's responsibility to assist patients to meet these needs and to gain the skills they require. During the surgical experience patients also learn skills that will help prevent postoperative complications such as pneumonia. Learning is an important part of the patient's care, and this learning is generally assisted by nurses.

REASONS FOR SURGERY

Surgical procedures can be considered to be optional, elective, or urgent. *Optional surgery* is requested by the patient, but it is not necessary for health. Usually an operation such as facial plastic surgery is optional and is done for psychologic reasons. *Elective surgery* is that which the patient chooses to have, such as straightening a bent finger. It is performed for his or her well-being but is not absolutely necessary. *Urgent surgery* is that which is required for the patient's health, such as the removal of an inflamed appendix. There are different types of urgent surgery, such as for the person who is hemorrhaging internally.

The reasons for an operation vary considerably. Some reasons are as follows:

1. *Diagnostic* surgery enables the surgeon to confirm a diagnosis. Sometimes a specimen of tissue is sent to a hospital laboratory during the operation, and the diagnosis determines how the surgeon will proceed.

2. *Exploratory* surgery is frequently performed to confirm the extent of a pathologic process and sometimes to confirm a diagnosis.

3. *Ablative* surgery is the removal of diseased organs, such as an inflamed appendix.

4. *Reconstructive* surgery is the repair of tissues whose function or appearance is damaged, such as a vaginal repair.

5. *Constructive* surgery is the repair of a congenitally malformed organ or tissue, such as the repair of a harelip.

6. *Palliative* surgery relieves the symptoms of a disease process, such as an intestinal bypass to relieve the symptoms of intestinal obstruction.

THE LEGAL ASPECTS OF SURGERY

Prior to any surgical procedure patients must sign a surgical permit (see Figure 37-1). Signing a form protects patients from having any surgical procedure they do not want or do not know about. It also protects the hospital and the health personnel from a claim by patients or family that permission was not granted.

The patient should have a full explanation before signing the form. Adults sign their own consent forms unless they are mentally incompetent or unconscious, in which cases a parent or guardian must sign for them. For children under 18 years of age the consent form must be signed by an adult, preferably a relative. If a minor's parents cannot be found, a court order can be obtained to permit surgery. The consent form becomes a part of the patient's record and goes to the operating room with the patient.

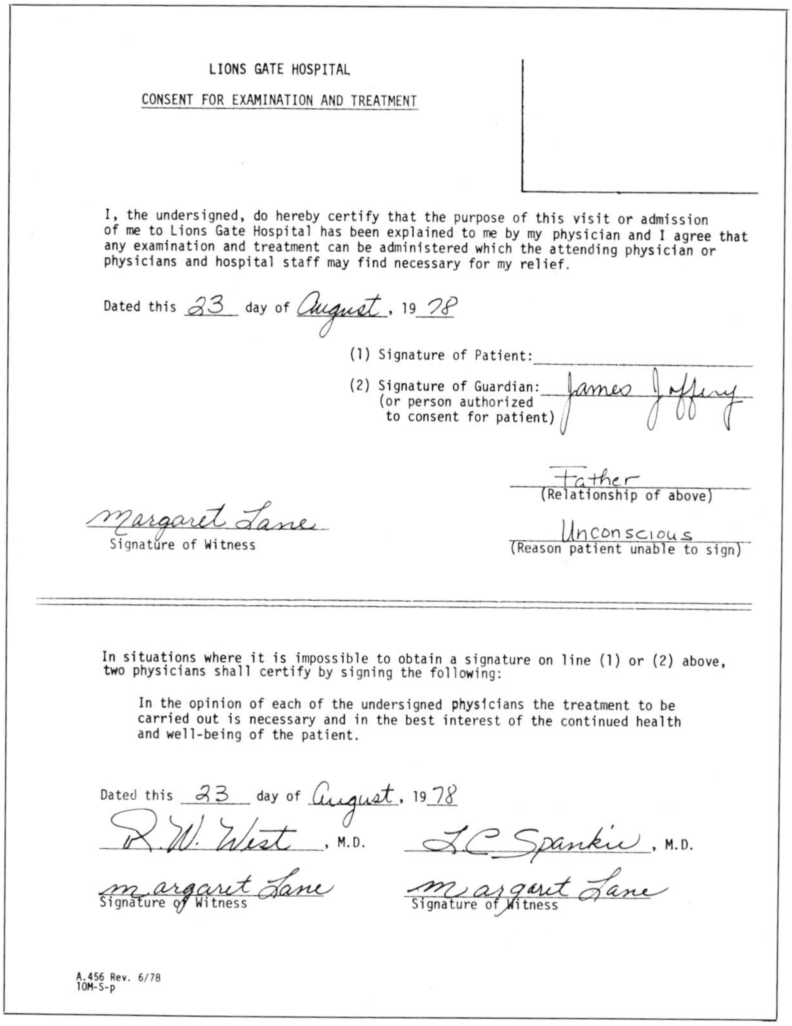

LIONS GATE HOSPITAL

CONSENT FOR EXAMINATION AND TREATMENT

I, the undersigned, do hereby certify that the purpose of this visit or admission of me to Lions Gate Hospital has been explained to me by my physician and I agree that any examination and treatment can be administered which the attending physician or physicians and hospital staff may find necessary for my relief.

Dated this _23_ day of _August_, 19 _78_

(1) Signature of Patient: _____

(2) Signature of Guardian: _James Joffrey_
(or person authorized
to consent for patient)

Margaret Lane
Signature of Witness

Father
(Relationship of above)

Unconscious
(Reason patient unable to sign)

In situations where it is impossible to obtain a signature on line (1) or (2) above, two physicians shall certify by signing the following:

In the opinion of each of the undersigned physicians the treatment to be carried out is necessary and in the best interest of the continued health and well-being of the patient.

Dated this _23_ day of _August_, 19 _78_

R.W. West, M.D.   _L C Spankie_, M.D.

Margaret Lane   _Margaret Lane_
Signature of Witness   Signature of Witness

A.456 Rev. 6/78
10M-S-p

Figure 37-1.   A sample consent form for surgery and treatment. (Courtesy Lions Gate Hospital; North Vancouver, B.C.)

ASSESSING A PATIENT PREOPERATIVELY

The degree of risk involved in a surgical procedure is affected by a number of factors: (a) age, (b) nutritional status, (c) fluid and electrolyte balance, (d) general health, (e) the use of medications, and (f) mental health, including attitude.

Age

The very young and the elderly are greater surgical risks than children and adults. The greatest difference in physiologic response compared to an adult is seen in the neonate. Factors that affect the risk are the neonate's circulation, which is largely central, and renal function, which is not fully developed un-

til about 6 months of age. The neonate can respond to an additional need for oxygen only by an increased respiratory rate, and limited blood volume results in a limited fluid reserve. The loss of 30 cc of blood from a neonate is the equivalent of an 850 cc loss from a 200 lb. man (Goulding, et al. 1965:84–85).

For the elderly person, surgery also has an additional risk. Circulation is frequently impaired by arteriosclerosis and limited cardiac function. Energy reserves are frequently limited, and hydration and the nutritional status are often poor. In addition, elderly people can be highly sensitive to medications frequently used preoperatively and postoperatively such as morphine sulfate and the barbiturates.

Nutritional Status

The two nutritional problems that can affect the surgical risk are obesity and malnutrition due to protein, iron, and vitamin deficiencies. Obesity can result in a deferment of surgery unless it is an emergency. Obese patients have an overburdened heart, and often their blood pressures are elevated. In addition, an abundance of fatty tissue around an incision makes suturing difficult, and it is particularly prone to infection. Nutritional deficiencies are seen particularly among the elderly and the chronically ill. Protein is needed for wound healing; vitamins are essential for wound healing and blood clotting (vitamin K).

Fluid and Electrolyte Balance

Dehydration and hypovolemia predispose the person to problems during surgery (see Chapter 30, "Assessment of the Dehydrated Person"). Electrolyte imbalances often accompany fluid imbalances. Imbalances in calcium, magnesium, potassium, and hydrogen ions are of particular concern in surgery (see Chapter 30).

General Health

The general health of a person also affects the operative risk. The presence of an infectious process or any pathophysiology of a body process increases the risk. Of particular concern are upper respiratory tract infections, which, together with a general anesthetic, can affect the respiratory function adversely.

Other problems such as a recent myocardial infarction or any cardiovascular disease can make surgery more dangerous than usual. Renal function is essential for the excretion of body wastes (see Chapter 27, "Assessment of Urinary Elimination"). Metabolic and liver function affect healing and the detoxification and elimination of medications. Un-

treated diabetes mellitus predisposes the person to infection and impaired tissue healing. Impaired liver function reduces the ability of the liver to detoxify drugs and to metabolize carbohydrates, proteins, and fats. A person with abnormal blood coagulation may have serious bleeding, which can become a hemorrhage and result in shock.

The Use of Medications

The regular use of certain medications can increase the operative risk. Some of these medications are as follows:

1. Anticoagulants, which increase the blood coagulation time.
2. Tranquilizers, which can increase hypotension and thus contribute to shock.
3. Depressants such as heroin, which decrease central nervous system responses.
4. Antibiotics that are incompatible with anesthetic agents, resulting in untoward reactions.
5. Diuretics, which can create electrolyte (especially potassium) imbalances.

Mental Health and Attitude

Extreme anxiety can increase the surgical risk. The person's anxiety is not always related to the seriousness of the surgical procedure. The surgeon needs to know about a person who believes that he or she will die prior to the surgery. In some instances professional counseling and a delay in the surgery is indicated.

Patients who have been poorly adjusted for some period of time may find that they cannot cope with the additional stress of surgery. People who are able to cope only at a minimal level in a stable, familiar environment can develop full neuroses or psychoses postoperatively.

PREOPERATIVE NURSING INTERVENTION

Most of a patient's special preoperative needs are related to a general concern for enhancing and maintaining the patient's safety and emotional security. Surgery is a stressor, and a patient can be expected to react to this stressor physiologically and emotionally (see Chapter 8, "Signs of Increased Stress").

Health Status

Careful determination of the patient's health status is important. Anesthetics depress physiologic functions, including those of the cardiovascular, respiratory, urinary, and central nervous systems. Therefore assessment of their level of function is important. Chest roentgenograms are made prior to admission in many hospitals as a part of the data related to respiratory function. Vital signs are taken and recorded, and special tests such as a urinalysis, blood grouping, and blood coagulation time are also completed prior to surgery.

Nutrition and Hydration

Adequate hydration and nutrition are necessary for normal physiologic functioning and specifically for the healing process. Recording any signs of malnutrition is important. Weighing the patient and recording the weight provides one measure of nutrition.

Anesthetics depress gastrointestinal functioning, and there is a danger of vomiting and aspirating vomitus during administration of a general anesthetic. The patient is therefore usually required to fast at least six to eight hours preoperatively. The patient and family need to understand the necessity of fasting, and usually food and fluids are removed from the bedside as a precaution. A fasting sign is placed at the bed the evening before surgery. Because a patient's mouth will feel dry, a mouthwash can be used frequently during the fasting period. If the patient does take food or fluids during the fasting period, this must be reported to the surgeon before the operation.

Freedom from Infection

The skin can never be completely free of microorganisms, but it can be rendered relatively free by general hygienic measures, antimicrobial agents, and removal of hair. The day before surgery, the patient should bathe as a general hygenic measure. A cap is placed over the hair prior to surgery, and the patient wears a clean gown to the operating room. A local skin preparation is done, the hair is removed, and an antimicrobial agent is applied (see "Surgical Skin Preparation" in this chapter).

Respiratory Process

A general anesthetic irritates the mucous membrane and can increase the production of mucus, which will need to be removed by deep breathing and coughing. Deep breathing permits the exchange of air in the lungs, minimizing the stagnation of fluid and the subsequent development of pneumonia. Coughing also removes lung fluid and thus helps to prevent penumonia and atelectasis. *Atelectasis* is the collapse of lung tissue often due to bronchial obstruction, which can be caused by thick secretions. Patients are taught to cough and deep breathe preoperatively. The coughing needs to be deep, reaching into the lungs and not merely the throat.

Learning to turn and to move in bed can also help prevent lung complications. By moving from side to side, both lungs become aerated, and any mucus is more readily coughed up.

Procedure 37-1. Learning Deep Breathing and Coughing

Action	Explanation
1. Encourage deep breathing every hour during the waking hours.	To facilitate a wide exchange of gases. To maximize the amount of oxygen available to the cells. To prevent hypostatic pneumonia.
2. Deep breathing consists of about five deep respirations.	Patient takes one deep breath and holds it for about three seconds before expiring.
3. When teaching deep breathing, demonstrate what is meant. Outline the number of deep breaths and frequency. Explain the importance of the exercises in terms appropriate for the patient.	
4. Teach the patient to cough.	Take a deep breath. Hold the breath for about three seconds. Cough at least twice.
5. Show the patient how to support a surgical wound with both hands when coughing and deep breathing.	To lessen discomfort.

Rest

Body cells require a period of decreased activity to restore themselves; therefore prior to surgery most patients will take a sedative. This should be given after all preoperative preparation has been carried out and the environmental stimuli are minimal. The preoperative medication is usually ordered by the anesthetist.

On the day of surgery the patient will also be given a medication, such as meperidine (Demerol) or atropine, that acts as a respiratory depressant, prevents laryngospasm, and dries secretions. Patients need to be cautioned to remain in bed after sedation. A call light should be placed nearby, and often siderails are raised. The patient also needs to understand not to smoke during this drowsy state. Some agencies suggest no smoking at least eight hours prior to a general anesthetic to reduce respiratory irritation.

Preventing Discomfort and Trauma

The patient may need to be assisted to void immediately preoperatively. This should empty the urinary bladder; therefore involuntary voiding under anesthesia is less likely, and in abdominal surgery the bladder is less likely to be punctured. The amount voided is recorded on the patient's record.

Because anesthesia produces muscular relaxation and reflexes disappear, an enema is usually given the evening prior to surgery to empty the colon of feces. Another practice designed to prevent trauma is the removal of dentures and any prostheses. These can become dislodged during administration of the anesthetic, and dentures could lodge in the patient's throat. Makeup and nailpolish are removed so that the patient's color can be quickly assessed. The nail beds are very sensitive and indicate a lack of oxygen quickly by becoming cyanotic.

Emotional Security

Patients will need an explanation of what will happen, and it should be adjusted to their needs. The patient who will have any tubes needs to know this beforehand. The unknown is a source of anxiety; therefore by knowing what will happen most people feel more secure. It is important for the nurse to be sensitive to a patient's concerns. Fear is manifested in a number of ways. Some patients are overly talkative, others withdraw, and others are inappropriately cheerful.

The nurse must find out what the surgery means to the patient and to the family. In some instances self-image may be threatened by disfigurement or impaired bodily function (see Chapter 35, "Intervening in Problems of Body Image"). Nurses should listen carefully to patients and not dismiss their fears by saying "Everything will be all right." Often a nurse can clarify misconceptions and relieve anxiety. By listening carefully, a nurse can often assist patients to talk their fears through.

Children require explanations that are meaningful to them. The nurse should introduce information at a speed that keeps their attention but does not overwhelm them. A child should see the anesthetic machine and try on the mask. The postanesthesia room will also need to be explained; it can be referred to as the "wake-up room." The nurse can also explain about discomfort, using words that the child understands such as "sore tummy." All postoperative care should be explained. Most important, children need to know when their parents will come (Luciano 1974:65).

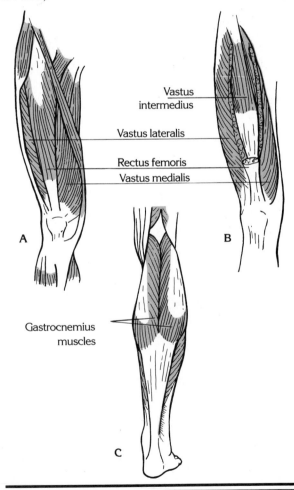

Figure 37-2. The quadriceps and gastrocnemius muscles are exercised preoperatively and postoperatively.

Preventing Complications Postoperatively

Leg exercises can assist in the prevention of thrombophlebitis due to slowed circulation (venous stasis) and inactivity postoperatively. The ultimate concern of thrombophlebitis is the formation of thrombi, which can become emboli and lodge in an artery such as the coronary and pulmonary, causing death.

Leg exercises have been discussed in Chapter 23. The leg exercises described here need to be learned preoperatively and practiced postoperatively. The exercises include contracting and relaxing the quadriceps and gastrocnemius (calf) muscles as well as the smaller muscles of the feet and toes. (See Figure 37-2 for quadriceps and gastrocnemius muscles.)

The patient flexes the knees and then extends them, pressing the back of the knees into the bed. Then the legs are raised with the knees extended. If unable to do this, the patient can alternately contract and relax the quadriceps muscles. Leg exercises also should include the gastrocnemius muscles, which are also alternately contracted and relaxed. Finally, toe and foot exercises, which stimulate circulation in those areas, include flexion, extension, and rotation of the feet.

Many hospitals have preoperative routines that nurses follow to ensure that patients have complete preoperative preparation. These routines vary from one agency to another, and students are advised to be familiar with the practices of the hospital in which they are nursing (see Procedure 37-2).

Procedure 37-2.   Preoperative Nursing Intervention

Action	Explanation
Day Before Surgery	
1. The patient signs a consent form.	To protect the rights of the patient, the physician, and the hospital.
2. A medical and nursing history is taken and placed on the patient's record.	This may not be done in emergencies.
3. Laboratory tests are done.	Urinalysis, hemoglobin, and cross matching for blood are carried out in most hospitals.
4. Surgical skin preparation is done.	The physician orders skin preparation.
5. The large bowel is evacuated.	An enema is given on the physician's order.
6. Deep breathing, coughing, and leg exercises are taught.	The patient can do these postoperatively to prevent pneumonia and thrombophlebitis.
7. Infections, respiratory disorders, elevated temperature, or unusual skin conditions are reported to the physician.	These may necessitate postponing surgery because of possible infection or respiratory problems.
8. The anesthesiologist visits the patient and orders preoperative medications.	Includes evening preoperative medication and immediately before surgery.
9. The patient fasts six to eight hours prior to surgery.	
10. The patient is told the time of surgery and what to expect; this explanation is adjusted to the patient's needs.	
Day of Surgery	
1. Vital signs are taken before surgery. Any abnormality is reported to the surgeon.	To serve as a base for comparison postoperatively.

Procedure 37-2.   Cont'd.

2. The patient has a complete bath unless this was done the evening before.	See agency policy.
3. Remove dentures, contact lenses, combs, pins, nail polish, and lipstick.	
4. Remove all jewelry.	In some hospitals a wedding band can be taped to the finger unless breast or chest surgery is planned. After this surgery the arms and hands may become edematous for a short time.
5. The patient voids before taking a sedative. Report if the patient is unable to void.	Record the amount voided. An empty bladder decreases the danger of injury during surgery and prevents voiding while under the anesthetic.
6. Assist the patient to put on OR (operating room) socks, cap, and gown.	
7. Take the blood pressure and record it.	
8. Give the patient preoperative sedation as prescribed.	
9. Note on the front of the patient's record any physical handicap such as blindness or the presence of hearing aid or religious medals.	Religious medals may be left on.
10. Disconnect the gastric tube if the patient has had one inserted.	Cover the end of the tube with 4 × 4 gauze.
11. Complete the preoperative check list.	Many hospitals have check lists as a guide to complete preoperative care.

SURGICAL SKIN PREPARATION

The purpose of preparing the skin before surgery (preoperative skin preparation) is to reduce the number of microorganisms present and consequently reduce the chance of an infection.

The actual area to be prepared is generally larger than that required for the incision. This minimizes the number of microorganisms in the areas adjacent to the incision. Many hospitals have policies to guide the nurse as to the area of preparation for various operations. For example, for breast and chest surgery the area of preparation can extend from the neck to below the waist, past the midline on the anterior and posterior surfaces of the torso, and the surfaces of the arm to below the elbow on the affected side. In some settings, special preparations such as pHisohex are used. In some hospitals, electric clippers are used rather than a razor and shaving cream. Each hospital has its own policies regarding skin preparation for surgery.

Another variation of the skin preparation technique is the use of an antiseptic solution to cleanse the area after the shave; in some places this cleansing is repeated every 4 hours during the waking hours until 2 hours before surgery. The area may be wrapped in sterile towels between cleansings, and sterile gloves and sterile technique are employed during the skin preparation.

Procedure 37-3.   Skin Preparation Preoperative

Action	**Explanation**
Assemble Equipment	
Dry Shave	
1. Electric clippers.	Make sure heads are sharp and teeth are not broken.
2. Scissors.	For long hair if needed.
3. Check the physician's order and the area to be prepared.	
Wet Shave	
1. Skin preparation set.	This contains a disposable razor, compartmented basin, moisture-proof drape, hexachlorophene soap, sponge, cotton-tipped applicators, wash cloth, and towel.
2. Warm Water.	
3. Light.	
Prepare Skin	
Dry Shave	To reassure the patient. To identify the patient.
1. Explain to the patient what you plan to do. Adjust the explanation to the patient's needs.	Expose only a small area necessary for the shave. Shave about 6 inches at a time.
2. Drape the patient.	
3. Make sure the area is dry.	Pressure can cause abrasions, particularly over bony prominences.
4. Shave with clippers; do not apply pressure.	
Wet Shave	
1. Explain to the patient as for a dry shave.	Expose only a small area as necessary for the shave. Shave about 6 inches at a time.
2. Drape the patient.	
3. Lather the area.	Hold the skin taut. The razor is held at about a 45° angle to the skin and moved in the direction the hair is growing. See Figure 37-3.
4. Shave.	

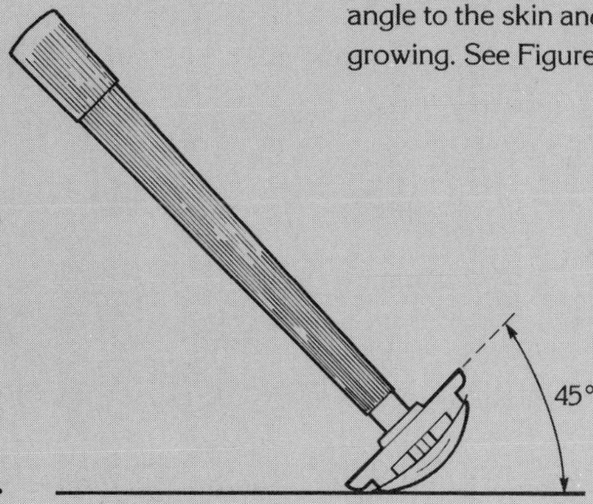

45°

Figure 37-3.

Procedure 37-3.   Cont'd.

5. Rinse the area and pat it dry.

6. Repeat steps 3 to 5 until the entire designated area
    has been prepared and no hair is visible.

7. Have the skin preparation checked by the nurse in   The orderly in charge will check male perineal prepara-
    charge.   tions.

8. Record the preparation on the patient's chart.

Procedure 37-4.   Skin Preparation Areas

Action   **Explanation**

Lower Extremities (Hip and Thigh)

Shave from the waistline to 6 inches below the knee;
from 2 inches past midbuttock to 2 inches past mid-
abdomen. Include a complete perineal shave.

Indications

1. Fractured femur.

2. Any upper leg or thigh surgery.

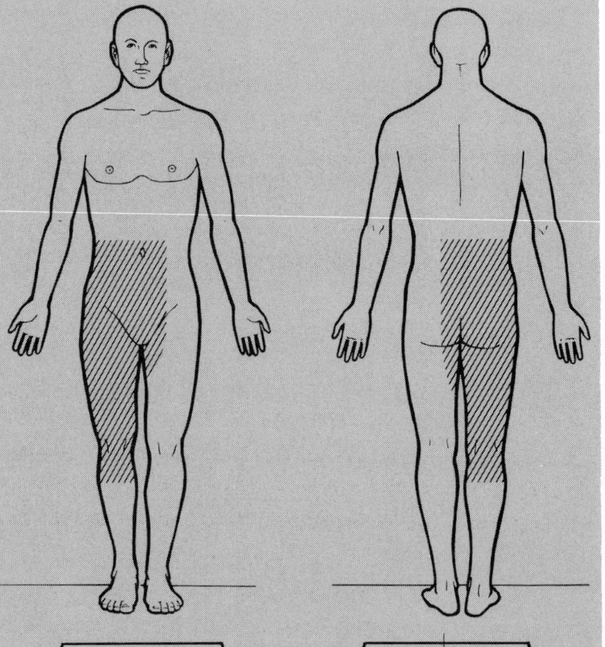

Figure 37-4.

Lower Extremeties (Knee)

Shave the entire leg from the ankle to the groin.
Indications

1. Meniscectomy.

2. Knee prostheses.

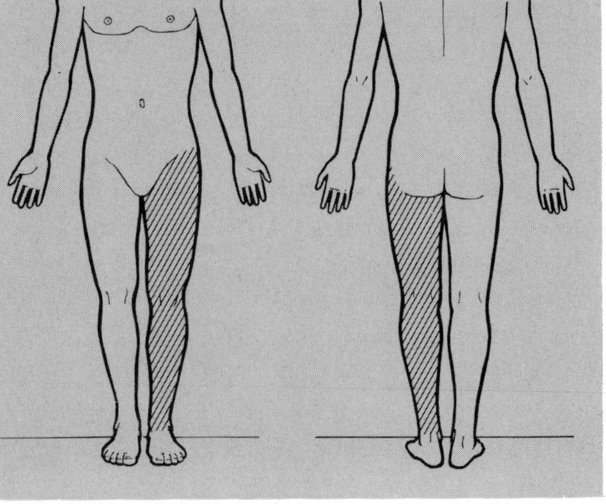

Figure 37-5.

Lower Extremities (Lower Leg or Foot)

Shave the entire foot and leg to 8 inches above the knee. Clean and trim nails and remove nail polish.
Indications

1. Open reductions of the tibia and fibula.

2. Ankle surgery.

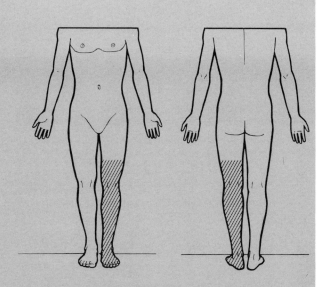

Figure 37-6.

Lower Extremities (Foot)

Shave the entire foot and leg to the midcalf. Clean and trim the nails and remove nail polish.

Indications

1. Bunions.

2. Ingrown toenails.

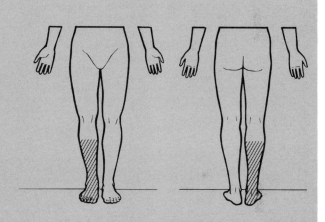

Figure 37-7.

Lower Extremities (Complete Lower Extremities)

Shave the entire leg and foot extending up to a point above the umbilicus, including a complete perineal shave.

Indications

1. Femoral arterial graft.

2. Ligation and stripping of varicose veins.

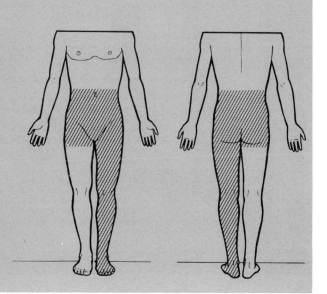

Figure 37-8.

Procedure 37-4. Cont'd.

Abdominal and Leg

Prepare the entire abdomen from axillae margins to the bedline and extending down affected side to below the knee and to the midthigh on the other leg. On the back include buttocks, backs of legs as above, and a complete perineal preparation.

Indications

1. Femoral-popliteal artery

2. Common iliac artery surgery.

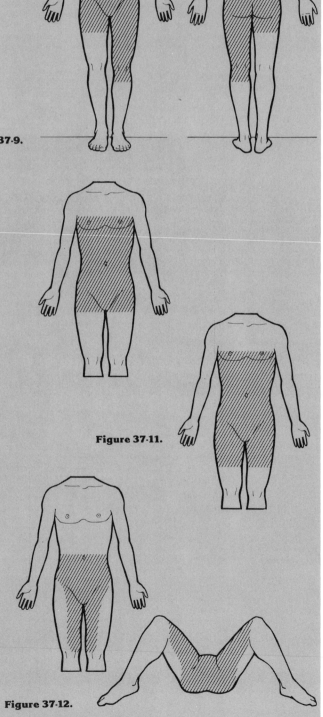

Figure 37-9.

Abdominal (Incision above the Umbilicus)

Prepare the entire abdomen from the axillae martins, including all visible pubic hair and to the bedline on the lateral aspects of the patient.

Indications

1. Cholecystectomy.

2. Gastrectomy.

3. Bowel resections. Figure 37-10.

Abdominal (Incision below the Umbilicus)

Prepare the entire abdomen from the nipple line to the midthigh. Include all visible pubic hair when the legs are together. Prepare to the bedline on each side.

Indications

1. Appendectomy.

2. Hernia repairs.

Figure 37-11.

Perineal

Prepare pubes, perineum, and inner side of thighs and buttocks.

Indications
1. Rectal surgery.

2. Vaginal surgery.

3. Prostatectomy. Figure 37-12.

Kidney

Prepare from 2 inches past the midline of the abdomen to 2 inches past the midline of the back, from the nipple line to the pubes including visible pubic hair when the legs are together. Include an axilla shave.

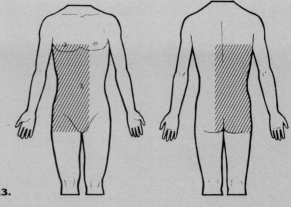

Figure 37-13.

Back (Cervical Spine)

Prepare 1 inch above the external occipital pro-tuberance to the midlumbar area of the back and to the bedline on both sides.

Indication   **Figure 37-14.**

    Cervical spine surgery (posterior).

Back (Posterior Thoracic and Lumbar Spine)

Prepare from the hairline to the bedline on both sides.

Indications
1. Thoracic spine surgery.

2. Lumbar spine surgery.   **Figure 37-15.**

Spinal Surgery

Prepare the back from the axillary line to the midthigh and to the bedline on each side.

Indications
1. Intractable pain.

2. Spinal tumors

3. Spina bifida.

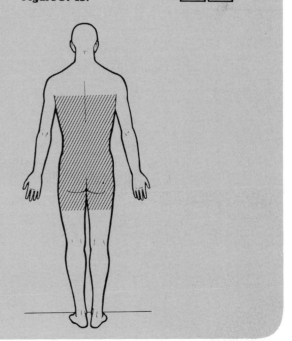

Figure 37-16.

Procedure 37-4.   Cont'd.

Chest

Prepare from the nipple line of the opposite breast over the affected breast to the midline of the back, from the shoulder to the umbilicus, and the whole arm from the shoulder to 1 inch below the elbow. Include an axilla shave.

The physician may order a complete chest shave (both sides and both shoulders).

Indications

1. Breast surgery.

2. Chest surgery.

3. Closed heart surgery.

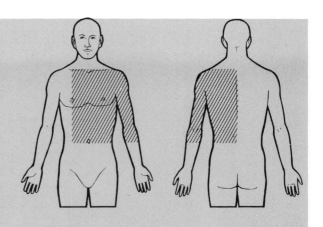

Figure 37-17.

Neck

Prepare from the chin to the nipple line and from the right shoulder to the left shoulder.

Indication

Thyroid surgery.

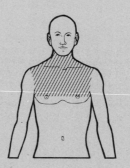

Figure 37-18.

Chest (for open heart surgery)

Prepare from the chin to the midthigh and to each bedline. Include both axillae and visible pubic hair.

Indication

Open heart surgery.

Upper Extremities

Remove rings, cleanse and trim nails, and remove polish. The identification bracelet should be on the unoperative arm. Prepare the whole arm and hand up to the shoulder.

Indications

1. Forearm surgery.

2. Hand surgery.

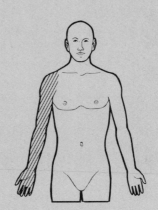

Figure 37-19.

Upper Arm

Prepare from 2 inches past the midline on the back to 2 inches past the midline of the chest. Include the shoulder, axilla, and arm to 2 inches below the elbow.

Indication

Shoulder surgery.

Figure 37-20.

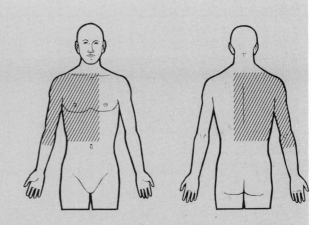

Elbow

Prepare from the shoulder to and including the hand. Include an axilla shave.

Indication

Elbow surgery.

Upper Extremity (Entire)

Prepare from 2 inches past the midline on the back to 2 inches past the midline on the chest. Include the complete shoulder, axilla, whole arm, hand.

Indications

Fracture of the Humerus.

Head

Check with the physician about the exact area to be prepared. Cut long hair with clippers. Shaving may be done in the operating room before the operation. All hair is to be saved and given to the patient upon discharge.

Indication

Craniotomy.

Head (Nasal)

Male patients shave the morning of surgery. This includes the mustache. Prepare from the bridge of the nose on both sides of the face to the ears and under the chin. Cut hairs as far up the nares as possible.

Indications

1. Submucous resections.

2. Removal of polyps.

Head (Mastoid and Ear)

Prepare 2 to 3 inches behind the ear. Clip all visible hair around the external auditory meatus. Comb lacquer into long hair to the midline on the operative side; hold the hair with bobby pins. Repeat on the morning of surgery and remove the pins.

Figure 37-21.

Skin or Bone Graft

Prepare as directed by the physician.

Procedure 37-5.   Insertion of a Levin Tube

Some patients, such as those who will have gastric or duodenal surgery, require the insertion of a Levin (gastric) tube preoperatively. The tube is usually inserted to remove fluid and flatus from the stomach, thereby preventing nausea, vomiting, and distention when peristaltic action has been reduced after surgery.

Action	Explanation
Assemble Equipment	
1. Gastric tube.	
2. Solution basin.	To prepare the gastric tube (see step 11).
3. Lubricant.	To lubricate the tube prior to insertion.
4. Bib or towel for the patient; glass of water and drinking straw.	Protective measure for the patient. To assist the patient to swallow the tube.
5. 20 to 50 ml syringe with adapter	To withdraw stomach contents after insertion.
6. Kidney basin.	To collect gastric contents.
7. Facial tissue.	As required for the patient.
8. Clamp or hemostat (optional).	To clamp the tube after insertion.
9. Adhesive tape.	To secure the tube to the face.
10. Safety pin and elastic band.	To secure the nasogastric tube to the patient's gown.

Some places may have gastric trays that include most of the above items.

Action	Explanation
11. Prior to insertion:	
a. Plastic tubes should be placed in a solution of warm water.	To make the tube more flexible for insertion.
b. Rubber tubes should be placed on ice.	To stiffen the rubber tube for easier insertion.
To Insert a Gastric Tube	
1. Explain to the patient what you plan to do. Adjust the explanation to the patient's needs.	To reassure the patient and to identify the patient. Inserting a gastric tube is not painful, but it is unpleasant because the gag reflex is stimulated during the insertion.
2. Assist the patient to a high Fowler's position. The patient's head may be supported on pillows, hyperflexed or hyperextended.	Gravity helps the passage of the tube. The patient will make this choice.
3. Determine the length of tube to insert by using the tube to measure the distance from the patient's ear lobe to the tip of the nose and then from the tip of the nose to the patient's umbilicus. (See Figure 37-22.)	The distance from nares to stomach varies in individual patients.
4. Lubricate the tip of the tube well with a water-soluble lubricant.	This kind of lubricant will dissolve if the tube enters the lungs accidentally. An oil-base lubricant such as petroleum jelly will not dissolve.
5. Insert the tube into the right or left naries. Slight pressure is sometimes required to pass the tube into the nasopharynx. Some patients may tear from the eyes at this point.	The patient may indicate a preference. Never force the tube if there is an obstruction. A natural body response.

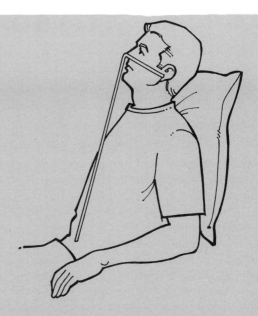

Figure 37-22.

6. Once the tube has reached the oropharynx (throat), encourage the patient to drink and swallow. If the patient is fasting for surgery, only a small amount of water should be taken. The water will be quickly removed after the tube is inserted. The patient may gag and retch at this point. If the patient coughs or chokes, withdraw the tubing slightly until coughing subsides and then try again to pass the tube.

The patient will know when to begin; the patient will feel the tube if conscious. Swallowing assists the passage of the tube. Concentration of the patient on swallowing often prevents gagging.

Coughing or choking indicates that the tube has entered the trachea instead of the esophagus. There is no cause for alarm or panic.

7. Cooperatively with the pateint, pass the tube 2 to 4 inches with each swallow until the indicated length is inserted.

8. To ensure the position of the tube in the stomach:

   a. Aspirate stomach contents with a syringe.

   If fluid is removed, the assumption is that the tube is in the stomach. Stomach contents may be clear or yellow with mucus.

   b. Inject 10 ml of air into the tube, and listen at the epigastric area with a stethoscope for gurgling.

   c. Ask the patient to hum.

   A patient cannot hum if the tube is in the lungs.

   d. Place the end of tube in a glass of water and expect no or few bubbles.

   If bubbles appear steadily from the tube, particularly on exhalation, it is probably in the lungs.

   e. Hold the tube end to your ear and expect no sound.

   A crackling noise can indicate that the tube is in the lungs.

9. Secure the tube in place:

   a. Tape the tube comfortably to the bridge of the nose and then across the cheek or forehead (avoid the eyebrow).

   Avoid pulling up on the nostril.

   b. For preoperative patients apply a plastic specimen bag and elastic band over the end of tube.

   c. If ordered, attach the tube directly to a suction.

TYPES OF ANESTHESIA

There are three types of anesthesia: general, regional, and local.

General Anesthesia

With general anesthesia the patient loses all sensation and consciousness. A general anesthetic acts by blocking the awareness centers in the brain. It can be administered by intravenous infusion, inhalation, or rectal induction.

A general anesthetic has a number of advantages. The respirations and cardiac function are readily regulated because the patient is unconscious rather than awake and anxious. The anesthesia can be adjusted to the length of the operation and the age and physical status of the patient. Its chief disadvantage is respiratory and circulatory depression. (See Table 37-1 for stages of anesthesia.)

Regional Anesthesia

In regional anesthesia painful sensations in one area of the body are reduced by blocking sensory impulses to the brain. A number of methods are employed, such as spinal anesthesia, nerve block, and epidural block. In spinal anesthesia a lumbar puncture is performed (see "Lumbar Puncture" in Chapter 38). The physician then injects the anesthesia into the spinal canal (subarachnoid space). Commonly used anesthetic agents are procaine hydrochloride (Novocain) and tetracaine hydrochloride (Pontocaine).

A *nerve block* is the injection of an anesthetic agent such as tetracaine into a nerve plexus such as the brachial plexus, which results in anesthetizing the arm. An *epidural block* is used commonly in obstetrics. It is the injection of an anesthetic agent between a lumbar interspace but extrathecally. A *caudal* anesthetic is similar to an epidural anesthetic except that the needle is inserted through the sacral hiatus into the caudal canal (see Figure 37-23).

Local anesthesia desensitizes a small tissue area. It may be sprayed on the skin or mucous membrane or injected into tissue. Cocaine is commonly used in a

Table 37-1.   Stages of General Anesthesia

Stage 1	Patient appears drowsy and dizzy.
Stage 2	Patient loses consciousness. Patient can be excited and can move during the initial part of this stage.
Stage 3	This is the stage of relaxation. Reflexes are lost and vital functions are depressed. It is during this stage that surgery is performed.
Stage 4	This is a dangerous stage, when vital functions are too depressed. Patients normally do not enter this stage.

4% to 10% solution to anesthetize the eye and mucous membranes. Tetracaine and lidocaine (Xylocaine) are commonly used anesthetic agents, which are injected. The chief advantage of this method is that it acts quickly and has few side effects.

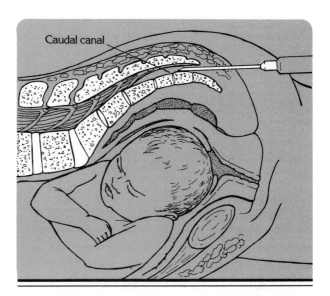

Figure 37-23.   The insertion of a needle into the caudal canal.

SURGICAL PROCEDURES

There are thousands of surgical procedures performed in hospitals. Some patients have day surgery: they come to the hospital on the day of the operation and leave the same day after the operation. Other surgical procedures necessitate a longer hospital stay from a few days to several weeks. To understand what a surgical procedure means, nurses can be guided by specific suffixes and prefixes and commonly used medical terms. The student is referred to the Appendix for commonly used prefixes and suffixes.

ASSESSING A PATIENT POSTOPERATIVELY

An immediate postoperative assessment involves four aspects:

1. Adequate respiratory function.
2. Adequate cardiovascular function.
3. Balanced fluid and electrolytes.
4. A safe environment with physical and emotional comfort (McConnell 1977:34).

Immediate nursing intervention after surgery is usually carried out in the hospital recovery room (postanesthetic room, PAR). Here nurses have special skills required to assist patients who are recovering from anesthetics and surgery. Once a patient's condition has stabilized, he or she will then return to a clinical nursing area; a day surgery patient will return home.

After a general anesthetic, patients awaken in the following sequence: respond to stimuli, drowsy, awake but not oriented, alert and oriented (McConnell 1977:34). The return of the patient's reflexes such as swallowing and gagging indicates that the anesthesia is wearing off. A patient who has an airway will probably spit it out (see "Artificial Oropharyngeal Airways" in Chapter 28). The patient will then become gradually oriented to person, place, and last to time.

Adequate Respiratory Function

Inadequate respirations are the most common emergency in the recovery room. Respirations should be assessed as to rate, depth, quality, and chest movement (see "Respirations" in Chapter 13). These need to be compared with the patient's normal respirations recorded on the chart. The patient's color should also be assessed for any cyanosis. When the patient is unconscious, a lateral of Sims's position without a pillow and with the head slightly extended and face down is preferred. Gravity keeps the tongue from falling backward and occluding the air passages, and mucus and vomitus can drain freely. Once the patient's reflexes return, another position may be normally assumed such as a back-lying position.

Adequate Cardiovascular Function

Cardiovascular function is assessed by measuring the blood pressure and assessing the pulse. Postoperative hypotension can be a problem as a result of some anesthetic agents and muscle relaxants. Analgesics can further produce hypotension, and their administration needs to be evaluated carefully. If the blood pressure drops more than 20 mm Hg after surgery, the physician needs to be notified. Dressings need to be checked regularly for bleeding or undue fluid loss.

Balanced Fluid and Electrolytes

During surgery aldosterone production is increased, resulting in the body's conservation of sodium and fluid. Therefore care must be taken not to overload the body with fluid; however, at the same time blood pressure must be maintained.

Safe Environment

A safe environment is one in which patients cannot harm themselves. Siderails need to be raised on the bed and warmth provided. Often notifying the family that the patient is well is comforting to the family and the patient. If the patient is experiencing pain, the location needs to be assessed and often an analgesic given. Pain can be frightening to people.

A safe environment is also free of pathogenic microorganisms. Postoperative patients are particularly prone to infection because of their weakened condition, and the presence of an open wound provides an opportunity for microorganisms to enter the body.

POSTOPERATIVE NURSING INTERVENTION

Once patients are awake and have a stable condition, they are normally transferred back to the nursing unit. Upon arrival each patient's condition needs to be carefully assessed. Checking-in practices generally involve taking vital signs, including blood pressure, checking dressings for bleeding or drainage, checking intravenous infusion for rate and any interstitial infiltration, checking drainage tubes for patency, and checking the physician's orders in regard to care.

Postoperative care is designed to assist patients meet their physiologic and psychologic needs and to prevent any complications.

Respiratory Needs

The patient will have learned deep breathing and coughing techniques preoperatively. These should be carried out hourly during the waking hours. Early ambulation will also assist deep breathing. For patients who cannot get out of bed, a bed-sitting position permits the greatest lung expansion, and assisting the patient to turn from side to side every 2 hours helps total lung expansion. In some settings intermittent positive pressure breathing (IPPB) is routinely given to patients to ensure optimum lung expansion (see "Intermittent Positive Pressure Breathing Therapy" in Chapter 28).

Atelectasis is a respiratory complication that can occur any time postoperatively. It is caused by mucous plugs, which result from a number of factors such as atropine, which makes mucus tenacious and thick, and narcotics, which can suppress the cough reflex. The symptoms of atelectasis are marked dyspnea, cyanosis, pleural pain, prostration, and tachycardia.

Another respiratory complication that can develop 1 to 2 weeks postoperatively is *hypostatic pneumonia*. This pneumonia is caused by inadequate aeration of lung tissue. Mucous membranes and capillary blood become congested in one part of the lung, and an infectious process results when microorganisms from the upper respiratory tract invade the area. Immobility and inadequate lung expansion can contribute to hypostatic pneumonia.

Circulatory Needs

Maintaining blood circulation is essential to recovery. A number of measures can assist the maintenance of adequate circulation. Leg exercises were learned preoperatively and need to be carried out every hour during the waking hours. Early ambulation also encourages circulation. For persons who have any cardiovascular disease, bandaging the legs may be indicated to support the superficial veins. Adequate fluid intake prevents the concentration of the blood. Another nursing measure of importance is

to avoid the use of pillows or rolls under the patient's knees because the pressure can constrict the blood vessels and slow circulation to and from the lower legs.

The circulatory complications to be avoided are shock, thrombophlebitis, and phlebothrombosis. *Shock* or cardiovascular collapse can be caused by many factors, but the most common postoperative one is blood loss. Shock is manifested by low blood pressure, rapid thready pulse, shallow rapid respirations, and cold clammy skin. Vital signs should be checked frequently (every 15 minutes) until they are stable and then regularly (every three hours) for several days, and dressings must be checked for blood oozing regularly. Other complications are *thrombophlebitis* (inflammation of a vein followed by development of a blood clot) and *phlebothrombosis* (intravascular clotting with marked inflammation of a vein). In thrombophlebitis the clots are firmly attached to the vein, and they can increase in size until the vessel lumen is occluded. In phlebothrombosis the clots are soft and loosely attached; they can become detached and as an embolus go to the lung (pulmonary embolism) or to the heart (coronary embolism). The signs of an embolus are startling. The patient experiences a sharp stabbing pain, becomes breathless, cyanotic, and anxious. If death does not occur within half an hour the patient may recover. The causes of thrombophlebitis and phlebothrombosis are the slowing of the blood flow, increased blood concentration, and injury to a vein such as can occur from the pressure of a pillow under the knees.

Urinary Needs

With the administration of an anesthetic the urinary bladder tone is temporarily depressed, but it usually returns six to eight hours after surgery. Some patients experience difficulty voiding after surgery of the rectum, vagina, or lower abdomen. This is thought to be due to spasm of the bladder sphincter. If a patient has not voided eight hours after surgery, this needs to be reported and urinary retention suspected. Nurses need to be aware of retention with overflow and the signs that indicate this condition (frequent voiding or voiding small amounts). Measuring the patient's fluid intake and output can provide the nurse with an indication of urinary adequacy. In some instances urinary bladder catheterization is indicated if other measures are not successful in stimulating voiding (see "Assistance to Maintain Normal Voiding Patterns" in Chapter 27).

Gastrointestinal Needs

Postoperatively most patients will complain of thirst; they will say that their mouth is dry and sticky. The reasons for this feeling of thirst are the fasting period preoperatively, the preoperative medication such as atropine or hyoscine, and the loss of body fluid because of blood loss, perspiration, and perhaps vomiting. The patient who can have fluids by mouth should first take only sips of water because of limited tolerance. If patients cannot take fluid by mouth, they may be permitted ice chips to suck (check the physician's order), or mouth care is indicated (see "Oral Hygiene" in Chapter 20).

Nausea and vomiting can also occur postoperatively. This is often due to the type of anesthetic, a side effect of a medication, intestinal activity, or stress. A patient who expects to vomit after surgery probably will. The nurse should initially assess the reason for the nausea. If it is due to the anesthesia, provide mouth care and withhold fluids temporarily. If it is due to a medication, note the time of nausea in relation to the medications, and notify the physician. Lying quietly and taking deep breaths will also help prevent vomiting.

Abdominal distention is very common after surgery. It is primarily due to the slowing of the bowel peristalsis because of the anesthesia and trauma to the bowels during surgery. Often food and fluids are not given to the patient until peristalsis has returned to normal. For nursing intervention in regard to distention see "Nursing Intervention for Flatulence" in Chapter 26. In addition, nurses should observe and report the passage of flatus and encourage peristalsis by ambulation, exercise, turning frequently in bed, and providing food and fluids when the patient is ready.

The discomfort due to distention can be relieved by the following:

1. Rectal tube.
2. Carminative enema. See "Enemas" in Chapter 26.
3. Suppository.
4. Analgesic.
5. Reducing anxiety, thus reducing the amount of air that is swallowed and relaxing the anal sphincter to ease passage of flatus.

Relief from Pain

Pain is often feared by patients who have surgery. It is usually greatest 12 to 36 hours postoperatively and

Table 37-2.   ABC's of Recovery

A	Ambulation	Dangling
		Standing
		Walking
B	Breathing and coughing	Deep breathing and coughing every hour
C	Comfort	Analgesics
		Moving
D	Drink and drain	Fluid intake and output
E	Exercise	Leg exercises
		Moving
F	Food and flatus	Return of peristalsis
		Exercise

generally starts decreasing on the second day. Usually patients will have analgesics administered the first day, in many cases every 4 hours. By the second day they are given less frequently, and by the third day most patients require only oral analgesics. The amount of pain experienced is the same for all persons; that is, the same intensity causes the same perception. However, the reaction to pain varies considerably among individual patients. These reactions are learned responses, and it is important that the nurse accept these responses. The signs of acute pain are pallor, perspiration, and tenseness (see "Assessment of Pain" in Chapter 24). For methods of relieving pain see "Nursing Interventions to Relieve Pain" in Chapter 24. See Table 37-2 for the ABC's of recovery.

Safety

If the patient has an open wound, it is important that sterile technique be used for dressing changes. To prevent respiratory tract infections patients should not be in contact with a person who has an infection such as a cold.

The feeling of safety also includes the perception of competency of the nursing personnel. Nursing intervention needs to be provided competently and on time. Patients feel greatly reassured when a nurse answers a light promptly and follows through with the care planned. These actions of the nurse will reassure a patient and the family. Thus anxiety is relieved when they feel that the patient is being competently cared for.

SUMMARY

There are many reasons for surgery and many kinds of operations. Nurses should know why a patient is having an operation. The reason is important in appreciating the patient's point of view and concerns. Before any surgical procedure it is necessary to have a consent form signed. For persons under 18 years of age consent must be signed by an adult, preferably a relative.

Preoperatively a patient's needs are assessed relative to age, nutritional status, fluid and electrolyte balance, general health, medication use, and mental health. A nurse's observations should be recorded and any unusual observation reported to the surgeon. Preoperative nursing intervention is designed to promote the patient's recovery postoperatively and to avoid complications. Learning deep breathing, coughing, and leg exercises are important aspects of preoperative care. Most patients will require a skin preparation preoperatively, and some patients will need to have a gastric tube inserted.

When the anesthetist visits the patient preoperatively, he or she will discuss the administration of an anesthetic and order the preoperative medications. After the surgery, most patients will go to a recovery room where they will wake up. Once patients are awake and their conditions have stabilized they will return to the nursing unit for postoperative care.

Postoperative nursing care is oriented toward maintaining the patient's physiologic and psychologic homeostasis. The patient may need assistance from nurses to meet respiratory, circulatory, and urinary needs. Most patients fear pain, and it is important to use analgesics wisely to avoid severe pain but not to depress vital physiologic functions.

The length of stay in a hospital for surgery is generally shorter than it was ten years ago. Patients are encouraged to ambulate early and keep their muscle tone. A recent trend is the day surgery patient who comes to the hospital for an operation and goes home that same day. Some agencies have special day-care centers for the care of these patients. In some pediatric settings, parents are encouraged to attend the day-care center and assist with their child's care.

SUGGESTED ACTIVITIES

1. Select a patient who is anticipating surgery. Plan and provide the preoperative nursing required.

Observe the patient in the recovery room after the surgery. Compare your assessment with the nurse's assessment.

2. Plan the nursing care for a patient who is 2 days postoperative. Identify the patient's needs, and plan to assist the patient with these needs.

3. Interview a patient who had an operation a week or more ago. What concerns did the patient have? How did nursing personnel assist with these needs?

SUGGESTED READINGS

Goulding, E. J. et al. October, 1965. The newborn: his response to surgery. *American Journal of Nursing* 65:84–87.

   The authors describe the special postoperative concerns for the newborn. Blood loss and preventing aspiration are discussed.

Luciano, Kathy. November, 1974. The who, when, where, what and how of preparing children for surgery. *Nursing '74* 4:64–65.

   The article discusses the special preoperative preparation needed by children. Practical guides are provided for nurses in regard to appropriate vocabulary to use when providing information to children.

Mezzanotte, Elizabeth J. January, 1970. Group instruction in preparation for surgery. *American Journal of Nursing* 70:89–91.

   Preoperative group instruction for a selected group of patients anticipating abdominal surgery is discussed. A sample patient instruction sheet is included.

SELECTED REFERENCES

Collart, Marie, and Brenneman, Janice K. October, 1971. Preventing postoperative atelectasis. *American Journal of Nursing* 71:1982–1987.

Goulding, E. J., et al. October, 1965. The newborn: his responses to surgery. *American Journal of Nursing* 65:84–87.

Hardgrove, Carol, and Rutledge, Ann. May, 1975. Parenting during hospitalization. *American Journal of Nursing* 75:836–838.

Healy, Kathryn M. January, 1968. Does preoperative instruction make a difference? *American Journal of Nursing* 68:62–67.

Laird, Mona. August, 1975. Techniques for teaching pre and post operative patients. *American Journal of Nursing* 75:1338–1340.

Libman, Robert H., and Keithley, Joyce. April, 1975. Relieving airway obstruction in the recovery room. *American Journal of Nursing* 75:603–605.

Luciano, Kathy. November, 1974. The who, when, where, what and how of preparing children for surgery. *Nursing '74* 4:64–65.

McConnell, Edwina A. March, 1977. After surgery. *Nursing 77* 7:32–39.

McConnell, Edwina A. September, 1975. All about gastrointenstinal intubation. *Nursing 75* 5:30–37.

McConnell, Edwina A. September, 1977. Ensuring safer stomach suctioning with a Salem sump tube. *Nursing 77* 7:54–57.

CHAPTER 38

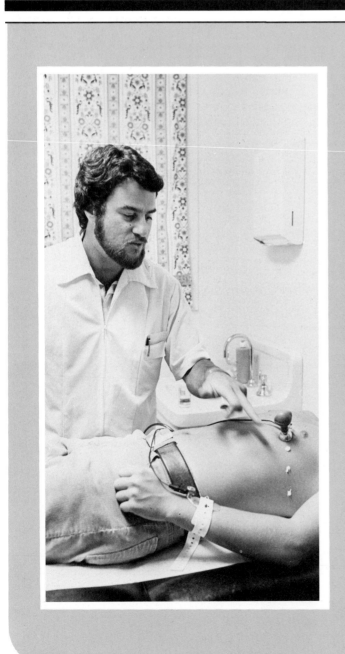

TESTS AND TREATMENTS

GENERAL NURSING GUIDELINES

EXAMINATIONS THAT MEASURE AND RECORD ELECTRICAL IMPULSES

EXAMINATIONS INVOLVING VISUAL INSPECTION

EXAMINATIONS INVOLVING ROENTGENOGRAPHY (X-RAY)

EXAMINATIONS INVOLVING RADIOACTIVE SUBSTANCES

LUMBAR PUNCTURE

ABDOMINAL PARACENTESIS

THORACENTESIS

PERICARDIAL ASPIRATION

BONE MARROW BIOPSY

GASTRIC ANALYSIS

TESTS

OBJECTIVES

- Discuss the psychologic preparation of the patient and family.

- Prepare a patient physically for a specific examination.

- Assemble the equipment for an examination.

- Plan and implement care for a patient during and after an examination.

- Care for the specimen after an examination.

- Describe the purpose and the technique for each of the following examinations or treatments.
  a. electrocardiogram
  b. electroencephalogram
  c. electromyogram
  d. bronchoscopy
  e. laryngoscopy
  f. gastroscopy
  g. cystoscopy
  h. proctoscopy, sigmoidoscopy, colonoscopy
  i. upper GI series
  j. barium enema
  k. cholecystogram
  l. angiogram
  m. myelogram
  n. abdominal paracentesis
  o. thoracentesis
  p. pericardial aspiration
  q. bone marrow biopsy
  r. gastric analysis

- List the criteria by which the effectiveness of each of the above treatments or examinations can be evaluated.

Assisting with tests and treatments is a dependent nursing function; the test or treatment is generally ordered by a physician. The nurse's function focuses on two aspects: the patient and family and the test being conducted. Tests and treatments are frightening to many people. Their fear is generally related to pain that might be experienced, the results of the test, and how they will handle both of these. The unknown enhances this fear. It is important for the nurse to be aware of the particular needs of patients and their families and to assist them to meet these needs.

The nurse also has a responsibility in regard to the test or treatment itself. It is frequently a nursing function to assemble the equipment when the technique is to take place in a clinical nursing unit or a physician's office. The nurse is also responsible for assessing the patient during the procedure and after it. Many tests and treatments require special nursing intervention afterward to minimize untoward reactions. The nurse is the person who is often responsible for the success of these procedures. A well-prepared patient is more likely to have a successful test or treatment with minimal discomfort.

The diagnostic aspect of tests often requires the services of a number of health personnel. Some of these are specialists in laboratory tests, radiologic or roentgenographic techniques, and cardiac testing. The nurse has a coordinating function in regard to these various personnel and their services. It is the nurse who will assist in their scheduling and who will assist the patient with this schedule.

GENERAL NURSING GUIDELINES

Prepare the Patient and Family Psychologically

The patient and possibly the family will need an explanation of what the test or treatment is and what will happen. This explanation needs to be adjusted to the patient's needs. A small child will require a different explanation than a curious adult. Some persons want to know every detail, but others only need a general explanation. It is important that the nurse be honest with the patient; if there is to be an instant of sharp pain, it is better to say this rather than to overlook it.

Often patients want to know where the test will take place, who will do it, how long will it last, and when will the results be available. The latter is a most important question, often associated with fear. The nurse can give the best answer based upon experience and the physician's opinion. If the results are delayed, it is important that this be followed up and the patient given an explanation.

As a general rule it is wise not to offer information about possible complications and severe reactions, but if the patient asks, the questions should be answered honestly. The facts need to be presented objectively and accurately without exaggeration. For a child who is undergoing tests the family will probably require assistance. By being able to anticipate when they can visit and how the patient will feel, they will be better able to offer support.

Prepare the Patient Physically

For some tests special preparation is required, such as a cleansing enema before a barium enema or sedation before a bronchoscopy. In some instances special lighting and drapes are required at the patient's unit. Just before a treatment such as a paracentesis the patient will need to assume a special position. The provision of a sedation or a tranquilizer is often a nursing judgment when they are ordered prn (when needed). It is important that the nurse be sensitive to the patient's emotions and aware of excessive anxiety.

Assemble Equipment

It is usually a nursing responsibility to assemble the equipment for any tests and treatments carried out at a patient's bedside in a hospital or in an adjacent clinical treatment room. When a patient goes to another unit such as the radiology department, assembling the equipment is the responsibility of that department. It is also a nursing responsibility to maintain the sterility of sterile equipment.

Many hospitals today use prepackaged disposable sets, which require a minimum of setting up. The set should be checked to see that all required equipment is there. If the nurse is unsure, it is important to check the agency policy and procedure and make any adjustments to the set.

During the Procedure: Assist the Patient

During the treatment or test it is important for the nurse to observe the patient and provide emotional support. The observations need to include any signs of distress such as pallor, profuse sweating, nausea, accelerated pulse, or acute pain. Any of these signs need to be reported to the person conducting the procedure immediately. The nurse can support the patient by providing some information such as, "It will only be 2 more minutes," "The needle is all the way in now," or "You won't feel any additional discomfort." Sometimes asking the patient questions can distract him or her and relieve anxiety; however, it is important that the nurse be sensitive to the patient's needs in this regard.

During the Procedure: Assist with the Procedure

In some instances the nurse is required to hand the person carrying out the procedure additional equipment or to make notes such as writing down the spinal fluid pressure during a lumbar puncture. It is important to be alert to any needs in relation to the treatment and to anticipate these whenever possible.

After the Procedure: Assist the Patient and Support the Family

After the procedure the nurse's first responsibility is to assist the patient to a comfortable position or in some instances, such as a lumbar puncture, to a dorsal recumbent position. If family members are waiting, they need to be told when it is completed and that they can see the patient. It is best to remove the equipment before visitors enter because of the anxiety some equipment such as long needles can elicit.

Care of Equipment and Specimens

After the test or treatment the equipment is returned to the appropriate area and disposed of according to agency policy. Equipment that is not disposed of is washed and rinsed and placed in the area for further care.

Any specimen must be appropriately labeled. In a hospital this usually includes the patient's name, identification number, and date. Some specimens require special care if they are not sent directly to the laboratory. Some urine specimens are refrigerated, and some feces specimens must be kept warm so that microorganisms such as parasites can be identified.

Recording

After the procedure, the nurse is responsible for the recording on the patient's record. This needs to include the treatment or test performed, the time, who carried it out, whether a specimen was taken, any specific information such as spinal fluid pressures, and the patient's response.

Nursing Evaluation after the Procedure

It is important that the nurse evaluate the patient's condition after any test or treatment. The time interval will depend upon the patient's reaction to the test. Even if there have been no untoward reactions, the patient's condition needs to be evaluated, for example, ½ hour afterward, and any adjustments made in care. Some patients feel nauseated half an hour after a procedure such as a thoracentesis.

EXAMINATIONS THAT MEASURE AND RECORD ELECTRICAL IMPULSES

There are a number of machines that measure and record electrical impulses. The *electrocardiograph* receives impulses from the heart, the *electroencephalograph* from the brain, and the *electromyograph* from muscles. With all these machines electrodes are attached to the body part. The electrodes pick up the electrical activity and transfer this on paper in the form of a graph such as an *electrocardiogram* (graph of electrical impulses from the heart, also called an *ECG* or *EKG).* The graph reading can also be shown on an oscilloscope screen.

Electrocardiogram

The electrodes from an electrocardiograph are attached to leads, which in turn are attached to the

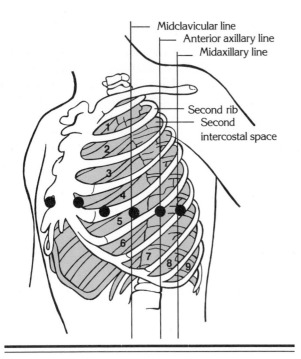

Figure 38-1. The placement of electrodes upon the chest of an adult for an electrocardiogram.

machine. The electrodes are attached to the person's body by paste, suction cups, or tape. One electrode is attached to each lower limb, and a fifth electrode is moved to different positions on the chest. It is customary to use six standard positions over the heart. The first position is on the right sternal border, then they follow the general outline of the heart around to the left sternal border, then laterally as far as the midaxillary line. (See Figure 38-1.)

The heart muscle is said to be *polarized* or charged when it is in a state of rest. When the muscle

cells of the ventricles and the atria contract, they *depolarize* or lose their charge. During a resting stage they regain their electrical charge or *repolarize*. Depolarization and repolarization are recorded on an electrocardiogram.

The heartbeat is normally initiated at the *sinoatrial (SA) node,* which is located in the upper aspect of the right atrium. The SA node is often referred to as the pacemaker of the heart. The impulse radiates over the atria, causing them to contract. It is then picked up by the *atrioventricular (AV) node,* which is situated at the base of the atrial septum. The impulse then travels down two bundle branches from the AV node, which have numerous fibers, referred to as *Purkinje fibers* or the Purkinje system, throughout the ventricles of the heart. As the impulse travels throughout this system the ventricles contract or depolarize. Figure 38-2 shows a normal electrocardiogram and indicates times of depolarization and repolarization. The P wave arises when the impulse from the SA node causes the atria to contract or depolarize. The QRS wave occurs with contraction and depolarization of the ventricles. The T wave represents the resting or repolarization of the ventricles. Repolarization of the atria occurs during the QRS segment of the graph; it is normally not seen on an ECG. The ECG is normally produced on finely lined paper. The horizontal lines represent the voltage of the electrical impulse, and the vertical lines represent time. (See Figure 38-3.) With cardiac pathologic conditions the graph waves can be abnormal in size, position, and form.

Patients who require ECGs may go to a special department of a hospital or laboratory. If the patient is very ill, there are portable ECG machines that can be brought to a bedside in a home or hospital. Con-

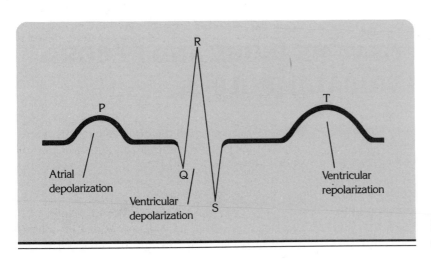

Figure 38-2. A normal electrocardiograph.

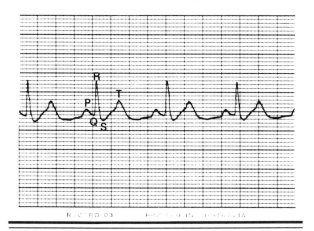

Figure 38-3. A graph of a normal elctrocardiogram reading.

tinual monitoring of the heart is often done for persons who are critically ill. In this case the machine is called a *cardiac monitor*, and the cardiac waves show up on an oscilloscope, usually on the machine.

Having an electrocardiogram taken is painless and usually takes about 10 minutes. Some physicians include an electrocardiogram as part of a routine physical examination for patients over 40 years of age. No special preparation is required before the test.

Electroencephalogram

Electrodes from an electroencephalograph are attached to the machine by leads and to the person's scalp with paste or small needles. The patient lies in a dorsal recumbent position in a darkened room. The patient may be asked to take deep breaths (*hyperventilate*), and readings may also be taken while asleep. If the latter is required, the test may take 2 hours; otherwise it may last no more than ½ to 1 hour. The test is normally painless, although the patient may feel occasional pinpricks if the needle electrodes are used in the scalp.

Preparation for an EEG varies. Some agencies advise that the patient not take stimulants such as coffee or depressants such as alcohol the day of the test. Usually no medications are taken prior to the test, and the hair is shampooed and should be free of any preparations such as spray.

Electromyogram

An electromyogram records the electrical potential created by the contraction of a muscle. Two electrodes are attached to the skin over the muscle with paste or small needles. This test is used to discern muscle abnormalities such as *fasciculation* (abnormal contraction involving the whole motor unit).

EXAMINATIONS INVOLVING VISUAL INSPECTION

A number of examinations involve looking at an interior part of the body with a lighted instrument.

Bronchoscopy

A lighted instrument, a *bronchoscope*, is used to visualize the bronchi of the lungs. The examination is referred to as a *bronchoscopy*. Prior to the procedure the patient usually fasts for 6 hours and is given a sedative. If a general anesthetic is given, routine preoperative care is given (see Chapter 37). Dentures are removed prior to the examination.

If a general anesthetic is not given, a local anesthetic will be sprayed on the patient's pharynx to prevent gagging. The bronchoscope is then inserted to visualize the bronchi. In some instances a section of tissue may be taken for biopsy. After this examination, the patient should not take food or fluids until the local anesthetic has worn off and the gag reflex

has returned, otherwise the patient could aspirate food and fluid. The possible complications are bleeding due to damaged tissue, laryngospasm, and respiratory distress. A *bronchogram* is a roentgenogram (x-ray film) of the bronchial tree after an iodized oil dye has been instilled. A general anesthetic is usually given for this.

Laryngoscopy

A *laryngoscope* is a lighted instrument used to visualize the larynx. The examination is called a *laryngoscopy*. The preparation is similar to that for a bronchoscopy; local or generalized anesthetic can be used. A biopsy may be taken during the examination.

Precautions afterward include withholding food and fluids until the gag reflex is restored after a local anesthetic. The complications to observe for include bleeding due to tissue damage and laryngogospasm.

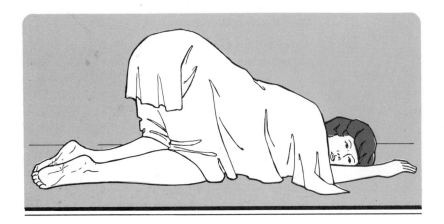

Figure 38-4. The knee-chest position commonly used for examinations of the rectum and colon.

Gastroscopy

A *gastroscopy* is the visualization of the interior of the stomach with a lighted instrument called a *gastroscope*. The preparation and care of the patient are the same as in a bronchoscopy. An *esophagoscopy* is the examination of the esophagus with a lighted instrument; it is similar to a gastroscopy.

Cystoscopy

Cystoscopy is the visualization of the interior of the urinary bladder with a lighted instrument called a *cystoscope*. Usually a general anesthetic is given, and the preparation is similar to that for a bronchoscopy. During a cystoscopy ureteral catheters may be inserted up the ureters into each kidney. Contrast medium is then injected into the kidneys. This procedure is known as a *retrograde pyelogram*. The x-ray film will show the kidney calices, the kidney pelvis, the ureters, and the urinary bladder. When a pyelogram is to be carried out, the intestines need to be free of feces and gas. This is done through the administration of laxatives and enemas. An *intravenous pyelogram* is the injection of dye into the arterial system for circulation to the kidneys; it shows the same structures as in a retrograde pyelogram. This examination does not require an anesthetic and normally takes about one hour.

It is advised to encourage fluids to decrease irritation and the possibility of infections after a cystoscopy. No special intervention is indicated after a pyelogram.

Proctoscopy, Sigmoidoscopy, and Colonoscopy

A *proctoscopy* is the examination of the rectum with a lighted instrument (*proctoscope*). A *sigmoidoscopy* is the examination of the sigmoid colon and the rectum with a lighted instrument (*sigmoidoscope*). A *colonoscopy* is the examination of the entire colon (large bowel) with a lighted instrument (*colonoscope*).

Preparation generally includes laxatives or enemas begun the evening before to clear the bowel of feces. General anesthesia is usually not used, although the patient may experience some discomfort. The patient assumes a knee-chest position for the examination (see Figure 38-4). After these examinations, bleeding because of tissue trauma needs to be watched for.

EXAMINATIONS INVOLVING ROENTGENOGRAPHY (X-RAY)

There are a wide variety of roentgenographic (x-ray) examinations, some of which involve the simple projection of a body part upon a film. Because of the density of body parts such as bones, a view can be projected onto x-ray film by view taking. The particular view is usually requested by a physician. Other roentgenograms (x-ray films) require the use of contrast media because otherwise the body part such as a

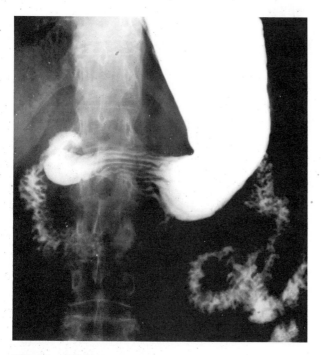

Figure 38-5. An X-ray of the stomach and duodenum using barium as the contrast medium.

gallbladder will not show up. The pyelogram is one of these which has already been discussed.

Upper GI Series (Stomach, Esophagus, Duodenum)

For roentgenogram of the upper gastrointestinal tract the tract must be free of food and fluid; therefore the patient takes nothing by mouth (food or fluid) after midnight. The patient drinks a barium solution, and roentgenograms are taken outlining the organs (see Figure 38-5). Some barium solutions have a slight flavor such as chocolate. The solution is thick, and about one glass is swallowed.

After the examination the patient is advised to take a laxative to eliminate the barium before it hardens in the gastrointestinal tract.

Barium Enema (Lower GI Series)

For a roentgenogram of the large intestine the lower bowel is first filled with barium. This is instilled by enema, and the patient will be asked to change position several times in order for the barium to reach all parts of the colon. The patient has laxatives and an enema starting the evening before the examination.

Precautions after the examination are the same as for an upper gastrointestinal series.

Cholecystogram and Cholangiogram

These are roentgenograms of the gallbladder (*cholecystogram*) and the bile ducts (*cholangiogram*). Before these tests the person takes no food or fluids after midnight. For the cholecystogram a fat-free meal is taken the previous evening, and contrast pills are also ingested. The contrast medium is excreted through the gallbladder; therefore roentgenograms are taken to see whether the dye is present in the gallbladder. A fatty meal is then taken by the patient, and more roentgenograms are taken to observe the function of the gallbladder. A cholangiogram is generally done during surgery. The dye is injected into the bile ducts, and roentgenograms are then taken.

There is no unusual intervention required, although the patient may experience some burning when the dye is excreted in the urine after a cholecystogram.

Angiogram

An *angiogram* visualizes the veins and arteries, often in an organ such as the heart but also in major vessels such as the femoral arteries. The patient takes nothing by mouth after midnight of the evening before. A catheter is threaded into an artery, contrast dye is injected, and roentgenograms are taken of the circulation. Nursing observations need to include any indications of thrombus formation or bleeding from the site of the injection. An *arteriogram* is the same as an angiogram but applies specifically to arterial circulation.

Myelogram

A *myelogram* is the examination of the spinal canal through the injection of dye into the spinal canal. A lumbar puncture (see "Lumbar Puncture" in this chapter) is performed; some spinal fluid is removed and replaced by dye. The patient is usually on a tilt table so that the head can be lowered and the dye permitted to ascend to the desired level. Roentgenograms are taken of the spinal canal. Preparation beforehand includes nothing by mouth after midnight and a sedative before the examination. After the myelogram the patient is advised to remain in a prone position (see "Lumbar Puncture").

For a *pneumoencephalogram* air is injected into the spinal canal instead of dye. The air rises to the ventricles of the brain, and roentgenograms are taken showing the outlines of the ventricles. After this examination, headache frequently occurs until all the air has been absorbed.

EXAMINATIONS INVOLVING RADIOACTIVE SUBSTANCES

For some examinations radioactive substances are injected or ingested. These substances have an affinity for specific tissues, such as iodine 131 for the thyroid gland. The tissue is then scanned, and the radioactive substance will provide an indication of its absorption by the tissue. For example, a tumor of the thyroid may show up as tissue that did not absorb the radioactive iodine as well as the thyroid tissue. The amount of radiation is minimal and is considered to be harmless. A number of scans are done; some of the most common are the brain scan, liver scan, and lung scan. For all of these examinations no special preparation is required. The examination is painless. The radioactive material is injected intravenously, and a machine moving back and forth over the body area picks up the radioactivity and transmits it to graph paper.

LUMBAR PUNCTURE

A *lumbar puncture* (spinal tap) is the insertion of a needle into the subarachnoid space of the spinal canal. Cerebrospinal fluid (CSF) is formed through the choroid villi in each of the brain's four ventricles. The fluid normally circulates freely through the ventricles, the subarachnoid space, and the central canal of the cord. It is absorbed into the venous circulation through villi from the arachnoid layer, which extend into the superior sagittal sinus.

Lumbar punctures are carried out for the following diagnostic and therapeutic reasons:

1. To obtain a specimen of cerebrospinal fluid.
2. To test the pressure of the cerebrospinal fluid.
3. To relieve the pressure from cerebrospinal fluid.
4. To inject a medication, dye, or air into the spinal canal.

A lumbar puncture is carried out by a physician. The nurse's function is to assist the patient and the physician.

Equipment

The lumbar puncture is a sterile technique requiring sterile equipment and supplies. Many hospitals have disposable kits for lumbar punctures. The equipment required is sterile sponges, disinfectant, needles (no. 21 and 24) 1.75 cm (¾ inch) and syringes, local anesthetic, sterile gloves, mask, lumbar puncture needle 5 to 12.5 cm (2 to 5 inches) depending upon the age and size of the patient (infants require a 5 cm [2 inch] needle), specimen tubes if needed, adapters for needles, manometer to measure spinal fluid pressure, three-way stopcock, and a container for discarded materials.

Prior to the start of the lumbar puncture the patient assumes a position arching the back. The nurse

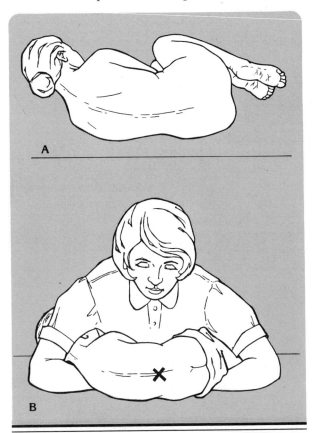

Figure 38-6.   Position of the patient for a lumbar puncture. **A,** Adult; and **B,** child.

can assist the patient to maintain this position by supporting the back of the patient's neck and the knees (see Figure 38-6). Many agencies have sterile fenestrated drapes, which the physician places over the area after scrubbing and gloving.

Site

The site of a lumbar puncture is usually between the third and fourth or the fourth and fifth vertebrae (see Figure 38-7). The fourth lumbar interspace is most commonly used on adults, but the site is usually lower for infants and small children because the spinal cord extends almost into the sacral region.

Technique

The physician applies a disinfectant to the area and then injects the local anesthetic. The needle is then inserted into the intravertebral space. The ma-

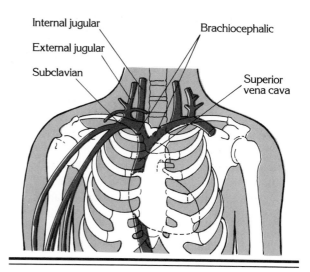

Figure 38-8.   A diagram showing the position of the internal jugular veins.

nometer is usually attached initially to obtain a pressure. The physician may wish to perform the Queckenstedt-Stookey test while the manometer is attached. Pressure is placed on both internal jugular veins (see Figure 38-8), often by the nurse, and normally the manometer will register an increased pressure. This is because the pressure impeded the flow of spinal fluid temporarily. A specimen may be taken at this time, and a medication can be introduced *intrathecally* (into the spinal canal). The physician will remove the spinal needle; sometimes a final spinal fluid pressure is taken first. The patient is then assisted to a comfortable position, usually dorsal recumbent or prone, until the spinal fluid has been replaced. Some physicians suggest elevating the foot of the bed. The patient can expect to maintain one of these bed positions for at least 24 hours. The patient can also expect some backache and headache for a few days after a lumbar puncture. Minimal environmental stimuli will assist the patient.

After a lumbar puncture the nurse gathers up the equipment and labels the specimen, which is sent to the laboratory. Normal cerebrospinal fluid is a clear, colorless fluid. The presence of blood may appear as a reddish color, and the presence of an infection can be manifested by cloudy fluid.

Recording after a lumbar puncture includes time, the lumbar puncture, the name of the physician, the color and consistency of the fluid, the amount taken for a specimen, initial and final pressures, medications, injections, and the response of the patient.

Nursing intervention after a lumbar puncture includes decreasing environmental stimuli, assisting

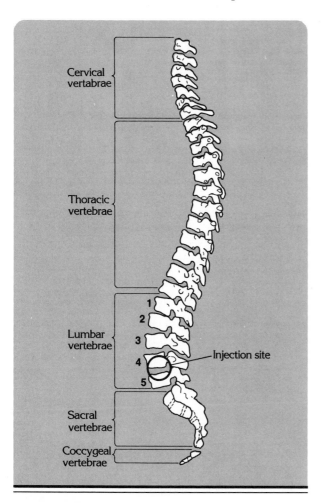

Figure 38-7.   A diagram of the vertebral column indicating the sites used for a lumbar puncture.

the patient to maintain the bed position described, and observations for shock (pallor, accelerated pulse rate, or excessive perspiration).

Cisternal Puncture

A *cisternal puncture* is similar to a lumbar puncture except that the physician inserts a needle into the subarachnoid space of the cisterna magna (see Figure 38-9). For this technique the patient acutely flexes the neck to permit the insertion of the needle between the first cervical vertebra and the rim of the foramen magnum. A cisternal puncture is done for a ventriculogram and pneumoventriculogram. A *ventriculogram* is a roentgenogram of the ventricles of the brain after the introduction of an opaque dye. A *pneumoventriculogram* is a roentgenogram of the ventricles of the brain after the introduction of air.

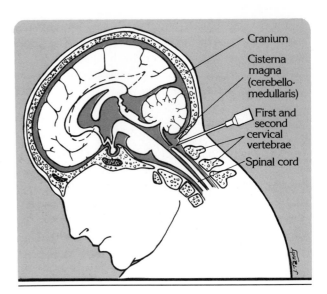

Figure 38-9.   The insertion of a needle into the subarachnoid space of the cisterna magna.

ABDOMINAL PARACENTESIS

An *abdominal paracentesis* is the removal of fluid from the peritoneal cavity. When a large amount of fluid collects in the cavity, the condition is called *ascites.* Normally there is just sufficient fluid present to lubricate the surface of the peritoneum and prevent friction between the peritoneum and the tissues with which it comes in contact. Normally the fluid formed is absorbed into the lymph circulation through lymph vessels in the peritoneum; however, in some conditions excessive fluid is formed, which the lymph system is unable to handle. Methods of treatment include restriction of fluids, low sodium intake, administration of diuretics, and occasionally an abdominal paracentesis. A paracentesis is also carried out for diagnostic purposes. A specimen of peritoneal fluid may be examined for abnormal constituents such as red blood cells and white blood cells.

Equipment

The abdominal paracentesis is a sterile technique requiring sterile equipment and supplies. Sets are usually available, and they need to contain disinfectant, sponges, local anesthetic, syringe and no. 24 and 22 needles to administer the anesthetic, sterile gloves, dressings, and the aspirating set. The latter generally includes a receptacle for the fluid, tubing, and a trocar and cannula. A *trocar* is a sharp-pointed instrument often used with a cannula. A *cannula* is a tube that can

be inserted into body cavities; a trocar fits inside the cannula and provides the sharp point for insertion. Plastic tubing can often thread through the trocar, ensuring slow drainage of the fluid. If the abdomen is to be entered solely to obtain a specimen, a long aspirating needle is used rather than a trocar. In this instance an incision is not made; therefore a scalpel, sutures, and needle holder are not required as they are when the paracentesis is done to drain fluid. A sterile fenestrated drape is frequently applied by the physician after gloving.

Prior to the start of the abdominal paracentesis the patient should empty the bladder to avoid puncturing it when the trocar is inserted. If the patient is unable to void, the physician needs to be informed of this before starting. The position of choice for an abdominal paracentesis is a sitting one so that the force of gravity and the pressure of the abdominal organs can help the flow of the fluid (see Figure 38-10).

Site

A common site is midway between the symphysis pubis and the umbilicus on the midline. The patient needs to be supported in the sitting position. The procedure itself is usually not painful; however, the patient may feel faint as a result of released abdominal pressure. Draining ascitic fluid is done slowly to minimize this shock.

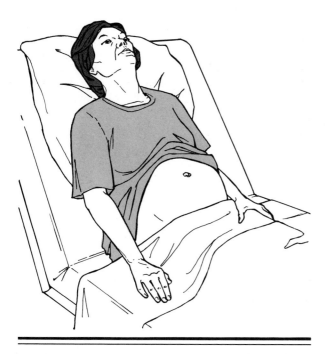

Figure 38-10.   The sitting position assumed by a patient who is having an abdominal paracentesis.

Technique

The physician paints the area with disinfectant, anesthetizes the area, and then makes a small incision at the site. The trocar and cannula are inserted, the trocar is removed, and the plastic tubing is threaded through the cannula into the abdominal cavity. The other end of the tubing is placed in the container to collect the fluid.

The nurse needs to observe the patient carefully during the procedure for signs of shock such as pallor, accelerated pulse rate, sweating, and *syncope* (fainting). After the paracentesis is completed, the cannula and tubing are removed, and a small dressing is placed over the incision. The wound may be sutured. Often patients feel more comfortable wearing an abdominal binder after a paracentesis because it provides support.

Observation of the patient for signs of shock needs to be continued after the procedure. The release of pressure results in redistribution of circulating fluids, and this can result in inadequate cerebral and peripheral circulation.

After an abdominal paracentesis the nurse gathers up the equipment and labels the specimen, which is sent to the laboratory. Normal ascitic fluid is clear, serous, and light yellow. The protein content is normally low. A record is made of the time, treatment, name of the physician, color and consistency of the fluid, amount of fluid removed, and the response of the patient.

Nursing intervention after an abdominal paracentesis includes assessing blood pressure, pulse, and respirations, as well as taking body weight. The latter gives a measure of the amount of fluid removed.

THORACENTESIS

A *thoracentesis* is the withdrawal of fluid from the pleural cavity. Pleural fluid is removed for both diagnostic and therapeutic purposes. A specimen can be analyzed for the presence of microorganisms such as pneumococci or streptococci. Aspiration may be indicated to relieve pain, dyspnea, and other symptoms of pressure. Normally there is just sufficient fluid present to lubricate the pleura so that they can move freely. The pleural cavity is a potential space where the pressure is a negative one.

Equipment

The equipment required for a thoracentesis includes local anesthetic, needle and syringe for its administration (see "Lumbar Puncture"), disinfectant, gauze swabs, aspirating set, airtight drainage receptacle, suction machine or pump to obtain a negative pressure in the drainage receptacle, sterile gloves, mask, and discard container. This is also a sterile procedure, and all supplies and equipment need to be sterile with the exception of the drainage container and suction.

Prior to the start of the procedure the nurse should establish a negative pressure in the drainage receptacle. The pressure needs to be greater than that in the pleural space (–4 mm of mercury) so that the fluid will drain into the container. Fluid flows from an area of high pressure to one of lesser pressure. The negative pressure also prevents air from entering the pleural space to cause a pneumothorax (accumulation of air in the pleural cavity), which could cause a lung to collapse. The thoracentesis needle can be attached to the container through tubing and a stopcock. A syringe can be attached to the stopcock to obtain a specimen.

Site

The patient assumes a supported sitting position with the arm across the chest or over the head to spread the ribs (see Figure 38-11, *A*). Another position is the side-lying recumbent position on the affected side. The arm on that side is held above the head. Some patients sit leaning forward over pillows or an overbed table (see Figure 38-11, *B*).

The site of insertion is selected by palpation. It is important that it be below the level of the fluid. A site in the lower posterior chest is often used to remove fluid and one in the upper anterior chest to remove air.

Technique

The physician applies disinfectant to the site and injects local anesthetic. The aspirating needle, which is attached to the adapter, is inserted through the intercostal space into the pleural cavity. The adapter is in a closed position so that no air will enter the pleural cavity. The tubing from the vacuum bottle is attached to the needle. The adapter and stopcock (on the container) are opened, producing a suction between the pleural cavity and the container. This suction pulls the fluid from the cavity.

It is important that the patient not cough during this procedure. If the patient has to cough, the physician will close the adapter and withdraw the needle a little so that it will not puncture a lung. If a sterile specimen is required, the physician can withdraw it with a syringe attached to the adapter.

Throughout a thoracentesis it is important to observe the patient for any untoward reactions such as color, pulse, and respiratory rates. The sudden withdrawal of fluid may cause fainting, or puncturing a blood vessel could cause a lung to collapse.

After all the fluid has been withdrawn, pressure is applied, and a sterile dressing or a sealing fluid or both are applied over the site. The nurse records the time, treatment, name of the physician, amount, color, and consistency of the fluid, and the response of the patient.

Nursing intervention after a thoracentesis includes observation of the patient's respirations, particularly noting excessive coughing or the presence of any blood-tinged sputum *(hemoptysis)*. If the thora-

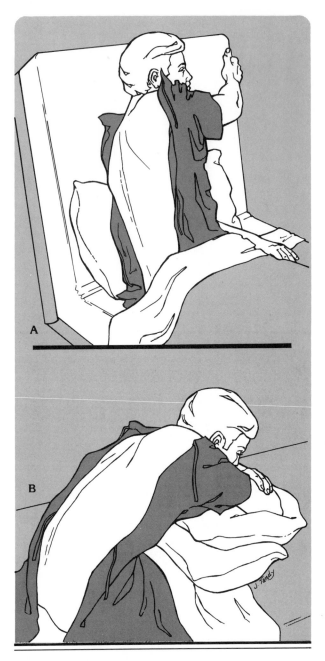

Figure 38-11. The two positions commonly assumed by patients having a thoracentesis. **A,** Arm above head; and **B,** sitting and leaning forward over pillows.

centesis has been successful, the patient will probably experience a sense of relief because respirations will be easier.

PERICARDIAL ASPIRATION

A *pericardial aspiration* is the removal of fluid from the pericardial sac. It is usually carried out either to relieve pressure upon the heart or to obtain a specimen for diagnostic purposes. Normally there are only about 15 to 30 ml of a clear, light yellow fluid present in the pericardial sac. The patient assumes a sitting position so that the fluid will fill the base of the sac by gravity.

The required equipment is similar to that used for a thoracentesis except that because the amount of fluid is small, a syringe attached to a stopcock can be used to provide the suction. The aspirating needle is usually inserted in the fourth, fifth, or sixth intercos-

tal space to the left edge of the sternum in an adult. For an infant and child the heart assumes other positions (see "The Heart" in Chapter 14).

During and after the aspiration the patient's pulse, color, and breathing need to be assessed carefully. The technique is recorded as for a thoracentesis.

BONE MARROW BIOPSY

To *biopsy* is to remove a specimen of tissue from the body for examination. A bone marrow biopsy or aspiration is the removal of a specimen of bone marrow for examination. It is done to assist in the diagnosis of diseases of the blood and the blood-forming organs. The bones used are the iliac crest, posterior superior iliac, spine, and, most commonly, the sternum.

The equipment and technique are similar to those of a paracentesis. After local anesthetic a needle is introduced into the marrow cavity of the bone, and

a small amount of bone marrow is aspirated. After the needle is withdrawn, a small sterile dressing is placed over the site. The specimen is put in a small container especially for bone marrow or on glass slides.

In spite of a local anesthetic two aspects of the technique are painful: entering into bone and aspirating the marrow. Patients need to be told that this will hurt for a short time. After a bone marrow aspiration, patients usually do not require special nursing intervention.

GASTRIC ANALYSIS

A *gastric analysis* is the examination of gastric contents. The stomach contents are usually removed by a nurse and examined in a laboratory.

A gastric tube is inserted through the nose into the stomach (see Procedure 37-5). Once the tube is in place the stomach contents are removed with a syringe. The number of specimens and frequency with which they are taken will vary with the agency. All analyses require a fasting specimen, and some provide a test meal. After completion of the test the

tube is removed. Although this test is not painful, it is unpleasant for many people. The insertion and removal of the gastric tube often stimulates the gag reflex, and the presence of the tube can be irritating to the nose and throat.

A gastric analysis is usually done to determine the volume and the acidity of the contents. Interpretation of the results can assist in the diagnosis of conditions such as pernicious anemia and gastric ulcers.

TESTS

There are a large number of tests carried out in laboratories to assist physicians in the diagnosis and treatment of patients. The tests carried out by the nurse in a clinical setting have been discussed previously in the appropriate chapter. The nurse is sometimes also responsible for taking specimens, which are sent to a laboratory for assessment. (See "Care of Equipment and Specimens" in this chapter.) Laboratory tests can be grouped in the following manner.

1. Hematologic tests determine blood factors such as bleeding time, coagulation, and white blood cell count.

2. Microbiologic tests determine and identify any microorganisms present in tissues or body fluid.

3. Biochemistry of blood plasma and serum tests include the determination of the presence and amounts of chemical constituents such as blood amylase, copper, or bicarbonates.

4. Urine value tests include testing for such factors as aldosterone, calcium, and creatinine.

5. Tests are made for other body fluids, including cerebrospinal fluid, sputum, and ascitic fluid.

Nurses are referred to laboratory policy and procedure manuals of their agency for guidance in the method of collecting specimens and the precautions to take.

After a laboratory has examined a specimen, a report form is filled out and returned to the physician. On a hospital unit this report will be placed on the patient's record and added to the data about the patient's health status. Normal laboratory values vary according to the type of test performed. Therefore nurses should be guided by the normals provided by the specific laboratory when assessing these reports. Laboratory reports frequently use special abbreviations (see the Appendix).

SUGGESTED ACTIVITIES

1. Interview a patient who has had a test or treatment such as a spinal tap or paracentesis. What was the patient told beforehand, and what would the patient have liked to know? Discuss your findings in a group of students who have interviewed other patients.

2. For a patient who will be having a test or treatment, plan nursing intervention related to that patient's needs. Establish evaluative criteria related to the patient's response after the test and to the effectiveness of the test or treatment.

SUGGESTED READINGS

Luciano, Kathy, and Shumsky, Claire J. January, 1975. Pediatric procedures: the explanation should always come first. *Nursing 75* 5:49–52.

The importance of explanations to children together with how to do this are discussed. The need to reassure infants and toddlers and their parents is important. The ways of communicating with examples are provided for each age group.

Van Meter, Margaret, and Lavine, Peter G. April, 1975. What every nurse should know about EKGs. *Nursing 75* 5:19–27.

Included are the interpretation of EKG readings, the twelve-lead system, and types of rhythms. The electrical physiology of the heart's conduction system is explained on pages 26 and 27.

SELECTED REFERENCES

Asbury, A. J. July 5, 1973. Electronic equipment in nursing. *Nursing Times* 69:861–863.

Beaumont, Estelle. April, 1975. Diagnostic kits. *Nursing 75* 5:28–33.

Blackwell, Carol Ann. February, 1975. PEG and angiography: a patient's sensations. *American Journal of Nursing* 75:264–266.

French, Ruth M. 1975. *Guide to diagnostic procedures.* 4th ed. New York: McGraw-Hill Book Co.

Lamb, Joann. November, 1977. Intra-arterial monitoring: rescinding the risks. *Nursing 77* 7:65–71.

Marici, Frank N. October, 1973. The flexible fiberoptic bronchoscope. *American Journal of Nursing* 73:1776–1778.

Neufeld, A. H. February, 1974. Clinical laboratory procedures. *The Canadian Nurse* 70:25–44.

Shearer, D., et al. January, 1975. Preparing a patient for E.E.G. *American Journal of Nursing* 75:63–64.

APPENDICES

APPENDIX A
COMMONLY USED ABBREVIATIONS

abd	abdomen	ARM	artificial rupture of membranes (obstetrics)
ABO	the main blood group system	ASHD	arteriosclerotic heart disease
a.c.	before meals (*ante cibum*)	A-V	atrioventricular
Ac.	acid	A & W	alive and well
A-C	anti-inflammation corticoids	ax	axillary (armpit)
ACD	acid-citrate-dextrose	AZ	Aschheim-Zondek test for pregnancy
ACTH	adrenocorticotropic hormone		
ADH	antidiuretic hormone		
ADL	activities of daily living		
ad lib.	as desired (*ad libitum*)	Ba	barium
adm	admitted or admission	BBB	bundle branch block
AFB	acid-fast bacillus	BCG	BCG vaccine; ballistocardiograph
A/G	albumin-globulin ratio		
$AgNO_3$	silver nitrate	BE	barium enema
alk.	alkaline	b.i.d.	twice daily (*bis in die*)
AM	morning (ante meridiem)	BM (bm)	bowel movement
amb	ambulatory	BMR	basal metabolic rate
amp	ampule	BP	blood pressure
amt	amount	BPH	benign prostatic hypertrophy
AP	anteroposterior	BRP	bathroom privileges
A & P	auscultation and percussion; anterior and posterior repair	BS	blood sugar; breath sounds
		BSP	bromosulfophthalein (sulfobromophthalein)
approx	approximately (about)		
aq.	water (*aqua*)	BT	bleeding time
aq. dest.	distilled water (*aqua destillata*)	BUN	blood urea nitrogen

C (c̄)	with		diff.	differential
C	Celsius, centigrade		dil.	dilute
Ca	calcium		dist	distilled
CA (Ca)	cancer, carcinoma		DOA	dead on arrival
C_1, C_2, C_3	cervical vertebrae		dr	dram; drain; drainage
cap.	capsule		Dr	doctor
CBC	complete blood count		DR	dressing room; delivery room
CBD	common bile duct		drsg	dressing
CBR	complete bed rest		Dx	diagnosis
cc	cubic centimeter			
CC	chief complaint		ECG (EKG)	electrocardiogram
CCF	cephalin cholesterol flocculation (liver test)		ECD	expected date of confinement
			ECT	electroconvulsive therapy
CCU	coronary care unit		EDD	expected date of delivery
CD	communicable disease		EDTA	ethylenediaminetetraacetic acid
cg	centigram		EEG	electroencephalogram
CHF	congestive heart failure		EENT	eye, ear, nose, and throat
Cl	chlorine		e.g.	for example (*exempli gratia*)
CNS	central nervous system		ENT	ear, nose, and throat
c/o	complains of		EOM	extraocular movements
comp.	compound		eos.	eosinophil
conc	concentrated		ER	emergency room
CPD	cephalopelvic disproportion		ESP	extrasensory perception
CPK	creatine phosphokinase		ESR	erythrocyte sedimentation rate
Cr	chromium		et al	and others (*et alii*)
C & S	culture and sensitivity		etc	et cetera
CS	cesarean section		EUA	examination under anesthetic
CSF	cerebrospinal fluid		exam	examination
CSR	central supply room			
CST	convulsive shock therapy		F	Fahrenheit
Cu	copper		FBS	fasting blood sugar
CV	cardiovascular; cell volume		Fe	iron
CVA	cerebrovascular accident		FH	family history
CVI	cell volume index		FHS	fetal heart sound; follicle-stimulating hormone
CVP	central venous pressure			
CVS	cardiovascular system		fld	fluid
Cx	cervix			
Cysto	cystoscopy examination		G	gravida
CZI	crystalline zinc insulin		GA	gastric analysis; general anesthetic
			GB	gallbladder
DAT	diet as tolerated		GC (Gc)	gonococcus (gonorrhea)
dc (disc)	discontinue		GI	gastrointestinal
D & C	dilation and curettage		GIT	gastrointestinal tract
DD	differential diagnosis		Gm (gm)	gram
dg	decigram		GP	general practitioner
Dg	decagram (dekagram)		gr	grain

gtt	drops (*guttae*)		IV	intravenous
GU	genitourinary		IVP	intravenous pyelogram
GUT	genitourinary tract			
Gyn	gynecology		JVD	jugular venous distention
h.(hr)	hour		K	potassium
Hb (Hg, Hgb)	hemoglobin		kg	kilogram
HCl	hydrochloric acid		17KS	17-ketosteroids
hct	hematocrit		KUB	kidney, ureter, and bladder
HCVD	hypertensive cardiovascular disease			
			L	lumbar; left; liter
H & E	hematoxylin and eosin stain		L1, L2, L3, etc.	lumbar vertebrae
l7HC	l7-hydroxycorticoids		L & A	light and accommodation
HCG	human chorionic gonadotropic hormone		Lab	laboratory
			Lap	laparotomy
hg	hectogram		LBBB	left bundle branch block
Hg	mercury		LDH	lactic dehydrogenase
Hgb	hemoglobin		LE	lupus erythematosus
5HIAA	5-hydroxyindoleacetic acid		LH	luteinizing hormone
H_2O	water		liq	liquid
h/o	history of		LLE	left lower extremity
HPI	history of present illness		LLL	left lower lobe
hr	heart rate		LLQ	left lower quadrant
h.s.	hour of sleep		LMP	last menstrual period
ht	height; hematocrit		LNMP	last normal menstrual period
Hx	history		LOA	left occiput anterior
			LP	lumbar puncture
ICDH	isocitric dehydrogenase		LSK	liver, spleen, kidneys
ICU	intensive care unit		lt	left
id	the same (*idem*)		LUE	left upper extremity
ID	intradermal		LUL	left upper lobe
I & D	incision and drainage		LUP	left upper quadrant
i.e.	that is (*id est*)		LVH	left ventricular hypertrophy
Ig	immunoglobulin		lymph.	lymphocyte
IM	intramuscular			
inf	infusion		μg	microgram
inj	injection		m	meter or minim
invol	involuntary		M	thousand
I & O	intake and output		MCH	mean corpuscular hemoglobin
IOP	intraocular pressure		MCHC	mean corpuscular hemoglobin concentration
IPPA	inspection, palpitation, percussion, and auscultation		MCL	midclavicular line
			MCU	maximum care unit
IPPB	intermittent positive pressure breathing		MCV	mean corpuscular volume
			meds	medications
IQ	intelligence quotient		mEq	milliequivalent
irrig	irrigation		mEq/L	milliequivalent per liter
IU	international unit			

mg	milligram	os	mouth
MH	marital history	OS	left eye (oculus sinister)
MI	myocardial infarction	Osm	one osmotically active unit (molecule or ion) per liter
mid	middle		
min	minute or minim	OT	occupational therapy
mixt	mixture	OU	both eyes (oculus uterque)
ml	milliliter	oz	ounce
mm	millimeter		
MM	mucous membrane	p̄	after
mod	moderate	P	pulse, para
mOsm	milliosmole	PA	posteroanterior; pernicious anemia
MS	multiple sclerosis; musculoskeletal		
		Pap	Papanicolaou's smear test
MSL	midsternal line	Path	pathology
MSU	midstream úrine	PBI	protein bound iodine
myelo.	myelocyte	p.c.	after meals (post cibum)
		P_{CO_2}	partial pressure of carbon dioxide
N	nitrogen; normal		
Na	sodium	PE (Px)	physical examination
NAD	no abnormality detected	Ped (Peds)	pediatrics
NB	note carefully (nota bene); newborn	per	by or through
		PERLA	pupils equal and reactive to light and accommodation
neg	negative		
neuro	neurology	PET	preeclampsic toxemia
neut.	neutrophil, a variety of white blood cells	Pg	picogram
		P.H.	past history
ng	nanogram	pH	hydrogen ion concentration
nil	none	physio	physiotherapy
no. (#)	number	PI	present illness
noct	at night	PID	pelvic inflammatory disease
NPN	nonprotein nitrogen	pl. ct.	blood platelet count
NPO (NBM)	nothing by mouth	PM	afternoon (post meridiem)
NS (N/S)	normal saline	PMI	point of maximal impulse
nsq	not sufficient quantity	p.o.	by mouth (per os)
NYD	not yet diagnosed	P_{O_2}	partial pressure of oxygen
		pop	plaster of Paris
ō	none	postop	postoperative(ly)
O_2	oxygen	premed	pre medication
OB (obst)	obstetrics	preop	preoperative(ly)
od	daily	prep	preparation
OD	right eye (oculus dexter); overdose	p.r.n.	when necessary (pro re nata)
		Prog	prognosis
o.h.	every hour	pro time	prothrombin time
OOB	out of bed	PSP	phenolsulfonphthalein
OPD	outpatient department	psych	psychiatry (psychology)
Ophth	ophthalmology	pt (Pt)	patient
O.R.	operating room	PT	physical therapy (physical therapist)
Ortho	orthopedics		

PUO	pyrexia of unknown origin
PVD	peripheral vascular disease
PZI	protamine zinc insulin
q.	every (*quaque*)
q.d.	every day (*quaque die*)
q.h. (.q1h.)	every hour (*quaque hora*)
q.2h., q.3h., etc.	every 2 hours, 3 hours, etc.
q.h.s.	every night at bedtime
q.i.d.	four times a day (*quater in die*)
qns	quantity not sufficient
q.s.	sufficient quantity
R	right; respiration; rectal
RBBB	right bundle branch block
RBC (rbc)	red blood cells
req	requisition
RF	rheumatoid factor
Rh	Rhesus, the Rh factor of blood
Rh Neg	Rhesus factor negative
RISA	radioiodinated serum albumin
R & L	right and left
RLE	right lower extremity
RLL	right lower lobe
RLQ	right lower quadrant
RML	right middle lobe
RR	respiratory rate
Rt (rt)	right
RUE	right upper extremity
RUL	right upper lobe
RUQ	right upper quadrant
Rx	take, therapy
S ($\bar{s}$)	without (*sine*)
sang	sanguineous
SB	sternal border
SC	subcutaneous
SG	specific gravity
SGOT	serum glutamic-oxaloacetic transaminase (now known as aspartate aminotransferase)
SGPT	serum glutamic-pyruvic transaminase (now known as alanine aminotransferase)
SI	seriously ill
Sig.	let it be labeled, write on label (*signa*)
SMR	submucous resection

SOA	swelling of ankles
SOB (sob)	shortness of breath
soda bicarb	sodium bicarbonate
Sol (sol)	solution
Solv	dissolve
s.o.s.	if necessary (*si opus sit*)
spec	specimen
Sp gr	specific gravity
SR (sed rate)	sedimentation rate
SS (ss)	soap solution, soap suds (enema)
$\bar{s}\bar{s}$	one half
staph	staphylococcus
stat.	at once, immediately (*statim*)
st dr	straight drainage
STS	serologic test for syphilis
Strep	streptococcus
subcu	subcutaneous
subling	sublingual (under the tongue)
supp.	suppository
Sx	symptoms
syr	syrup
T & A	tonsillectomy and adenoidectomy; tonsils and adenoids
T_3	an in vitro test for thyroid function
T_4	a test for thyroxine, the thyroid hormone
tab	tablet
TAB	typhoid, parathyroid A, and parathyroid B
TB	tuberculosis
t.i.d.	three times a day (*ter in die*)
TL	team leader
TLC	tender loving care
TNR	tonic neck reflex
To	telephone order
TPI	*Treponema pallidum* immobilization
TPR	temperature, pulse, and respiration
TSH	thyroid-stimulating hormone
TUPR	transurethral prostatic resection
TUR	transurethral resection
U	unit
U/A	urinalysis
ung	ointment

Ur. Ac.	uric acid	vo	verbal order
URI	upper respiratory infection	VS (vs)	vital signs
UTI	urinary tract infection		
vag	vaginal	WBC	white blood cells
VD	venereal disease	WF	white female
VDRL	venereal disease research labora-tory (test for syphilis)	WM	white male
		WNL	within normal limits
viz	namely (*videlicet*)	WR	Wassermann reaction
VMA	vanilymandelic acid	wt	weight

APPENDIX B   MEDICATIONS AND TREATMENTS: ABBREVIATIONS AND LATIN DERIVATIONS

Abbreviation	Explanation	Latin word	Example of administration time
a.c.	before meals	ante cibum	0700, 1100, and 1700 hours
ad lib.	freely, as desired	ad libitum	
agit.	shake, stir	agita	
aq.	water	aqua	
aq. dest.	distilled water	aqua destillata	
b.i.d.	twice a day	bis in die	0900 and 2100 hours
c̄	with	cum	
cap.	capsule	capsula	
comp.	compound	compositus	
dil.	dissolve, dilute	dilatus	
elix.	elixir	elixir	
h.	an hour	hora	
h.s.	at bedtime	hora somni	
M. or m.	mix	misce	
no.	number	numerus	
non rep.	do not repeat	non repetatur	
p.o.	by mouth	per os	
OS or o.l.	left eye	oculus sinister or laevus	
OD	right eye	oculus dexter	
o.u.	each eye	oculus uterque	
p.c.	after meals	post cibum	0900, 1300, and 1900 hours
p.r.n.	when needed	pro re nata	
q.	every	quaque	
q.d.	every day	quaque die	

Abbreviation	Explanation	Latin word	Example of administration time
q.a.m. (o.m.)	every morning	quaque ante meridiem (omni mane)	1000 hours
q.h. (qlh.oh)	every hour	quaque omni hora (omni hora)	
q.2h.	every 2 hours	quaque 2 hora	0800, 1000, 1200 hours, etc.
q.3h.	every 3 hours	quaque 3 hora	0900, 1200, 1500 hours, etc.
q.4h.	every 4 hours	quaque 4 hora	1000, 1400, 1800 hours, etc.
q.6h.	every 6 hours	quaque 6 hora	0600, 1200, 1800, 2400 hours
q.h.s. (o.n.)	every night	quaque hora somni (omni nocte)	
q.i.d.	four times a day	quater in die	1000, 1400, 1800, 2200 hours
q.o.d.	every other day		0900 hours on odd dates
q.s.	sufficient quantity	quantum satis	
rept.	may be repeated	repetatur	
Rx	take	recipe	
s̄	without	sine	
Sig. or S.	label	signa	
s.o.s.	if it is needed	si opus sit	
ss	a half	semis	
stat.	at once	statim	
sup. or supp.	suppository		
susp.	suspension		
t.i.d.	three times a day	ter in die	1000, 1400, and 1800 hours
tr. or tinct.	tincture	tinctura	

APPENDIX C   COMMONLY USED PREFIXES AND SUFFIXES AND COMBINING FORMS

Prefix	Meaning	Prefix	Meaning
a, an, ar	without or not	amyl	starch
ab	away from	ante	before, forward
acro	extremities	anti	against, counteracting
ad	toward, to	bi	double
adeno	glandular	bili	bile
aero	air	bio	life
ambi	around, on both sides	bis	two

Appendices

Prefix	Meaning	Prefix	Meaning
brachio	arm	intra	within
brady	slow	intro	in, within, into
broncho	bronchi	juxta	nearness, closeness
cardio	heart	laryngo	larynx
cervico	neck	latero	side
chole	gall or bile	lapar	abdomen
cholecysto	gall bladder	leuk	white
circum	around	macro	large, big
co	together	mal	bad, poor
contra	against, opposite	mast	breast
costo	ribs	medio	middle
cyto	cell	mega (megalo)	large, great
cysto	bladder	meno	menses
demi	half	mono	single
derma	skin	multi	many
dis	from	myelo	bone marrow, spinal cord
dorso	back	myo	muscle
dys	abnormal, difficult	neo	new
electro	related to electricity	nephro	kidney
en	into, in, within	neuro	nerve
encephal	brain	nitro	nitrogen
entero	pertaining to the intestine	noct	night
equi	equal	non	not
eryth	red	ob	against, in front of
ex	out, out of, away from	oculo	eye
extra	outside of, in addition to	odonto	tooth
ferro	iron	ophthalmo	eye
fibro	fiber	ortho	straight, normal
fore	before, in front of	os	mouth, bone
gastro	stomach	osteo	bone
glosso	tongue	oto	ear
glyco	sugar	pan	all
hemi	half	para	beside, accessory to
hemo	blood	path	disease
hepa (hepato)	liver	ped	child, foot
histo	tissue	per	by, through
homo	same	peri	around
hydro	water	pharyngo	pharynx
hygro	moisture	phlebo	vein
hyper	too much, high	photo	light
hypo	under, decreased	phren	diaphragm, mind
hyster	uterus	pneumo	air, lungs
ileo	ileum	pod	foot
in	in, within, into	poly	many, much
inter	between	post	after

Prefix	Meaning	Suffix	Meaning
pre	before	cele	tumor, swelling
proct	rectum	centesis	surgical puncture to remove fluid
pseudo	false		
psych	mind	cide	killing, destructive
pyel	pelvis of the kidney	cule	little
pyo	pus	cyte	cell
pyro	fever	ectasia	dilating or stretching
quadri	four	ectomy	excision, surgical removal of
radio	radiation	emia	blood
re	back, again	esis	action
reno	kidney	form	shaped like
retro	backward	genesis (genetic)	formation, origin
rhin	nose	graph	writing
sacro	sacrum	ism	condition
salpingo	fallopian tube	itis	inflammation
sarco	flesh	ize	to treat
sclero	hard, hardening	lith	stone, calculus
semi	half	lithiasis	presence of stones
sex	six	lysis	disintegration
skeleto	skeleton	megaly	enlargement
steno	harrowing, constriction	meter	instrument that measures
sub	under	oid	likeness, resemblance
super	above, excess	oma	tumor
supra	above	opathy	any disease of
syn	together	orrhaphy	surgical repair
tachy	fast	osis	disease, condition of
thyro	thyroid, gland	ostomy	to form an opening or outlet
trache	trachea	otomy	to incise
trans	across, over	pexy	fixation
tri	three	phage	ingesting
ultra	beyond	phobia	fear
un	not, back, reversal	plasty	plastic surgery
uni	one	plegia	paralysis
uretero	ureter	rhage	hemorrhage
urethro	urethra	rhea	excessive discharge
uro	urine, urinary organs	rhexis	rupture
vaso	vessel	scope	lighted instrument for visual examination

Suffix	Meaning	Suffix	Meaning
able	able to	scopy	to examine visually
algia	pain	stomy	to form an opening
		tomy	incision into
		uria	urine

APPENDIX D SYMBOLS

>	greater than
<	less than
=	equal
↑	increased
↓	decreased
♀	female
♂	male
°	degree
#	number, fracture
ℨ	dram
℥	ounce
×	times
@	at

APPENDIX E EQUIVALENTS

Metric Equivalents

Weights

1 picogram	$= 10^{-12}$ gm
1 nanogram	$= 10^{-9}$ gm
1 microgram	$= 10^{-3}$ mg $= 10^{-6}$ gm
1 milligram	$= 1000$ micrograms $= 10^{-6}$ gram
1 centigram	$= 10$ milligrams $= 10^{-1}$ decigrams $= 10^{-2}$ gram
1 decigram	$= 100$ milligrams $= 10$ centigrams $= 10^{-1}$ gram
1 gram	$= 1000$ milligrams $= 100$ centigrams $= 10$ decigrams
1 kilogram	$= 1000$ grams

Volume

1 milliliter	$= 1$ gram
1 liter	$= 1$ kilogram $= 1000$ grams (milliliters)

924

Approximate Weight Equivalents: Metric and Apothecaries' Systems

Metric	Apothecaries'	Metric	Apothecaries'
0.1 mg	1/600 grain	60 mg	1 grain
1.12 mg	1/500 grain	100 mg (0.1 gm)	1 1/2 grains
0.15 mg	1/400 grain	150 mg (0.15 gm)	2 1/2 grains
0.2 mg	1/300 grain	200 mg (0.2 gm)	3 grains
0.25 mg	1/250 grain	300 mg (0.3 gm)	5 grains
0.3 mg	1/200 grain	400 mg (0.4 gm)	6 grains
0.4 mg	1/150 grain	500 mg (0.5 gm)	7 1/2 grains
0.5 mg	1/120 grain	600 mg (0.6 gm)	10 grains
0.6 mg	1/100 grain	1 gram	15 grains
0.8 mg	1/80 grain	1.5 gm	22 grains
1 mg	1/60 grain	2 gm	30 grains
1.2 mg	1/50 grain	3 gm	45 grains
1.5 mg	1/40 grain	4 gm	60 grains (1 dram)
2 mg	1/30 grain	5 gm	75 grains
3 mg	1/20 grain	6 gm	90 grains
4 mg	1/15 grain	7.5 gm	120 grains (2 drams)
5 mg	1/12 grain	10 gm	2½ drams
6 mg	1/10 grain	30 gm	1 ounce (8 drams)
8 mg	1/8 grain	500 gm	1.1 pounds
10 mg	1/6 grain	1000 gm	2.2 pounds (1 kilogram)
12 mg	1/5 grain		
15 mg	1/4 grain		
20 mg	1/3 grain		
25 mg	3/8 grain		
30 mg	1/2 grain		
40 mg	2/3 grain		
50 mg	3/4 grain		

Approximate Volume Equivalents: Metric, Apothecaries', and Household Systems

Metric	Apothecaries'	Household
0.06 ml	1 minim ( )	1 drop (g +)
0.3 ml	5 minims	
0.6 ml	10 minims	
1 ml	15 minims	15 drops
2 ml	30 minims	
3 ml	45 minims	
4 ml	60 minims (1 fluid dram)	60 drops (1 tsp)
8 ml	2 fl. drams (f)	2 teaspoons
15 ml	4 fl. drams	4 tsp. (1 tbsp)
30 ml	8 fl. drams (1 fl. ounce) (f)	2 tablespoons

Metric	Apothecaries	House-hold
60 ml	2 fl. ounces	
90 ml	3 fl. ounces	
200 ml	6 fl. ounces	1 teacup
250 ml	8 fl. ounces	1 large glass
500 ml	16 fl. ounces (1 pint)	1 pint
750 ml	1½ pints	
1000 ml (1 liter)	2 pints (1 quart)	1 quart
4000 ml	4 quarts	1 gallon

GLOSSARY

abduction movement of a bone away from the midline of the body.

abrasion an open wound that occurs as a result of friction.

abscess a localized collection of pus and/or disintegrating body tissues.

abstracting 1) forming a summary; 2) isolating or considering separately a particular aspect of an object.

acapnia a decreased level of carbon dioxide in the blood.

acatalasia a disease characterized by the absence of the enzyme catalase, occurring mostly in Japanese people.

accommodation (Piaget) the process of change whereby a person's cognitive processes are sufficiently matured enabling the solving of problems that could not be solved previously.

acetone a flammable, colorless liquid with an ethereal odor used as a solvent or to cleanse the skin before injections.

acetylcholine an acetic acid ester of choline with a function in the transmission of nerve impulses.

acholic deficiency of bile.

acidosis (acidemia) a condition resulting from excessive acid in the blood; blood pH is below 7.35.

acne an inflammatory condition of the sebaceous glands most commonly seen in adolescents and young adults.

acromion (acromial process) the lateral projection of the scapula extending over the shoulder joint.

active exercise exercise for which the individual supplies the energy, rather than the nurse or therapist; compare with passive exercise.

acupuncture a Chinese practice of piercing specific superficial nerves with needles, often to treat pain.

acute 1) sharp or severe; 2) a severe condition with a sudden onset and short course (as opposed to *chronic*).

adaptation (Piaget) the coping behavior of a person who has the ability to handle the demands of the environment.

adaptive (defense) mechanisms learned behaviors that assist an individual to adjust to the environment.

addiction a state of dependence upon a drug or some habit.

adduction movement of a bone toward the midline of the body.

adenohypophysis the anterior part of the pituitary gland.

adhesion a fibrous band or structure by which parts are abnormally held together.

adipose fat; fatty nature.

adolescence a period of life beginning with the appearance of secondary sex characteristics and terminating with somatic growth, usually between ages 11 and 19.

adrenal gland an endocrine gland that is located on the superior aspect of the kidney.

adrenalin a trademark name for preparations of epinephrine.

927

adrenocortical   arising from the cortex of the adrenal gland.

adrenocorticotrophic hormone (ACTH)   one hormone produced by the pituitary gland that stimulates the adrenal cortex to produce hormones.

aerobe   a microorganism that lives and grows in the presence of oxygen.

affective   pertaining to or arising from a feeling, emotion, or mental state.

agglutinogen   a substance that acts as an antigen and stimulates the production of agglutinin.

air hunger   dyspnea occurring in paroxysms.

alarm reaction (Selye)   the initial reaction of the body to a stressor.

albuminuria   the presence of albumin in the urine.

aldosterone   a hormone produced by the adrenal cortex that regulates the level of sodium in the body.

alignment   the position of body parts that facilitates body function.

alkalosis (alkalemia)   a condition resulting from excessive alkali (base) in the blood; blood pH is above 7.45.

alveolus   any of a number of types of tiny sac-like dilatations or cavities in the body.

ambulate (ambulation)   to walk; the act of walking.

amino acid   one of a group of organic acids containing nitrogen. These are considered to be the components of proteins.

amphetamine   a drug used to stimulate the central nervous system.

ampule   a glass container that can be sealed to preserve a medication or solution.

anabolism   a process whereby simple substances are converted by the body cells into more complex substances.

anaerobe   a microorganism that lives and grows in the absence of oxygen.

anal incontinence   loss of the voluntary ability to control fecal and gaseous discharges through the anal sphincter.

anal stage (Freud)   stage of human development usually occurring during the second and third years.

analgesic   a pain relieving agent.

anaphylaxis   an extreme allergic reaction to a foreign protein or substance.

anasarca   generalized edema throughout the body.

anatomic position   position of normal body alignment.

andropause (climacteric)   the period of change in men when sexual activity decreases.

androsperm   sperm bearing a Y chromosome.

anemia   a condition in which the blood is deficient in red blood cells or hemoglobin.

aneroid   containing no liquid.

anesthesia   loss of sensation or feeling; in particular, induced loss of the sense of pain.

angiogram   a diagnostic measure enabling visualization of the veins and arteries by introduction of a radioactive dye.

angstrom (Å)   a unit of wavelength of the electromagnetic spectrum.

anilingus   anal stimulation provided orally.

anion   an ion carrying a negative charge.

ankylosis   stiffening or immobility of a joint as a result of disease, injury, or surgery.

anogenital   referring to the area around the anus and the genitals.

anorexia   lack of appetite.

anorexia nervosa   a psychologic condition in which the person eats little or nothing leading to emaciation.

anoxemia   a condition in which the level of oxygen in the blood is below normal.

anoxia   lack or absence of oxygen in body tissues.

antecubital   located in front of the elbow.

anthelmintic   an agent capable of destroying worms.

antibiosis   an antagonistic association between organisms.

antibiotic   a substance produced by microorganisms that has the capacity to inhibit the growth of or kill other microorganisms.

antibody   an immunoglobulin which combines with a specific antigen to combat infection, harmful bacteria, or toxins.

antidiuretic hormone (ADH)   a hormone released by the posterior pituitary gland which controls water reabsorption from the kidney tubules; also referred to as vasopressin.

antigen   a substance capable of inducing the formation of antibodies and of reacting in a specific manner with the antibodies so induced.

anti-inflammatory corticoid (A-C)   a substance which counteracts or suppresses inflammation.

antipyretic   a substance that is effective in treating burns.

antiseptic   an agent that inhibits the growth of microorganisms.

antiserum (immune sera)   a serum that contains antibodies.

anuria   a condition in which the kidneys produce no urine.

anus   the posterior opening of the gastrointestinal tract.

anxiety   mental uneasiness owing to an impending or anticipated threat often associated with physiologic changes such as increased pulse rate and sweating.

apathy   the lack of interest or feeling.

Apgar score   the system of numerically scoring the condition of a newborn infant.

aphasia   the inability to communicate by speech, signs, or writing resulting from an injury or disease.

apical beat   the heart beat as heard over the apex of the heart.

apical-radial pulse   the simultaneous measurement of the apical beat and the radial pulse.

apnea   the cessation of breathing.

apocrine gland   a large sweat gland whose duct usually opens into a hair follicle.

appendicitis   an inflammation of the appendix.

areola   the circular area of different color around a central point such as the circular pigmented area surrounding the nipple of the breast.

arrector pili muscles   smooth muscles in the skin attached to the hair follicles.

arrhythmia   an irregularity in the rhythm of a heart beat.

arteriogram   a diagnostic measure enabling visualization of the arteries by the introduction of a radioactive dye.

arteriosclerosis   a condition in which the walls of the arteries become hardened and thickened.

Aschheim-Zondek test (AZT)   a test for pregnancy whereby a specimen of urine from a female is injected into a female mouse.

ascites   the accumulation of fluid in the abdominal cavity.

asepsis   the absence of all disease-producing microorganisms.

asphyxia   a condition resulting from a lack of oxygen in the inspired air.

aspiration   1) the act of inhalation; 2) the removal of fluids or gases from a cavity by suction.

assimilation (Piaget)   the process whereby humans are able to encounter and react to new situations by using the mechanisms they already possess.

astigmatism   an unequal curvature of the refractive surfaces of the eye.

astringent   an agent that causes contraction; usually applied topically.

asymmetric   absence of symmetry; dissimilarity of corresponding organs on opposite sides of the body.

atelectasis   collapse of lung tissue.

atony   lack of normal muscle tone.

atresia   absence, closure, or degeneration of a passageway or cavity such as occurs to the primordial follicles of the ovaries.

atrioventricular (AV) node   neuromuscular tissue of the heart at the base of the atrium that conveys impulses to the ventricles.

atrioventricular valves   cardiac valves between the atria and the ventricles; also referred to as the tricuspid and the mitral valve.

atrophy   the wasting away or decrease in size of a body part.

attenuate   to make thin or to weaken.

audit   a methodical examination and review.

auditory   related to or experienced through hearing.

auricle   chamber of the ear or the heart.

auscultation   the practice of examining the body by listening to body sounds.

autoantigen   an antigen that is immunogenic in the body in which it originates.

autonomic   self-controlling; capable of independent function.

autonomy   the quality or state of being independent and self-directed without outside control.

autopsy   postmortem examination of a body.

Babinski (plantar) reflex   the normal downward bending of the toes elicited upon stroking the sole of the foot.

bactericide   a bacteria-destroying agent.

bacteriostatic   inhibiting the multiplication and growth of bacteria.

Balkan frame   a metal frame extending lengthwise over a bed and supported at either end for the purpose of attaching splints or providing a means of mobility to bedridden patients.

bandage   a material used to wrap or bind a body part.

barbiturate   a drug commonly used as a hypnotic and sedative.

Bard-Parker forceps   a type of transfer forceps commonly used to handle sterile supplies.

barium   a metallic element commonly used in solution as a contrast medium for x-ray of the gastrointestinal tract.

barrier technique (medical asepsis)   medical practices used to control the spread of pathogenic microorganisms and assist with their destruction.

basal metabolic rate   the rate at which energy is expended to maintain body functions by a body at rest.

basilic vein   a superficial vein which arises on the ulnar side of the dorsum of the hand, goes up the forearm and joins the brachial vein to form the axillary vein.

bereavement   loss of a loved one by death.

beriberi   a condition due to the deficiency of thiamine (vitamin B_1).

bilirubin   red pigment in the bile.

binder   a kind of abdominal bandage.

biology   the science of life and living organisms.

biopsy   the removal and examination of tissue from the living body.

biorhythm   an inner rhythm that appears to control a variety of biologic processes.

bleb   a flaccid skin vesicle usually filled with fluid.

blister   a collection of fluid between the epidermis and the dermis.

blood pressure   the pressure of the blood as it pulsates through the arteries.

body mechanics   the movement and coordination of the body in response to stimuli, and the body's efforts to maintain its balance while it responds.

body temperature   the internal temperature of the human body.

bolus   a mass of food or pharmaceutical preparation ready to be swallowed or a mass passing along the gastrointestinal tract; a concentrated mass of pharmaceutical preparation given intravenously.

brachial pulse   a pulse located on the inner side of the biceps muscle just below the axilla.

bradycardia   an abnormally slow heart rate, less than 60 beats per minute.

bradypnea   abnormally slow breathing, less than 10 respirations per minute.

Braxton Hicks' contractions   painless intermittent contractions of the uterus during pregnancy.

bronchodilator   an agent which dilates the bronchi of the lungs.

bronchogram   an x-ray of the bronchial tree using an iodized oil dye as the contrast medium.

bronchoscope   a lighted instrument used to visualize the bronchi of the lungs.

bronchoscopy   a visual examination of the bronchi.

bronchus   a large air passage of the lungs.

bubbling   gurgling sounds during breathing.

buffer   an agent or system that tends to maintain constancy or that prevents changes in chemical concentration of a substance.

cachexia   a state of malnutrition and general ill health.

calculus   a stone composed of minerals that is formed in the body, for example, a renal calculus formed in the kidney.

callus   hyperplasia or thickening of the horny layer of the epidermis, usually due to friction.

calorie   a unit of heat, usually a small calorie which is the amount of heat required to raise the temperature of 1 gm of water 1°C; a large calorie is the amount of heat required to raise the temperature of 1 kg of water 1°C.

calyx (calix)   a cup-shaped organ or cavity.

cannula   a tube with a lumen which is inserted into a cavity or duct and often fitted with a trocar during insertion.

canthus   the angle formed by the upper and lower eyelids; each eye has an inner and outer canthus.

capillary action   the movement of fluid in a tube; caused by the adhesion of the fluid to the wall of the tube.

capsule   1) a soft soluble container for a medication; 2) an anatomical structure enclosing an organ or part of the body.

carbaminohemoglobin the chemical combination of carbon dioxide and hemoglobin.

carbohydrate a nutrient composed of carbon, hydrogen, and oxygen, for example, starches and sugars.

cardiac arrest a sudden termination of the cardiac function.

cardiac monitor a machine which measures and records the heart function.

caries tooth decay; also applies to the decay of bone.

carina the ridge or junction where the main bronchi meet the trachea.

carminative relieving flatulence.

carotid receptors nerve endings found in the carotid bodies and carotid sinuses; sensitive to blood pH, changes in blood pressure, and excessive blood CO_2.

carrier a person who is not ill but who carries microorganisms which can be transmitted to others.

catabolism a destructive process whereby complex substances are broken down into simpler substances.

cataract an opacity of the lens of the eye.

catarrh inflammation of the mucous membrane with a discharge.

cathartic a drug that induces evacuation of the bowels.

catheter a flexible, tubular instrument used to introduce or withdraw fluids from a body cavity.

cation a positively charged ion.

cauda a tail or tail-like appendage.

cellular (intracellular) fluid fluid found within a cell.

cellulitis inflammation of cellular tissue.

cementum a bone-like connective tissue surrounding the root of a tooth.

centigrade (Celcius) a metric temperature scale in which the interval between two established points is divided into 100 equal units; $1°C = 1.8°F$.

cerebrospinal fluid fluid contained within the four ventricles of the brain, the subarachnoid space, and the central canal of the spinal cord.

cerumen the wax-like material found in the external auditory canal.

cervix the neck of the uterus that extends into the vagina and serves as a passageway between the two organs.

Chadwick's sign change in the appearance of the mucous membrane of the vagina during pregnancy in which it becomes bluish or violet in color.

chancre a papular lesion (sore) occuring at the entry of infection in some diseases; primary sore of syphilis.

cheilosis cracks or scaling at the corners of the lips.

chemical thermogenesis the production of heat by chemical means.

chemoreceptor a receptor which is sensitive to chemical substances.

chemotaxis the movement of a cell or an organism in response to a chemical gradient.

Cheyne-Stokes breathing rhythmic waxing and waning of respirations from very deep respirations to very shallow and temporary apnea.

chill shivering and shaking of the body with involuntary contractions of the voluntary muscles.

cholangiogram x-ray of the biliary tract involving the injection of a dye.

cholecystogram an x-ray of the gall bladder.

chordotomy surgical severing of the anterolateral nerve tracts of the spinal cord.

chorionic gonadotropin (HCG) hormone produced by the placenta.

chorionic somatomammotropin (human placental lactogen) hormone secreted by the placenta which influences fetal growth.

choroid plexus projections of the pia mater into the ventricles of the brain which secrete cerebrospinal fluid.

chromosome a structure in the nucleus of a cell which contains DNA and transmits genetic information.

chronic persisting over a long period of time.

chyme the semifluid material produced by gastric digestion of food in the stomach.

cicatrix scar; the new tissue formed when a wound heals.

cicatrization the formation of a scar.

cilia hairlike projections of the respiratory mucous membrane.

circadian rhythm rhythmic repetition of certain phenomena each 24 hours.

circulatory overload a state occurring when the intravascular fluid compartment contains more fluid than normal.

circumcision surgical removal of part or all of the foreskin of the penis, usually performed during infancy.

circumduction the movement of the distal part of the bone in a circle, with the proximal end remaining fixed.

cisterna a space that is enclosed and serves as a reservoir for body fluid.

cisternal puncture the insertion of a needle into the subarachnoid space of the cisterna magna.

civil action legal action between two or more individuals.

civil (private) law rules that regulate or control relationships between people rather than between persons and governments.

clavicle the bone commonly known as the collar bone; it articulates with the scapula and the sternum.

clean free of disease producing microorganisms.

clean technique a technique that maintains freedom from disease producing microorganisms.

climacteric the point in development when reproduction capacity in the female terminates (menopause) and the sexual activity of the male decreases.

clitoris a small round mass of erectile tissue located behind the junction of the labia minora in the female; homologous with the penis in the male.

closed wound a wound in which there is no break in the skin.

coagulate to clot.

coccidiomycosis a fungus disease with an acute, benign respiratory infection in the primary stage and a virulent, progressive secondary stage.

cognition the process of knowing, including judgment and awareness.

cohesion a force which causes particles to unite.

coitus sexual intercourse; a term of Latin derivation meaning "a coming together."

coitus interruptus a method of contraception in which the penis is withdrawn prior to the ejaculation of semen.

collagen a protein found in connective tissue.

colloid matter that is distributed throughout a medium in a state preventing its passage through a semipermeable membrane.

colonoscope an instrument used to visualize the interior of the colon.

colonoscopy the visual examination of the interior of the colon with a lighted instrument.

colostomy a surgically-made opening where the colon opens on the body surface.

colostrum a yellow, milky fluid secreted by the mammary glands a few days before or after birth.

coma a state of unconsciousness in which the person does not respond to environmental stimuli.

combustible a characteristic of a substance whereby it can burn; flammable.

comedo (blackhead) a plug in an excretory duct in the skin that contains microorganisms and shedded keratin; blackhead.

commode a portable, chair-like structure used as a toilet.

common law unwritten laws that are binding and upheld by precedent cases rather than statutes.

communicable disease a disease that can spread from one person to another.

compensation a psychologic phenomenon in which a person substitutes one behavior trait for a less adequate characteristic.

compliance expansibility or stretchability.

compress a pad or cloth that is applied to the body, sometimes medicated.

concave hollowed or rounded inward.

concurrent disinfection measures taken while a patient is infectious to control the spread of the microorganisms.

conditioning learning in which a response is elicited by a neutral stimulus that has been previously presented accompanying a stimulus that originally elicited the response.

condom a sheath or cover, usually made of rubber or plastic, worn over the penis during coitus to prevent conception or infection.

conduction the transfer of heat, sound, or nervous impulses by molecular interaction.

confused a mental state in which a person appears bewildered and may make inappropriate statements and answers to questions.

congenital existing at, and often before, birth.

congestion the excessive accumulation of blood in a part of the body.

consciousness a person's normal state of awareness of the environment.

constipation   the passage of small, dry, hard stools or the passage of no stool for a period of time.

constitutional law   laws stated in federal, state, and/or provincial constitutions.

consumer   a person who uses a service or a product.

contact   a person who has been near an infected person and thus exposed to the pathogenic microorganisms.

contaminate   to make unclean or unsterile; to soil.

contraception   the prevention of fertilization of the ovum by any method.

contract   an agreement between two or more competent persons, upon sufficient consideration, to do or not do some lawful act.

contracture   the permanent shortening of a muscle.

contusion   a closed wound that occurs as a result of a blow from a blunt instrument.

convection   the transfer of heat by movement of a liquid or gas.

conversive heat   heat that results from the conversion of a primary source of energy.

convex   curved or rounded as the external surface of a sphere.

coping (mental adaptive) mechanisms   those mechanisms used by individuals to adapt to environmental stressors and to preserve the individual's self-esteem and sense of security.

copulation   sexual intercourse; a term derived from Latin meaning "coupling or joining."

corn   a hardening and thickening of the skin forming a conical mass pointing downward into the corium.

corneal reflex   irritation of the cornea resulting in a reflex closing of the eyelids.

corpus albicans   a mass of white, scarred tissue that replaces the corpus luteum when fertilization does not occur.

corpus luteum   a yellow body formed in the graafian follicle after the ovum is discharged.

corticoid   a term applied to hormones of the adrenal cortex or substances with similar activity.

cortisone   a hormone produced by the adrenal cortex which has anti-inflammatory properties and also is involved in the metabolism of glycogen to glucose.

counterirritant   an agent that produces an irritation with the intent of relieving some other problem.

creatinine   a nitrogenous waste which is excreted in the urine.

cremaster   inner layer of striated muscle and connective tissue in the scrotum.

crepitation (crèps)   dry, crackling sound.

crisis (of a fever)   the sudden reduction of a fever.

crown (of a tooth)   the portion of a tooth that is covered by enamel.

crutch paralysis   damage to the nerves of the axillae due to pressure.

cryptorchidism   failure of the testes to descend from the abdominal cavity to the scrotal sac(s).

crystalline amino acids   refined protein used in hyperalimentation.

culture   1) the cultivation of microorganisms or cells in a special growth medium; 2) a system within a society of acquired and transmitted standards in regard to judgments, beliefs, and conduct.

cultural shock   the shock which can occur when an individual changes quickly from one social setting to another.

cumulative effect   the total effect of accumulated portions.

cunnilingus   oral stimulation of the clitoris and labia by a partner.

curet   a spoon-shaped instrument used for removing material from a body cavity.

curettage   removal of material from the wall of a cavity, for example, the uterus, with a curet.

cyanosis   a bluish tinge of the skin and mucous membranes due to excessive concentration of reduced hemoglobin in the blood.

cyst   an enclosed cavity or sac lined by epithelium and containing liquid or semi-solid material.

cystitis   inflammation of the urinary bladder.

cystocele   protrusion of the urinary bladder through the vaginal wall.

cystoscope   lighted instrument used to visualize the interior of the urinary bladder.

cystoscopy   an examination of the urinary bladder with a lighted instrument.

dandruff   a dry scaly material shedded from the scalp.

data base (baseline data)   all information known about a patient.

debilitated   having lost strength.

debridement to remove foreign and dying tissue from a wound so that healthy tissue is exposed.

decibel a unit used to measure or describe sound.

deciduous teeth the first teeth which are replaced by permanent teeth.

decisional law those laws determined by courts which rule on cases, rather than by statutes.

decoding the process receiving a communication and converting the message into understandable terms.

decubitus ulcer an ulcer produced by prolonged pressure.

defamation communication in writing (libel) or spoken word (slander) that is injurious to the reputation of a person.

defecation the discharge of feces from the bowels.

defense mechanism see adaptive mechanism.

dehiscence a splitting open; a rupture.

dehydration (anhydration) lack of sufficient fluid in the body.

delirious experiencing mental confusion, restlessness, and incoherence.

demineralization the excessive loss of minerals or inorganic salts.

demography statistical study of the population.

demulcent a drug which coats the bowel, thus protecting the lining.

denial a defense mechanism in which events, actions, or such are unconsciously denied.

deoxyribonucleic acid (DNA) a nucleic acid found in all living cells; it is the carrier of genetic information.

dependent nursing functions activities of a nurse as a result of a physician's order.

depolarize to reduce toward a nonpolarized state; loss of charge.

depression 1) a psychiatric syndrome involving sadness and dejection, often accompanied by physiologic change; 2) a decrease of functional activity, as in depression of sensorium.

dermis the inner layer of the skin; also called the corium.

detrusor muscle the three layers of smooth muscle which make up the urinary bladder.

detumescence the process of returning to a flaccid state such as the penis following ejaculation.

development an individual's increasing capacity and skill in functioning, related to growth.

developmental crisis a crisis which occurs as a result of stressors impeding development.

developmental tasks skills and behavior patterns learned during development.

diagnosis determination of the nature of a disease.

diapedesis the movement of blood corpuscles through the blood vessel wall.

diaphoresis profuse perspiration.

diarrhea the passage of liquid feces and an increased frequency of defecation.

diastolic blood pressure the pressure of the blood within the blood vessels when the ventricles of the heart are relaxed or dilated.

diathermy the production of heat in the body tissues by high-frequency electric currents.

dietitian a person who specializes in the science of nutrition.

diffusion 1) the process of spreading freely; 2) dialysis through a membrane.

digital performed with the finger.

diploid number the term used to describe the original number of chromosomes in all cells of the body (23 pairs).

diplopia double vision.

direct nursing activities activities of a nurse that are carried out in the presence of the patient.

disease a morbid (unhealthful) process having definite symptoms.

disequilibrium a disturbed state of equilibrium, either mental or physical.

disinfection (disinfectant) to render pathogenic microorganisms harmless.

disorientation a state of mental confusion; loss of bearings, time, place.

displacement a mental mechanism in which an emotional reaction is transferred from one object to another.

distal farthest from the point of reference.

distention the state of being enlarged.

diuresis the increased (excessive) production of urine.

diuretic an agent which increases the production of urine, thereby decreasing the body's fluid retention.

dorsal referring to the back.

dorsal recumbent a back lying position.

dorsalis pedis pulse a pulse located on the instep of the foot.

dressing   a material used to cover and protect a wound.

drive   the force which activates human impulses.

drug (medication)   a chemical compound taken by humans and animals for the purpose of disease prevention, cure, relief or to affect the structure or function of the body.

drug allergy   a hypersensitivity to a drug.

duodenocolic reflex   mass peristaltic movement of the colon stimulated by the presence of chyme in the duodenum.

dura (dura mater)   the outermost, fibrous membrane covering the brain and spinal cord.

dyspareunia   pain experienced by a woman during intercourse.

dysphagia   difficulty or inability to swallow.

dysphasia   difficulty speaking.

dyspnea   difficult or labored breathing.

dysuria   difficulty voiding (urinating) or pain upon voiding.

ecchymosis   a small hemorrhagic spot in the skin or mucous membrane, larger than a petechia.

echolalia   the repetition by a person of words addressed to him or her.

ecology   the study of man's relationship with the environment.

ectoderm   the outermost of the three primary germ layers of the embryo.

ectopic pregnancy   implantation of the fertilized ovum outside of the uterus.

edema   excess fluid in the interstitial compartment.

edentulous   without teeth.

effector organ   an organ which acts (produces output) to alter the environment.

efferent   conveying away from the center.

ego   that part of the psyche which maintains its identity; the conscious sense of self.

egocentricity (egocentricism)   the quality of being centered around self, having ideas which center upon self.

ejaculation   expulsion of semen out of the aroused penis.

ejaculatory ducts   short tubes that pass through the prostate gland and terminate in the urethra.

Electra complex   the female child's attraction to her father; compare with Oedipus complex.

electrocardiograph   a machine which measures and records impulses from the heart on a graph called an electrocardiogram (ECG, EKG).

electroencephalograph   a machine which measures and records impulses from the brain on a graph called an electroencephalogram (EEG).

electrolyte   a compound which in an aqueous solution is able to conduct an electric current.

electromyograph   a machine which measures and records impulses from the muscles on a graph called an electromyogram (EMG).

emaciation   excessive thinness.

embolus   1) a clot in a blood vessel which has moved from its place of origin; 2) a clot or other plug, such as an air embolus, obstructing a blood vessel.

embryo   the derivitive of a fertilized ovum that develops into the offspring.

emesis   vomiting.

emigration   the movement of leukocytes through the walls of small blood vessels.

emmetropia   the state when the rays of light entering the eye come to focus exactly on the retina.

emollient   an agent which soothes and softens, often oily substances.

empacho   a Chicano term for a disease seen primarily in children that includes a swollen abdomen as a result of intestinal blockage.

empathy   seeing or feeling a situation the way another person sees or feels it.

empirical   by observation or experience.

emulsion   a preparation in which one liquid is distributed throughout another.

enamel   the hard, inorganic substance which covers the crown of a tooth.

encoding   the selection of specific signs and symbols to transmit a message.

endemic   present in a community all the time.

endoderm (entoderm)   the innermost of the three primary germ layers of the embryo.

endogenous   developing from within.

endometrium   the inner mucous membrane lining of the uterus.

endothelium   the layer of endothelial cells found lining the blood vessels, cavities of the heart, and serous cavities.

enema   a solution which is injected into the rectum and sigmoid colon.

engorgement excessive fullness of an organ or passage.

enteric-coated a special coating used for tablets and capsules which prevents release of the drug until it is in the intestines.

enteritis inflammation of the small intestine.

enteroclysis the injection of a nutrient or drug into the colon.

enterostomy an opening through the abdominal wall into the intestines.

enuresis involuntary urination.

environment all conditions which make up the internal and external surroundings for an individual; external factors and internal influences.

epidemic occurrence of a disease in many people at the same time or in rapid succession in an area.

epidemiology the study of the occurrence and distribution of disease.

epidermis the outermost layer of the skin.

epididymis a highly coiled duct between the seminiferous tubules of the testes and the vas deferens.

epidural outside the dura.

epinephrine a hormone produced by the medulla of the adrenal glands; also manufactured artificially.

epistaxis nosebleed.

equilibrium a state of balance.

erection (penile) lengthening, widening, and hardening of the penis as it becomes congested with blood during sexual arousal.

erotic stimuli sensations that cause sexual arousal.

errogenous sexually sensitive.

eructation belching; bringing up gas or wind from the stomach through the mouth.

erythema redness of the skin.

esophagoscopy visual examination of the interior of the esophagus.

espanto a Chicano term for a disease in which the individual is frightened by seeing supernatural spirits or events.

estrogen a female sex hormone formed by the ovaries, adrenal cortex, the testes, and fetoplacental organ.

ethics rules or principles which govern right conduct.

ethnic relating to races or to large groups of people with common traits and customs.

ethnoscience systematic study of the way of life of a designated cultural group in order to obtain accurate data regarding behavior, perceptions, and interpretations of the universe.

etiology cause.

eupnea normal respiration that is quiet, rhythmic, and effortless.

eversion turning outward.

excoriation the loss of superficial layers of skin.

excreta waste products eliminated by the body.

expected date of confinement (EDC) expected date of the birth of a baby.

expectorate the act of spitting up mucus or other materials.

expiration the outflow of air from the lungs to the atmosphere.

extended family includes the nuclear family and other relatives such as uncles, aunts, grandparents, and such.

extension increasing the angle of a joint (between two bones).

extensor (muscle) a muscle that acts to straighten a joint.

extracellular outside the cells.

extrathecal outside the sheath, as in outside the spinal canal.

extravasation the escape of blood from a vessel into the body tissues.

exudate material such as fluid and cells which has escaped from blood vessels and is deposited in tissues or on tissue surfaces.

Fahrenheit the temperature scale in which the freezing point of water is 32° and the boiling point 212°; abreviated F and Fahr.

fasciculation abnormal contraction involving the whole motor unit of a muscle.

fastigium the highest point.

fasting abstinence from eating.

fat 1) adipose tissue; a whitish-yellow tissue forming soft pads between various body organs and which serves as an energy reserve; 2) an ester of glycerol with fatty acids.

fecal impaction a mass of hardened putty-like feces in the folds of the rectum.

feces (stool) excreta discharged by the large intestine.

feedback 1) the response to some of a system's output as intake for the purpose of exerting some influence over a process; 2) in the communication process, it is the response.

fellatio the act of stimulating the male genitalia by oral means such as licking, blowing, or sucking.

felony crimes of a serious nature punishable by imprisionment.

femoral anteversion the forward tipping or tilting of the femur.

femoral pulse the pulse found in the groin at the midpoint of the inguinal ligament.

fenestrated perforated as to provide a window or opening.

fetal heart beat the heart beat of the fetus as heard through the maternal abdominal wall.

fetal phase the stage of development from 8 or 12 weeks after conception until birth.

fetus the unborn offspring in the postembryonic state of development.

fever elevated body temperature.

fibrillation (muscle) involuntary contractions of a muscle.

fibrin an insoluble protein formed from fibrinogen during the clotting of blood.

fibroplasia the formation of fibrous tissue.

figure-of-eight bandage a bandage turn usually used for flexed joints in which the bandage makes a figure-of-eight around and over the joint.

first intention healing primary healing which occurs in a wound when the tissue surfaces have been approximated.

fissure a groove or deep fold, such as an anal fissure.

fistula an abnormal communication or passage usually between two organs or between an organ and the body surface.

flatulence the presence of excessive amounts of gas (flatus) in the intestines.

flatus gas or air in the stomach or intestines.

flexion decreasing the angle of a joint (between two bones); the act of bending.

flexor (muscle) a muscle which acts to bend, as in flexion.

flush transient redness of the skin, often of the face and neck.

focus the point of convergence of light rays or sound waves.

Follicle (hair) a tubular sturcture in the skin which encloses hair.

follicle stimulating hormone (FSH) hormone produced by the anterior pituitary gland (adenohypophysis) which stimulates the development of the ovarian follicle.

fomite an inanimate object which harbors pathogenic microorganisms and is capable of transmitting an infection.

fontanelle a soft spot, such as one of the spaces in the skull of an infant, which has a membranous covering.

footboard a board placed at the foot of a bed against which a patient can brace his feet.

forcep an instrument with two blades and a handle used to handle sterile supplies and to compress or grasp tissues.

foreplay purposeful physical contact or petting that increases sexual arousal prior to intercourse; also referred to as precoital stimulation.

foreskin the skin of the shaft of the penis; also referred to as prepuce.

formal operations stage (Piaget) the fourth cognitive developmental stage during 11 to 15 or 16 years.

formulary a collection of prescriptions and formulas.

Fowler's position a bed-sitting position.

fracture board a support placed under the mattress of a bed to give it added support.

friction rubbing; that force which opposes motion.

frigidity a low or non-detectable sex drive, usually applied to females.

frontal plane the plane which divides the body into ventral and dorsal sections.

frustration increased emotional tension due to inability to meet goals.

fulcrum the fixed point of a lever.

gastric pertaining to the stomach.

gastrocolic reflex increased colonic peristalsis after food has entered the stomach.

gastroenteritis inflammation of the stomach and the intestines.

gastroscope a lighted instrument used to visualize the interior of the stomach.

gastroscopy the examination of the stomach with a lighted instrument.

gastrostomy a surgical opening which leads directly into the stomach.

gavage administration of nourishment to the stomach through a tube; forced feeding.

gender role encompasses all that a person says or does to indicate whether the person is male or female.

gene the biologic unit of heredity located on a chromosome.

general adaptation syndrome (GAS) a general response of the body to a stressor.

genital stage the final stage of maturity of the adult according to Freud.

genitalia the reproductive organs, usually the external reproductive organs.

geriatrics the branch of medicine pertaining to elderly people.

germicide an agent that kills pathogenic (disease) microorganisms.

gerontology the study of all aspects of problems of the aging.

gingiva the gum.

gingivitis inflammation of the gum.

glossitis inflammation of the tongue.

glottis the vocal apparatus of the larynx.

glucocorticoid a corticoid substance which increases gluconeogenesis, thus raising liver glycogen.

glycerol the alcohol component of fats.

glycogen the chief carbohydrate stored in humans.

glycosuria (glucosuria) the presence of glucose in the urine.

gonad an ovary or testis.

gonorrhea a sexually transmitted (venereal) infection due to the *Neisseria gonorrhoeae*.

good samaritan act the law that protects physicians and nurses when rendering aid to a person in an emergency.

Goodell's sign the softening of the cervix during pregnancy.

gout a condition characterized by excessive uric acid in the blood.

granulation tissue tissue formed in a wound which is not healing by first intention.

gravity the force which pulls objects towards the center of the earth.

grief emotional suffering often caused by bereavement.

growth 1) an increase in weight and height; an increase in physical size; 2) the proliferation of cells.

guilt the painful, emotional feeling associated with transgression of moral-ethical beliefs.

gustatory referring to the sense of taste.

gynecology the branch of medicine which deals with processes of the female reproductive tract.

gynosperm sperm bearing an X chromosome.

halitosis foul odor of the breath.

hallucination distortions of sensory perceptions; hearing or seeing voices or things which do not exist.

hallucinogens drugs which cause distortion of the sensory perception.

haploid number refers to the number of chromosomes (23 single) found in sperm and egg cells.

health a state of being physically fit, mentally stable, and socially comfortable; encompasses more than the state of being free of disease.

health continuum a continuum (continuous process) with high level wellness at one end and death at the other.

health maintenance organization (HMO) an organization which provides a wide range of health services on a fixed contract basis, usually geared to preventive medicine.

health practitioner a person whose activities provide a health care service.

health team a group of individuals with varying skills whose cooperative efforts are designed to assist people with their health.

hectic (septic) fever an intermittent fever with wide variations in the body temperature and in which the temperature is normal sometime during each 24-hour period.

Hegar's sign the softening of the lower portion of the uterus during pregnancy.

hemangioma newly formed blood vessels which form a benign tumor.

hematemesis vomiting blood.

hematocrit the percentage proportion of red blood cell mass to whole blood.

hematoma a collection of blood in a tissue, organ, or space owing to a break in the wall of a blood vessel.

hematuria blood in the urine.

hemiplegia the loss of movement on one side of the body.

hemoglobin the red pigment contained in red blood cells which carries oxygen.

hemoglobinuria hemoglobin in the urine.

hemoptysis the presence of blood in the sputum.

hemorrhage the escape of blood from the blood vessels.

hemorrhoids a condition resulting from distended veins in the rectum.

hemosiderosis an increase in the amount of iron stored in the tissues without tissue damage.

hemostat a small instrument used to constrict blood vessels.

hemothorax a collection of blood in the thoracic cavity.

herb a leafy plant which does not have a wood stem and is valued for its medicinal, savory, or aromatic qualities.

herbalist an herb doctor; one who prescribes herbs for treating people.

Hering-Breuer reflex a reflex that inhibits inspiration.

hex a jinx; a spell imposed in witchcraft.

hirsutism abnormal hairiness, particularly in women.

holism refers to a theory that the whole must be viewed as the sum of its parts; in health, this means the whole person (that is, physical and emotional being) must be treated as one.

holophrastic speech a type of speech in which one word expresses a whole sentence.

homeostasis the state of physiologic and psychologic stability in the body.

homogamy 1) inbreeding; 2) reproduction resulting from the union of two identical cells.

hormone a chemical substance produced by the body that has certain regulatory effects.

human chorionic gonadotropin (HCG) a hormone produced by the placenta; it functions to maintain the intactness of the ovary.

human placental lactogen (chorionic somatomammotropin) a hormone secreted by the placenta that influences growth of fetal cells and prepares the breasts for lactation.

humanism an interest in or devotion to human welfare.

humidity the degree of moisture, particularly the moisture in the air.

hunger an unpleasant sensation caused by deprivation of something, especially food.

hyaluronidase an enzyme found in tissues; it catalyzes hydrolysis of hyaluronic acid, the cement substance of tissues.

hydration the act of combining with water, or causing to combine with water.

hydraulics the branch of physics which deals with the physical actions of liquids.

hydrocortisone an adrenocortical steroid produced by the adrenal glands or produced synthetically.

hydrolysates relatively crude proteins.

hydrometer an instrument used to determine the specific gravity of a fluid.

hydrostatic pressure the pressure a liquid exerts on the sides of the container within which it is contained.

hygiene the science of health and its preservation.

hymen a vascularized, membranous fold partly closing the vaginal orifice.

hyperalgesia extreme sensitivity to pain.

hyperalimentation intravenous administration of nutrients; parenteral nutrition.

hypercalcemia an excessive amount of calcium in the blood.

hyperemia an excessive amount of blood in a body part.

hyperextension excessive extension, or stretching of a joint.

hyperglycemia an increased concentration of glucose in the blood.

hyperkalemia an excessive amount of potassium in the blood.

hypernatremia an elevated level of sodium in the blood plasma.

hyperopia a condition in which the rays of light entering the eye come to focus behind the retina; farsightedness.

hyperplasia an abnormal increase in the number of cells in a tissue or an organ.

hyperpnea an abnormal increase in the rate and the depth of respirations.

hyperreflexia an exaggeration of the reflexes.

hypersensitivity an exaggerated response of the body to a foreign substance.

hypersomnia uncontrollable drowsiness.

hypertension persistent elevated arterial blood pressure.

hyperthermia an abnormally high body temperature, sometimes induced as a therapeutic measure.

hypertonic solution solutions with a greater tonicity than blood.

hypertonicity excessive muscle tone or activity.

hypertrophy an abnormal increase in the size of a tissue or organ as a result of an increase in the size of the cells.

hyperventilation an increase in the amount of air in the lungs characterized by prolonged deep breaths.

hypervolemia an abnormal increase in the body's blood volume.

hypnosis an abnormally induced passive state in which an individual responds to suggestions which do not conflict with the person's conscious or unconscious desires.

hypnotic a drug that induces sleep.

hypocalcemia a decreased amount of calcium in the blood serum.

hypochloremia a reduced concentration of chlorides in the blood.

hypodermis (subcutaneous) the layer of tissue beneath the dermis.

hypodermoclysis the introduction of fluid into the subcutaneous tissues.

hypofibrinogenemia a deficiency of fibrinogen in the blood.

hypoglycemia a reduced amount of glucose in the blood.

hypokalemia a reduced amount of potassium in the blood.

hyponatremia a below normal amount of sodium in the blood plasma.

hypostatic pneumonia a condition caused by stagnation of fluids produced by the inactivity of the lungs.

hypotension abnormally low arterial blood pressure.

hypothalamus that part of the brain which forms the floor and part of the wall of the third ventricle.

hypothermia an abnormally low body temperature, often induced as a therapeutic measure.

hypotonicity decreased muscle tone.

hypoventilation a reduction in the amount of air entering the lungs, characterized by shallow respiration.

hypovolemia an abnormally decreased amount of blood plasma.

hypoxemia a reduced level of oxygen in the blood.

hypoxia a reduced level of oxygen in the body tissues.

hysterectomy the surgical removal of the uterus.

id the unconscious part of the personality that contains primitive desires and urges and is ruled by the pleasure principle.

identification a mental mechanism by which one feels or thinks as another person.

idiosyncratic effect different, unexpected, or individual effect from the normal one that is usually expected from a medication; unpredictable and unexplainable symptoms occur.

illness sickness or deviation from a healthy state or the normal functioning of the total person.

illusion false interpretation of some stimulus.

imagination a creation of the mind; the act of forming a mental image of something not present to stimulate the senses.

imitation copying the behaviors and attitudes of another person.

immobility the prescribed or unavoidable restriction of movement in any area of the patient's life.

immunity protection from a particular disease by natural endowed resistance or by developing the resistance after exposure to a disease agent.

immunoglobulin a part of the body's serum proteins; also referred to as immune bodies or antibodies.

impaction a condition of being firmly wedged or lodged, with usual reference to feces.

imperforate abnormally closed; used to describe an opening, such as an anus or a hymen, that is not open.

impotence the inability to achieve or to maintain an erection sufficiently to perform intercourse.

inattentive the inability to focus one's mind upon an aspect of the environment or upon a specific idea.

incision a cut or wound that is intentionally made, such as during surgery.

incoherent   actions or speech lacking cohesion, orderly continuity, relevance, or consistency.

incontinence   the inability to restrain urine or feces (anal incontinence).

incubation period   the time between the entrance of the pathogen into the body and the onset of the symptoms of the infection.

infarct   a localized area of necrosis (dead cells) usually owing to obstructed arterial blood flow to the part.

infection   the invasion of the body by pathogenic organisms and the subsequent physiologic reaction of the body to these organisms.

infestation   the invasion of the body by insects, mites, and/or ticks.

infiltration   the diffusion or deposition into the tissues of substances that are not normal to it.

inflammation   the tissue response to injury of cells or cell destruction.

infradian rhythm   a biorythm which cycles monthly, such as the human menstrual cycle.

infrared heat   a radiant type of heat capable of penetrating body tissues to a depth of 10 mm; sources of infrared rays include heat lamps and incandescent light bulbs.

infusion   the introduction of fluid into a vein or another part of the body for therapeutic purpose.

ingestion   the act of taking in food or medication.

inhalation (inspiration)   the breathing in of air or other substances into the lungs.

inhalation therapist   respiratory technologist skilled in therapies used in the care of patients with respiratory problems.

inorganic   having no organs or not of organic origin; used in chemistry to describe acids or compounds that do not contain carbon.

insensible perspiration   unnoticeable sweating since it evaporates immediately once it reaches the surface of the skin.

insertion   attachment, such as that of skeletal muscle on the bone it moves when contracted, or that of the umbilical cord to fetal membranes.

insomnia   the inability to obtain sufficient sleep.

inspection   visual examination to detect features perceptible to the eye.

inspiration   the act of drawing air into the lungs.

inspiratory capacity   tidal volume and inspiratory reserve volume.

instillation   dropping or inserting liquid into a cavity, such as the bladder or the eye.

insulator   a substance or material that inhibits conduction, for example, heat or electricity.

integument   the skin or covering of the body.

intelligence   term used to describe the functioning of the mind, specifically the combination of judgment, memory, imagination, and reasoning.

intercostal   between the ribs.

interdigital   between the digits (toes and fingers).

intermittent (quotidian) fever   a fever that recurs daily.

intern   a graduate of a basic health program who is taking planned practical experience usually in order to obtain a license to practice, such as, nursing, medicine.

internal feedback   positive or negative responses from the self to the communication one gives either in writing or verbally.

interstitial   between the cells of the body's tissues.

interview   a structured consultation used to obtain information or to evaluate the progress of a person.

intestinal distention (tympanites)   stretching and inflation of the intestines due to the presence of air or gas.

intraarterial   within or inside an artery.

intracellular   within a cell or cells.

intractable pain   pain that is resistant to cure or relief.

intradermal (intracutaneous)   within the dermis.

intralipid   fat solutions that can be given in superficial veins.

intramuscular   within or inside muscle tissue.

intraosseus   within the bone.

intrapleural pressure   pressure within the pleural cavity.

intrapulmonic pressure   pressure within the lungs.

intrathecal   within a sheath, such as the spinal canal.

intrauterine   inside the uterus.

intravascular   within a blood vessel, usually arterial.

intravenous   within a vein.

intravertebral   within the vertebrae (intraspinal).

introjection   the acceptance and incorporation of

the patterns, attitudes, and ideals of another person as one's own.

introversion   the directing of one's energy and interest towards one's self.

intubation   insertion of a tube.

inunction   rubbing of the skin with an ointment.

inversion   a turning inward.

involution   a rolling or turning inward of a particular organ or the entire body such as occurs with the uterus after the fetus is expelled or with the bodily changes that occur in old age.

inward rotation   a turning towards the midline such as occurs with the hip joint.

ion   an atom or group of atoms that carry a positive or negative electric charge; also referred to as an electrolyte.

irradiation   exposure to penetrating rays such as x-rays, gamma rays, infrared rays, or ultraviolet rays.

irrational   a state of being confused as to time, place, and/or person.

irrigation   the washing of a body cavity or a wound.

irritant   a substance that stimulates unpleasant responses, that is, irritates.

ischemia   the lack of blood supply to a body part.

isolation   the setting apart or segregation of patients with communicable diseases.

isometric   pertains to the same measure or length; used commonly to describe exercises that do not change the length of the muscle (static muscle exercises).

isotonic   the term used to compare solutions of the same strength or concentration.

isotonic exercise   active exercise involving muscle contractions in which there is a marked shortening of muscle length.

isthmus   a narrow passage connecting two larger parts of an organ.

jargon   the technical or idiomatic terminology characteristic of a particular group.

jaundice   a syndrome involving hyperbilirubinemia and the deposit of bile pigment in the skin and mucous membranes, resulting in the patient appearing yellowish.

Kelly forcep   a type of hemostat.

keratin   a protein found in the skin, hair, nails, horny tissue, and the enamel of teeth.

keratosis   a horny growth, such as a callus or wart.

keratotic   pertaining to keratosis.

ketone   any compound containing the carbonyl group, CO, and having hydrocarbon groups attached to the carbonyl group.

kilocalorie   the amount of heat required to raise the temperature of 1 kg of water 1°C.

kilogram   a unit of weight equal to 1000 gm or approximately 2.2 lb.

kinesiology   the study of the motion of the human body.

kinesthesia   the sense of awareness of the position and the movement of the body parts.

Kosher   sanctioned by Jewish law.

Kussmaul's breathing (Kussmaul-Klien respiration)   a dyspnea occurring in paroxysms.

kwashiorkor   a condition occurring in children after weaning as a result of protein and calorie malnutrition; evidenced by growth failure, pot belly, edema, and mental apathy.

labia majora   the two longitudinal folds or lips of skin extending downward and backward from the mons pubis that protect the vaginal and urethral orifices.

labia minora   small folds of skin lying between the labia majora and the vaginal opening.

labored breathing   difficult or dyspneic breathing.

laceration   a wound in which the tissues have been torn.

lactase   an enzyme that acts as a catalyst to convert lactose into glucose and galactose.

lactase deficiency   a condition which occurs in Asians and black Americans.

lactate   a salt of lactic acid.

lactation   the secretion of milk, or the period of secretion.

lactiferous   conveying or producing milk.

lactose   a carbohydrate found in milk.

lalling   repetitive sounds infants make based upon what they hear.

lanugo   fine hair on the shoulders, back, and sacrum of the fetus.

laryngeal stridor   a harsh, crowing sound due to laryngeal obstruction.

laryngoscope   a lighted instrument used to visualize the larynx.

laryngoscopy   a visual examination of the larynx.

laryngospasm   spasmodic closure of the larynx.

latency period (Freud)   the school-age years (6 to 12 years).

lateral   to the side, away from the midline.

lavage   the washing of an organ, as for example the stomach.

laxative   a medication that stimulates bowel activity.

legumes   the fruit or pod of a leguminous plant, such as peas or beans.

lesion   the traumatic or pathologic interruption of a tissue or the loss of function of a body part.

leukocyte   white blood cell.

leukocytosis   an increase in the number of white blood cells.

lever   a firm bar which revolves around a fixed point.

liability   the legal responsibility of a person to account for wrongful acts by making financial restitution.

libel   defamation by means of print, writing or pictures.

libido   sexual desire; psychic energy (Freud); the energy from primitive impulses.

license   a legal document permitting a person to offer his skills and knowledge to the public in a particular area.

life expectancy   the age to which a person is expected to live.

lifestyle   the values and behaviors adopted by an individual for daily living.

ligament   a band of fibrous tissue that connects bones or cartilages and supports joints.

lightening   the descent of the uterus into the pelvic cavity which usually occurs two to three weeks before labor begins.

liniment   an oily liquid used on the skin.

local adaptation syndrome (LAS)   the reaction of one organ or body part to stress.

lochia   the vaginal discharge which occurs during the first week or two after the birth of a baby.

lordosis   the anterior concavity in the curvature of the cervical and lumbar spine when viewed from the side.

lotions   liquids which often carry an insoluble powder.

lumbar puncture   the insertion of a needle into the subarachnoid space at the lumbar region.

lumen   a channel within a tube such as the channel of an artery in which blood flows.

lung recoil   the tendency of lungs to collapse away from the chest wall.

lymphadenitis   inflammation of the lymph nodes.

lymphangitis   the inflammation of a lymphatic vessel or vessels.

lymphatic   referring to lymph or lymph vessels.

lysis (of a fever)   the gradual reduction of an elevated body temperature to normal.

lysosome   a minute body found in many types of cells; it is involved in intracellular digestion.

lysozyme   an enzyme that is present in saliva and tears and functions as an antibacterial agent.

maceration   the wasting away or softening of a solid as if by the action of soaking; often used to describe degenerative changes and eventual disintegration.

macrophage   a large phagocytic cell that destroys microorganisms or harmful cells.

malaise   a general feeling of being unwell or indisposed.

mal de ojo   a cultural disease of Chicanos believed to result from a person admiring a part of another person's body, such as the eyes.

malingering   the willful and fraudulent feigning of the symptoms of illness to obtain a consciously desired goal.

malnutrition   any disorder connected with nutrition.

malpractice   negligence applied to a professional action, such as professional misconduct or lack of skill.

mammary glands   breast tissues which secrete for the nourishment of the young.

mandatory licensure   governing laws that insist that all persons who practice in a particular field, such as nursing, must be licensed.

manslaughter   a felony in which an unlawful killing is committed without previous intent.

marasmus   condition of children under one year as a result of protein and calorie malnutrition; evidenced by wasting, wrinkled skin, thinness, eyes appearing large.

margination   the aggregating or lining up of substances along a surface or edge; used to describe the lining up of white blood cells against the wall of a blood vessel during the inflammatory process.

marihuana   an intoxicating agent from the leaves and flowers of the plant *Cannabis sativa;* commonly used in cigarettes and inhaled as smoke.

mastectomy   surgical removal of the breast.

masticate   to chew, as to chew food.

matriarchy   a system in which the mother is considered to be head of the house or family.

matrilineal   relating to descent through the female line.

masturbation   self stimulation of the genitals or other body parts to evoke erotic pleasure.

maturation   the process of becoming mature or fully developed.

meatus   an opening.

meconium   a dark green, mucilaginous material found in the intestines of the newborn.

medical asepsis   clean technique which limits the spread of pathogenic microorganisms.

melanin   the dark pigment of the skin and hair.

menarche   the first menstrual period occurring sometime between the ages of nine and seventeen.

menopause   cessation of menstruation in the human female that occurs usually around the age of 45 to 50 years.

menses   menstrual flow.

mental defense mechanism   mental coping processes used by all persons to adapt to life situations and to protect self esteem.

mental well-being   a state of feeling contentment, peace of mind, and satisfaction with living and life.

meosis   a specialized type of cell division that occurs with sperm and egg cells.

mesoderm   the middle layer of the three primary developmental germ layers in the embryo; lies between the entoderm and the ectoderm.

microglia   a type of nerve tissue that has migratory cells which act as phagocytes to the waste products of nerve tissues.

microorganism   a minute (usually microscopic) living organism.

micturition   the process of emptying the urinary bladder; also referred to as voiding or urination.

milia   plural for milium; small whitish nodules of the skin; usually are cysts of the sebaceous glands or hair follicles.

milliequivalent   the number of grams of a solute that is contained in one milliliter of a normal solution; abbreviated mEq.

milliliter   a unit of volume in the metric system approximating one cubic centimeter; abbreviated ml.

mineralocorticoid   a steroid hormone of the adrenal cortex that acts to retain sodium in the body and to excrete potassium.

minim   a unit of liquid measure equal to 0.0616 ml.

misdemeanor   crimes of less serious nature than felony and punishable by fines or short term imprisonment or both.

mitosis   process of cell division.

mongolian spots   dark bluish areas on the buttocks or backs of non-white babies that usually disappear spontaneously in the first year.

mons pubis   a pillow of adipose tissue situated over the symphysis pubis and covered by coarse hair; also referred to as the mons veneris.

Montgomery's glands   sebaceous glands in the areola of the nipple which become enlarged and prominent during pregnancy.

Montgomery straps   tie tapes used to hold dressings in place.

morbidity   the condition of being diseased.

morning sickness   the nausea and vomiting which occurs frequently in the mornings during the first trimester of pregnancy.

Moro's reflex   the startle reflex of infants in which the arms and legs are extended outward and retracted in response to a sudden stimulus such as a loud noise.

mortality   the death rate.

mucin   the chief constituent of mucus.

mucolytic   the act of destroying or dissolving mucus.

mucus   the lubricating, free slime of the mucous membranes.

muscular strain   the overstretching or overexertion of muscles.

myelogram   an x-ray of the spinal cord.

myocardial infarction   cardiac tissue necrosis resulting from obstruction of the blood flow to the area.

myocardium   the heart muscle; the middle layer of the heart tissue.

myometrium the middle, thick, smooth muscle layer of the uterus.

myopia near-sightedness.

narcolepsy a condition in which an individual experiences an uncontrollable desire for sleep, or attacks of sleep which occur at certain intervals.

narcotic a drug that induces insensibility and stupor at the same time relieving pain.

nasopharynx the upper part of the pharynx which adjoins the nasal passage.

naturopath a nonmedical practitioner who practices therapy involving such things as light, heat, water, but no drugs.

nausea the urge to vomit.

nebulizer an atomizer or sprayer.

necessary cause one factor which must be present for a specific disease to occur.

necrosis nonliving cells or tissue in contact with living cells.

negative feedback system a common control mechanism of the body that causes a reduction in hormone output.

negligence the failure to do something that a reasonable person would do, or doing something that a reasonable, prudent person would not do; careless workmanship.

neonatal mortality infant death within twenty-eight days of birth.

neoplasm any growth that is new and abnormal.

nephritis the inflammation of a kidney.

nephron the functional unit of the kidney.

nephrosis a disease of the kidney.

nervousness a state of being readily excited, irritated, or uneasy.

neurogenous arising in the nervous system.

neurohypophysis the posterior part of the pituitary gland.

neurologic pertaining to the nervous system.

neuron a nerve cell and its processes; the functional unit of the nervous system.

nocturia (nycturia, nocturnal frequency) increased urinary frequency at night that is not a result of increased fluid intake.

nocturnal enuresis involuntary urination at night.

non-pathogen a microorganism that does not cause disease.

nonverbal communication (body language) communication other than verbal, including gestures and posture.

norm an ideal or fixed standard.

normal saline an isotonic concentration of salt (NaC1) solution.

nosocomial referring to or originating in a hospital or similar institution, such as a nosocomial disease.

nuclear family the family unit composed of parents and children.

nursing audit the review of a patient's charts for evidence of nursing competency.

nutrient an organic or inorganic substance found in food and which is digested and absorbed in the gastrointestinal tract and then used in the body's metabolic processes.

nutritionist an individual who is a specialist in food and nutrition.

obese excessively fat; overweight.

objective symptom evidence of disease or body dysfunction that can be observed and described by others.

obligatory heat the heat produced by the body as a result of the metabolism of food.

obstetrics the branch of medicine dealing with the birth process and those related events which precede and follow it.

occult hidden.

occupational therapist an individual who assists a person with skills related to activities of daily living.

Oedipus complex (Freud) the male child's attraction for his mother and accompanying hostile attitudes toward his father; compare with Electra complex.

ointment a semisolid preparation applied externally to the body.

olfactory referring to the sense of smell.

oliguria the production of abnormally small amounts of urine by the kidneys.

open wound a wound in which the continuity of the skin or mucous membrane has been interrupted.

ophthalmoscope a lighted instrument used to examine the interior of the eye.

oral referring to the mouth.

oral stage (Freud) that stage of development which occurs during the first year.

organic referring to an organ or organs.

orgasm the climax of sexual excitement in which a feeling of physiologic and psychologic release occurs; characterized by rhythmic spasmodic contractions of the genitals.

orgasmic dysfunction the inability of females to achieve orgasm.

orgasmic platform an increase in size of the outer one-third of the vagina and the labia minora during precoital stimulation.

orientation awareness of time, place, and person.

orifice the external opening (entrance or outlet) of any body cavity such as the vagina, urethra, anus.

origin (of a muscle) the fixed or least moveable point of attachment to a bone.

oropharynx that aspect of the pharynx which lies between the upper aspect of the epiglottis and the soft palate.

orthostatism erect standing posture of the body.

orthopnea the ability to breathe only in the upright position of sitting or standing.

orthostatic hypotension low blood pressure in a standing position.

osmosis the passage of a solvent through a semi-permeable membrane from the lesser concentration to the greater concentration of the two solutions.

osmotic pressure the amount of required pressure to exactly oppose osmosis.

osseous pertaining to bone.

ossification the formation of bone or bony substance.

osteomalacia the softening of the bones.

osteoporosis the demineralization of bone.

otoscope the instrument used to examine the ear.

outward rotation turning away from the midline.

ovary female gonad (sexual gland); ova are formed in the two ovaries.

overbed cradle a frame placed over a patient while in bed to protect the body from contact with the upper bedclothes.

overnutrition the over-supply of calories.

ovulation the discharge of a mature ovum from the graafian follicle of the ovary.

ovum the female reproductive cell (egg) which becomes the embryo after fertilization.

oxyhemoglobin the compound of oxygen and hemoglobin.

oxytocin a hormone secreted by the posterior pituitary gland.

packing the act of filling an open wound with a material such as gauze.

pain a basically unpleasant sensation, localized or general, mild or intense, which represents the suffering induced by the stimulation of specialized nerve endings; may be threatened, or fantasied; may be induced by disease, injury, or mental derangement caused by disease or injury.

pain perception threshhold the amount of stimulation required for pain to be perceived.

palliative affording relief but not cure.

pallor the absence of normal skin coloration.

palmar grasp reflex a reflex normally present in the newborn in which the fingers will curl around a small object placed in the palm of the hand.

palpation an act of feeling with the hands, usually the fingers.

pandemic an epidemic disease that is widespread.

panic severe anxiety.

Papanicolaou (Pap) smear a method of taking sample cells from the cervix for microscopic examination to detect malignancy.

papule a small round elevation of the skin.

paracentesis the insertion of a needle into a cavity (usually the abdominal cavity) to remove fluid.

paralysis the impairment or loss of motor function of a body part.

paramedical having some connection with the practice of medicine.

paraplegia paralysis of the lower part of the body (including the legs) in which both motor function and sensation are affected.

parasite a plant or animal which lives on or within another living organism.

parasympathetic (craniosacral) nervous system a branch of the autonomic nervous system.

parathyroid hormone the hormone, produced by the parathyroid glands, that regulates the calcium and phosphorus levels in the body.

parenchyma the functional or essential elements of an organ.

parenteral 1) that which occurs outside the alimentary tract; 2) injection into the body through some route other than the alimentary canal, for example, intravenous.

paresthesia an abnormal sensation of burning or prickling.

paronychia an inflammation of the folds of tissue around a fingernail.

parotid glands large salivary glands in front of the ears.

parotitis inflammation of the parotid gland.

paroxysm a sudden attack or sharp reoccurrence; a spasm.

passive exercise exercise in which the energy is not provided by the patient (as it is in active exercise).

passivity lethargic; receptive to outside influence; lacking energy or will.

patency wide open; not clogged or shut.

pathogen a microorganism or material that produces disease.

pathogenic that which is capable of producing disease.

pathology a branch of medicine concerned with the nature of disease.

patient a person who is seeking assistance for an illness or injury.

patient advocate a person who speaks on behalf of a patient and can intercede on the patient's behalf.

patriarchy a system in which the father is considered to be the head of the house or family.

patrilineal relating to descent through the male line.

pediculosis a condition of infestation with lice.

peer review review by persons of equal standing.

penetrating wound a wound created by an instrument which penetrated deeply through the skin or mucous membranes into the tissues.

penis the male copulatory organ; functions also as the organ for urine excretion.

penrose drain a flexible, rubber drain.

perception 1) the process of understanding something new and then making it part of one's previous experience or knowledge; 2) a person's awareness and identification of a person, thing, or situation.

percussion the act of striking a body area with sharp blows as an aid to diagnosing a condition by the sounds produced.

pericardial aspiration the removal of fluid from the pericardial sac via an inserted needle.

peridontal disease disease occurring in the tissues around the teeth.

perimetrium the thin, outer, serous layer of the uterus.

perineum the area between the anus and the posterior aspect of the genitalia.

periorbital around the eye socket.

periosteum the tough, fibrous membrane surrounding a bone.

periostitis inflammation of the periosteum.

peripheral at the edge or outward boundary.

peristalsis the propulsive waves of the intestine.

peritoneal cavity the area between the layers of the peritoneum; a potential space.

peritoneum the serous membrane lining the abdominal cavity.

peritonitis inflammation of the peritoneum.

permissive licensure the policy by which practitioners do not require licensure to practice but are not protected by the licensing body.

perspiration the saline fluid secreted by the sweat glands for the purpose of excretion and cooling the body.

petechiae tiny, purplish-red spots resulting from intradermal or submucous hemorrhage.

pH symbol used to express the measure of alkalinity or acidity of a solution by relating hydrogen ion concentration of the solution to that of a given solution.

phagocyte a cell that ingests microorganisms and other cells or foreign particles.

phagocytosis the act of engulfing microorganisms, other cells, or foreign particles by phagocytes.

phallic state (Freud) the stage of development during the fourth and fifth years.

phantom pain pain which remains after the cause has been removed, such as pain perceived in a foot after the leg has been amputated.

pharmacist an individual who is licensed to prepare and dispense drugs and to make up prescriptions.

pharmacology a science which deals with the actions of drugs upon living animals and humans.

pharmacopoeia a book containing a list of products used in medicine including their description and formulas.

pharmacy 1) the art of preparing and dispensing medicines; 2) the place where medicines are prepared and dispensed.

phlebitis inflammation of a vein.

phlebothrombosis intravascular clotting with marked inflammation of a vein.

phlebotomy opening a vein to remove blood.

physiatrist a physician who specializes in rehabilitation medicine using physical aids such as light, heat, apparatus.

physical pertaining to the body or to physics.

physical well being a state of having physical needs met appropriately for homeostasis.

physiologic concerned with body function.

physiology the science concerned with the functioning of living organisms and their parts.

physiotherapist (physical therapist) a member of the health team who provides assistance to patients who have problems related to the musculoskeletal system.

pica a craving to eat unnatural substances during pregnancy, some psychologic conditions, or extreme malnutrition.

pinna the part of the ear which projects outside the head.

placebo an inactive, harmless substance given to a patient for a variety of reasons, one of which is to determine the effectiveness of the preparation during controlled studies.

placenta the tissue which is attached to the wall of the uterus and through which the fetus receives nourishment; after the child is born it is expelled as the "afterbirth."

plantar flexion movement of the foot so that the toes point downward.

plantar reflex a reflex of the newborn that occurs when pressure is applied to the ball of the foot; the toes promptly flex.

plaque a film of mucus and bacteria which forms on the teeth.

plasma the portion of the blood which is fluid.

pleura the serous membrane which lines the thoracic cavity.

pleural cavity a potential space between the layers of pleura.

pleural rub (friction rub) coarse, leathery, or grating sound produced by the pleurae rubbing together.

pneumoencephalogram the x-ray of the cerebrospinal spaces after the introduction of air.

pneumothorax the presence of gas or air in the pleural cavity.

pneumoventriculogram the x-ray of the ventricles of the brain after the introduction of oxygen.

polarity the presence of two opposite poles.

poliomyelitis an acute viral disease which may involve paralysis.

polydipsia excessive thirst.

polyneuritis inflammation of many nerves.

polypnea an abnormal increase in the respiratory rate.

polyunsaturated fatty acid fatty acids which contain two or more double bonds such as linoleic and arachidonic acids.

polyuria (diuresis) production of abnormally large amounts of urine by the kidneys.

POMR see problem oriented medical record.

popliteal referring to the posterior aspect of the knee.

population density the number of people per square mile of a given area.

positive feedback a control or regulating mechanism of the body which causes the production of additional hormone.

positivism the state of being positive; a theory that positive knowledge is based upon nautral phenomena as verified by empirical sciences.

posterior fornix (of the vagina) a vault-like space at the posterior aspect of the vagina.

postovulatory after ovulation; synonyms are secretory or luteal when used to describe the last half of the menstrual cycle.

postpartum occurring after childbirth.

posture the bearing and position of the body; the relative arrangement of the various parts of the body.

potency power; the ability of the male to perform the sexual act.

precedent the first case that establishes a common law.

precordium the area over the heart or stomach.

preeclampsia a toxemia of late pregnancy.

prelinguistic sounds made by an infant which are not related to language.

premature ejaculation the inability to control ejaculation prior to satisfaction of the partner or before 30 seconds to one minute after intromission into the vagina.

pre-operational stage (Piaget) the phase of cognitive development which occurs during three to seven years.

preoptic center the nerve center anterior to the optic center.

preovulatory before ovulation; as related to menses, the average 14 days from the first day of menstrual flow; synonyms are proliferative or follicular.

prepuberty the period preceding puberty.

prepubic urethra that part of the male urethra which is inferior to the pubis.

presbyobia (hyperopia) long-sightedness that can result in old age.

prescription the written direction for the preparation and administration of a remedy.

previable a fetus incapable of extrauterine life.

primary care a type of practice in which the first person to meet the patient, for example, the nurse, assumes responsibility for patient care.

primary union (wound healing) healing that involves the production of minimal scar tissue.

primordial follicle primitive sac or cavity of the ovary that contains the ovum.

principle a fundamental law or doctrine.

privileged communication information given to a professional person, for example, a physician.

problem oriented medical record (POMR) a method of written communication which all members of the health disciplines use together.

proctoclysis a slow instillation of fluid into the rectum.

proctoscope a lighted instrument used to visualize the interior of the rectum.

proctoscopy the visualization of the interior of the rectum with a lighted instrument.

prodromal stage a period of illness during which there are some early manifestations of the illness.

progesterone a hormone produced by the ovaries, placenta, and the adrenal cortex.

prognosis the medical opinion in regard to the outcome of a disease.

prolactin a hormone from the anterior pituitary which stimulates lactation.

proliferation rapid reproduction of parts, cells, or new parts.

pronation moving the bones of the forearm so that the palm of the hand is moved from anterior to posterior while in anatomic position.

prone lying with the face downward; having the palm of the hand turned downward.

prophylaxis preventive treatment; prevention of disease.

proprioceptor a sensory receptor which receives stimuli from within the organism.

prostate gland a gland around the base of the urethra of the male.

prostectomy the removal of the prostate gland.

prosthesis an artificial part such as an eye, leg, or dentures.

prostration extreme exhaustion.

protein any of the large, complex compounds containing essential elements; the major constituent of protoplasm; essential to body maintenance.

proteinuria protein in the urine.

proximal closer to the point of attachment or to the point of reference.

pruritis intense itching.

psychiatry the branch of medicine which deals with disorders that are behavioral, emotional, or mental.

psychology the science concerned with the mind and mental processes.

psychomotor motor effects related to cerebral or psychic activity.

psychosomatic 1) concerning the mind and the body; 2) emotional disturbances manifested by physiologic symptoms.

ptyalin an enzyme occurring in saliva.

ptyalism excessive secretion of saliva.

puberty the age during which the reproductive organs become active and secondary sex characteristics develop.

public law rules regulating relationships between individuals and government.

puerperium that period of time from delivery to about six weeks after delivery of an infant.

949

pulmonary capacity   combination of two or more pulmonary volumes.

pulse   the rhythmic, recurrent wave of blood created by the contraction of the left ventricle of the heart.

pulse deficit   the difference between the apical rate and the radial pulse rate.

pulse pressure   the difference between the systolic and diastolic blood pressures.

pulse rate   the number of pulse beats per minute.

pulse volume   the force of the blood with each pulse beat.

puncture (stab) wound   a wound made by a sharp instrument penetrating the skin and underlying tissues.

pupil   the opening at the center of the iris of the eye.

Purkinje fibers   fibers leaving the atrioventricular node of the heart.

purulent   containing pus.

pus   a thick liquid resulting from inflammation; composed of cells, liquid, microorganisms, and tissue debris.

pustule   a small elevation of the skin or mucous membrane or a clogged pore or follicle containing pus.

putrid   rotten.

pyelogram   a roentgenogram of the kidney and ureter, showing the pelvis of the kidney.

pyemia   a generalized, persistent blood poisoning.

pyogenic   pus-producing.

pyrexia   a fever; an elevated body temperature.

pyrogen   a substance which produces a fever.

pyuria   pus in the urine.

quadriplegia   the paralysis of all four limbs.

rabbi   a Jew ordained for professional religious leadership.

radial pulse   the pulse point located where the radial artery passes over the radius of the arm.

radiation therapy   therapy administered by x-rays, radium, or other radioactive substances.

radiology technologist   a member of the health team who takes roentgenograms and assists with other related tests.

radiopaque   the property of blocking the passage of radiant energy, such as x-rays.

rale   an abnormal sound of respiration resembling rattling or bubbling, usually heard on inspiration during ausculation.

rationalization   a mental mechanism of giving socially acceptable reasons for one's behavior.

reaction formation   a mental mechanism whereby a person assumes an attitude which is the opposite of a repressed socially unacceptable impulse.

readiness   the state of being ready; used to describe the developmental maturation and growth necessary prior to being able to perform some activities such as walking.

receptor   the terminal of a sensory nerve which is sensitive to specific stimuli.

recreational therapist   a member of the health team who assists patients with activities for recreation.

rectocele   proctocele; a protrusion of part of the rectum into the vagina.

rectum   the distal portion of the large intestine.

reduced hemoglobin   hemoglobin which has released its oxygen.

referred pain   pain which is perceived to be in one area but the source of which is another area.

reflex   an involuntary activity in response to a stimulus.

reflexive vocalization   nondescriptive sounds infants make in response to various stimuli and environmental conditions.

reflexogenic erection   erection of the penis that occurs without apparent sexual stimuli.

regeneration   the renewal of cells or tissues as a result of lost or damaged cells or tissues.

regimen   a regulated pattern of activity.

regression   a mental mechanism of reverting to a previously acceptable behavior or state.

rehabilitation   the restoration of a person who is ill or injured to the highest possible capacity.

relapsing fever   a fever in which the temperature returns to normal for one or more days between periods of fever.

REM   rapid eye movement.

remittent fever   a fever in which there is a wide range of temperatures over a 24-hour period, all of which are elevated above normal.

renal   relating to the kidney.

renal dialysis a process in which blood flows from an artery through an artificial membrane where impurities are removed, and then returns to the patient through a vein.

renal pelvis the funnel-shaped upper end of each ureter.

repression a mental mechanism of unconscious forgetting of problems or experiences.

residual urine the amount of urine remaining in the bladder after voiding.

residual volume (air) the amount of air remaining in the lungs after a forceful exhalation.

resistive behaviors those behaviors which inhibit involvment, cooperation, or change.

respiration the transport of oxygen from the atmosphere to the body cells, and the transport of carbon dioxide from the cells back to the atmosphere.

respiratory technologist a person who provides diagnostic and therapeutic measures for patients who have respiratory problems.

rest a state of repose after exertion.

resuscitation the act of reviving a patient from death or unconsciousness, including cardiac massage and artificial respiration.

retching the involuntary attempt to vomit without producing emesis.

retention (urine) a condition in which urine accumulates in the bladder and is not excreted.

retraction the act of drawing back.

retroperitoneal behind the peritoneum.

rhonchus a snoring sound, a rattling in the throat; coarse, dry, wheezy or whistling sound heard chiefly upon expiration.

rickets a disorder resulting from a deficiency of vitamin D.

rigor mortis the stiffening of the body after death.

ritualistic behavior (ritualism) a series of repetitive acts performed compulsively to relieve anxiety.

roentgen the unit of measurement of γ or χ radiation.

roentgenogram a film produced by photography with roentgen rays.

role the pattern of behavior expected of an individual in a situation or particular group.

rooting reflex a reflex in the newborn in which stimulation of the side of the cheek or lip causes the infant to turn his head toward the stimulus.

rotation turning in a circular movement around a fixed axis.

rubefacient reddening of the skin; a substance which reddens the skin.

ruga a ridge or fold of linings of organs such as the vagina or the stomach.

sagittal parallel to the long axis of the body.

sanguineous bloody.

saphenous vein either of two superficial veins of the leg; the greater one extends from the foot to the inguinal region, while the lesser one extends from the foot up the back of the leg to the knee joint.

sarcoidosis a disease in which all affected tissues develop epithelioid cell tubercles; commonly affected organs are the lymph nodes, liver, spleen, lungs, skin, eyes, and small bones in the feet and hands.

saturated fat fat that is saturated with hydrogen; commonly found in animal fats such as meat, butter, and eggs.

scab the crust over a superficial wound.

scapula shoulder blade; flat, triangular bone at the back of the shoulder.

sclerosis process of hardening that occurs from inflammation and from disease of the interstitial substance; used to describe hardening of nervous tissues and arterioles.

scored marked with measuring notches or lines.

scrotum the sac suspended down and behind the penis that contains and protects the testes.

scultetus binder abdominal binder applied in strips that overlap each other.

scurvy a condition resulting from vitamin C deficiency.

sebaceous oil-secreting.

sebum the oil-like secretion of sebaceous glands.

secretion a special product produced by a gland such as saliva from the salivary glands.

sedative an agent that tends to calm or to tranquilize.

self-actualization the term used by Abraham Maslow to describe the highest level of personality development.

semen seminal plasma combined with sperm.

semicircular canal half-circle–shaped passages in the inner ear that control the sense of balance by the effect of fluid moving against hair-like nerves.

semilunar valves half-moon–shaped valves that guard the entrances from the cardiac ventricles into the aorta and pulmonary trunk.

seminal plasma substances produced by the seminal vesicles, prostate, and Cowper's glands that energize the sperm and enhance their transport.

seminiferous tubules highly coiled tubes that manufacture sperm within each testes.

senility feebleness or loss of mental, emotional, or physical control that occurs in old age.

sensitivity capability of responding to a stimulus, such as bacteria responding to a specific antibiotic.

sensorimotor state the initial phase of cognitive development described by Piaget that occurs between the ages of 0 to 2 years.

sensoristasis the need for sensory stimulation.

sensory deficit partial or complete impairment of any sensory organ.

sensory deprivation an underabundance of sensory stimulation or an alteration of the impulses that are conveyed from the sensory organs to the higher centers of the brain.

sensory overload an overabundance of sensory stimulation.

septic produced by putrefaction or decomposition.

septic (hectic) fever intermittent fever characterized by wide fluctuations and periods when it falls to normal or below normal levels each day.

sero-sanguinous comprised of serum and blood.

serum the clear portion of animal fluid; the liquid part of blood as contrasted to the solid particles.

sex chromosome pair the pair of chromosomes, one from the sperm and one from the ovum, that determine whether the person's gonads develop into testes or ovaries; designated as XX or XY.

sex-typed behavior the action that typically elicits different rewards for one sex or the other.

sexual differentiation biologic sex determination in which male genitalia or female genitalia develop during fetal life.

sexual diphormism the physical and psychologic differences between males and females in any given species.

shivering invlountary contraction or twitching of the muscles as with coldness.

shock the state of acute peripheral circulatory failure.

sickle cell anemia a genetic defect of hemoglobin synthesis that accounts for abnormally crescent-shaped erythocytes; common to blacks.

side effect outcomes that are not intended, such as unintended actions or complications of a drug.

sigmoidoscopy examination of the interior of the sigmoid colon by the use of an endoscope (sigmoidoscope).

Sim's position semiprone position.

sings healing ceremonies or rituals carried out by the native Indians.

sinoatrial (SA) node the pacemaker of the heart; atypical muscle fibers in the right atrium of the heart where the rhythm of contraction is initiated.

slander defamation by the spoken word; untruthful statements causing ridicule or contempt.

slipper pan a bedpan that has one end flattened to ease the placing of it under the patient.

smear a specimen for microscopic study that is prepared by spreading the substance thinly over a glass slide.

smegma a cheesy material that accumulates from a mixture of the oil sceretions of the glans penis and dead tissue cells.

social pertaining to sociology, the science dealing with social relations and phenomena.

social worker an individual who assists persons and families with their social problems.

socialized speech the exchange of thoughts between individuals that includes questions, answers, commands, and criticisms of others.

sociology the study of social relationships and social institutions such as marriage or family structure.

sociopath a person who is unable to follow societies' moral and ethical standards.

somatic referring to the physical body.

somnambulism habitual sleep-walking.

sordes the accumulation of foul matter on the teeth and lips.

souffle a blowing sound heard by auscultation.

spasm involuntary contraction of a muscle or muscle group.

specific gravity   the weight of a substance, such as urine, compared to the weight of an equal volume of some other substance used as a standard, such as water; the specific gravity of water is 1.

speculum   an instrument used to open or distend a body orifice for the purpose of viewing an internal cavity.

sperm   the male germ cell that unites with the ovum in sexual reproduction.

spermacide   foams, jellies, or creams inserted into the vagina before intercourse to chemically destroy the sperm.

sphincter   a ringlike muscle that closes or constricts a natural orifice.

sphygmomanometer   the instrument used to measure arterial blood pressure.

spinothalmic tract   nerve pathway that ascends from the lower level of the spinal cord to the higher levels in the brain.

spiral bandage   a bandage applied to parts of the body extremities that are of uniform circumference.

spiral reverse bandage   a bandage applied to extremities of the body that are not of uniform circumference.

spirometry   measurement of the pulmonary capacities.

spore   the reproductive component of a microorgansim.

sprain   injury of the ligaments and associated structures of a joint by wrenching or twisting; associated structures include tendons, muscles, nerves, and blood vessels.

sputum   the mucus secretion from the lungs, bronchi, and trachea that is ejected through the mouth.

stab wound   see puncture wound.

stamina   staying power or endurance.

stammer   involuntary repetitions and stops in vocal utterances.

standard   a measure of quantity, quality, weight, extent, or value that is set up as a rule by authority.

stasis   stagnation or stoppage of flow of body fluids, such as intestinal or vascular fluids; a state of equilibrium.

stat   slang for at once; immediately; derived from the Latin word "statim," meaning immediately.

statutory law   a law passed by legislature (that is, state, provincial, or federal).

stenosis   constriction or narrowing of a body canal or opening.

stereotype   1) something held in common by the members of a group that conforms to a fixed or molded pattern; 2) oversimplified judgment or attitude about a person or group.

sterile   free from microorganisms and their pathogenic byproducts.

sterilization   1) the process by heat or chemical means that destroys all microorganisms; 2) the process that renders an individual incapable of reproduction, such as vasectomy or tubal ligation.

sternum   the breast bone.

stertor   snoring or sonorous respiration.

stethoscope   instrument used to auscultate sounds produced within the body.

stimulus   anything that arouses or incites action of a receptor.

stomatitis   inflammation of the mouth specifically the mucous lining.

stool (feces)   excreted waste products from the large intestine.

stopcock   a valve that controls the flow of fluid through a tube.

strabismus   crossed eyes or squint.

strain (of a muscle)   overexertion or overstretching of a muscle or part of a muscle.

stress   any physical or psychologic condition or situation that causes tension in the body and requires it to adapt.

stressor   any factor that produces stress or alters the body's equilibrium.

striae gravidarum   colorless streaks or lines similar to scars on the abdomen, breasts, or thighs caused by pregnancy; stretch marks.

stricture   a narrowing of a passageway or canal.

stridor   a shrill harsh sound heard during inspiration.

stroke volume   the amount of blood ejected from the heart with each ventricular contraction.

stroma   tissue that forms the framework or structure of an organ.

stupor   partial or nearly complete unconsciousness characterized by lethargy and reduced responsiveness to stimulation.

stuttering   a speech problem evidenced by the repetition of letters or words and prolonged pauses in between.

subarachnoid space the area below the arachnoid membrane which lies between the dura mater and the pia mater.

subcutaneous (hypodermic) beneath the layers of the skin.

subjective data symptoms of dysfunction or disease that are perceived only by the person involved, such as pain or nausea.

sublimation the channeling of unacceptable desires into socially acceptable forms of behavior.

sublingual located under the tongue.

suborbital beneath the cavity or orbit.

subscapular located below the scapula.

substitution replacing one thing by another; a mental defense mechanism in which unattainable or unacceptable goals are replaced by ones that are attainable or acceptable.

suctioning aspiration of secretions by a catheter connected to a suction machine or wall outlet.

sudoriferous glands glands that produce sweat.

superego an unconscious part of the psyche that monitors the id and the ego; concerned primarily with ethics, conscience, and social standards.

supination turning the palm upwards, or lying on the back.

supine a lying position with the face upwards.

support system those activities and people who can assist a person at a time of stress.

suppository a solid cone-shaped medicated substance that is inserted into the vagina, rectum, or urethra.

suppression 1) sudden stoppage of an excretion such as urine; 2) a mental mechanism whereby unpleasant feelings and experiences are kept from conscious awareness.

suppuration the formation of pus.

suprapubic above the pubic arch.

supraoptic the area above the eye.

supraorbital above the orbit of the eye.

surfactant lipoprotein mixture in the alveoli.

surgical asepsis (sterile technique) those measures that render and maintain objects free from all microorganisms (pathogens and nonpathogens).

surgical scrub a thorough chemical and mechanical cleansing procedure of the hands, wrists, and forearms in which the hands are held higher than the elbows.

susto a Chicano folk disease of emotional origin.

suture surgical stitch used to close accidental or surgical wounds.

sympathetic nervous system the thoracolumbar branch of the autonomic nervous system.

symphysis pubis the fibrocartilagenous line of union of the bodies of the pubic bones.

symptom (covert data) see subjective data.

synapse the junction between two neurons where the nerve impulses are transmitted from one neuron to another.

syncope faintness or temporary loss of consciousness.

syndrome a group of signs and symptoms resulting from a single cause; constitutes a typical clinical picture, such as the shock syndrome.

synergist an agent that enhances the action of another so that their combined effect is greater than either individual agent.

synovial joint a freely movable joint surrounded by a capsule enclosing a cavity that contains a transparent viscid fluid.

synthesis the process of putting together the elements or parts of a whole.

syphilis contagious venereal disease transmitted principally by coitus.

systemic pertains to the body as a whole.

systolic blood pressure the pressure exerted by the blood in the arteries when the ventricles contract.

tablet a medication in solid form which may be compressed and molded.

tachycardia an accelerated heart rate of over 100 beats per minute in an adult.

tachypnea an abnormally accelerated respiratory rate.

tactile pertaining to the sense of touch.

Talmud the authoritative body of Jewish tradition.

Taoism Chinese mystical philosophy.

tartar the film formed on teeth; dental calculus.

T-binder a cloth material shaped in a T and often used to retain dressings in the genital region.

technical assault   assault without the intent to injure, such as when giving a hypodermic injection.

temporal pulse   a pulse point where the temporal artery passes over the temporal bone of the skull.

tenacious   adhesive.

tenesmus   straining; painful ineffective straining at stool or urine.

testes   the male gonads.

testosterone   a testicular hormone that stimulates the growth and development of the genital organs and secondary sexual male characteristics.

tetany   a syndrome manifested by muscle twitching, cramps, convulsions, and sharp flexion of the wrist and ankle joints.

thalamus   the larger and middle portion of the diencephalon of the brain.

therapeutic environment   an environment which is supportive of health or the restoration of health.

therapy   remedial treatment.

thermal trauma   injury caused from excessive heat or cold.

thoracentesis   the insertion of a needle into the pleural cavity for diagnostic or therapeutic purposes.

thrombophlebitis   the inflammation of a vein followed by the development of a blood clot.

thrombosis   the development of a blood clot.

thrombus   a solid mass of blood constituents which forms in the heart or blood vessels.

thyrotrophic hormone or thyroid stimulating hormone (TSH)   a hormone produced by the anterior pituitary gland that stimulates the thyroid gland to produce its hormone thyroxine.

thyroxine   the hormone produced by the thyroid gland.

tidal volume   the volume of air that is normally inhaled and exhaled.

tinnitus   a ringing or buzzing sensation in the ears.

tissue turgor   normal skin fullness and resilience.

tolerance   the ability to endure without ill effects, often with reference to taking medications.

tonic neck reflex   a reflex in the newborn, alternately called the fencing reflex; the arm and leg on the side to which the head is forcibly turned are extended while the opposite limbs are flexed.

tonsillectomy   the surgical removal of a tonsil or tonsils.

tonus   slight continual contraction of muscles.

topical   external application such as to skin, mucous membrane, or conjunctiva.

tourniquet   a device, such as a rubber strip, that is wrapped around a body area to compress the blood vessels.

toxemia   a generalized intoxication due to the absorption of toxins in the body.

toxemia of pregnancy   a metabolic disturbance during pregnancy.

toxin   a poison which may be produced by some microorganisms, animals, and plants.

toxoid   a modified exotoxin which is no longer toxic but still has the ability to stimulate the production of antibodies.

trachea   a membranous tube composed of cartilage descending from the larynx and branching into the left and right bronchi.

tracheostomy   the surgical opening into the trachea through the neck.

traction   the act of pulling or exerting a force along an axis.

transudation   the passage of serum or other body fluid through a membrane or tissue.

transverse plane   the plane which is at right angles to the long axis.

trauma   injury.

tremor   involuntary muscle contraction such as quivering, twitching, or convulsion.

trendelenburg position   the position in which the patient's head is lower than his feet when lying on his back.

trimester   the period of three months.

trocar   an instrument; a cannula with a sharp pointed plate for entering body cavities.

troche   lozenge.

tubal ligation   a surgical tying of the fallopian tubes rendering the female sterile.

tumor   a growth of tissue in which the cells multiply in an uncontrolled and progressive manner.

tunica dartos   the middle layer of smooth muscle and tough connective tissue in the scrotum.

tympanites   the distention of the abdomen due to the presence of gas or air in the intestines or peritoneal cavity.

ulcer a localized sloughing of skin tissue or mucous membrane commonly associated with varicosities or hyperactivity of the gastrointestinal tract.

Ultradian rhythm a rhythm which cycles during minutes or hours.

ultrasound high-frequency mechanical radiant energy.

ultraviolet radiation between the violet rays and the roentgen rays with powerful chemical properties.

umbilicus the navel; that which was the site for the attachment of the umbilical cord in a fetus.

unconscious incapable of responding to sensory stimuli; insensible.

undernutrition inadequate caloric intake.

universal donor a person with type O blood.

unpalatable distasteful, unpleasant to the taste.

untoward adverse.

urban relating to or constituting a city.

urea a substance found in urine, blood, and lymph; the main nitrogenous substance in blood.

urea frost the appearance of the skin when the salt crystals remain after the evaporation of the sweat in urhidrosis.

uremia the retention in the blood of excessive amounts of the byproducts of protein metabolism.

ureter the fibrous, muscular tube extending from the kidneys to the urinary bladder.

urethra the canal extending from the urinary bladder to the outside of the body.

urethritis inflammation of the urethra.

urgency the feeling one must void.

urhidrosis a condition in which urinous materials are present in the sweat, such as uric acid and urea present in sweat.

urinalysis the analysis of urine by physical, chemical, or microscopic means.

urobilin the oxydized form of urobilinogen found in feces and occasionally in urine.

urticaria a condition in which the skin has a vascular reaction with smooth, reddened, slightly elevated patches which are itchy.

uterus the womb; the hollow, muscular organ in the female in which the fertilized ovum normally becomes imbedded and develops.

uvula a small fleshy mass projecting from the soft palate above the base of the tongue.

vaccine a suspension of killed, attenuated, or living microorganisms administered to prevent or treat an infectious disease.

vagina the canal in the female extending from the vulva to the cervix.

vaginismus irregular and involuntary contraction of the muscles around the outer third of the vagina during coitus.

vaporization (evaporation) the conversion of a solid or liquid into a gas.

varicosity the state of swollen, distended, and knotted veins, especially in the legs.

vas deferens a long tube that extends from the scrotum, curves around the urinary bladder and empties into the ejaculatory ducts.

vasectomy ligation and cutting of the vas deferens rendering the male sterile.

vasoconstriction a decrease or narrowing in the caliber (lumen) of blood vessels, especially of the arterioles.

vasodilatation an increase or widening in the caliber (lumen) of the blood vessels, particularly of the arterioles.

vector animals or insects that transfer pathogens from one host to another.

vehicle a transporting agent or medium.

vellus the fine body hair that appears after the lanugo disappears and persists until puberty.

ventilation (of the lungs) the act of breathing.

ventral located towards the front as related to the anatomic position; anterior; the opposite of dorsal.

ventricle a small cavity such as those located in the brain or the heart.

ventriculography radiologic examination of the ventricles of the brain following the insertion of air or other radiopaque medium.

vermin external animal parasites such as ticks, lice, and fleas.

vernix caseosa cheesy substance covering the skin of the fetus.

vertigo dizziness.

vestibule a space at the entrance to another structure, such as the cleft between the labia that contains the vaginal orifice, urethral orifice, and hymen.

viable capable of living; used to describe a fetus that is able to live outside the uterus.

vial a small glass bottle with a rubber stopper.

virulence the degree of pathogenicity of a microorganism.

virus minute infectious agents smaller than bacteria.

viscera large interior organs in body cavities such as the liver or stomach; singular organ is a viscus.

visceral pain pain originating from the viscera.

viscosity the quality of being gummy or sticky.

vital capacity tidal volume plus the inspiratory reserve volume and the expiratory reserve volume.

vital (cardinal) signs measurements of physiologic functioning, specifically temperature, pulse, and respirations.

vitamins organic chemical substances essential for normal metabolism and life; found in natural foods.

voiding excreting body wastes, particularly urine.

volatile substances that evaporate rapidly.

vomitus material vomited; emesis.

voodoo practice of witchcraft or magic.

vulva the external female genitalia that surround the vaginal orifice and the urethra; also referred to as the pudendum.

wheeze whistling respiratory sound on expiration.

xanthoma plaques of fatty substances in the skin, usually yellow in color.

xiphoid process the lower part of the sternum.

x-rays visualization of body parts on film by the use of roentgen rays.

yang a positive force in Chinese folk medicine that regulates health; represents the male, warmth, light, and fullness.

yin a negative force in Chinese folk medicine that regulates health; represents the female, coldness, darkness, and emptiness.

zygote the fertilized ovum.

INDEX